Abbreviation	Definition
NP	nasopharyngeal
NPV	negative-pressure ventilation
O_2	oxygen
O_2Hb	oxygenated hemoglobin
OH^-	hydroxide ions
OHDC	oxyhemoglobin dissociation curve
P	pressure
ΔP	change in pressure
P_{50}	PO_2 at which 50% saturation of hemoglobin occurs
P_{100}	pressure on active inspiration measured at 100 ms
PA	alveolar pressure
Pa	arterial pressure
PA	pulmonary artery
$P(A\text{-}a)O_2$	alveolar-to-arterial partial pressure of oxygen
$PACO_2$	partial pressure of carbon dioxide in the alveoli
$PaCO_2$	partial pressure of carbon dioxide in the arteries
Palv	alveolar pressure
PAO_2	partial pressure of oxygen in the alveoli
PaO_2	partial pressure of oxygen in the arteries
PaO_2/F_IO_2	ratio of arterial PO_2 to F_IO_2
PaO_2/P_AO_2	ratio of arterial PO_2 to alveolar PO_2
PAP	pulmonary artery pressure
$\overline{P}AP$	mean pulmonary artery pressure
$P(a\text{-et})CO_2$	Arterial to end-tidal partial pressure of carbon dioxide also, a-et PCO_2
PAGE	perfluorocarbon-associated gas exchange
Paug	pressure augmentation
PAV	proportional assist ventilation
PAWP	pulmonary artery wedge pressure
Paw	airway pressure
$\overline{P}aw$	mean airway pressure (also P$\overline{aw}$)
Pawo	airway opening pressure
PB	barometric pressure
Pbs	pressure at the body's surface
PCEF	peak cough expiratory flow
PC-CMV	pressure-controlled continuous mandatory ventilation
PC-IMV	pressure-controlled intermittent mandatory ventilation
PCIRV	pressure-controlled inverse-ratio ventilation
PCO_2	partial pressure of carbon dioxide
PCV	pressure-controlled ventilation
PCWP	pulmonary capillary wedge pressure
$PCWP_{tm}$	transmural pulmonary capillary wedge pressure
PDA	patent ductus arteriosus
PEA	pulseless electrical activity
$P\overline{e}CO_2$	partial pressure of mixed expired carbon dioxide
PEEP	positive end expiratory pressure
$PEEP_E$	extrinsic PEEP (set-PEEP)
$PEEP_I$	intrinsic PEEP (auto-PEEP)
$PEEP_{total}$	total PEEP (the sum of intrinsic and extrinsic PEEP)
PEFR	peak expiratory flow rate
P_{ES}	esophageal pressure
$P_{ET}CO_2$	partial pressure of end-tidal carbon dioxide; also $PetCO_2$
P_{FLEX}	pressure at the inflection point of a pressure/volume curve
P_{GA}	gastric pressure
P_{high}	high pressure during APRV
PHY	permissive hypercapnia
PIE	pulmonary interstitial edema
PIF	pulmonary interstitial fibrosis
P_{Imax}	maximum inspiratory pressure; also MIP, MIF, NIF
P_{inside}	inside pressure
$P_{intrapleural}$	intrapleural pressure; also P_{pl}
P_IO_2	partial pressure of inspired oxygen
PIP	peak inspiratory pressure; also P_{peak}
P_L	transpulmonary pressure
P_{low}	low pressure during APRV
PLV	partial liquid ventilation
P_M	mouth pressure
P_{mus}	muscle pressure
PO_2	partial pressure of oxygen
$P_{outside}$	pressure outside
P_{peak}	peak inspiratory pressure; also PIP
PPHN	persistent pulmonary hypertension of the newborn
P_{pl}	intrapleural pressure
$P_{plateau}$	plateau pressure
ppm	parts per million
PPV	positive-pressure ventilation
PRA	plasma renin activity
PRVC	pressure-regulated volume control
PS	pressure support
P_{set}	set pressure
PSmax	maximum pressure support
PSV	pressure support ventilation
psi	pounds per square inch
psig	pounds per square inch gauge
P_{TA}	transairway pressure
$PtcCO_2$	transcutaneous PCO_2
$PtcO_2$	transcutaneous PO_2
P_{TM}	transmural pressure
P_{TR}	transrespiratory pressure
P_{TT}	transthoracic pressure; also P_w
PV	pressure ventilation
PVC(s)	premature ventricular contraction(s)
P_vO_2	partial pressure of oxygen in mixed venous blood
PVR	pulmonary vascular resistance
PVS	partial ventilatory support
P_w	transthoracic pressure; also P_{TT}
Q2H	every two hours
$\dot{Q}_T$	cardiac output
$\dot{Q}_S/\dot{Q}_T$	shunt
R	respiratory exchange ratio
RAM	random-access memory
RAP	right atrial pressure
R_{aw}	airway resistance
RCP	respiratory care practitioner
RDS	respiratory distress syndrome
Re	Reynolds' number
R_E	expiratory resistance
REE	resting energy expenditure
R_I	inspiratory resistance
ROM	read-only memory
RQ	respiratory quotient
RT	respiratory therapist
RV	right ventricle or residual volume
RVP	right ventricular pressure
RVEDP	right ventricular end-diastolic pressure
RVEDV	right ventricular end-diastolic volume
SA	sinoatrial
SaO_2	arterial oxygen saturation
S.I.	systéme Internationale (international system)
SIMV	synchronized intermittent mandatory ventilation
Sine	sinusoidal
sp.	species
sPEEP	spontaneous PEEP
SpO_2	oxygen saturation measured by pulse oximeter
STPD	standard temperature, pressure saturated; zero degrees Celsius, 760 mm Hg, dry
SV	stroke volume
SVC	slow vital capacity
$S_{\bar{v}}O_2$	mixed venous oxygen saturation
SVN	small-volume nebulizer
SVR	systemic vascular resistance
T	temperature
TCPL	time-cycled, pressure-limited
TCT	total cycle time
T_E	expiratory time
TGI	tracheal gas insufflation
T_I	inspiratory time
tid	three times a day
T_I/TCT	duty cycle
T_{high}	time for high-pressure delivery in APRV
T_{low}	time for low-pressure delivery in APRV
TLC	total lung capacity
torr	measurement of pressure equivalent to mm Hg
TPTV	time-triggered, pressure-limited, time-cycled ventilation
U	unit
UN	urinary nitrogen
$\dot{V}$	volume; volt(s)
$\dot{V}$	flow
$\dot{V}_A$	alveolar ventilation per minute
VA	venoarterial
VAI	ventilator-assisted individuals
VAPS	volume-assured pressure support
VC	vital capacity; volume-cycled
V_C	volume lost to tubing compressibility
VC-CMV	volume-controlled continuous mandatory ventilation
VC-IMV	volume-controlled intermittent mandatory ventilation
VCIRV	volume-controlled inverse-ratio ventilation
$\dot{V}CO_2$	carbon dioxide production per minute
V_D	volume of dead space
$\dot{V}_D$	dead space ventilation per minute
V_{Dalv}	alveolar dead space
V_{Danat}	anatomical dead space
V_{Dmech}	mechanical dead space
$\dot{V}_E$	minute ventilation
VEDV	ventricular end-diastolic volume
$\dot{V}O_2$	oxygen consumption per minute
VS	volume support
V_T	tidal volume
V_D/V_T	ratio of dead space to tidal volume
vol%	volume per 100 mL of blood
V/Q	ventilation/perfusion ratio
VV	volume ventilation; also venovenous
W	work; watt(s)
WOB	work of breathing
WOBi	imposed work of breathing
y	year(s)

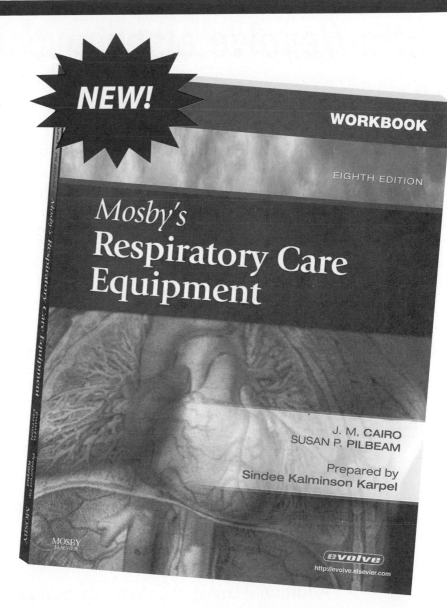

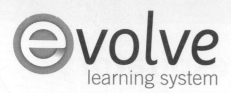
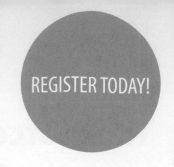
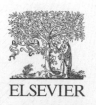

EIGHTH EDITION

Mosby's Respiratory Care Equipment

J.M. Cairo, PhD, RRT, FAARC

Dean of the School of Allied Health Professions
Professor of Cardiopulmonary Science, Physiology, and Anesthesiology
Louisiana State University Health Sciences Center
New Orleans, Louisiana

Susan P. Pilbeam, MS, RRT, FAARC

Clinical Applications Specialist
Maquet, Inc
St. Augustine, Florida

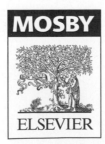

MOSBY

ELSEVIER

11830 Westline Industrial Drive
St. Louis, Missouri 63146

MOSBY'S RESPIRATORY CARE EQUIPMENT   ISBN: 978-0-323-05176-7

Library of Congress Cataloging-in-Publication Data

Cairo, Jimmy M.
   Mosby's respiratory care equipment.—8th ed. / J.M. Cairo, Susan P. Pilbeam.
     p. ; cm.
   Includes bibliographical references and index.
   ISBN-13: 978-0-323-05176-7 (hardcover : alk. paper)
   ISBN-10: 0-323-05176-6 (hardcover : alk. paper)
   1. Respiratory therapy—Equipment and supplies.   2. Respiratory intensive care—Equipment and supplies. I. Pilbeam, Susan P., 1945– II. Title. III. Title: Respiratory care equipment.
   [DNLM: 1. Respiratory Therapy–instrumentation. WF 26 C136m 2010]
   RC735.I5R4728 2010
   615.8'36028—dc22

2008053643

Publisher: Jeanne Wilke
Managing Editor: Billi Sharp
Senior Developmental Editor: Mindy Hutchinson
Publishing Services Manager: Julie Eddy
Project Manager: Marquita Parker
Designer: Paula Catalano

Printed in Canada

Last digit is the print number: 9 8 7 6 5 4 3 2

To Rhonda and Allyson
JMC

To Bob and Laura
SPP

Contributors

Charles G. Durbin Jr., MD, FAARC

Professor of Anesthesiology and Surgery
Medical Director, Respiratory Care
University of Virginia Health Sciences Center
Charlottesville, Virginia

James Fink, MS, RRT, FAARC

Fellow, Respiratory Science
Nektar Therapeutics
Mountain View, California

Ashley M. Shilling, MD

Assistant Professor of Anesthesiology
University of Virginia Health Sciences Center
Charlottesville, Virginia

Steven E. Sittig, RRT-NPS

Assistant Professor of Anesthesiology
College of Medicine
Mayo Clinic
Rochester, Minnesota

Kenneth F. Watson, MS RRT

Staff Respiratory Therapist
Children's Hospital
Boston, Massachusetts

Reviewers

Kelli Chronister, RRT, MS

Director of Clinical Education
Respiratory Care Program
Cuyahoga Community College
Parma Heights, Ohio

Julie Hopwood, MS, RRT, RCP

Director of Clinical Education
Respiratory Therapy Program
Central Piedmont Community College
Charlotte, North Carolina

James Knight, Ed.D, RRT

Associate Professor and Director, Clinical Education
Division of Respiratory Care
Long Island University
Brooklyn, New York

David Lucas, MS, RRT-NPS, AE-C

Program Manager
Respiratory Care and Polysomnography
Cuyahoga Community College
Parma Heights, Ohio

Tim OptHolt, Ed.D, RRT, AE-C, FAARC

Professor of Cardiorespiratory Care
University of South Alabama
Mobile, Alabama

Bill Pruitt, MBA, RRT, CPFT, AE-C

Instructor, Cardiorespiratory Care
University of South Alabama
Mobile, Alabama

Chris Russian, M.Ed, RRT, RPSGT

Assistant Professor
Department of Respiratory Care
Texas State University-San Marcos
San Marcos, Texas

Preface

"Information is not knowledge; knowledge is not wisdom."

This simple, but profound quote, which paraphrases a verse from T.S. Elliot's poem *The Rock*, is used often by scientists who study computer modeling and artificial intelligence to describe the learning hierarchy. It is also a fitting description of the challenges that every student faces in education. We are presented with a staggering volume of information that must be integrated into a working knowledge, usually in a relatively short amount of time. Assimilation of wisdom, in contrast, requires a personal dedication to the idea of lifelong learning. Our goal in writing this textbook was to provide guidance for students who choose to confront these challenges and embark on an educational journey to master the discipline of respiratory therapy.

FEATURES

In the eighth edition of *Mosby's Respiratory Care Equipment*, we have renewed our commitment to provide an up-to-date and comprehensive review of the devices and techniques used by respiratory therapists to diagnose and treat patients with cardiopulmonary dysfunction. As in previous editions, we have tried to present the material in a concise and readable fashion. You will notice throughout the text that we have used a number of pedagogical aids to assist the reader in mastering the material that is presented including:

- Brief subject outlines
- Measurable learning objectives
- Lists of relevant key terms
- Current AARC clinical practice guidelines
- Updated reference lists, including computer and internet resources, to reinforce the use of evidence based practices.
- "Clinical Rounds" have been updated and expanded to present practical scenarios that are encountered by respiratory therapists.
- Bulleted "Key Points" conclude each chapter to emphasize specific concepts presented in the chapter.
- National Board for Respiratory Care-style questions are included at the end of each chapter to allow the reader to test their comprehension of the subject matter.
- Figures, boxes, and tables have been updated when necessary and every effort has been made to assure that the photographs and illustrations are descriptive and easy to follow.

ORGANIZATION

The structure of the text has been maintained to follow a typical progression through a respiratory therapy educational program. We have added several new authors who we believe give a fresh perspective on key topics covered in the text.

- Chapter 1 includes a review of the basic physical principles that the reader will encounter in later chapters.
- Chapters 2 and 3 provide a detailed discussion of the devices and concepts that are used in the medical gas therapy.
- Chapter 4, similarly, describes the concepts and equipment that are used in the administration of humidity and aerosol therapy.
- Chapter 5 provides a concise review of microbiological principles and infection control procedures that apply to respiratory care equipment. This chapter includes the most current recommendations from the Centers for Disease Control and Prevention to reduce the risk of infection to patients and healthcare providers.
- Chapter 6 presents a clinically useful approach to airway management. It includes an extensive review of the indications, application, contraindications, and complications associated with the use of various artificial airways and the related ancillary equipment.
- Chapter 7 describes lung expansion and bronchial hygiene devices, including incentive spirometers and chest physiotherapy equipment.
- Chapters 8, 9, and 10 provide an overview of devices and techniques that are routinely used to assess patients with cardiopulmonary dysfunction.
  - Chapter 8 discusses the devices and techniques used to measure physiologic function in the pulmonary diagnostic laboratory and at the bedside.
  - Chapter 9 provides a description of the equipment and techniques used to perform electrocardiography and hemodynamic monitoring.
  - Chapter 10 includes information about invasive and noninvasive techniques and equipment used to measure and monitor arterial blood gases.

The chapters on mechanical ventilators have been updated to include the most current information available to us.

- Chapter 11 reviews basic technical operation and physical function of ventilator components and includes coverage of such subjects as current descriptions of the types of breath delivery and ventilator mode classification, ventilator graphics, and high-frequency ventilators. As in previous editions of this text, we have not attempted to cover management of the patient-ventilator system, which is handled in our other textbook on mechanical ventilation.*

- Chapters 12, 13, and 14 provide a systematic review of the various ventilators that are used in clinical practice.
  - o Chapter 12 reviews multipurpose ventilators that are primarily used for ICU patients.
  - o Chapter 13 provides an update on mechanical ventilators used in pediatric and neonatal care and also includes the neonatal and pediatric application of the general use ICU ventilators.
  - o Chapter 14 focuses on those ventilators and devices that are used in patient transport, ventilation in the home setting, and noninvasive devices.

Readers will find that we did not attempt to include every commercially available ventilator, but rather we have chosen to present those devices which are currently the most commonly used in clinical practice. In addition, content on older model ventilators may be found on the Evolve Resources accompanying this text. Ventilators included on the website may still be in clinical use, but their use has declined significantly or are no longer produced or supported by the manufacturer. As we stated in previous editions of this text, it is reasonable to assume that one or more new ventilators will be introduced shortly after this book is published.

The final chapter of *Mosby's Respiratory Care Equipment* contains a conceptual approach to the diagnosis of sleep related disorders. This approach focuses on a discussion of the physiology of sleep, pathophysiologic findings associated with sleep apnea, as well as behavioral and electrographic criteria used to diagnose the presence of a sleep-related disorder. Many respiratory therapy educational programs now offer certificate programs in polysomnography. This chapter is not intended to be a compendium of sleep medicine but rather an overview of the equipment and procedures commonly used in sleep laboratories.

We have incorporated a number of valuable suggestions that we received from our colleagues who used the 7th edition of this text in teaching in respiratory therapy programs and from the students that they mentor. Our hope is that this book will continue to be a useful resource for students and practitioners involved in care of patients with cardiopulmonary dysfunction.

LEARNING AIDS

Workbook

New to this edition is the *Workbook for Mosby's Respiratory Care Equipment*, authored by Sindee Kalminson Karpel. It is an invaluable resource for students; providing the reinforcement and practice necessary for students to succeed in their study of respiratory care. The more difficult concepts from the text are broken down through a variety of exercises including crossword-puzzles, short-answer, and fill-in-the-blank questions tied to each objective, critical thinking/essay questions, NBRC-type questions, helpful websites, and more.

Evolve Resources—http://evolve. elsevier.com/Cairo/

Evolve is an interactive learning environment designed to work in coordination with this text. Instructors may use Evolve to provide an Internet-based course component that reinforces and expands the concepts presented in class. Evolve may be used to publish the class syllabus, outlines, and lecture notes; set up "virtual office hours" and e-mail communication; share important dates and information through the online class calendar; and encourage student participation through chat rooms and discussion boards. Evolve allows instructors to post exams and manage their grade books online.

For the Instructor

For the instructor, Evolve offers valuable resources to help them prepare their courses including:
- Over 1,500 questions in ExamView
- An image collection of the figures from the book available in jpeg and PowerPoint formats
- An Instructor's Manual

For Students

For students, Evolve offers valuable resources to help them succeed in their courses including:
- Suggested Answers to Clinical Rounds
- Answers to Assessment Questions
- Answer Key to the *Workbook for Mosby's Respiratory Care Equipment*
- Additional General-Use Ventilators
- Additional Transport, Home-Care and Alternative Ventilators
- Infectious Disease PowerPoint Presentation
- Weblinks

For more information, visit http://evolve.elsevier.com/ Cairo/ or contact an Elsevier sales representative.

---

*Pilbeam SP, Cairo JM: Mechanical Ventilation—Physiological and Clinical Application, ed 4, St. Louis, 2006, Mosby.

Acknowledgments

We wish to thank Steve Sittig, RRT-NPS, FAARC, Ken Watson, MS, RRT, Charles Durbin, MD, Ashley Shilling, MD, and Jim Fink, MS, RRT, FAARC. We would like to offer a special thanks to all of the manufacturers and distributors represented in this text and for their tremendous cooperation. They include Kerry Ross, Marketing Products Manager, VIASYS, a division of Cardinal Health; Mike Tracy, Senior product Specialist, Robyn Whalen, Director of Marketing and Nancy Hemmert, Regional Sales Associate, Dräger Medical; Melissa Turner, Clinical Support Specialist, and Paul Garbarini, Clinical Operations Manager, Hamilton Medical; Cyndy Miller, Director of Clinical Education, Jim Seeley, Product Manager, Newport Medical Instruments; Gary S Milne, Senior Clinical Marketing Specialist, David Hyde, Senior Clinical Research Specialist, Puritan Bennett Ventilators, a division of Covidien; and, Barbara Sullivan, Education Manager, Respironics, a division of Phillips.

Steve Sittig, RRT-NPS, FAARC, who authored chapter 14, wanted to thank Jeff Ward MS RRT, FAARC, Colleen Upton RRT, Frank Milano RN, RRT and Carrie Massey RRT, AE-C for their technical assistance and support with this chapter.

We would also like to thank the following individuals who graciously offered assistance during this project. They include Michael G. Levitzky, PhD, John Zamjahn, PhD, RRT, Andrew Pellett, PhD, RCVT, Martha Baul, Lindsey Paige NesSmith, Jessica Knox Haines.

We want to express our sincere appreciation to Mindy Hutchinson for providing guidance throughout this endeavor, and to Marquita Parker, Paige Wilke, and Kia Michalegko for their assistance during the final manuscript preparation.

Jim Cairo
New Orleans, Louisiana

Sue Pilbeam
St. Augustine, Florida

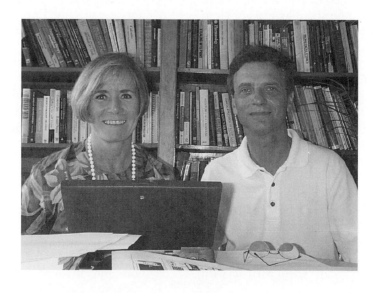

Contents

AARC Clinical Practice Guideline Excerpts

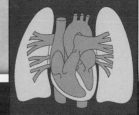

Chapter 1

Basic Physics for the Respiratory Therapist

J.M. CAIRO

Physics is the most fundamental and all-inclusive of all the sciences, and has had a profound effect on all scientific development. In fact, physics is the present-day equivalent of what used to be called natural philosophy, from which most of our modern sciences arose. Students of many fields find themselves studying physics because of the basic role it plays in all phenomena.

Richard P. Feynman
Six Easy Pieces[1]

OUTLINE

Energy and Matter
  Energy and Work
  Kinetic and Potential Energy
States of Matter
  Change of State
Physical Properties of Matter
  Temperature
  Pressure
  Density
  Buoyancy
  Viscosity
  Surface Tension
The Gas Laws
  Boyle's Law
  Charles' and Gay-Lussac's Laws
  Combined Gas Law

Dalton's Law of Partial Pressures
Avogadro's Law
Laws of Diffusion
Fluid Mechanics
  Patterns of Flow
  Poiseuille's Law
  Reynolds' Number
  Bernoulli Principle
  Venturi Principle
  Coanda Effect
Principles of Electricity
  Principles of Electronics
  Ohm's Law
  Electrical Circuits
  Electrical Safety
  Preventing Electrical Hazards

OBJECTIVES

Upon completion of this chapter, you will be able to:
· Differentiate between kinetic and potential energy.
· Compare the physical and chemical properties of the three primary states of matter.
· Explain why large amounts of energy are required to accomplish the changes associated with solid-liquid and liquid-gas phase transitions.
· Convert temperature measurements from the Kelvin, Celsius, and Fahrenheit temperature scales.
· Define pressure and describe two devices commonly used to measure it.
· List various pressure equivalents for 1 atmosphere (atm).
· Calculate the density and specific gravity of liquids and gases.
· Explain how changes in pressure, volume, temperature, and mass affect the behavior of an ideal gas.
· Calculate the partial pressure of oxygen in a room air sample of gas obtained at 1 atm.
· List the physical variables that influence the flow of a gas through a tube.
· Explain how the pressure, velocity, and flow of a gas change as it moves from a part of a tube with a large radius to another part with a small radius.
· Describe the Venturi and Coanda effects and how both can be used in the design of respiratory care equipment.
· State Ohm's law and relate how changes in voltage and resistance affect current flow in a direct-current series circuit.
· Describe three strategies that can be used to protect patients from electrical hazards.

KEY TERMS

absolute humidity
acoustics
adhesive forces
ammeter
amorphous solids
ampere
Archimedes' principle
atomic theory
atoms
Avogadro's number
boiling point
Boltzmann's Universal Gas
   Constant
buoyancy
Celsius
cohesive forces
compounds
condensation
critical point
critical pressure
critical temperature
diffusion
dipole-dipole interactions
electricity and magnetism
electromotive force

elements
evaporation
Fahrenheit
fluidic
freezing point
gravitational potential
   energy
horsepower
hydrogen bonding
hydrometer
insulators
joules
Kelvin
kilowatt
kinetic energy
kinetic theory
latent heat
macroshock
mechanics
melting point
microshock
mixtures
molecules
Newton
ohm

Ohm's law
optics
potential energy
power
Rankine
relative humidity
resistors
semiconductors
sublimation
supercooled liquids
Système International
thermistor
thermodynamics
thermometers (electrical and
   nonelectrical)
Van der Waals forces
vaporization
vapor pressure
vapors
volt
voltmeter
watts
weight density
Wheatstone bridge

Physics is the branch of science that deals with the interactions of matter and energy. Classical physics comprises the fields of **mechanics, optics, acoustics, electricity** and **magnetism,** and **thermodynamics.** The laws of classical physics describe the behavior of matter and energy under ordinary, everyday conditions. Modern physics, which began at the end of the nineteenth century, seeks to explain the interactions of matter and energy under extraordinary conditions, such as in extreme temperatures or when moving near the speed of light. Modern physics also is concerned with the interactions of matter and energy on a very small scale (i.e., nuclear and elementary particle physics). It is noteworthy that, at the subatomic level, the laws of classical physics governing space, time, matter, and energy are no longer valid.

A knowledge of the principles of classical physics is fundamental to a clear understanding of the ways various types of respiratory care equipment operate. Indeed, this chapter began with a quote from Nobel laureate Richard Feynman to underscore the fact that physics not only is part of the foundation of respiratory care, it serves the same function for all the clinical sciences.

This chapter presents a review of classical physics applicable to respiratory care equipment. It is not intended to present a compendium of physics, but rather focuses on how these physical principles are commonly encountered in respiratory care equipment. Several physics textbooks are included in the References list at the end of the chapter to facilitate a more detailed study of physics.[2-4]

ENERGY AND MATTER

Energy and Work

The concepts of energy and work are closely related. In fact, energy usually is defined as the ability to do work, where work (W) equals the product of a force (F) acting on an object to move it a distance (d), or

$$W = F \times d$$

Note that this definition is more specific than our everyday description of work. In everyday life, we say that work is anything that requires the exertion of effort. In physics, work is performed only when the effort produces a change in the position of the matter (i.e., the matter moves in the direction of the force). In the **Système International** (SI) of measurements, energy and work are expressed in **joules** (J), where 1 J equals the force of 1 Newton (N) acting on a 1-kilogram (kg) object to move it 1 meter (m). **Power** (P), which is a measure of the rate at which work is being performed (P = W/t), is expressed in **watts** (W), with 1 W equivalent to 1 J/second. Because the watt is a relatively small number, we rely more on the **kilowatt** (kW), which equals 1000 watts (e.g., a 2-kW motor can perform work at a rate of 2000 J/second). Another common term used for power is **horsepower** (hp). Approximately, 1 hp equals 746 W of power, or 0.746 kW.

The energy required to perform work can exist in various forms, including mechanical energy, thermal energy, chemical energy, sound energy, nuclear energy, and electrical energy. According to the law of conservation of energy, energy cannot be created or destroyed but can only be transferred. For example, a fossil fuel such as coal, which is a form of chemical energy, can be converted to electrical energy, which in turn can provide the power to operate a fan or compressor. Therefore, we can think of work as the transfer of energy by mechanical means. As such, mechanical energy usually is divided into two categories: **kinetic energy** and **potential energy.**

Kinetic and Potential Energy

Kinetic energy is the energy an object possesses when it is in motion; potential energy is stored energy, or the energy that an object possesses because of its position. The kinetic energy (KE) of an object can be quantified with the formula

$$KE = 1/2(mv^2)$$

where m is the mass of the object and v is the velocity at which it is traveling. Intuitively, one might guess that the greater the mass, the greater the kinetic energy. It is not necessarily obvious that the kinetic energy of the substance increases to a greater extent with similar increases in the velocity at which the object is traveling. In fact, looking at the formula, one can see that kinetic energy increases exponentially when velocity increases. That is, kinetic energy is proportional to the square of the velocity at which the object is moving (e.g., a twofold increase in mass increases the kinetic energy twofold, and a twofold increase in velocity results in a fourfold increase in the kinetic energy).

Potential energy can be thought of as the energy an object has by virtue of its position. For example, a weight raised above your head has the potential to exert a force when it falls. The energy the weight gains as it falls is the result of gravity. (In this example, however, potential energy is more correctly referred to as **gravitational potential energy**.) The amount of potential energy (PE) an object has can be calculated as

$$PE = mgh$$

where m is the mass of the object, g is the force of gravity (32 feet/sec^2), and h is the height the object is raised. Potential energy also can be stored in a compressed spring or a chemical bond. With a spring, energy is required for compression. This elastic PE is then converted into kinetic energy when the spring is allowed to uncoil. Petroleum reserves of coal, oil, and gas, which represent chemical PE stores, can be converted to KE when chemical bonds are broken to provide the power required to operate lights, automobiles, and other devices we use in our daily lives.

STATES OF MATTER

Matter generally is defined as anything that has mass and occupies space. The **atomic theory,** which is the result of the work of John Dalton (1766-1844), states that all matter is composed of tiny particles, called **atoms.** Although it can appear in various forms, all matter is made up of only about 100 different types of atoms, called **elements.**[5,6] These elements can combine in fixed proportions to form **molecules,** which in turn can form **compounds** and **mixtures.**

All matter can exist in three distinct states: solid, liquid, and gas. The physical properties of each of these states can be explained by the **kinetic theory,** which states that the atoms and molecules that make up matter are in constant motion. The schematic in Figure 1-1 illustrates the three states of matter. Solids usually are characterized as either crystalline or amorphous. Notice that crystalline solids are highly organized structures in which the atoms and molecules are arranged in a lattice. **Amorphous solids,** such as glass or margarine, have constituent particles that are less rigidly arranged. Amorphous solids sometimes are called **supercooled liquids** because of this random arrangement.

Of the three states of matter, solids have the least amount of kinetic energy. Most of their internal energy is PE that is contained in the intermolecular forces holding the individual particles of solids together. In solids these forces are strong enough to limit the motion of the atoms and molecules to what appear to be vibrations or oscillations about a fixed point. Because of these features, solids are characterized as incompressible substances that can maintain their volume and shape.

Like solids, liquids have attractive forces, but the cohesive forces in liquids are not as strong. Liquid molecules have greater freedom of movement and more kinetic energy than do molecules of solids. Illustrating exactly how liquid particles move is difficult, but one can envision that these particles are able to slide past each other, which gives liquids *fluidity*, or the ability to flow. Although the intermolecular forces holding liquids together are relatively weak compared with those in solids, these forces lend enough cohesiveness to liquid molecules to allow them to maintain their volumes. Liquids essentially are incompressible; that is, a liquid can be made to occupy a smaller volume only if an incredible amount of force is exerted upon it.

Gases have extremely weak, if any, cohesive forces between their constituent particles. Therefore, gases have

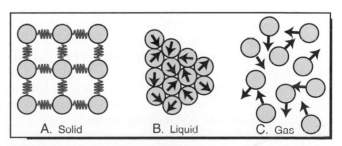

FIGURE 1-1 Simplified models illustrating the three states of matter. **A,** Solid. **B,** Liquid. **C,** Gas.

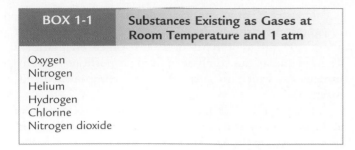

BOX 1-1	Substances Existing as Gases at Room Temperature and 1 atm

Oxygen
Nitrogen
Helium
Hydrogen
Chlorine
Nitrogen dioxide

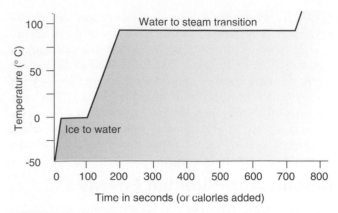

FIGURE 1-2 Energy-temperature relationship for the conversion of solid ice to liquid water to steam. Energy is added at a rate of 1 cal/sec. (Redrawn from Nave CR, Nave BC: *Physics for the health sciences*, ed 3, Philadelphia, 1985, WB Saunders.)

the greatest amount of KE of the three states of matter, and their PE is minimal compared to that of the other two states of matter. The motion of the atoms and molecules that make up gases is random. Gases do not maintain their shapes and volumes, but rather expand to fill the available space. Gases are similar to liquids in that the particles composing them can move freely, thus giving gases the ability to flow. For this reason, gases and liquids are described as *fluids.*

Box 1-1 lists some of the more common substances that normally exist as gases at room temperature. Most of the gases encountered in everyday life [i.e., nitrogen (N_2), oxygen (O_2), carbon dioxide (CO_2), and carbon monoxide (CO)] are colorless and odorless; a notable exception is nitrogen dioxide (NO_2), an atmospheric pollutant that is dark brown and has a pungent odor. The properties of individual medical gases are discussed in Chapter 2.

Change of State

It should be apparent from the discussion so far that the physical state of any substance is determined from the relation of its kinetic energy content and the potential energy stored in its intermolecular bonds. Changes of state involve the interconversion of solids, liquids, and gases, which can be accomplished by altering the relationship between the KE and PE of a substance, such as by changing its temperature (i.e., by adding or removing heat). Consider the example of converting the solid form of water (ice) to liquid and then to steam. Adding heat to ice increases the kinetic activity (i.e., vibration of the water molecules) in the ice, thus melting or weakening the intermolecular attractive forces and producing liquid water. (Freezing, which is the opposite of melting, can be accomplished by transferring the KE of a substance to its surroundings, such as when a substance is exposed to cold temperatures.) Adding more heat causes the liquid water molecules to move more vigorously and escape into the gaseous state, or vaporize **(evaporation).** The temperature at which a solid converts to a liquid is a substance's **melting point.** (Note that the **freezing point** is the same temperature as the melting point; that is, the temperature at which a liquid is changed to a solid state.) The temperature at which a liquid converts to a gaseous state is its **boiling point.**

Figure 1-2 shows the phase changes associated with the conversion of 1 gram (g) of ice to steam.[7] As heat is added, ice begins to change to liquid at a temperature of 0° C.

Note that although the addition of heat effects a change in state, the temperature of the water does not change immediately (i.e., there is a plateau in temperature). The temperature changes only after all of the ice is converted to liquid. The amount of heat that must be added to a substance to cause a complete change of state is called the **latent heat** of fusion and is expressed in calories per gram (cal/g). Therefore, the amount of heat that must be added to effect the change from solid to liquid is called the *latent heat of melting.* In the case of water, approximately 80 calories (cal/g) of ice must be added to liquefy ice completely when the temperature reaches 0° C. After the ice has been completely liquefied, the temperature will increase 1° C per second if heat continues to be added at a rate of 1 cal/sec. This same type of phenomenon occurs at the substance's boiling point when water is converted to steam. The amount of heat that must be supplied to change liquid to steam completely (i.e., vaporize water) is the latent heat of **vaporization.** As one can see, a considerably greater amount of heat (540 cal/g) must be added to convert water to steam compared with the amount of heat that must be added to melt ice into water. More energy is required in the process of vaporization because intermolecular forces essentially must be removed to allow the molecules to break loose and enter into the gaseous state.[8] Table 1-1 lists the melting and boiling points for some commonly used substances, along with the latent heats of fusion and vaporization.

Sublimation

Under certain conditions, solid molecules can completely bypass the liquid state and change to gas. This process, called **sublimation,** occurs when the heat content of a substance increases to a point at which the molecules in the solid state gain enough energy to break loose and enter the gaseous state while remaining below its melting point. The conversion of solid carbon dioxide (i.e., dry ice) to gaseous carbon dioxide is the most common example of this process.

TABLE 1-1

Melting and Boiling Points and Latent Heats of Fusion and Vaporization of Some Common Substances

Substance	Melting Point (°C)	Heat of Fusion (cal/g)	Boiling Point (°C)*	Heat of Vaporization (cal/g)
Water	0	80	100	540
Ammonia	−75	108.0	−33	327
Ethyl alcohol	−114	26	78	204
Nitrogen	−210	6.2	−196	48
Oxygen	−219	3.3	−183	51
Lead	327	5.9	1620	208
Mercury	−39	2.7	357	68

*At standard atmospheric pressure of 760 mm Hg.

From Scanlan CL, Spearman CB, Sheldon RL: *Egan's fundamentals of respiratory care,* ed 6, St Louis, 1995, Mosby.

Evaporation and Condensation

The conversion of a liquid to the gaseous state has been discussed in terms of boiling (e.g., the transition from water to steam occurs at a temperature of 100°C). Although it may not be obvious, this phase transition (evaporation) begins at temperatures between 0°C and 100°C. Evaporation occurs when some of the liquid molecules gain enough kinetic energy to break through the surface of the liquid and convert to free gaseous molecules. The rate of evaporation increases with an increase in temperature, an increase in surface area, or a decrease in pressure.

Two forces must be overcome for evaporation to occur: the mass attraction of the molecules for each other (i.e., **dipole-dipole interactions, hydrogen bonding,** and **Van der Waals forces**) and the pressure of the gas above the liquid. We can enhance the process of evaporation either by increasing the kinetic energy of the liquid molecules or by reducing the pressure above the liquid. Raising the temperature of a liquid increases the velocity and the force of the molecules hitting each other and moves them farther apart. This increased kinetic activity increases the force that these molecules possess as they hit the surface of the liquid, thus allowing the liquid molecules to escape more easily and frequently.

Vapor pressure is a measure of the force that molecules exert as they hit the surface of a liquid and escape into the gaseous phase. The concept of vapor pressure can be used to define the boiling point of a liquid in more precise terms; that is, the boiling point is the temperature at which the vapor pressure of a liquid equals the atmospheric pressure. Reducing the pressure above the liquid lowers its boiling point, because the forces opposing the escape of molecules from the liquid are decreased. This concept explains why water boils at a lower temperature at high altitudes. It also explains the process of freeze-drying as a means of food preservation; the food is placed in a vacuum, which reduces the opposition that liquid molecules must overcome to evaporate, thereby boiling off any liquid present.

The opposite of evaporation is **condensation,** which is simply defined as the conversion of a substance from a gas to a liquid. In evaporation, heat energy is removed from the air surrounding a liquid and transferred to the liquid, thus cooling the air. In contrast, during condensation, heat is removed from the liquid and transferred to the surrounding air, warming it. Box 1-2 contains an example of how evaporation and condensation can affect a person's daily life.

BOX 1-2   Evaporation and Condensation

A fairly common example that can be used to illustrate concepts of evaporation and condensation relates to the water vapor content, or humidity, of the air surrounding us. This concept is obvious to anyone who has ever spent a hot August day somewhere in the southern part of the United States, such as New Orleans. As stated in the section on evaporation, one of the main factors influencing evaporation is temperature. Increasing the temperature increases water evaporation (in New Orleans, the water is from the lakes and bayous surrounding the city) by increasing the molecular activity of the water and increasing the capacity of the air to hold water vapor. If the actual amount of water vapor in the air is to be measured, the water vapor content must be determined. The amount or weight of water that can be contained (to capacity) in the air is called the **absolute humidity** and is expressed in grams of water vapor per cubic meter (g/m³) or milligrams per liter (mg/L). (The absolute humidity can be measured, or it can be computed with tables supplied by the U.S. Weather Bureau.[8]) Note that at a temperature of 37°C (98.6°F), a typical temperature in New Orleans during August, air that is 100% saturated will contain 43.8 mg of water per liter of air. In most cases the air is not fully saturated but only 90% saturated with water vapor; that is, it contains only 0.90 × 43.80 mg/L, or 39.42 mg of water in every liter of air. For this reason, the National Weather Service chooses to report the **relative humidity,** or the ratio of actual water content to its saturated capacity, at a given temperature (in this case, the relative humidity would be 90%).

One might ask how condensation can be included in this example, but consider that late in the afternoon, it is not uncommon for rain to fall in New Orleans. The rain occurs because the air cools (the sun begins to set), and the capacity of the air to hold water decreases. This decreased capacity to hold water vapor causes condensation, and rain results.

Evaporation and condensation are essential components of respiration. Specifically, effective ventilation requires a balance between the evaporation and condensation of the moisture of respired gases so that the airway mucosa are not dried and irritated. Therapeutic procedures, such as administration of dry medical gases or insertion of an endotracheal tube into a patient's airway to provide mechanical ventilatory support, can severely interfere with the body's ability to maintain this balance. The potential problems associated with bypassing the body's mechanisms for humidifying inspired gases can be minimized by ensuring that all gases delivered to the patient are adequately humidified. Devices such as humidifiers, hygroscopic condenser filters, or artificial noses can be used to ensure adequate humidification of inspired gases. These concepts are revisited in our discussion of humidity and aerosol therapy (see Chapter 4).

Critical Temperature and Critical Pressure

When a liquid is placed in a closed container, the force of the molecules trying to escape from the liquid eventually equilibrates with the force or pressure of the liquid molecules that have entered into the gaseous state, and no more liquid molecules will escape. If the temperature of the liquid is raised, however, the velocity at which its molecules are traveling will increase, whereas the mass attraction between its constituent molecules is reduced. Raising the temperature also increases the capacity of the air above the liquid to hold liquid vapor. Thus the vapor pressure also increases with increases in temperature, necessitating a higher opposing force to equilibrate the molecule's escape from the liquid state. At its boiling point, the force of the molecules in the liquid equals the surrounding pressure, and the molecules may fail to escape. Therefore, in essence, the boiling point is the temperature at which the force exerted by the molecule of the liquid trying to escape equals the forces opposing its escape (i.e., atmospheric pressure and mass attraction). As gas molecules are heated above the boiling point, the force (pressure) required for converting them back to a liquid also increases. Ultimately, a temperature is reached above which gaseous molecules of a substance cannot be converted back to a liquid, no matter what pressure is exerted on them. This temperature is called the **critical temperature**[7]. Therefore, the critical

temperature can be thought of as the highest temperature at which a substance can exist in a liquid state. **Critical pressure** is the pressure that must be applied to the substance at its critical temperature to maintain equilibrium between the liquid and gas phases.[8] The term **critical point** is used to describe the critical temperature and the critical pressure of a substance. Substances that exist as liquids at ambient conditions have critical temperatures that are greater than room temperature (i.e., 20° C to 25° C). Substances that normally exist as gases at ambient conditions have critical temperatures that are usually well below room temperature. (Table 1-2 lists critical temperatures and pressures of some commonly encountered substances.)

Two commonly encountered substances can be used to demonstrate the principles of critical temperature and critical pressure. Water, for example, boils at 100° C and has a critical temperature of 374° C. At temperatures below 100° C, water exists as a liquid. As its temperature is raised above 100° C, water converts to a gas, steam. Between 100° C and 374° C, steam can be converted back into liquid by applying progressively greater amounts of pressure to it. In fact, to maintain equilibrium between the liquid and gaseous states of water at 374° C, 218 atm of pressure must be applied. Furthermore, above 374° C, water can exist only as a gas—no matter how much pressure is applied. Oxygen has a boiling point of −183° C and a critical temperature of about −119° C. At temperatures below −183° C, oxygen can exist as a liquid. After its temperature is raised above −183° C, liquid oxygen becomes a gas. At temperatures between −183° C and −119° C, the gaseous oxygen can be converted back to a liquid by compression. As with water, greater amounts of pressure must be applied to cause this conversion until the critical temperature of −119° C is reached. At oxygen's critical temperature, a pressure of 49.7 atm must be applied to maintain equilibrium between the gaseous and liquid phases of oxygen. After the temperature is raised above the critical temperature, oxygen cannot be converted to a liquid, no matter how much pressure is applied to it.

Application of the concepts of critical temperature and critical pressure can be seen in medical gas therapy. As is discussed in chapters 2 and 3, medical gases can be supplied in cylinders and bulk storage systems. Substances such as nitrous oxide and carbon dioxide have critical tem-

---

TABLE 1-2

Critical Temperatures and Pressures Required to Maintain the Liquid State of Gases at Room Temperature

Gas	Critical Temperature		Critical Pressure		Approximate Pressure in Commercial Cylinder at Room Temperature	
	°C	°F	atm	psi	atm	psig
Cyclopropane	125	257	54.2	797	5.4	79
Nitrous oxide	36.5	97.7	71.8	1054	50.6	745
Carbon dioxide	31.1	87.9	73.0	1071	57.0	838

From Scanlan CL, Spearman CB, Sheldon RL: *Egan's fundamentals of respiratory care*, ed 6, St Louis, 1995, Mosby.

peratures above room temperature and thus can exist as **vapors** (i.e., as a mixture of liquid and gas when placed in a compressed-gas cylinder [gases and vapors are discussed in the next section of this chapter]). Air, oxygen, and helium, on the other hand, have critical temperatures well below room temperature and exist as gases when placed under pressure in a compressed-gas cylinder. Liquid air and oxygen, which must be kept at very low temperatures (i.e., below their boiling points), are stored in specially insulated containers. When needed, the liquid oxygen or air is allowed to exceed its critical temperature and convert to gas.[8]

Gases Versus Vapors

A gas is a state of matter that is above its critical temperature. Free molecules of the same substance below its critical temperature are a vapor. Simply stated, a vapor is the gaseous form of any substance that can exist as a liquid or a solid at ordinary pressures and temperatures. For example, under conditions of 1 atm and a room temperature of 25° C, oxygen exists in the gaseous state because it is above its critical temperature (−119° C); it therefore is classified as a true gas. Water, on the other hand, is below its critical temperature (374° C) and is considered a vapor. Water vapor can be converted back to liquid or ice if sufficient pressure is applied.

Two commonly used vapors are carbon dioxide and nitrous oxide. Both of these substances can be converted to liquid at room temperature if enough pressure is applied. In fact, both gases are supplied to hospitals in pressurized cylinders in which most of the vapor is converted to liquid. As is discussed in Chapter 2, the amount of CO_2 or N_2O remaining in cylinders containing substances below their critical temperature (liquids) must be determined by weighing the cylinders instead of reading the pressure level within the cylinder. Gases such as oxygen, nitrogen, and helium are examples of substances that usually are supplied in compressed-gas cylinders above their critical temperatures. In these cases, the pressure gauge gives an accurate estimate of the amount of gas remaining in the cylinder.

PHYSICAL PROPERTIES OF MATTER

Temperature

As already stated, temperature is a measure of the average kinetic energy of the molecules of an object[9]; however, it is also a measure of the relative warmth or coolness of a substance. Recall that adding heat to a substance changes its physical properties. This phenomenon of changing physical properties can be used in temperature measurements and in designing temperature scales.[10]

Thermometers are devices used to measure temperature. They are made with materials that undergo physical changes as their temperature changes. Thermometers generally are classified as **nonelectrical** and **electrical**

thermometers.[10] The most commonly used nonelectrical devices are mercury and alcohol thermometers. Resistance thermometers, thermistors, and thermocouples are examples of electrical thermometers.

The mercury thermometer is probably the best-known example of a nonelectrical thermometer. This device is the product of Gabriel Daniel Fahrenheit's work on temperature measurement during the early part of the eighteenth century. Fahrenheit (1686-1736) used mercury because he found that it expanded and contracted as its temperature changed. He constructed the first thermometer and ultimately the first mercury temperature scale (i.e., the Fahrenheit temperature scale).

Electrical thermometers operate on the principle that the electrical resistance of metal increases linearly with increases in temperature.[10] A typical resistance thermometer consists of a platinum wire resistor, a battery, and an ammeter for measuring current flow. Because the amount of current flowing through the platinum wire is directly related to the resistance of the wire, the ammeter can detect temperature changes by measuring the changes in current flow that occur when the resistor's temperature is changed.*

Another common example of an electrical thermometer is the **thermistor.** It is typically a metal oxide bead whose resistance changes according to its temperature. An ammeter connected to an electrical circuit measures temperature in a manner similar to that described for the resistance thermometer. Thermistors are incorporated into a number of medical devices, including mechanical ventilators, spirometers, capnographs, and metabolic monitors. Thermistors are also an integral part of the balloon-flotation catheters used with thermodilution cardiac output monitors. All of these devices are discussed in more detail in Chapters 8 and 9, in which monitoring of physiologic function is considered.

Temperature Scales

A temperature scale is constructed by choosing two reference temperatures and dividing the difference between these points into a certain number of degrees. The size of the degree depends on the particular temperature scale being used. The most common reference temperatures are the melting point of ice and the boiling point of water, because recognizable changes take place and thus can be given a value against which other temperatures can be measured.

Three temperature scales are routinely used in science and medicine: the absolute **(Kelvin)** scale, the **Celsius** scale, and the **Fahrenheit** scale. A fourth temperature scale, the **Rankine** scale, is used in the engineering

---

*Actually, the electrical circuit consists of multiple **resistors** arranged in a configuration called a *Wheatstone bridge.* The principles of electronics are discussed later in this chapter. See Box 1-6 for a brief description of a Wheatstone bridge circuit.

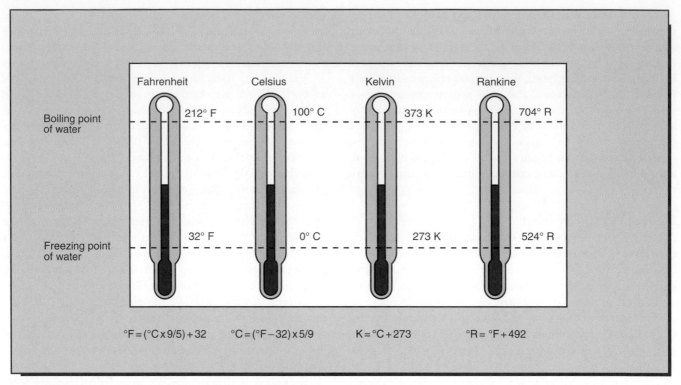

FIGURE 1-3 Temperature scales.

sciences.[7] Figure 1-3 shows the scalar relationships between the Kelvin, Celsius, Fahrenheit, and Rankine scales.

The SI units for temperature are based on the Kelvin scale, with the zero point equal to 0 K or absolute zero, and the boiling point equal to 100 K. Theoretically, absolute zero is the temperature at which all molecular motion stops. Notice that the Kelvin scale is described as a centigrade scale because there are 100 divisions between the freezing and boiling points of water.

The metric or centimeter-gram-second (cgs) system is based on the Celsius scale, which can also be characterized as a centigrade scale. In the Celsius scale, the freezing point for water is designated as 0° C, whereas the boiling point of water equals 100° C. It is important to recognize that although the Celsius and Kelvin scales are both considered centigrade scales, the same temperature has a different value on each. Notice in Figure 1-3 that a temperature of 0 K (i.e., absolute zero, or the temperature at which all the kinetic activity of a substance stops) corresponds to a temperature of −273° C, and that the zero point on the Celsius scale (0° C; i.e., the freezing point of water) therefore corresponds to a temperature of 273 K on the Kelvin scale. Similarly, the boiling point of water on the Celsius scale (100° C) corresponds to a temperature of 373 K.

The Fahrenheit scale, which is used in the British, or foot-pound-second (fps), system, sets the freezing point of water at 32° F and the boiling point of water at 212° F. The Fahrenheit scale has 180 divisions between the freezing and the boiling points of water and therefore cannot be considered a centigrade scale.

Box 1-3 contains formulae for converting temperatures between the various scales. As is seen later in this chapter, the Kelvin scale is used when the gas and other physical laws are described. Also, although increased emphasis is placed on the use of the Celsius scale in the scientific literature and clinical medicine, clinicians in the United States continue to use the Fahrenheit scale for recording patient temperatures.

Pressure

When gas molecules collide with solid or liquid surfaces, they exert a pressure. Pressure (P) is usually defined as the force that a gas exerts over a given area (P = Force/Area). Pressure measurements are reported in a variety of units, including pounds per square inch (psi, or lb/in^2), millimeters of mercury (mm Hg), torr, centimeters of water (cm H_2O), and kilopascals (kPa).[11] Box 1-4 contains formulae for converting pressure units.

Atmospheric pressure is the pressure atmospheric gases exert on objects within the Earth's atmosphere. It exists because the gases that make up the atmosphere are attracted to the Earth's surface by gravity, thus forming a column of air around the Earth. Atmospheric pressure is highest near the Earth's surface; at sea level, atmospheric pressure equals 760 mm Hg. As you move away from the earth's core, the atmospheric pressure decreases because of a reduction in the force of gravity pulling air molecules toward the Earth. For example, the atmospheric pressure in Chicago, which is located at sea level, averages around 760 mm Hg. The atmospheric pres-

BOX 1-3   Temperature Scales

CONVERSIONS BETWEEN THE KELVIN AND CELSIUS SCALES

$$K = °C + 273$$
$$°C = K - 273$$

Example 1
37° C equals how many Kelvin?
$$K = 37°C + 273$$
$$= 310 K$$
(Note that Kelvin is not preceded by the symbol for degrees.)

Example 2
373 K equals how many degrees Celsius?
$$°C = 373 K - 273$$
$$= 100°C$$

CONVERSIONS BETWEEN THE CELSIUS AND FAHRENHEIT SCALES

$$°C = 5/9 \ (°F - 32)$$
$$°F = (9/5 \times °C) + 32$$

Example 1
98.6° F equals how many degrees Celsius?
$$°C = 5/9 \ (98.6°F - 32)$$
$$= 5/9 \ (66.6)$$
$$= 37°C$$

Example 2
25° C equals how many degrees Fahrenheit?
$$°F = (9/5 \times 25) + 32$$
$$= 45 + 32$$
$$= 77°F$$

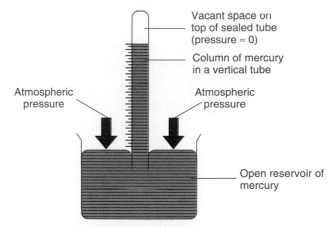

FIGURE 1-4 A mercury barometer. (From Eubanks DH, Bone RC: *Comprehensive respiratory care*, ed 2, St Louis, 1990, Mosby.)

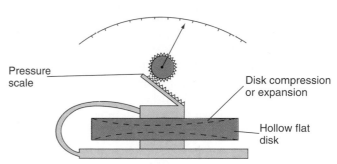

FIGURE 1-5 An aneroid barometer. (From Eubanks DH, Bone RC: *Comprehensive respiratory care*, ed 2, St Louis, 1990, Mosby.)

BOX 1-4   Pressure Conversions

Pressure can be measured in a variety of units, including:
- Centimeters of water (cm H_2O)
- Millimeters of mercury (mm Hg), or torr
- Pounds per square inch (lb/in², or psi)
- Atmospheres (atm)
- Kilopascals (kPa)

The following formulae enable conversions between these units:
- cm H_2O × 0.7355 = mm Hg (torr)
- mm Hg (torr) ÷ 0.7355 = cm H_2O
- cm H_2O × 0.098 = kPa
- kPa ÷ 0.098 = cm H_2O
- mm Hg × 0.1333 = kPa
- kPa ÷ 0.1333 = mm Hg
- mm Hg ÷ 760 = atm
- atm × 14.7 = lb/in² (psi)

sure in Denver, which is located 1 mile above sea level, averages about 630 mm Hg.

Atmospheric pressure can be measured with a barometer similar to the one shown in Figure 1-4. The mercury barometer, which was invented by Evangelista Torricelli (c. 1608-1647), is the most commonly used device for measuring atmospheric pressure. (Torricelli was the first person to recognize the existence of atmospheric pressure;

the pressure measurement *torr* is named in his honor.) The mercury barometer uses the weight of a column of mercury to equilibrate with the force of the gas molecules hitting the surface of a mercury reservoir. A column is completely filled with mercury and erected with its open end below the surface of a mercury reservoir. The mercury in the column tries to return to the reservoir as a result of gravity. The force, which gas molecules exert as they hit the surface of the reservoir, counteracts the force of gravity and pushes the mercury upward in the tube. The atmospheric pressure equals the height of the mercury column.

The aneroid barometer (Figure 1-5) measures atmospheric pressure by equilibrating the atmospheric gas pressure with a mechanical force, or the expansion force of an evacuated metal container. As atmospheric pressure increases, the pressure on the surface of the metal container tends to compress it. The change in the container's dimensions is recorded by a gearing mechanism, which changes the location of an indicator on the recording dial. Likewise, a decrease in atmospheric pressure surrounding the container allows the metal container to expand toward its normal shape.

Density

Density (d) is the measure of a substance's mass per unit volume under specific conditions of pressure and temperature, or

$$d = Mass/Volume$$

For measurements taken near the surface of the Earth, mass may be replaced by a substance's weight, so that **weight density** (d_w) equals weight divided by its volume, or

$$d_W = Weight/Volume$$

As one travels away from the surface of the Earth, the force of gravity diminishes, and thus the relationship between mass and weight changes (i.e., as the force of gravity decreases, so does weight, even though mass stays the same).

For solids and liquids, density can be expressed in grams per liter (g/L) or in grams per cubic centimeter (g/cm^3). The density of gases is also expressed in grams per liter. Because of the influence of pressure and temperature on the density of gases, density is calculated under standard temperature and pressure conditions. Note that standard temperature and pressure (STPD) is defined as 0° C, 760 mm Hg, and dry. The density of gases is covered in more detail with the discussion of Avogadro's law later in this chapter.

Buoyancy

When an object is immersed in a fluid, it appears to weigh less than it does in air. This effect, **buoyancy,** can be explained by the **Archimedes' principle.**[7-9] This principle states that when an object is submerged in a fluid, it will be buoyed up by a force equal to the weight of the fluid that is displaced by the object. The weight of the displaced liquid can be calculated as the product of the volume (V) of displaced liquid and the weight density (d_w) of the liquid:

$$F_{buoyancy} = V \times d_W$$

Consider what happens when an object is submerged in water. Water has a weight density of 1 g/cm^3. If the weight density of the object being submerged is less than the weight density of water, the object will float. If the weight density of the submerged object is greater than that of water, the object will sink. Figure 1-6 illustrates a practical example of this concept. In this case, the weight density of a block of Styrofoam is considerably less than that of a block of lead. It should be apparent from this example that the Styrofoam has a weight density less than water and therefore floats, whereas the block of lead has a weight density greater than water and consequently sinks.

Measurement of the specific gravity of a liquid or gas represents another practical application of the Archimedes principle. Specific gravity is a comparison of a substance's weight density relative to a standard. For liquids, water is used as the standard, and gases are compared with oxygen

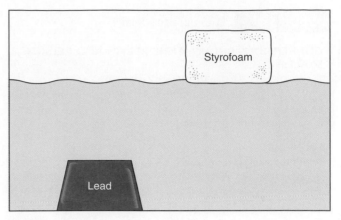

FIGURE 1-6 A practical example of buoyancy. Notice that the block of Styrofoam floats because its weight density is less than that of water, whereas the block of lead sinks because its weight density is greater than the weight density of water.

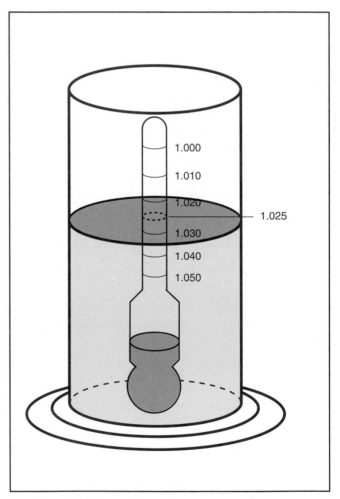

FIGURE 1-7 A hydrometer for measuring specific gravity. (Modified from Nave CR, Nave BC: *Physics for the health sciences,* ed 3, Philadelphia, 1985, WB Saunders.)

or hydrogen.[6] The device shown in Figure 1-7, a **hydrometer,** is used clinically to measure the weight density or specific gravity of liquids, such as urine. The density of a liquid is measured by the level at which the hydrometer floats in the liquid. Thus if the liquid is very dense, the hydrometer floats near the surface, because only a small volume of liquid needs to be displaced to equal the weight of the hydrometer. Conversely, as the density of the liquid decreases, the hydrometer sinks to the bottom of the beaker containing the liquid. Notice in Figure 1-7 that the specific gravity can be read from the tube. Thus a reading of 1.025 indicates that the liquid weighs 1.025 times more than water.[8]

Viscosity

Viscosity can be defined as the force opposing deformation of a fluid. The viscosity of a fluid depends on its density and on the cohesive forces between its constituent molecules (i.e., as the cohesive forces of a fluid increase, so does its viscosity).

Viscosity is manifest differently in liquids and gases.[9] The viscosity of a liquid is primarily determined by the cohesive forces between its molecules, whereas the viscosity of a gas is determined by the number of collisions of the gas molecules. For example, raising the temperature of a liquid such as cooking oil weakens the cohesive forces between its molecules and decreases its viscosity. As the oil is heated and its temperature increases, it flows more freely than at a lower temperature (e.g., room temperature). Conversely, increasing the temperature of a gas increases its kinetic energy (i.e., the frequency of collisions of its constituent molecules). The greater number of collisions results in a higher internal friction and thus an increase in viscosity.

Viscosity is an important factor to consider when describing laminar, or streamlined, flow. The way viscosity influences fluid mechanics, specifically as it relates to Poiseuille's law, is discussed later in this chapter.

Surface Tension

Before the phenomenon of surface tension is described, the difference between **adhesive** and **cohesive forces** should be discussed. Adhesive forces are attractive forces between two different kinds of molecules. Cohesive forces, on the other hand, are attractive forces between like kinds of molecules. The difference between these two forces can be envisioned by taking two dishes and filling one with water and the other with mercury. If a paper towel is gently submerged into each liquid, the results will be different. When the towel is placed in the water dish, it absorbs the water. This is because the attractive, adhesive forces between the molecules of the towel and the water are greater than the attractive forces of the water molecules for each other. When the towel is submerged in the mercury dish, it does not absorb the mercury, because the attractive, cohesive forces between the mercury molecules are greater than the attractive forces between the molecules of the towel and the mercury. Box 1-5 presents another application involving adhesive and cohesive forces.

Surface tension is generated by the cohesive forces between liquid molecules at a gas-liquid interface or at the interface of two immiscible (i.e., unable to mix) liquids,

The properties of adhesion and cohesion can be demonstrated by placing liquid in a small-diameter glass tube, such as those shown in the figure. Notice that at the top of the column of liquid, the liquid forms a curved surface, or *meniscus*. In tube A, which contains water, the meniscus is concave; however, in tube B, which contains mercury, the meniscus is convex. In tube A the meniscus is turned up because the attractive, adhesive forces between the water and the glass cause the water to adhere to the wall of the tube. In tube B the meniscus is turned down because the cohesive forces within the mercury are stronger than the adhesive forces between the mercury and the glass.

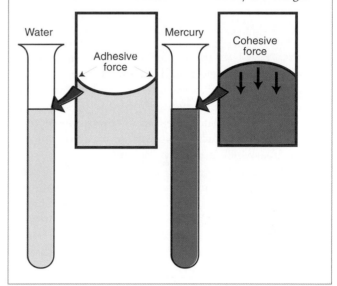

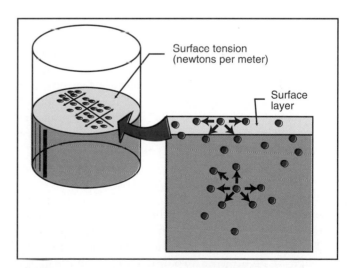

FIGURE 1-8 The molecular basis for surface tension. See text for explanation.

such as oil and water. Figure 1-8 illustrates the molecular basis of surface tension at a gas-liquid interface. At some depth, the molecules within a liquid are attracted equally from all sides, whereas the molecules near the surface experience unequal attractions.[10] Notice that near the surface of the liquid, some of the forces in the liquid act in a direc-

TABLE 1-3

Examples of Surface Tension

Substance	°C	Surface Tension (dyn/cm)
Water	20	73
Water	37	70
Tissue fluid	37	50
Whole blood	37	58
Plasma	37	73
Ethyl alcohol	20	22
Mercury	17	547

From Scanlan CL, Wilkins RL, Stoller JK: *Egan's fundamentals of respiratory care*, ed 7, St Louis, 1999, Mosby.

tion that is parallel to the surface, whereas others are drawn toward the center of the liquid mass by this net force. The forces acting parallel to the surface of the liquid cause the liquid to behave as though a film is present at the gas-liquid interface. The forces drawn toward the center of the liquid tend to reduce its exposed surface to the smallest possible area, which is usually a sphere.

We can measure the surface tension of a liquid by determining the force that must be applied to produce a "tear" in this film.[7] As such, in the SI system of measurements, surface tension usually is expressed in dynes per centimeter (dyn/cm). Table 1-3 lists surface tensions for several liquids commonly encountered in respiratory care. Note that the surface tension of a given liquid varies inversely with its temperature. Thus surface tension decreases as the temperature of a liquid increases.

Laplace's Law

As just stated, surface tension forces cause a liquid to have a tendency to occupy the smallest possible area, which usually is a sphere. The pressure within a liquid sphere should be influenced both by the surface tension forces offered by the liquid and by the size of the sphere. Indeed, Pierre-Simon Laplace (1749-1827), a French astronomer and mathematician, found that pressure within a sphere is directly related to the surface tension of the liquid and inversely related to the radius of the sphere, or

$$P = 2(ST/r)$$

where P is the pressure within the sphere, ST is the surface tension of the liquid, and r is the radius of the sphere.

The examples in Figure 1-9 should help to illustrate this principle. In Figure 1-9A, two droplets of water are shown. One droplet has a radius of 2 cm, and the other droplet has a radius of 4 cm. If we assume that the surface tension is equal in both droplets (i.e., the surface tension of water is 73 dyn/cm), then the pressure in the smaller droplet is twice that of the larger droplet.

Now consider what happens when the surface tension of the smaller droplet is reduced, for example, by adding a surface-active agent (i.e., soap) to the water. As shown in Figure 1-9B, the surface tension of the larger water

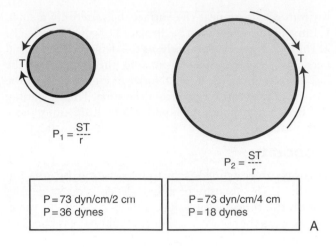

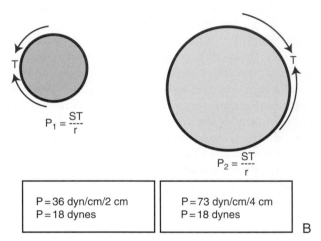

FIGURE 1-9 Laplace's law. **A,** Water bubble. **B,** Soap bubble. See text for discussion.

droplet remains at 73 dyn/cm, but the surface tension of the smaller soap bubble is reduced to half as much (36 dyn/cm). By a simple calculation, one can see that the pressures within the two spheres are now equal.

Applications of Laplace's law can be found in the discussion of aerosol therapy in Chapter 4. As will be seen, surface tension explains why liquid particles retain their spherical shape when suspended in an aerosol suspension.

THE GAS LAWS

The gas laws presented in this section are important generalizations about the macroscopic behavior of gaseous substances. These laws can be seen as summaries of numerous experiments that were conducted over the course of several centuries. The importance of these laws in the development of physics and chemistry is undeniable, and their relevance to the practice of respiratory care cannot be overstated.

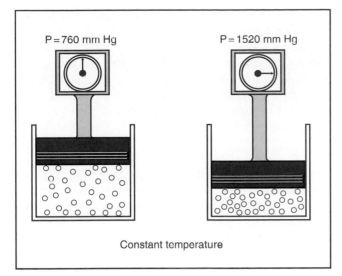

FIGURE 1-10 Boyle's law. (Redrawn from Levitzky MG, Cairo JM, Hall SM: *Introduction to respiratory care*, Philadelphia, 1990, WB Saunders.)

Boyle's Law

Robert Boyle (1627-1691), a British chemist, was the first scientist to investigate the pressure-volume relationships of a gas sample systematically. Boyle found that the volume a gas occupies when it is maintained at a constant temperature is inversely proportional to the absolute pressure exerted on it, or

$$V = 1/P, \text{ or } V = k(1/P)$$

Figure 1-10 illustrates Boyle's law. Note that the absolute pressure of a gas equals the atmospheric pressure plus the pressure measured with a gauge. For example, the pressure of a gas compressed into a 10-L tank is measured as 29.4 psi. The absolute pressure of the gas equals the atmospheric pressure (14.7 psi) plus the gauge pressure of 29.4 psi. Thus the absolute pressure of the gas is 44.1 psi.

Boyle's law can be expressed in a more useful form:

$$V_1 P_1 = V_2 P_2, \text{ or } V_1/V_2 = P_2/P_1$$

which allows an unknown volume or pressure to be calculated when the other variables are known. For example, one can solve for an unknown volume by rearranging the equation to read

$$V_2 = V_1 P_1/P_2$$

Applications of Boyle's law can be found in a number of topics included in this text, such as the mechanics of ventilation, medical gas therapy, blood gas measurements, and pulmonary function testing, which includes spirometry and body plethysmography (see Clinical Rounds 1-1).

Charles' and Gay-Lussac's Laws

Jacques Charles (1746-1823), a French chemist, is recognized as the first scientist to demonstrate experimentally how the volume of a gas varies with changes in temperature. He showed that the volume of a given amount of gas

CLINICAL ROUNDS 1-1

A snorkel diver is preparing to descend in a freshwater pond to a depth of 66 feet. At sea level, his lungs contain about 3000 ml of air. What will happen to the gas volume in his lungs as he descends to 33 feet and then to 66 feet below the surface of the pond? Remember that atmospheric pressure at sea level equals 1 atm and increase by 1 atm for every 33 ft that the diver descends below the surface.

See Evolve Resources for answer.

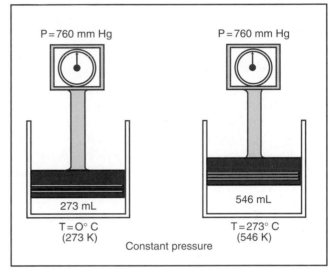

FIGURE 1-11 Charles' law. (Redrawn from Levitzky MG, Cairo JM, Hall SM: *Introduction to respiratory care,* Philadelphia, 1990, WB Saunders.)

held at a constant pressure increases proportionately with increases in the temperature of the gas (Figure 1-11).[12] The relationship between volume and temperature can be explained by the fact that as the temperature of the gas increases, the kinetic energy of the gas molecules increases. This increased kinetic energy content causes the gas molecules to move more vigorously, therefore the gas expands. Conversely, as the temperature of the gas decreases, its molecular activity diminishes, and the gas volume contracts.

William Thomson (Lord Kelvin, 1824-1907) realized the significance of these findings and suggested that there should theoretically be a temperature at which all molecular activity ceases and the associated gas volume is zero. This temperature is called *absolute zero* and has been calculated to be −273.15° C. Although the absolute zero of any substance has not been achieved in a laboratory setting, this temperature serves as a starting point for the Kelvin temperature scale. As mentioned earlier, 1° C corresponds to 1 K. Also, notice that temperature is expressed without degrees in the Kelvin scale (e.g., 0 K equals −273.15° C). Based on the work of Kelvin, Charles' law now is stated thus: when the pressure of a gas is held constant, the volume of a gas varies directly with its absolute temperature expressed in Kelvin, or

$$V/T = k, \text{ or } V_1/T_1 = V_2/T_2$$

Therefore, doubling the absolute temperature of a gas increases the volume of the gas twofold. Conversely, reducing the temperature of a gas by half decreases the volume of the gas by half.

Joseph Gay-Lussac (1778-1850) extended Charles' work by showing that if the volume of a gas is held constant, the gas pressure rises as the absolute temperature of the gas increases, or

$$P/T = k, \text{ or } P_1/T_1 = P_2/T_2$$

Figure 1-12 illustrates Gay-Lussac's law. An example of Gay-Lussac's law that might be encountered in clinical practice can be found in Clinical Rounds 1-2.

Combined Gas Law

In the discussions of the gas laws so far, it has been assumed that one or more of the variables in each law were constant. For example, Boyle's law describes the relationship between pressure and volume when temperature is constant. Charles' law specifies the relationship between temperature and volume when pressure is constant; and Gay-Lussac's law describes the relationship between temperature and pressure when volume is constant.

The combined gas law describes the macroscopic behavior of gases when any or all of the variables change simultaneously. As such, the combined gas law states that the absolute pressure of a gas is inversely related to the volume it occupies and directly related to its absolute temperature, or

$$PV/T = nR$$

where n is the number of moles of gas (a mole is a quantity of substance with a mass equal to its molecular weight expressed in grams), and R is **Boltzmann's universal gas constant**.[3,7,8]

A more practical expression of the combined gas law equation that is used throughout this text is

$$P_1V_1/T_1 = P_2V_2/T_2$$

In this form of the combined gas law, the gas constant (R) and the number of moles of gas (n) are not included, because it is assumed that they will not be affected by changes in pressure, volume, and temperature. Clinical Rounds 1-3 presents an example of a calculation using this form of the combined gas law.

Applications of the combined gas law are found throughout this text. Pressure, volume, and temperature corrections are used extensively in arterial blood gas measurements (see Chapter 10) and during pulmonary function testing (see Chapters 8 and 9).

Dalton's Law of Partial Pressures

Dalton's law states that the sum of the partial pressures of a gas mixture equals the total pressure of the system. Furthermore, the partial pressure of any gas within a gas mixture is proportional to its percentage of the mixture.[7,8] The partial pressure of a gas in a mixture can be calculated by multiplying the total pressure of the mixture by the percentage of the mixture that the gas in question occupies. For example, the partial pressure of oxygen in room air when the barometric pressure equals 1 atm (760 mm Hg) can be calculated by multiplying the total barometric pressure by the percentage of oxygen in the room air. (Note that oxygen makes up approximately 21% of the atmosphere, or 0.21.) Therefore

$$PO_2 = (760)(0.21)$$
$$PO_2 = 159.6 \text{ mm Hg}$$

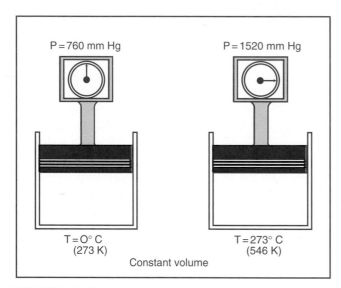

FIGURE 1-12 Gay-Lussac's law. (Redrawn from Levitzky MG, Cairo JM, Hall SM: *Introduction to respiratory care,* Philadelphia, 1990, WB Saunders.)

CLINICAL ROUNDS 1-2

An alarm signals that a fire has broken out in the basement of the hospital. Although the fire is confined to an area approximately 300 feet from the room where the compressed gas cylinders are stored, you are asked to move the cylinders to a safer location. Why is it necessary to move the cylinders?

See Evolve Resources for answer.

CLINICAL ROUNDS 1-3

What is the new volume of a 6 L gas sample existing at 273 K and 760 mm Hg when it is heated to 37° C (310 K) and subjected to 3 atm (2280 mm Hg) of pressure?

See Evolve Resources for answer.

Continuing with this example, the total atmospheric pressure equals the sum of the partial pressures for oxygen (21%), nitrogen (78%), carbon dioxide (0.03%), and other trace gases (~0.7%), or

$$P_B = PO_2 + PN_2 + PCO_2 + P(\text{trace gases})$$
$$P_B = (760)(0.21) + (760)(0.78) + (760)(0.0003) + (760)(0.07)$$
$$P_B = 760 \text{ mm Hg}$$

It should be noted that water vapor pressure does not follow Dalton's law, because such pressure primarily depends on temperature. Because water vapor displaces the partial pressure of other gases, the water vapor pressure (PH_2O) must be subtracted from the total pressure of the gas mixture when the partial pressure of a gas saturated with water vapor is calculated. For example, to calculate the partial pressure of oxygen in a sample of gas that is saturated with water vapor at 37° C, the following formula* is applied:

$$PO_2 = (P_B - PH_2O)(F_iO_2)$$
$$PO_2 = (760 \text{ mm Hg} - 47 \text{ mm Hg})(0.21)$$
$$PO_2 = 149.73 \text{ mm Hg}$$

Avogadro's Law

Avogadro's law states that equal volumes of gas at the same pressure and temperature contain the same number of molecules. It is based on the work of Amedeo Avogadro (1776-1856), who determined that 1 gram molecular weight (gmw), or mole, of any gas occupies 22.4 L at a temperature of 0° C (273 K) and a pressure of 1 atm. Subsequently, it was determined that 1 mole of gas at this volume contains 6.02×10^{23} molecules **(Avogadro's number).** For example, 1 mole of oxygen (mw = 32 g) occupies a volume of 22.4 L and contains 6.02×10^{23} molecules when measured at 0° C (273 K) and 1 atm.

A practical application of Avogadro's law is seen in the calculation of gas densities and specific gravity. The density of a gas per unit volume can be calculated with the following formula:

$$\text{Density} (g/L) = \text{mw of gas} / 22.4 \text{ L}$$

The specific gravity of a gas is defined as the ratio of the density of a gas relative to the density of a standard gas, such as air, oxygen, or hydrogen. Figure 1-13 shows the specific gravity of several gases used in respiratory care and anesthetics.

Laws of Diffusion

Up to this point, the discussion of gases has focused on the ability of a gas to expand and to be compressed. Another property that must be discussed in any analysis of gas

TABLE 1-4	
Water Vapor Pressure and Content at Selected Temperatures and 760 mm Hg	
° C	**Vapor Pressure (mm Hg)**
0	4.58
10	9.21
11	9.84
12	10.52
13	11.23
14	11.99
15	12.79
16	13.63
17	14.53
18	15.48
19	16.48
20	17.54
21	18.65
22	19.83
23	21.07
24	22.38
25	23.76
26	25.21
27	26.74
28	28.35
29	30.04
30	31.82
31	33.70
32	35.66
33	37.73
34	39.90
35	42.18
36	44.56
37	47.07
38	49.70
39	52.44
40	55.32

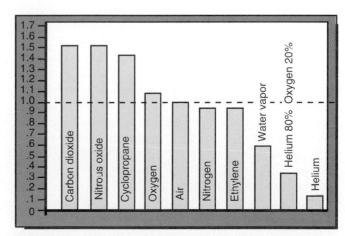

FIGURE 1-13 Specific gravity for several gases that are used in respiratory care and anesthetics. Comparisons have been made with air at 25° C and 1 atm. (Redrawn from Adriani J: *The chemistry and physics of anesthesia,* ed 3, Springfield, Ill, 1979, Charles C Thomas.)

*Note that the vapor pressure of water at 37° C is 47 mm Hg. Table 1-4 lists the vapor pressures for water at selected temperatures.

behavior is **diffusion,** which can be defined as the net movement of gas molecules, by virtue of their kinetic properties, from an area of high concentration to an area of low concentration. Graham's law, Henry's law, and Fick's law are used to describe diffusion and its applications in respiratory care.

Graham's Law

In 1832, Thomas Graham (1805-1869) stated that when two gases are placed under the same temperature and pressure conditions, the rates of diffusion of the two gases are inversely proportional to the square root of their masses, or

$$r_1/r_2 = \sqrt{M_2/M_1}$$

where r_1 and r_2 represent the diffusion rates of the respective gases, and M_1 and M_2 are the molar masses.

If the mass of a gas is considered directly proportional to its density at a constant temperature and pressure, then

$$r_1/r_2 = \sqrt{d_2/d_1}$$

where d_1 and d_2 are the densities of the gases in question.

Henry's Law

When a gas is confined in a space adjacent to a liquid, a certain number of gas molecules dissolve in the liquid phase. Joseph Henry (1797-1878) found that for a given temperature, the mass of a gas that dissolves (and does not combine chemically) in a specified volume of liquid is directly proportional to the product of the partial pressure of the gas and its solubility coefficient, or

$$c \propto P \times S$$

where c is the molar concentration (in mol/L) of the dissolved gas, P is the pressure (in atm) of gas over the liquid, and S is the solubility coefficient (also known as Bunsen's coefficient) for the gas in that particular liquid (in L/atm or L/mm Hg). The solubility of a gas in a liquid is equal to the volume of gas (in liters) that will saturate 1 L of liquid at standard temperature and pressure (0° C and 1 atm). In respiratory care, Henry's law is encountered in discussions of the solubility of gases, such as oxygen, in blood. In these cases, we express the solubility of a gas in milliliters of gas dissolved in milliliters of blood. For example, it is known that 0.023 mL of oxygen dissolves in every milliliter of blood at a temperature of 38° C and 1 atm of pressure.

Fick's Law of Diffusion

Thus far we have limited our discussion to the rate of diffusion of one gas into another gas and the diffusion rate of a gas into a liquid. In respiratory care, the diffusion of gases across semipermeable membranes (e.g., the diffusion of oxygen and carbon dioxide across the alveolar-capillary membrane) is also a concern.[12,13] A semipermeable membrane is not freely permeable to all components of a

mixture. Thus the membrane may be impermeable to a substance because of its size or chemical composition (e.g., electrical charge).

Adolph Fick (1829-1901) stated that the flow of a gas across a semipermeable membrane per unit time ($\dot{V}$gas) into a membrane fluid phase is directly proportional to the surface area (A) available for diffusion, the partial pressure gradient between the two compartments (ΔP), and the solubility of the gas (S). This flow is inversely proportional to the square root of the molecular weight of the gas ($\sqrt{MW}$) and the thickness of the membrane (T) (Figure 1-14). Fick's law can be shown as

$$\dot{V}gas = A \times S \times \Delta P \div \sqrt{MW} \times T$$

Considering that the diffusivity of a gas equals its solubility divided by the square root of its molecular weight, or

$$D = S \div \sqrt{MW}$$

where D is the diffusivity, S is the solubility, and MW is the molecular weight, then Fick's law can be restated as

$$\dot{V}gas = A \times D \times DP/T$$

Test your understanding of the laws of diffusion by answering the question in Clinical Rounds 1-4.

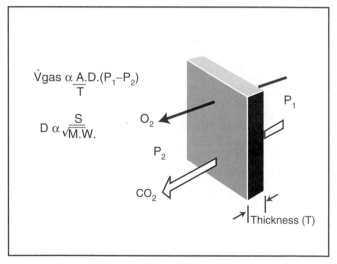

FIGURE 1-14 Fick's law of diffusion. (Modified from West JB: *Respiratory physiology: the essentials,* ed 3, Baltimore, 1985, Williams & Wilkins.)

CLINICAL ROUNDS 1-4

Using Fick's law of diffusion, describe several conditions in which the diffusion of oxygen across the alveolar-capillary membrane is reduced.

See Evolve Resources for answer.

FLUID MECHANICS

Fluid mechanics is the branch of physics dealing with the properties and behavior of fluids in motion. This field involves fluid dynamics, which is subdivided into hydrodynamics (the study of liquids in motion) and aerodynamics (the study of gases in motion). With diffusion, gas movement was described as being the result of the spontaneous intermingling of the individual gas molecules as a result of random thermal motion. In the section that follows, bulk gas flow is discussed; this deals with the transport of whole groups of molecules (i.e., a volume of gas) from one location to another, rather than the movement of individual gas molecules.

Patterns of Flow

This text is concerned primarily with the flow of fluids through various types of tubes. Whether this flow involves the movement of liquids or gases, all fluid flow may be characterized as laminar, turbulent, or transitional in nature. Figure 1-15 shows the three types of flow.

In laminar flow, the fluid flows in discrete cylindrical layers, or streamlines.[8] Laminar flow normally is associated with the movement of fluids through tubes with smooth surfaces and fixed radii. With laminar flow, the pressure required to produce a given flow is directly related to the viscosity of the fluid and the length of the tube and inversely related to the radius of the tube. These relationships are discussed in detail in the section on Poiseuille's law.

With turbulent flow, the movement of fluid molecules becomes chaotic and the orderly pattern of concentric layers seen with laminar flow is lost. As will be seen, Poiseuille's law cannot be used to predict the amount of pressure required for a given flow when turbulence is present. When turbulence is present, the pressure required to produce a given flow is influenced less by the viscosity of the fluid and more by its density. Additionally, the driving pressure required to achieve a given flow is proportional to the *square* of the flow. Turbulent flow occurs when the velocity at which the fluid is moving increases sharply, when the tube's radius varies, and when tubes have rough, uneven surfaces. The likelihood of turbulent flow developing can be predicted by Reynolds' number, which is discussed shortly.

Transitional flow is simply a mixture of laminar and turbulent flows. In cases when laminar flow predominates, the driving pressure varies linearly with the flow. When turbulent flow dominates, the driving pressure varies with the *square* of the flow. Transitional flow typically occurs at points where tubes divide into one or more branches. Figure 1-15 illustrates the types of flow that can be observed as gas flows into the lungs. Gas flow in the larger airways is turbulent, but laminar flow predominates in the smaller airways. Transitional flow (or tracheobronchial flow, as it appears in Figure 1-15) occurs at points where the airways divide (e.g., where the mainstem bronchi divide into the lobar bronchi).

Poiseuille's Law

When one considers the flow of a liquid or gas through a tube, two factors must be taken into account: the driving pressure forcing the fluid through the tube (i.e., the pressure gradient) and the resistance the fluid must overcome as it flows through the tube. Jean L.M. Poiseuille (1797-1869), a French physiologist, described the interrelationships between pressure, flow, and resistance for a liquid flowing through an unbranched, rigid tube with the following formula:

$$\Delta P = \dot{Q} \times R$$

where ΔP is the pressure gradient from the beginning to the end of the tube ($P_1 - P_2$), $\dot{Q}$ is the flow of the liquid through the tube, and R is the resistance opposing the flow of the liquid. (Note that in discussions of the mechanics of breathing, $\dot{Q}$ is replaced with $\dot{V}$, which is used to symbolize the flow of a gas.) The pressure gradient can be described as the difference in pressure at the entrance of the tube and the exit point, or $P_1 - P_2$. Poiseuille found that the factors determining resistance to flow include the viscosity of the fluid and the length and radius of the tube, or

$$R = (8\eta l)/(\pi r^4)$$

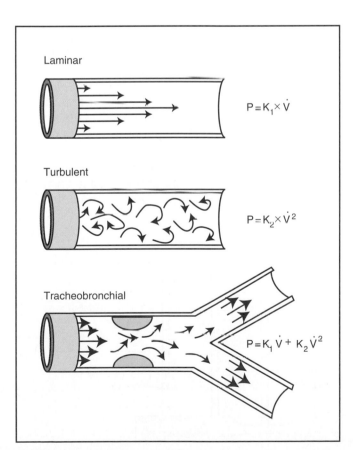

Laminar

$$P = K_1 \times \dot{V}$$

Turbulent

$$P = K_2 \times \dot{V}^2$$

Tracheobronchial

$$P = K_1 \dot{V} + K_2 \dot{V}^2$$

FIGURE 1-15 Three patterns of flow: laminar, turbulent, and transitional.

where η is the viscosity of the liquid, l is the length of the tube, and r is the radius of the tube. Incorporating these findings, Poiseuille's law can be rewritten as

$$\Delta P = \dot{Q} \times [(8\eta l)/(\pi r^4)]$$

Based on these equations, the following can be stated:
1. The more viscous a fluid, the greater the pressure gradient required to cause it to move through a given tube.
2. The resistance offered by a tube is directly proportional to its length; the pressure required to achieve a given flow through a tube must increase in direct proportion to the length of the tube.
3. Because the resistance to flow is inversely proportional to the fourth power of the radius, small changes in the radius of a tube cause profound decreases in the flow of the fluid through the tube. For example, decreasing the radius by one half increases the resistance 16-fold.

Applications of Poiseuille's law are found in the discussion related to medical gas therapy, physiologic pressure monitoring, and mechanical ventilation.

Reynolds' Number

As was discussed earlier, fluid flow becomes turbulent when the velocity at which the liquid or gas molecules are traveling increases sharply. Several other factors also can produce turbulent flow, including changes in the density and viscosity of the gas or in the radius of the tube. These factors can be combined mathematically to determine Reynolds' number:

$$N_R = v \times d \times (2r/\eta)$$

where v is the velocity of flow, r is the radius of the tube, and d and η are the density and viscosity of the gas, respectively. Note that the Reynolds number does not have units. Turbulent flow predominates when the Reynolds number exceeds 2000, although turbulent flow may occur at lower Reynolds' numbers when the surface of the tube is rough or irregular.[8,14]

Turbulent flow is produced by an increase in the linear velocity of the gas, the density of the gas, or the radius of the tube; it also can be produced by reductions in the viscosity of the gas. Applications of the Reynolds number are seen in the discussions of the mechanics of breathing and mechanical ventilation later in this text.

Bernoulli Principle

The Bernoulli principle is the result of work by Daniel Bernoulli (1700-1782), a Swiss mathematician who stated that as the forward velocity of a gas (or liquid) moving through a tube increases, the lateral wall pressure of the tube decreases.[7,15] This can be demonstrated with an apparatus such as the one in Figure 1-16, which consists of a fluid flowing through a tube with a series of manometers attached to its wall. The manometers register the lateral wall pressure as the fluid flows through the tube. Notice that as the fluid flows through a tube of uniform diameter, a progressive drop in pressure occurs over the length of the tube. The gradual decrease in pressure can be determined by looking at the first three manometers in Figure 1-16. Notice that as the fluid flows through a constriction in the tube, the pressure in the fourth manometer shows an even greater drop in pressure. If it is assumed that the total flow of liquid is the same before and after the constriction, then the flow of liquid must accelerate as it enters the constriction. Therefore, it is reasonable to assume that the drop in fluid pressure is directly related to the increase in fluid speed.

Venturi Principle

The Venturi principle, which is related to the work of Bernoulli, was first described by Giovanni Venturi (1746-1822) and can be illustrated with an apparatus such as the one in Figure 1-17. Notice that this apparatus is similar to the tube used to explain the Bernoulli principle. The Venturi principle states that the pressure that has dropped as the fluid flows through a constriction in the tube can be restored to the preconstriction pressure if a gradual dilation occurs in the tube distal to the constriction. Note that

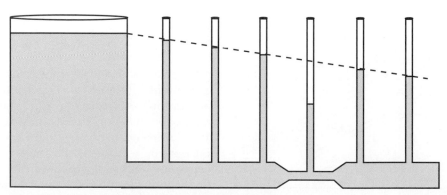

FIGURE 1-16 The Bernoulli principle. (Redrawn from Nave CR, Nave BC: *Physics for the health sciences,* ed 3, Philadelphia, 1985, WB Saunders.)

the gradual dilation of the tube must have an angle of divergence that is less than or equal to 15 degrees.[7,8,16]

Venturi tubes are used in many devices in respiratory care. Air entrainment masks, aerosol generators, and humidifiers are the most common examples. With these devices, a lateral port just distal to the constriction is used to entrain the second gas or a liquid into the main gas flow. The increased gas flow is accommodated by a gradual dilation of the tube downstream of the constriction. Other applications of the Venturi principle are described throughout this text.

Coanda Effect

The Coanda effect, which is also based on the Bernoulli principle, is illustrated in Figure 1-18. As was previously explained, the lateral wall pressure of the tube decreases when the fluid flows through a narrowing of the tube because of the increased forward velocity of the fluid flow. If the wall does not have a side port for entraining another fluid, the low pressure adjacent to the wall draws the stream of fluid against the wall. When a specially contoured tube, such as the one in Figure 1-18, is attached distal to the narrow part of the tube, the flow exiting the narrow part of the tube tends to adhere to the wall of the contoured tube because of two factors: a negative pressure is generated past the constriction, thus drawing the fluid toward the curved extension; and the ambient pressure opposite the extension pushes the fluid stream against the wall, where it remains locked until interrupted by a counterforce, such as a pulse of air.[8] Using these findings, Coanda was able to demonstrate that with careful placement of the postconstriction extensions, he could deflect a stream of air through a full 180-degree turn by extending the wall contour.[10]

The Coanda effect is the basis for **fluidic** devices used in several mechanical ventilators (see Chapter 12). Such devices use gates that are regulated by gas flow from side jets, which operate on the principle that pulses of air are used to redirect the original gas stream. The main advan-

tage of using these fluid logic devices is that they have fewer valves and moving parts that can break (i.e., gas flow is regulated by gas jets, not typical mechanical metal or plastic valves). The primary disadvantage is that these devices consume more gas than more conventional devices because gas flow is used to power the various fluid logic gates. Chapter 11 includes an extensive discussion of fluidic elements used in mechanical ventilators.

PRINCIPLES OF ELECTRICITY

Many respiratory care devices are powered by electricity and in many cases are also controlled by computers that use solid-state electronic circuitry. Mechanical ventilators, blood gas analyzers, physiologic transducers and monitors, cathode ray tube displays, and strip chart and X-Y recorders are some examples.[8] Because of the importance of these devices in respiratory care, a basic understanding of electronics and electrical safety is essential.

Principles of Electronics

Electricity is produced by the flow of electrons through a conductive path or circuit. This flow, electric current, is influenced by (1) the force pushing the electrons through a conductive path (i.e., electromotive force or voltage) and

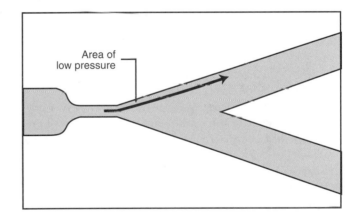

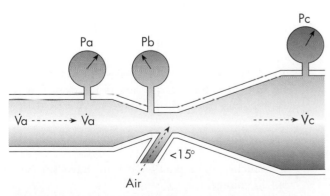

FIGURE 1-17 The Venturi principle. See text for discussion. (From Scanlan CL, Wilkins BL, Stoller JK: *Egan's fundamentals of respiratory care,* ed 7, St Louis, 1999, Mosby.)

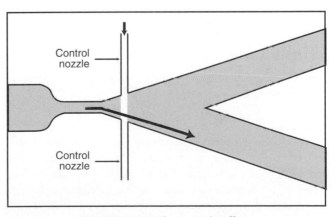

FIGURE 1-18 The Coanda effect.

(2) the resistance the electrons must overcome as they flow through the conductive path.

Electric current, which is symbolized as I, can be measured with an **ammeter.** The standard unit of measurement of electric current is the **ampere** (A), where 1 A is equivalent to 6.25×10^{18} electrons passing a point in 1 second. (Note that in electronics, the term *coulomb* is used as a shorthand notation for 6.25×10^{18} electrons. Thus 1 A equals 1 coulomb per second). Amperes can be subdivided into smaller quantities, such as milliamperes (mA, or milliamp) and microamperes (μA or microamp), using scientific notation. For example, 1 mA is 1/1000 of an ampere, and 1 μA is 1/1,000,000 of an ampere. Ammeters typically have scales calibrated in amperes, milliamperes, and microamperes.

As previously stated, voltage is the electrical force (more correctly termed **electromotive force,** or emf) that drives electrons through the conductive path. In most physics textbooks, voltage is also described as the potential difference between two points. Voltage sources include batteries, hydroelectric generators, solar cells, and piezoelectric crystals. Voltage is measured using a **voltmeter;** the standard unit of measurement for voltage is the **volt** (V), which can be defined as the electrical potential required for 1 A of electricity to move through 1 **ohm** (Ω) of resistance. As with amperes, volts can be subdivided into smaller units, such as millivolts (mV) and microvolts (μV).

Resistance in electric circuits, as with resistance in fluid circuits, is the opposition to flow. Resistance, which is measured in ohms, is a property of a conductor that is influenced by the conductor's chemical composition or specific resistance (ρ), as well as by its length and cross-sectional area. Most metals and salt solutions are good conductors (i.e., they offer low resistance to current flow). With regard to physical dimensions, the resistance of a conductor increases as its length increases or its cross-sectional area decreases. Rubber, plastic, and glass are poor conductors, because they offer high resistance to current flow. Because these materials are such poor conductors, they can be used as protective coverings on conductive wires; they therefore are often called **insulators. Semiconductors** are materials with conductivity characteristics that are intermediate between conductors and insulators. Semiconductors can be found in thermistors, and photodetectors often are used in diagnostic equipment.

Ohm's Law

The relationships among current, voltage, and resistance can be explained with **Ohm's law:**

$$V = I \times R$$

According to Ohm's law, voltage and current are directly related, which simply means that if the resistance is constant, increases in voltage cause increases in current flow. Conversely, decreases in source voltage cause a reduction in current flow (assuming resistance is constant). Now consider how changes in resistance affect current flow. If voltage is held constant, increases in resistance cause a decrease in current flow, whereas decreases in resistance cause an increase in current flow. Thus current and resistance are inversely related.

It should be apparent from this discussion that any one variable can be solved for if the other two are known. Thus, by rearranging the above equation, the current can be solved for:

$$I = V/R$$

Similarly, resistance can be solved for with the following rearrangement:

$$R = V/I$$

It is important to grasp these concepts to understand circuit analysis. These principles will now be applied in an analysis of simple electric circuits.

Electrical Circuits

An electrical circuit consists of a voltage source, a load, and a conductive path. An applied voltage causes a current to flow through a conductive path containing one or more loads before returning to the voltage source.

Electrical circuits can be classified as series circuits and parallel circuits. Notice that in a series circuit, the current flows through one path. The current flows from the voltage source through the conductor and through a series of resistive loads, which are arranged end to end (i.e., through R_1 then R_2, and so on), and then back to the voltage source. In contrast, the parallel circuit may be depicted as two or more series circuits connected to a common voltage source.

One must keep in mind several principles when analyzing series and parallel circuits. These principles, which are referred to as Kirchhoff's laws, provide the framework for performing circuit analysis.

Kirchhoff's laws governing series circuits may be summarized as follows:

1. A series circuit can have one or more voltage sources. The total source voltage equals the sum of the individual sources if their direction of polarity is the same.
2. In a series circuit, current is the same through all components.
3. The total resistance in a series circuit can be computed by finding the sum of all resistance in the circuit. That is, $R_T = R_1 + R_2 + R_3$, and so on.
4. The sum of voltage drops across resistance in the circuit equals the applied voltage, or $V_T = IR_1 + IR_2 + IR_3$, and so on.

Parallel circuits must adhere to the following guidelines:

1. All branches of a parallel circuit have the same applied voltage.
2. Each branch of a parallel circuit may have a different current flow, depending on the resistance of the branch.

3. The total current flowing through a parallel circuit can be computed by finding the sum of the currents flowing through the various branches of the circuit. Thus, $I_T = I_1 + I_2 + I_3$, and so on.

4. The total resistance in a parallel circuit can be computed by finding the sum of the reciprocals for each resistance. That is, $R_T = 1/(1/R_1 + 1/R_2 + 1/R_3,$ and so on).

Box 1-6 provides a description of a **Wheatstone bridge** circuit. This type of circuitry is widely used in medical instrumentation, such as oxygen analyzers and strain gauge pressure transducers. These devices are discussed in more detail in Chapters 8 and 9.

Electrical Safety

Electrical accidents occur when current from an electrical device interacts with body tissue, impairing physiologic function. It is important to recognize that electrical hazards exist only when the current path through the body is complete. That is, two connections to the body are required for an electrical shock to occur.[8,14] One connection (the "hot" wire) brings the current to the body, and the second connection (the neutral wire) completes the circuit by sending the charge to a point of lower potential or ground.

The extent of impairment depends on the amount of current flowing through the body, the duration the current

---

| BOX 1-6 | Electrical Circuit Analysis: The Wheatstone Bridge |

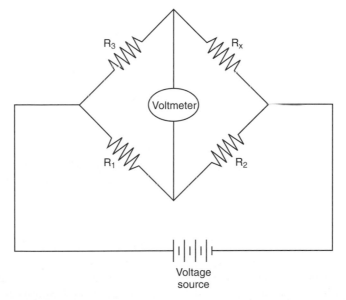

The Wheatstone bridge is a series-parallel circuit that consists of a direct current (DC) voltage source (e.g., a battery) and a galvanometer that connects two parallel branches containing four resistors (R_1, R_2, R_3, and R_X). The values of R_1 and R_2 are known, and R_3 is a calibrated variable resistance, for which the current value may be read from a dial on the galvanometer. The unknown resistor (R_X) is connected to the fourth side of the circuit. As the resistance of the unknown resistor changes (e.g., changes in the resistance of R_X occur when the physical dimensions of the wire are altered, such as when pressure is applied to the resistance wire), the variable resistance of R_3 is adjusted until the galvanometer reads zero.

The Wheatstone bridge circuit actually was first described by Samuel Hunter Christie in 1833. Sir Charles Wheatstone was later responsible for developing practical uses for the circuit. For example, the Wheatstone bridge is ideal for measuring small changes in resistance; it therefore can be used in devices such as the strain gauge pressure transducer, which is used to measure blood pressure in the critical care setting.

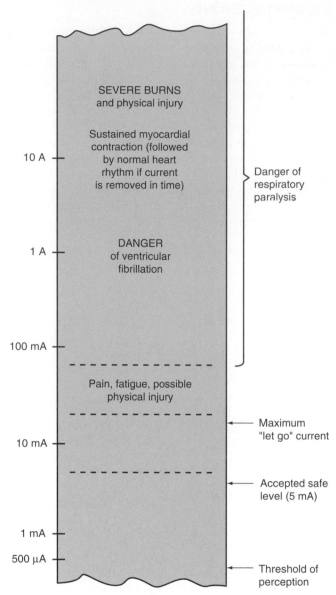

FIGURE 1-19 Physiologic effects of electrical current associated with a 1-second external contact with a 110 VAC current at 60 Hz. (Redrawn from Cromwell L, Weibell FJ, Pfeiffer EA: *Biomedical instrumentation and measurements,* ed 2, 1980, Reprinted by permission of Pearson Education, Inc. Upper Saddle River, NJ.)

is applied, and the path the current takes through the body.[8] Figure 1-19 shows the approximate current ranges and the physiologic effects of a 1-second exposure to various levels of 110 V, 60 Hz alternating currents applied externally to the body.[14]

Two types of electric shock hazards usually are described: **macroshock** and **microshock.** A macroshock occurs when a relatively high current is applied to the body surface. Generally, a current of 1 mA is required to elicit a macroshock. A microshock occurs when a low current (usually less than 1 mA) is allowed to bypass the body surface and flow directly into the body.

Electric current can damage body tissues by causing thermal burns and inadvertently stimulating excitable tissue, such as cardiac muscle. Burns are caused when electric energy dissipates in body tissues, causing the temperature of the tissues to rise. If the temperature gets high enough, it can cause burns. Inadvertent stimulation of excitable tissue can occur when an extraneous electric current of sufficient magnitude causes local voltages that can trigger action potentials. Action potentials triggered in sensory nerves cause a tingling sensation that is associated with electric shock. Action potentials generated in motor nerves and muscles result in muscle contractions, which, if the intensity of the stimulation is high enough, can cause tetanus or sustained contraction of the muscle.

It should be noted that the heart is the organ most susceptible to electrical hazards. Its susceptibility to electrical hazards arises from the fact that when current exceeds a certain value, extra systolic contractions can occur in cardiac muscle. Further increases in current can cause the heart to fibrillate and ultimately can cause sustained myocardial contraction.

Preventing Electrical Hazards

Various strategies should be used to reduce the likelihood of electrical accidents. These include ensuring proper grounding of medical equipment, installing ground-fault circuit interrupters, and avoiding contact with transcutaneous conductors.[14]

Grounding

The principle of the grounding protection method for medical equipment is to provide a low-resistance conductive path that allows most fault current to bypass the patient and return to ground. In cord-connected electrical equipment, this ground connection is established by a third round or U-shaped contact in the plug.

It is important to recognize that grounding is effective only if a good ground connection exists. Worn or broken wires, inadvertent disconnection of ground wires from receptacles, and deliberate removal of ground contacts from plugs interfere with the protection associated with grounding. Because conventional receptacles, line cords, and plugs do not hold up to hospital use, most manufacturers provide hospital-grade receptacles and plugs that must meet Underwriters' Laboratory specifications. Hospital-grade receptacles and plugs usually can be identified by a green dot.[14]

Ground-Fault Circuit Interrupters

Normally, all the power entering a device through the hot wire returns through the neutral wire. Circuit interrupters monitor the difference between the hot and neutral wires of the power line with a differential transformer and an electrical amplifier. When this difference exceeds a predetermined level (e.g., 5 mA), as occurs when the current bypasses the neutral wire and flows through the patient, the power is interrupted by a circuit breaker. Notice that this interruption occurs rapidly so that the patient does not encounter any harmful effects.

Avoiding Contact with Transcutaneous Conductors

The resistance offered by the skin represents the greatest part of the body's electrical resistance.[16] This resistance can be significantly reduced by permeating the skin with conductive fluid, by cuts and abrasions to the epithelium, or by the introduction of needles through the skin's surface. Electrically conductive catheters inserted through a vein or artery can also bypass the natural electrical resistance offered by the skin.

It should be apparent from the discussion so far that these conditions can place patients in compromised states and make them susceptible to microshock hazards. These hazardous effects can be lessened if all electrical devices used with a microshock-sensitive patient are well insulated and connected to outlets with a common low-resistance ground.[8] Additionally, devices should be inspected regularly for frayed or bare wires.

KEY POINTS

- Kinetic energy is the energy that an object possesses when it is in motion; potential energy is stored energy, or the energy that it possesses because of its position.
- The physical and chemical properties of all matter can be explained by the kinetic theory. The physical state of any substance is determined by the relationship between its kinetic energy content and the potential energy stored in its intermolecular bonds.
- Changes in state involve the interconversion of solids, liquids, and gases, which can be accomplished by altering the relationship between the substance's kinetic and potential energies.
- The amount of heat that must be added to effect the change of a solid to a liquid (latent heat of fusion) or a liquid to a gas (latent heat of vaporization) depends the intermolecular attractive forces that must be overcome.
- Three temperature scales are routinely used in science and medicine. The SI units for temperature are based on the Kelvin scale, whereas the metric unit for temperature is the Celsius scale. The Fahrenheit scale is used in the British system of units.
- The Kelvin scale is used when describing physical laws and the Celsius and Fahrenheit scales are used to quantify temperature measurements in the scientific literature and clinical medicine.
- Pressure is defined as the force that a gas exerts over a given area, or $P = F/A$. The pressure units most often used in respiratory care include mm Hg, cm H_2O, torr, kPa, and lb/in^2.
- The density of a substance is a measure of its mass or weight per unit volume under standard conditions of temperature and pressure (STPD). The specific gravity of a liquid or gas is a comparison of its weight density relative to a standard, such as water in the case of a liquid or oxygen in the case of gas.

- The gas laws are important generalizations about the behavior of gases. The combined gas law expresses the relationship between V, P, T, and mass for any gas. Applications of the combined gas law can be found in blood gas and pulmonary function measurements.
- According to Dalton's law, the partial pressure of a gas is the absolute pressure of that gas in a multiple gas mixture. For example, the partial pressure of oxygen in room air can be calculated by multiplying the barometric pressure by the 0.21 or the percentage of oxygen that makes up room air.
- Poiseuille's law can be used to demonstrate that the flow of gas through a tube is directly proportional to the pressure gradient from the beginning to the end of the tube and inversely related to the resistance to flow. The resistance is determined by the length and radius of the tube and the viscosity of the gas flowing through the tube.
- The Bernoulli principle states that the lateral wall pressure of a tube decreases as the forward velocity of the fluid moving through the tube increases.
- The Venturi principle states that the pressure drop that occurs as a fluid flows through a constriction in a tube can be restored to the preconstriction level if the tube gradually dilates distal to the constriction.
- The Coanda effect, which is a variation on the Bernoulli principle, is the basis for fluidic gates, which are used in the design of mechanical ventilators.
- Ohm's law describes the relationship between voltage, current, and resistance in an electrical circuit. As such, Ohm's law states that the total current flow through a circuit is directly proportional to the total applied voltage and inversely related to the total resistance of the circuit.
- The most effective methods for reducing the likelihood of electrical accidents include using proper grounding of all electrical equipment, installing ground-fault circuit interrupters, and avoiding transcutaneous conductors.

ASSESSMENT QUESTIONS

See Evolve Resources for answers.

1. Convert the following temperatures:
   a. _____ °C = 102° F
   b. 25° C = _____ ° F
   c. _____ K = 98.6° F
   d. 37° C = _____ K

2. Perform the following pressure conversions:
   a. _____ kPa = 30 cm H_2O
   b. _____ mm Hg = 1033 cm H_2O
   c. 20 cm H_2O = _____ mm Hg
   d. _____ lb/in^2 = 2 atm

3. Calculate the partial pressures of each of the following gases in room air when the barometric pressure is 760 mm Hg (assume that room air contains 21% oxygen, 78% nitrogen, and 0.03% carbon dioxide):
   a. PO_2 = _____ mm Hg
   b. PN_2 = _____ mm Hg
   c. PCO_2 = _____ mm Hg

4. What is the total pressure of a gas mixture if PO_2 = 90 mm Hg, PCO_2 = 40 mm Hg, PN_2 = 573 mm Hg, and PH_2O = 47 mm Hg?
   a. 573 mm Hg
   b. 713 mm Hg
   c. 750 mm Hg
   d. 760 mm Hg

5. A compressed-gas cylinder at 760 mm Hg and 25° C is moved into a room where the temperature is 38° C. What is the new pressure of the cylinder, assuming that the volume of gas within the cylinder remains constant?

6. A patient's lung capacity is measured as 6 L at an initial temperature of 25° C and an ambient pressure of 760 mm Hg. What will the new volume be if the temperature increases to 37° C and the pressure to 1520 mm Hg?

7. Calculate the densities of oxygen and carbon dioxide. The molecular weight of oxygen is 32 gmw, and the molecular weight of carbon dioxide is 44 gmw.

8. According to Poiseuille's law, the gas flow through a tube is inversely proportional to the:
   I. length of the tube
   II. driving pressure of the gas through the tube
   III. viscosity of the gas
   IV. radius of the tube
      a. I and III only
      b. II and IV only
      c. I, II, and III only
      d. II, III, and IV only

9. Which of the following will increase the flow of a gas across a semipermeable membrane, according to Fick's law of diffusion?

   I. Increasing the surface area of the membrane
   II. Increasing the partial pressure gradient of the gas across the membrane
   III. Increasing the density of the gas
   IV. Increasing the thickness of the membrane
      a. I and II only
      b. III and IV only
      c. I, II, and III only
      d. II, III, and IV only

10. Which of the following variables will lead to an increase in turbulent airflow?
    I. Increased density of the gas
    II. Decreased linear velocity of the gas flow
    III. Increased radius of the conducting tube
    IV. Decreased viscosity of the gas
       a. I and III only
       b. II and IV only
       c. I, II, and III only
       d. I, III, and IV only

11. What is the total current flowing through a DC circuit containing a 100 V power source and a total resistance of 50 Ω?

12. List three strategies that can be used to protect patients from electrical hazards.

13. Calculate the energy cost of operating a 1000 W air compressor for 24 hours if the electrical energy cost is 10 cents per kilowatt-hour.

14. Macroshock can occur when a person has a 1-second external contact with a 110 VAC current at 60 Hz. What is generally considered the minimum current the person must contact to experience macroshock?
    a. 100 μA
    b. 1 mA
    c. 10 mA
    d. 1 A

15. A respiratory therapist traveling from Chicago, Illinois, to Denver, Colorado, notices that he becomes short of breath while walking to the luggage area of the airport. His wife, who is also a respiratory therapist, comments that his breathlessness is due to the thinness of the air in Denver. He says that he knew that could explain the breathlessness, but he also remembered that the air in Denver contains 21% oxygen, just like in Chicago. Bemused by his comment, his wife asks him what is the PO_2 of the air in Denver. Note that the barometric pressure in Denver was recorded as 630 mm Hg.
    a. 147 mm Hg
    b. 132 mm Hg
    c. 122 mm Hg
    d. 90 mm Hg

References

1. Feynman R: *Six easy pieces,* Reading, Mass, 1995, Addison-Wesley.
2. Krauskoff KB, Beiser A: *The physical universe,* ed 10, New York, 2005, McGraw-Hill.
3. Asimov I: *Understanding physics,* New York, 1993, Barnes & Noble Books.
4. Bevelacqua JJ: *Basic health physics,* New York, 1999, Wiley-Interscience.
5. Chang R: *Chemistry,* ed 9, New York, 2006, McGraw-Hill.
6. Lide DR, editor: *Handbook of chemistry and physics,* ed 87, Cleveland, 2006, Chemical Rubber Co.
7. Nave CR, Nave BC: *Physics for the health sciences,* ed 3, Philadelphia, 1985, WB Saunders.
8. Scanlan CL: Physical principles in respiratory care. In Scanlan CL, Spearman CB, Sheldon RL, editors: *Egan's fundamentals of respiratory care,* ed 7, St Louis, 1999, Mosby.
9. Wojciechowski WV: *Respiratory care sciences: an integrated approach,* ed 4, Albany, NY, 2005, Delmar.
10. Davis PD, Parbrook GD, Kenny GNC: *Basic physics and measurement in anaesthesia,* ed 5, Oxford, 2003, Butterworth-Heinemann.
11. Adriani J: *The chemistry and physics of anesthesia,* ed 3, Springfield, Ill, 1979, Charles C Thomas.
12. Levitzky MG: *Pulmonary physiology,* ed 7, New York, 2007, McGraw-Hill.
13. Guyton AC, Hall JE: *Textbook of medical physiology,* ed 11, Philadelphia, 2005, WB Saunders.
14. Cromwell L, Weibell FJ, Pfeiffer EA: *Biomedical instrumentation and measurements,* ed 2, Englewood Cliffs, NJ, 1980, Prentice-Hall.
15. Levitzky MG, Cairo JM, Hall SM: *Introduction to respiratory care,* Philadelphia, 1990, WB Saunders.
16. Kacmarek RM, Mack CM, Dimas S: *The essentials of respiratory care,* ed 4, St Louis, 2005, Mosby.

Internet Resources

American Association for Respiratory Care: http://www.aarc.org
American Physical Society: http://www.aps.org
How Things Work—Louis A. Bloomfield: http://howthingswork.virginia.edu
Physics Reference Guide: http://www.physlink.com
The Internet Public Library: http://www.ipl.org
Oracle Think Quest Education Foundation: http://www.thinkquest.org
United States Library of Medicine: http://www.nlm.nih.gov
University of Winnipeg Introductory Physics Notes: http://theory.uwinnipeg.ca/physics/
Virtual Physics Laboratory: http://jersey.uoregon.edu/vlab

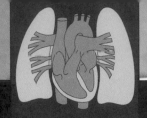
Manufacture, Storage, and Transport of Medical Gases

J.M. CAIRO

OUTLINE

Properties of Medical Gases
Air
Oxygen (O_2)
Carbon Dioxide (CO_2)
Helium (He)
Nitric Oxide (NO)
Nitrous Oxide (N_2O)

Storage and Transport of Medical Gases
Cylinders
Liquid Oxygen Systems
Medical Air Supply
Central Supply Systems
Piping Systems
Station Outlets
Oxygen Concentrators

OBJECTIVES

Upon completion of this chapter, you will be able to:
· Describe the chemical and physical properties of the medical gases most often encountered in respiratory care.
· Identify various types of medical gas cylinders (e.g., Types 3, 3A, 3AA, and 3AL).
· Identify the following cylinder markings: Department of Transportation (DOT) specifications, service pressure, hydrostatic testing dates, manufacturer's identification, ownership mark, serial number, and cylinder size.
· List the color codes used to identify medical gas cylinders.
· Discuss United States Pharmacopeia (USP) purity standards for medical gases.
· Compare the operation of direct-acting cylinder valves with that of diaphragm-type cylinder valves.
· Explain the American Standards Association (ASA) indexing, the Pin Index Safety System (PISS), and the Diameter Index Safety System (DISS).
· Identify and correct a problem with cylinder valve assembly.
· Calculate the gas volume remaining in a compressed-gas cylinder and estimate the duration of gas flow based on the cylinder's gauge pressure.
· Describe the components of a bulk liquid oxygen system and discuss the recommendations of the National Fire Protection Association (NFPA) for the storage and use of liquid oxygen in bulk systems.
· Discuss the operation of a portable liquid oxygen system and describe NFPA recommendations for these systems.
· Calculate the duration of a portable liquid oxygen supply.
· Identify three types of medical air compressors and describe the operational theory of each.
· Summarize NFPA recommendations for medical air supply safety.
· Compare continuous and alternating central supply systems.
· Identify a DISS station outlet and a quick-connect station outlet.
· Compare the operational theory of a membrane oxygenator with that of a molecular sieve oxygenator.

KEY TERMS

alternating supply systems
American Standards Association (ASA) indexing
check valves
continuous supply systems
cryogenic
Diameter Index Safety System (DISS)
diaphragm compressors
diaphragm valves
direct-acting valves

fractional distillation
fusible plugs
Joule-Kelvin (Joule-Thompson) effect
liquefaction
molecular sieves
oxygen concentrators
physical separation
Pin Index Safety System (PISS)
piston compressors

pressure swing adsorption (PSA) method
quick-connect adapters
rotary compressors
rupture disks
semipermeable membranes
spring-loaded devices
Thorpe tube flowmeter
volume-pressure constant
Wood's metal

Compressed gases are routinely used in the diagnosis and treatment of patients with cardiopulmonary dysfunction. The appropriate quality, purity, and potency of these medical gases are subject to government regulations. These regulations, along with recommendations proposed by the Compressed Gas Association (CGA) and other private agencies, provide guidelines for the manufacture, storage, and transport of compressed gases. As such, the primary purpose of these guidelines is to protect public safety. Respiratory therapists should be familiar with these regulations, as well as the indications, contraindications, and adverse effects associated with breathing medical gases.

PROPERTIES OF MEDICAL GASES

Air

At normal atmospheric conditions, air is a colorless, odorless gas mixture that contains varying amounts of water vapor. For practical purposes, we can assume that atmospheric air contains about 78% nitrogen and 21% oxygen by volume. Trace gases, including argon, carbon dioxide, neon, helium, methane, krypton, nitrous oxide, and xenon, make up the remaining 1% of atmospheric air. Table 2-1 shows a typical analysis of dry air at sea level.

Air is a nonflammable gas, but it supports combustion. It has a density of $1.2 \, kg/m^3$ at $21.1°C$ ($70°F$) and 760 mm Hg.[1] Because air is used as a standard for measuring the specific gravity of other gases, it is assigned a value of 1 at $21.1°C$ and 1 atmosphere (atm).[1] At its freezing point, $-195.6°C$ ($-320°F$), air is a transparent liquid with a pale bluish cast.

Compressed air is prepared synthetically from nitrogen and oxygen and shipped as a gas in cylinders at high pressure. Liquid air can be obtained through a process called **liquefaction** and shipped in bulk in specially designed **cryogenic** containers. For many medical applications, air is filtered and compressed at the point of use. The theory of operation of portable air compressors is described later in this chapter.

TABLE 2-1		
Composition of Room Air		
Component	% by Volume	% by Weight
Nitrogen	78.084	75.5
Oxygen	20.946	23.2
Argon	0.934	1.33
Carbon dioxide	0.0335	0.045
Neon	0.001818	—
Helium	0.000524	—
Methane	0.0002	—
Krypton	0.000114	—
Nitrous oxide	0.00005	—
Xenon	0.0000087	—

From the Compressed Gas Association: *Handbook of compressed gases,* ed 3, New York, 1990, Van Nostrand Reinhold.

Oxygen (O₂)

Oxygen is an elemental gas that is colorless, odorless, and tasteless at normal temperatures and pressures. It makes up 20.9% of the Earth's atmosphere by volume and 23.2% by weight. It constitutes about 50% of the Earth's crust by weight. Oxygen is slightly heavier than air, having a density of $1.326 \, kg/m^3$ at $21.1°C$ and 760 mm Hg (specific gravity = 1.105).[1] At temperatures less than $-183°C$ ($-300°F$), oxygen exists as a pale bluish liquid that is slightly heavier than water.

Oxygen is classified as a nonflammable gas, but it readily supports combustion (i.e., the burning of flammable materials is accelerated in the presence of oxygen). Some combustibles, such as oil and grease, burn with nearly explosive violence if ignited in the presence of oxygen.[1] All elements except the inert gases combine with oxygen to form oxides; oxygen therefore is characterized as an oxidizer.

The two methods most commonly used to prepare oxygen are the **fractional distillation** of liquid air and the **physical separation** of atmospheric air. The fractional distillation of liquid air, which relies on the **Joule-Kelvin** (or **Joule-Thompson**) **effect,** was introduced by Karl von Linde in 1907.[2] Box 2-1 describes the fractional distillation process; Figure 2-1 illustrates the components of a typical fractional distillation system. The fractional distillation process is used commercially to produce bulk oxygen,

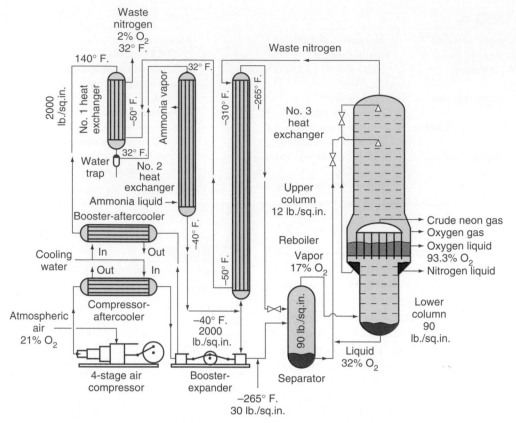

FIGURE 2-1 Fractional distillation apparatus for producing liquid oxygen. (Courtesy Nellcor Puritan Bennett, Pleasanton, Calif.)

BOX 2-1	Fractional Distillation of Liquid Air

1. Room air is drawn through scrubbers to remove dust and other impurities.
2. Air is cooled to near the freezing point of water (0° C) to remove water vapor.
3. Air is compressed to 200 atm, causing the temperature of the gas mixture to increase.
4. Compressed air is cooled to room temperature by passing nitrogen through coils surrounding the gas mixture.
5. As the temperature drops, the gas mixture expands. The temperature achieved is less than the critical temperature of nearly all gases in air, and a liquid gas mixture is produced.
6. The liquid air is transferred to a distilling column, where it is warmed to room temperature. As the air warms, various gases boil off as their individual boiling points are reached.
7. Liquid oxygen is obtained by maintaining the temperature of the gas mixture just below the boiling point of oxygen (−183° C, or −297.3° F at 1 atm).
8. The process is repeated until the liquid oxygen mixture is 99% pure with no toxic impurities.
9. The liquid oxygen is transferred to cold converters for storage and later transported either in bulk as a liquid or in compressed-gas cylinders as a gas.

which can be stored as a liquid in cryogenic storage tanks or converted into a gas and shipped in metal cylinders.

The physical separation of atmospheric air is accomplished with devices that use **molecular sieves** and **semipermeable membranes** to filter room air. These devices, called **oxygen concentrators,** are used primarily to provide enriched oxygen mixtures for oxygen therapy in the home care setting. The operation of oxygen concentrators is discussed in more detail later in this chapter.

Carbon Dioxide (CO$_2$)

Carbon dioxide is a colorless, odorless gas at normal atmospheric temperatures and pressures. It has a density of 1.833 kg/m^3 at 21.1° C and 1 atm; it therefore is about 1.5 times heavier than air (specific gravity = 1.522).[1] Carbon dioxide is nonflammable and does not support combustion or life.

Carbon dioxide can exist as a solid, liquid, and gas at a temperature of −56.6° C (−69.9° F) and a pressure of 60.4 psig (the triple point* of CO$_2$).[1] At temperatures and pressures below its triple point, carbon dioxide exists as a solid ("dry ice") or a gas, depending on the temperature. At temperatures and pressures above its triple point but below

*The triple point is a specific combination of temperature and pressure in which a substance can exist in all three states of matter in a dynamic equilibrium.

its critical temperature (31.1° C [87.9° F]), carbon dioxide can exist as a liquid or as a gas. Therefore, when carbon dioxide is stored at these temperatures in a pressurized container, such as a metal cylinder, the liquid and gaseous forms of carbon dioxide exist in equilibrium. Above 31.1° C, carbon dioxide cannot exist as a liquid, regardless of the pressure.[1]

Unrefined carbon dioxide can be obtained from the combustion of coal, natural gas, or other carbonaceous fuels.[1] Carbon dioxide can also be obtained as a byproduct in the production of ammonia, lime, and kilns, among other products. Purified carbon dioxide is prepared through the liquefaction and fractional distillation processes.

Solid carbon dioxide is used to refrigerate perishable materials while in transport (e.g., food and laboratory specimens). Liquid carbon dioxide can be used as an expendable refrigerant[1] and is used extensively as a fire-extinguishing agent in portable and stationary fire-extinguishing systems. Gaseous carbon dioxide is used in food processing (e.g., carbonation of beverages) and water treatment and as a growth stimulant for plants.[1]

Carbon dioxide is used for the treatment of singultus (hiccups) and as a stimulant/depressant of the central nervous system (CNS). It also is used as a standard calibration gas for blood gas analyzers, transcutaneous partial pressure of carbon dioxide (PCO_2) electrodes, and capnographs. Because carbon dioxide cannot support life, it must be combined with oxygen before it can be administered to patients. Carbon dioxide/oxygen mixtures (carbogen mixtures) are prepared by combining 5% to 10% carbon dioxide with 90% to 95% oxygen. The U.S. Food and Drug Administration (FDA) purity standard requires that carbon dioxide used for medical purposes be 99% pure.[3]

Helium (He)

Helium is the second-lightest element, having a density of 0.165 kg/m^3 at 21.1° C and 1 atm (specific gravity = 0.138).[1] It is an inert gas that has no color, odor, or taste. Helium is only slightly soluble in water and is a good conductor of heat, sound, and electricity.[4]

Helium occurs naturally in the atmosphere in very small quantities (see Table 2-1). It can be prepared commercially from natural gas, which contains as much as 2% helium.[1] Helium can also be obtained by heating uranium ore. Purity standards for the preparation of helium require that commercially available helium be 95% pure. Helium is chemically and physiologically inert and is classified as a nonflammable gas that will not support combustion or life. Note that breathing 100% helium can lead to severe hypoxemia. Because of its low density, He is combined with oxygen (i.e., heliox is a mixture of 80% helium and 20% oxygen)* to deliver oxygen therapy to patients with

*Heliox mixtures containing 70% helium and 30% oxygen, and 60% helium and 40% oxygen, are also available. It is important to mention that with an 80:20 mixture the actual heliox flow is 1.8 times greater than the flow indicated on an oxygen-calibrated flowmeter.

severe airway obstruction (i.e., it decreases the work of breathing by decreasing turbulent airflow).[3] It also is used in pulmonary function testing to measure residual volume and diffusing capacity.

Nitric Oxide (NO)

Nitric oxide is a diatomic molecule that exists as colorless gas with a slight metallic odor at room temperature. It is nonflammable and will support combustion. It has a density of 1.245 kg/m^3 and a specific gravity of 1.04 (at 21.1° C, 760 mm Hg).[1] Nitric oxide is highly unstable in the atmosphere and can exist in three biologically active forms in tissues: as nitrosonium (NO^+), as nitroxyl anions (NO^-), and as a free radical ($NO^·$).

In the presence of air, nitric oxide combines with oxygen to form brown fumes of nitrogen dioxide (NO_2), a strong oxidizing agent. It is not corrosive, and most structural materials are unaffected; in the presence of moisture, however, it can form nitrous and nitric acids, both of which can cause corrosion. Nitric oxide and nitrogen dioxide combined form a potent irritant that can cause chemical pneumonitis and pulmonary edema.[4]

Nitric oxide can be prepared by oxidizing ammonia at high temperatures (500° C) in the presence of a platinum catalyst or by reducing acid solutions of nitrates.[1] Chemiluminescent analysis is used to determine the final concentration of nitric oxide and nitrogen dioxide, with a stated accuracy of 62% (see Chapter 8 for a discussion of chemiluminescent analysis of nitric oxides). Nitric oxide is supplied with nitrogen in compressed-gas aluminum alloy cylinders.[5] Before 1997, nitric oxide was supplied in cylinders with a volume capacity of 152 ft^3 with 660 CGA valve outlets. It now is supplied in smaller cylinders (82 ft^3) with 626 CGA valve outlets.

Although nitric oxide is toxic in high concentrations, experimental results suggest that low doses are a powerful pulmonary vasodilator.[5] Very low concentrations (2 to 80 parts per million [ppm]) combined with oxygen have been used successfully to treat persistent pulmonary hypertension of the newborn (PPHN)[6] and adult respiratory distress syndrome.[7] Although many investigators have suggested that inhalation of low-dose nitric oxide is relatively safe, special precautions apply. Specifically, the levels of nitrogen dioxide and nitrogen trioxide, as well as the patient's methemoglobin levels, should be monitored throughout the procedure.[5]

Nitrous Oxide (N₂O)

Nitrous oxide is a colorless gas at normal temperatures and atmospheric pressures. It is odorless, tasteless, and nonflammable but will support combustion and is slightly soluble in water, alcohol, and oils. Nitrous oxide is noncorrosive and therefore may be stored in commercially available cylinders. Because it is an oxidizing agent, it will react with oils, grease, and other combustible materials.

Nitrous oxide is prepared commercially by the thermal decomposition of ammonium nitrate and as a byproduct of the adipic acid manufacturing processes.[1] At elevated temperatures (>649° C), it decomposes into nitrogen and oxygen.

Nitrous oxide is used primarily as a CNS depressant (i.e., an anesthetic). It is a potent anesthetic when administered in high concentrations; in low concentrations, other depressant drugs must be used concomitantly to achieve effective anesthesia. (Nitrous oxide often is called "laughing gas," a term coined in 1840.[8]) Note that inhalation of nitrous oxide without provision of a sufficient oxygen supply may cause brain damage or can be fatal.

Long-term exposure of health care workers to nitrous oxide has been associated with adverse side effects, including neuropathy and fetotoxic effects (spontaneous abortion).[1] The National Institute of Occupational Safety and Health has recommended limits on exposure to nitrous oxide for health care providers working in surgical suites and dental offices. Systems that trap exhaled nitrous oxide are used to capture any unused gas, preventing inadvertent exposure of health care workers.

Table 2-2 provides a summary of the properties of commonly used medical gases. Clinical Rounds 2-1 provides an exercise to help you test your understanding of the medical gases just discussed.

CLINICAL ROUNDS 2-1

Based on the discussion of compressed gases, name the appropriate gas for each of the following situations:
Use as a refrigerant.
For reducing the work of breathing in a patient with airway obstruction.
To treat hypoxemia in a patient with chronic obstructive pulmonary disease.
For reducing pulmonary vasoconstriction, such as occurs in PPHN.

See Evolve Resources for answer.

STORAGE AND TRANSPORT OF MEDICAL GASES

Medical gases can be classified as nonliquefied and liquefied. Nonliquefied gases are stored and transported under high pressure in metal cylinders. Liquefied gases are stored and transported in specially designed bulk liquid storage units. The design of compressed-gas cylinders, bulk storage containers, and their valve outlets, as well as their transportation, testing, and periodic examination, are subject to national standards and regulations.[9,10] Box 2-2 presents a list of agencies that provide recommendations and regulations for the manufacture, storage, transport, and use of medical gases.

Cylinders

Metal cylinders have been used for storing compressed gases since 1888.[10] Federal regulations issued by the DOT require that all cylinders used to store and transport compressed gases conform to well-defined specifications. These specifications, along with recommendations from the NFPA and the CGA, provide industry standards for cylinder design and maintenance and the safe use of compressed gases. Appendix 2-1 contains a summary of NFPA and CGA recommendations for compressed-gas cylinders.

Construction and Maintenance of Compressed-Gas Cylinders

Compressed-gas cylinders are constructed of seamless, high-quality steel, chrome-molybdenum, or aluminum that is either stamped into shape using a punch press die or spun into shape by wrapping heated steel bands around specially designed molds. The bottom of the cylinder is welded closed, and the top of the cylinder is threaded and fitted with a valve stem (Figure 2-2).

Type 3AA cylinders are produced from heat-treated, high-strength steel; type 3A cylinders are made of carbon-steel (non–heat treated). Type 3AL cylinders are con-

TABLE 2-2

Properties of Commonly Used Medical Gases

Medical Gas	Chemical Symbol	Molecular Weight	PHYSICAL CHARACTERISTICS			Boiling Point	Critical Temperature	Physical State	Combustion Characteristics
			Color	Odor	Taste				
Air	Air	28.97	Colorless	Odorless	Tasteless	−194.3	−140.6	Gas/liquid	NF/SC
Oxygen	O_2	31.99	Colorless	Odorless	Tasteless	−182.9	−118.4	Gas/liquid	NF/SC
Carbon dioxide	CO_2	44.01	Colorless	Odorless	Slightly acid	−29.0	+31.0	Liquid/gas	NF
Carbon monoxide	CO	28.01	Colorless	Odorless	Tasteless	−191.5	−140.2	Gas	F
Nitrous oxide	N_2O	44.01	Colorless	Odorless	Tasteless	−88.5	+36.4	Liquid/gas	NF
Nitric oxide	NO	30.01	Colorless	Slightly metallic	Tasteless	−151.8	−92.9	Gas	NF
Helium	He	4.00	Colorless	Odorless	Tasteless	−268.9	−267.0	Gas	NF

NF, Nonflammable; *SC*, supports combustion; *F*, flammable.

BOX 2-2	Agencies Regulating the Manufacture, Storage, and Transport of Medical Gases

REGULATING AGENCIES

Center for Devices and Radiological Health (CDRH)
An agency of the Food and Drug Administration (FDA) that provides standards for medical devices.

Department of Health and Human Services (HHS)
Department of the federal government that oversees health care delivery in the United States. Formerly known as the Department of Health, Education, and Welfare (HEW).

Department of Transportation
Provides regulations for the manufacture, storage, and transport of compressed gases. Before 1967, this responsibility was vested in the Interstate Commerce Commission (ICC).

Environmental Protection Agency (EPA)
Government agency that establishes standards and administers regulations concerning potential and actual environmental hazards.

Food and Drug Administration (FDA)
An agency of the Department of Health and Human Services (HHS) that sets purity standards for medical gases.

Occupational Safety and Health Administration (OSHA)
An agency of the Department of Labor that oversees safety issues related to the work environment.

Transport Canada (TC)
Canadian government agency that administers regulations concerning the manufacture and testing of compressed-gas cylinders and their distribution.

RECOMMENDING AGENCIES

American National Standards Institute (ANSI)
Private, nonprofit organization that coordinates the voluntary development of national standards in the United States. Represents the United States' interests in international standards.

American Society of Mechanical Engineers (ASME)
Issues information on the design, manufacture, and structural standards for components of central piping systems.

Compressed Gas Association (CGA)
Comprises companies involved in the manufacture, storage, and transport of all compressed gases. Provides standards and safety systems for compressed-gas systems.

International Organization for Standardization (ISO)
International agency that provides standards for technology.

National Fire Protection Association (NFPA)
Independent agency that provides information on fire protection and safety.

United States Pharmacopeia/National Formulary (USP/NF)
A not-for-profit private organization founded to develop officially recognized quality standards for drugs, including medical gases.

Z-79 Committee
ANSI committee for establishing standards for anesthetic and ventilatory devices, including anesthetic machines, reservoir bags, tracheal tubes, humidifiers, nebulizers, and other oxygen-related equipment.

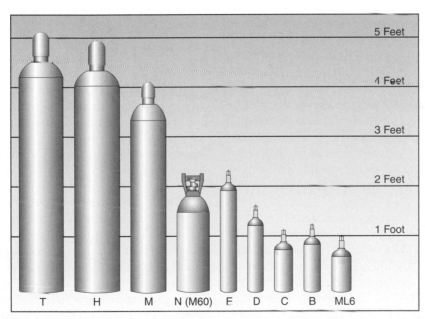

FIGURE 2-2 Various types of high-pressure cylinders used in medical gas therapy. (From Hess D, MacIntyre N, Adams A et al: *Respiratory care, principles and practice,* Philadelphia, 2002, WB Saunders.)

structed of specially prescribed seamless aluminum alloys. Type 3 cylinders, which are made of low-carbon steel, are no longer produced. Note that the steel used in the construction of cylinders must meet the chemical and physical standards set by the DOT. (In Canada, the specifications for the construction of cylinders are set by Transport Canada.[8])

Compressed-gas cylinders should be capable of holding up to 10% more than the maximum filling pressure as marked.[11,12] This added capacity is required because of variations in cylinder pressure that occur with changes in ambient temperature. The Bureau of Explosives, an agency of the U.S. Department of the Treasury, requires that all cylinders contain a pressure-relief mechanism to prevent explosion.[13]

Types 3AA and 3A cylinders must be hydrostatically reexamined every 10 years to determine their expansion characteristics. (The asterisk following the reexamination date on the cylinder markings [see Figure 2-4] indicates that the cylinder must be retested every 10 years.[11]) Type 3AL cylinders must be reexamined every 5 years to test their expansion characteristics. Hydrostatic examination involves measuring a cylinder's expansion characteristics when it is filled to a pressure of five thirds its working pressure. This examination consists of placing a cylinder filled with water in a vessel that is also filled with water. When pressure is applied to the interior of the cylinder, the cylinder expands, displacing water from the jacket surrounding the cylinder. The volume of water displaced when pressure is applied equals the total expansion of the cylinder. The permanent expansion of the cylinder equals the volume of water displaced when the pressure is released. This information is used to calculate the elastic expansion of the cylinder, which is directly related to the thickness of the cylinder. Increases in the elastic expansion of a cylinder indicate a reduction in the wall thickness. Reductions in wall thickness can occur when the cylinder is physically damaged or is subject to corrosion.[8]

Filling of Medical Cylinders

As you might expect, filling and refilling a medical gas cylinder is a potentially dangerous process. The DOT, the FDA, and the U.S. Pharmacopeia/National Formulary (USP/NF) have established a series of guidelines (i.e., good manufacturing practices) that set strict controls over large commercial cylinder filling operations, as well as small home medical equipment dealers refilling relatively small numbers of cylinders.[8] Companies performing cylinder filling and refilling procedures must register with the FDA, which monitors compliance through biannual on site inspections.

Good manufacturing practices are designed to ensure that only properly trained individuals are involved in the refilling process and that the procedure is performed using certified equipment. These guidelines also specify that only safe and clean cylinders can be refilled. Gases used in this process must meet USP/NF standards for purity, and each cylinder must have a current, intact label that is readable and meets FDA and DOT regulations. In addition, each batch of cylinders must be identified by an assigned lot number that is traceable if recall is necessary.

The process of filling and refilling gas cylinders involves four steps: (1) cylinder prefill inspection, (2) cylinder filling, (3) postfill procedures, and (4) appropriate documentation.[8] Cylinder prefill inspection focuses on removal of any residual gas before refilling, visual inspection of each cylinder for any signs of damage, verification that the last

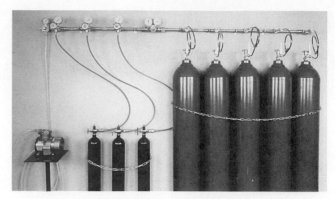

FIGURE 2-3 Example of a transfilling manifold.

hydrostatic testing date does not exceed DOT retest criteria, and ensuring that the cylinder is properly labeled. As mentioned, cylinder refilling must be done with certified equipment. Cylinders are attached to a specially designed manifold (Figure 2-3) that allows for cylinder evacuation before filling of the cylinder from a gas supply source. Gas from the supply source is introduced into the cylinders at a controlled flow that permits a filling rate of no more than 200 psig/min until the permitted full pressure is attained. (Note that the full pressure is corrected for temperature so that the accurate volume is present at standard temperature and pressure [STP] conditions.[8]) Once the cylinders are filled, the valves of the cylinders are closed and removed from the manifold. A postfill procedure is then performed on each cylinder to ensure that the cylinder valve does not leak and that the cylinder's contents meet the minimum purity standards set by the USP/NF. Documentation of each of the previous steps and the signature of the individual who filled the cylinders must be recorded in a transfilling log. Company records should also include daily calibration of the oxygen analyzers used to test the purity of the cylinders' contents, along with evidence that the manifold and gauges are inspected according to an established schedule.

Cylinder Sizes and Capacities

Table 2-3 summarizes the weights and volume capacities of various cylinders and gases used in respiratory care. The most commonly used cylinders for medical gas therapy are the E and H types. D cylinders are used for the storage of nitric oxide.

E cylinders frequently are used as a source of oxygen in emergency situations (e.g., cardiopulmonary resuscitation [CPR] carts) and for transporting patients requiring oxygen therapy. These smaller cylinders also store gases used in anesthetics, as well as calibration gases for portable diagnostic equipment (e.g., capnographs and pulse oximeters).

H cylinders are used as the primary source of oxygen and other medical gases in smaller hospitals that do not have bulk liquid systems (see the following section). Hospitals and other facilities with bulk liquid oxygen systems use these larger cylinders as a secondary or reserve source

TABLE 2-3

Physical Characteristics of Common-Sized Aluminum and Steel Cylinders

	ALUMINUM							STEEL				
	B or M6	ML6	C or M9	D	E	N or M60	M or MM	D	E	M	H	T
Service pressure (psig)	2216	2015	2015	2015	2015	2216	2216	2015	2015	2015	2265	2400
Height without valve (inches)	11.6	7.7	10.9	16.5	25.6	23	35.75	16.75	25.75	43	51	55
Diameter (inches)	3.2	4.4	4.4	4.4	4.4	7.25	8	4.2	4.2	7	9	9.25
Weight without valve (pounds)	2.2	2.9	3.7	5.3	7.9	21.7	38.6	7.9	11.3	58	117	139
Capacity at Listed Pressure at STPD												
Oxygen (cubic feet)	6	6	9	15	24	61.4	122	15	24	110	250	300
Oxygen (Liters)	170	170	255	425	680	1738	3455	425	680	3113	7075	8490

STPD, Standard temperature and pressure, dry.
From Hess D, MacIntyre N, Mishoe S et al: *Respiratory care: principles and practice,* St Louis, 2002, WB Saunders.

of medical gases. Large cylinders are frequently used for home care patients who need long-term oxygen therapy. These larger cylinders are also routinely used to store the calibration gases required in the blood gas and pulmonary function laboratories.

Cylinder Identification

Cylinders are engraved with information that is designed primarily to identify where the cylinder was manufactured, the type of material used in its construction (i.e., 3AA, 3A, or 3AL), the service pressure of the cylinder, the date of its original hydrostatic test, and its reexamination dates.[1] Additionally, the manufacturer's name, the owner's identification number, and the size of cylinder are usually engraved on the cylinder. Figure 2-4 shows the standard markings that appear on compressed-gas cylinders. Note that a "+" following the stamped hydrostatic examination date indicates that the cylinder complied with requirement of the examination. A "+" does not follow the reexamination date on aluminum cylinders.

Medical gas cylinders are color coded for easy identification. Table 2-4 shows the color codes prescribed by the U.S. National Formulary.[3] Generally, these colors conform to an international cylinder color-coding system. Two major exceptions in the international system are oxygen cylinders, which are painted white, and compressed-air cylinders, which are painted yellow or black and white. Cylinders containing gas mixtures (e.g., helium-oxygen and carbon dioxide-oxygen) are divided into two categories of color coding, each based on the percentage of gases contained. For example, cylinders of carbon dioxide–oxygen mixtures that contain more than 7% carbon dioxide are predominantly gray with the shoulder of the tank painted green. Cylinders containing carbon dioxide–oxygen mixtures with less than 7% carbon dioxide are predominantly green with a gray shoulder. Helium-oxygen cylinders containing more than 80% helium are painted brown

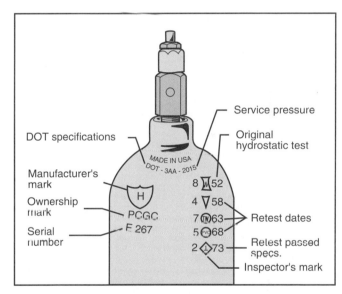

FIGURE 2-4 Standard markings for compressed-gas cylinders. (Modified from Nellcor Puritan Bennett, Pleasanton, Calif.)

with a green shoulder. Cylinders of helium-oxygen mixtures containing less than 80% helium (balanced with oxygen) are predominantly green with a brown shoulder.

Color codes are only a guide; printed labels are still the primary means of identifying the contents of a gas cylinder. Figure 2-5 is a standard label for an oxygen cylinder. The CGA and the American Standards Association (ASA) specify that all labels should include the name and chemical symbol of the gas in the cylinder. The label should also show the volume of the cylinder (in liters) at a temperature of 21.1° C (70° F).[1] Generally, labels also include any specific hazards related to use of the gas and precautionary measures and instructions in case of accidental exposure or contact with the contents.

The FDA requires that compressed gases used for medical purposes meet certain minimum requirements for

TABLE 2-4

Color Codes for Medical Gases

Gas	Chemical Symbol	Purity*	Color Code
Air	—	99.0%	Yellow or black and white[†]
Carbon dioxide	CO_2	99.0%	Gray
Carbon dioxide/oxygen	CO_2/O_2	99.0%	Gray and green[‡]
Cyclopropane	C_3H_6	99.0%	Orange
Ethylene	C_2H_4	99.0%	Red
Helium	He	99.0%	Brown
Helium/oxygen	He/O_2	99.0%	Brown and green[‡]
Nitrogen	N_2	99.0%	Black
Nitrous oxide	N_2O	97.0%	Light blue
Nitric oxide	NO	99.0%	Teal and black
Oxygen	O_2	99.0%	Green or white[†]

*National Formulary Standards.
[†]International color code.
[‡]Always check labels to determine the percentages of each gas.

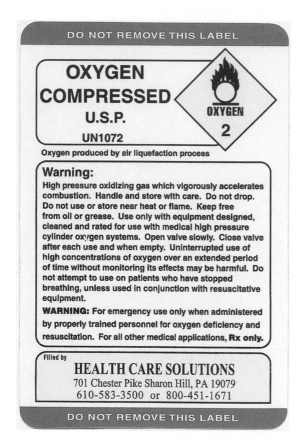

FIGURE 2-5 Example of compressed-gas cylinder labeling. (From Hess D, MacIntyre N, Adams A et al: *Respiratory care: principles and practice,* Philadelphia, 2002, WB Saunders.)

purity, and the purity of the gas must be indicated on the label identifying the contents of the cylinder. These standards are listed in the USP/NF (see Table 2-4 for a list of these purity requirements). The FDA also requires that the names of the manufacturer, packer, and distributor be included on the label.

Cylinder Valves

Cylinder valves are control devices that seal the contents of a compressed cylinder until it is ready for use. A cylinder valve is composed of the following parts:

1. A chrome-plated, brass body
2. A threaded inlet connector for attachment to the cylinder
3. A stem that opens and closes the cylinder when turned by a handwheel or handle
4. An outlet connection that allows for attachment of regulators and pressure-reducing valves
5. A pressure-relief valve

Figure 2-6 shows the two types of cylinder valves affixed to compressed medical gas cylinders: **direct-acting valves** and **diaphragm valves.** A direct-acting valve (Figure 2-6A) contains two fiber washers and a Teflon packing to prevent gas leakage around the threads. The term *direct-acting* is derived from the arrangement of movements in the valve wheel. These movements are directly reflected in the valve seat because it is one piece moved by threads. Direct-acting valves can withstand high pressures (i.e., more than 1500 psi).

Diaphragm valves (Figure 2-6B) use a threaded stem in place of the packing found on the direct-acting valves. The stem is separated from the valve seat and spring by two diaphragms, one made of steel and one made of copper. When the stem is turned counterclockwise and raised because of the threading, the diaphragm is pushed upward with the stem by the valve seat and spring, causing the valve to open. Turning the stem clockwise resets the diaphragm and closes the valve.

Diaphragm valves have several advantages: (1) the valve seat does not turn and therefore is resistant to scoring, which could cause leakage; (2) no stem leakage can occur because of the diaphragm; and (3) the stem can be opened with a partial rotation rather than with two turns of the wheel, as in direct-acting valves. Diaphragm valves generally are preferable when pressures are relatively low (i.e., less than 1500 psi). They also are ideal for situations in

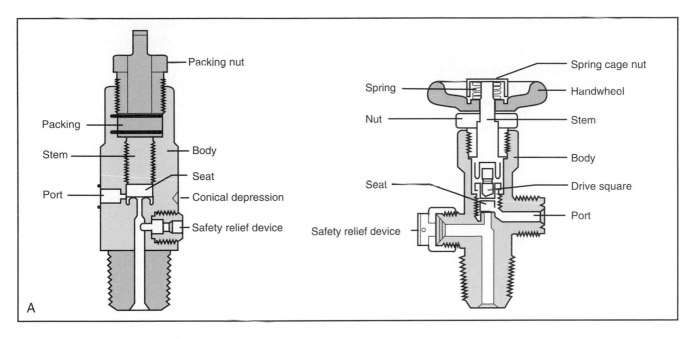

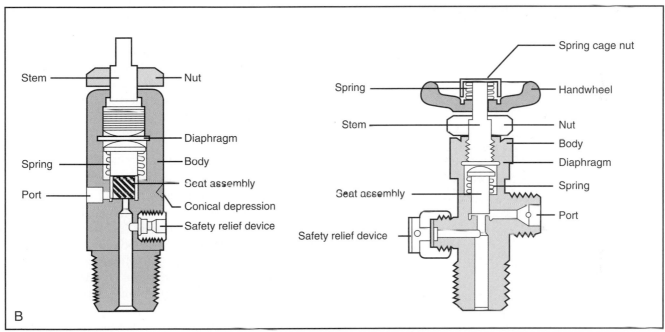

FIGURE 2-6 Cylinder valves. **A,** Direct-acting valve. **B,** Diaphragm valve. (Courtesy Nellcor Puritan Bennett, Pleasanton, Calif.)

which no gas leaks can be allowed, such as with flammable anesthetics.

Pressure-Relief Valves

Figure 2-7 illustrates three types of pressure-relief mechanisms: **rupture disks, fusible plugs,** and **spring-loaded devices.**[1] A rupture disk (also called a *frangible disk*) is a thin, metal disk that ruptures or buckles when the pressure inside the cylinder exceeds a certain predetermined limit. A fusible plug is made of a metal alloy that melts when the temperature of the gas in the tank exceeds a predetermined temperature. Fusible plugs operate on the principle that as the pressure in a tank increases, the temperature of the gas

increases, causing the plug to melt. After the plug melts, excess pressure is released.* Spring-loaded devices are designed to release excessive cylinder pressure and reseal, preventing further release of gas from the cylinder after the cause of the excessive pressure is removed.[1] With these devices, a metal seal is held in place by an adjustable spring. The amount of pressure required to force the seal open depends on the tension of the spring holding the metal seal in place. Spring-loaded devices usually are more sus-

*A commonly used metal alloy is called **Wood's metal;** fusible plugs made of this alloy generally have melting temperatures of 208° to 220° F (9°C to 104°C).

ceptible to leakage around the metal seal than are rupture disks and fusible plugs.[1] Note that spring-loaded devices may also be affected by changes in environmental conditions (i.e., freezing conditions can cause these devices to stick). Rupture disks and fusible plugs are often incorporated into smaller cylinders, whereas spring-loaded devices are found on larger cylinders.[8]

Safety Systems

Outlet connections of cylinder valves are indexed according to standards designed by the CGA and adopted by the ASA and the Canadian Standards Association. American Standard connections are noninterchangeable to prevent the interchange of regulating equipment between gases that are not compatible.

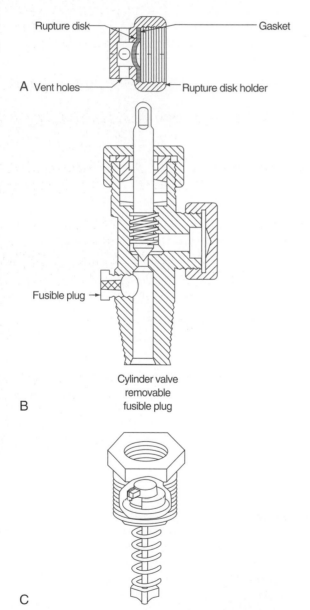

FIGURE 2-7 Pressure-relief valves. **A,** Rupture (frangible) disks. **B,** Fusible plug. **C,** Spring-loaded device. (Redrawn from the Compressed Gas Association: *Handbook of compressed gases,* ed 3, New York, 1990, Van Nostrand Reinhold.)

American Standard indexing includes separate systems for large and small cylinders. Large cylinder valve outlets and connections (e.g., for sizes H and K) are indexed by thread type, thread size, right- or left-handed threading, external or internal threading, and nipple-seat design.[12] Figure 2-8 illustrates the American Standard connections for medical gases that are commonly used in respiratory care. Look at the oxygen connection shown in this figure. The diameter of the cylinder's outlet is listed in thousandths of inches (e.g., the oxygen connection is 0.903 inch). The letters following these numbers indicate the type of threading used (i.e., right-handed [RH] versus left-handed [LH]). The abbreviations *Ext* and *Int* specify whether the threads are external or internal. Note that the connections for oxygen and other life support gases are right-handed and external. The remaining information indicates whether the outlet requires a nipple attachment. Oxygen valves require a rounded nipple.

Small cylinders (e.g., sizes AA to E) with post type valves use a different American Standard indexing called the **Pin Index Safety System (PISS).** In this system, indexing is accomplished by the exact placement of two pins into holes in the post valve. Note that the hole positions are numbered from 1 to 6; each medical gas uses a specified pin sequence. Figure 2-9 shows the different combinations used to differentiate the most common medical gases. For example, the pins for an oxygen regulator must be placed in the 2 and 5 positions for it to attach to the oxygen cylinder's post valve. Cylinder regulators are discussed in Chapter 3.

Setting Up and Troubleshooting Compressed-Gas Cylinders

Box 2-3 presents the steps that should be followed in setting up a compressed-gas cylinder.[14] The following is a list of simple suggestions that should be kept in mind in the handling of compressed-gas cylinders:

1. The cylinder's contents should be clearly labeled. If the contents of a cylinder are questionable, do not use it.
2. Full and empty cylinders should be appropriately labeled and kept separate.
3. Cylinder valves should be fully opened when in use and always closed when the gas contained in the cylinder is not being used. Cylinder valves should be closed if the cylinder is empty.
4. Large cylinders have a protective cap that fits over the valve stem. This cap should be kept on the cylinders when they are moved or stored. Small cylinders with PISS valve stems do not have protective caps but have an outlet seal that must be removed before the appropriate regulator is attached.
5. Regulators and other appliances intended for use with a specific gas should not be used with other gases.
6. Cylinders should be properly secured at all times, either in a stand, chained to a wall, or in a cart, to prevent them from tipping over.

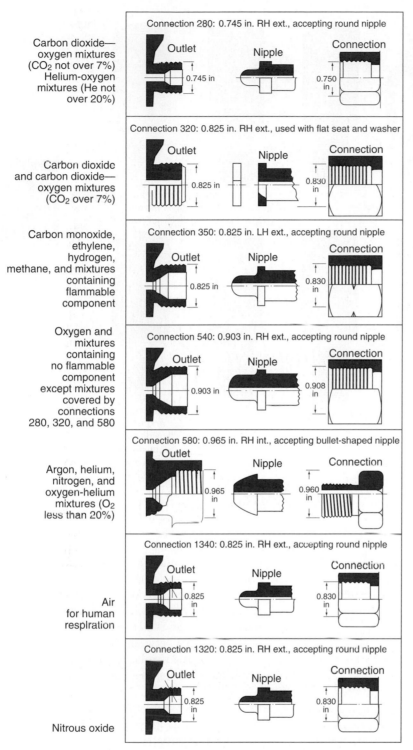

FIGURE 2-8 American Standard Indexing system for large cylinders. (Courtesy Datex-Ohmeda, Madison, Wis.)

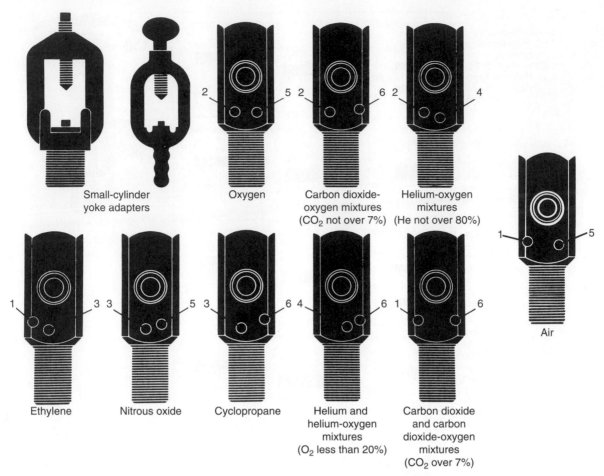

Small-cylinder
yoke adapters

Oxygen

Carbon dioxide-
oxygen mixtures
(CO_2 not over 7%)

Helium-oxygen
mixtures
(He not over 80%)

Ethylene

Nitrous oxide

Cyclopropane

Helium and
helium-oxygen
mixtures
(O_2 less than 20%)

Carbon dioxide
and carbon
dioxide-oxygen
mixtures
(CO_2 over 7%)

Air

FIGURE 2-9 Pin Index Safety System (PISS) for small cylinders. (Courtesy Datex-Ohmeda, Madison, Wis.)

BOX 2-3	**Procedure for Setting up a Compressed-Gas Cylinder**

1. Make sure the cylinder is properly secured.
2. Remove the protective cap or wrap and inspect the cylinder valve to ensure that it is free of dirt, debris, or oil.
3. Alert others nearby that you are about to "crack" the cylinder valve, making a loud noise. Turn the cylinder valve away from anyone present. Then quickly open and close the valve to remove dirt or small debris from the valve outlet.
4. Inspect the inlet of the device to be attached to ensure that it is free of dirt and debris.
5. Securely tighten—but do not force—the device onto the cylinder outlet. Use appropriate wrenches that are free of oil and grease; never use pipe wrenches. Remember to use only cylinder valve connections that conform to ANSI and PISS B57. Low-pressure, threaded connections must comply with DISS or must be noninterchangeable, low-pressure, quick-connecting devices. Never connect fixed or adjustable orifices or metering devices directly to a cylinder without a pressure-reducing valve.
6. Make sure the regulator or reducing valve is in the closed position and then slowly open the cylinder valve to pressurize the reducing valve or regulator that is attached. After pressurization has occurred, open the cylinder valve completely and turn it back a quarter- to half-turn to prevent "valve freeze" (i.e., the valve cannot be turned).

Most problems encountered with cylinders and regulators involve (1) gas leakage at the valve stem or in the regulator and (2) failure to achieve adequate gas flow at the cylinder regulator outlet. Leaks typically occur from large cylinders because of loose connections between the regulator and the cylinder valve. Gas leaks from small cylinders most often are associated with damage to the plastic washer that fits between the valve stem and the regulator. Gas leaks at the regulator outlet can be caused by a loose connection between the regulator and attached equipment (Clinical Rounds 2-2). Failure to achieve a desired gas flow from a cylinder regulator can result from inadequate pressure (e.g., low gauge pressure) or from an obstruction at the regulator outlet.

CLINICAL ROUNDS 2-2

A respiratory therapist "cracks" an H cylinder of oxygen and then attaches an oxygen regulator to the cylinder outlet. She slowly opens the valve stem and hears a sudden, loud hissing sound coming from the connection between the cylinder outlet and the regulator. What should she do?

See Evolve Resources for answer.

Determining the Volume of Gas Remaining in a Cylinder and the Duration of Cylinder Gas Flow

Calculation of the gas volume remaining in a cylinder requires a knowledge of either the pressure or the weight of the cylinder (see Table 2-3 for a list of values for commonly used medical gas cylinders). For nonliquefied gas cylinders (e.g., compressed air, oxygen, helium), the gas volume contained in a cylinder is directly related to the regulator's gauge pressure. Table 2-5 shows these **volume-pressure constants,** or "tank factors," for the more commonly used medical gas cylinders. The volume of gas remaining in a cylinder can then be calculated by multiplying the cylinder's volume-pressure constant by the gauge pressure. Box 2-4 presents an example of this calculation. The resultant volume can then be divided by the flow rate of gas being used to determine the duration of gas flow remaining in minutes.

Determining the gas volume remaining in a liquefied gas cylinder (e.g., carbon dioxide and nitrous oxide) is more of a challenge. The gas volume remaining in a liquefied gas cylinder cannot be determined by the method just described because the liquid remains in equilibrium with the gas above it until the liquid is depleted. The volume of liquefied gas remaining is best determined by weighing the cylinder before and after it is filled. Thus the volume of liquid gas remaining in the cylinder is directly related to the weight of the cylinder. After the volume is determined, the duration of gas flow can be calculated by dividing that volume by the flow rate of gas being used.

Liquid Oxygen Systems

Hospitals and larger health care facilities typically rely on bulk liquid supply systems for medical air and oxygen needs. The increased use of bulk liquid supply systems is the result of a couple of factors: (1) gases shipped in bulk are less expensive than gases shipped in cylinders, and (2) liquefied oxygen occupies a fraction of the space required to store gaseous oxygen. Note that gaseous oxygen occupies a volume 860 times that of liquid oxygen.

Construction of bulk gas systems is regulated by the NFPA and the American Society of Mechanical Engineers (ASME). The Bureau of Explosives provides regulations for the design and operation of pressure-release valves for these systems.[1,13]

Bulk Liquid Oxygen Systems

The NFPA defines a bulk oxygen system as more than 20,000 ft³ of oxygen (at atmospheric temperature and pressure), including unconnected reserves, that are on hand at a site.[13] Figure 2-10 shows the major components of a bulk oxygen system. It consists of an insulated reservoir, a vaporizer with associated tubing attached to the reservoir, a pressure-reducing valve, and an appropriate pressure-release valve. The reservoir stores a mixture of liquid and gaseous oxygen. The vaporizer acts as a heat exchanger, where heat is absorbed from the environment and used to warm the liquid oxygen to room temperature, thus forming

TABLE 2-5

Volume-Pressure Conversion Factors

Cylinder Size	Conversion Factor
E	622.0 L/2200 psi = 0.28
G	5264.0 L/2200 psi = 2.39
H or K	6900.0 L/2200 psi = 3.14

BOX 2-4 — Estimating the Duration of a Medical Gas Cylinder Supply

The amount of time it will take a cylinder filled with compressed gas to provide a set flow rate of gas can be calculated with the following formula:

$$\frac{\text{Cylinder pressure (psi)} \times \text{Cylinder factor*}}{\text{Flow rate of gas (L/min)}}$$
$$= \text{Duration of flow in minutes}$$

Example

You are asked to transport a patient who is receiving oxygen from a nasal cannula at 4 L/min. The pressure gauge on the cylinder reads 1800 psi. How long will the cylinder provide the appropriate oxygen flow?

1800 psi × (0.28) ÷ 4 L/min = 126 minutes, or about 2 hours

---

*The cylinder factor represents the relationship between the cylinder volume and the gauge pressure. For example, an E cylinder can hold 622 L of gas at a filling pressure of 2200 psi. The volume-pressure cylinder factor for E cylinders equals 622 L/2200 psi, or 0.28 L/psi. Table 2-5 shows the cylinder factors for the several commonly used cylinders.

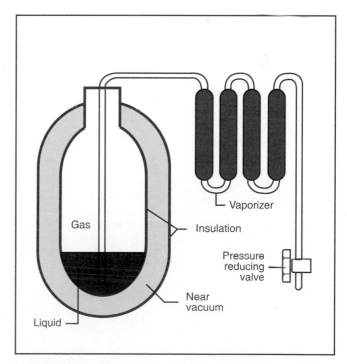

FIGURE 2-10 Components of a bulk oxygen supply system.

gaseous oxygen. The pressure-reducing valve serves to reduce the working pressure of the gas to a desired level (usually 50 psi for hospitals and other health care facilities) before it enters the hospital's compressed-gas piping system (see Figure 2-19 for a description of piping systems). The pressure-release valve allows some of the gas on top of the liquid to escape if the contents are warmed too much. This release of gas allows the gas within the container to expand, thus lowering the temperature (see Gay-Lussac's law in Chapter 1). This keeps the gas under pressure between its boiling point and its critical temperature, so that most of the reservoir's contents are maintained in the liquid state.

As previously stated, bulk reservoir systems must meet specifications established by the NFPA.[13] Appendix 2-2 contains a summary of the NFPA recommendations and regulations for bulk oxygen systems. Proper installment of these systems is critical to maintain public safety. Figure 2-11 shows the minimum distances between bulk oxygen storage facilities and other structures.

Portable Liquid Oxygen Systems

Smaller versions of the bulk oxygen system are available for the home care setting. A typical home liquid oxygen system consists of two components: a stationary base reservoir and a portable unit. The main unit contains a liquid

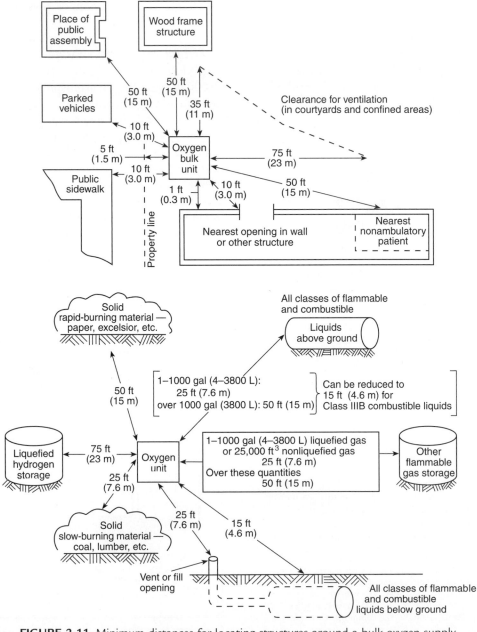

FIGURE 2-11 Minimum distances for locating structures around a bulk oxygen supply.

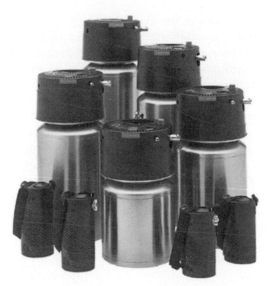

FIGURE 2-12 Stationary liquid oxygen reservoirs. (Courtesy Caire, Burnsville, Minn. In Hess DR, MacIntyre NR, Mishoe SC et al: *Respiratory care: principles and practice,* Philadelphia, 2002, WB Saunders.)

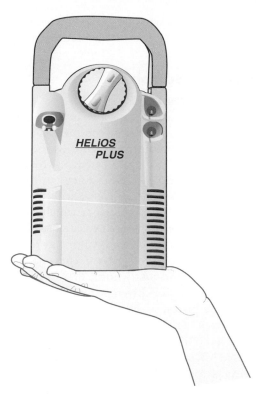

FIGURE 2-13 Portable Helios liquid oxygen system. This system uses an oxygen-conserving mechanism that relies on a demand valve, which delivers oxygen on inhalation and stops during exhalation. (Courtesy of Nellcor Puritan Bennett, Pleasanton, Calif.)

reservoir, a vaporizer coil, and a pressure-relief valve. Figure 2-12 shows various sizes of stationary liquid oxygen reservoirs that are available for the home care setting. The portable device is filled from the main unit.

Stationary reservoirs have capacities of 12 to 60 L of liquid oxygen, whereas portable units have capacities of 0.5 to 1.2 L.[8] Stationary reservoir systems can provide an economical source of oxygen for home care patients who require long term oxygen therapy. These systems generally can provide a reliable source of oxygen for 4 to 6 weeks, depending on the demand. Portable units can provide an 8- to 10-hour supply of oxygen for patients during times of greater mobility. Newer portable devices, such as the Helios unit shown in Figure 2-13 (Tyco Puritan Bennett, Pleasanton, California), weigh less than 4 pounds when filled and can provide continuous oxygen for 6 to 10 hours, depending on the flow rate used. As is discussed in Chapter 3, oxygen-conserving devices can increase the amount of time these smaller systems can provide oxygen. Box 2-5 explains how to calculate the duration of a liquid oxygen supply. Remember that the amount of time a supply will last depends on the weight of the liquid remaining in the reservoir—not the pressure, as for cylinders. Because 1 L of liquid oxygen weighs 2.5 pounds, the number of liters of liquid oxygen present can be calculated by dividing the weight of the liquid oxygen by 2.5. Considering that oxygen expands to 860 times its liquid volume at 25° C and 1 atm, the total volume of gaseous oxygen available can be calculated by multiplying the number of liters of liquid oxygen by 860. The amount of time in minutes that the supply will last can be determined by dividing this volume by the flow rate of the gas being delivered.

Most portable systems are designed to provide working pressures of approximately 20 psi. It is important to know

---

BOX 2-5	Calculating the Duration of a Liquid Oxygen Supply

1. A liter of liquid oxygen weighs 2.5 pounds, therefore:
   Liquid weight ÷ 2.5 = Number of liters of liquid oxygen
2. Gaseous oxygen occupies a volume that is 860 times the volume of liquid oxygen, therefore:
   Liters of liquid × 860 = Liters of gas
3. Duration of supply (minutes) = Gas supply remaining (in liters) ÷ Flow (L/min).

Example

How long would a liquid oxygen supply weighing 10 pounds last if a patient were receiving oxygen through a nasal cannula at 2 L/min?

Amount of gas (liters) = (10 pounds ÷ 2.5 lb/L) × 860
Amount of gas = 3440 L
Duration of supply (minutes) = Amount of gas ÷ Flow (in liters)
Duration of supply = 3440 L ÷ (2 L/min)
Duration of supply = 1720 minutes
or about 28 hours and 40 minutes

---

the operating pressure of the device before flowmeters or restrictors are attached to control gas flow out of the system. Failure to recognize the actual delivery pressure of these devices can result in injury to the patient or damage to the attached equipment. The actual flow delivered can be determined with a calibrated **Thorpe tube flowmeter** (see Chapter 3 for a discussion of flowmeters). Appendix 2-3 lists the NFPA safety recommendations for portable liquid oxygen systems.

Medical Air Supply

Portable Air Compressors

Compressed air is used to power many respiratory care devices. In many cases, air can be compressed at the point of administration by portable air compressors. Larger portable systems can produce compressed air with a standard working pressure of 50 psi; these units can therefore be used to power devices such as pneumatically powered ventilators. Smaller portable compressors, which are unable to achieve these high working pressures, are used for bedside applications (e.g., powering small-volume nebulizers).

Three types of compressors are currently available: piston, diaphragm, and rotary units. **Piston compressors** use the action of a motor-driven piston to compress atmospheric air. The piston is seated within a cylinder casing and is sealed to it with a carbon or Teflon ring. Figure 2-14 shows the operational principle of a typical piston air compressor used to power a mechanical ventilator. As the piston retracts, atmospheric air is drawn in through a one-way intake valve. When the piston protracts, the intake valve closes, and gas leaves through a one-way outflow valve. A small gas reservoir is placed in a coiled tube to allow the hot, compressed gas to cool to room temperature before it is delivered to the output valve. The reservoir also removes some of the humidity from the intake gas. Usually a water drain is located near the compressor's output, and a water trap should be placed between the output and the device to be attached to the compressor to prevent problems with moisture accumulation. Examples of portable piston compressors include the Bennett MC-1 and MC-2 compressors, the Ohio High Performance Compressor, and the Timemeter PCS-1 units.

Diaphragm compressors (Figure 2-15) use a flexible diaphragm attached to a piston to compress gas. As the piston moves down, the diaphragm is bent outward, and gas is drawn through a one-way valve into the cylinder. Upward movement of the piston forces the gas out of the cylinder through a separate one-way outflow valve. Examples of diaphragm compressors are the Air Shields Diapump and the DeVilbiss small nebulizer compressor.

Rotary compressors use a rotating vane to compress air from an intake valve. As the rotating vane turns, gas is drawn into the cylinder through a one-way valve (Figure 2-16). As the rotor turns, the gas is compressed as the oval-shaped cylinder becomes smaller. The compressed gas is then forced out of the compressor through another one-way outflow valve. Low-pressure, rotary compressors are used in ventilators such as the cardinal AVEA.

Bulk Air Supply Systems

Most bulk air systems use two compressors that can operate together or independently, depending on the demand for compressed air. Each compressor should also be able to deliver 100% of the average peak demand if the other compressor is turned off for maintenance or fails to operate. Box 2-6 summarizes the NFPA recommendations for safely operating medical air supply systems.

Air compressors used in bulk supply systems are usually piston or rotary compressors. Large piston compressors typically can provide a high-flow output and working pres-

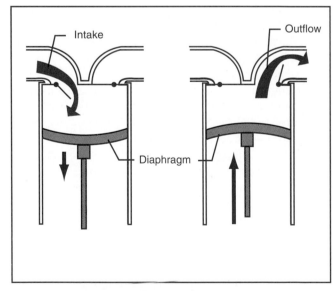

FIGURE 2-15 Diaphragm compressor.

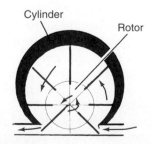

FIGURE 2-16 Rotary compressor.

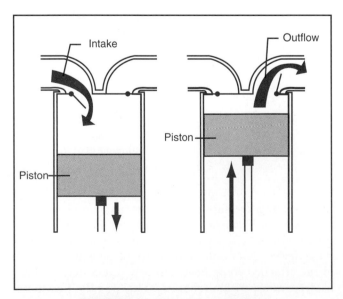

FIGURE 2-14 Piston air compressor.

BOX 2-6	National Fire Protection Association (NFPA) Recommendations for Medical Air Supply

1. The source of medical air must be from the outside atmosphere and should not contain contaminants such as particulate matter, odor, or other gases.
2. The air intake port must be located outdoors, above roof level, at a minimum distance above the ground and 10 feet from any door, window, or other intake opening in the building. Intake ports must be turned downward and screened.
3. Air taken into the system must contain no contamination from engine exhaust, fuel storage vents, vacuum system discharges, or other particulate matter, because odor of any type can be drawn into the system.
4. A minimum of two oil-free compressors must be duplexed together, with provisions for operating alternately or simultaneously, depending on the demand. Each compressor or duplex must be capable of maintaining the air supply to the system at peak demand.
5. Backflow through compressors that are cycled off must be prevented automatically.
6. Each duplex system should be provided with disconnection switches, motor-starting devices with overload protection, and a means of automatically alternating the compressor or compressors. Use of the compressors should be divided evenly, and automatic means of activating an additional compressor or compressors should be provided in case the supply source unit becomes incapable of maintaining adequate pressure.
7. Air storage tanks or receivers must have a safety valve, an automatic drain, a pressure gauge, and the capacity to ensure practical on-off operation.
8. The type of medical air compressor and the local atmospheric conditions govern the need for intake filters/mufflers, after-coolers for air dryers, and additional downstream regulators.
9. Antivibration mountings are to be installed (in accordance with the manufacturer's recommendations) under the components and flexible couplings that connect the air compressors, receivers, and intake and supply lines.
10. A maintenance program must be established following the manufacturer's recommendations.

From the Compressed Gas Association: *Handbook of compressed gases*, ed 3, New York, 1990, Van Nostrand Reinhold.

sures of at least 50 psi. A reservoir is incorporated into the design of the compressor unit to accommodate varying peak flow needs. The reservoir receives the compressed air and stores it at a higher pressure than in the piping system. A dryer attached to the outflow of the reservoir removes humidity (from refrigeration) from the air entering the piping system. A reducing valve on the reservoir outflow line reduces the pressure to 50 psi or the desired working pressure. In most cases, a pneumatic sensing unit turns off the compressor when the reservoir pressure reaches a preset high level. This sensing unit also turns the compressor back on when the reservoir pressure falls below 50 psi.

High-pressure rotary units require a liquid sealant to produce high pressures efficiently. These systems typically include a reservoir for storing gas under high pressure, a dryer to remove humidity, and a pressure-relief valve to control the output pressure of the compressed gas. A pneumatic sensing unit, such as those used in piston compressors, is also used to maintain a constant working pressure of 50 psi and to prevent unnecessary high pressures.

Central Supply Systems

Hospitals and other health care facilities, such as free-standing clinics, rehabilitation centers, and diagnostic laboratories, typically rely on central supply systems to provide medical gases to multiple sites in the institution.

Large hospitals usually rely on continuous supply systems. A **continuous supply system** contains two sources of gas supply, one of which serves as a reserve source for use only in an emergency.[13] The primary source is usually a large liquid oxygen or air reservoir, whereas the reserve supply is a smaller liquid reservoir or a bank of compressed-gas cylinders. The primary source must be refilled at regular intervals. NFPA regulations require that the reserve supply contain an average day's supply of oxygen. The NFPA also requires that these systems include a pressure regulator, **check valves,** and a pressure-relief valve between each gas supply and main piping system.

Alternating supply systems usually consist of two banks of cylinders, one designated as the primary source and the other as the secondary source. Each bank of cylinders must contain a minimum of two cylinders or at least an average day's supply of oxygen or air. After the primary source is depleted or unable to meet system demands, the secondary system automatically becomes the primary source of oxygen or air. The empty bank is simply refilled or replaced. As a safety feature, an actuating switch must be connected to the master control panel to indicate when the change to the secondary bank is about to occur.[13] Check valves are installed between each cylinder and the manifold to prevent loss of gas from the manifold cylinders in the event the pressure-relief devices on an individual cylinder function or a cylinder lead fails.

Figure 2-17 shows an alternating system that contains liquid oxygen cylinders as the primary and secondary oxygen sources, along with a reserve oxygen supply of compressed-gas cylinders. The reserve supply is used only when the primary and secondary sources are unable to supply system demands.[13] Note that the system must contain check valves and pressure-relief devices between the gas source and the main supply line. As with the previously described alternating system, an actuating switch signals when the changeover from the primary to the secondary source occurs.

Piping Systems

Gases stored in central supply units are distributed to various sites or zones in a hospital or health care facility via a piping system such as the one shown in Figure 2-18. NFPA regulations govern the construction, installation, and testing of these systems.[13] Pipes used to transport gases must be seamless type K or L (ASTMB-8) copper

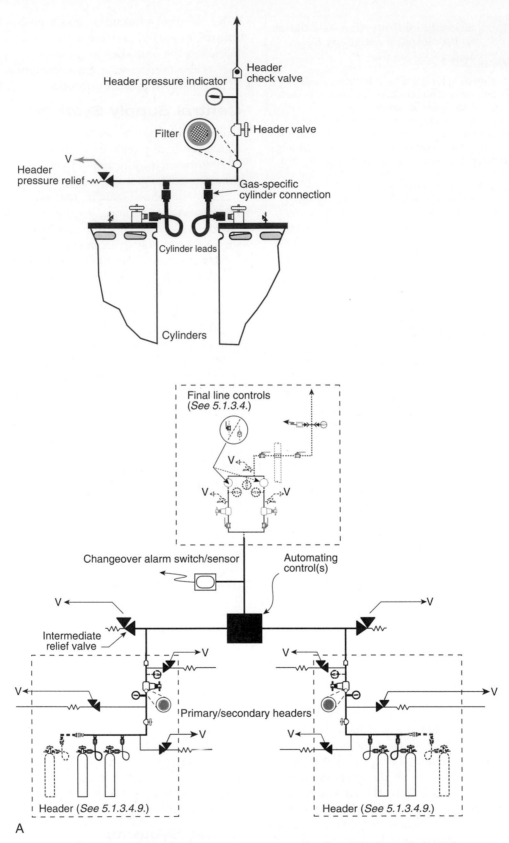

FIGURE 2-17 Systems for medical air or oxygen. **A,** Header for cryogenic gas in containers.

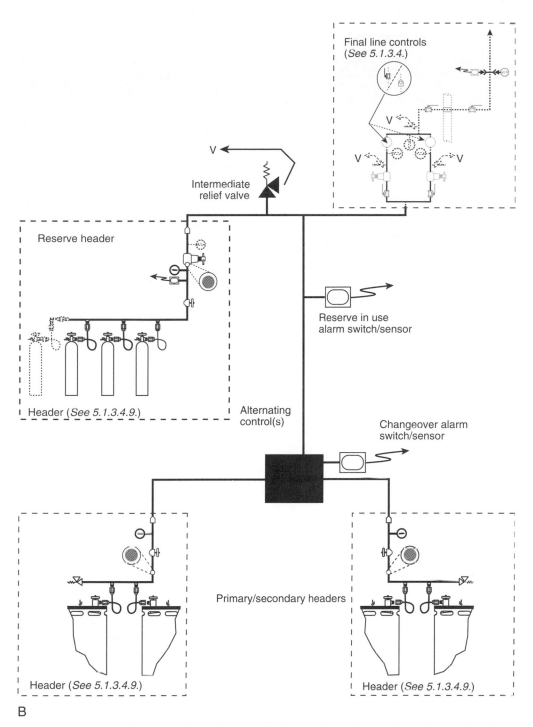

Final line controls
(*See 5.1.3.4.*)

V

Intermediate
relief valve

Reserve header

Reserve in use
alarm switch/sensor

Alternating
control(s)

Changeover alarm
switch/sensor

Header (*See 5.1.3.4.9.*)

Primary/secondary headers

Header (*See 5.1.3.4.9.*)

Header (*See 5.1.3.4.9.*)

B

FIGURE 2-17 cont'd B, Typical supply source for cryogenic gas in containers. (Reproduced with permission from NFPA99: Health Care Facilities, Copyright © 2005, National Fire Protection Association. This reprinted material is not the complete and official position of the NFPA on the referenced subject, which is represented only by the standard in its entirety.)

tubing or standard weight brass pipe. The size of the pipes must be sufficient to maintain proper delivery volumes and to conform to good engineering practices. The gas contents of the pipeline must be labeled at least every 20 feet and at least once in each room or story through which the pipeline travels.

Pressure-regulating devices located between the bulk and the main supply lines must be capable of maintaining a minimum delivery pressure of 50 psi to all station outlets at the maximum delivery line flow. Pressure-relief valves should be installed downstream from the main-line pressure regulator. A pressure-relief valve should also be installed upstream of any zone valve to prevent excessive pressure in a zone where the shutoff valve is closed. All pressure-relief valves are set 50% higher than the system working pressure (e.g., 75 psi for a 50-psi system pressure).

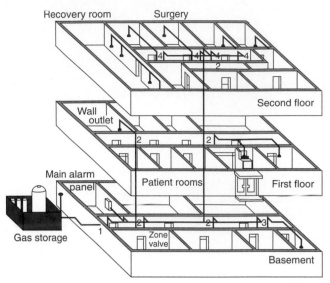

FIGURE 2-18 Hospital piping system. Zone valves must be placed (1) at the entrance to the hospital, (2) at each riser, (3) at each branch supplying an area, and (4) at each operating room. (Courtesy Nellcor Puritan Bennett, Pleasanton, Calif.)

CLINICAL ROUNDS 2-3

A fire breaks out on the north wing of the fifth floor of the hospital where you work. How should you respond to this emergency?

See Evolve Resources for answer.

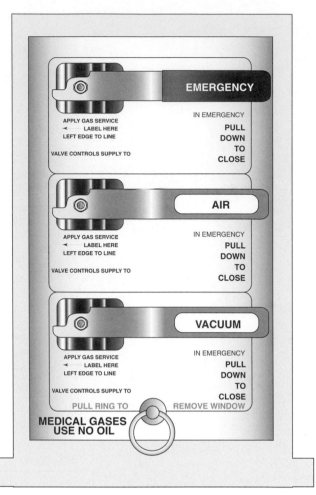

FIGURE 2-19 Zone shutoff valves for a bulk oxygen supply.

As previously stated, piping systems in hospitals are organized into zones, which allow for quick isolation of all independent areas if maintenance is required. In case of fire, affected zones can be isolated, preventing the problem from spreading to other areas of the hospital (Clinical Rounds 2-3). Shutoff valves are located at the point where the mainline enters the hospital, at each riser, and between each zone and the main supply line. Zone shutoff valves for oxygen must be located outside of each critical care unit. Shutoff valves for every oxygen or nitrous oxide line must also be located outside of each surgical suite.

Shutoff valves generally are located in a large box with removable windows large enough to permit manual operation of the valve. They should be installed at a height where they can be operated from the standing position in an emergency. All valves must be labeled as shown in Figure 2-19.

Piping systems must be tested for leaks and to ensure that gas supply lines have not become crossed. Visual inspection of the system can identify obvious problems, such as worn or loose connections; damaged pipes; pipes soiled with oil, grease, or other oxidizable materials; and crossing of gas supplies (e.g., crossing of compressed air and oxygen supply lines). Crossing of supply lines can be checked by reducing the system pressure to atmospheric and then purging each supply line separately with oil-free

dry air or nitrogen. Whether the gas lines are crossed can also be determined by analyzing gas samples from the appropriate station outlets. Gases used to purge the supply lines should be passed through a white filter at a flow of 100 L/min to determine whether the purge gas is clean and odor free. The content of gas lines should be tested for purity with the appropriate gas analysis.

All medical gas supply lines should have alarm systems that alert hospital personnel of system malfunctions (e.g., loss of system pressure, change from the primary system supply source to the secondary and reserve supplies, and reduction in reserve supply below an average day's amount). Alarm panels should include visual and audible alerting signals and should be placed in locations that allow continuous surveillance (e.g., in the engineering department of the hospital). Alarm systems should also be located in critical care areas where life support systems (e.g., mechanical ventilators) are used. The Joint Commission on Accreditation of Healthcare Organizations mandates a written policy for responding to alarms and requires that personnel working in areas where alarms are located be instructed in how to respond.[14] Failure to respond appropriately can result in disaster. Response plans should include ensuring that all patient equipment

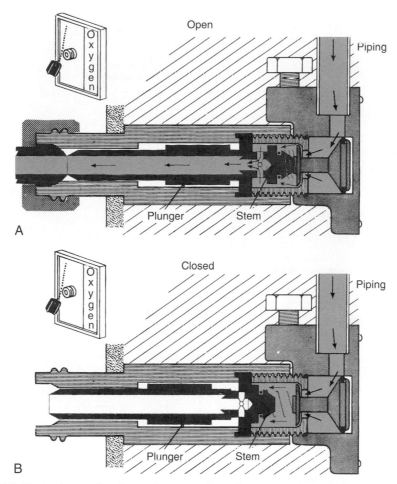

FIGURE 2-20 Station outlets for a Diameter Index Safety System (DISS). (Courtesy Nellcor Puritan Bennett, Pleasanton, Calif.)

is working properly and that appropriate personnel (i.e., respiratory care services and engineering) are immediately notified.

Station Outlets

Station outlets provide connections for gas delivery devices, such as flowmeters and mechanical ventilators. These outlets consist of a body mounted to the supply line, an outlet faceplate, and primary and secondary check valves, which are safety valves that open when the delivery device's adapter is inserted into the station outlet and close automatically when the adapter is disengaged from the outlet. Station outlets must not be supplied directly from a riser unless they are supplied through the manual shutoff valve located in the same story as the outlet. Outlet faceplates must be labeled with the name or symbol of the delivered gas. They may also be color coded for easy identification.

Station outlets are designed with safety systems that prevent the connection of incompatible devices. Two safety systems are currently available: the **Diameter Index Safety System (DISS)** and **quick-connect adapters.** Figure 2-20 shows an outlet that uses DISS. This system, which was designed by the CGA, uses noninterchangeable, threaded fittings to connect gas-powered devices to station outlets. Each outlet must be fitted with a cap on a chain or installed in a recessed box that is equipped with a door to protect the outlet when not in use. Outlets typically are located about 5 feet above the floor or are recessed to prevent physical damage to the valve or control equipment. Delivery lines that serve anesthetic devices must have a backflow of gas into the system, and the check valves must be able to hold a minimum of 2400 psi.[1,13,15]

Figure 2-21 shows a schematic of a quick-connect connection, and Figure 2-22 shows examples of quick-connect adapters. These connections use a plunger that is held forward by a spring to prevent gas from leaving the outlet. Insertion of the appropriate adapter pushes the plunger backward, allowing gas to flow into the striker and into the equipment attached to the adapter. When the adapter is removed, the spring resets the plunger and closes the outlet.

Oxygen Concentrators

Oxygen concentrators are devices that produce enriched oxygen from atmospheric air. They provide an alternative

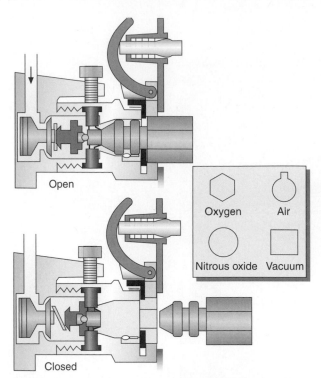

FIGURE 2-21 Schematic of a typical quick-connect station outlet. (From Hess DR, MacIntyre NR, Mishoe SC et al: *Respiratory care: principles and practice*, Philadelphia, 2002, WB Saunders.)

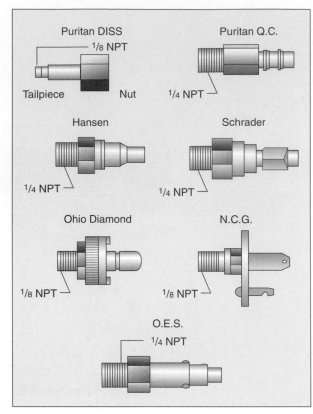

FIGURE 2-22 Examples of various quick-connect adapters from different manufacturers and suppliers.

to compressed-gas cylinders, particularly in the delivery of respiratory therapy to home care patients. Two types of concentrators are currently available: those using semipermeable plastic membranes and those using molecular sieves.

Concentrators using semipermeable membranes to separate oxygen from room air are composed of plastic membranes containing pores that are 1 mm in diameter (1 mm = 1/25,000 in). Atmospheric gases diffuse through the membrane at different rates. The rate at which a gas diffuses depends on its diffusion constant and solubility for the plastic membrane and the pressure gradient for the gas across the membrane. A diaphragm compressor is used to provide a constant vacuum across the membrane.

Oxygen and water vapor diffuse through these membranes faster than nitrogen. Generally, a constant flow of humidified 40% oxygen can be provided at a flow of 1 to 10 L/min.[16] Figure 2-23 is a functional diagram of an oxygen concentrator that uses a semipermeable membrane.

Figure 2-24 shows a typical oxygen concentrator that relies on molecular sieves to produce an enriched oxygen mixture. Such systems use a compressor to pump room air at pressures of 15 to 25 psig to one of two sets of sieves. Nitrogen is removed by passing room air through sodium-aluminum silicate (zeolite) pellets, producing an enriched oxygen mixture. It is important to mention that nitrogen and other gases absorbed by the zeolite pellets must be purged to ensure that the unit functions properly. In the **pressure swing adsorption (PSA) method,** intermittent pressurization of one of the sieve beds occurs while the other bed is purged to remove any absorbed gases and moisture.

The concentration of oxygen leaving the system depends on the flow rate set. For example, at flows less than 6 L/min, the gas contains about +/−93% oxygen.[8] Note that flowmeters calibrated for low inlet pressures must be used to ensure accurate delivery of oxygen to the patient, because the outlet pressure from these concentrators is approximately 5 to 10 psig. Examples of molecular sieve concentrators include the AirSep NewLife, LifeStyle, and FreeStyle, and VisionAire oxygen concentrators, and the DeVilbiss 303 DS/DZ and 515 DS/DZ oxygen concentrators.

Figure 2-25A shows a typical compact oxygen concentrator (VisionAire) used for home care treatment of patients requiring long-term oxygen therapy. The NewLife oxygen concentrator (AirSep Corp., Buffalo, New York) shown is equipped with alarms that signal power failure, high and low pressure, and low oxygen concentration. At just 30 lbs and providing nearly silent operation at 40 decibels, the industry's most compact in-home oxygen concentrator is also the most power efficient at 290 watts. Figure 2-25B shows a portable oxygen concentrator that permits greater mobility for patients requiring long-term oxygen therapy. The FreeStyle unit shown can be powered by an internal battery, an AC power supply, a DC power supply, or an optional rechargeable battery belt that can be used in combination with the unit's internal battery. The battery belt pack, when used with a fully charged internal battery, can supply power to the unit for up to 10 hours between charges.

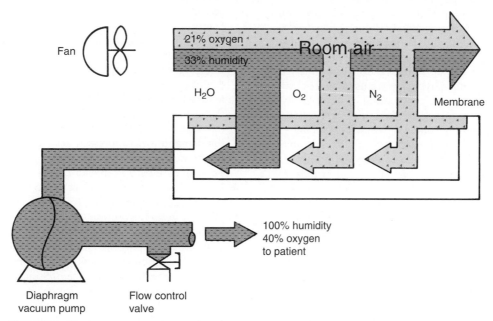

FIGURE 2-23 Oxygen concentrator that uses a semipermeable membrane. (Courtesy Oxygen Enrichment, Schenectady, NY.)

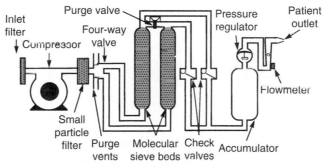

FIGURE 2-24 Oxygen concentrator that relies on a molecular sieve.

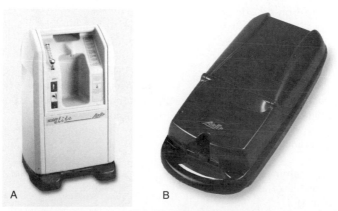

FIGURE 2-25 A, Stationary oxygen concentrator for home care patients. **B,** Lightweight portable oxygen concentrator. (Courtesy AirSep, Buffalo, NY.)

KEY POINTS

▶ An understanding of the properties of the commonly used medical gases is essential for safe and effective use of these agents in the clinical setting.

▶ Medical gases typically are classified as nonliquefied and liquefied. Nonliquefied gases are stored and transported under pressure in metal cylinders; liquefied gases are stored and transported in specially design bulk storage units.

▶ Compressed-gas cylinders are available in a variety of sizes. Smaller cylinders typically are used as a portable source of oxygen in emergency situations and for transporting patients requiring O_2 therapy. Larger cylinders are used as a primary source of medical gases in medical facilities that do not have bulk storage units.

▶ The contents of compressed-gas cylinders must be easily identifiable. Standard labels should include the name and chemical symbol of the gas in the cylinder, along with information about hazards associated with use of the gas. The label should also include information about precautionary measures that should be taken when exposure to the contents leads to an adverse reaction.

▶ The volume of gas remaining in a cylinder and the duration of cylinder gas flow can easily be determined if one knows the cylinder gauge pressure and the cylinder's volume-pressure factor. To determine the volume of gas in a cylinder containing liquefied gas (e.g., carbon dioxide or nitrous oxide cylinders), one must weigh the cylinder, because a liquid remains in equilibrium with gas above it until the liquid is depleted.

▶ Bulk liquid storage systems for medical gases are cost-effective and require considerably less space than compressed-gas cylinders. Lightweight portable units are particularly advantageous for patients who require long-term oxygen therapy.

▶ Compressed air is used to power many respiratory care devices, ranging from small handheld nebulizers to pneumatically powered ventilators. Bulk systems for hospitals and other health care facilities use multiple compressors that operate together or independently, depending on the demand for compressed air. In many cases, such as the home care setting, air can be compressed at the point of care by portable air compressors.

▶ Hospitals and other health care facilities typically rely on central supply systems to provide medical gases to multiple sites in the institution. Gases are stored in central supply units and distributed to the various sites through standardized piping systems. Alarm panels and shutoff valves throughout the facility allow continuous surveillance and control of the system. Standardized station outlets provide connections for gas delivery devices, such as flowmeters and mechanical ventilators.

▶ Oxygen concentrators are an effective alternative to compressed-gas cylinders for home care patients.

ASSESSMENT QUESTIONS

See Evolve Resources for answers.

1. Which of the following is classified as a nonflammable gas that does not support combustion?
   a. Oxygen
   b. Carbon dioxide
   c. Helium
   d. Nitric oxide

2. Medical gas cylinders are color coded for easy identification. E cylinders of carbon dioxide are painted:
   a. Yellow
   b. Green
   c. Black
   d. Gray

3. A respiratory therapist is having trouble attaching a regulator to an E cylinder. One possible cause might be:
   a. The outlet threads of the cylinder do not match the threads of the regulator.
   b. The regulator diaphragm is jammed.
   c. The pin positions of the regulator are not the same as those on the cylinder.
   d. The cylinder has not been cracked.

4. Bulk liquid oxygen supplies should not be closer than _____ to public sidewalks.
   a. 2 feet
   b. 4 feet
   c. 7 feet
   d. 10 feet

5. Calculate the duration of the liquid oxygen supply if the liquid supply weighs 30 pounds and the oxygen demand is 4 L/min.
   a. 10 hours
   b. 23 hours
   c. 35 hours
   d. 43 hours

6. What is the duration of oxygen flow from an H cylinder containing 1200 psi of oxygen when the flow to a nasal cannula is 4 L/min?
   a. 9 hours, 42 minutes
   b. 12 hours, 15 minutes
   c. 15 hours, 42 minutes
   d. 16 hours, 10 minutes

ASSESSMENT QUESTIONS—cont'd

7. Large piston air compressors used in bulk supply systems typically can provide working pressures of:
   a. 50 psi
   b. 75 psi
   c. 100 psi
   d. 120 psi

8. Alternating supply systems for medical gases that are used in hospitals should include a reserve supply for oxygen in case the primary system fails. How much reserve oxygen should be available?
   a. An average 8-hour supply
   b. An average day's supply
   c. An average 3-day supply
   d. An average week's supply

9. Oxygen concentrators that use semipermeable membranes usually can provide what percentage of oxygen at flows of 1 to 10 L/min?
   a. 24%
   b. 40%
   c. 60%
   d. 100%

10. The percentage of oxygen delivery provided by molecular sieve O_2 concentrators depends on which of the following factors?
    I. The size of the concentrator
    II. The rate of gas flow
    III. The temperature of the refrigeration unit
    IV. The age of the sieve beds
       a. II only
       b. II and IV only
       c. I, II, and III only
       d. I, II, and IV only

11. The pressure inside a cylinder increases dramatically when the cylinder is exposed to extremely high temperatures. What prevents cylinders with frangible disks from exploding when exposed to extremely high temperatures?
    a. The frangible disk ruptures from the increased pressure, allowing gas to escape from the cylinder.
    b. The cylinder stem blows off when the temperature reaches 200° F.
    c. The stem diaphragm ruptures, allowing gas to escape.
    d. The frangible disk melts when the temperature reaches 100° F.

12. A respiratory therapist is checking cylinder markings to determine whether any of the cylinders need to be tested. The labeling reads as follows:
    9   83+
    6   94+
    This information indicates:
    a. The cylinder is due for retesting.
    b. The time between the test dates shown exceeds recommendations.
    c. The cylinder is made of aluminum.
    d. The owner of the cylinder.

13. Before using an H cylinder of oxygen, a respiratory therapist opens it, and gas at high pressure comes out of the cylinder outlet. Which of the following statements is true?
    a. This was an accident and should not be repeated.
    b. Allowing gas to escape from the cylinder lets the therapist smell the gas to ensure that it is oxygen.
    c. This action clears debris from the connector.
    d. This action should be performed after a regulator is attached to the cylinder outlet.

14. A respiratory therapist is helping design a new hospital wing. Which of the following agencies should be contacted so that the piping system of oxygen and air is correctly installed?
    a. NFPA
    b. FDA
    c. HHS
    d. DOT

15. A hospital uses a large air compressor system to supply air through its piped gas lines. This gas will be free of pollutants found in the local environment. True or false? Why?

References

1. Compressed Gas Association: *Handbook of compressed gases,* ed 4, New York, 1999, Van Nostrand Reinhold.
2. Dorsch JA, Dorsch SE: *Understanding anesthesia equipment: construction, care, and complications,* ed 5, Baltimore, 2008, Williams & Wilkins.
3. Kacmarek RM, Dimas S, Mack CW: *The essentials of respiratory care,* ed 4, St Louis, 2005, Elsevier-Mosby.
4. Wilkins RL, Stoller JK, Scanlon C: *Egan's fundamentals of respiratory care,* ed 8, St Louis, 2003, Mosby.
5. Gardenshire DS: *Rau's respiratory care pharmacology,* ed 6, St Louis, 2007, Elsevier.
6. Kinsella JP, Neish SR, Dunbar I et al: Clinical response to prolonged treatment of persistent pulmonary hypertension of the newborn with low doses of inhaled nitric oxide, *J Pediatr* 123:103, 1993.
7. Gerlach H, Pappert D, Lawandowski K, et al: Long term inhalation with evaluated low doses of nitric oxide for improvement of oxygenation in patients with adult respiratory distress syndrome, *Intensive Care Med* 19:443, 1993.

8. Hess D, MacIntyre N, Mishoe S et al: *Respiratory care: principles and practice,* Philadelphia, 2002, WB Saunders.

9. Schreiber P: *Anesthetic equipment,* New York, 1972, Springer-Verlag.

10. McPherson S: *Respiratory care equipment,* ed 5, St Louis, 1995, Mosby.

11. Code of Federal Regulations: Title 49, Parts 1-199, Washington, DC, 1974, US Government Printing Office.

12. National Fire Protection Association: *Standard for health care facilities,* (ANSI/NFPA 99), New York, 2002, The Association.

13. Blaze C: *Quick reference to respiratory care equipment assembly and troubleshooting,* St Louis, 1995, Mosby.

14. Klein BR, editor: *Health care facilities handbook,* ed 4, Quincy, Mass, 1993, National Fire Protection Association.

15. Lampton LM: Home and outpatient oxygen therapy. In Harchear RE, Rhodes MI, editors: *Chronic obstructive lung disease: clinical treatment and management,* St Louis, 1978, Mosby.

16. Kacmarek RM: Delivery systems for long-term oxygen therapy, *Respir Care* 45:84, 2000.

Internet Resources

American Association for Respiratory Care: http://www.aarc.org

Compressed Gas Association: http://www.cganet.com

GasNet—Global Anesthesiology Server Network: http://gasnet.med.yale.edu

Joint Commission on Health Care Organizations: http://www.jcaho.org

Mallinckrodt: http://www.mallinckrodt.com

National Fire Protection Association: http://www.nfpa.org

Ohmeda Medical: http://www.ohmedamedical.com

US Food and Drug Administration: http://www.fda.gov

National Fire Protection Association (NFPA) and Compressed Gas Association (CGA) Recommendations for Compressed-Gas Cylinders

STORAGE

1. Storage rooms must be dry, cool, and well-ventilated. Cylinders should not be stored in an area where the temperature exceeds 51.67° C (125° F).
2. No flames should have the potential of coming in contact with the cylinders.
3. The storage facility should be fire resistant where practical.
4. Cylinders must not be stored near flammable or combustible substances.
5. Gases that support combustion must be stored in a separate location from those that are combustible.
6. The storage area must be permanently posted.
7. Cylinders must be grouped by content.
8. Full and empty cylinders must be segregated in the storage areas.
9. Below-ground storage should be avoided.
10. Cylinders should never be stored in the operating room.
11. Large cylinders must be stored upright.
12. Cylinders must be protected from being cut or abraded.
13. Cylinders must be protected from extreme weather to prevent rusting, excessive temperatures, and accumulations of snow and ice.
14. Cylinders should not be exposed to continuous dampness or corrosive substances that could promote rusting of the cylinder and its valve.
15. Cylinders should be protected from tampering.
16. Valves on empty cylinders should be kept closed at all times.
17. Cylinders must be stored with protective caps in place.
18. Cylinders must not be stored in a confined space, such as a closet or the trunk of a car.

TRANSPORTATION

1. If protective valve caps are supplied, they should be used whenever cylinders are in transport and until they are ready for use.
2. Cylinders must not be dropped, dragged, slid, or allowed to strike each other violently.
3. Cylinders must be transported on an appropriate cart secured by a chain or strap.

USE

1. Before connecting equipment to a cylinder, make sure that connections are free of foreign materials.
2. Turn valve outlet away from personnel and crack cylinder valve to remove any dust or debris from outlet.
3. Cylinder valve outlet connections must be American Standard or CGA pin indexed, and low-pressure connections must be CGA diameter indexed.
4. Cylinders must be secured at the administration site and not to any movable objects or heat radiators.
5. Outlets and connections must be tightened only with appropriate wrenches and must never be forced on.
6. Equipment designed to use one gas should not be used with another.
7. Never use medical cylinder gases when contamination by backflow of other gases may occur.
8. Regulators should be off when the cylinder is turned on, and the cylinder valve should be opened slowly.
9. Before equipment is disconnected from a cylinder, the cylinder valve should be closed and the pressure released from the device.
10. Cylinder valves should be closed at all times except when in use.
11. Do not transfill cylinders, because this is hazardous.

12. Cylinders may be refilled only if permission is secured from the owner.
13. Cylinders must not be lifted by the cap.
14. Equipment connected to cylinders containing gaseous oxygen should be labeled: OXYGEN—USE NO OIL.
15. Enclosures intended to contain patients must have the minimum text regarding NO SMOKING, and the labels must be located (1) in a position to be read by the patients and (2) on two or more opposing sides visible from the exterior. It should be noted that oxygen hoods fall under the classification of oxygen enclosures and require these labels as well. In addition, another label is required that instructs visitors to get approval from hospital personnel before placing toys in an oxygen enclosure.
16. High-pressure oxygen equipment must not be sterilized with flammable agents (e.g., alcohol and ethylene oxide), and the agents used must be oil free and nondamaging.
17. Polyethylene bags must not be used to wrap sterilized, high-pressure oxygen equipment because when flexed, polyethylene releases pure hydrocarbons that are highly flammable.
18. Oxygen equipment exposed to pressures of less than 60 psi may be sterilized with either a nonflammable mixture of ethylene oxide and carbon dioxide or with fluorocarbons.
19. Cylinders must not be handled with oily or greasy hands, gloves, or clothing.
20. Never lubricate valve outlets or connecting equipment. (Oxygen and oil under pressure cause an explosive oxidation reaction.)
21. Do not flame test for leaks. (Usually a soap solution is used.)
22. When a cylinder is in use, open the valve fully and then turn it back a quarter- to a half-turn.
23. Replace the cap on an empty cylinder.
24. Position the cylinder so that the label is clearly visible. The label must not be defaced, altered, or removed.
25. Check the label before use; it should always match the color code.

26. No sources of open flames should be permitted in the area of administration. A NO SMOKING sign must be posted at the administration site. It must be legible from a distance of 5 feet and displayed in a conspicuous location.
27. Inform all area occupants of the hazards of smoking and of the regulations.
28. Equipment designated for use with a specific gas must be clearly and permanently labeled accordingly. The name of the manufacturer should be clearly marked on the device. If calibration or accuracy depends on gas density, the device must be labeled with the proper supply pressure.
29. Cylinder carts must be of a self-supporting design with appropriate casters and wheels, and those intended for use in surgery where flammable anesthetics are used must be grounded.
30. Cold cylinders must be handled with care to avoid hand injury resulting from tissue freezing caused by rapid gas expansion.
31. Safety-relief mechanisms, uninterchangeable connections, and other safety features must not be removed or altered.
32. Control valves on equipment must be closed both before connection and when not in use.

REPAIR AND MAINTENANCE

1. Use only the service manuals, operator manuals, instructions, procedures, and repair parts that are provided or recommended by the manufacturer.
2. Allow only qualified personnel to maintain the equipment.
3. Designate and set aside an area clean and free of oil and grease for the maintenance of oxygen equipment. Do not use this area for the repair and maintenance of other types of equipment.
4. Follow a scheduled preventive maintenance program.

National Fire Protection Association (NFPA) Recommendations and Regulations for Bulk Oxygen Systems

1. Containers that are permanently installed should be mounted on noncombustible supports and foundations.

2. Liquid oxygen containers should be constructed from materials that meet the impact test requirements of paragraph UG-48 of the ASME Boiler and Pressure Vessel Codes, Section VII, and must be in accordance with DOT specifications and regulations for 4 L liquid oxygen containers. Containers operating above 15 psi must be designed and tested in accordance with the ASME Boiler and Pressure Vessel Code, Section VII, and the insulation of the liquid oxygen container must be of noncombustible material.

3. All high-pressure gaseous oxygen containers must comply with the construction and test requirements of ASME Boiler and Pressure Vessel Code, Section VIII.

4. Bulk oxygen storage containers must be equipped with safety-release devices as required by ASME Code IV and the provisions of ASME S-1.3 or DOT specifications for both the container and safety releases.

5. Isolation casings on liquid oxygen containers shall be equipped with suitable safety-release devices. These devices must be designed or located so that moisture cannot either freeze the unit or interfere in any manner with its proper operation.

6. The vaporizing columns and connecting pipes shall be anchored or sufficiently flexible to provide for expansion and contraction as a result of temperature changes. The column must also have a safety-release device to properly protect it.

7. Any heat supplied to oxygen vaporizers must be done in an indirect fashion, such as with steam, air, water, or water solutions that do not react with oxygen. If liquid heaters are used to provide the primary source of heat, the vaporizers must be electrically grounded.

8. All equipment composing the bulk system must be cleaned to remove oxidizable material before the system is placed into service.

9. All joints and connections in the tubing should be made by welding or using flanged, threaded slip, or compressed fittings; and any gaskets or thread seals must be of suitable substance for oxygen service. Any valves, gauges, or regulators placed into the system must be designed for oxygen service. The piping must conform to ANSI B 31.3; piping that operates below −20° F must be composed of materials meeting ASME Code, Section VIII.

10. Storage containers, piping valves, and regulating equipment must be protected from physical damage and tampering.

11. Any enclosure containing oxygen control or operating equipment must be adequately ventilated.

12. The location shall be permanently posted to indicate OXYGEN—NO SMOKING—NO OPEN FLAMES or an equivalent warning.

13. All bulk systems must be regularly inspected by qualified representatives of the oxygen supplier.

14. Weeds and tall grass must be kept a minimum of 15 feet from any bulk oxygen container. The bulk oxygen system must be located so that its distance provides maximum safety for other areas surrounding it. The minimum distances for location of a bulk oxygen system near the following structures (see Figure 2-11) are as follows:

a. 25 Feet from any combustible structure.

b. 25 Feet from any structure that consists of fire-resistant exterior walls or buildings of other construction that have sprinklers.

c. 10 Feet from any opening in the adjacent walls of fire-resistant structures.

d. 25 Feet from flammable liquid storage above ground that is less than 1000 gallons in capacity, or 50 feet from these storage areas if the quantity is in excess of 1000 gallons.

e. 15 Feet from an underground flammable liquid storage that is less than 1000 gallons, or 30 feet from one in excess of 1000 gallons capacity. The distance from the oxygen storage containers to connections used for filling and venting of flammable liquid must be at least 25 feet.

f. 25 Feet from combustible gas storage above ground that is less than 1000 gallons capacity, or 50 feet from the storage of over 1000 gallons capacity.

g. 15 Feet from combustible liquid storage underground and 25 feet from the vent or filling connections.

h. 50 Feet from flammable gas storage less than 5000 ft^3; 90 feet from flammable gas in excess of 5000 ft^3 NTP.

i. 25 Feet from solid materials that burn slowly (e.g., coal and heavy timber).

j. 75 Feet away in one direction and 35 feet away at an approximately 90-degree angle from confining walls unless they are made from a fire-resistant material and are less than 20 feet high. (This is to provide adequate ventilation in the area in case venting occurs.)

k. 50 Feet from places of public assembly.

l. 50 Feet from nonambulatory patients.

m. 10 Feet from public sidewalks.

n. 5 Feet from any adjoining property line.

o. Must be accessible by a mobile transport unit that fills the supply system.

15. The permanent installation of a liquid oxygen system must be supervised by personnel familiar with the proper installation and construction as outlined in the NFPA 50.

16. The oxygen supply must have an inlet for the connection of a temporary supply in emergency and maintenance situations. The inlet must be physically protected to prevent tampering or unauthorized use and must be labeled EMERGENCY LOW-PRESSURE GASEOUS OXYGEN INLET. The inlet is to be installed downstream from the main supply line shutoff valve and must have the necessary valves to provide the emergency supply of oxygen as well as isolate the pipeline to the normal source of supply. There must be a check valve in the main line between the inlet connection and the main shutoff valve and another check valve between the inlet connection and the emergency supply shutoff valve. The inlet connection must have a pressure-relief valve of adequate size to protect the downstream piping from pressures in excess of 50% above normal pipeline operating pressure.

17. The bulk oxygen system must be mounted on noncombustible supports and foundations.

18. A surface of noncombustible material must extend at least 3 feet beyond the reach of liquid oxygen leaks during system operation or filling. Asphalt or bitumastic paving is prohibited. The slope of the area must be considered in the sizing of the surface.

19. The same type of surface must extend at least the full width of the vehicle that fills the bulk unit and at least 8 feet in the transverse direction.

20. No part of the bulk system should be underneath electrical power lines or within reach of a downed power line.

21. No part of the system can be exposed to flammable gases or to piping containing any class of flammable or combustible liquids.

22. The system must be located so as to be readily accessible to mobile supply equipment at ground level, as well as to authorized personnel.

23. Warning and alarm systems are required to monitor the operation and condition of the supply system. Alarms and gauges are to be located for the best possible surveillance, and each alarm and gauge must be appropriately labeled.

24. The master alarm system must monitor the source of supply, the reserve (if any), and the mainline pressure of the gas system. The power source for warning systems must meet the essentials of NFPA 76 A.

25. All alarm conditions must be evaluated and necessary measures taken to establish or ensure the proper function of the supply system.

26. Two master alarm panels, with alarms that cannot be canceled, are to be located in separate locations to ensure continuous observation. One signal must alert the user to a changeover from one operating supply to another, and an additional signal must provide notification that the reserve is supplying the system.

27. If check valves are not installed in the cylinder leads and headers, another alarm signal should be initiated when the reserve reaches a 1-day supply.

28. All piping systems must have both audible and visible signals that cannot be canceled to indicate when the mainline pressure increases or decreases 20% from the normal supply pressure. A pressure gauge must be installed and appropriately labeled adjacent to the switch that generates the pressure alarm conditions.

29. All warning systems must be tested before being placed in service or being added to existing service. Periodic retesting and appropriate recordkeeping are required.

National Fire Protection Association (NFPA) Safety Recommendations and Regulations for Portable Liquid Oxygen Systems

1. Liquid oxygen units will vent gas when not in use, creating an oxygen-enriched environment. This can be particularly hazardous in the following situations:
   a. When the unit is stored in a closed space.
   b. When the unit is tipped over.
   c. When the oxygen is transferred to another container.
2. Liquid oxygen units should not be located adjacent to heat sources, which can accelerate the venting of oxygen.
3. The unit surface should not be contaminated with oil or grease.
4. Verify the contents of liquid containers when setting up the equipment, changing the containers, or refilling the containers at the home.
5. Connections for containers are to be made with the manufacturer's operating instructions.
6. The patient and family must be familiar with the proper operation of the liquid devices, along with all precautions, safeguards, and troubleshooting methods.
7. Transfill one unit from another in compliance with CGA pamphlet P-26, "Transfilling of Low Pressure Liquid Oxygen to be Used for Respiration," and in accordance with the manufacturer's operating instructions.
8. All connections for filling must conform to CGA V-1, and the hose assembly must have a pressure release set no higher than the container's rated pressure.
9. Liquid containers must have a pressure release to limit the container pressure to the rated level, and a device must also be incorporated to limit the amount of oxygen introduced into a container to the manufacturer's specified capacity.

10. Delivery vehicles should be well vented to prevent the buildup of high oxygen levels, and transfilling should take place with the delivery vehicle doors wide open.
11. "No Smoking" signs must be posted, and there can be no sources of ignition within 5 feet.
12. The transfiller must affix the labels required by DOT and FDA regulations, and records must be kept stating the content and purity. Instructions must be on the container, and the color coding and labeling must meet CGA and NFPA standards.
13. All devices used with liquid oxygen containers must be moisture free, and pressure releases must be positioned correctly to prevent freezing and the buildup of high pressures.
14. When liquid oxygen is spilled, both the liquid and gas that escape are very cold and will cause frostbite or eye injury. When filling liquid oxygen containers, wear safety goggles with side shields, along with loose-fitting, properly insulated gloves. High-top boots with cuffless pants worn outside of the boots are recommended.
15. Items exposed to liquid oxygen should not be touched, because they can not only cause frostbite, they can stick to the skin. Materials that are pliable at room temperature become brittle at the extreme temperatures of liquid oxygen.
16. If a liquid oxygen spill occurs, the cold liquid and resulting gas condense the moisture in the air, creating a fog. Normally the fog will extend over an area larger than the area of contact danger, except in extremely dry climates.
17. In the event of a spill, measures should be taken to prevent anyone from walking on the surface or wheeling equipment across the area for at least 15 minutes.

All sources of ignition must be kept away from the area.

18. Liquid oxygen spilled onto asphalt or oil-soaked concrete constitutes an extreme hazard because an explosive reaction can occur.

19. If liquid oxygen or gas comes in contact with the skin, remove any clothing that may constrict blood flow to the frozen area. Warm the affected area with water at about body temperature until medical personnel arrive. Seek immediate medical attention for eye contact or blistering of the skin.

20. Immediately remove contaminated clothing and air it away from sources of ignition for at least an hour.

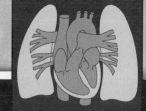

Chapter 3

Administering Medical Gases: Regulators, Flowmeters, and Controlling Devices

J.M. CAIRO

OUTLINE

Regulators and Flowmeters
  Regulators
  Flowmeters
Devices for Administering Medical Gases
  Oxygen Therapy
  Hyperbaric Oxygen Therapy

Nitric Oxide Therapy
Helium-Oxygen (Heliox) Therapy
Carbon Dioxide–Oxygen (Carbogen)
  Therapy

OBJECTIVES

Upon completion of this chapter, you will be able to:
· Compare the design and operation of single-stage and multistage regulators.
· Identify the components of preset and adjustable regulators.
· Explain the operational theory of a Thorpe tube flowmeter, a Bourdon flowmeter, and a flow restrictor.
· Demonstrate a method for determining whether a flowmeter is pressure compensated.
· Compare low-flow and high-flow oxygen delivery systems.
· Name several commonly used low-flow oxygen delivery systems.
· Discuss the advantages and disadvantages of oxygen-conserving devices.
· Explain the operational theory of air entrainment devices.
· Compare the operation of oxygen blenders with that of oxygen mixers and adders.
· Describe the physiologic effects of hyperbaric oxygen therapy.
· List the indications and contraindications of nitric oxide therapy.
· Describe the appropriate use of mixed gas (e.g., heliox, carbogen) therapy.

KEY TERMS

adjustable, multiple-orifice flow
  restrictors
adjustable regulators
Boothby-Lovelace-Bulbulian
  (BLB) mask
Bourdon flowmeters
carbogen
fixed-orifice flow restrictors
flow restrictors
French

heliox
high-flow (fixed-performance)
  oxygen delivery system
low-flow (variable-performance)
  oxygen delivery system
monoplace hyperbaric chamber
multiplace hyperbaric chamber
multistage regulators
mustache cannula
non–pressure-compensated

oxygen adder
oxygen blender
pendant cannula
preset regulators
pressure-compensated
pulse-demand oxygen delivery
  system
single-stage regulators
Thorpe tube flowmeters

Administering medical gases is one of the primary responsibilities of respiratory therapists. This responsibility stems from work that began in several eighteenth century physiology laboratories and came to fruition in the clinical settings of the mid–twentieth century. Barcroft, Davies and Gilchrist, Barach, Petty, and others made significant contributions to the theory and practice of oxygen therapy by designing apparatuses to deliver oxygen to dyspneic patients.[1,2] Cogent studies performed by these and other scientists demonstrated the value of oxygen therapy and laid the foundation for respiratory care professions.

As the responsibilities of respiratory therapists continue to grow, all practitioners must understand the principles of oxygen therapy, as well as other forms of medical gas therapy, including nitric oxide and hyperbaric oxygen therapy. Therefore, this chapter reviews the operational principles of devices commonly used to administer medical gases.

REGULATORS AND FLOWMETERS

Regulators (or reducing valves) are devices that reduce high-pressure gases from cylinders or bulk storage units to lower working pressures, usually to 50 psi. Flowmeters are devices that control and indicate the gas flow delivered to patients.

Regulators

Regulators generally are classified as **single-stage** or **multistage.** They can be further divided into preset and **adjustable regulators.** Preset regulators deliver a specific outlet pressure; adjustable regulators can deliver a range of outlet pressures.

Single-Stage Regulators

Figure 3-1 shows the components of a typical preset single-stage regulator, which consists of a body that is divided in half by a flexible metal diaphragm. The area above the diaphragm is a high-pressure chamber. The lower chamber has a spring attached to the lower surface of the diaphragm and is exposed to ambient pressure. A valve stem attached to the upper half of the diaphragm sits on the high-pressure inlet to the upper chamber. Note that excess pressures in the upper chamber can be released through a pressure-relief valve, which opens if the regulator malfunctions and the pressure inside the high-pressure chamber rises to 200 psig.

The gas flow into the high-pressure side of the regulator depends on the effects of two opposing forces: gas pressure above the diaphragm and spring tension below the diaphragm. When the force offered by the high-pressure gas above the diaphragm equals the force offered by spring tension, the diaphragm is straight and the inlet valve is closed. If the force offered by the spring exceeds the force offered by the gas pressure, the spring expands the diaphragm and opens the inlet valve.

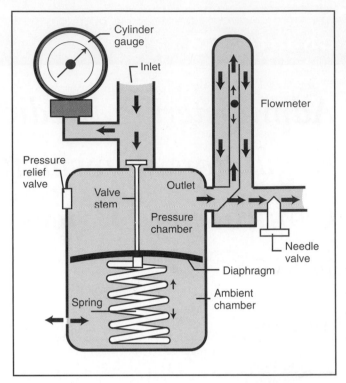

FIGURE 3-1 Components of a single-stage regulator. (Redrawn from Persing G: *Entry level respiratory care review,* Philadelphia, 1992, WB Saunders.)

For a preset single-stage regulator, the spring tension is calibrated to deliver gas at a preset pressure (usually 50 psig). Adjustable regulators, such as the one shown in Figure 3-2, allow the operator to adjust the spring tension (and thus control the outlet pressure) by using a threaded hand control attached to the spring-diaphragm apparatus. Most adjustable regulators can be set to deliver pressures between 0 and 100 psig.

Multistage Regulators

Multistage regulators are simply two or more single-stage regulators in a series. Figure 3-3 is a schematic of a two-stage regulator. Notice that the tension of the spring in the first stage of the regulator is usually preset by the manufacturer, but the spring tension in the second stage typically is adjustable. Each stage of the regulator contains a pressure-relief valve to release excess pressure if a malfunction occurs in either stage. (The number of stages of a regulator can be determined by counting the number of pressure-relief valves on the regulator.)

Multistage regulators operate on the principle that gas pressure is gradually reduced as gas flows from a high-pressure source through a series of stages to the outlet. For example, gas from a compressed cylinder (e.g., 2200 psig) enters the first stage of a two-stage regulator, and the gas pressure is reduced to an intermediate pressure (e.g., 700 psig). This lower pressure gas then enters the second stage of the regulator, where the gas pressure is further reduced to the desired working pressure (e.g., 50 psig) before the gas reaches the outlet.

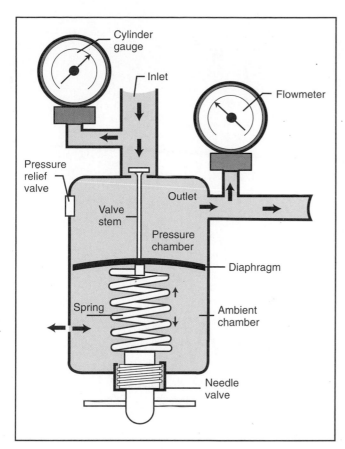

FIGURE 3-2 Components of an adjustable single-stage regulator. (Redrawn from Persing G: *Entry level respiratory care review,* Philadelphia, 1992, WB Saunders.)

Multistage regulators can control gas pressures with more precision than single-stage regulators because the pressure is reduced gradually. Additionally, multistage regulators produce gas flow that is much smoother than that from single-stage regulators. Multistage regulators are more expensive and larger than single-stage regulators, therefore they usually are reserved for tasks requiring precise gas flow (e.g., research purposes).

Flowmeters

As mentioned previously, flowmeters are devices that control and indicate flow. Three types usually are described: **Thorpe tube flowmeters, Bourdon flowmeters,** and **flow restrictors.**

Thorpe Tube Flowmeters

Thorpe tubes are the most common flowmeters used in respiratory care. As Figure 3-4 shows, these devices consist of a tapered, hollow tube engraved with a calibrated scale (usually in L/min), a float, and a needle valve for controlling the flow rate of gas. (Flowmeters used in neonatal and pediatric care may be calibrated in mL/min.) The flow rate of gas delivered is read by locating the float on the calibrated scale. It is important to use the center of the float as the reference point when reading flow rates on the cali-

brated scale. This is particularly evident when trying to adjust flows of 1 to 3 L/min.

The operational principle for these devices can be explained as follows: As gas flows through the unit, it pushes the ball float higher. As the ball float moves higher in the tube, more gas is allowed to travel around it as a result of the gradually increasing diameter of the indicator tube. The height that the ball float is raised depends on the force of gravity pulling down on it and the force of the molecules trying to push it up. The ball float rises until enough molecules can go around it to restore the equilibrium between gravity and the number of molecules hitting the bottom of the ball float.

Back Pressure Compensation. Thorpe tube flowmeters usually are described as **pressure compensated** or **non–pressure compensated.** On pressure-compensated flowmeters (Figure 3-5), the needle valve controlling gas flow out of the flowmeter is located distal to the Thorpe tube. This arrangement allows the pressure in the indicator tube to be maintained at the source gas pressure (i.e., 50 psig). Pressure-compensated flowmeters provide accurate estimates of flow, regardless of the downstream pressure. (Note that pressure-compensated flowmeters indicate actual flow unless the source gas pressure varies, the flowmeter is set to deliver a higher flow than is actually available from its source gas supply, or the float in the tube is not set in a vertical position.[1]) The following example may help illustrate how these devices operate: When a restriction or high-resistance device is attached to a pressure-compensated flowmeter, the pressure gradient between the source gas pressure and the outlet pressure is decreased. The float within the Thorpe tube registers the true gas flow out of the flowmeter, because back pressure created by downstream resistance increases only the pressure distal to the needle valve. It should be apparent, however, that if the back pressure exceeds the source gas pressure (e.g., 50 psig), gas flow stops.

With non–pressure-compensated flowmeters (Figure 3-6), the needle valve is located before the indicator tube. Restriction or high-resistance devices attached to the outlet of a non–pressure-compensated Thorpe tube flowmeter create back pressure, which is transmitted back to the needle valve. Because the needle valve is located proximal to the Thorpe tube, the back pressure causes the float to fall to a level that indicates a flow lower than the actual flow.

Pressure-compensated flowmeters usually are labeled as such on the back of the flowmeter. A flowmeter can also be determined to be pressure compensated if the following test is performed: With the needle valve closed, the flowmeter is plugged into a high-pressure gas source (i.e., bulk storage wall outlet). If the float in the indicator tube jumps and then falls to zero, the flowmeter is pressure compensated. This float movement occurs because the source gas must pass through the indicator tube before it reaches the needle valve.[1]

The most common problem associated with Thorpe tube flowmeters is gas leakage resulting from faulty valve

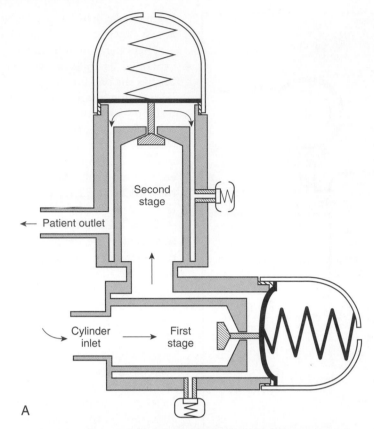

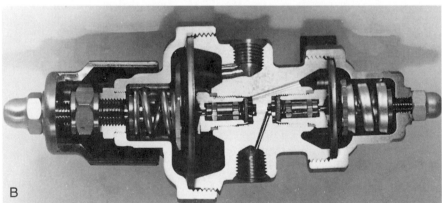

A

B

FIGURE 3-3 A, Multistage reducing valve. A double-stage valve is functionally two single-stage reducing valves in tandem. Gas enters the first stage (first reducing valve), and its pressure is lowered. Gas then enters the second stage (second reducing valve), and the pressure is lowered to the desired working pressure (usually 50 psig). A three-stage reducing valve has one more reducing valve in the series. **B,** National double-stage reducing valve. (Courtesy National Welding Equipment Co., Richmond, Calif.)

seats. This problem usually is detected when the flowmeter is turned off completely but gas can be heard continuing to flow from the flowmeter outlet; these flowmeters should be replaced.

Bourdon Flowmeters

As Figure 3-7 shows, the Bourdon flowmeter is actually a reducing valve that controls the pressure gradient across an outlet with a fixed orifice. The operational principle of this device is simple: as the driving pressure is increased, the flow from the flowmeter outlet increases.

The flow rate of gas can be measured because the Bourdon flowmeter gauge is calibrated in liters per minute. As long as the pressure distal to (i.e., downstream from) the orifice remains atmospheric, the indicated flow is accurate. As resistance to flow increases, the indicated flow reading becomes inaccurate (i.e., these devices are not back pressure compensated). Figure 3-8 shows how increasing resistance at the gas outlet affects the flow reading. Note that although the outlet becomes totally occluded, the flow reading remains constant. Figure 3-9 shows a commonly used Bourdon flowmeter.

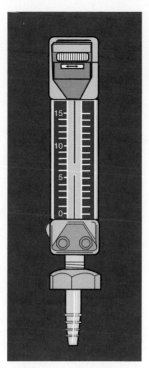

FIGURE 3-4 Thorpe tube flowmeter.

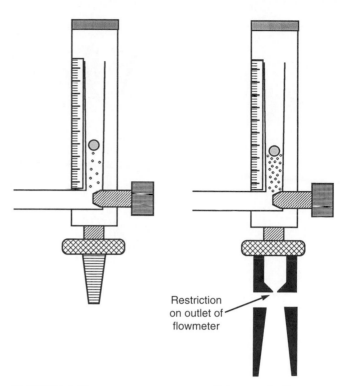

FIGURE 3-6 Non–pressure-compensated Thorpe tube flowmeter.

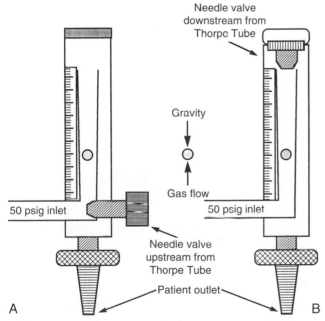

FIGURE 3-5 A, Non–pressure-compensated Thorpe flowmeter. **B,** Pressure-compensated Thorpe flowmeter. The two opposing forces are (1) gravity pulling the float downward and (2) the driving pressure of the gas flow pushing the float upward. When these two forces reach a balance (equilibrium), the float remains stationary, "floating" in the gas column. Because the gas column consists of a tapered tube, as the gas flow increases and the float is displaced upward, greater volumes of gas pass by the float and enter the patient outlet. Needle valve placement determines whether the device is back pressure compensated.

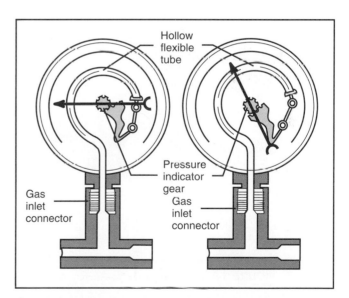

FIGURE 3-7 Schematic of a Bourdon flowmeter. (Redrawn from Ward JJ: Equipment for mixed gas and oxygen therapy. In Barnes TA, editor: *Core textbook of respiratory care practice,* ed 2, St Louis, 1994, Mosby.)

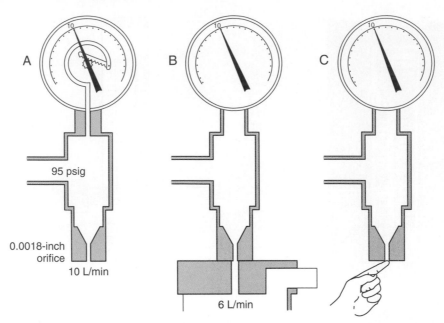

FIGURE 3-8 A, Bourdon gauge operating under normal conditions. The actual flow delivered equals the flow registered on the flowmeter. **B,** The effect when resistance is added downstream of the flowmeter at the outlet. Notice that the flow registered on the flowmeter is higher than the actual flow. **C,** Complete occlusion of the outlet has a similar effect; that is, the flow registered on the flowmeter is erroneously high. (Courtesy Nellcor Puritan Bennett, Pleasanton, Calif.)

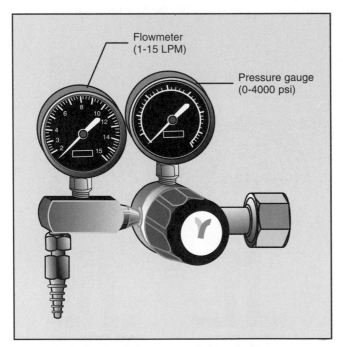

FIGURE 3-9 Bourdon gauge flowmeter.

Flow Restrictors

Flow restrictors operate on the same principle as Bourdon flowmeters (i.e., the gas flow through these devices can be increased by raising the driving pressure across a fixed resistance). Like Bourdon flowmeters, flow rate readings are inaccurate when resistance increases downstream from the gas outlet. The two types of flow restrictors are **fixed-orifice** and **adjustable, multiple-orifice** models (albeit fixed-orifice devices are no longer manufactured). The adjustable, multiple-orifice flow restrictor uses a series of calibrated openings in a disk that can be adjusted to deliver different flows. As with the fixed-orifice flow restrictor, the operating pressure is crucial to the accuracy of the device. Figure 3-10 shows an example of a variable-orifice flow restrictor.

For these devices to function properly, it is essential that the appropriate operating pressure be used. Some of the devices are designed for use with hospital gas sources (i.e., 50-psi gas sources), and others are designed to work on portable liquid oxygen equipment used in the home care setting (i.e., 20-psi gas source).

DEVICES FOR ADMINISTERING MEDICAL GASES

Oxygen Therapy

The goal of oxygen therapy is to treat or prevent hypoxemia. Many different devices can be used to achieve this goal in spontaneously breathing patients. It is important that respiratory therapists understand how to select and assemble these devices and ensure that they are working properly. The American Association for Respiratory Care has developed clinical practice guidelines for oxygen administration in acute care facilities, alternative site health care (e.g., extended care) facilities, and the home setting.[3-5] These guidelines inform practitioners of indications, contraindications, precautions, and possible complications of oxygen therapy. Each guideline lists the devices that can be used to administer oxygen to spontaneously breathing patients,

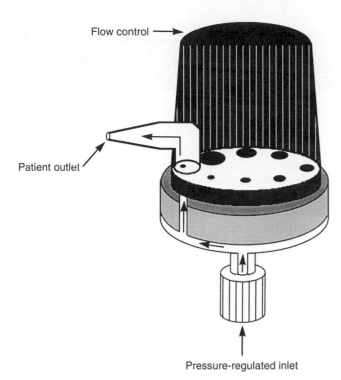

Flow control →

Patient outlet

Pressure-regulated inlet

FIGURE 3-10 Schematic of a variable-orifice flow restrictor. These devices use a series of calibrated ports to deliver a set flow at a designated pressure. Per the requirements of the National Fire Protection Agency (NFPA), the delivery pressure is included on the restrictor label.

along with a brief description of criteria that should be used to assess the need for and the outcome of oxygen therapy. These guidelines should be reviewed and used as a resource in the treatment of patients who require oxygen therapy. Clinical Practice Guidelines 3-1 and 3-2 summarize guidelines for oxygen therapy for adults in acute care and alternative site health care facilities. Clinical Practice Guideline 3-3 summarizes the guidelines for oxygen therapy for neonatal and pediatric patients.

Low-Flow versus High-Flow Devices

Oxygen therapy systems generally are classified as **low-flow (variable performance)** and **high-flow (fixed performance)** devices.[4,5] The terms *low flow* and *variable performance* are used because these devices supply oxygen at flow rates that are lower than a patient's inspiratory demands; therefore, varying amounts of room air must be added to provide part of the inspired volume. Low-flow devices deliver fractional inspired oxygen (F_IO_2) levels that can vary from 0.22 to approximately 0.8, depending on the patient's inspiratory flow and tidal volume and the oxygen flow used. Nasal cannulas and catheters (Historical Note 3-1), transtracheal catheters, simple oxygen masks, partial rebreathing reservoir masks, and nonrebreathing reservoir masks are examples of low-flow oxygen therapy devices.

High-flow, or fixed performance, devices provide oxygen at flow rates high enough to completely satisfy a patient's inspiratory demands. Such devices supply the inspiratory demands of the patient either by entraining fixed quanti-

ties of ambient air or by using high-flow rates and reservoirs. The most important characteristic of high-flow devices is that they can deliver fixed F_IO_2 levels (i.e., from 0.24 to 1), regardless of the patient's breathing pattern. Air entrainment masks, incubators, oxygen tents, and oxygen hoods are high-flow systems. High-volume aerosol devices and humidifiers that are used to provide continuous humidification through face masks and tracheostomy collars incorporate air entrainment devices and thus can also be considered high-flow oxygen therapy devices.

A common misconception is that low-flow systems can deliver only a low F_IO_2 and high-flow systems can deliver only a high F_IO_2. As will be seen, both low- and high-flow systems can deliver a wide range of F_IO_2 levels. Do not confuse the terms *low-flow* and *high-flow* with the terms *low F_IO_2* and *high F_IO_2*.

Low-Flow Devices
Nasal Cannulas
Nasal cannulas (Figure 3-11) are used extensively to treat spontaneously breathing, hypoxemic patients in emergency departments, in general and critical care units, during exercise in cardiopulmonary rehabilitation, and for long-term oxygen therapy in the home care setting.[2,6] The standard nasal cannula is a blind-ended, soft plastic tube with two prongs that fit into the patient's external nares. The prongs are approximately 1/2-inch long and can be straight or curved. The cannula is held in place either with an elastic band that fits over the ears and around the head or with two small-diameter pieces of tubing that fit over the ears and can be tightened with a bolo tie–type device that fits under the chin. Cannulas are available in infant, child, and adult sizes.

The most common problems with nasal cannulas are related to (1) nasopharyngeal-mucosal irritation, (2) twisting of the connective tubing between the patient and the oxygen flowmeter, and (3) skin irritation at pressure points where the tubing holding the cannula in place touches the patient's face and ears. Irritation of the nasal mucosa and the paranasal sinuses occurs most often when high-flow rates of oxygen are used. The problem appears to be greater with nasal cannulas that use straight rather than curved prongs. With straight prongs, oxygen flow is directed toward the superior aspects of the nasal cavity, which promotes turbulent flow; with curved prongs, oxygen entering the nose is directed across the nasal turbinate, thus enhancing laminar flow as the gas flows through the nasal cavity. Twisting of connective tubing is an insidious problem that is difficult to prevent. Avoiding excessive lengths of connective tubing and periodically checking for patency appear to be the most reliable means of dealing with this problem. The problems of skin irritation and pressure point soreness can be minimized by placing cotton gauze padding between the tubing and the patient's face and ears.

For adult patients, nasal cannulas theoretically can produce F_IO_2 levels of 0.24 to 0.44 at oxygen flow rates of 1 to 6 L/min. Oxygen flows higher than 6 L/min delivered

Oxygen Therapy for Adults in the Acute Care Facility—2002 Revision and Update

Clinical Practice Guideline 3-1

■ DEFINITION/DESCRIPTION

Oxygen therapy is the administration of oxygen at concentrations greater than ambient air with the intent of treating or preventing the symptoms and manifestations of hypoxia. The procedure addressed is the administration of oxygen therapy in the acute care facility other than with mechanical ventilators and hyperbaric chambers.

■ INDICATIONS

· Documented hypoxemia. Defined as a decreased PaO_2 in the blood below normal range (i.e., $PaO_2 <$ 60 mm Hg or $SaO_2 < 90\%$ in patients breathing room air, or with a PaO_2 or SaO_2 below desirable range for the specific clinical situation.
· An acute situation in which hypoxemia is suspected; substantiation of hypoxemia is required within an appropriate period after initiation of therapy.
· Severe trauma.
· Acute myocardial infarction.
· Short-term therapy (postanesthesia) or surgical intervention.

■ PRECAUTIONS AND/OR COMPLICATIONS

· With a $PaO_2 \geq 60$ mm Hg, ventilatory depression may occur in spontaneously breathing patients with a chronically elevated $PaCO_2$.
· With an $F_IO_2 \geq 0.50$, absorption atelectasis, oxygen toxicity, and/or depression of ciliary and/or leukocyte function may occur.
· Bacterial contamination associated with certain nebulization and humidification systems is a possible hazard.
· Oxygen should be administered with caution to patients suffering from paraquat poisoning and those receiving bleomycin.
· During laser bronchoscopy, minimal levels of supplemental oxygen should be used to avoid intratracheal ignition.

■ LIMITATIONS

· Oxygen therapy has only limited benefit for the treatment of hypoxia resulting from anemia and may be of limited benefit with circulatory disturbances.
· Oxygen therapy should not be used in lieu of, but in addition to, mechanical ventilation when ventilatory support is indicated.

■ MONITORING

· Patient monitoring should include clinical assessment along with oxygen tension or saturation measurements. This should be done at the following times: when therapy is initiated; within 12 hours of initiation of therapy for F_IO_2 levels < 0.40; within 8 hours for F_IO_2 levels ≥ 0.40; within 72 hours of an acute myocardial infarction; within 2 hours for patients diagnosed with chronic obstructive pulmonary disease (COPD).
· All oxygen delivery systems should be checked at least once per day. More frequent checks with calibrated analyzers are indicated for systems susceptible to variations in the F_IO_2.

Modified from the American Association for Respiratory Care: Clinical practice guideline: oxygen therapy for adults in the acute care facility—2002 revision and update, Respir Care 47:717, 2002.

with a traditional nasal cannula system do not produce a significantly higher F_IO_2 and are poorly tolerated by patients because they cause nasal bleeding and drying of the nasal mucosa. For neonates, oxygen flows of 0.25 to 2 L/min can produce F_IO_2 levels of 0.35 to 0.7.[5,6] Keep in mind that the actual F_IO_2 delivered is influenced by the patient's tidal volume and respiratory rate and whether breathing is occurring predominantly through the nose or the mouth.

Table 3-1 lists the approximate F_IO_2 levels delivered by flow rates of 1 to 6 L/min to an adult patient. Generally,

the F_IO_2 increases by about 4% for each liter of flow increase. A problem-solving exercise for calculating the approximate F_IO_2 when using a variable-performance device such as a nasal cannula is provided in Clinical Rounds 3-1. It should be emphasized that this is simply an estimate and that the actual delivered F_IO_2 for any given oxygen flow rate may be significantly different.[2] In a clinical setting, adjusting the flow rate of oxygen delivered to the patient is generally an empirical process (i.e., it is adjusted according to the patient's oxygen needs). This empiric approach should be based on observations of the patient's breathing pattern

Oxygen Therapy in the Home or Alternative Site Health Care Facility—2007 Revision and Update

Clinical Practice Guideline 3-2

■ SETTING

This guideline is confined to oxygen administration in the home or in an alternative site health care facility (i.e., skilled nursing facility, extended care facility).

■ INDICATIONS: DOCUMENTED HYPOXEMIA

· In adults, children, and infants older than 28 days: As evidenced by a $PaO_2 \leq 55$ mm Hg or an $SaO_2 \leq 88\%$ in patients breathing room air, or a PaO_2 of 56 to 59 mm Hg or an SaO_2 or $SpO_2 \leq 89\%$ in association with specific clinical conditions (e.g., cor pulmonale, congestive heart failure, or erythrocythemia with a hematocrit > 56%).

· Some patients may not demonstrate a need for oxygen therapy at rest but become hypoxemic during ambulation, sleep, or exercise. Oxygen therapy is indicated during these specific activities when the SaO_2 is shown to fall to $\leq 88\%$.

■ PRECAUTIONS AND COMPLICATIONS

Precautions and complications are the same as those cited for oxygen therapy in the acute care setting.

■ RESOURCES

· Low-flow oxygen devices, such as nasal cannulas, transtracheal oxygen catheters, pulse-dose oxygen delivery devices, demand oxygen delivery systems, oxygen reservoir cannulas.

· High flow oxygen devices, such as tracheostomy collars and T-tube adapters that are associated with high-flow supplemental oxygen systems.

· Oxygen supply systems, including oxygen concentrators, liquid oxygen systems, and compressed gas cylinders.

■ MONITORING

· Initial and ongoing clinical assessment of the patient should be performed by a licensed and/or credentialed respiratory therapist or other professional functioning within the scope of practice required by the state standards under which the professional is licensed.

· Baseline oxygen tension and/or saturation levels must be measured before oxygen therapy is started; these measurements should be repeated when clinically indicated or to follow the course of the disease as determined by the attending physician.

· SpO_2 should be measured to determine the appropriate oxygen flow and pulse-dose or demand oxygen delivery settings for sleep, exercise, or ambulation.

· Oxygen therapy should be administered in accordance with the physician's prescription.

■ INFECTION CONTROL

Normally, low-flow oxygen systems without humidifiers do not present a clinically important risk of infection and need not be routinely replaced. High-flow systems that use heated humidifiers or aerosol generators, especially when applied to patients with artificial airways, should be cleaned and disinfected on a regular basis.

Modified from the American Association for Respiratory Care: Clinical practice guideline: oxygen therapy in the home or alternative site health care facility—2007 revision and update, **Respir Care 52:1063, 2007.**

and level of comfort, as well as pulse oximetry or arterial blood gas data, if available.

A relatively new approach for delivering a high F_IO_2 (>0.6) via nasal cannula has been introduced by Salter Labs (Arivin, California) and Vapotherm (Annapolis, Maryland).[7] The Salter Labs high-flow system can provide nonheated, humidified oxygen at flows up to 15 L/min (F_IO_2 > 0.6) and a relative humidity of 72% to 78%. The Vapotherm 2000i system can deliver heated and humidified oxygen (relative humidity of 99%) at flows of 5 to 40 L/min and an F_IO_2 greater than 0.9.

CLINICAL ROUNDS 3-1

A Simple Method for Estimating the Theoretical F_IO_2

A 150-pound, spontaneously breathing patient is receiving oxygen at the rate of 6 L/min through a nasal cannula. The patient's tidal volume is 500 mL, and the respiratory rate is 20 breaths per minute (inspiratory time = 1 second; expiratory time = 2 seconds). Estimate the theoretical F_IO_2.

See Evolve Resources for the answer.

Selection of an Oxygen Delivery Device for Neonatal and Pediatric Patients—2002 Revision and Update

Clinical Practice Guideline 3-3

■ **DEFINITION/DESCRIPTION**

The administration of supplemental oxygen to neonatal and pediatric patients requires the selection of an oxygen delivery system that suits the patient's size and needs and the therapeutic goals.

■ **INDICATIONS**

· Documented hypoxemia.
· An acute situation in which hypoxemia is suspected or in which suspected regional hypoxia may respond to an increase in PaO_2. Verification of the PaO_2 level is required within an appropriate period after initiation of therapy.

■ **CONTRAINDICATIONS**

· No specific contraindications exist to the delivery of oxygen when indications are judged to be present.
· Nasal cannulas and nasopharyngeal catheters are contraindicated in patients with nasal obstruction (e.g., nasal polyps, choanal atresia).
· Nasopharyngeal catheters are contraindicated in patients with maxillofacial trauma and in those with or suspected of having a basal skull fracture or coagulation problems.
· It is the expert opinion of the Clinical Practice Guideline Steering Committee (2002) that nasopharyngeal catheters are not appropriate for oxygen administration in the neonatal population.

■ **HAZARDS/PRECAUTIONS/POSSIBLE COMPLICATIONS**

· The etiology of retinopathy of prematurity, especially the role of oxygen, is controversial. Care should be taken when supplemental oxygen is provided to preterm infants (<37 weeks' gestation). It is suggested that oxygen supplementation should not result in a $PaO_2 > 80$ mm Hg.
· Administration of supplemental oxygen to patients with certain congenital heart lesions (e.g., hypoplastic left heart, single ventricle) may cause an increase in alveolar oxygen tension and compromise the balance between pulmonary and systemic blood flow.
· Administration of supplemental oxygen to patients suffering from paraquat poisoning or to patients receiving certain chemotherapeutic agents (e.g., bleomycin) may result in pulmonary complications (e.g., oxygen toxicity and pulmonary fibrosis).
· Stimulation of the superior laryngeal nerves in an infant may cause alterations in the respiratory pattern if the gas flow from the oxygen source is cool and is directed at the infant's face.
· Inappropriate selection of the fractional delivered oxygen concentration (F_DO_2) or oxygen flow may result in hypoxemia or hyperoxemia.
· Skin irritation can result from material used to secure the cannula or from local allergic reaction to polyvinyl chloride. Improper sizing can lead to nasal obstruction or irritation.
· Displacement can lead to loss of oxygen delivery.
· Inadvertent continuous positive airway pressure (CPAP) may be administered, depending on the size of the nasal cannula, the gas flow, and the infant's anatomy.
· Irritation can result if flows are excessive; improper insertion can cause gagging and nasal or pharyngeal trauma; improper sizing can lead to nasal obstruction or irritation.
· Excessive secretions and/or mucosal inflammation can result.
· Skin irritation may result from material used to secure the cannula and/or from local allergic reaction to polyvinyl chloride.
· Excessive flow may cause gastric distention.
· Transtracheal catheters may be associated with an increase risk of infection compared to nasal cannulas and catheters.
· Aspiration of vomitus may be more likely with oxygen masks. Rebreathing of CO_2 may occur if the total O_2 flow to the mask is inadequate.
· It is the expert opinion of the Clinical Practice Guideline Steering Committee (2002) that partial rebreathers or nonrebreathers are not appropriate for the neonatal population.

Selection of an Oxygen Delivery Device for Neonatal and Pediatric Patients—2002 Revision and Update—cont'd

■ LIMITATIONS

· *Nasal cannulas:* Changes in minute ventilation and inspiratory flow affect air entrainment and result in fluctuations in F_IO_2. Prongs are difficult to keep in position, particularly with small infants. The effect of mouth versus nose breathing on the F_IO_2 remains controversial. Use may be limited by the presence of excessive mucus drainage, mucosal edema, or a deviated septum. Maximum flow should be limited to 2 L/min in infants and newborns. Care should be taken to keep the cannula tubing and straps away from the neck to prevent airway obstruction in infants. Discrepancies between the set and the delivered flow can occur in the same flowmeter at different settings and among different flowmeters. Discrepancies in flow and oxygen concentration between set and delivered values can occur in low-flow blenders at flows below the recommended range of the blender.

· *Nasopharyngeal catheters:* This method is less commonly used because of the complexity of care. The F_IO_2 is difficult to control and measure. The effect of mouth versus nose breathing on the F_IO_2 remains controversial. Use may be limited by excessive mucus drainage, mucosal edema, or the presence of a deviated septum. The catheter should be cleared frequently to prevent occlusion of the distal holes. Patients should be observed for evidence of catheter occlusion, and the catheter should be alternated between nares every 8 to 12 hours and changed daily. Catheter sizes smaller than 8 F are less effective in oxygen delivery. Lower oxygen concentrations are delivered if the catheter is placed in the nose rather than in the pharynx. Low-flow flowmeters (<3 L/min) should be used. Discrepancies between the set and the delivered flow can occur in the same flowmeter at different settings and among different flowmeters. Discrepancies in flow and oxygen concentration between the set and delivered values can occur in low-flow blenders at flows below those recommended by the manufacturer.

· *Transtracheal catheters:* This method is less commonly used because of the complexity of care. Frequent medical monitoring is required, and replacement catheters are costly. Increased time is needed for candidate evaluation and teaching.

· *Masks:* Masks provide a variable F_IO_2, depending on the inspiratory flow and the construction of the mask's reservoir. Masks are not recommended when precise concentrations are required. Also, they are confining and may not be well tolerated; they interfere with feeding; they may not be available in sizes appropriate for all patients; and they require a minimum flow, per the manufacturer's instructions, to prevent possible rebreathing of CO_2. The maximum F_IO_2 attainable with a simple nonrebreathing or partial rebreathing mask in neonates, infants, and children has not been well documented. The performance of air entrainment masks may be altered by resistance to flow distal to the restricted orifice (resulting in a higher F_DO_2 and a lower total flow delivered). The total flow from air entrainment masks at settings greater than 0.40 may not equal or may exceed the patient's inspiratory flow. Performance is altered if the entrainment ports are blocked.

· *Hoods:* O_2 concentrations may vary within the hood. O_2 concentrations should be measured as near the nose and mouth as possible. Opening of any enclosure reduces the O_2 concentration. For infants and children confined to hoods, nasal O_2 may need to be supplied during feeding and nursing care. Flows greater than 7 L/min are required to wash out CO_2. Devices can be confining and isolating. Concentration in a hood can be varied from 0.21 to 1.0. The temperature of the gases in the hood should be maintained to provide a neutral thermal environment. High gas flows may produce harmful noise levels.

■ ASSESSMENT OF NEED

Need is determined by measurement of inadequate oxygen tensions and saturations by invasive or noninvasive methods and/or the presence of clinical indicators as previously described. Supplemental oxygen flow should be titrated to maintain adequate oxygen saturation as indicated by pulse oximetry SpO_2 or appropriate arterial or venous blood gas values.

■ MONITORING

· Clinical assessment should include but should not be limited to cardiac, pulmonary, and neurologic status and apparent work of breathing; noninvasive or invasive measurement of oxygen tensions or saturation should be performed within 1 hour of initiation of therapy in any neonate treated with oxygen.

· All oxygen delivery systems should be checked at least once each day. More frequent checks by calibrated analyzer are necessary in systems susceptible to variation in oxygen concentration or that are applied to patients with artificial airways. Continuous analysis is recommended in hoods. Oxygen should be analyzed as close as possible to the infant's face.

· All heated delivery systems should be monitored continuously for temperature.

Modified from the American Association for Respiratory Care: Clinical practice guideline: selection of an oxygen delivery device for neonatal and pediatric patients—2002 revision and update, Respir Care 47:707, 2002.

HISTORICAL NOTE 3-1

Nasal Catheters

Nasal catheters were introduced by Lane in 1907.[1,6] It is important to recognize that although these devices are still available, they are used infrequently. Nasal catheters consist of a hollow, soft plastic tube that contains a blind distal tip with a series of holes. They are available in 8 to 10 French (F) for children and 12 to 14 F for adults.

Note that the term **French** is a method of sizing catheters according to the outside diameter (OD). Each unit in the French scale is approximately 0.33 mm; a 10 F tube, therefore, has an outside diameter of 3.3 mm.

The catheter can be placed with relative ease and minimal patient discomfort if done properly. First, it should be coated with a water-soluble lubricant and its patency should be checked (by observing whether oxygen flows through it unobstructed). Once the patency has been confirmed, the catheter is inserted into an external naris and advanced along the floor of the nasal cavity until it can be seen at the back of the patient's oropharynx. It should then be positioned just behind the uvula. For blind insertion, the distance the catheter must be inserted can be estimated by measuring the distance from the tip of the patient's nose to the earlobe; this length can then be marked on the catheter with a small piece of surgical tape. The catheter can be held in place by taping it to the nose.

Nasal catheters can deliver an F_IO_2 of approximately 0.22 to 0.35 when the oxygen flow is set at 2 to 5 L/min. A higher F_IO_2 can be obtained by increasing the oxygen flow to the patient. Notice that the actual F_IO_2 varies considerably, depending on the patient's tidal volume and respiratory rate and whether respiration occurs primarily through the nose or the mouth.

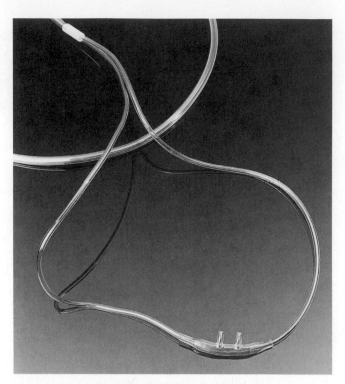

FIGURE 3-11 Nasal cannula.

TABLE 3-1

Guidelines for Estimating F_IO_2 with Low-Flow Oxygen Delivery Systems

100% Oxygen Flow Rate (L/min)	F_IO_2
Nasal Cannula or Catheter	
1	0.24
2	0.28
3	0.32
4	0.36
5	0.40
6	0.44
Oxygen Mask	
5-6	0.40
6-7	0.50
7-8	0.60
Mask with Reservoir Bag	
6	0.60
7	0.70
8	0.80
9	0.80+
10	0.80+

F_IO_2, Fractional inspired oxygen.
From Shapiro BA, Peruzzi WT, Templin R, et al: *Clinical application of blood gases,* ed 5, St Louis, 1994, Mosby.

Figure 3-12 shows the components of the Vapotherm 2000i system. The core of the system uses a *vapor transfer cartridge,* which allows water vapor to be added to the oxygen flow via a semipermeable membrane. The manufacturer reports that the pores of the membrane are less than 0.1 μm in diameter and thus are small enough to prevent the transfer of bacteria into the gas stream.

Oxygen-Conserving Devices. Transtracheal oxygen (TTO) catheters, reservoir cannulas, and **pulse-demand oxygen delivery systems** are recent developments that have significantly improved the delivery of oxygen therapy, especially with regard to conserving oxygen supplies during long-term oxygen therapy.

Transtracheal Catheters. The concept of TTO therapy was first described by Heimlich in 1982.[8] The guiding principle for such oxygen therapy is that oxygen delivered directly into the trachea should provide the patient with adequate oxygen while reducing the amount of oxygen used; that is, direct delivery of oxygen into the trachea reduces dilution with room air on inspiration because the upper airways (the anatomic reservoir) are filled with oxygen. Consequently, lower oxygen flows from the source gas (e.g., 0.25 to 2 L/min) are required to achieve a desired level of oxygenation. Indeed, TTO catheters can produce overall oxygen savings of 54% to 59%.[1]

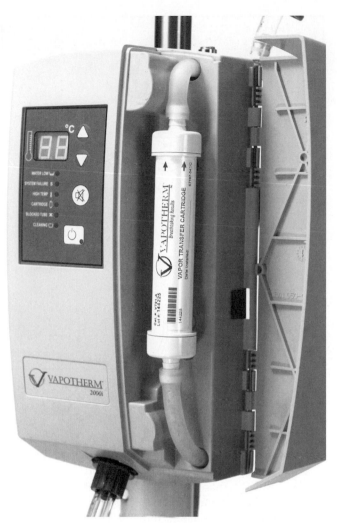

FIGURE 3-12 A, Vapotherm vapor transfer cartridge. **B,** Frontal view of the Vapotherm 2000i. (Courtesy Vapotherm, Annapolis, Md.)

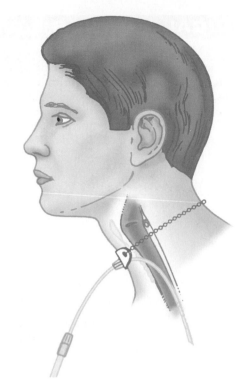

FIGURE 3-13 Transtracheal catheter. (From Wilkins RL, Stoller JK, Kacmarek RM: *Egan's fundamentals of respiratory care,* ed 9, St Louis, 2009, Mosby.)

Catheter placement requires minor surgery. A small, plastic stent is inserted into the patient's trachea between the second and third tracheal rings.[1,9] The stent remains in place for about a week to ensure that a permanent tract is formed between the trachea and the outer skin. Removal of the stent is accomplished over a guide wire. After the stent is removed, a 9 F Teflon catheter is inserted into the tract over the guide wire. The catheter is held in place with a neck chain to prevent inadvertent dislodgment or removal (Figure 3-13). It is recommended that catheters be replaced at 90 days or sooner, before they become cracked, kinked, or occluded by pus or mucus.[1,9,10] Patients must be taught the proper care of these devices to prevent complications. Routine care should include cleaning, lavage, and use of a cleaning rod to remove mucus that can occlude the lumen of the catheter.[9,10]

As previously stated, transtracheal catheters reduce oxygen costs by requiring lower oxygen flows to prevent hypoxemia. Therefore, patients can purchase smaller, lighter cylinders or reservoirs for greater convenience. The use of special low-flow regulators or flow restrictors may also lead to greater cost savings.[1,10] Other important advantages of transtracheal catheters include improved patient compliance with oxygen therapy because of cosmetic appearance (these devices are relatively inconspicuous), increased patient mobility, and the avoidance of nasal irritation associated with the use of nasal cannulas. Finally, it should be mentioned that TTO devices use standard oxygen therapy equipment; this is important because if a problem arises with the catheter, emergency equipment (e.g., a conventional nasal cannula) can easily be set up and used by the patient.

The primary disadvantage of transtracheal catheters is complications associated with minor surgery (i.e., hemoptysis, infection, and subcutaneous emphysema).[9,10] Mucous obstruction and occlusion of the distal end of the tube can also cause complications; however, these can be minimized with proper care, including saline instillation and periodic clearing of the catheter lumen with a guide wire or cleaning rod. Clinical Rounds 3-2 presents a common example of how TTO can increase patient compliance with oxygen therapy.

Reservoir Cannulas. Two commercially available reservoir cannulas are the **mustache cannula** (Figure 3-14) and the **pendant cannula** (Figure 3-15). The mustache cannula can hold about 20 mL of gas. During the early part of exhalation, gas derived from the patient's dead space inflates the reservoir. As exhalation continues, oxygen from the source gas (e.g., 100% oxygen from a 50-psi source)

CLINICAL ROUNDS 3-2

A home care patient who requires continuous oxygen therapy is instructed to use a nasal cannula at a flow of 2 L/min. After a short period, the patient is admitted to the hospital with signs of hypoxemia. When asked if he had been using the prescribed oxygen, the patient explains that he used it only intermittently because it was uncomfortable, and furthermore he felt self-conscious about wearing the equipment in public. What would you suggest to help this patient overcome the problems he described?

See Evolve Resources for the answer.

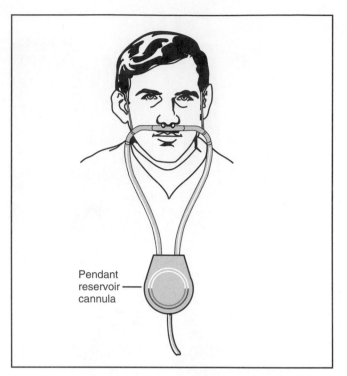

FIGURE 3-15 Pendant reservoir cannula.

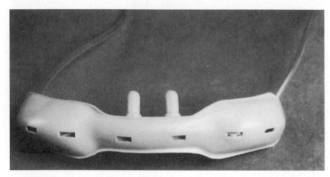

FIGURE 3-14 Mustache reservoir cannula. (Courtesy Chad Therapeutics, Chatsworth, Calif.)

flows into the lateral aspects of the cannula, forcing the dead space gas medial and out of the nasal prongs and filling the reservoir with 100% oxygen. On inspiration, the initial part of the inhaled gas entering the patient's airway is drawn from this reservoir. As the reservoir collapses, the device functions like a conventional nasal cannula. Thus the reservoir adds 20 mL of 100% oxygen as a bolus in addition to the continuous oxygen flow from the supply source. The added bolus of gas reduces the amount of oxygen that must be derived from the continuous flow source to achieve a desired F_IO_2.

Pendant cannulas operate in a similar manner, except that the reservoir is attached with connective tubing that serves as a conduit to a pendant that hangs below the chin. The added tubing between the reservoir and the pendant increases the amount of gas that can be stored, therefore these types of devices can hold nearly 40 mL of 100% oxygen. As with mustache cannulas, the main advantage of these devices is their ability to conserve gas flow.

Mustache and pendant cannulas can significantly reduce oxygen supply use compared with continuous flow nasal cannulas. Studies indicate that mustache and pendant systems may reduce oxygen supply use by 50%,[11] although the cost of reservoir cannulas is higher than that of standard nasal cannulas. Also, many patients feel that mustache cannulas are heavier, larger, and more obvious

than conventional nasal cannulas. Pendant cannulas, however, can be concealed by the patient's clothing.

Pulse-Demand Oxygen Delivery Systems. As the name implies, pulse-demand oxygen delivery systems deliver oxygen to the patient on demand; that is, they provide oxygen only during inspiration. Electronic, fluidic, and combined electronic-fluidic sensors are used to control gas delivery to the patient. Demand systems can operate with nasal catheters, nasal cannulas, and transtracheal catheters.[11,12] Figure 3-16 is a schematic of a demand system for a nasal cannula.[1] With this type of system, oxygen is delivered to the patient only after a sufficient inspiratory effort is made (i.e., <–1 cm H_2O). After it is activated, the demand valve opens, delivering oxygen at a preset flow rate; it closes during exhalation to conserve oxygen. Because the demand valve connects directly to the oxygen source (50 psig), it replaces the flowmeter used with continuous flow cannulas. Note that demand systems can function as pulsed or continuous flow sources of oxygen. Settings allow the operator to select the equivalent of 1 to 5 L/min of oxygen flow from a conventional flowmeter. Shigeoka and Bonnekat[12] calculated that a patient receives about 17 mL of oxygen at the 1 L/min setting, 35 ml at the 2 L/min setting, 51 mL at the 3 L/min setting, and so on. It should be pointed out that oxygen delivered from these devices is not humidified, because the system is delivering small pulses of oxygen. Humidification is not necessary because drying of the mucous membranes, as might occur with continuous flow delivery systems, does not occur with these devices.

A common problem with demand devices is improper placement of the sensor; this can result in interference with

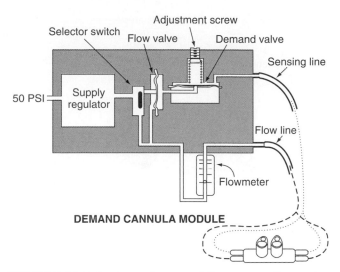

FIGURE 3-16 Pulse-demand oxygen delivery system for nasal cannula. (Redrawn from Barnes TA: *Core textbook of respiratory care practice,* ed 2, St Louis, 1994, Mosby.)

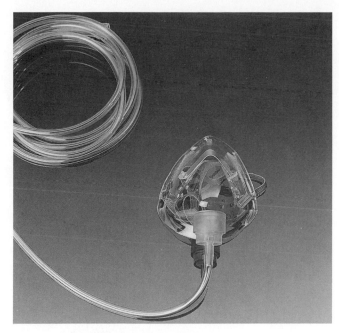

FIGURE 3-17 Simple oxygen mask.

detection of an inspiratory effort, malfunction of the demand (solenoid) valve, and inadequate inspiratory flows. Improper placement of the sensor and malfunction of the demand valve usually can be detected by careful observation of the patient during the initial set-up. Determining the adequacy of inspiratory flow requires feedback from the patient, either through verbal comments or oximetric analysis.

Simple Oxygen Mask. Although modern oxygen masks are made of different materials from those used in earlier masks, their overall design has hardly changed since their introduction in the late eighteenth century.[6] Modern oxygen masks, such as the one shown in Figure 3-17, are cone-shaped devices that fit over the patient's nose and mouth and are held in place with an elastic band that fits around the patient's head. During inspiration, the patient draws gases both from oxygen flowing into the mask through small-bore tubing connected to the base of the mask and from room air via ports on the sides of the mask. These ports also serve as exhalation ports. A typical adult oxygen mask has a volume of approximately 100 to 200 mL and may be thought of as an extension of the anatomic reservoir, because the patient inhales its contents during the early part of inspiration. As such, simple oxygen masks can deliver higher F_IO_2 levels than nasal cannulas because of a "reservoir effect." Note that the oxygen flow into the mask must be sufficient to wash out exhaled carbon dioxide, which can accumulate in this potential reservoir.

Generally, simple oxygen masks can deliver an F_IO_2 of 35% to 50% at oxygen flows of 5 to 10 L/min. The F_IO_2 actually delivered to the patient depends on the flow of oxygen to the mask, the size of the mask, and the patient's breathing pattern (see Table 3-1 for a list of approximate F_IO_2 levels for flows of 5 to 8 L/min). Simple oxygen masks are reliable and easy to set up. Disposable plastic masks are available in infant, child, and adult sizes. They are ideal for delivering oxygen during minor surgical procedures and emergency situations.

However, the use of oxygen masks has several disadvantages. For example, the delivered F_IO_2 can vary significantly, which limits the use of these devices for patients who require well-defined inspired oxygen concentrations. Carbon dioxide rebreathing can occur if the oxygen flow to the mask is not sufficient to wash out the patient's exhaled gases. For this reason, it generally is recommended that the minimum flow set on an oxygen mask should be 5 L/min. Oxygen masks are confining and may not be well tolerated by some patients. Furthermore, they must be removed during eating, drinking, and facial and airway care. Patients often complain that oxygen masks cause skin irritation, especially when they are tightly fitted. Finally, aspiration of vomitus may be more likely when the mask is in place.

Partial Rebreathing Masks. The partial rebreathing mask is derived from the **Boothby-Lovelace-Bulbulian (BLB) mask,** which was introduced by Boothby and associates in 1940.[13] As Figure 3-18 shows, the partial rebreathing mask consists of a facepiece, which is similar to the simple oxygen mask described previously, and a reservoir bag that is attached to the base of the mask. In a typical adult partial rebreathing mask, the reservoir bag has a volume capacity of about 300 to 500 mL. Gas flow from the oxygen source is directed into mask and the reservoir via small-bore tubing that connects at the junction of the mask and bag.

The operational theory of these devices is fairly straightforward. When the patient inhales, gas is drawn from the bag, the source gas flowing into the mask, and potentially from the room air through the exhalation ports. As the patient exhales, the first third of the exhaled gas fills the

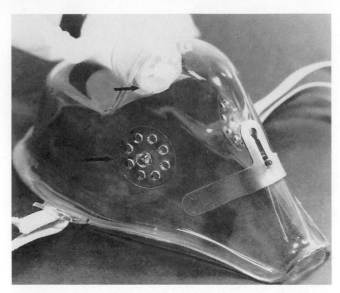

FIGURE 3-18 Partial rebreathing mask. (From Gilmore TJ, Shoup CA: *Laboratory exercises in respiratory care*, ed 3, St Louis, 1988, Mosby.)

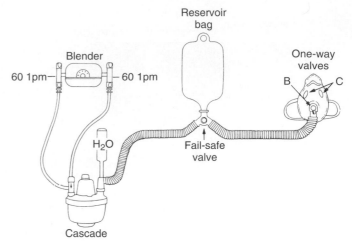

FIGURE 3-19 Nonrebreathing mask. (From Foust GN et al: *Chest* 99:1346, 1991.)

reservoir bag, and the last two thirds of the exhaled gas are vented through the exhalation ports. Notice that the volume that fills the reservoir bag is roughly equivalent to the volume of the patient's anatomic dead space volume. Because the volume that fills the reservoir bag represents gas that has not participated in gas exchange, it has a high partial pressure of oxygen (PO_2) and a low partial pressure of carbon dioxide (PCO_2). The patient inhales this gas mixture during the next breath.

Partial rebreathing masks can deliver an F_IO_2 of 0.4 to 0.6 for oxygen flows of 6 to 8 L/min (see Table 3-1). The actual percentage of oxygen delivered is also influenced by the patient's ventilatory pattern. Note that the minimum flow of oxygen should be sufficient to ensure that the bag does not completely deflate when the patient inhales (i.e., the flow should be sufficient to maintain the reservoir bag at least one-third to one-half full on inspiration).[4,14] Partial rebreathing masks are available in child and adult sizes.

Nonrebreathing Masks. Nonrebreathing masks look very similar to partial rebreathing masks except that they have two types of valves attached to the mask as Figure 3-19 illustrates, the first set of valves is a one-way valve (B) located between the reservoir bag and the base of the mask. This valve allows gas flow to enter the mask from the reservoir bag when the patient inhales and prevents gas flow from the mask back into the reservoir bag during the patient's exhalation, as occurs with the partial rebreathing mask. The second set of valves is at the exhalation ports (C). These one-way valves prevent room air from entering the mask during inhalation and allow the patient's exhaled gases to exit the mask on exhalation. As with the partial rebreathing mask, the flow of oxygen to the mask should be sufficient to maintain the reservoir bag at least one-third to one-half full on inspiration.

Nonrebreathing masks theoretically can deliver 100% oxygen, assuming that the mask fits snugly on the patient's face and the only source of gas being inhaled is derived from the oxygen flowing into the mask-reservoir system. In actual practice, disposable nonrebreathing masks can deliver an F_IO_2 of 0.6 to 0.8.[14] The discrepancy between disposable nonrebreathing masks and the original BLB masks is primarily related to the fact that manufacturers usually supply disposable masks with one of the exhalation valves removed. The valve is removed as a precaution in case the oxygen flow to the mask is interrupted or inadequate for the patient's needs (i.e., according to safety regulations, the patient must still be able to entrain room air if source gas flow is interrupted). Original BLB masks contain a spring-disk safety valve that opens if oxygen flow to the mask is interrupted.

Nonrebreathing masks are effective for administering a high F_IO_2 to spontaneously breathing patients for short periods. Prolonged use of these masks can be associated with valve malfunctions (i.e., sticking as a result of moisture accumulation or deformity from wear).

High-Flow Oxygen Systems
Air Entrainment Masks

Air entrainment masks are the result of the pioneering work of Barach and associates[15,16] and Campbell[17] from the 1930s to the 1960s. Figure 3-20 is a schematic of a typical air entrainment mask. It consists of a plastic mask connected to a jet nozzle, which is encased within a plastic housing that contains air entrainment ports. Oxygen flowing through the nozzle "drags" in room air through the entrainment ports as a result of viscous, shearing forces between the gas exiting the jet nozzle outlet and the surrounding ambient air.[18] The concentration of oxygen delivered to the patient, therefore, depends on the flow of oxygen exiting the jet nozzle, the size of the jet nozzle outlet, and the size of the entrainment port.

For most commercially available masks, the oxygen concentration is varied by changing the size of the nozzle outlet or the entrainment ports. The flow of oxygen to the

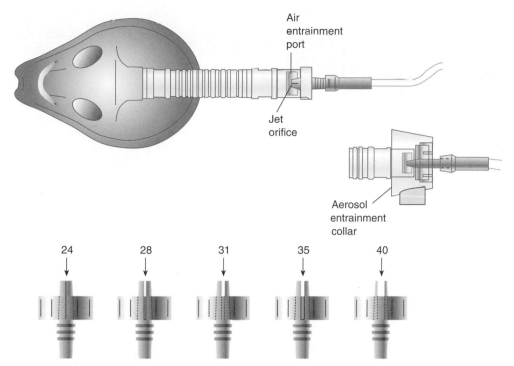

FIGURE 3-20 Schematic of the components of an air entrainment mask. The aerosol collar allows high humidity or aerosol entrainment from an air source. (Modified from Kacmarek RM: In-hospital O_2 therapy. In Kacmarek RM, Stoller JK, editors: *Current respiratory care*, Toronto, 1988, BC Decker.)

nozzle is constant and set to a minimum value, usually 2 to 10 L/min. Note that partial obstruction of oxygen flow downstream of the jet orifice or partial obstruction of the entrainment ports reduces the amount of room air entrained, thus raising the F_IO_2 of the delivered gas.[19-21]

Figure 3-21 presents a simple method for calculating the air:oxygen entrainment ratio and the total gas flow delivered for a given F_IO_2.[20] Table 3-2 presents a list of the air:oxygen entrainment ratios required to achieve a given F_IO_2, showing that the total flow of gas delivered is greater for a low F_IO_2 than for a high F_IO_2. Air entrainment masks function much better as fixed-performance devices at a low F_IO_2 (less than 0.4) than at a higher F_IO_2 (greater than 0.4).[19,21,22] The discrepancy between the set F_IO_2 and the actual delivered F_IO_2 is exaggerated by abrupt increases in inspiratory flow. Campbell and Minty[23] suggest that many commercially available masks produce a variable F_IO_2 when patients generate high inspiratory flows because of insufficient mask volume.

Air entrainment masks are excellent for providing oxygen therapy to hypoxemic patients with chronic obstructive pulmonary disease (COPD); these patients typically require a fixed F_IO_2 between 0.24 and 0.35.[17] The total flow of gas delivered by such masks (oxygen plus air) for lower F_IO_2 levels usually is sufficient to meet the peak inspiratory flow requirements of these patients. Supplemental humidification of the delivered gas usually is not required when the oxygen flow is low (i.e., less than 4 L/min) because the oxygen flow is a small percentage of the total flow. Increased moisture can be delivered by attaching

a compressed, air-driven aerosol to the air entrainment port via an open plastic collar (such collars work best with masks that have large air entrainment ports[20]). Alternatively, high humidity can be delivered with a fixed F_IO_2 with large-volume aerosol nebulizers and humidifier units that use air entrainment devices, which can provide increased levels of moisture at several fixed oxygen percentage settings (e.g., 0.4, 0.6, and 1). A number of appliances, including aerosol masks, face tents, T-tubes, and tracheostomy collars, can be used to deliver these moisture-rich gases. Care should be taken not to allow moisture to accumulate in the tubing downstream from the air entrainment device. Accumulated moisture acts as an obstruction, which can reduce the amount of room air entrained and raise the F_IO_2 delivered to the patient. Notice that the total flow of gas provided by this type of apparatus may not be sufficient to meet patients' high ventilatory demands. Thus the F_IO_2 may vary considerably in these situations, because the patient is forced to entrain room air to meet increased ventilatory needs.[24,25] Large-volume nebulizers and humidifiers are discussed in more detail in Chapter 4.

Oxygen Hoods. Oxygen hoods were introduced in the 1970s as a means of maintaining a relatively constant F_IO_2 to infants requiring supplemental oxygen. Figure 3-22 shows a disposable hood used to deliver oxygen therapy to neonatal pediatric patients. It is a clear plastic enclosure that is placed around the patient's head. Fixed oxygen concentrations (from an air entrainment device or an oxygen-air blender [see the section on oxygen blenders later in this chapter]) can be connected to the hood via an inlet port at

$$O_2 \text{ flow} = \frac{\text{Total flow} \times (FIO_2 - 0.2)}{0.8}$$

EXAMPLE:
Known: Total flow = 10 L/min
$\qquad FIO_2 = 0.4$

$$O_2 \text{ flow} = \frac{10 \times (0.4 - 0.2)}{0.8}$$

$$O_2 \text{ flow} = \frac{10 \times 0.2}{0.8}$$

$$O_2 \text{ flow} = \frac{2}{0.8}$$

$$O_2 \text{ flow} = 2.5 \text{ L/min}$$

(Air flow = Total flow − O_2 flow)

$$FIO_2 \text{ flow} = \frac{O_2 \text{ flow} + (0.2 \times \text{Air flow})}{\text{Total flow}}$$

EXAMPLE:
Known: O_2 flow = 2.5 L/min
$\qquad$ Air flow = 7.5 L/min
$\qquad$ Total flow = 10 L/min

$$FIO_2 = \frac{2.5 + (0.2 \times 7.5)}{10}$$

$$FIO_2 = \frac{2.5 + 1.5}{10}$$

$$FIO_2 = \frac{4}{10}$$

$$FIO_2 = 0.4$$

$$\text{Total flow} = \frac{O_2 \text{ flow} \times 0.8}{FIO_2 - 0.2}$$

EXAMPLE:
Known: O_2 flow = 2.5 L/min
$\qquad FIO_2 = 0.4$

$$\text{Total flow} = \frac{2.5 \times 0.8}{0.4 - 0.2}$$

$$\text{Total flow} = \frac{2}{0.2}$$

$$\text{Total flow} = 10 \text{ L/min}$$

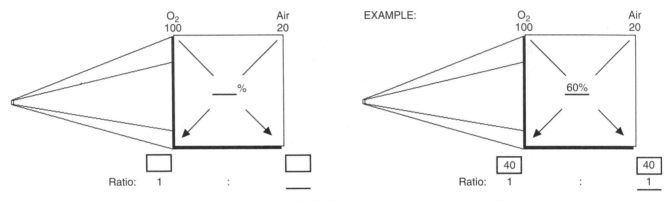

FIGURE 3-21 Method of calculating air : oxygen entrainment ratios.

TABLE 3-2

Approximate Entrainment Ratios for Commonly Used Oxygen Concentrations*

Oxygen Percentage	Air : Oxygen Ratio	Total Parts[†]
100	0:1	1
70	0.6:1	1.6
60	1:1	2
50	1.7:1	2.7
40	3:1	4
35	5:1	6
30	8:1	9
28	10:1	11
24	25:1	26

*Assuming the F_1O_2 is 20.9%.
[†]Total parts × Oxygen flow = Total flow estimate.

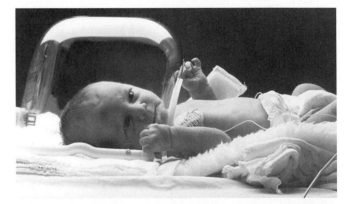

FIGURE 3-22 Oxygen hood. (Courtesy Utah Medical Products Inc., Midvale, Utah.)

the rear of the hood. The flow rate of gas entering the hood is set to ensure that the exhaled carbon dioxide is flushed out (i.e., the flow rate should be approximately 5 to 10 L/min).

The F_1O_2 must be measured intermittently or monitored continuously with an oxygen analyzer. Several studies have shown that in hoods, the oxygen seems to be layered, with the highest concentration near the bottom of the hood. The partial pressure of oxygen in the arteries (PaO_2) should also be measured by arterial blood gas analysis at regular intervals. The noise levels inside some oxygen hoods can present problems, and every effort should be made to minimize this effect.[26]

Incubators. Incubators, along with oxygen tents, can be classified as environmental delivery systems because they provide large volumes of oxygen-enriched gas to the atmosphere immediately surrounding the patient. The first incubator was designed by Denuce in 1857.[20] Several years later (c. 1880), Tarnier designed an enclosed incubator to provide a warm environment for premature infants.[20] Current incubators (Figure 3-23) allow for variable control of the environmental temperature, humidity, and F_IO_2. The temperature and humidity of the gas in the incubator are regulated by a servo-controlled mechanism connected to a fan that circulates environmental gas over heating coils and a blow-by humidifier. Supplemental oxygen can be provided by connecting a heated humidifier directly to the incubator.

The F_IO_2 is controlled with an air entrainment apparatus that allows the selection of high and low F_IO_2 levels. Generally, when the air entrainment port remains open, an F_IO_2 of 0.4 or less is delivered. The port must be occluded for delivery of higher F_IO_2 levels. The port is opened and closed by moving an occluder attached to a red metal flag. This feature is incorporated into the design of the system to alert the medical staff that high concentrations of oxygen are being delivered.

It is important to remember that the actual concentration of oxygen delivered to the patient can vary considerably when the enclosure is opened for nursing care procedures. Because of the variability in oxygen concentrations that can occur when oxygen is provided through the incubator's oxygen inlet, oxygen may need to be delivered directly to the infant via an oxygen hood placed directly over the infant's head inside the incubator.[9] Regardless of the method used to deliver oxygen to the infant, the actual F_IO_2 in the incubator should be measured intermittently or continuously monitored. Additionally, blood gases should be sampled at regular intervals to ensure that the infant is receiving the appropriate oxygen therapy. The partial pressure of arterial oxygen should be monitored in infants receiving oxygen therapy. High PaO_2 values in these patients are associated with a high incidence of retinopathy and loss of sight.

Recent studies have demonstrated that noise levels in incubators can be quite high.[26] Although noise may be a difficult problem to control, every effort must be made to minimize it inside these devices.

Oxygen Tents. Sir Leonard Hill is credited with being the first clinician to use the oxygen tent,[3] but Alvin Barach improved the operation of these devices by conditioning the air inside the tent.[4] (Barach accomplished this early form of air conditioning by adding a fan to circulate the air over a cooling tower containing ice.) During the early 1900s, oxygen tents were often used to provide oxygen to hypoxemic adults and children. Currently, oxygen tents are used primarily for pediatric patients who require enriched oxygen and high humidity levels. Today's oxygen tents can provide environmental control of (1) oxygen concentration, (2) humidity, and (3) temperature (Figure 3-24). The F_IO_2 and the humidity content delivered to the patient are controlled by a high-flow aerosol unit, which is incorporated into the tent. Ultrasonic nebulizers (see Chapter 4) can also be used to increase the humidity inside the tent. The temperature is controlled with refrigeration coils containing Freon. These systems typically can reduce the temperature inside the tent from 10° to 12° F below room temperature.

Oxygen Proportioners
Oxygen Adders

The simplest example of an oxygen proportioner is an oxygen adder, such as the one shown in Figure 3-25.

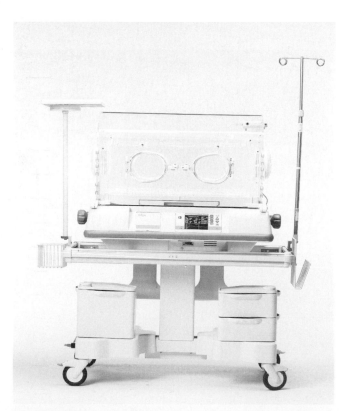

FIGURE 3-23 Infant incubator. (Courtesy Dräger Medical AG & Co., Lübeck, Germany.)

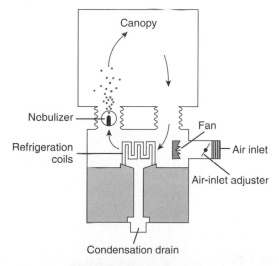

FIGURE 3-24 Oxygen tent.

Although these devices are not commonly used clinically, the principle of operation can be used to describe how oxygen proportioners work. The typical oxygen adder system consists of two flowmeters, one attached to an oxygen supply and the other attached to an air supply. The outputs of the two flowmeters are directed to humidifiers and then to the patient via any of the delivery systems previously described. The F_IO_2 of the gas delivered to the patient depends on the ratio of air:oxygen flow. The concentration can be calculated using the same principle as for calculating air:oxygen entrainment ratios for air entrainment masks. For example, if the air and oxygen flowmeters are each set to deliver 15 L/min, the ratio is 1:1, which corresponds to an F_IO_2 of 0.6. However, if the air flowmeter is set to 15 L/min and the oxygen flowmeter is set to 5 L/min, the air:oxygen entrainment ratio is 3:1, corresponding to an F_IO_2 of 0.4 (see Table 3-2).

Oxygen Blenders and Mixers. A more sophisticated device for accomplishing air-oxygen mixing is the **oxygen blender** (or oxygen mixer). Figure 3-26 shows a typical oxygen blender and its components. Compressed air and oxygen from a high-pressure source enter a chamber, where the pressures of the two gases are equalized. An alarm system is incorporated into the design of these devices to alert the practitioner if the pressures of the source gases are not comparable (i.e., the air and oxygen pressures differ by greater than 10 psi). Unequal source gas pressures can cause the blender to malfunction and deliver unreliable F_IO_2 levels. Unequal pressures are remedied by reducing the higher pressure gas to match the lower pressure gas, which is usually 50 psig. The gases then are routed to a precise metering device that controls the amount of each gas reaching the outlet. This metering device can be adjusted with a rotary mixing control knob on the faceplate. Turning the knob counterclockwise reduces the amount of oxygen reaching the outlet, thereby reducing the delivered F_IO_2. Conversely, turning the knob clockwise reduces the amount of air reaching the outlet, increasing the F_IO_2.

Oxygen blenders are a reliable means of providing a variety of F_IO_2 levels. Flowmeters can be connected to the blender's outlet, as can ventilators or any other devices that use 50-psig source gas. Because moisture and particulate matter introduced into the blender by the source gases can cause the blender to malfunction, it is important to filter the gas before it enters the blender housing.

Hyperbaric Oxygen Therapy

Hyperbaric oxygen therapy exposes patients to a pressure greater than atmospheric pressure while they breathe 100% oxygen, either continuously or intermittently. Historically, hyperbaric therapy has been used most often to treat individuals with decompression sickness and air embolism associated with deep sea diving. More recently, it has been used successfully to treat patients with a variety of disorders, including carbon monoxide poisoning and smoke inhalation, anaerobic infections refractory to conventional therapy, thermal injuries, skin grafts, and refractory osteomyelitis. Although hyperbaric oxygen therapy has increased significantly during the past decade, its use is somewhat limited, because it is expensive to purchase and maintain hyperbaric units. A brief discussion of the physiologic basis of hyperbaric oxygen therapy and a description of the equipment required follow. For a more detailed analysis of hyperbaric oxygen therapy, the reader should consult the references at the end of this chapter.[27-29]

Physiologic Principles

Effects on Respiratory Function

Exposure to elevated barometric pressures during hyperbaric oxygen therapy can directly affect a number of physiologic parameters related to respiration, including lung volume, arterial and alveolar partial pressures of oxygen,

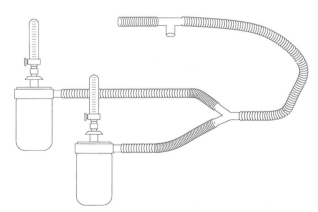

FIGURE 3-25 Schematic of an oxygen adder. (From Wilkins RL, Stoller JK, Scanlan CL: *Egan's fundamentals of respiratory care,* ed 8, St Louis, 2003, Mosby.)

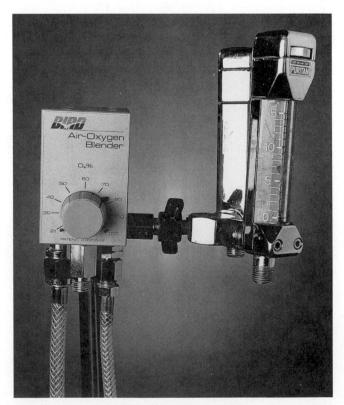

FIGURE 3-26 Oxygen blender.

the temperature of the gases breathed, and the work of breathing.

Lung Volumes. The effects on lung volume can be explained by Boyle's law, which states that if the temperature of a gas remains constant, the volume of a gas is inversely related to its pressure. That is, as pressure exerted on the container increases, the gas volume decreases. Therefore, when a person is exposed to elevated pressures, the gas volume contained in any body cavity tends to be compressed. For example, as the ambient pressure is doubled (1520 mm Hg, or 2 atm), the air volume in the lung is reduced to one half of what it would occupy at a normal ambient pressure (760 mm Hg, or 1 atm). Figure 3-27 shows the pressure-volume relationships typically encountered during hyperbaric oxygen therapy.

Alveolar and Arterial Partial Pressures of Oxygen. The effect of increased ambient pressure on the partial pressure of alveolar oxygen (P_AO_2) can be explained by Dalton's law, which states that the total pressure of a gas mixture, such as air, equals the sum of the partial pressures of each of the constituent gases in the mixture. Considering that air is 21% oxygen and 79% nitrogen, then ambient air (assuming that the barometric pressure is 760 mm Hg) has a partial oxygen pressure (PO_2) of about 160 mm Hg (0.21×760 mm Hg) and a partial nitrogen pressure of about 600 mm Hg (0.79×760 mm Hg). This same logic can be applied to the alveolar air equation for calculating the P_AO_2:

$$P_AO_2 = (P_{bar} - P_{H_2O})F_IO_2 - P_aCO_2 \div 0.8$$

Therefore, if the barometric pressure (P_{bar}) equals 760 mm Hg, the P_{H_2O} equals 47 mm Hg, the P_aCO_2 equals 40 mm Hg, and the F_IO_2 equals 0.21, the P_AO_2 would be

about 100 mm Hg. Consider the case if the barometric pressure is doubled to 1520 mm Hg, or 2 atm. If all other variables in the equation remain constant, the P_AO_2 would equal 333 mm Hg.

Henry's law is used to explain the changes in the PaO_2 that occur with exposure to elevated ambient pressures. The law states that the degree to which a gas enters into physical solution in body fluids is directly proportional to the partial pressure of gas to which the fluid is exposed. Remember that Henry's law states that the relative quantities of gas entering a fluid are related to the pressure of gas exerted on the fluid and the solubility of the gas in the fluid in question. Oxygen's solubility in plasma is about 0.003 vol % (milliliters of oxygen/100 mL of whole blood) for every 1 mm Hg of PaO_2. If it is assumed that the ventilation-perfusion relationship for a patient's lungs is normal, the PaO_2 would be slightly less than 100 mm Hg when the patient is breathing room air at 1 atm. Furthermore, the PaO_2 would be approximately 333 mm Hg for breathing room air when the ambient pressure is increased to 2 atm. Then it can be calculated that as the PaO_2 increases from about 100 mm Hg (at 1 atm) to approximately 333 mm Hg (at 2 atm), the amount of dissolved oxygen increases from 0.3 vol % (100 mm Hg × 0.003 vol %/mm Hg) to 1 vol % (333 mm Hg × 0.003 vol %/mm Hg). As can be seen, the oxygen-carrying capacity of plasma increases considerably under hyperbaric conditions. Therefore, it is reasonable to assume that this form of therapy is beneficial in the treatment of patients with abnormally functioning hemoglobin and consequently a reduced ability to carry oxygen attached to hemoglobin, such as occurs with carbon monoxide poisoning.

Gas Temperatures. According to Gay-Lussac's law, if the volume of a gas remains constant, a direct relationship exists between the absolute pressure of a gas and its temperature. It is reasonable to suggest that if the volume of a hyperbaric chamber remains constant, increasing the pressure would raise the temperature inside the chamber. (Indeed, this problem should limit the usefulness of this form of therapy.) In practice, gas temperature changes encountered during hyperbaric therapy are easily controlled by regulating the rates at which pressures are increased and decreased, the temperature of the air used for compression and decompression, and the flow rate of ventilation used to dissipate heat.[28,29]

Work of Breathing. As the barometric pressure increases, the density of the gas being breathed also increases. The increase in gas density results in an increased work of breathing, which is not noticeable and can easily be accommodated in normal patients. In patients with reduced lung reserves, however, this increased work may present problems and require ventilatory support. It also is important to recognize that many ventilators malfunction when placed in a hyperbaric chamber.[30]

Vascular Function. Several studies have demonstrated that hyperbaric oxygen therapy increases the synthetic ability of tissues by increasing collagen deposition, thus enhancing the growth of new blood vessels in damaged

Depth in feet	Pressure in ATA	Relative volume	Relative diameter
0	1	100%	100%
33	2	50%	79.3%
66	3	33.3%	69.3%
99	4	25%	63%
132	5	20%	58.5%
165	6	16.6%	55%

FIGURE 3-27 Pressure-volume relationships during hyperbaric oxygen therapy. (Redrawn from Davis JC, Hunt TK: *Hyperbaric oxygen therapy,* Kensington, Md, 1977, Undersea Medical Society.)

tissues and the revascularization of these tissues.[27] This effect has been used to successfully treat patients with skin grafts.

Immunologic Function. It is well established that leukocyte function is enhanced during hyperbaric oxygen therapy. This improved function is thought to be related to an increase in the oxygen available for microbicidal metabolism (i.e., H_2O_2, OH^-). Coupled with this enhanced microbicidal activity of leukocytes, oxygen appears to directly inhibit the growth of certain bacteria, particularly those involved in anaerobic infections, such as *Clostridia* sp., which are responsible for gas gangrene.

Equipment

Hyperbaric chambers generally are classified as either monoplace or multiplace units (Figure 3-28). **Monoplace hyperbaric chambers** are categorized by the National Fire Protection Association (NFPA) as Class B chambers and are rated for single occupancy.[28] Several models of monoplace units are available commercially. Although

they differ considerably in appearance, they all use the same principle of operation, generally relying on a single gas source for compression and respiration. Some newer systems provide connections for a separate source gas for respiration.

A typical chamber generally is about 8 to 10 feet long and 3 feet in diameter. The outer shell of the unit is constructed of steel and clear, double-thick acrylic. Some newer units contain a separate chamber compartment to accommodate attendants working with the patient. Most units are mounted on wheels for portability, but they usually are treated as stationary systems and are placed in a room designated for the purposes of hyperbaric therapy.

Multiplace hyperbaric chambers are walk-in units that provide enough space to allow two or more patients to be treated simultaneously. They vary in size (2 to 13 occupants) but usually contain a main chamber for treating patients and a smaller chamber that allows attendants to enter and leave without altering the pressure in the main chamber. Multiplace chambers provide two gas sources,

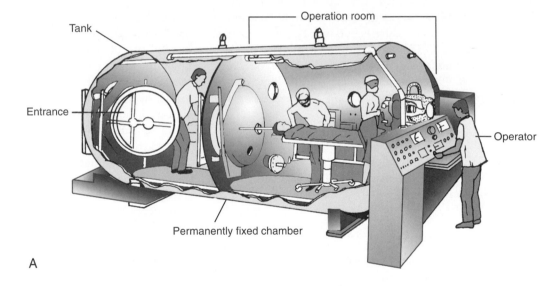

A

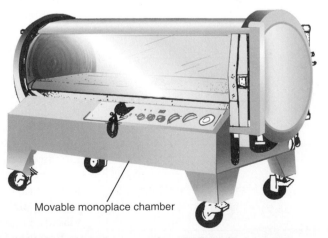

B

FIGURE 3-28 Schematics of a multiplace **(A)** and a monoplace **(B)** hyperbaric oxygen chamber. (From Wilkins RL, Stoller JK, Kacmarek RM: *Egan's fundamentals of respiratory care,* ed 9, St Louis, 2009, Mosby.)

one for compression and one for respiration. Hyperbaric oxygenation is achieved by having the patient breathe oxygen by mask or through a specially designed hood while exposed to elevated barometric pressures in the compressed air chamber. Treatment schedules (i.e., the amount of time the patient breathes 100% oxygen versus air) are tailored to the specific needs of the patient. Generally, patients are placed on schedules in which intermittent air breathing periods of 5 minutes or longer are programmed approximately every 20 minutes. This intermittent air breathing is used to prevent oxygen toxicity.

Monitoring Devices. All hyperbaric facilities should have the capability to monitor the oxygenation status of patients undergoing hyperbaric oxygen therapy. Transcutaneous monitoring has proven to be valuable in assessing the overall oxygenation status of a patient undergoing this treatment. Selective placement of the probe also can provide information on the localized effects of hyperbaric oxygen therapy on ischemic tissue.

Arterial blood gas monitoring can provide information on the oxygenation status of patients receiving hyperbaric therapy and is also an indication of their ventilatory status. Arterial blood samples can be drawn from patients and removed from the chamber for analysis. Care must be taken to ensure that the sample remains tightly sealed until it is analyzed. Transcutaneous monitoring and arterial blood gas analysis are discussed further in Chapters 8 and 10.

Indications and Contraindications for Hyperbaric Oxygen Therapy

As stated previously, hyperbaric oxygen therapy is most often associated with the treatment of individuals who have experienced decompression sickness and other maladies associated with deep-sea diving. Box 3-1 lists several other conditions that have been successfully treated with this type of oxygen therapy.[31-33] Although the effectiveness of hyperbaric oxygen therapy may vary among patients, those with any of these conditions should respond to it.

Box 3-2 lists some of the known contraindications to hyperbaric oxygen therapy. The only absolute contraindication is pneumothorax. If pneumothorax occurs during hyperbaric treatment, chest tubes should be inserted immediately; failure to treat pneumothorax can have dire consequences. The other conditions listed are relative contraindications. Note that serious problems can arise when patients with obstructive bronchial disease caused by asthma, bronchitis, or emphysema are treated with hyperbaric therapy. Gas trapping can result in barotrauma. Similarly, patients who have upper respiratory infections and nasal congestion usually are unable to clear their ears during compression and decompression and thus are prone to eardrum rupture during treatment.

Nitric Oxide Therapy

As was discussed in Chapter 2, nitric oxide has been shown to be a potent pulmonary vasodilator. It has been used

---

BOX 3-1	Indications for Hyperbaric Oxygen Therapy

- Air embolism
- Carbon monoxide poisoning
- Cyanide poisoning
- Decompression sickness
- Gas gangrene
- Refractory anaerobic infections
- Refractory osteomyelitis
- Skin grafts
- Thermal burns
- Wound healing

BOX 3-2	Contraindications for Hyperbaric Oxygen Therapy

- Congenital spherocytosis
- High fevers
- Hypercapnia (>60 mm Hg)
- Obstructive airway disease
- Optic neuritis
- Pneumothorax
- Seizure disorders
- Sinusitis
- Upper respiratory infections
- Viral infections

From Kindall EP: Clinical hyperbaric oxygen therapy. In Bennett P, Elliot D, editors: *Physiology and medicine of diving*, ed 4, Philadelphia, 1993, WB Saunders.

---

successfully to treat persistent pulmonary hypertension of the newborn,[31,34] as an adjunct to the treatment of congenital cardiac defects, to reverse pulmonary vasoconstriction associated with adult respiratory distress syndrome, and possibly to reverse the bronchoconstriction induced by histamine and methacholine.[35-38]

Nitric oxide is supplied as a compressed gas mixture of nitric oxide and nitrogen (minimum purity 99%) in cylinders constructed of aluminum alloy.[39] It is supplied this way because it is a highly reactive molecule that is rapidly oxidized to nitrogen dioxide in the presence of oxygen and to nitric acid in the presence of water. Nitrogen dioxide and nitric acid are toxic if inhaled. In low concentrations they can cause a chemical pneumonitis; higher concentrations can cause lung injury, such as pulmonary edema, which ultimately can lead to death.[31,40]

The therapeutic dose of nitric oxide is 2 to 80 ppm.[39] Figure 3-29 shows a commercially available nitric oxide delivery system manufactured by Ohmeda, Datex-Ohmeda (GE Healthcare, Piscataway, NJ). The INOmax® DS (delivery system) delivers INOmax® (nitric oxide) for inhalation into the inspiratory limb of the patient breathing circuit in a way that provides a constant concentration of nitric oxide (NO), as set by the user, throughout the inspired breath (Figure 3-29). Using a dual channel design, the first channel utilizes a delivery CPU, flow controller and an injector module to ensure the accurate delivery of NO. The

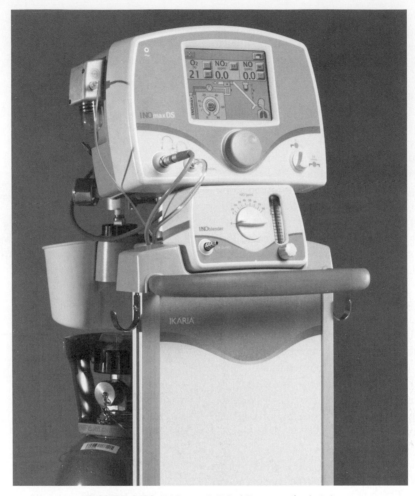

FIGURE 3-29 INOmax® DS. (Courtesy Ikaria®.)

specially designed injector module enables tracking of the ventilator flow waveforms and the delivery of a synchronized and proportional dose of NO. The second channel is the monitoring system, utilizing a separate monitor CPU, electrochemical gas sensors and a graphically enhanced user interface. Integrated monitoring and alarm systems allow for continuous monitoring of inspired O_2, NO_2, and NO. Several alarm systems are available to alert staff members when problems arise, including alarms for high and low nitric oxide, high nitrogen dioxide, and high and low oxygen. Other alarms can be set to notify the user when source gas pressure is lost, the electrochemical cells fail, and calibration is required.[39]

Helium-Oxygen (Heliox) Therapy

Helium-oxygen **(heliox)** mixtures have been used on a limited basis to treat patients with airway obstruction.[41-43] Specifically, heliox has been used to manage asthmatic patients with acute respiratory failure, to treat postextubation stridor in pediatric trauma patients, as an adjunct in the treatment of pediatric patients with refractory croup, to administer anesthetic gases to patients with small-diameter endotracheal tubes, and to provide ventilatory support for patients with severe airway obstruction caused by chronic bronchitis and emphysema.[44-47]

Heliox mixtures are supplied in compressed-gas cylinders. Three concentrations are generally available: an 80%:20% (helium:oxygen) mixture, a 70%:30% mixture, and a 60%:40% mixture. As was stated in Chapter 2, the benefit of breathing heliox is related to its lower density compared with pure oxygen or air. Remember that the density of an 80%:20% (helium:oxygen) mixture is 0.43 g/L, and that 100% oxygen has a density of 1.43 g/L. Therefore, an 80%:20% mixture is 1.8 times less dense than 100% oxygen. A 70%:30% mixture of heliox has a density of 0.55 g/L and is therefore 1.6 times less dense than 100% oxygen, and a 60%:40% mixture has a density of 0.58 g/L and is 1.4 times less dense than 100% oxygen.* The lower density promotes laminar flow and reduces the amount of

---

*The density of a helium-oxygen mixture can be calculated using the following relationships: The density of 100% helium is 0.179 g/L, and the density of 100% oxygen is 1.43 g/L. Therefore, the density of an 80%:20% heliox mixture equals (0.8 × 0.179 g/L) + (0.2 × 1.43 g/L), or 0.43 g/L.

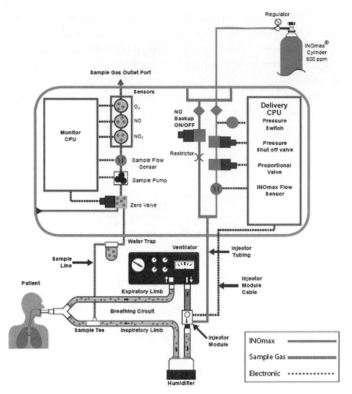

FIGURE 3-30 Schematic illustrating the principle of operation of the INOmax DS. (See text for description.) (Courtesy Ikaria®.)

TABLE 3-3

Heliox Correction Factors for Oxygen Flowmeters

Helium:Oxygen Ratio	Correction Factor
80:20	1.8 × liter flow
70:30	1.6 × liter flow
60:40	1.4 × liter flow

Modified from Myers TR: Use of heliox in children, *Respir Care* 51:619, 2006.

CLINICAL ROUNDS 3-4

You are the therapist on call when an asthmatic patient is admitted to the emergency department of the hospital. The attending physician requests that you administer heliox containing 30% oxygen to the patient. While you are administering the gas from a cylinder labeled 70%:30% (helium:oxygen), the patient becomes progressively more dyspneic and cyanotic. What should you do?

See Evolve Resources for the answer.

BOX 3-3	Clinical Manifestations of Carbon Dioxide Toxicity*

· Extrasystole (premature ventricular contractions)
· Flushed skin
· Full and bounding pulse
· Hypertension
· Muscle twitching

*Note that hypercapnia cannot be reliably diagnosed on clinical examination only. Arterial blood gases (measurement of the partial pressure of arterial carbon dioxide) should be determined in case of doubt.

CLINICAL ROUNDS 3-3

You are asked to set up a large-volume nebulizer for the treatment of a patient with an acute asthma exacerbation. The attending physician asks you to use an 80%:20% heliox gas mixture as the driving gas for nebulizing the β_2-bronchodilator. What is the actual flow of gas being administered to the patient if the set flow on the oxygen flowmeter used is 10 L/min?

See Evolve Resources for the answer.

turbulent flow. This relationship is important to remember when administering heliox because the actual flow rate of gas delivered is greater than the set flow. Table 3-3 presents a list of correction factors that can be applied to calculate the actual flow when a typical oxygen flowmeter is used to deliver a heliox mixture. (Clinical Rounds 3-3 presents an example of this concept.)[48]

Heliox usually is administered to intubated patients with an intermittent positive pressure device. For nonintubated patients, a well-fitted, nonrebreathing mask attached to a reservoir bag should be used. The flow rate of gas should be high enough to prevent the reservoir bag from collapsing during inspiration. Nasal cannulas are ineffective for delivering heliox because of leakage. Large-volume enclosures, such as hoods, also are unsatisfactory because helium tends to concentrate at the top of these devices.

It is important to monitor the fractional concentration of oxygen delivered to the patient when a heliox mixture is administered. In some cases, commercial cylinders containing helium and oxygen may be "unmixed" (i.e., because of the difference in densities between helium and oxygen, a layering effect can occur). If a sufficient amount of oxygen is not mixed with the helium breathed by the patient, hypoxemia can result.[49] (Clinical Rounds 3-4 presents a problem-solving exercise involving heliox therapy.)

Carbon Dioxide–Oxygen (Carbogen) Therapy

Carbon dioxide–oxygen mixtures (**carbogen**) are used to treat hiccoughs and carbon monoxide poisoning, as a stimulant/depressant of ventilation, and to prevent the complete washout of carbon dioxide during cardiopulmonary bypass. The frequency of this procedure is limited because of the adverse effects associated with breathing elevated concentrations of carbon dioxide. Box 3-3 lists the clinical manifestations of carbon dioxide toxicity.

Carbogen is supplied in compressed-gas cylinders as either 5%:95% (carbon dioxide:oxygen) or 7%:93% (carbon dioxide:oxygen). It can be administered to patients with a nonrebreathing mask connected to a reservoir bag. The mask should fit snugly on the patient's face, and the flow rate of gas should be high enough to prevent the bag from collapsing when the patient inhales.

To prevent adverse reactions when this type of therapy is administered, it is essential to monitor the patient's pulse, blood pressure, and respiration, as well as mental status. Pulse, arterial blood pressure, and minute volume normally increase as the patient breathes carbogen, but the rapidity and level of these changes depend on the concentration of the mixture. Changes occur faster and the effects are greater if the patient breathes a 7%:93% (carbon dioxide:oxygen) mixture than with a 5%:95% mixture. The treatment should be stopped immediately if any of the monitored parameters increase or decrease abruptly or significantly.

KEY POINTS

▶ Multistage regulators can control gas pressures with more precision than single-stage regulators because the pressure is reduced gradually. Additionally, multistage regulators produce a much smoother gas flow than do single-stage regulators.

▶ Flowmeters are devices that control and indicate flow. Pressure-compensated Thorpe tube flowmeters, the most commonly used flowmeters in respiratory care, provide accurate estimates of flow, regardless of the downstream pressure. Bourdon flowmeters and adjustable, multiple-orifice flow resistors are actually reducing valves that control the pressure gradient across an outlet with a fixed orifice.

▶ Oxygen therapy systems generally are classified as *low-flow (variable performance)* and *high-flow (fixed performance)* devices. Low-flow devices are also called *variable-performance devices* because they supply oxygen at flow rates that are lower than a patient's inspiratory demands. High-flow (fixed-performance) devices provide oxygen at flow rates high enough to satisfy the patient's inspiratory demands. Examples of low-flow devices include nasal cannulas, simple oxygen masks, and partial rebreathing masks. The most common example of a high-flow device is the air entrainment mask.

▶ Hyperbaric oxygen therapy exposes patients to a pressure greater than atmospheric pressure while they breathe 100% oxygen either continuously or intermittently. Hyperbaric oxygen therapy is indicated for air embolism, carbon monoxide poisoning, and decompression sickness and as an adjunct in the treatment of gas gangrene, refractory osteomyelitis, and wound healing.

▶ Nitric oxide delivery systems are designed for use with most conventional critical care ventilators and can be adapted for use with both adult and pediatric ventilators. Nitric oxide therapy has been shown to be effective in the treatment of persistent pulmonary hypertension of the newborn, as an adjunct to the treatment of congenital cardiac defects, and as a means to reverse pulmonary vasoconstriction associated with adult respiratory distress syndrome.

▶ Heliox has been successfully used in the management of airflow obstructive diseases. It has been used successfully to improve oxygen delivery and as an adjunct to aerosol therapy in spontaneously breathing patients with acute asthmatic exacerbations and refractory croup. Heliox also has been used to administer anesthetic gases to patients with small-diameter endotracheal tubes and to provide ventilatory support for patients with severe lower airway obstruction.

ASSESSMENT QUESTIONS

See Evolve Resources for answers.

1. Describe an easy method of determining the number of stages in a multistage regulator.

2. Which of the following devices is/are considered high-flow (fixed performance) oxygen delivery system(s)?
   I.   Nasal cannula
   II. Nasal catheter
   III. Air entrainment mask
   IV. Partial rebreathing mask
      a. I and II only
      b. I, II, and III only
      c. III only
      d. I, II, III, and IV

3. Which of the following statements is true regarding back pressure–compensated flowmeters?
   a. The needle valve is positioned before the indicator tube.
   b. High-resistance devices attached to these flowmeters cause erroneously high flow readings.
   c. Faulty valve seats do not affect flow readings.
   d. Gas flow from these flowmeters stops if resistance creates a back pressure that exceeds the source gas pressure.

4. Which of the following are advantages of using TTO therapy catheters?
   I. They do not require periodic replacement.
   II. The incidence of infection is considerably lower than with other low-flow oxygen devices.
   III. They require lower oxygen flows to achieve a given F_1O_2 than do standard nasal cannulas.
   IV. They are less obtrusive (i.e., more cosmetically pleasing) than nasal cannulas.
      a. I and III only
      b. II and III only
      c. III and IV only
      d. II, III, and IV only

5. What is the air:oxygen entrainment ratio for delivering 40% oxygen through an air entrainment mask?
   a. 2:1
   b. 1:2
   c. 1:3
   d. 3:1

6. Studies have shown that mustache and pendant cannulas can reduce the cost of oxygen therapy by as much as:
   a. 10%
   b. 30%
   c. 50%
   d. 80%

7. What is the approximate partial pressure of inspired oxygen of room air if the barometric pressure is raised to 2 atm?
   a. 150 mm Hg
   b. 300 mm Hg
   c. 200 mm Hg
   d. 1520 mm Hg

8. Hyperbaric oxygen therapy is indicated for:
   I. Air embolism
   II. Hypercapnia (>60 mm Hg)
   III. Carbon monoxide poisoning
   IV. Sinusitis
      a. I and III only
      b. II and IV only
      c. I, II, and III only
      d. II, III, and IV only

9. Administration of heliox can be an effective form of therapy in which of the following situations?
   I. Managing postextubation stridor in pediatric trauma patients
   II. Providing ventilatory support for patients with severe airway obstruction resulting from chronic bronchitis and emphysema
   III. Administering anesthetic gases to patients with small-diameter endotracheal tubes
   IV. Delivering oxygen therapy to asthmatic children
      a. I and II only
      b. I and III only
      c. I, II, and III only
      d. I, II, III, and IV

10. You are asked to administer a helium-oxygen mixture to an asthmatic patient who is admitted to the emergency department with acute respiratory distress. Which of the following devices is the most appropriate method of delivering this form of medical gas therapy?
    a. air entrainment mask
    b. partial rebreathing mask
    c. nasal cannula
    d. nonrebreathing mask

11. Which of the following is an indication for nitric oxide therapy?
    I. It has been used successfully to treat persistent pulmonary hypertension of the newborn.
    II. It can be used as an adjunct to the treatment of congenital cardiac defects.
    III. It can be used to reverse pulmonary vasoconstriction associated with adult respiratory distress syndrome.
    IV. It can be used to treat refractory croup.
       a. I and III only
       b. II and IV only
       c. I, II, and III only
       d. I, II, III, and IV

12. The gas flow delivered to a patient receiving a 70%:30% (helium:oxygen) mixture is indicated on the standard oxygen flowmeter as 10 L/min. What is the actual gas flow delivered to the patient?
    a. 5.6 L/min
    b. 6.25 L/min
    c. 16 L/min
    d. 18 L/min

13. When carbogen is administered, which of the following vital signs should be monitored?
    I. Pulse
    II. Blood pressure
    III. Respirations
    IV. Mental status
       a. I and II only
       b. I and III only
       c. I, III, and IV only
       d. I, II, III, and IV

14. Which of the following statements are true regarding nitric oxide therapy?
    I. Nitric oxide is a potent vasoconstrictor.
    II. Nitric oxide is supplied in compressed-gas cylinders constructed of steel.
    III. Nitrogen dioxide and nitric oxide are toxic if inhaled.
    IV. The therapeutic dose of nitric oxide is 2 to 80 ppm.
       a. I and II only
       b. II and III only
       c. III and IV only
       d. I, III, and IV only

15. Which of the following would be considered clinical manifestations of carbon dioxide toxicity?
    I. Hypertension
    II. Bounding pulse
    III. $PaCO_2$ > 70 mm Hg
    IV. Multiple premature ventricular contractions
       a. I and II only
       b. II and III only
       c. I, II, and III only
       d. I, II, III, and IV

References

1. Ward JJ: Equipment for mixed gas and oxygen therapy. In Barnes TA, editor: Core *textbook of respiratory care practice,* ed 2, St Louis, 1994, Mosby.
2. Petty TL: Historical highlights of long-term oxygen therapy, *Respir Care* 45:29, 2000.
3. American Association for Respiratory Care: Clinical practice guideline: oxygen therapy in the home or alternative site health care facility—2007 revision and update, *Respir Care* 52:1063, 2007.
4. American Association for Respiratory Care: Clinical practice guideline: oxygen therapy for adults in the acute care facility—2002 revision and update, *Respir Care* 47:717, 2002.
5. American Association for Respiratory Care: Clinical practice guideline: selection of an oxygen delivery device for neonatal and pediatric patients—2002 revision and update, *Respir Care* 47:707, 2002.
6. Vain NE, Prudent LM, Stevens DP, et al: Regulation of oxygen concentrations delivered to infants by nasal cannulas, *Am J Dis Child* 143:1458, 1989.
7. Waugh JB, Granger WM: An evaluation of two new devices for nasal high-flow gas therapy, *Respir Care* 49:902, 2004.
8. Heimlich HJ: Respiratory rehabilitation with a transtracheal oxygen system, *Ann Otol Rhinol Laryngol* 91:643, 1982.
9. Saponsnick AB, Hess D: Oxygen therapy: administration and management. In Hess D, MacIntyre N, Adams A et al: *Respiratory care: principles and practice,* Philadelphia, 2002, WB Saunders.
10. Johnson JT, Dauber JH, Hoffman LA, et al: Transtracheal delivery of oxygen: efficacy and safety for long-term continuous therapy, *Ann Otol Rhinol Laryngol* 100:108, 1991.
11. Tieb BL, Lewis MI: Oxygen conservation and oxygen conserving devices, *Chest* 92:263, 1987.
12. Shigeoka JW, Bonnekat HW: The current status of oxygen-conserving devices, *Respir Care* 30:833, 1985.
13. Boothby VM, Lovelace WR, Bulbulian AH: I. Oxygen administration: the value of high concentration of oxygen for therapy. II. Oxygen for therapy and aviation: an apparatus for the administration of oxygen or oxygen and helium by inhalation. III. Design and construction of the masks for oxygen inhalation apparatus, *Proc Mayo Clinic* 13:641, 1938.
14. Kacmarek RM: Methods of oxygen delivery in the hospital, *Probl Respir Care* 3:563, 1990.
15. Barach AL, Eckman BS: A physiologically controlled oxygen mask apparatus, *Anesthesiology* 2:421, 1941.
16. Barach AL: Symposium: inhalation therapy historical background, *Anesthesiology* 23:407, 1962.
17. Campbell EJM: A method of controlling oxygen administration which reduces the risk of carbon dioxide retention, *Lancet* 2:12, 1960.
18. Scacci R: Air entrainment masks: jet mixing is how they work; the Bernoulli and Venturi principles are how they don't, *Respir Care* 24:928, 1979.
19. Cohen JL, Demers RR, Sakland M: Air entrainment masks: a performance evaluation, *Respir Care* 22:279, 1977.
20. McPherson S: *Respiratory care equipment,* ed 5, St Louis, 1995, Elsevier-Mosby.
21. Wilkins RL, Stoller JK, Scanlan CL: *Egan's fundamentals of respiratory care,* ed 8, St Louis, 2003, Elsevier-Mosby.
22. Cox D, Gilbe C: Fixed performance oxygen masks, *Anesthesiology* 36:958, 1981.
23. Campbell EJM, Minty KB: Controlled oxygen at 60% concentration, *Lancet* 2:1199, 1976.
24. Fourst GN, Potter MA, Wilons MD, et al: Shortcomings of using two jet nebulizers in tandem with an aerosol face mask, *Chest* 99:1346, 1991.
25. Kuo CD, Lin SE, Wang JH: Aerosol, humidity, and oxygen levels, *Chest* 99:1325, 1991.
26. Mishoe SC, Brooks CW, Dennison FH et al: Octave waveband analysis to determine sound frequencies and intensities produced by nebulizers and humidifier used with hoods, *Respir Care* 40:1120, 1995.
27. Harch PG, McCulllough V: *The oxygen revolution,* New York, 1007, Hatherleigh.
28. Kindall EP: Clinical hyperbaric oxygen therapy. In Bennett P, Elliott D, editors: *The physiology and medicine of diving,* ed 4, Philadelphia, 1993, WB Saunders.
29. Moon RE, Camporesi EM: Clinical applications of hyperbaric oxygen therapy, *Probl Resp Care* 4:176, 1991.
30. Gallagher TJ, Smith RA, Bell GC: Evaluation of mechanical ventilators in a hyperbaric environment, *Space Environ Med* 49:375, 1978.
31. Lustbader D, Fein A: Other modalities of oxygen therapy: hyperbaric oxygen, nitric oxide, and ECMO, *Resp Care Clin North Am* 6:659, 2000.
32. National Heart, Lung and Blood Institute (NHLBI) Workshop Summary: Hyperbaric oxygenation therapy, *Am Rev Resp Dis* 144:1414, 1991.
33. Myers RAM, Snyder SK, Lindberg S, et al: Value of hyperbaric oxygen in suspected carbon monoxide poisoning, *JAMA* 246:2478, 1981.
34. Craig J, Mullins D: Nitric oxide inhalation in infants and children: physiologic and clinical implications, *Am J Crit Care* 4:43, 1995.
35. Roberts JD, Lang P, Bigatello LM: Inhaled nitric oxide in congenital heart disease, *Circulation* 87:447, 1993.
36. Bone RC: A new therapy for the adult respiratory distress syndrome, *N Engl J Med* 328:431, 1993.
37. Bigatello LM, Hurford WE, Kacmarek RM, et al: Prolonged inhalation of low concentrations of nitric oxide in patients with severe adult respiratory distress syndrome: effects on pulmonary hemodynamics and oxygenation, *Anesthesiology* 80:761, 1994.
38. Brown RH, Zerhouni EA, Hirshman C: Reversal of bronchoconstriction by inhaled nitric oxide: histamine versus methacholine, *Am J Resp Crit Care Med* 150:233, 1994.
39. Hess D, Ritz R, Branson RD: Delivery systems for inhaled nitric oxide, *Resp Care Clin North Am* 3:371, 1997.
40. Hess DH, Bigatello LM, Hurford WE: Toxicity and complications of inhaled nitric oxide, *Resp Care Clin North Am* 3:487, 1997.
41. Barach AL: The therapeutic use of helium, *JAMA* 107:1273, 1935.
42. Hess SE, Fink JB, Venkastaraman ST et al: The history and physics of heliox, *Respir Care* 51:608, 2006.
43. Kim K, Saville AL, Sikes KL et al: Heliox-driven albuterol nebulization for asthma exacerbations: an overview, *Respir Care* 51:613, 2006.
44. Stillwell PC, Quick JD, Munro PR, et al: Effectiveness of open-circuit and Oxy-Hood delivery of helium-oxygen, *Chest* 95:1222, 1989.
45. Skrinskas GJ, Hyland RH, Hutcheon MA: Using helium-oxygen mixtures in the management of acute upper airway obstruction, *Can Med Assoc J* 128:555, 1983.
46. Kemper KJ, Ritz RH, Benson MS, et al: Helium-oxygen mixtures in the treatment of postextubation stridor in pediatric patients, *Crit Care Med* 19:356, 1991.
47. Nelson DS, McClellan L: Helium-oxygen mixtures as adjunctive support for refractory viral croup, *Ohio State Med J* 78:729, 1982.
48. Myers TR: Use of heliox in children, *Respir Care* 51:619, 2006.
49. Emergency Care Research Institute: Cylinders with unmixed helium-oxygen, *Health Devices* 19:146, 1990.

Internet Resources

American Association for Respiratory Care (Clinical Practice Guidelines): http://www.aarc.org

The American College of Hyperbaric Medicine: http://www.hyperbaricmedicine.org

American Lung Association: http://www.lungusa.org

Global Anesthesiology Server Network: http://gasnet.med.yale.edu

Joint Commission on Accreditation of Healthcare Organizations: http://www.jcaho.org

Mallinckrodt: http://www.mallinckrodt.com

Medexplorer (search engine for medicine): http://www.medexplorer.com

The Undersea and Hyperbaric Medical Society: http://www.uhms.org

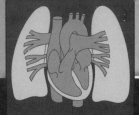

CHAPTER 4

Humidity and Aerosol Therapy

JIM FINK

OUTLINE

Humidity Therapy
Physiologic Control of Heat and Moisture Exchange
Indications for Humidification and Warming of Inspired Gases
Types of Humidifiers
Heat and Moisture Exchangers
Problem Solving and Troubleshooting for Humidification Systems

Selecting the Appropriate Humidity and Bland Aerosol Therapy
Aerosol Therapy
Characteristics of Therapeutic Aerosols
Hazards of Aerosol Therapy
Aerosol Drug Delivery Systems
New Nebulizer Designs
Selecting an Aerosol Drug Delivery System
Special Considerations

OBJECTIVES

Upon completion of this chapter, you will be able to:
· Differentiate humidity from aerosol.
· Differentiate the roles of humidity and aerosol in respiratory care.
· Describe the mechanisms of humidification.
· Describe the natural physiologic humidification process throughout the respiratory tract.
· Identify the indications, contraindications, and hazards associated with humidity therapy.
· Describe how various types of humidifiers work.
· Compare and contrast low-flow and high-flow humidifiers.
· Explain the importance of monitoring and maintaining humidity therapy.
· Describe the physical characteristics of an aerosol.
· Discuss factors that influence aerosol deposition.
· Describe the therapeutic indications for aerosol therapy.
· Identify special considerations for administering aerosol therapy.
· Determine the optimum technique for administering aerosol: small-volume nebulizer, large-volume nebulizer, pressurized metered-dose inhaler, or dry powder inhaler.
· Explain how pneumatic, ultrasonic, and vibrating mesh aerosol generators work.
· Discuss criteria for device selection.
· Describe how each type of device should be set up, used, and maintained.

KEY TERMS

absolute humidity
adiabatic
aerosol
aerosol output
aging
atomizer
baffle
body temperature and pressure saturated (BTPS)
breath-actuated nebulizer
breath-enhanced nebulizer
brownian motion

bubble humidifier
chlorofluorocarbons (CFCs)
condensation
deposition
diffusion
dry powder inhaler (DPI)
emitted dose
evaporation
fine-particle fraction (FP)
geometric standard deviation (GSD)

heat and moisture exchangers (HMEs)
heated wires
heterodisperse
humidifier
humidity
humidity deficit
hydrofluoroalkane
hydrophobic
hygrometer
hygroscopic
inertial impaction

KEY TERMS—cont'd

inhaled mass
inhaler
inspissated
International Organization for
    Standardization (ISO)
isothermic saturation boundary
    (ISB)
large-volume jet nebulizer
large-volume nebulizer (LVN)
mass median aerodynamic
    diameter (MMAD)

monodisperse
nebulizer
passover humidifier
piezoelectric ceramic
    transducer
pressurized metered-dose
    inhaler (pMDI)
relative humidity (RH)
residual drug volume
respirable mass
sedimentation

servo-controlled systems
small-volume nebulizer
    (SVN)
spacer
therapeutic index
ultrasonic nebulizer (USN)
vibrating mesh
volume median diameter
    (VMD)
wick humidifier

Vapors and mists have been used for thousands of years to treat patients with respiratory diseases. Respiratory therapists use these treatments routinely at the bedside in the form of water vapor **(humidity),** bland water aerosols, and active medicated aerosols. This chapter reviews the principles, methods, and devices typically used to deliver humidity and aerosol therapy.

Humidity is water that exists in the form of individual molecules in the vaporous or gaseous state. Molecules of water (0.001 μm) are much smaller than medical aerosols, which can range from 0.2 to 50 μm. A vapor consists of individual free molecules of a substance that exist below its critical temperature; humidity, therefore, often is described as water vapor. An **aerosol** is a suspension of solid or liquid particles in a gas. Aerosols occur in nature as pollens, spores, dust, smoke, smog, fog, and mist.[1] Medical aerosols, which are generated with an **atomizer,** a **nebulizer,** or an **inhaler,** can be used to deliver bland water solutions to the respiratory tract or to administer drugs to the lungs, throat, or nose for both local and systemic effects.

Water vapor exerts a pressure (P_{H2O}) that results from the continuous random movement of water molecules (i.e., kinetic activity). As the temperature of a gas increases, water vapor pressure also increases because gas molecules move faster, resulting in a greater number of molecular collisions. As molecular collisions increase, kinetic activity increases, and water molecules leave the liquid state and evaporate (i.e., enter into a vaporous, or molecular, state).

As discussed in Chapter 1, the energy required to vaporize a liquid is called the *latent heat of vaporization.* As water is heated to its boiling point and molecules leave the liquid state, water vapor is produced. The boiling point of water is influenced by the pressure above the water's surface. If this pressure increases, the boiling point increases (this is the principle by which pressure cookers and steam autoclaves work). Similarly, if the pressure decreases, the boiling point decreases (this is the reason water boils faster at a lower temperature in the mountains). **Evaporation** occurs when liquid molecules near the surface contain enough kinetic energy to break free and enter a vaporous state, reducing the volume and energy contained in the liquid.

BOX 4-1	Calculating the Relative Humidity

The actual water content (absolute humidity) of a sample of room air is measured with a hygrometer and is found to be 12 mg/L. If the room air temperature is 20° C (68° F), what is the relative humidity?

STEP 1
Refer to Table 4-1, locate 20°C, and note the water content, which is the maximum amount of water a gas sample at this temperature can hold.

STEP 2
The relative humidity (RH) is the ratio of the actual amount of water in the gas sample (content) to the amount the gas sample can hold when saturated with water vapor (capacity). To calculate the relative humidity, divide the content by the capacity:

$$\frac{\text{Measured humidity (content)}}{\text{Water capacity}} \times 100 = \text{Relative humidity}$$

$$\frac{12 \text{ mg/L}}{17 \text{ mg/L}} = 71\%$$

STEP 3
Interpret the answer. In this case, the room air is holding 71% of what it is capable of holding at 20° C.
    What would the RH be at body temperature?

Humidity usually is described in terms of *absolute humidity* or *relative humidity.* **Absolute humidity** is the actual content or weight of water present in a given volume of gas (expressed in grams per cubic meter [g/m³] or milligrams per liter [mg/L]). **Relative humidity (RH)** is the ratio of the actual content or weight of the water present in a gas sample relative to the sample's capacity to hold water at that temperature. The RH is calculated by dividing the amount of water in the gas (content) by the amount of water the gas can hold at that temperature (capacity). This ratio is expressed as a percentage and can be calculated using humidity measurements of weight (mg/L) or partial pressure (P_{H2O}). Box 4-1 shows an example of how to calculate the relative humidity.

Humidity can be measured with a **hygrometer.** Hygrometers can work on a variety of principles. For example, a psychrometer uses two thermometers (one wet and one dry). The device is rotated rapidly through the air to ventilate the wet and dry bulbs of the thermometers. The difference between the temperatures measured with the two thermometers is used to calculate the relative humidity. Electronic hygrometers use a transducing element with electrical properties that change with water content. Some electronic hygrometers have sensors small enough to be used to monitor humidity and temperature in a ventilator circuit. However, some problems exist with this technology, and once saturated, these hygrometers are not reliable for reporting changes in humidity over time. At best, they should be used only for spot checks.

When the amount of water a gas contains is equal to the gas's capacity to hold water, the RH is 100% and the gas is saturated. Table 4-1 shows the relationship between absolute humidity and water vapor pressure at various temperatures when the gas is saturated with water. Note that at sea level, a gas at **body temperature and pressure saturated (BTPS)** has a water vapor pressure of 47 mm Hg and contains 43.9 mg of water per liter of gas. As is discussed later in this chapter, these are the conditions found in the lung under normal circumstances.

It is important to understand that when the absolute humidity is held constant, increasing the temperature of the gas decreases the RH, because the higher temperatures increase the gas's capacity to hold water. In contrast, a decrease in the temperature of the gas decreases the gas's capacity to hold water. Water molecules in excess of the amount of water vapor the saturated gas can hold combine

to condense into liquid droplets. In nature, this is described as *fog formation*. The liquid particles suspended in gas (aerosols) continue to collect water molecules, growing larger and heavier. As the particles collide and coalesce (on each other and on surfaces), they condense, fall out of suspension, and form larger bodies of liquid.

In many respiratory care devices, this **condensation** can accumulate in the lowest point of delivery tubing, and it must be removed to eliminate the possibility of the water obstructing the gas delivery tube, disrupting gas and humidity delivery to the patient.

HUMIDITY THERAPY

Humidity therapy involves adding water vapor to inspired gas. An understanding of the respiratory system's control of heat and moisture exchange is essential for determining the need for and the appropriate level of humidity therapy.

Physiologic Control of Heat and Moisture Exchange

Heat and moisture exchange is one of the primary functions of the respiratory tract.[1] The upper airways add heat and humidity to inspired gases during inhalation and cool and reclaim water during exhalation. The nasal mucosa is kept moist by secretions from mucous glands, goblet cells, transudation of fluid through cell walls, and condensation of exhaled humidity. The vascular mucosa lining the sinuses, trachea, and bronchi promote effective heat transfer by serving as an active energy source for heating and humidifying inspired gases. The tortuous path of gas through the turbinates increases contact between the inspired air and the mucosa. As the inspired air enters the nose, it is warmed by convection and picks up water vapor from the moist mucosal lining by evaporation, thus cooling the mucosal surface.

During exhalation, the expired gas transfers heat back to the cooler tracheal and nasal mucosa by convection. As the saturated gas cools, the water vapor in the exhaled gas condenses because it holds less water vapor, and water is reabsorbed by mucus (rehydration). In cold environments, the formation of condensate may exceed the ability of mucus to reabsorb water (resulting in a "runny nose"). The mouth is less efficient than the nose because of the relatively low ratio of gas volume to moist surface area of the less vascular squamous epithelium lining the oropharynx and hypopharynx. When a person inhales through the mouth at normal room temperature, temperatures at the hypopharynx are about 3° C lower and the RH is about 20% less than when a person inhales through the nose. During exhalation, the mouth is much less efficient than the nose at reclaiming heat and water.[2]

As Figure 4-1 shows, the **isothermic saturation boundary (ISB)** is the point where inhaled gas reaches saturation (100% relative humidity at a body temperature of 37° C); this point typically is 5 cm below the carina.[3] Below the

TABLE 4-1

Absolute Humidity and Water Vapor Pressure at Various Temperatures when the Gas Is Saturated with Water

Temperature (°C)	Absolute Humidity (mg/L)	Water Vapor Pressure (mm Hg)
19	16.3	16.5
20	17.3	17.5
21	18.4	18.6
22	19.4	19.8
23	20.6	21.0
24	21.8	22.3
25	23.0	23.7
26	24.4	25.1
27	25.8	26.7
28	27.2	28.3
29	28.8	29.9
30	30.4	31.7
31	32.0	33.6
32	33.8	35.5
33	35.6	37.6
34	37.6	39.8
35	39.6	42.0
36	41.7	44.4
37	43.9	46.9
38	46.2	49.5
39	48.6	52.3
40	51.1	55.1
41	53.7	58.1

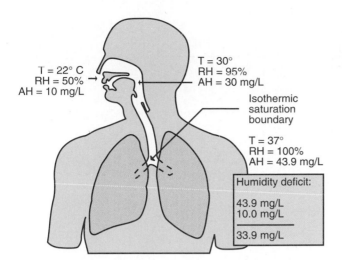

FIGURE 4-1 When a person breathes typical ambient air, the upper airway adds 20 mg/L of water vapor and the lower airway adds 13.9 mg/L. If all that humidity were exhaled, this would represent a 33.9 mg/L humidity deficit.

BOX 4-2	Clinical Signs and Symptoms of Inadequate Airway Humidification

- Atelectasis
- Dry, nonproductive cough
- Increased airway resistance
- Increased incidence of infection
- Increased work of breathing
- Substernal pain
- Thick, dehydrated secretions

BOX 4-3	Humidity Requirements for Gas Delivery at Various Sites in the Upper and Lower Airway

GAS DELIVERED TO THE NOSE OR MOUTH
50% relative humidity with an absolute humidity level of 10 mg/L at 22° C

GAS DELIVERED TO THE HYPOPHARYNX
95% relative humidity with an absolute humidity level of 28 to 34 mg/L at 29° to 32° C

GAS DELIVERED TO THE MIDTRACHEA
100% relative humidity with an absolute humidity level of 36 to 40 mg/L at 31° to 35° C

ISB, temperature and relative humidity remain constant (BTPS). Temperature and humidity decrease with inspiration and increase with exhalation. The ISB shifts deeper into the lungs when a person inhales through the mouth; breathes cold, dry air through an artificial tracheal airway; or simply increases the minute ventilation. Prolonged and severe shifts of the ISB can damage the airways and compromise the body's normal heat and moisture exchange mechanisms.

Indications for Humidification and Warming of Inspired Gases

The primary goal of humidification is to maintain normal physiologic conditions in the airways. Proper levels of heat and humidity help ensure normal functioning of the mucociliary transport system. When the airways are exposed to relatively cold, dry air, ciliary motility is reduced and the airways become more irritable. The production of mucus increases, and pulmonary secretions become thick and **inspissated.** The hazards of breathing dry gas are even greater when the upper airway is bypassed, as occurs with endotracheal intubation[4]; prolonged breathing of improperly conditioned gases through a tracheal airway can lead to serious consequences. Box 4-2 provides a summary of the signs and symptoms associated with breathing cold, dry gases.

When the relative humidity of inspired gas is greater than 60% of BTPS conditions, no injury is believed to occur in normal lungs.[5,6] As Figure 4-1 shows, the targeted level of heat and humidity depends on the site of gas delivery (e.g., nose/mouth, hypopharynx, or trachea). Box 4-3 summarizes the recommended humidity levels for administering medical gases based on current standards.[7,8]

In addition to maintaining normal humidity levels in the airway, warm, humidified gases are used to raise the core temperature of hypothermic patients, to prevent intraoperative hypothermia, and to alleviate bronchospasm in patients with reactive airways when they breathe cold air.[9-12] Cool, humidified gas often is used with bland aerosol delivery to treat upper airway inflammation caused by croup, epiglottitis, and postextubation edema.

Types of Humidifiers

A **humidifier** is a device that adds molecular water to gas. This occurs by means of evaporation of water from a surface, such as a reservoir, a wick, or a sphere of water in suspension (i.e., aerosol). Box 4-4 summarizes the various factors that can affect the quality of a humidifier's performance. These factors include (1) temperature, (2) surface area, (3) time of contact, and (4) thermal mass.

Humidifiers generally are classified as active and passive devices. Figure 4-2 shows the three primary types of active humidifiers: (1) bubble, (2) aerosol, and (3) passover, which includes wick and membrane devices. The most common examples of a passive humidifier are **heat and moisture exchangers (HMEs).** Design and performance requirements for all medical humidifiers are established by the American Society for Testing and Materials (ASTM).[13]

Bubble Humidifiers

Bubble humidifiers direct gas through a tube or channel into the bottom of a water reservoir, where the gas stream produces bubbles that rise through the water and pass through the device outlet to the patient (Figure 4-3). The

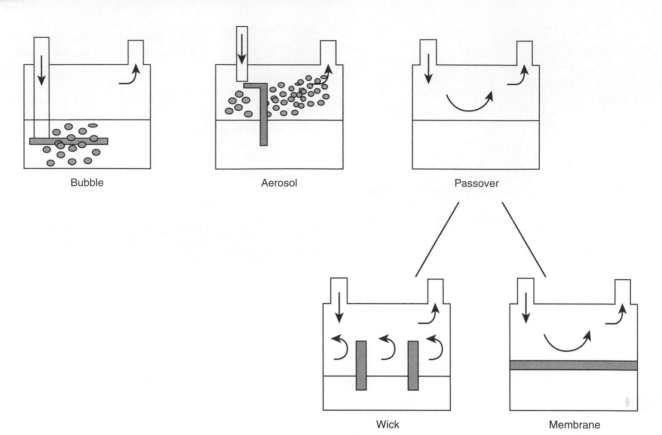

FIGURE 4-2 Primary types of active humidifiers. Gas passes through the water (bubble) or around drops of water (aerosol), or gas passes over the surface of water (passover), a saturated material (wick), or a semipermeable membrane (membrane).

BOX 4-4	Physical Principles Governing Humidifier Function

- *Temperature:* The higher the temperature of a gas, the more water vapor it can hold (increased capacity). The colder the gas, the less water vapor it can hold.
- *Surface area:* The greater the surface area of contact between water and gas, the more opportunity for evaporation to occur.
- *Contact time:* The longer a gas remains in contact with water, the greater the opportunity for evaporation to occur. For example, the slower the gas flow through a heated body of water or chamber, the more heat and water vapor are transferred to the gas. In contrast, a humidifier that fully heats and humidifies gas at low to moderate flows may fail to maintain that level of humidity with high peak flows.
- *Thermal mass:* The greater the mass of water or the core element of a humidifier, the greater its capacity to hold and transfer heat. As heat is transferred from the thermal mass, the differential between the core and the gas is reduced, and the speed of heat transfer is reduced.

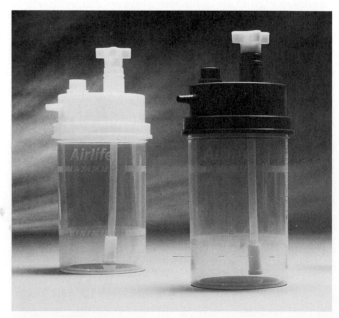

FIGURE 4-3 Bubble humidifier. (Courtesy Cardinal Health, McGraw, Illinois.)

gas within the bubbles is humidified as the bubbles rise to the water's surface. Increasing the height of the water column above the gas outlet increases the humidity content of the bubbles by allowing a longer contact time.

Standard low-flow bubble humidifiers incorporate pressure-relief gravity or spring-loaded valves that release high pressures (above 2 psi) to prevent bursting of the humidifier bottle and warn of flow path obstruction. Humidifier pop-off valves typically provide both audible and visible alarms, which automatically resume normal operation once the excess pressure has been vented.[13] If the system is obstructed at or near the patient interface and the pop-off sounds, the system is leak free; failure of the pop-off valve to produce an alerting sound may indicate a leak (or a faulty pop-off valve).

Unheated bubble humidifiers are commonly used with low-flow oral-nasal oxygen delivery systems when the goal is to raise the water vapor content of the gas to ambient levels. An unheated bubble humidifier can provide an absolute humidity level of 10 to 20 mg/L.[14-16] An absolute humidity of 10 mg/L in a gas corresponds to a 50% RH at standard room temperatures, but only a 20% RH at BTPS. Notice that as gas flow increases, the reservoir cools by as much as 10° C, thus limiting the effectiveness of providing humidity at flow rates higher than 10 L/min.

Bubble size is governed by the design of the gas outlet at the bottom of the capillary tube. A device with an open lumen makes larger bubbles than one that uses a diffuser made of plastic foam, porous metal, or a plastic or metal mesh (Figure 4-4). Diffuser humidifiers are designed to create a large number of small bubbles, allowing a greater surface area for gas and water interaction.[8] (It is important to recognize that although larger bubbles have greater surface area, the greater internal volume of these bubbles produces a lower surface to volume ratio than smaller bubbles.)

Adding heat to a bubble humidifier increases the absolute humidity in the gas. However, in bubble humidifiers designed for low-flow oxygen applications, condensation can occur with heating, and liquid droplets can form in the narrow tubing, obstructing the gas pathway. Condensate therefore is an important issue with any heated humidification system. This problem can be partially averted by using large-bore (10- to 22-mm internal diameter [ID]) corrugated tubing, which results in a less immediate risk of obstruction, and by placing a water trap at the lowest point of the tubing circuit to collect condensate. **Heated wires** also can be added to the circuit to minimize the formation of condensate.

High-flow bubble humidifiers are available for use during mechanical ventilation. They were designed to accommodate flow rates of gas delivered up to 100 L/min. It is worth mentioning that absolute humidity decreases during periods of peak flow with these devices. Consequently, the absolute humidity of gas passing through a heated humidifier can change during the course of an individual breath. Manufacturers have attempted to address this issue by using 22-mm ID inlet and outlets ports on high-flow humidifiers. In addition, these devices typically have shallower reservoirs than low-flow humidifiers, and they use bubble diffusers, which allow for a greater air-liquid interface. Note that the system compensates for the reduced water contact time by heating the reservoir (up to 50° C). Figure 4-5 shows how the exiting gas cools as it passes through a 6-foot corrugated aerosol tube to the patient and yet still is 37° C at the patient's airway. Because the gas in the standard corrugated aerosol tubing is hotter than the ambient air surrounding it, the gas cools as it travels through the 5- to 6-foot inspiratory limb of the ventilator circuit. Water content drops from 84 mg/L to 44 mg/L as vapor, the difference forming condensate in the circuit tubing. High-flow humidifiers do not typically have internal pop-off valves.

Aerosol Generators

Humidity is simply water in the gas phase; a bland aerosol, however, consists of liquid particles suspended in a gas providing both humidity and additional liquid applied locally to the airway. Bland aerosol therapy involves the delivery of sterile water or hypotonic, isotonic, or hypertonic saline aerosols. The American Association for Respiratory Care (AARC) has published a Clinical Practice Guideline on Bland Aerosol Administration.[17] Devices used to generate bland aerosols include large-volume jet nebulizers and ultrasonic nebulizers. Aerosol delivery systems can include a variety of direct airway appliances, such as aerosol face masks, tracheostomy masks, face tents, and enclosures such as mist tents.

Large-Volume Jet Nebulizers. A **large-volume jet nebulizer** is the device most commonly used to generate bland aerosols. Liquid particle aerosols are generated by passing gas at a high velocity through a small "jet" orifice (Figure 4-6). The resulting low pressure generated at the

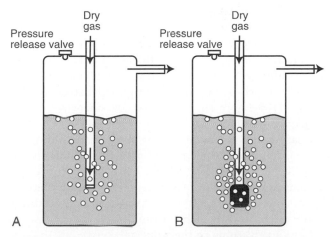

FIGURE 4-4 Bubble humidifiers pass gas under the surface of the water using an open lumen **(A)** or a diffuser **(B)**. Diffusers tend to make smaller bubbles with a higher surface to volume ratio for humidification.

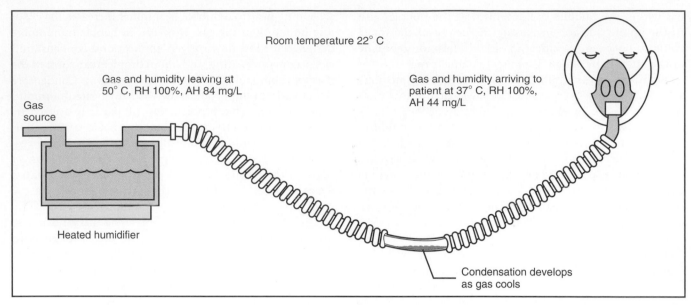

Room temperature 22° C

Gas and humidity leaving at
50° C, RH 100%, AH 84 mg/L

Gas and humidity arriving to
patient at 37° C, RH 100%,
AH 44 mg/L

Gas
source

Heated humidifier

Condensation develops
as gas cools

FIGURE 4-5 Condensation forms in a gas delivery tube as heated humidity is cooled by ambient conditions surrounding the tube. As the temperature of the gas cools (up to 1° C per foot of 22-mm corrugated tubing), excess water leaves the gas and accumulates in the gravity-dependent loops of the delivery tubing.

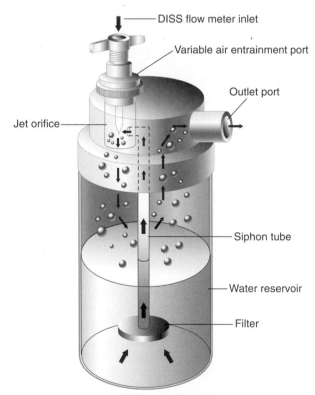

DISS flow meter inlet

Variable air entrainment port

Outlet port

Jet orifice

Siphon tube

Water reservoir

Filter

FIGURE 4-6 Diagram of a large-volume jet nebulizer with a variable entrainment port. (From Wilkins RL, Stoller JK, Kacmarek RM: *Egan's fundamentals of respiratory care,* ed 9, St Louis, 2009, Mosby.)

jet draws fluid from the reservoir up to the top of a siphon tube, where it is sheared off and shattered into liquid particles (i.e., the Bernoulli principle). The larger, unstable particles fall out of suspension and strike the internal surfaces of the device and the fluid surface, a process called *baffling*. The smaller particles remaining in suspension leave the nebulizer through the outlet port and are carried in the gas stream.

Jet nebulizers typically operate at a flow of 6 to 15 L/min; however, higher flows may be required to meet a patient's inspiratory needs. Devices with air entrainment ports can be used to increase inspiratory flows by allowing for air mixing (Figure 4-7). Also, various levels of fractional inspired oxygen (F_iO_2) can be achieved with these devices. Closed dilution nebulizers use a primary gas to drive the jet nebulizer, and a second gas inlet port can be used to add gas to the nebulizer at a rate greater than 40 L/min (Figure 4-8). Depending on the design, input flow, and air entrainment setting, the total water output of an unheated, large-volume jet nebulizer can vary from 26 to 35 mg H_2O/L. If the device is heated, the output increases to 33 to 55 mg H_2O/L, mainly because of increased vapor capacity.[18,19]

Heating options include a hot plate, wraparound, yolk (collar), or immersion element (Figure 4-9). Unfortunately, many of these devices do not have **servo-controlled systems** to regulate the delivery temperature and therefore do not shut down when the reservoir empties. In addition, failure of the heating element can cause a loss of heating, without any warning to the clinician.

Babington Nebulizer. In this type of nebulizer, fluid is spread over the surface of a glass sphere and struck by compressed gas passing from the inside of the sphere

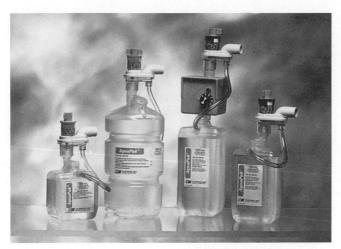

FIGURE 4-7 Hudson RCI Prefilled Precision Nebulizer. (Courtesy Hudson Respiratory Care, Temecula, California.)

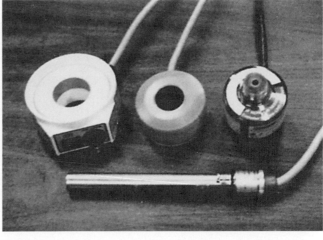

FIGURE 4-9 Heaters used with large-volume nebulizers. (From Scanlan CL, Wilkins RL, Stoller JK: *Egan's fundamentals of respiratory care,* ed 7, St Louis, 1999, Mosby.)

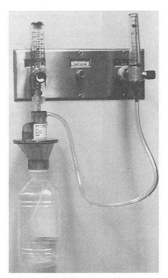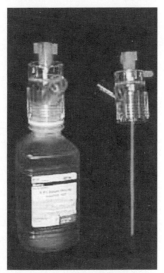

FIGURE 4-8 Two models of closed dilution nebulizers. The primary gas is delivered to the jet, which delivers limited flows up to 40 L/min; the secondary gas port allows additional flow up to 80 L/min. The ratio of oxygen to airflow determines the oxygen concentration and total flow to the patient. (Courtesy Vital Signs, a GE Healthcare company.)

FIGURE 4-10 Diagram of a Babington nebulizer.

through one or more orifices on its surface. The liquid is sheared from the thin layer and directed against a **baffle** (Figure 4-10). The Hydrosphere and the Solosphere, two models of large-volume Babington nebulizers, are no longer manufactured. These devices generated aerosol with a relatively small particle size (less than 2 µm) and had a relatively high aerosol output.

Spinning Disk Devices. Sometimes referred to as a *centrifugal nebulizer,* the spinning disk nebulizer is a mechanical aerosol generator. It operates on the principle that a spinning disk with a hollow shaft draws liquid from the reservoir (Figure 4-11). As the liquid leaves the shaft, it is spread across the top of the disk and contacts a system of

baffles attached to the disk, producing an aerosol. This mechanism is used in many commercially available, large-volume room humidifiers intended for home use.

Larger versions of spinning disk nebulizers (2- to 3-L reservoirs) are used to deliver bland aerosols into mist tents. These enclosure systems can generate flow rates greater than 20 L/min, with water outputs as high as 5 mL/min (300 mL/hr). Because heat buildup is a problem in enclosures, these systems are always unheated.

Ultrasonic Nebulizers. An **ultrasonic nebulizer (USN)** is an electrically powered device that uses a **piezoelectric ceramic transducer** that vibrates at 1.3 to 2.3 mHz (Figure 4-12). These vibrations are transmitted through a liquid to create a cavitation in the liquid, forming a standing wave or "geyser" that sheds aerosol droplets. The vibrational energy is transmitted through a water-filled couplant

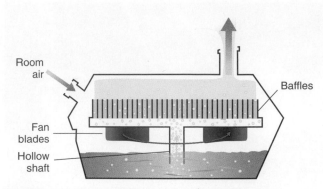

FIGURE 4-11 Diagram of a spinning disk large-volume nebulizer.

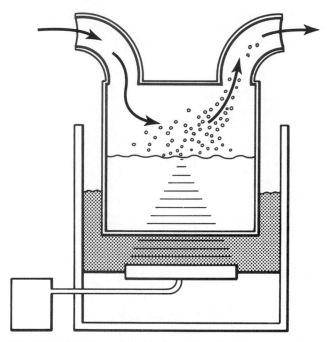

FIGURE 4-12 Ultrasonic nebulizer. High-frequency sound waves from a transducer are transmitted through a tap water couplant to the medication cup, where the fluid forms standing waves, producing aerosol. A gas source (e.g., a fan or compressed gas) is used to move the aerosol from the unit to the patient. (From Barnes TA: *Core textbook for respiratory care practice,* ed 2, St Louis, 1994, Mosby.)

reservoir or directly to a drug solution chamber. Although gas is not required to generate the aerosol, gas flow is required to convey the aerosol particles from the nebulizer to the patient. Some large-volume USNs use a built-in fan to direct room air through the nebulizer chamber. The airflow can be adjusted by changing the fan speed or by using a simple damper valve. As an alternative, compressed anhydrous gases can be delivered to the chamber inlet through a flowmeter. If necessary, the clinician can precisely control the delivered oxygen concentration by attaching a flowmeter with an oxygen blender or air entrainment system to the chamber inlet.

The size of the particles produced by a USN is inversely proportional to the transducer's signal frequency, which is set by the manufacturer. The rate of aerosol production is directly related to the signal's amplitude. In some large-volume USNs, the signal amplitude can be adjusted by the clinician. The flow and amplitude settings interact to determine the density of the aerosol (mg/L) and the total water output (mL/min) (Figure 4-13). At a given amplitude setting, the greater the flow through the chamber, the less dense the aerosol. Conversely, low flows result in higher density aerosols. The total aerosol output (mL/min) is greatest when both flow and amplitude are set at the maximum level. Using these settings, some units can achieve a total water output as high as 7 mL/min. High density and high aerosol output make the large-volume USN a valuable clinical tool for inducing sputum specimens for diagnostic analysis. USNs yield a higher quantity and quality of sputum for analysis than other nebulizers, but at some cost in increased airway reactivity.[20]

It is important to recognize that the particle size, aerosol density, and output of USNs are also affected by the relative humidity of the carrier gas. Because of the considerable energy required to generate aerosols with a USN, the temperature of the solution increases by as much as 20° C during use of the device.

USNs marketed as "cool mist" devices are sold as room humidifiers for home use. The wet, large-volume reservoirs of these devices can easily become contaminated, resulting in airborne transmission of pathogens. Care should be taken to ensure that these units are cleaned according to the manufacturer's recommendations and that water is discarded from the reservoir periodically between cleanings. In the absence of a manufacturer's recommendation, these units should undergo appropriate disinfection at least every 6 days. As is discussed later in this chapter, passover and wick humidifiers present less risk of cross-contamination than does a USN used as a room humidifier.

Patient Interface Appliances. Airway appliances used to deliver bland aerosol therapy include the aerosol mask, face tent, T-tube, and tracheostomy mask. In all cases, large-bore tubing (22-mm ID) is used to minimize flow resistance and prevent occlusion by condensate. The aerosol mask and face tent are used with patients who have intact upper airways. T-tubes and tracheostomy masks are used for patients who have been intubated with an endotracheal tube or who have a tracheostomy tube in place. Tracheostomy masks can be used only for patients with tracheostomies.

For short-term therapy in patients with intact upper airways, the aerosol mask is the device of choice. However, some patients cannot tolerate masks and may do better with a face tent. No data are available to support preferential use of an open aerosol mask versus a face tent.

Although the T-tube is the most common application for tracheostomy patients, unless moderate to high F_IO_2 levels are needed, a tracheostomy mask may be a better

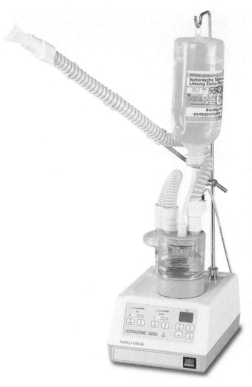
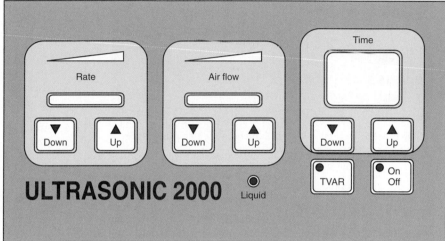

FIGURE 4-13 The Ultrasonic 2000, a large-volume ultrasonic nebulizer, which has controls for adjusting the fan flow and the nebulizer output rate. (Courtesy Nouvag AG, Goldach, Switzerland.)

choice. Unlike T-tubes, tracheostomy masks exert no traction on the airway, and they allow secretions and condensate to escape from the airway, reducing airway resistance.

A limitation of standard aerosol masks is the large venting holes that allow room air to be inhaled, which dilutes the gas and aerosol delivered. As mentioned previously, standard large-volume nebulizers do not have sufficient output to match the peak inspiratory flow of many patients. Aerosol masks can be modified by adding 6-inch sections of the 22-mm ID aerosol tubing to the ports, which provides a small reservoir when peak inspiratory flow exceeds gas flow delivered to the mask (Figure 4-14). An alternate strategy is to increase the aerosol output to the patient by setting up two aerosol devices in tandem and connecting them by a T-piece to the aerosol mask (Figure 4-15).

Box 4-5 provides a step-by-step approach to setting up a large-volume jet nebulizer. (See Clinical Rounds 4-1.)

Mist Tents and Hoods. Infants and small children may not easily tolerate direct airway appliances such as masks, therefore enclosures such as mist tents and aerosol hoods are used to deliver bland aerosol therapy to these patients. Recent studies have shown that in infants, aerosol hoods can provide aerosol delivery with an efficiency similar to that of a properly fitted aerosol mask, with less discomfort for the patient.

Because mist tents were used for more than 40 years mainly to treat croup, clinicians often still refer to these

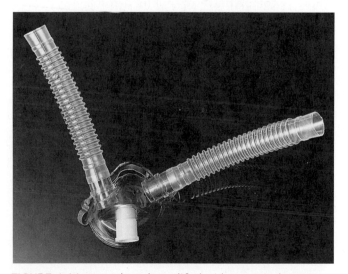

FIGURE 4-14 Aerosol mask modified with two 6-inch sections of 22-mm ID aerosol tubing. Each 6-inch section has a 50-mL internal volume.

devices as "croup tents." The use of this device to treat croup patients is based on the theory that a cool mist promotes vasoconstriction, reduces edema, and diminishes upper airway obstruction.

Mist tents and hood enclosures present two major problems for many patients: carbon dioxide (CO_2) buildup and heat retention. The buildup of CO_2 can be reduced by providing sufficiently high gas flow rates. High flows of

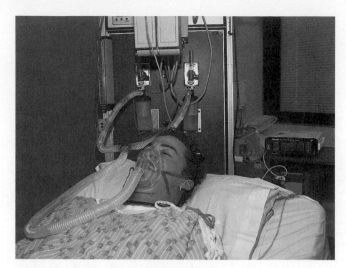

FIGURE 4-15 Two entrainment large-volume nebulizers are combined to create a high-flow system.

fresh gas circulate continually through the enclosure and "wash out" carbon dioxide while helping maintain the desired oxygen concentrations. Heat retention is handled differently by each manufacturer. Some devices (e.g., the Maxicool) use high flows of fresh gas to prevent heat buildup. Others incorporate a separate cooling device. Some tent devices (e.g., the Air Shields Croupette) use a simple ice compartment to cool the aerosol.

The Ohmeda Ohio Pediatric Aerosol Tent (Figure 4-16) and the Mistogen CAM-2M Tent use electrically powered refrigeration units to cool the circulating air. The cooling from these refrigeration units produces a great deal of condensation, which must be drained into a collection bottle outside the tent. The problem was resolved in the Mistogen CAM-3M Tent through the use of a thermoelectric cooling system, in which an electric current passing through a semiconductor augments heat absorption and release. As warm air is taken from the tent, heat is transferred and released in the room while cool air is returned to the tent.

Problem Solving and Troubleshooting for Bland Aerosol Systems. The most common problems with bland aerosol delivery systems involve infection control, environmental safety, inadequate mist production, overhydration, bronchospasm, and noise.

Infection control can be aided by rigorous adherence to infection control guidelines, especially those covering equipment processing. For example, water should be changed regularly, and the couplant compartments and nebulizer chambers of USNs should be disinfected or replaced regularly. Careful compliance with these measures helps minimize the risks involved in the use of aerosol systems.

Environmental safety concerns regarding secondhand and exhaled aerosol arise mainly when aerosol therapy is prescribed for immunosuppressed patients or patients who have been diagnosed with active tuberculosis. Respira-

BOX 4-5	Setting Up a Cool or Heated Air Entrainment Large-Volume Jet Nebulizer

1. Obtain the appropriate equipment:
   Oxygen flowmeter
   Nebulizer
   Large-bore corrugated tubing
   Drain bag
   Appropriate patient interface (i.e., aerosol mask, face tent, tracheostomy collar, or T-piece)
   Oxygen analyzer
   Thermometer (heated aerosol)
   Heating device (heated aerosol)
2. Attach flowmeter to 50-psi outlet.
3. Assemble the nebulizer. Aseptically fill the device with sterile water for inhalation if it was not prefilled.
4. Attach the nebulizer to the flowmeter.
5. Attach the large-bore corrugated tubing to the nebulizer.
6. Position the tubing so the drain bag is in the lowest position.
7. Attach the patient interface.
8. Turn on the gas flow to the nebulizer and adjust the entrainment collar to the appropriate fractional delivered oxygen (F_DO_2). Verify the F_DO_2 with the oxygen analyzer and adjust the entrainment collar as necessary to obtain the F_DO_2.
9. Make sure that the device is producing an adequate gas flow and then apply the interface to the patient. Confirm adequacy of the gas flow by observing the aerosol escaping from the patient interface; the aerosol should not completely disappear during inspiration. If total flow remains inadequate (as demonstrated by complete disappearance of the aerosol during inspiration), increase the oxygen flow to the nebulizer. If the total flow continues to be inadequate and the oxygen flow is at maximum level, change the device to an injection nebulizer or a high-flow heated humidifier.
10. If a heated aerosol is clinically indicated, add the appropriate heating device to the nebulizer. Place a thermometer close to the patient interface and verify that the aerosol has been warmed to a safe operating temperature.

CLINICAL ROUNDS 4-1

After abdominal surgery, a 50-year-old man is brought to the recovery room and started on an aerosol mask at an F_IO_2 of 0.5. While performing your initial assessment of this patient, you notice that his respiratory rate is 20 breaths per minute and he shows signs of respiratory distress. You also note that during inspiration, the aerosol stops flowing from the mask. How would you remedy this situation to ensure that the patient is receiving 50% oxygen?

See Evolve Resources for the answer.

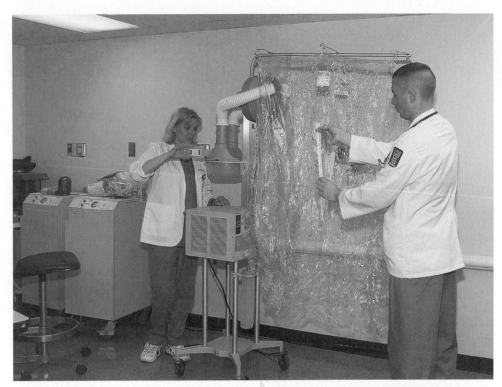

FIGURE 4-16 For this large aerosol tent, a large-volume reservoir and jet nebulizer have been integrated with a compressor-driven cooling unit to dissipate heat buildup in the tent.

tory therapists may be at increased risk for developing asthma-like symptoms, attributed in part to secondhand exposure to aerosols such as ribavirin. To minimize the risk, all clinicians should strictly follow the standards and airborne precautions established by the Centers for Disease Control and Prevention (CDC).

Inadequate mist production is a common problem with all nebulizer systems. With pneumatically powered jet nebulizers, poor mist production can be caused by inadequate input flow of driving gas, loose connections that cause a leak between the source gas and the nebulizer input, siphon tube obstruction, or jet orifice misalignment. Except for inadequate driving gas flow and loose connections, these problems require repair or replacement of the unit. For USNs that are not functioning properly, the electrical power supply (cord, plug, and fuse or circuit breakers) should be checked first. The clinician then should confirm that (1) carrier gas is actually flowing through the device and (2) the amplitude, or output, control is set above minimum. If the unit still has no visible mist output, the clinician should inspect the couplant chamber to confirm that the device has been filled to the proper level and that the nebulizer cup or crystal is free of any visible dirt, debris, or corrosion. Finally, the clinician must make sure that the solution in the couplant chamber meets the manufacturer's specifications (some units do not function properly with distilled water).

Overhydration is a potentially serious problem for patients treated with heated jet nebulizers and USNs.

Because large-volume USNs are capable of high water outputs, they should never be used for continuous therapy. The risk of overhydration is greatest for infants, small children, and those with preexisting fluid or electrolyte imbalances. Even if used only to meet BTPS conditions, bland aerosol therapy effectively eliminates insensible water loss through the lungs and thus should be equated to a daily water gain (approximately 200 mL/day for the average adult). Another complication associated with overhydration is the potential for inspissated pulmonary secretions to swell after high-density aerosol therapy, which ultimately can lead to worsening airway obstruction. Careful patient selection and monitoring can prevent most potential problems with overhydration.

Bland water aerosols can cause bronchospasm in some patients. In fact, ultrasonic nebulization of distilled water is used in some pulmonary function laboratories to provoke bronchospasm and to assess bronchial hyperactivity.[21] To avoid this complication at the bedside, the clinician should always review the patient's history and diagnosis before administering any bland aerosol, especially a hypotonic water solution. As indicated in the AARC Clinical Practice Guideline, patients receiving continuous bland aerosol therapy initially should be monitored closely (including breath sounds and subjective response) and reevaluated every 8 hours or with any change in the patient's clinical condition.[17] If bronchospasm occurs during therapy, treatment must be stopped immediately, oxygen must be provided, and appropriate bronchodilator therapy should be initiated as soon as possible. If the physician still requests bland aerosol therapy for such a patient, pretreatment with a bronchodilator may be required. Also, these patients may better tolerate isotonic solutions (0.9% saline) than water.

A problem unique to large-volume air entrainment jet nebulizers is the noise they generate, especially at high flows. The American Academy of Pediatrics recommends that sound levels be kept below 58 dB to prevent hearing loss in infants cared for in incubators and oxygen hoods. Because a number of commercially available nebulizers exceed this noise level when in operation, careful selection of equipment is necessary.

Passover Humidifiers

A **passover humidifier** directs gas over a liquid or a liquid-saturated surface. The three common types of passover humidifiers are (1) simple reservoir models, (2) wick units, and (3) membrane devices.

The simple reservoir model directs gas over the surface of a volume of water or fluid. The surface for gas-fluid interface is limited. These systems typically are used to provide heated humidified gases during mechanical ventilation. Figure 4-17 shows the Fisher & Paykel MR 850. Passover humidifiers are also used for noninvasive nasal continuous positive airway pressure or bilevel ventilation.

In a **wick humidifier,** gas passes over or through water-saturated material. Figure 4-18 shows a cross section of a wick humidifier designed for placement in a ventilator circuit. The wick (a cylinder of absorbent material) is placed upright with the gravity-dependent end in a water reservoir and surrounded by a heating element. Capillary action continually draws up water from the reservoir and keeps the wick saturated. As dry gas enters the chamber, it flows around the wick, quickly picking up heat and moisture, leaving the chamber fully saturated with water vapor. No bubbling occurs, therefore no aerosol is produced. The Hudson RCI Conchatherm IV (Hudson Respiratory Care, Temecula, California) is an example of this type of humidifier (Figure 4-19).

In a membrane humidifier, the water is separated from the gas stream by a **hydrophobic** membrane. Water vapor molecules can pass through the membrane, but liquid water (and pathogens) cannot. As with wick humidifiers, bubbling and aerosol generation do not occur. Moreover, if a membrane humidifier were to be inspected while in use, no liquid water would be seen in the humidifier chamber.

The Vapotherm 2000i (Vapotherm, Stevensville, Maryland) is a membrane cartridge system (see Figure 3-12). It can heat and humidify oxygen at flows up to 40 L/

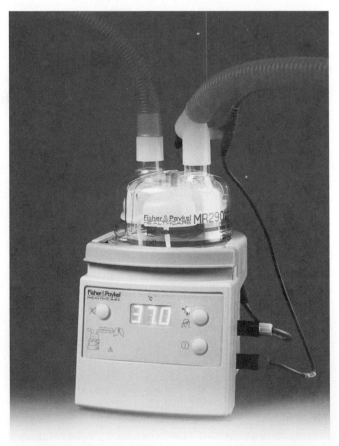

FIGURE 4-17 Fisher & Paykel MR 850 heated humidifier. (Courtesy Fisher & Paykel Healthcare, Irvine, California.)

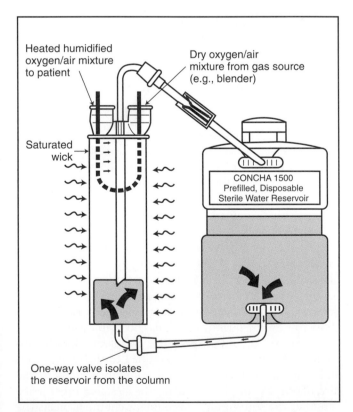

FIGURE 4-18 The low-compliance Conchacolumn with water reservoir assembly. Water enters the bottom of a metal column and saturates an absorbent wick lining the column. The column is inserted into a wraparound heating element. (Redrawn from Hudson Respiratory Care, Temecula, California.)

The SCT 2000 heating element, as well as the Hydrate device (Figure 4-20), represent a relatively new technology that was introduced with the Hydrate. It uses C-force technology based on capillary force vaporization (CFV) (Vapore, Alameda, California, www.vapore.com). The capillary force vaporizer is a thin film, high surface area boiler that combines capillary force and phase transition to impart pressure onto an expanding gas (water vapor) and ejects it. The CFV is driven by software that controls a heater element and water flow. The disk, which is 19 mm in diameter, can deliver up to 2.2 mg/min of water vapor at 37° C. The single-patient use C-force device, which includes the CFV disk mounted in a plastic housing, can be used for mechanical ventilation or high-flow gas. The unit includes a PC board, temperature probe, water and gas flow connecters, and a cable to the controller (Hydrate). Data from prototypes suggest that the temperature can be regulated from 33° to 41° C for flows from 2 to 40 L/min.[32,33]

Humidifier heating systems generally have a controller that regulates the power to the heating element. In the simplest systems, the controller monitors the heating element, varying the delivered current to match either a preset or an adjustable temperature. These systems might use a thermistor placed at the outlet of the humidifier, with the heater set to control output temperature. Servo-controlled heating systems monitor the temperature at the humidifier's outlet and at the patient's airway using a thermistor probe. The controller then adjusts heater power to achieve the desired airway temperature. Both types of controller units usually incorporate alarms and an alarm-activated heater shutdown function.

Reservoir and Feed Systems

Manual Systems

Simple large reservoir systems may be manually refilled with sterile or distilled water. It is important to recognize that manually refilling the reservoir can change the reservoir temperature. Opening the reservoir for refilling can also interrupt mechanical ventilation and increase the risk of cross-contamination. Changing water levels alter the gas compression factor and thus the delivered volume during mechanical ventilation, a critical factor during mechanical ventilation of the neonate.

Gravity Feed System. A small inlet port in the wall of the humidifier chamber attached to a gravity-fed water bag allows refilling without interruption of ventilation. Such systems still require constant checking and manual replenishment by opening the line valve or clamp. If not checked regularly, the reservoir in these systems can go dry, placing the patient at risk.

Automatic feed systems avoid the need for constant checking and manual refilling of humidifiers. The simplest type of automatic feed system is the level-compensated reservoir (see Figure 4-18). In these systems, an external reservoir is aligned horizontally with the humidifier, maintaining relatively consistent water levels between the reservoir and the humidifier chamber. The addition of a siphon

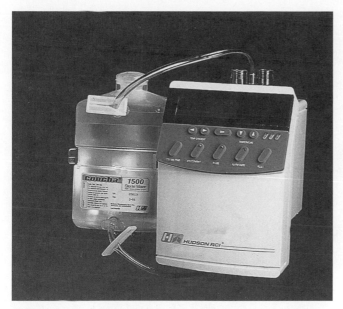

FIGURE 4-19 Hudson RCI Conchatherm IV Heater Humidifier. (Courtesy Hudson Respiratory Care, Temecula, California.)

min. This system has been used to provide high-flow oxygen via nasal cannula to a range of patients from infants to adults. The manufacturer maintains that this technology allows molecular water vapor to pass into the gas stream but prevents direct contact between the water source and breathing gas, thereby creating a bacterial filter. The Hummax II (Metran Medical Instruments, Saitama, Japan) consists of a heated wire and polyethylene microporous hollow fiber placed in the tubing of the inspiratory circuit so that water vapor is delivered throughout the circuit.

Humidifier Heating Systems

Six types of heating elements and strategies are currently available:

- A hot plate element at the base of the humidifier (e.g., the SCT 2000 [Vital Signs, Inc. Totawa, NJ] and the Fisher & Paykel MR 850 [Fisher and Paykel Healthcare Panmure, Auckland, New Zealand]).
- A wraparound element that surrounds the humidifier chamber (e.g., the Conchatherm IV [Hudson] and the Vapotherm [Vapotherm, Stevensville, MD]).
- A yolk (or collar) element that sits between the water reservoir and the gas outlet.
- An immersion heater, with the element actually placed in the water reservoir (e.g., Cascade humidifier [Puritan Bennett, Nellcor Puritan Bennett Yorba Linda, California]).
- A heated wire in the inspiratory limb that warms a saturated wick or hollow fiber (e.g., Anamed [Vital Signs, Inc. Totawa, NJ] and Hummax II [Metran, Chome, Kawaguchi]).
- A thin film, high surface area boiler (e.g., Hydrate [Pari Respiratory Equipment, Midlothian, Virginia]).

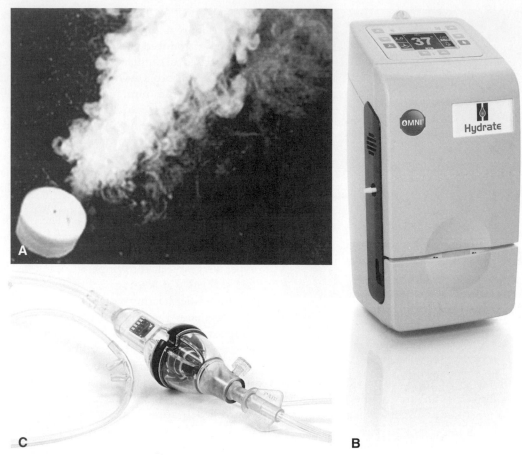

FIGURE 4-20 Hydrate humidification system for high-flow oxygen. (From Wilkins RL, Stoller JK, Kacmarek RM: *Egan's fundamentals of respiratory care,* ed 9, St Louis, 2009, Mosby.)

tube allows the low-compliance Conchacolumn to maintain the same water level independent of the water level in the reservoir.

Flotation valve controls can be used to maintain the fluid volume of the humidifier. In flotation systems, a float rises and falls with the water level. If the water level falls below a preset value, the float opens the feed valve; as the water rises back to the set fill level, the float closes the feed valve (Fisher and Paykel 290 chamber, Panmure, Auckland, New Zealand). Membrane humidifiers typically do not require a sophisticated flow control system. Because the liquid water chamber underlying the membrane cannot overfill, membrane humidifiers require only an open gravity feed system to ensure proper function.

Condensation. In standard heated humidifier systems, saturated gas cools as it leaves the point of humidification en route to the patient. As the gas cools, its water vapor capacity decreases, resulting in condensation, or "rain out." Factors that influence the amount of condensation include (1) the temperature difference across the system (humidifier to airway); (2) the ambient temperature; (3) the gas flow; (4) the set airway temperature; and (5) the length, diameter, and thermal mass of the breathing circuit.

Consider the following example, which illustrates how condensation forms in a ventilator circuit: Gas flowing from the ventilator to the patient is cooled as it flows through the circuit. To compensate for this cooling, the humidifier temperature must be set to a higher level (50° C) than that desired at the airway. At 50° C, the humidifier fully saturates the gas to an absolute humidity of 84 mg/L of water. The capacity of the gas to hold water vapor decreases as cooling occurs along the tubing path. By the time the gas reaches the patient, its temperature has dropped to 37° C, and it is capable of holding only 44 mg/L of water vapor. Although BTPS conditions have been achieved, 40 mg/L, half the total output of the humidifier (84 − 44 mg/L = 40 mg/L), has condensed in the inspiratory limb of the circuit.

Condensation can disrupt or occlude gas flow through the circuit, potentially altering the F_1O_2 or ventilator function (or both), and it may even be aspirated by the patient. Typically, patients contaminate ventilator circuits within hours, and condensate is colonized with bacteria that can pose an infection risk.[22] To avoid problems in this area,

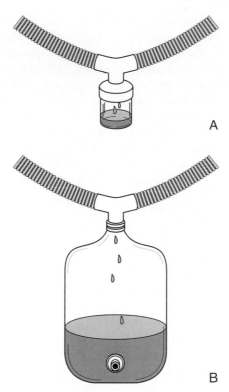

FIGURE 4-21 When condensate forms, the ribs in the 22-mm ID corrugated tubing catch and hold it, and overflow tends to pool in the tubing. Placement of a trap (A) or drain bag (B) at the low point of the circuit prevents condensate from obstructing the tubing.

health care personnel should treat all breathing circuit condensate as infectious waste.

To reduce the negative impact of condensate, circuits must be positioned to drain condensate away from the patient, and excess condensate must be drained from the circuit on a regular basis (Figure 4-21). Water traps placed at low points in the circuit (both the inspiratory and expiratory limbs of ventilator circuits) allow emptying without disruption of ventilation. Several approaches can be used to collect condensate. Large-bore, corrugated tubing and small-volume taps can help minimize early pooling, which can obstruct the tubing. Small-volume traps can also help minimize pooling of condensate, and do not cause large changes in ventilator circuit compliance. Some have spring-loaded valves that maintain a closed circuit during emptying. Drain system bags can collect large volumes of condensate over time, and the bag can be drained without breaking the ventilator circuit; however, the compressible volume may change a great deal.

It is worth mentioning that nebulizers with medication reservoirs below the aerosol generator that are placed in the ventilator circuit can act as a water trap, collecting contaminated condensate. This presents considerable risk that contaminated aerosols can be generated and pathogens delivered to the deep lung. To minimize this risk, nebulizers should be placed in a superior position so that any condensate travels downstream from the nebulizer. In addition, these nebulizers should be removed from the ventilator circuit between treatments. They should be rinsed and air-dried or disposed of and replaced, if necessary.

Some other techniques that can be used to deal with the potential problems associated with condensation include adding insulation or increasing the thermal mass of the circuit and using coaxial circuits. With the insulation technique, condensation is reduced because the circuit is kept at a constant temperature. In a coaxial circuit, the inspiratory limb of the ventilator circuit is within the expiratory limb, which insulates the inspiratory limb with the ambient air (i.e., the warm exhaled gas surrounds the inspiratory limb, reducing the temperature gradient). These circuits have been more popular for use with anesthesia ventilators, but they are gaining some acceptance for use in the intensive care unit (ICU).

Heated wire circuits, which are quite common in the ICU, offer another approach to addressing the problems associated with condensation. Placing wire heating elements in the ventilator circuit allows the gas delivered to the patient to remain at a constant temperature. Most heated wire circuits use a dual control mechanism with two temperature sensors, one that monitors the temperature of the gas leaving the humidifier and the other placed at or near the patient's airway (Figure 4-22). The controller regulates the temperature difference between the humidifier output and the patient's airway. When heated wire circuit are used, the humidifier heats gas to a lower temperature (32° to 40° C) than it does with conventional circuits (45° to 50° C). Management of this temperature gradient is critical to proper humidification. When the humidifier is warmer than the circuit, rain out occurs. When the circuit is warmer than the humidifier output, the inspired gas will not be fully saturated and a **humidity deficit** can be created. Notice that heated wire circuits can produce unwanted levels of condensate. Fine tuning with the temperature differential is important. An additional strategy is to provide absorptive material in the inspiratory limb of the ventilator circuit, which acts as a wick warmed by the heated wire system (e.g., Fisher & Paykel and Anamed Vital Signs, Totawa, NJ).

The use of heated wire circuits in the treatment of neonates is complicated by the use of incubators and radiant warmers. Incubators provide a warm environment surrounding the child, and radiant warmers use radiant energy to warm objects that intercept radiant light. In both cases, a temperature probe placed in the heated environment will affect the humidifier's performance, resulting in reduced humidity received by the patient. Therefore, temperature probes should always be placed outside the radiant field or incubator (Figure 4-23).

Heat and Moisture Exchangers

The heat and moisture exchanger, or artificial nose, is classified as a passive humidifier. Like the nose, an HME captures exhaled heat and moisture and uses it to heat and humidify the next inspiration (Figure 4-24). Unlike the nose, with its rich vasculature and endothelium, most HMEs do not actively add heat or water to the system.

HMEs have been used successfully to meet the short-term humidification needs of spontaneously breathing and mechanically ventilated patients with endotracheal and tracheostomy tubes.[23] Earlier methods of classifying HMEs included (1) simple condenser humidifiers, (2) **hygroscopic** condenser humidifiers, and (3) hydrophobic condenser humidifiers.

Simple HMEs contain a condenser element with high thermal conductivity, usually consisting of metallic gauze, corrugated metal, or parallel metal tubes with or without an additional fibrous element. On inspiration, inspired air cools the condenser element. On exhalation, expired water vapor condenses directly on the element's surface and warms it. On the next inspiration, cool, dry air is warmed and humidified as its passes over the condenser element. Simple condenser humidifiers are only able to recapture less than 50% of a patient's exhaled moisture (50% efficiency). Fibrous material aids in moisture retention and reduces pooling of condensate. Moisture output ranges from 10 to 14 mg H_2O/L. The addition of filtering capability to the HME has increased its efficiency. These heat and moisture exchanging filters (HMEFs) have an increased internal surface area of the medium and can provide a moisture output in the range of 18 to 28 mg H_2O/L.

Hygroscopic heat and moisture exchangers (HHMEs) provide higher efficiency by (1) using a condensing element of low thermal conductivity (e.g., paper, wool, or foam) and (2) impregnating this material with a hygroscopic salt (calcium or lithium chloride). During exhalation, some water vapor condenses on the cool condenser element, whereas other water molecules bind directly to the hygroscopic salt. During inspiration, the lower water vapor pressure in the inspired gas liberates water molecules directly

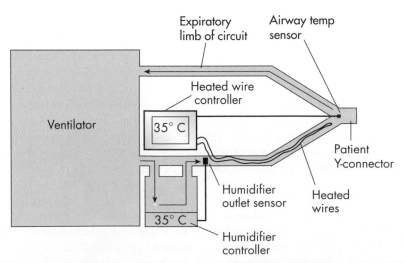

FIGURE 4-22 A heated wire circuit in the inspiratory limb of the gas delivery tube. (From Wilkins RL, Stoller JK, Kacmarek RM: *Egan's fundamentals of respiratory care,* ed 9, St Louis, 2009, Mosby.)

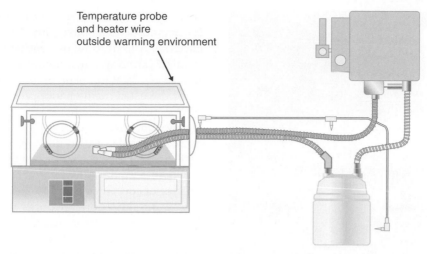

FIGURE 4-23 Neonatal breathing circuit configuration with incubator. The temperature probe is placed outside the warming environment, and an unheated portion of the inspiratory circuit passes into the incubator and attaches to the Y-piece. (From Wilkins RL, Stoller JK, Kacmarek RM: *Egan's fundamentals of respiratory care,* ed 9, St Louis, 2009, Mosby.)

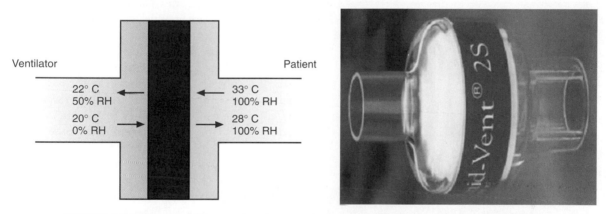

FIGURE 4-24 Diagram of heat and moisture exchanger with changes in temperature and relative humidity (RH) as gas passes from the patient to the ventilator circuit during exhalation *(left)* and from the vent to the patient during inhalation *(right)*. (Courtesy Telefax Medical, Research Triangle Park, NC.)

from the hygroscopic salt, without cooling. These devices typically achieve approximately 70% efficiency. Moisture output ranges from 22 to 34 mg H_2O/L.

Hygroscopic heat and moisture exchanging filters (HHMEFs) combine the HHME with a water-repellent and often electrostatically charged medium with a large surface area with filtration capabilities and low thermal conductivity. The filter medium often is placed between the HHME and the ventilator circuit. In efficiency, these devices are comparable to hygroscopic condenser humidifiers; they offer a small increase in moisture output but with increased airway resistance. Examples of several different types of HMEs are shown in Figure 4-25.

Design and performance standards for HMEs are set by the **International Organization for Standardization (ISO).**[24] Ideally, an HME should operate at 70% efficiency

or better (providing at least 30 mg/L of water vapor). HMEs use standard connections, have a low compliance, and add minimal weight, dead space, and flow resistance to a breathing circuit.[25] HMEs come in a broad range of shapes and sizes. The moisture output of HMEs tends to fall at high volumes and high rates of breathing. In addition, high inspiratory flows and high F_IO_2 levels can reduce the HME's efficiency.[25] When an HME is dry, resistance across most devices is minimal. However, because of water absorption, HME flow resistance increases after several hours' use.[26,27] In some patients the increased resistance imposed by the HME may not be well tolerated, particularly if the underlying lung disease already causes increased work of breathing.

Because HMEs eliminate the problem of breathing circuit condensation, many consider these devices (espe-

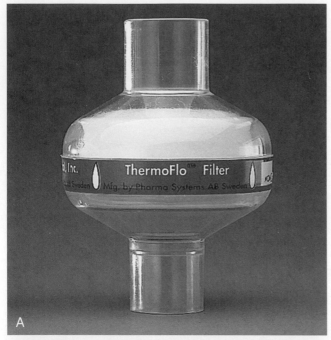

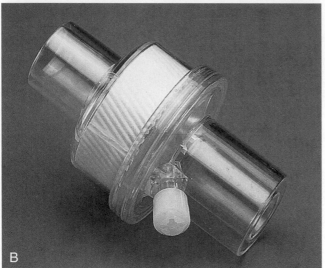

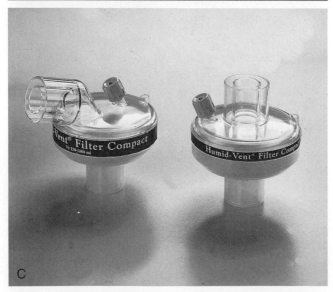

FIGURE 4-25 Heat and moisture exchangers are available in a variety of shapes, sizes, and types.

cially HMEs with hydrophobic filters) to be helpful in preventing nosocomial infections. Although HMEs show less bacterial colonization of ventilator circuits than active humidification systems, circuit colonization plays a minor role in the development of nosocomial infections, provided the usual maintenance precautions are applied.[28]

The position of the HME relative to the patient's airway can affect the device's ability both to heat and humidify inhaled gas. Intuitively, placing the HME directly at the patient airway would seem to be best; however, secretions can occlude an HME attached directly to the airway. The use of equipment such as closed suction catheters and airway monitor ports requires placement of the HME closer to the ventilator circuit's Y-piece. Inui et al. tested the performance of HMEs placed in two different positions: directly at the airway (10 cm from an endotracheal tube) and proximal to the ventilator circuit.[27] Both HMEs tested performed best at the airway, although one model did not perform adequately at either site. The other HME model exceeded recommended performance standards (equal to or greater than 30 mg/L absolute humidity and 30° C) at both sites. Clinicians should select the HME that performs adequately when placed at the intended site.

Although use of HMEs has been associated with thickened secretions in some patients, the incidence of endotracheal tube (ETT) occlusion is lower with HMEs than when heated humidifiers are used.[29] HMEs are not recommended for use with infants for several reasons. HMEs add 30 to 90 mL of mechanical dead space, often exceeding the tidal volume of a 5-kg infant (25 mL). Uncuffed endotracheal tubes in small infants allow a portion of exhaled gas to leak around the tube, bypassing the HME and reducing its ability to capture exhaled heat and humidity. The provision of heated humidity at temperatures under 35° C has been associated with narrowing and obstruction of ETTs in infants. A simple clinical algorithm can help determine when use of an HME is appropriate (Figure 4-26).

HMEs have been developed for use by patients with a tracheostomy who no longer require mechanical ventilation but only room air or low-flow oxygen. Devices to fit on an ETT vary by design, but they typically allow an inlet port for low-flow oxygen and in some cases have silicon suction ports that act as one-way valves.

Patients who no longer need an artificial airway and can breathe through an open stoma may benefit from HMEs like the one shown in Figure 4-27. This combines the benefit of heat and humidity with the filtration of gross particulates from inhaled gas.

Active Heat and Moisture Exchangers

Active HMEs add humidity or heat (or both) to inspired gas by chemical or electrical means. These devices have been shown to be equivalent to mainstream active humidifiers in both in vitro and in vivo use. Active HMEs add weight and complexity at the patient airway.

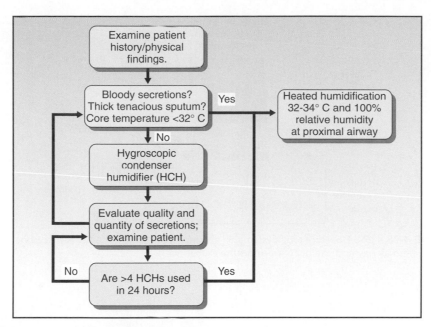

FIGURE 4-26 Clinical algorithm for use of a heat and moisture exchanger. (From Hess DR, MacIntyre NR, Mishoe SC et al: *Respiratory care: principles and practices,* Philadelphia, 2002, WB Saunders.)

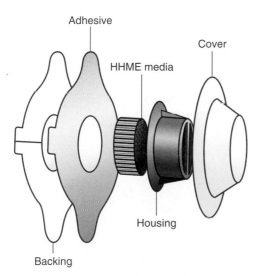

FIGURE 4-27 Components of a hygroscopic heat and moisture exchanger (HHME) for use with a tracheal stoma.

The Humid-Heat (Louis Gibeck AB, Upplands Väsby, Sweden) consists of a supply unit with a microprocessor, water pump, and a humidification device, which is placed between the Y-piece and the endotracheal tube. The humidification device is based on a hygroscopic HME, which absorbs expired heat and moisture and releases it into the inspired gas. External heat and water are then added to the patient side of the HME so that the inspired gas should reach 100% humidity at 37° C (44 mg H_2O/L of air). The external water is delivered to the humidification device via a pump onto a wick and then evaporated into the inspired air by an electrical heater. The microprocessor controls the water pump and the heater by an algorithm using the minute ventilation (which is fed into the microprocessor) and the airway temperature measured by a sensor mounted in the flex-tube on the patient side of the humidification device.

The HME Booster (King Systems, Noblesville, Indiana), which was designed for use as an adjunct to a passive HME, consists of a T-piece containing an electrically heated element (Figure 4-28). The heating element heats water so that water vapor passes into the airway between the artificial airway and the ETT, through a Gore-Tex membrane and aluminum. Water is fed to the heater from a gravity feed bag via a flow regulator that limits flow to 10 mL/hr. The heater operates at 110° C and adds 3 to 5.5 mg/L of humidity and 3° to 4° C to inhaled gas compared to an HME alone. It is designed for patients with minute volumes of 4 to 20 L, and it is not appropriate for use with pediatric patients or infants.

Box 4-6 presents information about the contraindications to use of these devices.

Setting Humidification Levels

The American National Standards Institute (ANSI) recommends that the minimum level of humidity for intubated patients exceed 30 mg/L; however, the ANSI has not recommended an optimum level of humidification for nonintubated patients. One suggestion is to deliver the temperature and level of humidity for normal conditions at the point where the gas enters the airway. For example,

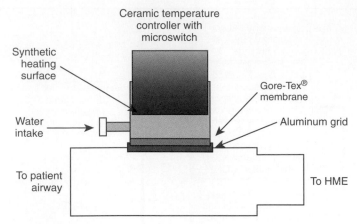

FIGURE 4-28 HME-Booster (King Systems) is a membrane humidifier that is placed between the patient's airway and the heat and moisture exchanger.

air entering the carina typically has a humidity level of 35 to 40 mg/L. Studies have suggested that operating a humidifier at a temperature under 32° C for adults and 35° C for infants can lead to increased airway plugging. Furthermore, active heated humidifiers may perform differently under the same conditions. Nishida et al.[30] compared the performance of five active humidifiers (MR 290 with MR 730, MR 310 with MR 730,* ConchaTherm IV,[†] and Hummax II[‡]), which were set to maintain the temperature of the airway opening at 32° and 37° C under a variety of ventilator parameters. The greater the minute ventilation, the lower the humidity delivered with all the devices except the Hummax II. When the devices' airway temperature control was set at 32° C, neither the ConchaTherm IV, the MR 310, nor the MR 730 delivered 30 mg/L of vapor, the minimum level recommended by the ANSI. These results point up the need to set humidifiers to maintain airway temperatures in the range of 35° to 37° C.

The appropriate temperature and humidity of inspired gas delivered to mechanically ventilated patients with artificial airways are the subject of controversy. The current AARC Clinical Practice Guideline recommends a temperature of 33° ± 2° C and a minimum humidity level of 30 mg/L. Williams et al.[31] suggest that inspired gas be delivered at 37° C with 100% relative humidity and a water vapor level of 44 mg/L to prevent complications. Theoretically, optimum humidity improves mucociliary clearance. To guide practitioners in the use of humidity therapy for patients receiving ventilatory support, AARC has a published Clinical Practice Guideline on Humidification during Mechanical Ventilation.[7]

*MR 290, MR 310, and MR 30 from Fisher and Paykel Healthcare, Inc Saguna Hills, Calif.
[†]ConchaTherm IV from Hudson RCI, Temecula, Calif.
[‡]Hummax II from Metran Medical Inst. Mfg., Co., Ltd, Saitama, Japan.

BOX 4-6	Contraindications to Use of a Heat and Moisture Exchanger

- Increased volume of secretions
- Thick, dehydrated secretions
- Hypothermia
- Large tidal volumes (>700 ml)
- Small tidal volume (V_T) with large-rebreathed-volume heat and moisture exchanger (HME) (i.e., HME volume > 30% of V_T)
- Uncuffed endotracheal tubes
- Large leak around an endotracheal tube, such as might occur with a large bronchopleurocutaneous fistula or leaking endotracheal tube cuff
- Exhaled V_T < 70% of inhaled V_T
- HME cannot be placed between nebulizer and airway during aerosol therapy.
- HME cannot be used with heated humidification.

Problem Solving and Troubleshooting for Humidification Systems

Common problems with humidification systems include dealing with condensation, preventing cross-contamination, and ensuring proper conditioning of the inspired gas.

Cross-Contamination

Aerosol and condensate from ventilator circuits are known sources of bacterial colonization.[22] However, advances in both circuit and humidifier technology have reduced the risk of nosocomial infection with the use of these systems. Wick or membrane passover humidifiers prevent the formation of bacteria-carrying aerosols. Heated wire circuits reduce the production and pooling of condensate within the circuit. In addition, the high reservoir temperatures in humidifiers are bacteriocidal.[32] In fact, in ventilator circuits using wick humidifiers with heated wire systems, circuit contamination usually occurs from the patient to the circuit rather than vice versa.

For decades the traditional way to minimize the risk of circuit-related nosocomial infection in critically ill patients receiving ventilatory support was to change the ventilator tubing and its attached components every 24 hours. It is now known that frequent ventilator circuit changes actually increase the risk of nosocomial pneumonia.[33] Current research indicates that minimal risk of ventilator-associated pneumonia exists with weekly circuit changes and that circuits may not need to be changed at all.[33,34] In addition, substantial cost savings can accrue with less frequent circuit changes.

Monitoring Proper Conditioning of the Inspired Gas

All respiratory therapists are trained to measure patients' F_IO_2 levels regularly and, in ventilatory care, to monitor selected pressures, volumes, and flows. However, few clinicians take the steps needed to ensure proper conditioning of the inspired gas received by their patients. The most accurate and reliable way to ensure that patients receive gas at the expected temperature and humidity level is to measure these parameters. Portable, battery-operated digital hygrometer-thermometer systems are available for less than $300 and are invaluable for ensuring proper conditioning of the inspired gas. These devices should be as common at the bedside as oxygen analyzers.

Many heated wire humidification systems have a humidity control. However, this control does not reflect either the absolute or the relative humidity, but only the temperature differential between the humidifier and the airway sensor. If the heated wires are set warmer than the humidifier, less RH is delivered to the patient. To ensure that the inspired gas is properly conditioned, clinicians should always adjust the temperature differential to the point where a few drops of condensation form near the patient's Y. Lacking direct measurement of humidity, observation of this minimal condensate is the most reliable indicator that the gas is fully saturated at the specified temperature. If condensate cannot be seen, there is no way of knowing the level of relative humidity without direct measurement; it could be anything from 99% to 0%! HME performance can be evaluated in a similar manner.[35]

Selecting the Appropriate Humidity and Bland Aerosol Therapy

Figure 4-29 presents a basic algorithm for selecting or recommending the appropriate therapy to condition a patient's inspired gas. Key considerations include (1) the gas flow, (2) the presence or absence of an artificial tracheal airway, (3) the character of the pulmonary secretions, (4) the need for and expected duration of mechanical ventilation, and (5) contraindications to use of an HME.

For delivering oxygen to the upper airway, the American College of Chest Physicians advises against using a bubble humidifier at flow rates of 4 L/min or less.[36] For the occasional patient who complains of nasal dryness or irritation when receiving low-flow oxygen, a humidifier should be added to the delivery system. Conversely, the relative inefficiency of unheated bubble humidifiers means that the clinician may need to consider heated humidification for patients receiving long-term oxygen at high flow rates (greater than 10 L/min without air entrainment).

HMEs provide an inexpensive alternative to heated humidifiers when used for ventilation of patients who do not have complex humidification needs. However, passive HMEs may not provide sufficient heat or humidification for long-term management of certain patients. When an HME is used, its selection should be based on the individual patient's ventilatory pattern, as well as the unit's performance, efficiency, and size. Moreover, all patients using HMEs should be reevaluated regularly so that the appropriateness of continued use can be confirmed.[37]

Clinical Rounds 4-2 presents an exercise to test your ability to select the appropriate device for patients requiring humidity therapy.

AEROSOL THERAPY

The goal of medical aerosol therapy is to deliver a therapeutic dose of a selected agent (i.e., drug) to the desired site of action.[38] The indications for delivering a particular agent depend on the condition being treated. For patients with pulmonary disorders, the administration of drugs by aerosol offers the advantage of achieving higher local drug

---

CLINICAL ROUNDS 4-2

Determine the best humidity device options for the following patients:

· Patient A: A 60-year-old patient with emphysema who is receiving oxygen via nasal cannula at 3 L/min.

· Patient B: A 48-year-old patient with chronic bronchitis who has been prescribed 35% oxygen.

· Patient C: A 28-year-old postoperative patient with an endotracheal tube in the surgical intensive care unit who is not expected to require the tube longer than 24 hours.

· Patient D: A 72-year-old woman with chronic obstructive pulmonary disease (COPD) and thick secretions who requires mechanical ventilation in the respiratory intensive care unit.

See Evolve Resources for the answer.

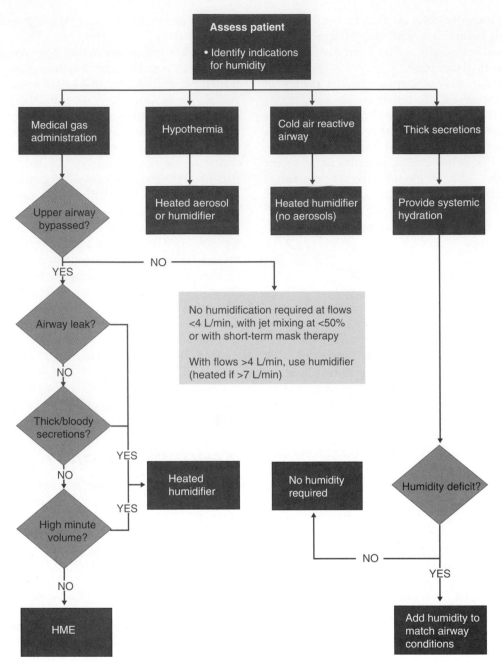

FIGURE 4-29 Algorithm for selecting the correct humidity and bland aerosol therapy. (From Wilkins RL, Stoller JK, Kacmarek RM: *Egan's fundamentals of respiratory care,* ed 9, St Louis, 2009, Mosby.)

concentrations in the lung with lower systemic levels compared to other forms of administration. Improved therapeutic action with fewer systemic side effects provides a higher **therapeutic index.**

Characteristics of Therapeutic Aerosols

Effective use of medical aerosols requires an understanding of the characteristics of aerosols and their effect on drug delivery to the desired site of action. Key concepts include aerosol output, particle size, and **deposition.**

Aerosol Output

Aerosol output is the mass of fluid or drug produced or emitted by a nebulizer. The **emitted dose** is the mass of drug leaving the mouthpiece of a nebulizer or inhaler as aerosol. Output is expressed as either the total mass emitted or as a percentage of the dose placed in the nebulizer. The output rate is the mass emitted per unit of time.

Aerosol output is measured by collecting the emitted aerosol on filters and measuring either the weight (gravimetric analysis) or the amount of drug (assay). Gravimetric measurements of drugs in aerosols are less reliable than drug assay techniques because weight changes caused by water evaporation cannot be differentiated from changes in drug mass.

Particle Size

Aerosol particle size depends on the method used to generate the aerosol, the substance nebulized, and the environmental conditions surrounding the particle. The unaided human eye cannot see particles less than 50 μm in diameter (the size of a small grain of sand). The most common laboratory methods used to measure aerosol particle size are liquid impingers, cascade impactors, and laser diffraction. Liquid impingers capture particles of different sizes on fluid placed in serial reservoirs. Cascade impactors collect aerosol particles of different size ranges on a series of stages or plates. For both methods, the mass of aerosol deposited is quantified by drug assay, and a distribution of particle sizes is calculated. With laser diffraction, a computer is used to estimate the range and frequency of droplet volumes crossing the laser beam.

Because medical aerosols contain particles of many different sizes (i.e., they are **heterodisperse**), the average particle size is expressed with a measure of central tendency, such as **mass median aerodynamic diameter (MMAD)** for cascade impaction or **volume median diameter (VMD)** for laser diffraction. These measurement methods may report different sizes for the same aerosol.

In an aerosol distribution with a specific MMAD or VMD, 50% of the particles are smaller and have less mass and 50% are larger and have greater mass. The variability of particle sizes in an aerosol distribution set at one standard deviation (SD) above or below the median (15.8% and 84.13% respectively) is the **geometric standard deviation (GSD)**. The greater the GSD, the wider the range of particle sizes and the more heterodisperse the aerosol. **Monodisperse** aerosols consisting of particles of similar size have a GSD less than or equal to 1.4. Nebulizers that produce monodisperse aerosols are used mainly in laboratory research and nonmedical industries.

Deposition

The **inhaled mass** is the amount of drug inhaled. It represents only a portion of the emitted dose. The **fine-particle fraction (FPF)** is the percentage of the aerosol small enough to have a good chance of depositing in lung (1 to 5 μm). The product of the inhaled mass multiplied by the fine-particle fraction is the **respirable mass.**

In **inertial impaction,** a particle of sufficient (relatively large) mass, which is moving in a gas stream that changes direction, tends to remain on its initial path and collide with the airway surface. This is the primary mechanism of deposition for particles larger than 5 μm. Inertia involves both mass and velocity. Turbulent flow patterns, obstructed or tortuous pathways, and inspiratory flow rates greater than 30 L/min are associated with increased inertial impaction.

Sedimentation occurs when aerosol particles settle out of suspension as a result of gravity. The greater the mass of a particle, the faster it settles. During normal breathing, sedimentation is the primary mechanism of deposition for particles 1 to 5 μm. Sedimentation occurs mostly in the central airways and increases with time.

Diffusion, or **brownian motion,** is the primary mechanism of deposition for small particles (less than 3 μm), mainly in the respiratory region, where bulk gas flow ceases and most aerosol particles reach the alveoli by diffusion. These aerosol particles have very low mass and are easily bounced around by collisions with carrier gas molecules. These random molecular collisions cause some particles to contact and become deposited on surrounding surfaces. Particles between 0.5 and 1 μm are so stable that most remain in suspension and are cleared with the exhaled gas, whereas particles smaller than 0.5 μm have a greater retention rate in the lungs. Fortunately, these small particles do not have much mass, therefore they represent only a small percentage of the total drug dose that is lost on exhalation (typically 1% to 5% of an inhaled drug).

Aging is the process by which aerosol particles grow, shrink, coalesce, and fall out of suspension over time. The way an aerosol ages depends on the composition of the aerosol, the initial size of its particles, the time in suspension, and the ambient conditions to which it is exposed. Aerosol particle size can decrease or increase as a result of evaporation or hygroscopic water absorption, respectively. The relative rate of particle size change is inversely proportional to the size of a particle, therefore small particles grow or shrink faster than larger particles.

Aerosol deposition is affected by the inspiratory flow rate and pattern, respiratory rate, inhaled volume, ratio of inspiratory time to expiratory time (I:E ratio), and breath-holding. Airway obstruction is one of the most important factors influencing aerosol deposition. Kim et al. demonstrated that total pulmonary deposition is greater in smokers and patients with obstructive airway disease than in healthy individuals.[39] Similarly, when inspiratory flow rates are constant, the deposition fraction of monodisperse aerosols increases with increased tidal volume, length of respiratory (inspiratory) period, and particle size.

Relatively simple in vitro models simulating a range of tidal volumes, inspiratory flow rates, I:E ratios, and respiratory rates have been useful in predicting the inhaled mass of drug and the relative performance of nebulizers.[40] Figure 4-30 summarizes the relationships between particle size and aerosol deposition in the respiratory tract. Notice that the depth of penetration and deposition of a particle in the respiratory tract tend to vary with size and tidal volume.[41]

Hazards of Aerosol Therapy

In addition to an adverse reaction to the medication administered, the hazards of aerosol therapy include infec-

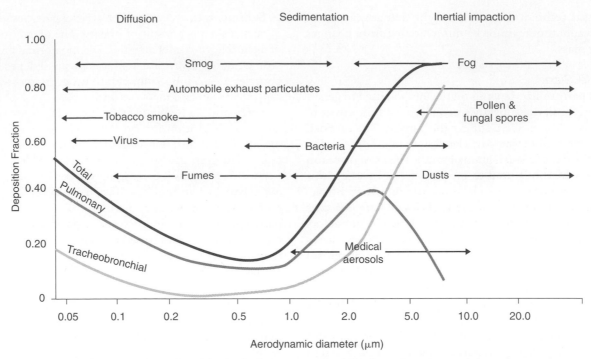

FIGURE 4-30 Range of particle size for common aerosols in the environment and the influence of particle size on diffusion, sedimentation, and inertial impaction. (Modified from Yu CP, Diu CK, Soong TT, et al: *Am Ind Hyg Assoc J* 40:999, 1979.)

tion, airway reactivity, systemic effects of bland aerosols, and drug concentration changes during nebulization.

Infection

Aerosol generators can contribute to nosocomial infections by allowing the airborne spread of bacteria. Common sources of bacteria include contaminated solutions (i.e., multiple-dose drug vials), caregivers' hands, and the patient's own secretions. The organisms most often associated with these types of nosocomial infections are gram-negative bacilli, particularly *Pseudomonas aeruginosa* and *Legionella pneumophila*.[42] According to CDC guidelines, nebulizers should be either sterilized between patients or replaced every 24 hours. In the home care setting, the generally accepted practice is to rinse the nebulizer with sterile water (not tap water) and air-dry it after each treatment.

Airway Reactivity

Cold and high-density aerosols can cause reactive bronchospasm and increased airway resistance.[43] Medications such as acetylcysteine, antibiotics, steroids, cromolyn sodium, ribavirin, and distilled water have been associated with increased airway resistance and wheezing during aerosol therapy. Administration of bronchodilators before or with administration of these agents may reduce the risk or duration of increased airway resistance.

The risk of inducing bronchospasm always should be considered when aerosols are administered. Monitoring for reactive bronchospasm should include peak flow measurements or measurement of the percentage of the forced

expiratory volume in 1 second (% FEV_1) before and after therapy; auscultation for adventitious breath sounds; observation of the patient's breathing pattern and overall appearance; and, the most essential part, communicating with the patient during therapy to determine the perceived work of breathing.[44]

Pulmonary and Systemic Effects

Aerosols have the potential to cause both local and systemic effects (i.e., effects at the site of delivery or effects caused by absorption into the systemic circulation). These effects largely depend on the drug concentration delivered, but they also may be associated with the size, temperature, and volumes of aerosols delivered.

As has already been mentioned, aerosols can have a local irritating effect, resulting in bronchospasm. Animal data indicate that long-term, continuous administration of bland aerosols can cause localized inflammation and tissue damage, atelectasis, and pulmonary edema. Continuous high-output aerosol administration also can increase the risks of overhydration and electrolyte disturbances, such as hypernatremia (the latter risks are especially important in pediatric patients).

Preliminary assessment, therefore, should balance the need versus the risk of aerosol therapy, especially among patients at high risk, such as infants, those prone to fluid and electrolyte imbalances, and patients with atelectasis or pulmonary edema. Care must be taken to ensure that patients are capable of clearing secretions once the secretions are mobilized by aerosol therapy. Appropriate airway clearance techniques should accompany any aerosol therapy designed to help mobilize secretions.

Drug Concentration Changes

During the evaporation, heating, baffling, and recycling of drug solutions undergoing jet or ultrasonic nebulization, the solute concentration may increase significantly.[45] This process may expose the patient to increasingly higher concentrations of the drug over the course of a therapeutic session. An increase in concentration, therefore, is time dependent, with the greatest effect occurring when medications are nebulized over extended periods. Although the clinical implications of this change in drug concentration have not been well documented, the clinician should keep this factor in mind during continuous aerosol drug delivery.

Aerosol Drug Delivery Systems

Aerosol generators in clinical use include pressurized metered-dose inhalers (pMDIs), dry powder inhalers (DPIs), jet nebulizers (small and large volume), ultrasonic nebulizers (USNs), hand-bulb atomizers (including nasal spray pumps), vibrating mesh nebulizers, and a number of emerging technologic devices. Device selection and proper operation can make the difference between successful and unsuccessful therapy; therefore, clinicians must have in-depth knowledge of the operating principles and performance characteristics of the various systems and how best to select and apply them.

Metered-Dose Inhalers

The **pressurized metered-dose inhaler (pMDI)** is the most commonly prescribed method of aerosol delivery. Pressurized MDIs are compact, portable, relatively easy to use, and offer multidose convenience. Unlike most nebulizers, the pMDI was developed as a drug/device combination, with the actuator boot and canister designed for the specific drug formulation and dose volume to be delivered. pMDIs can be used to administer short- and long-acting bronchodilators, anticholinergics, and steroids. Indeed, more formulations of these drugs are available for use by pMDI than for any other type of nebulizer.

Although pMDIs appear to be rather simple and relatively easy to use, they represent sophisticated technology and engineering and are often misused by patients. When properly used, pMDIs are at least as effective as other nebulizers for drug delivery. For this reason, pMDIs often are the preferred method for delivering bronchodilators to spontaneously breathing patients, as well as to those who are intubated and undergoing mechanical ventilation.[46]

Equipment Design. A typical pMDI consists of a pressurized canister that contains drug (a micronized powder or aqueous solution) in a volatile propellant combined with surfactants, dispersing agents, preservatives, and flavoring agents (Figure 4-31). The active drug represents 1% or less of the mixture emitted from the pMDI. **Chlorofluorocarbons (CFCs),** such as Freon, were the propellants

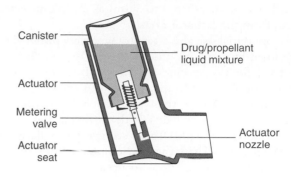

Metered Dose Inhaler

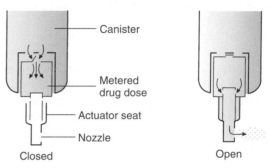

Metered Valve Function

FIGURE 4-31 Key components of a pressurized metered-dose inhaler. (From Rau JL Jr: *Respiratory care pharmacology*, ed 6, St Louis, 2002, Mosby.)

used in pMDIs since their introduction in 1956. However, because of Freon's contribution to the effects of global warming, other pMDI propellants have been developed, such as **hydrofluoroalkane** (HFA-134a). The most common dispersal agents are surfactants (e.g., soya lecithin, sorbitan trioleate, and oleic acid), which help keep the drug suspended in the propellant and lubricate the valve mechanism. Solvents used to dissolve the drug and surfactant include ethanol, glycerol, and propylene glycol.

A pMDI is designed to deliver smaller doses than nebulizers and dry powder inhalers. Metering valve volumes of 25 to 100 μL limit dose per actuation to typically 50 mcg to 5 mg, depending on the drug formulation. When the canister is inverted (nozzle down) and placed in its actuator, or "boot," the volatile suspension fills a metering chamber that controls the amount of drug delivered. Pressing down on the canister aligns a hole in the metering valve with the metering chamber. The high-propellant vapor pressure quickly forces the metered dose out through this hole and through the actuator nozzle.

Aerosol production takes approximately 20 milliseconds (msec). As the liquid suspension is forced out of the pMDI, it forms a plume, within which the propellants vaporize, or "flash." Once the pMDI is actuated, the initial velocity of this plume is high (greater than 30 m/sec), and the particles are large (35 μm). Within 0.1 second, the plume velocity decreases more than 50%, and propellant particle size reduces (to 3 to 5 µm) as the plume extends 10 cm from the actuator nozzle.[47]

Before initial use and after storage, every pMDI should be primed by actuating the device one to four times (see the label for the specific pMDI). Without priming, the initial dose actuated from a new pMDI canister contains less active substance than subsequent actuations.[48] A reduction in the emitted dose with the first actuation commonly occurs with a pMDI after storage, particularly when the pMDI is stored with the valve pointed in the downward position. This "loss of dose" from a pMDI occurs when drug particles rise to the top of the canister over time, like cream rising to the top of milk. This development is related to valve design and occurs when propellant leaks from the metering chamber during periods of nonuse (in as little as 4 hours).[48]

Improved metering valve designs have been developed for use with HFA propellants in an attempt to reduce these losses. Unlike CFC pMDIs that have not been used for 8 to 12 hours, pMDIs containing HFA propellants may not require wasting of dose for periods ranging from 2 days to 2 weeks. Each pMDI is different, therefore the clinician and the patient need to be aware of the priming requirements for the specific formulation being used.

Depending on the drug and the manufacturer, a pMDI may contain 60 to 240 doses. After the number of labeled doses has been administered, the pMDI may appear to contain as many as 20 to 60 additional doses. It is important to recognize that little or no medication may be delivered in these latter actuations as the doses decrease. (The term "tail-off effect" often is used to refer to the variability of drug dispensed toward the end of the canister's life; this can result in swings from normal to almost no dose emitted from one breath to the next.)

Historically, pMDIs have had no mechanism that tells the patient how many doses remain in the canister. As a result of this lack of a "dose counter," patients frequently use a pMDI long after any active medication remains in the canister. The only reliable way to track the remaining doses is to count the number of actuations. Some manufacturers' labels recommend floating the pMDI canister in water to estimate the percentage of medication remaining in the device; however, this may not provide an accurate estimate of the amount of drug remaining. Also, water can seep into the nozzle of the pMDI and impair its performance and output. The U.S. Food and Drug Administration (FDA) now requires all new pMDIs to include an accurate method of tracking the pMDI actuations used (Figure 4-32).

A cold ambient temperature (under 10° C) dramatically reduces the output of CFC pMDIs. This is an issue during cold weather, when people with asthma tend to keep their pMDIs in an outer coat pocket for easy access. Patients should be instructed to keep the pMDI closer to the body and to warm the pMDI to body temperature before inhalation by rubbing the canister with their hands. Reduction

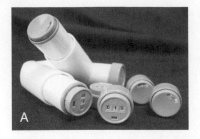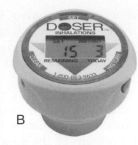

FIGURE 4-32 Dose counters mounted on top of a pMDI canister. **A,** AeroCount. **B,** Doser. (**A,** Courtesy Trudell Medical International, London, Ontario, Canada; **B,** courtesy Meditrack, Hudson, Mass.)

of dose at lower temperatures is less of an issue with the pMDIs that use HFA and other, newer propellants.[13]

Aerosol Delivery Characteristics. Pulmonary deposition ranges from 10% to 20% with a standard CFC pMDI.[49] Some pMDIs containing HFA propellants (e.g., QVAR, 3M, St. Paul, Minnesota) can produce deposition of as much as 50% of the emitted dose. Although pMDIs can produce particles in the respired range (MMAD of 3 to 6 µm), this transition occurs at approximately 10 cm from the nozzle.[48] Consequently, when pMDIs are used as directed, the initial velocity and larger particles that are generated when the device is placed between the lips result in approximately 80% of the dose being deposited in the oropharynx.

Techniques of Administration. Administration of aerosol drugs by pMDI is technique dependent. It has been estimated that as many as two thirds of patients and of health professionals who teach patients how to use a pMDI do not perform the procedure properly.[50] Preliminary patient instruction can last 10 to 30 minutes and should include demonstration, practice, and confirmation of patient performance (demonstration pMDIs with a placebo should be available from manufacturers for this purpose). Repeated instruction usually improves performance and can be performed on follow-up clinic or home visits. Repeat demonstrations may be required several times to ensure that the patient is using the device properly.

Box 4-7 outlines the recommended steps for self-administering a bronchodilator by a simple pMDI. The pMDI should be actuated at the beginning of a slow, deep inspiration. Hand-breath coordination problems include actuating the pMDI before or after the breath. Infants, young children, the elderly, and patients in acute distress may not be able to coordinate actuation of the pMDI with inspiration. The "cold Freon effect" occurs when the cold aerosol plume reaches the back of the mouth and the patient stops inhaling. All of these problems reduce aerosol delivery to the lung.

Most pMDI labels instruct patients to place the mouthpiece between the lips. Positioning the outlet of the pMDI approximately 4 cm (two fingers' width) in front of an open mouth with a low inspiratory flow rate can increase

BOX 4-7	Optimum Technique for Using a Simple Pressurized Metered-Dose Inhaler

1. Shake the inhaler well immediately before each use.
2. Remove the cap from the actuator mouthpiece.
3. Inspect the mouthpiece and clear it of any debris.
4. Shake the inhaler well and prime it by releasing 1 to 4 test sprays into the air, away from your face. (The inhaler should be primed before it is used for the first time and when it has not been used for longer than 1 day.)
5. Breathe out fully through your mouth.
6. Insert the mouthpiece fully into your mouth with the canister above the mouthpiece, and close your lips around the mouthpiece. Alternatively, place the mouthpiece 4 cm from your mouth. (NOTE: Do not use the latter technique with anticholinergic drugs.)
7. Depress the top of the metal canister at the beginning of a breath while breathing in deeply and slowly.
8. Hold your breath up to 10 seconds.
9. Repeat at 30- to 60-second intervals.
10. Replace the cap on the mouthpiece.
11. Clean the actuator mouthpiece at least once a week. Rinse it under running water, shake off the excess water, and allow the mouthpiece to air-dry.
12. Discard the canister after you have taken the labeled number of doses. Never immerse the canister in water to determine how full it is.

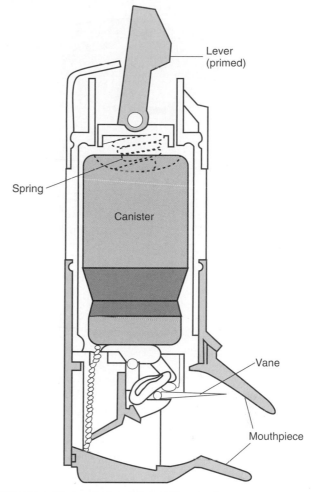

FIGURE 4-33 Autohaler pMDI. Lifting the lever compresses a spring, pressing the canister into the actuator boot and vane mechanism. As the patient inhales, the vanes move up and allow the pMDI canister to be pressed into the actuator, emitting a dose. (From Rau JL Jr: *Respiratory care pharmacology,* ed 6, St Louis, 2002, Mosby.)

the dose delivered to the lower respiratory tract of an adult from approximately 7% to 10% to 14% to 20%, as well as reduce oropharyngeal impaction.[51] However, this technique is more difficult for patients to perform reliably than is the closed mouth technique. Concerns have been raised about use of the open-mouth technique with ipratropium bromide, because poor coordination can result in the drug being sprayed into the eyes.

pMDI Accessory Devices

A variety of pMDI accessory devices have been developed to overcome problems such as hand-breath coordination, dose counting, and high oropharyngeal deposition.

Breath-actuated pMDIs. Breath-actuated pMDIs trigger during inhalation, reducing the need for the patient or caregiver to coordinate actuation with inhalation.[52] The Autohaler (3M, St. Paul, Minnesota), shown in Figure 4-33, is a flow-triggered pMDI designed to eliminate the need for hand-breath coordination by automatically actuating in response to the patient's inspiratory effort.[52] To use the Autohaler, a lever is cocked on top of the unit, which sets a downward spring force on the canister. Using a closed-mouth technique with the lips sealed, the patient inhales through the mouthpiece. As the flow rate exceeds 30 L/min, a vane releases the spring, forcing the canister down and actuating the pMDI. A limitation of this device is that it can only be breath actuated. Caution may be appropriate in ordering breath-triggered pMDIs for small children and patients prone to severe levels of airway obstruction. The

Easihaler (Glaxo Smith Kline Mississauga, Ontario, Canada), which is currently available in Europe and Canada, is a breath actuated pMDI that has been developed for use with a range of medications.

The MD Turbo (Respirics, Raleigh, North Carolina) is an accessory device that enables breath triggering with most pMDIs. The pMDI/actuator boot is placed in the device, and a spring-loaded mechanism is manually cocked before each actuation. An integrated LED dose counter lets the patient know when to reorder and replace the pMDI (Figure 4-34).

Spacers and Holding Chambers. A **spacer** or a valved holding chamber can reduce oropharyngeal deposition and the need for hand-breath coordination. A spacer is a simple, valveless extension device that adds distance between the pMDI outlet and the patient's mouth. This allows the aerosol plume to expand and the propellants to evaporate before the medication reaches the oropharynx.

Holding chambers allow exhaled aerosol to remain in a chamber and available to be inhaled with the next breath.

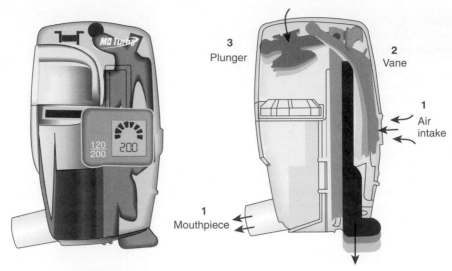

FIGURE 4-34 The MD Turbo is an accessory device that converts a standard pMDI with original boot into a breath-actuated device with a counter. As the patient inhales at the mouthpiece, *(1)* the pressure moves the vane, *(2)* releasing the spring latch, causing the plunger *(3)* to actuate the pMDI. The digital counter indicates the number of doses remaining. (Courtesy Respirics, Raleigh, NC.)

These devices provide less oropharyngeal deposition by retaining larger droplets and increasing respirable drug dosages. A holding chamber minimizes the cold Freon effect and any bad tastes associated with a drug. A valve may be incorporated into the holding chamber to prevent the chamber aerosol from being cleared on exhalation. This allows patients with small tidal volumes to empty the aerosol from the chamber with multiple successive breaths. These valved holding chambers enable infants, small children, and adults who cannot control their breathing pattern or who demonstrate poor hand-breath coordination to be treated effectively with pMDIs.

It is worth mentioning that multiple actuations of one or more drugs placed into a spacer can reduce both the total dose and the respirable dose of drug available for inhalation. The extent of these losses may vary for different drugs and spacer designs. Also, a pMDI drug administered with one type of accessory device may produce differences in the MMAD, GSD, and fine-particle fraction when used with a different accessory devices. Placement of a valve between the pMDI and the chamber and the mouthpiece also can affect drug delivery, because the valve acts as a **baffle,** reducing the size of particles inhaled. A simple tube spacer may reduce oral deposition by up to 90%, whereas a valved holding chamber can reduce oral deposition by 99%.

Another factor that can affect the performance of spacers and holding chambers is electrostatic charge. Electrostatic charges on the surface of a spacer or holding chamber attract and capture small aerosol particles, reducing the amount of respirable drug available to the lung. With repeated use (20 to 40 puffs), drug builds up on the wall of the chamber and the charge is dissipated, allowing more drug to be inhaled by the patient. Washing the chamber with water (without soap) reestablishes the electrostatic charge, making the device less effective until drug is deposited in the chamber and the static charge is once again reduced.[53] The use of conductive metal, paper, or nonelectrostatic plastic chambers or washing the plastic chamber periodically with deionizing detergent (e.g., dilute liquid dish soap) can overcome the loss of fine-particle mass caused by electrostatic charge and increase the inhaled mass from 20% up to 50% of the emitted dose of the pMDI, even in children.[53] Washing the chamber with conventional dishwashing soap reduces the static charge for up to 30 days.

Types of Spacers. Figure 4-35 shows examples of several commercially available spacers. Selection of the appropriate spacer should be based on the whether the patient requires a small-volume adapter, an open tube design, a bag reservoir, or a valved holding chamber. More than a dozen different devices, with volumes ranging from 15 to 750 mL, have been developed over the past 30 years.

Proper use of a simple open tube spacer requires some hand-breath coordination, because a momentary delay between triggering and inhalation of the discharged spray results in a substantial loss of drug and reduced lung delivery. Exhalation into a simple spacer after pMDI actuation clears the aerosol from the device and wastes most of the dose to the atmosphere. This reduction in dose also occurs with small-volume, reverse-flow spacers if no provision is made for "holding" the aerosol in the device. Box 4-8 outlines the proper technique for using a pMDI with a valved holding chamber.

Holding chambers with masks (Figure 4-36) are available for use in the care of infants, children, and adults who are unable to use a mouthpiece device because of their size, age, or level of hand-breath coordination. Holding cham-

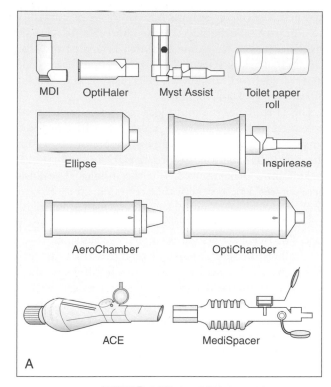

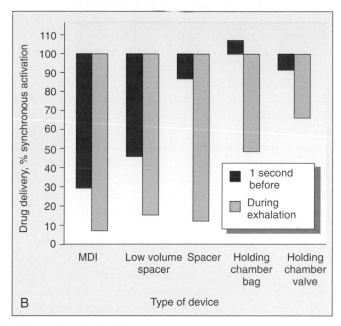

FIGURE 4-35 A, pMDI, low-volume spacers (Optihaler, Myst Assist), large-volume spacers (toilet paper roll, Ellipse), holding chamber bag (Inspirease), and valved holding chambers (AeroChamber, OptiChamber, ACE, and Medispacer). **B,** The percentage of inhaled mass with perfect technique was compared to actuation 1 second before inhalation *(solid bar)* and during exhalation *(clear bar).* Most of the dose is lost with the pMDI and the small-volume spacer. Valved holding chambers gave the highest dose under both conditions. (Modified from Wilkes W, Fink JB, Dhand R: Selecting an accessory device with a metered-dose inhaler: variable influence of accessory devices on fine particle dose, throat deposition, and drug delivery with asynchronous actuations from a metered-dose inhaler. *J Aerosol Med*, 2001.)

BOX 4-8	Technique for Using a Pressurized Metered-Dose Inhaler with a Valved Holding Chamber

1. Remove the caps from the boot of the pressurized metered-dose inhaler (pMDI) and from the valved holding chamber (VHC). Insert the inhaler into the VHC.
2. Shake the pMDI and chamber.
3. Actuate 1 dose into the chamber while breathing through the VHC.
4. Take a large breath and hold it for up to 10 seconds. If this is not possible, breathe through the VHC for several breaths (for adults, this should involve 1 to 3 tidal breaths; infants can take up to 10 breaths or 30 seconds with tidal breathing).
5. Repeat actuation at 30- to 60-second intervals.
6. Remove the pMDI from the VHC.
7. Replace the caps on the pMDI and VHC.
8. Store both the pMDI and VHC properly.
9. Periodically wash the VHC in warm, soapy water, rinse it, and allow it to air-dry.

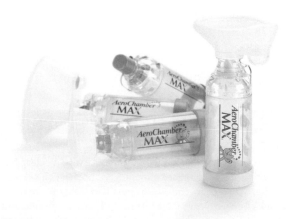

FIGURE 4-36 Mouthpiece masks are available in a range of sizes for use with valved holding chambers in infants through adults. (Courtesy Trudell Medical International, London, Ontario, Canada.)

bers are useful in the administration of steroids because deposition of the drug in the mouth is largely eliminated, and systemic side effects can be minimized.

Clinicians should choose a spacer that maximizes the delivery efficiency of the aerosol for the individual patient. Differences of twofold to threefold in the amount of drug available at the mouth have been measured among spacers currently used to treat infants. Spacers and holding chambers that use the manufacturer-designed boot that comes with the pMDI are more effective for a wider range of formulations than is a "universal adapter" that fits any pMDI canister. With solution HFA pMDIs, the diameter of the valve stem and actuator orifice is smaller than that of albuterol CFC pMDIs. When the HFA pMDI is used in an actuator designed for use with CFC pMDIs, output is reduced. When these HFA formulations are used with any particular spacer, it is important to know how comparable the available dose and particle size distribution are to the dose and particle size from an existing CFC pMDI.[48] Additional accessory devices for the pMDI include the Vent-Ease MDI adapter, which serves as a mechanical lever system to make actuation of the pMDI easier for patients with arthritic limitations. (See Clinical Rounds 4-3.)

Dry Powder Inhalers

As the name implies, **dry powder inhalers (DPIs)** are aerosol devices that deliver a drug in powder form. DPIs typically are breath-actuated dosing systems. The theory of operation for these devices is that the patient generates the aerosol by drawing air though a dose of finely milled drug powder with sufficient force to disperse and suspend the powder in the air. DPIs are relatively inexpensive, do not need propellants, and do not require the hand-breath coordination needed for pMDIs. Dispersion of the powder into respirable particles depends on the creation of turbulent flow in the inhaler. Turbulent flow is a function of the patient's ability to inhale the powder with a sufficiently high inspiratory flow rate.[54]

Equipment Design and Function. A number of different DPIs are available. Figure 4-37 shows the major components of a single-dose DPI and a multidose DPI. Early first-generation devices (e.g., Spinhaler, Rotahaler) dispense individual doses of drug from punctured gelatin

capsules. Multidose systems have since been introduced, including the Turbuhaler (Astra Draco, Lund, Sweden), Diskhaler (Glaxo Wellcome, Research Triangle Park, North Carolina), Diskus (Glaxo Wellcome), Handihaler (Boehringer Ingleheim, Ingleheim, Germany), and Aerolizer (Novartis, East Hanover, NJ).

The Turbuhaler is a multidose reservoir powder system preloaded with a quantity of pure drug sufficient for dispensing 200 doses of terbutaline sulphate or budesonide. The Diskhaler has drug in four or eight individual blister packets on a disk inserted into the inhaler. The Diskus incorporates a tape system that contains up to 60 sealed single doses. The Handihaler uses capsules containing individual doses and directions that require 10 steps per dose. The Aerolizer also uses single-dose capsules.

Small respirable-size particles tend to attract each other and aggregate. Passive dry powder dispensing systems use a carrier substance (lactose or glucose) mixed with the small particles of drug to enable the drug powder to disaggregate during inhalation. (Note that reactions to lactose or glucose appear to be fewer than reactions to the surfactants and propellants used in pressurized pMDIs.) The particle size of the dry powder particles of drug ranges from 1 to 3 μm, but the size of the lactose or glucose particles can range from approximately 20 to 65 μm; therefore, most of the carrier (up to 80%) is deposited in the oropharynx.

The performance of DPIs can be affected by the materials used in production and manufacturing. Optimum performance for each type of DPI occurs at a specific inspiratory flow rate. The fine-particle fraction of respirable drug from existing DPIs ranges from 10% to 60% of the nominal dose. The amount varies with inspiratory flow and device design. The higher the resistance or the greater the flow requirement of a DPI, the more difficult it is for a compromised or young patient to generate inspiratory flow sufficient to obtain the maximum dose of drug. The high peak inspiratory flow rates required to dispense the drug powder from most passive DPIs (greater than 60 L/min), result in a pharyngeal dose comparable with that received from a typical pMDI without an add-on device. If inhalation is not performed at the optimum inspiratory flow rate for a particular device, the dose of drug dispensed decreases and the particle size of the powder aerosol increases.[54] Finally, it should be evident that ambient humidity can affect drug delivery from DPIs. The emitted dose decreases in a humid environment, likely because of powder clumping. Exposure to humidity can affect dry powder in milliseconds. The higher the level of absolute humidity, the lower the dose emitted.

Despite the foregoing issues, DPIs in general are convenient and easy to use. Newer designs are being developed that provide aerosols with higher fine-particle fractions and more reproducible dosing, independent of inspiratory flow rate. For example, passive, or patient-driven, DPIs rely on the patient's inspiratory effort to dispense the dose. The result is differences in lung delivery and clinical response.

CLINICAL ROUNDS 4-3

You are called to the emergency department to deliver a medicated aerosol to a 6-year-old child who is alert but restless and complains of shortness of breath. The child's mother says that the child has had several "asthma attacks" since 1 year of age but that all have been mild and this is the first visit to a hospital. The emergency department physician asks you to suggest an appropriate aerosol device. What do you recommend?

See Evolve Resources for the answer.

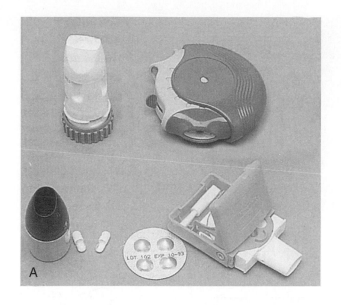

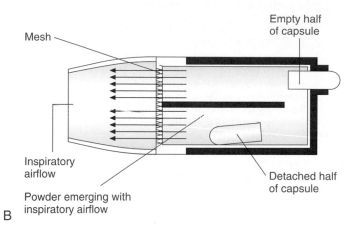

Mesh

Empty half
of capsule

Inspiratory
airflow

Powder emerging with
inspiratory airflow

Detached half
of capsule

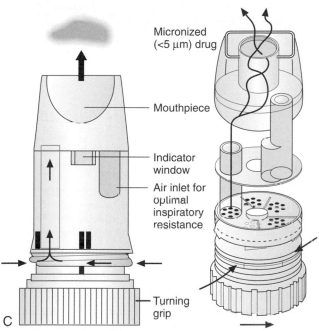

Micronized
(<5 µm) drug

Mouthpiece

Indicator
window

Air inlet for
optimal
inspiratory
resistance

Turning
grip

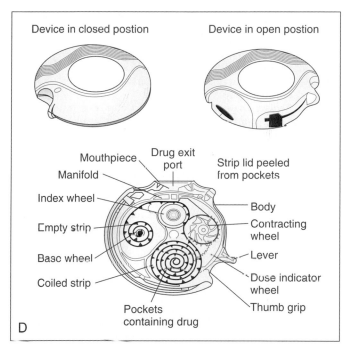

Device in closed postion

Device in open postion

Mouthpiece
Manifold
Index wheel
Empty strip
Base wheel
Coiled strip

Drug exit
port

Strip lid peeled
from pockets

Body

Contracting
wheel

Lever

Dose indicator
wheel

Thumb grip

Pockets
containing drug

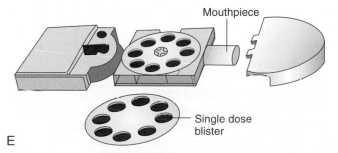

Mouthpiece

Single dose
blister

FIGURE 4-37 Dry powder inhaler **(A)** and diagrams of the Rotahaler **(B),** Turbuhaler **(C),** Diskus **(D),** and Diskhaler **(E).** (**A** Modified from Albert R, Spiro S, Jett J, editors: *Comprehensive respiratory medicine,* St Louis, 1999, Mosby; **B** to **E** modified from Dhand R, Fink JB: Dry powder inhalers, *Respir Care* 44(9):940-951.)

BOX 4-9	Technique for Using the Turbuhaler Dry Powder Inhaler

Priming instructions: Before using a new Turbuhaler for the first time:
1. Turn the cover and lift off.
2. Hold the inhaler upright.
3. Twist the brown grip fully to the right and then back again to the left.
4. Repeat.
5. The inhaler is ready to be used. (NOTE: It is not necessary to prime the inhaler again, even after a prolonged period of disuse.)

Steps for using the Turbuhaler:
1. Remove the cap from the inhaler (i.e., twist and lift off).
2. Keep the inhaler upright when loading (see step 3).
3. Rotate the grip counterclockwise as far as it will go, then back again until you hear a click.
4. Do not shake the inhaler after loading.
5. Exhale away from the mouthpiece.
6. Place the mouthpiece between your teeth and lips.
7. Inhale forcefully and deeply (you may not taste or feel medication).
8. Do not chew or bite on the mouthpiece.
9. Exhale away from the mouthpiece.
10. If more than one dose is required, repeat the previous steps.
11. Replace the cover on the inhaler and twist it to close.
12. Rinse your mouth with water; do not swallow.
13. Keep the inhaler clean and dry at all times.
14. Do not use the Turbuhaler if it is damaged or if the mouthpiece becomes detached.
15. Keep the device in a dry place at a controlled room temperature (i.e., 20° to 25° C [68° to 77° F]). Do not wash it.
16. When a red mark appears at the top of the window, the inhaler has 20 doses left. When the red mark reaches the bottom of the window, discard the device. Do not immerse it in water to determine whether it is empty.

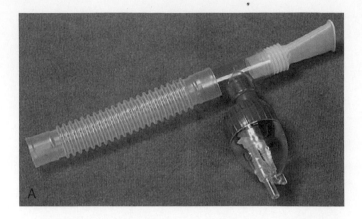

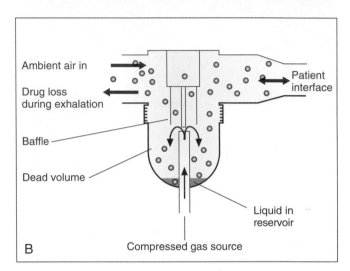

FIGURE 4-38 A, Small-volume jet nebulizer for liquid drug delivery. **B,** Schematic of a small-volume jet nebulizer. (From Hess DR, MacIntyre NR: *Respiratory care: principles and practices,* Philadelphia, 2002, WB Saunders.)

Active, or powered, DPIs, which disaggregate the powder before inhalation, are independent of patient effort. Active DPIs use an energy source to disaggregate the powder and suspend it into an aerosol, allowing the dose to be suspended independent of the patient's inspiratory flow rates. One example of an active DPI is the Exubra powder insulin delivery system (Pfizer, New York, NY). This device is manually powered, using pneumatic pressure to disperse the powder into a reservoir chamber from which the aerosol is inhaled.

Technique. The most critical factor in the use of a passive DPI is the need for high inspiratory flow. Patients must generate inspiratory flows of at least 40 to 60 L/min to produce a respirable powder aerosol. Because infants, small children (younger than 5 years), and those not able to follow instructions cannot develop flow this high, these patient groups cannot use DPIs effectively. Patients with severe airway obstruction also may not be able to achieve the required flow (DPIs therefore are not be used in the management of acute bronchospasm).

Although hand-breath coordination is not as important with DPIs as it is with pMDIs, exhalation into the device can result in loss of drug delivery to the lung. Some devices also require assembly, which can be cumbersome or difficult for some patients, especially those with arthritis. It is important that patients receive demonstrations with their inhalers and have the opportunity to assemble and use the DPI before self-administration. Box 4-9 outlines the basic steps in the use and care of the Turbuhaler DPI.

Small-Volume Nebulizers

Most modern jet nebulizers are powered by high-pressure air or oxygen provided by a portable compressor, compressed-gas cylinder, or 50-psi wall outlet. Because the nebulizers commonly used at home and in the hospital for drug administration have medication reservoirs of less than 10 mL, they are called **small-volume nebulizers (SVNs).** A number of factors can affect the performance of these devices, including nebulizer design, gas pressure, gas density, temperature and humidity, and medication characteristics.

Nebulizer Design. As shown in Figure 4-38, a typical SVN is powered by a high-pressure stream of gas directed through a restricted orifice (the jet). The gas stream leaving the jet passes the opening of a capillary tube immersed in solution. Because it produces low lateral pressure at the outlet, the high jet velocity draws the liquid up the capillary tube and into the gas stream, where it is sheared into filaments of liquid that break up into droplets. This primary spray produces a heterodisperse aerosol with droplets that range in size from 0.1 to 500 μm.[55] The droplets are directed against one or more baffles, which can include a sphere or plate placed in line with the jet flow. The internal walls of the nebulizer, the surface of the solution being nebulized, or the internal walls of the delivery system can serve the same purpose. In many designs, droplets that strike the baffles in the SVN return to the medication reservoir to be nebulized again.

Baffles are key elements in the design of SVNs. In jet nebulizers, well-designed baffling systems reduce both the MMAD and the GSD of the generated aerosol. Baffling also can occur unintentionally. Unintentional baffles are created by the angles within delivery tubing, by interfaces with other devices outside the aerosol generator, and by the surfaces of the upper airway itself.[56]

Residual drug volume, or dead volume, is the medication that remains in the SVN and cannot be nebulized.[57] The residual volume of a 3-mL dose varies from as little as 0.5 ml to more than 2.2 mL, which can be more than two thirds of the total dose. It should be obvious that the greater the residual drug volume, the more drug wasted

and the less efficient the delivery system. Residual volume also depends on the position of the SVN. Some SVNs stop producing aerosol when tilted as little as 30 degrees from vertical. Increasing the liquid volume in the SVN allows a greater proportion of active medication to be nebulized. For example, in a nebulizer with a residual volume of 1.5 mL, filling the device with 3 mL would leave only 50% of the nebulizer charge (nominal dose) available for nebulization. In contrast, filling the nebulizer with 5 mL would make 3.5 mL (or more than 70%) of the medication available for nebulization. To date, no significant difference in clinical response has been shown with varying diluent volumes and flow rates.

Continuous nebulization with conventional nebulizers emits aerosol throughout the respiratory cycle. Inhalation is less than 40% of the respiratory cycle, therefore more than 60% of the emitted aerosol is lost to the atmosphere. Lung delivery of 6% to 12% deposition has been measured in adults receiving continuous nebulizer therapy. Deposition in neonates and infants is less than 1%.

Breath-enhanced nebulizers generate aerosol continuously, using an inspiratory vent that allows the patient to draw in air through the nebulization chamber containing aerosolized drug. On exhalation, the inlet vent closes and aerosol exits by a one-way valve near the mouthpiece; this process increases the inhaled mass by as much as 50% over standard continuous nebulizers and reduces aerosol waste to the atmosphere. Figure 4-39 illustrates this principle and gives an example of a breath-enhanced nebulizer.

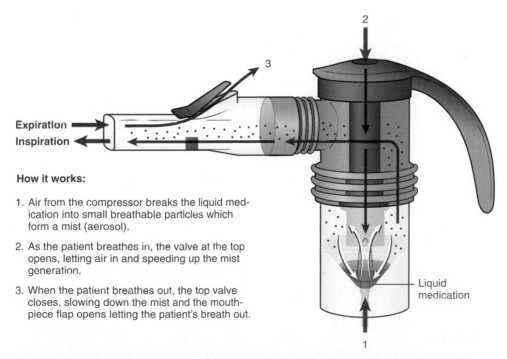

How it works:

1. Air from the compressor breaks the liquid medication into small breathable particles which form a mist (aerosol).

2. As the patient breathes in, the valve at the top opens, letting air in and speeding up the mist generation.

3. When the patient breathes out, the top valve closes, slowing down the mist and the mouthpiece flap opens letting the patient's breath out.

FIGURE 4-39 Operating principles of the Sprint (Pari Midlothran, VA) breath-enhanced nebulizer. (1) Gas enters through the jet, entrains fluid from the reservoir, and shears droplets into the baffler. (2) During inspiration, gas is inhaled both from the jet and through a valve at the top of the device. (3) During exhalation, gas passes through the valve on the mouthpiece while the jet continues to generate aerosol.

As was mentioned previously, **breath-actuated nebulizers** generate aerosol only during inspiration. This feature eliminates waste of aerosol during exhalation and increases the delivered dose threefold or more over continuous and breath-enhanced nebulizers. Breath-synchronized nebulization can increase the inhaled aerosol mass by threefold to fourfold over conventional continuous nebulization. Historically, this was accomplished with a patient-controlled finger port that directs gas to the nebulizer only during inspiration (Figure 4-40). Although this type of system wastes less of the drug being aerosolized, it can quadruple the treatment time and requires good hand-breath coordination.

The AeroEclipse BanII (Trudell Medical International, London, Ontario, Canada), shown in Figure 4-41, is a breath-actuated nebulizer with a spring-loaded, one-way valve design that draws a jet to the capillary tube during inspiration. Nebulization stops when the patient's inspiratory flow decreases below the threshold. Cessation of negative inspiratory pressure or flow allows the nebulizer baffle to move away from its position directly above the jet orifice, stopping nebulization. The AeroEclipse nebulizer also can be operated manually to synchronize aerosol on inspiration for use with infants and children too small to trigger the device. Although this device has a residual volume similar to that of other jet nebulizers, aerosol drug waste and contamination of the environment during the expiratory phase of the breathing cycle are greatly reduced.

The ProDose and INeb systems (Respironics, Concord, Calif.) (Figure 4-42) are examples breath-actuated jet nebulizers with adaptive aerosol delivery (AAD). As Figure 4-42 shows these devices monitor the pressure changes and inspiratory time for the patient's first three consecutive breaths.[62] The drug then is aerosolized for 50% of the inspiration during the fourth and all subsequent breaths. When

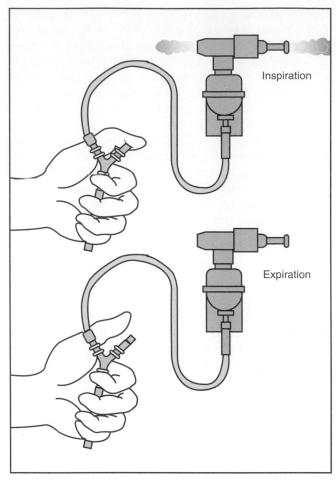

FIGURE 4-40 Use of a finger control to control regulate production during inspiration and expiration.

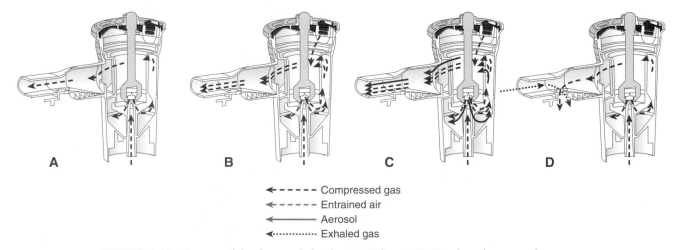

←----- Compressed gas
←----- Entrained air
←—— Aerosol
←·········· Exhaled gas

FIGURE 4-41 Diagram of the flow path for the AeroEclipse BAN II, a breath-actuated pneumatic nebulizer. **A,** Before inhalation, the actuator is up and compressed gas freely circulates with no aerosol produced. **B,** As the patient inhales, the actuator starts to move down. **C,** Negative pressure pulls the diaphragm down with the actuator, sealing around the nozzle cover and producing aerosol. **D,** The patient exhales through a valve in the mouthpiece; as the pressure increases, the diaphragm and actuator move up, stopping aerosol production. (Courtesy Trudell Medical International, London, Ontario, Canada.)

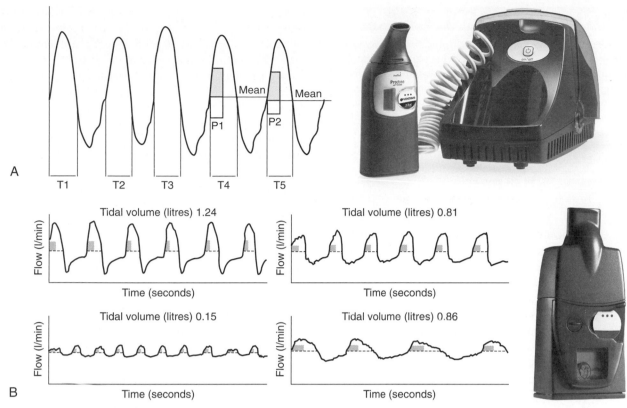

FIGURE 4-42 Adaptive aerosol delivery (AAD) delivers a precise, preset dose with variation between patients. A microprocessor tracks the patient's breathing pattern on a running average of the previous three breaths, generating aerosol for 50% of the predicted inspiration. **A,** The ProDose uses a compressor and jet nebulizer. **B,** The I Neb is a handheld unit that uses a vibrating mesh. (From Wilkins RL, Stoller JK, Kacmarek RM: *Egan's fundamentals of respiratory care,* ed 9, St Louis, 2009, Mosby.)

the patient's preestablished dose has been aerosolized, the system provides an audible signal indicating that treatment should be stopped and the remaining medication discarded. Built-in electronics monitor the patient's treatment schedules and delivered doses. The device is programmed with an externally applied chip that determines the inhaled dose for the specific drug used. By design, these breath-actuated devices are highly efficient at providing emitted aerosol to the lungs; however, the overall efficiency of the dose placed in the nebulizer is considerably less. A unit dose of drug may only need to be partly nebulized to achieve the intended dose, which leaves a large proportion of the drug in the reservoir.

The ProDose system consists of a compressor and a jet nebulizer. The I-Neb (see Figure 4-42) is a handheld AAD device that uses passive vibrating mesh technology with AAD. The I-Neb has been released for delivery of Ventavist, a form of inhaled prostacyclin used to treat primary pulmonary hypertension. As a drug-device combination, the I-Neb is available only for use with this one drug.

Flow. Droplet size and nebulization time are inversely proportional to gas flow through the jet. The higher the flow of gas to the nebulizer, the smaller the particle size generated and the shorter the time required for nebulizing the full dose of the drug. Nebulizers that produce smaller particle sizes by use of baffles, such as one-way valves, may reduce total drug output per minute compared with the same nebulizer without baffling. Consequently, these devices may require more time to deliver a standard dose of medication to the lungs.

Gas Source (Hospital versus Home). The driving pressure supplied to the nebulizer can affect particle size distribution and output. Higher driving pressures (and flows) result in smaller particle sizes, greater aerosol output, and shorter treatment times. A nebulizer that produces an MMAD of 2.5 µm when driven by a gas source of 50 psi at 6 to 10 L/min may produce an MMAD of more than 5 µm when operated on a home compressor (or ventilator), which can develop a pressure of only 10 psi. Using a driving pressure or flow that is too low can result in significantly decreased nebulizer output. Consequently, nebulizers used for home care should be matched to the compressor according to data supplied by the manufacturer so that the specific nebulizer used delivers the desired medications prescribed for the patient. In Europe, equipment manufacturers are required to characterize the performance of their nebulizer and compressor combinations using standardized methods so that consumers can compare the performance characteristics of a nebulizer with a particular compressor. Until such time as similar standards are required in the United States, clinicians should make every effort to determine whether the system prescribed meets these criteria.

Other concerns in the use of disposable nebulizers with compressors at home involve possible performance degradation of the plastic device with multiple uses. One study showed that repeated use did not alter the MMAD or output as long as the nebulizer was cleaned properly.[56] Failure to clean the nebulizer properly can result in degradation of performance as a result of clogging of the Venturi orifice (which reduces the output flow) and the buildup of electrostatic charge in the device. (See Clinical Rounds 4-4.)

Gas Density. The density of the driving gas affects both aerosol generation and the delivery of aerosols to the lungs. Lowering the density of a carrier gas reduces the amount of turbulent flow (i.e., lowers the Reynolds number), which results in less aerosol impaction in the upper airways. This phenomenon has been demonstrated with low-density helium-oxygen (heliox) mixtures. The lower the density of a carrier gas, the less aerosol impaction occurs as the gas passes through the upper airways, and the greater the deposition of aerosol in the lungs.[58] Heliox concentrations equal to or greater than 40% have been shown to increase aerosol delivery to obstructed airways and through an endotracheal tube by as much as 50%.[59] However, it is worth noting that when heliox is used to drive a jet nebulizer at standard flow rates, aerosol output is substantially less than with air or oxygen, and aerosol particles are considerably smaller. (Nebulizers driven with heliox typically require a twofold to threefold increase in flow to produce a comparable aerosol output.)

Humidity and Temperature. Humidity and temperature can affect particle size and the concentration of drug remaining in the nebulizer. Evaporation of water and **adiabatic** expansion of gas can reduce the temperature of an aerosol to as much as 10° C below the ambient temperature. This cooling may increase solution viscosity and reduce the nebulizer output.[60] Aerosol particles entrained into a warm and fully saturated gas stream increase in size. These particles can also coalesce (stick together), further increasing the MMAD and severely compromising the output of respirable particles. How much these particles enlarge depends primarily on the tonicity of the solution. Aerosol particles generated from isotonic solutions probably maintain their size as they enter the respiratory tract; particles generated from hypertonic solutions tend to enlarge, and evaporation can cause hypotonic droplets to shrink in size.

Characteristics of Drug Formulation. The viscosity and density of a drug formulation affect both output and particle size. Some drugs, such as antibiotics, are so viscous that they cannot be nebulized effectively in standard SVNs. This also is an issue with suspensions in which some aerosolized particles contain no active drug, and other, generally larger particles are required to carry the active medication.

Special Medication Delivery Issues for Infants and Children. Infants and small children require smaller minute volumes than adults, therefore they inhale a smaller proportion of a continuous nebulizer output.[63] For patients who can tolerate a mask, a medication nebulizer can be attached to an appropriately sized aerosol mask. Because the clinical response is the same to a mouthpiece or close-fitting mask treatment, patient compliance and preference should guide selection of the device. However, aerosol delivery to a patient is substantially reduced when a loosely fitting mask (leak greater than 1 cm) is used rather than a snug mask or mouthpiece.[64]

Blowing the aerosol into the face of an infant or a child is not a good aerosol delivery option for children who will not tolerate mask treatment (e.g., will not wear a close-fitting mask). This "blow-by" technique typically is performed by directing the aerosol from the nebulizer toward the patient's nose and mouth from several inches from the face. Studies suggest that very little drug enters the airway with this method. It may be more efficient to take the time to condition the patient to tolerate the mask or to deliver medication with a close-fitting mask when the patient is sound asleep.[65] A possible alternative to the blow-by technique is the PediNeb (Westmed Tucson, AZ), shown in Figure 4-43. The PediNeb is a pacifier that directs aerosol from a jet nebulizer toward the infant's nose. No published data are available, in vitro or otherwise, on the effectiveness of this device.

Crying greatly reduces lower airway deposition of aerosol medication. If a mask is not tolerated, other options should be considered. Aerosol hoods and tents have been used for aerosol delivery to small children, with good effect. In infants, a properly fitted hood can deliver a lung dose similar to that obtained with a tightly fitting mask;

however, hoods are rarely used for toddlers and older children.

For patients who will not tolerate a mask but will tolerate a nasal cannula, aerosol delivery with humidified gas via nasal cannula has been studied in vitro. Bhashyam et al.[66] passed 3 L/min of oxygen through the connector of a vibrating mesh nebulizer (Aeroneb, Solo) placed at the inlet of a heated humidifier with the outlet attached to a nasal cannula (Figure 4-44). They reported that 8% to 18% of the drug dose was delivered through an infant nasal cannula; 18% to 24% was delivered through a pediatric cannula; and 25% to 29% was delivered through an adult cannula. With a nebulizer producing a 5-μm VMD aerosol, the particles exiting the cannula were smaller than 2 μm. Particles of this size should readily pass through the nose and upper airways with little impact loss. Further in vivo studies are required to confirm the therapeutic benefits of this approach.

Technique. Box 4-10 outlines the optimum technique for using an SVN for aerosol drug delivery. A slow inspiratory flow optimizes aerosol deposition with an SVN; however, deep breathing and breath-holding during SVN therapy do little to enhance deposition over normal tidal breathing.[69] Because the nose is an efficient filter of particles larger than 5 mm, many clinicians prefer not to use a mask for SVN therapy. As long as the patient is mouth-breathing, little difference in the clinical response is seen between therapy given by mouthpiece and that given by mask. The selection of delivery method (mask or mouthpiece) should be based on the patient's ability, preference, and comfort.

Infection Control Issues. The CDC recommends that nebulizers be cleaned and disinfected (or rinsed with sterile water) and air-dried between uses.[70] Box 4-11 provides some useful recommendations for care of an SVN used in the home care setting.

Large-Volume Jet Nebulizers

A **large-volume nebulizer (LVN)** is used to provide continuous nebulization. The high-output, extended aerosol respiratory therapy nebulizers are examples of devices designed for this purpose. These nebulizers have a reservoir greater than 200 mL, and they can produce an aerosol with an MMAD of 2.2 to 3.5 μm. Actual output and particle size vary with the pressure and flow at which the nebulizer operates. As was already mentioned, a potential problem with continuous bronchodilator therapy (CBT) is increased drug concentration in the reservoir over time. Therefore, patients receiving CBT should be closely monitored for signs of drug toxicity (e.g., tachycardia and tremor).

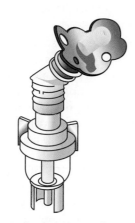

FIGURE 4-43 The PediNeb (Westmed Tucson, AZ) combines a pacifier with aerosol ports directed at the nares. No data are available to confirm the device's efficacy, and concerns have been raised about high ocular deposition.

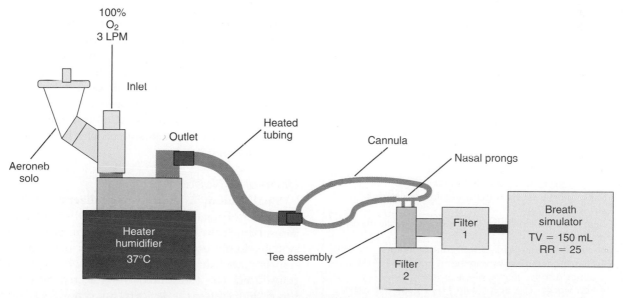

FIGURE 4-44 In vitro setup for testing aerosol delivery with a heated humidifier through a nasal cannula. The nebulizer is placed at the inlet of the humidifier, and the cannula is attached to a T-piece that allows aerosol to collect on filter 1 and condensate to collect on filter 2. This device can be used in infants, children, and adults.

BOX 4-10	Technique for Using a Small-Volume Nebulizer

1. Assemble the tubing or cable, the nebulizer, and the mouthpiece or mask.
2. Place the prescribed amount of medication in the nebulizer's reservoir.
3. For a pneumatic nebulizer:
   · Connect the tubing to the flowmeter or compressor.
   · Set the flow according to the manufacturer's recommendation (often 6 to 10 L/min).
4. For a vibrating mesh or small ultrasonic nebulizer:
   · Connect a clean nebulizer/medication reservoir to the mask or mouthpiece.
   · Attach the nebulizer/reservoir to the electronic controller.
   · Attach the nebulizer to a power source or make sure the device's battery has a sufficient charge.
5. Instruct the patient to sit in an upright position, as tolerated.
6. Apply the mouthpiece or mask and encourage the patient to breathe through the mouth. If an artificial airway is used, make sure the nebulizer is positioned appropriately and does not put undue pressure on the airway.
7. Encourage relaxed tidal breathing with low inspiratory flow rates and occasional deep breaths.
8. Operate the nebulizer in an upright position, 45 degrees from vertical.
9. Run the nebulizer until the onset of sputter or until aerosol is no longer produced.
10. At the conclusion of therapy, rinse, wash, disinfect, and air-dry the nebulizer/reservoir or dispose of it.
11. Do not submerge the electronic controller or compressor in water or disinfectant.
12. Store the nebulizer in a clean, dry place.

BOX 4-11	Cleaning and Disinfection of Nebulizers for Home Use

· After each use:
   · Disassemble the nebulizer and mouthpiece or mask.
   · Wash them in warm, soapy water.
   · Rinse with tap water.
   · Shake off the excess water.
   · Place the parts on a clean, absorbent towel and allow them to air-dry.
   · Reassemble the nebulizer and store it in a clean, dry place.
· Once a day:
   · After washing the nebulizer and mouthpiece or mask, place them in a disinfectant solution to soak for 1 hour.
   · Rinse with sterile or distilled water.
   · Shake off the excess water and allow the parts to air-dry.
   · Reassemble the nebulizer and store it in a clean, dry place.
· Some types of homemade disinfecting solutions:
   · 1 Ounce quaternary ammonium compound (QAC) to 1 ounce distilled water; discard weekly.
   · 1 Part vinegar (5% acetic acid) to 3 parts hot water; discard after each use.
   · 1 Teaspoon household chlorine bleach to 1 gallon of water; discard after use.

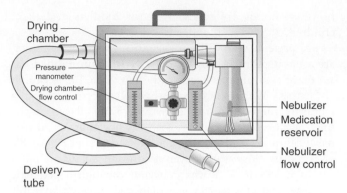

FIGURE 4-45 Small particle aerosol generator. (From Wilkins RL, Stoller JK, Kacmarek RM: *Egan's fundamentals of respiratory care,* ed 9, St Louis, 2009, Mosby.)

Another special purpose LVN is the small particle aerosol generator (SPAG) like the one shown in figure 4-45. The SPAG (ICN Pharmaceuticals, valeant Pharmaceuticals International, Aliso Viejo, CA) was designed specifically for administration of ribavirin (Virazole) to infants with respiratory syncytial virus infection. The SPAG incorporates a drying chamber with its own flow control to produce a stable aerosol. The SPAG reduces the medical gas source to as low as 26 psig with an adjustable regulator. The regulator is connected to two flowmeters that separately control flow to the nebulizer and the drying chamber. The nebulizer is in the medication reservoir, the fluid surface and wall of which serve as primary baffles. The aerosol enters the long, cylindrical drying chamber where the separate flow of dry gas reduces the particle size by evaporation, creating a monodisperse aerosol with an MMAD of 1.2 to 1.4 μm. Nebulizer flow should be maintained at approximately 7 L/min, with total flow from both flowmeters no lower than 15 L/min. The latest model operates consistently, even with back pressure, and can be used with masks, hoods, tents, or ventilator circuits. It is worth mentioning that when the SPAG is used to deliver ribavirin through a mechanical ventilation circuit, drug precipitation can jam breathing valves or occlude the ventilator circuit. This problem can be prevented by (1) placing a one-way valve between the SPAG and the circuit and (2) filtering out the excess aerosol particles before they reach the exhalation valve.[71]

Ultrasonic Nebulizers
Small-Volume Ultrasonic Nebulizers
A number of small-volume USNs have been marketed for aerosol drug delivery. Unlike the larger units, some of these systems do not use a couplant compartment; the medication is placed directly into the manifold on top of the transducer. The transducer is connected by cable to a power source; often the device is battery powered to increase portability. These devices have no blower; the patient's inspiratory flow draws the aerosol from the nebulizer into the lung.

Small-volume USNs have been promoted for administration of a wide variety of formulations, ranging from bronchodilators to anti-inflammatory agents and antibiotics.[73] Use of a small-volume USN may increase the available respirable mass for devices with less residual drug volume than SVNs. This may reduce the need for a large amount of diluent to ensure delivery of the drugs. The contained portable power source adds a great deal of convenience in mobility. However, these advantages are offset by relatively high purchase costs and poor reliability.

Some ventilator manufacturers (e.g., Siemens, Nellcor Puritan Bennett) have advocated the use of USNs for administration of aerosols during mechanical ventilation. Unlike SVNs, USNs do not add extra gas flow to the ventilator circuit during use. This feature reduces the need to change and reset ventilator and alarm settings during aerosol administration.[74]

Large-Volume Ultrasonic Nebulizers. Large-volume USNs are used mainly for bland aerosol therapy or sputum induction. These devices incorporate air blowers to carry the mist to the patient. Low flow through these large-volume USNs is associated with smaller particles and higher mist density. High flow yields larger particles and less density. Unlike jet nebulizers, the temperature of the solution placed in a USN increases during use. As the temperature increases, the drug concentration increases, as does the likelihood of undesirable side effects.

Atomizers and Spray Pumps

Hand-bulb atomizers (Figure 4-46) and nasal spray pumps are used to administer sympathomimetic, antimuscarinic, anti-inflammatory, and anesthetic aerosols to the upper airway (nasal passages, pharynx, and larynx). These agents are used to manage upper airway inflammation and rhinitis, to provide local anesthesia, and to achieve systemic

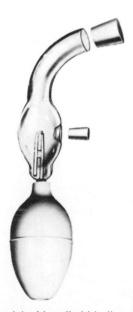

FIGURE 4-46 The original handheld bulb nebulizer manufactured by DeVilbiss. (Courtesy Sunrise Medical Home Healthcare, Longmont, Colo.)

effects. AARC has developed guidelines for the delivery of drugs to the upper airway.[74]

A nasal spray pump produces an aerosol suspension with a high MMAD and GSD, which are ideal for upper airway deposition. Nasopharyngeal deposition is greatest for particles 5 to 20 μm. Deposition with the hand-bulb atomizer applied to the nose occurs mostly in the anterior nasal passages, with clearance to the nasopharynx. The 100-μL puffs appear to deposit more medication than do 50-μL puffs, and deposition to a greater surface area occurs with a 35-degree spray angle than with a 60-degree angle.

Vibrating Mesh Nebulizers

Vibrating mesh (VM) nebulizers, are electromechanical devices that pass liquid through a mesh or aperture plate to form droplets. VM nebulizers rely on two different operating principles, which are classified as passive and active.[75]

Passive (static) VM nebulizers use an ultrasonic transducer or ultrasonic horn to generate vibrations of 180 kHz, which push liquid through the static mesh to produce aerosol that can be inhaled directly by the patient. The particles range in size from 3 to 6 μm. The passive vibrating mesh was first introduced on a limited basis in the 1980s by Omron Healthcare (Bannockburn, Illinois). It is now available in the Micro aire NEU-22 (Omron, Japan) and the I-Neb (Respironics).

Active VM nebulizers use a dome-shaped aperture plate containing 1000 to 4000 funnel-shaped, tapered apertures. The wide inlet of the aperture faces the reservoir of medication, and the narrow outlet determines the particle size produced. The domed aperture plate is attached to a flat disk, which is attached to a piezoelectric ceramic element that surrounds the aperture plate. Electricity applied to this element causes the aperture plate to vibrate at a frequency greater than 120 kHz (one tenth that of an ultrasonic nebulizer), moving the apertures up and down by 1 or 2 μm and creating a pumping action. The liquid is pumped through the apertures, where it is broken into fine droplets. The exit velocity of the aerosol is slow (less than 4 m/sec), and the particle size can range from 2 to 5 μm (MMAD), varying with aperture size of the specific nebulizer. Active VM aerosol generators can nebulize individual drops as small as 5 μL, with as little as 1 μL residual drug. Examples of active VM nebulizers are the Aeroneb Professional Nebulizer, Solo, and Go (Aerogen, Galway, Ireland) and the eFlow Rapid (Pari, Munich, Germany).

VM nebulizers can generate aerosol from a single drop of liquid and have residual drug volumes ranging from 0.1 to 1.2 ml, based largely on the design of the medication reservoir feeding the mesh. Unlike with jet and USN nebulizers, the mesh acts as a physical barrier between the drug in the medication reservoir and the body of the nebulizer in which the aerosol output is collected. This reduces the risk of exhaled pathogens contaminating the medication in the reservoir.

VM nebulizers do not require any propellants or gas and add no gas to the aerosol stream. This makes them attractive for use in closed systems, such as during mechanical ventilation. The piezoelectric and ultrasonic components are used to vibrate the mesh or push fluid through a mesh, rather than creating a standing wave in the medication, as happens in a USN. Compared to the USN, VM technology has lower residual drug volumes, requires less energy, generates less heat, and is more reliable for generation of suspensions and for extended use.

VM nebulizers are considerably more expensive than jet nebulizers but similar to USNs (Table 4-2). Mesh nebulizer are small, silent, portable, and compatible with use of a broad range of drug compounds. Delivery of a suspension can be less efficient with the VM nebulizer, because larger particles (larger than the mesh aperture diameter) are filtered out and do not reach the patient as aerosol.

Marketed mesh nebulizers for home use (Micro Aire NEU-22, Aeroneb Go, and eFlow Rapid) are probably similar in performance to the best of the breath-enhanced/breath-actuated pneumatic nebulizers in terms of inhaled drug mass and particle size. The Aeroneb Pro and Solo were both designed for hospital use and primarily targeted for use during mechanical ventilation. They have been shown in vitro to be more efficient than standard jet nebulizers.[76]

The I-Neb has been released only as a drug-device combination for use with Ventavist in the treatment of ambulatory patients with primary pulmonary hypertension. A variant of the Pari eFlow Nebulizer will be released with Aztreonam, an antibiotic used in the treatment of cystic fibrosis (CF).

New Nebulizer Designs[78]

The Respimat (Boehringer Ingelheim) is a disposable, multiple-dose, soft mist inhaler (Figure 4-47). It uses energy produced by spring compression to generate an aerosol from liquid solutions to produce a low-velocity spray (10 m/sec) with a single actuation. The small 11-µL dose is generated in 1.2 seconds to achieve 45% lung deposition. To operate the device, the patient places the Respimat in the mouth and presses a button to release the drug spray as the person begins a slow, deep inspiration. Although the Respimat requires hand-breath coordination, it produces lower oropharyngeal deposition than pMDIs or DPIs. The Respimat has been released in Europe for delivery of Tiotropium.

The Akita2 system (Activaero, Gemunden/Wohra, Germany) is a microprocessor-controlled system that integrates a breath-actuated aerosol generator (pneumatic or vibrating mesh) with a separate gas source to control the patient's inspiratory flow. Low inspiratory flows allow for prolonged inspirations, up to 12 seconds. Low inspiratory flow also reduces turbulence in the upper and middle airways, allowing a dramatic increase in aerosol delivered to the lung periphery. Breath parameters are set on the basis of the individual patient's pulmonary function and the intended target area for deposition. The Akita2 has been used in the treatment of patients with CF in Germany and currently is used in research applications for the delivery of specific drug formulations. The Akita2 is the first commercial liquid aerosol delivery system that provides an opportunity for controlled delivery of aerosols to different regions of the lung.

The AERx (Aradigm, Hayward, California) uses a drug solution in a unit-dose, sterile, preservative-free blister

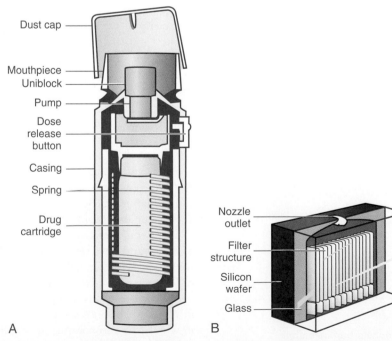

FIGURE 4-47 A, Respimat soft mist inhaler provides multidose convenience. **B,** Mechanical energy drives 11 µL of liquid medication through the Uniblock to generate aerosol.

TABLE 4-2

Comparison of Aerosol Generators Used to Administer Medications to the Lung

	MDI Alone	MDI with VHC	DPI	SVN	USN	VM
Flow independent	−	+++	−	+++	+++	+++
Volume independent	−	+++	−	+++	+++	+++
Coordination independent	−	+++	+++	+++	+++	+++
Low oral deposition	−−	+++	−−	+	+	+
Ease of use	++	+++	++	+++	++	+++
Portable	+++	++	+++	+	++	+++
Quick to administer	++	+++	+++	+	++	+++
Cost	+++	++	++	++	−−	−−
Low infection risk	+++	+++	+++	−−−	−−−	+
Effective with:						
Severe asthma	+	+++	+	+++	++	+++
Small children	−	+++	−−	+++	−	+++
Ventilators	−	++++	−−−	+	+++	+++
Unusual medication	−−	−−	−−	++	+	++

+, Positive characteristic; −, negative characteristic.

DPI, Dry powder inhaler; *MDI*, metered-dose inhaler; *MDI with VHC*, metered-dose inhaler with a valved holding chamber; *SVN*, small-volume nebulizer; *USN*, ultrasonic nebulizer; *VM*, vibrating mesh nebulizer.

pack containing 25 to 50 µL of fluid. The drug is extruded under pressure through a nozzle containing a number of small, precision-drilled holes that produce a fine, respirable spray on inhalation. The aerosolization nozzle is part of the disposable blister and is not reused. The dose from a single blister is metered in approximately 1.5 seconds. The emitted dose is more than 70% of the dose contained in the blister with an inspiratory flow rate range of 30 to 85 L/min. The AERx device has built-in electronic monitoring capabilities for measuring the inspiratory flow rate (IFR) during dosing and for triggering the dispensing the dose at the appropriate IFR for optimum delivery. The dose administered is logged to provide a record of treatments and an indication of patient compliance with therapy. The AERx device is in clinical trials in the United States.

Selecting an Aerosol Drug Delivery System

Selection of the most appropriate aerosol delivery system requires a knowledge of the advantages and disadvantages of the various systems currently available. Table 4-2 compares the pMDI, DPI, SVN, USN, and VM delivery systems. A comparison of aerosol distribution by device is shown in Figure 4-48.

The American College of Chest Physicians (ACCP) commissioned an extensive, evidence-based review of the literature to determine which types of aerosol delivery system were most effective. They concluded that pMDIs, DPIs, and nebulizers all work with comparable clinical results, as long as they are prescribed for the appropriate patients and are used properly.[78]

The AARC has published several clinical practice guidelines to guide practitioners in selecting the best aerosol delivery system for a given clinical situation. Summaries of

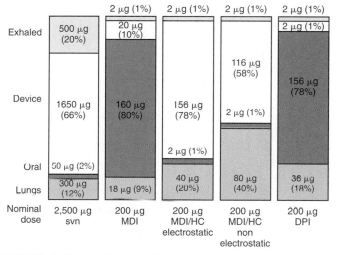

FIGURE 4-48 Distribution of albuterol via nebulizer, pMDI, pMDI with a holding chamber (electrostatic and nonelectrostatic), and DPI.

the various guidelines can be found in Clinical Practice Guidelines. Excerpts from three of these guidelines are included in Clinical Practice Guidelines 4-1 through 4-3.

A number of factors should be considered when selecting the appropriate aerosol delivery device for a particular patient: (1) the available drug formulation, (2) the desired site of deposition, (3) the patient's characteristics (age, acuity of respiratory problem, alertness, and ability to follow instructions), (4) the patient's ability to properly use the device, and (5) the patient's preference.[76]

For administration of maintenance therapy bronchodilators and anti-inflammatory agents to adults, a pMDI with a valved holding chamber is the most convenient, versatile, and cost-effective method. DPIs are gaining popularity as equivalent to pMDIs for maintenance therapy with available drugs for patients capable of generating an adequate inspiratory flow. In acute situations, when high or multiple doses are needed, or when adult patients are not able to follow instructions, an SVN or large-volume continuous nebulizer is an alternative.

An adult patient's preference must be considered, because a device that is not favored will not be used. USN and VM nebulizers may be the devices of choice when portability and short duration of therapy is desired; however, cost is often a mitigating factor in device selection. For ambulatory use, compressor-driven nebulizers often are the least expensive option.

Finally, it is important to state that the effectiveness of aerosol therapy (or any type of self-administered therapy) is greatly influenced by the patient's understanding of the procedure. Nearly all aerosol therapy is self-administered. Interestingly, many patients using aerosol devices report that they did not receive adequate instruction on how to use their equipment. Box 4-12 provides some suggestions for improving the effectiveness of patient education about aerosol therapy.

Special Considerations

Continuous Nebulization

Patients who come to the emergency department with a severe exacerbation of asthma or acute bronchospasm often have been taking their bronchodilator for 24 to 36

Selection of an Aerosol Delivery Device

Clinical Practice Guideline 4-1

■ **DESCRIPTION**

The device selected for administration of a pharmacologically active aerosol to the lower airway should produce particles with a mass median aerodynamic diameter (MMAD) of 1–3 μm. Such devices include pressurized metered-dose inhalers (pMDIs), pMDIs with accessory devices (e.g., spacers), dry powder inhalers (DPIs), small-volume nebulizers (SVNs), large-volume nebulizers (LVNs), and ultrasonic nebulizers (USNs). Note that this guideline does not address bland aerosol administration and sputum induction.

■ **INDICATIONS**

Aerosol delivery devices are needed to deliver aerosolized medications to the lower airways, such as β-adrenergic agents, anticholinergic agents (antimuscarinic), anti-inflammatory agents (e.g., corticosteroids), mediator-modifying compounds (e.g., cromolyn sodium), and mucokinetics.

■ **CONTRAINDICATIONS**

No contraindications exist to the administration of aerosols by inhalation, although contraindications may be posed by the substances being delivered. Package inserts should be consulted for product-specific contraindications.

■ **HAZARDS AND COMPLICATIONS**

1. Malfunction of the device or improper technique may result in the delivery of an incorrect dose of medication.
2. Complications of specific pharmacologic agents may occur.
3. Cardiotoxic effects of Freon have been reported as idiosyncratic responses that may be a problem with excessive use of an MDI.
4. Freon may harm the environment by its effect on the ozone layer.
5. Repeated exposure to aerosols has been reported to produce asthmatic symptoms in some caregivers.

■ **MONITORING**

1. Device performance
2. Device application technique
3. Patient response, including changes in vital signs

■ **INFECTION CONTROL**

1. Standard precautions for body substance isolation must be used.
2. SVNs and LVNs are for single-patient use or should be subjected to high-level disinfection between patients.
3. Published data establishing a safe use period for SVNs and LVNs are lacking; however SVNs and LVNs probably should be changed or subjected to high-level disinfection at about 24-hour intervals.
4. Medications should be handled aseptically. Medications from multidose sources in acute care facilities must be handled aseptically and discarded after 24 hours, unless the manufacturer's recommendations specifically state that medications may be stored longer than 24 hours. Tap water should not be used as a diluent.
5. MDI accessory devices are only for single-patient use. No documented concerns exist about contamination of medication in pMDI canisters. Cleaning of accessory devices is based on aesthetic criteria.

Modified from the American Association for Respiratory Care: Clinical practice guideline: selection of aerosol delivery device, Respir Care 37:891, 1992.

BOX 4-12	Teaching Patients Psychomotor Skills for Inhaler Use

1. Set aside uninterrupted time to complete the instruction.
2. Perform the demonstration in a suitable environment.
3. Have all necessary equipment and spares close at hand.
4. Engage the patient's attention.
5. Explain verbally what you will do and why.
6. Demonstrate the technique for using the inhaler, naming and explaining each step.
7. Repeat the demonstration without explanation (talking, although necessary in the previous step, interferes with correct timing and inspiratory maneuvers).
8. Repeat again with verbal comments.
9. Have the patient demonstrate the maneuver, including correct identification of inhalers and assembly of the inhaler/spacer combination.
10. Identify problems in performance, and repeat the instruction and patient return demonstration.
11. Ask the patient to verbalize the most important aspects of the procedure and those most troublesome.
12. Arrange for follow-up instruction. Assure the patient that some loss of skill over time is typical and can be corrected. Remind the patient to bring inhalers and spacers to every appointment.
13. Provide instruction to family or friends if requested.
14. Review and provide instructional leaflets or videos if available.

Modified from Coates VE: *Education for patients and clients,* London, 1999, Routledge.

Bland Aerosol Administration

Clinical Practice Guideline 4-2

■ DESCRIPTION

For purposes of this guideline, bland aerosol administration includes the delivery of sterile water or hypotonic, isotonic, or hypertonic saline in aerosol form. Bland aerosol administration may be accompanied by oxygen administration.

■ INDICATIONS

Cool, bland aerosol therapy is indicated primarily for upper airway administration; therefore an MMAD equal to or greater than 5 μm is desirable. The use of hypotonic and hypertonic saline is indicated primarily for inducing sputum specimens; therefore an MMAD of 1 to 5 μm is desirable. Heated bland aerosol is indicated primarily for minimizing humidity deficit when the upper airway has been bypassed; for this purpose, an MMAD of 2 to 10 μm is desirable. Specific indications include:

1. Upper airway edema (cool bland aerosol)
2. Laryngotracheobronchitis (LTB)
3. Subglottic edema
4. Postextubation management of the upper airway
5. Postoperative management of the upper airway
6. Bypassed upper airway
7. Need for sputum specimens

■ CONTRAINDICATIONS

1. Bronchoconstriction
2. History of airway hyperresponsiveness

■ HAZARDS AND COMPLICATIONS

1. Wheezing or bronchospasm
2. Bronchoconstriction when an artificial airway is used
3. Infection
4. Overhydration
5. Patient discomfort
6. Caregiver exposure to droplet nuclei of *Mycobacterium tuberculosis* or other airborne contagious organisms released through coughing, particularly during sputum induction

■ ASSESSMENT OF NEED

The presence of one or more of the following may be an indication for administration of a water or isotonic or hypotonic saline aerosol:

1. Stridor
2. Brassy, crouplike cough
3. Hoarseness after extubation
4. Diagnosis of LTB or croup

Continued

Bland Aerosol Administration—cont'd

5. Clinical history suggesting upper airway irritation and increased work of breathing (e.g., smoke inhalation)
6. Patient discomfort associated with airway instrumentation or insult
7. Need for sputum induction (e.g., for diagnosis of *Pneumocystis carinii* pneumonia or tuberculosis)

ASSESSMENT OF OUTCOME
The desired outcomes for administration of water or hypotonic or isotonic saline include:
1. Decreased work of breathing
2. Improved vital signs
3. Decreased stridor
4. Decreased dyspnea
5. Improved arterial blood gas values
6. Improved oxygen saturation, as indicated by pulse oximetry (SpO_2)

The desired outcome for administration of hypertonic saline is a sputum sample adequate for analysis.

MONITORING
The extent of patient monitoring should be determined by the stability and severity of the patient's condition. Monitoring may include:
1. Subjective patient responses of pain, discomfort, dyspnea, or restlessness
2. Heart rate and rhythm
3. Blood pressure
4. Respiratory rate, as well as the breathing pattern and use of accessory respiratory muscles
5. Breath sounds
6. Sputum production quantity, color, consistency, and odor
7. Pulse oximetry (if hypoxemia is suspected)

Respiratory Care 2003;48(5)529-533, 1993.

Selection of a Device for Aerosol Delivery to the Lung Parenchyma

Clinical Practice Guideline 4-3

DESCRIPTION
A device selected for administration of a pharmacologically active aerosol to the lung parenchyma should produce particles with an MMAD of 1 to 3 µm. Such devices include ultrasonic nebulizers (USNs), some large-volume nebulizers (LVNs) (e.g., the SPAG unit, which is intended only for ribavirin delivery), and some small-volume nebulizers (SVNs) (e.g., the Circulaire, Respirgard II, and Pari IS 2).

INDICATIONS
The indication for selecting a suitable device is the need to deliver a topical medication (in aerosol form) with a site of action in the lung parenchyma or that is intended for systemic absorption. Such medications may include antibiotics, antivirals, antifungals, surfactants, and enzymes.

CONTRAINDICATIONS
No contraindications exist to choosing an appropriate device for parenchymal deposition. Contraindications may exist related to the substances being delivered. Package inserts should be consulted for product-specific contraindications to medication delivery.

HAZARDS AND COMPLICATIONS
1. Device malfunction or improper technique may result in delivery of incorrect medication doses.
2. For mechanically ventilated patients, the nebulizer design and the characteristics of the medication may affect ventilator function (e.g., filter obstruction, altered tidal volume, decreased trigger sensitivity) and medication deposition.
3. Aerosols may cause bronchospasm or airway irritation, and complications related to specific pharmacologic agents can occur.

Selection of a Device for Aerosol Delivery to the Lung Parenchyma—cont'd

4. Exposure to medication should be limited to the patient for whom it has been ordered. Nebulizer medication released into the atmosphere from the nebulizer or the patient may affect health care providers and others near the treatment. For example, awareness has increased of the possible health effects of aerosols such as ribavirin and pentamidine. Anecdotal reports associate symptoms such as conjunctivitis, decreased tolerance of contact lenses, headaches, bronchospasm, shortness of breath, and rashes in health care workers exposed to secondhand aerosols. Similar concerns have arisen concerning health care workers who are pregnant or planning to become pregnant within 8 weeks of administration. The potential exposure effects of aerosolized antibiotics (which may contribute to the development of resistant organisms), steroids, and bronchodilators are less often discussed. Because the data are incomplete regarding adverse health effects on health care workers and those casually exposed, exposure should be minimized in all situations.

5. The Centers for Disease Control and Prevention recommend that:
   a. Warning signs should be posted in an easy to see location to apprise all who enter the treatment area of the potential hazards of exposure. Accidental exposures should be documented and reported according to accepted standards.
   b. Staff members who administer medications must understand the inherent risks of the medication and the procedures for disposing of hazardous waste safely. Department administrators should screen staff members for adverse effects of aerosol exposure and provide alternative assignments for those at high risk of such adverse effects (e.g., pregnant women or those with demonstrated sensitivity to the specific agent).
   c. Filters or filtered scavenger systems should be used to remove aerosols that are not considered safe.
   d. Booths or stalls should be used for sputum induction and administration of aerosolized medications in areas where multiple patients are treated. The booths or stalls should be designed to provide adequate airflow to draw aerosol and droplet nuclei from the patient into an appropriate filtration system with exhaust directed to an appropriate outside vent. Note that filters, nebulizers, and other contaminated components of the aerosol delivery system used with suspect agents (e.g., pentamidine and ribavirin) should be handled as hazardous waste. If scavenger systems or specially designed booths are not available, clinicians administering these treatments should wear personal protection devices to reduce exposure to the medication residues and body substances. These devices may include fitted respirator masks, goggles, gloves, gowns, and splatter shields.

■ MONITORING

1. Device and scavenging system performance
2. Device application technique
3. Patient response

Modified from the American Association for Respiratory Care: Clinical practice guideline: selection of a device for delivery of aerosol to the lung parenchyma, Respir Care 41:647, 1996.

---

hours without any relief of the symptoms. Giving nebulizer treatments with standard bronchodilator doses and repeating the treatments at increased frequency (up to every 15 minutes) until the symptoms are relieved can require hours of staff time.[81,82]

An alternative strategy for bronchodilator resuscitation in the emergency department involves administering higher than standard doses of albuterol in either a short or prolonged time frame. Nebulizing undiluted 0.5% albuterol can deliver similar amounts of bronchodilator in 8 to 20 breaths over 1 to 2 minutes as that delivered with a standard SVN dose that takes 10 to 15 minutes. The nebulizer should be filled with 2 to 3 ml of 0.5% albuterol to overcome the 1 to 1.5 mL of residual drug volume inherent in these nebulizers. Dosing often is done to effect or until adverse effects (tremor or tachycardia) are observed.

Several studies have looked at the use of breath-actuated nebulizers with undiluted 0.5% albuterol for 2 to 3 minutes versus a standard SVN with 3 mL of 0.083% albuterol.[78,82] These studies concluded that similar results can be achieved with shorter treatment with breath actuation. However, it is unclear whether a standard SVN with a 0.5% solution would have effects similar to those obtained with a breath-actuated nebulizer.

Use of a pMDI and valved holding chamber to deliver up to 12 puffs in less than 12 minutes has also been advocated. Actuations can be given as frequently as every 30 seconds. One protocol suggests starting with 4 or 5 puffs, waiting 5 minutes to determine the effect, and then adding 1 puff every minute up to 12 puffs. If these strategies fail to provide relief, continuous bronchodilator therapy can be used to provide a range of doses to be administered over extended periods until the patient is able to respond with the desired effect.

Continuous brochodilator therapy (CBT) can be administered with LVNs that can hold 10 to 200 ml or with SVNs with a continuous feed mechanism to fill the nebulizer (Figure 4-49). Dose output is based on the output rate of the nebulizer and the concentration of medication placed in the nebulizer. With jet nebulizers, changing the rate of gas driving the nebulizer can make small changes in the output rate, but larger changes in output require emptying the reservoir or feed system and using a new concentration. Output rates for SVNs and LVNs vary between devices of the same model (even within the same lot), therefore accurate delivery requires calculation of the actual output of the individual nebulizer and adjustment of the flow as required.

Use of a VM nebulizer with continuous feed allows dosing on a drop-by-drop basis. Although the VM nebulizer is operating continuously, it produces aerosol only when the drop of drug reaches the aerosol generator. Volumetric dosing allows a greater degree of control for changing dose rates by changing the drip rate of the drug into the nebulizer. For example, with a solution of 0.5% albuterol, the VM nebulizer can deliver 10 mg/hr at an infusion rate of 2 mL/hr, or 2 drops/min using a 60 drops/mL minidrip. To increase the dose to 15 mg, the infusion rate is increased to 3 mL/hr or 3 drops/min (20 mg/hr would be 4 mL/hr or 4 drops/min). As long as the infusion of drug to the nebulizer is less than the minimum output rate of the nebulizer, no buildup of medication in the reservoir should be seen.

Once CBT is started, the patient is carefully assessed every 30 minutes for the first 2 hours and thereafter every hour. A positive response is indicated by an increase in the peak expiratory flow rate (PEFR) of at least 10% after the first hour of therapy. The goal is at least 50% of the predicted value. For small children, improved oxygenation (oxygen saturation by pulse oximeter, or an SpO_2 greater than 92% on room air) with evidence of decreased work of breathing indicates a favorable response. Once the patient "opens up," intermittent SVN administration is resumed or a pMDI dose-response assessment is conducted. The patient must be observed for adverse drug responses, including worsening tachycardia, palpitations, and vomiting. In these situations, the attending physician must be contacted immediately. Clinical Rounds 4-5 provides a case presentation of a patient admitted to the emergency department with severe asthma.

CBT has been proven to be safe and effective for both adult and pediatric patients. To provide an extra margin of safety, some clinicians recommend that patients receiving CBT undergo continuous electrocardiographic monitoring and measurement of the serum potassium level every 4 hours.

CLINICAL ROUNDS 4-5

A patient with a tidal volume of 500 ml, an inspiratory time of 1 second, and an I:E ratio of 1:4 is receiving a continuous nebulizer treatment of 4 ml of normal saline with 2.5 mg of albuterol at an oxygen flow rate of 8 L/min. What is the patient's respiratory rate, minute volume, and F_IO_2? What percentage of the medication (or gas) leaving the nebulizer is inhaled?

If the patient begins 10-second inspiratory holds, what will happen to the respiratory rate, minute volume, and percentage of medication inhaled? What will happen to the F_IO_2?

See Evolve Resources for the answer.

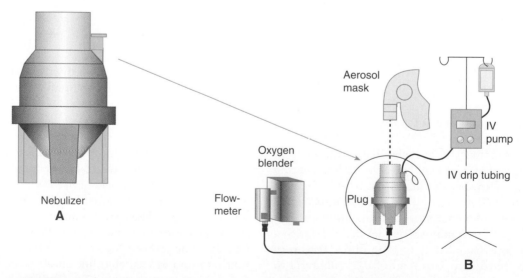

FIGURE 4-49 Intravenous drip for continuous nebulization. **A,** Small-volume nebulizer. **B,** Intravenous drip with blender, flowmeter, and drip. (From Wilkins RL, Stoller JK, Kacmarek RM: *Egan's fundamentals of respiratory care,* ed 9, St Louis, 2009, Mosby.)

Aerosol Administration to Intubated Patients[83]

Many patients undergoing mechanical ventilation receive aerosolized medications, with variable effects. The following sections cover techniques to optimize SVN, USN, VM nebulizer, and pMDI delivery to patients receiving ventilatory support. For all aerosol systems, HMEs should be considered a barrier to aerosol delivery and should not be placed between the aerosol generator and the patient. Also, active humidification should not be turned off during aerosol administration of standard medications.

Use of a SVN during Mechanical Ventilation

Aerosols administered by SVN to intubated patients receiving mechanical ventilation tend to be deposited mainly in the tubing of the ventilator circuit and expiratory filter. Under normal conditions with heated humidification and standard jet nebulizers, pulmonary deposition ranges from 1.5% to 3%. When the nebulizer output, humidity level, tidal volume, flow, and I:E ratio are optimized, deposition can increase to as much as 15%. Box 4-13 outlines the optimum technique for drug delivery by SVN to intubated patients undergoing mechanical ventilation. Although in vitro models using dry gas demonstrated up to 40% higher aerosol delivery compared to heated humidity, these effects have not been proven in patients, whereas the risks associated with administering cold, dry gas through an endotracheal tube have been demonstrated. If available with the specific ventilator, breath actuation can increase aerosol delivery by as much as 50%, but it may prolong the administration time by more than threefold.

Although some ventilators compensate for nebulizer gas flow entering the circuit, many do not. The additional flow of gas into the ventilator circuit may change the set flow and delivered volumes, as well as require adjustments to alarm settings both during and after nebulization. Smaller patients are affected to a greater extent when extra flow is added to the ventilator circuit. For example, 6 L/min of additional gas flow can more than double tidal volumes and inspiratory pressures, thus placing the patient at risk. The greatest risks are associated with changing ventilator parameters and not returning them to pretreatment levels after the treatment is completed and with interrupting ventilation while attaching and removing the SVN to the ventilator circuit. SVNs often are attached to the ventilator circuit with a standard 22-mm T adapter. Valved T adapters have been developed to allow SVN placement and removal without loss of pressure in the ventilator circuit. The risk also exists that condensate and secretions may drain into the nebulizer reservoir, which can contaminate the medication being delivered to the lungs.

BOX 4-13	Optimum Technique for Using a Small-Volume Nebulizer with Mechanical Ventilation

1. Assess the need for medication.
2. Establish the dose needed to compensate for decreased delivery (possibly 2 to 5 times the dose given to patients who are not ventilated).
3. Place the prescribed amount of drug in the small-volume nebulizer (SVN).
4. Place the SVN in the inspiratory line 12 to 18 inches from the patient Y. Check to make sure the circuit has no leaks.
5. Remove the heat and moisture exchanger (HME) from between the SVN and the patient; use an alternative form of humidification.
6. Consider placing a filter in the expiratory limb of the ventilator circuit to avoid loading the expiratory flow transducer with medications.
7. Connect the nebulizer to the nebulizer outlet port of the ventilator.
8. Use the ventilator nebulizer compressor if it meets the flow needs of the nebulizer and cycles on inspiration; otherwise, use continuous flow from an external 50-psi source with continuous gas flow to the nebulizer at 1 to 10 L/min; adjust the volume or pressure limit to compensate for additional flow during treatment.
9. Turn off the flowby or continuous flow function while nebulizing.
10. Tap the nebulizer periodically until all the medication has been nebulized.
11. Remove the nebulizer from the circuit. Rinse it with sterile water and air dry. Store the nebulizer in a clean bag between treatments or replace between treatments.
12. Check to make sure the ventilator circuit has no leaks. Return the ventilator and alarms to the previous settings.
13. Monitor the patient for an adverse response.
14. Assess the outcome of the treatment.

Use of a USN during Mechanical Ventilation

Aerosol administration by ultrasonic nebulizer can increase drug deposition during mechanical ventilation without the addition of gas into the ventilator circuit. The most efficient placement of the USN is in the upright position on the inspiratory limb at the Y near the patient. Unfortunately, the size and weight of USNs make this positioning difficult, especially with infant ventilators. USN typically are operated continuously and not breath actuated. Two examples of USNs used during mechanical ventilation are the SUN 345 (Maquet Bridgewater, NJ) and the EasyNeb (Covidien Norwalk, CT). The SUN 145 (Figure 4-50) operates with either an integrated module with the Maquet ventilator or as a stand-alone device. An on/off button turns on the nebulizer for 30 minutes, and a temperature override turns off the nebulizer if heats beyond a set temperature. (This means that nebulization may be interrupted without warning to the clinician.) The EasyNeb has a stand-alone power/timer box that is designed to be placed on the ventilator. Both nebulizers use a disposable, plastic, single patient use medication cup designed to separate medications from the liquid couplant conducting energy from the ultrasonic membrane. Couplant must be maintained at an adequate level; the nebulizer top and T-piece should be cleaned and sterilized between patient uses.

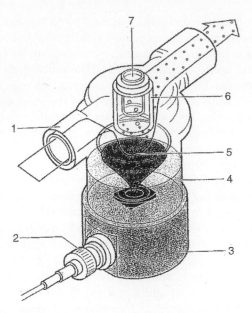

FIGURE 4-50 Maquet SUN 145 ultrasonic nebulizer with power control module. (1) Main gas flow connector; (2) power cable from ventilator; (3) ultrasonic generator; (4) couplant cup; (5) medication cup; (6) T-Piece adapter containing baffles; (7) injector membrane.

Use of a Vibrating Mesh Nebulizer during Mechanical Ventilation

Aerosol administration by VM nebulizer has been estimated to deliver greater than 10% deposition in both adults and infants without the addition of gas into the ventilator circuit. The low residual drug volume and small particle size are associated with higher efficiency. Two models of VM nebulizers are the Aeroneb Professional and the Aeroneb Solo. The Aeroneb Pro is a multiple patient use nebulizer designed to be autoclaved between patients. The Solo is a single patient use disposable nebulizer designed to remain in the ventilator circuit for up to 28 days. The Aeroneb Solo has a Luer lock adapter for use with a continuous infusion system, such as a syringe pump. Unlike with jet SVNs and USNs, the medication reservoir is above the circuit and separated from the ventilator tubing by the mesh, which reduces the risk of contamination or of contaminated aerosols being introduced into the ventilator circuit. Unlike with the SVN, VM aerosol generation characteristics are the same in air, oxygen, or helium-oxygen. Although the VM has 1000 apertures, no perceptible leakage occurs, even with heliox, when the nebulizer reservoir is open to the atmosphere. Thus the VM nebulizer can be opened and refilled without interrupting ventilation.

Use of a Pressurized Metered-Dose Inhaler in the Care of Intubated Patients Undergoing Mechanical Ventilation

In vitro studies have shown that effective aerosol delivery by pMDIs during mechanical ventilation can range from as little as 2% to as much as 98%.[89] Direct pMDI actuation

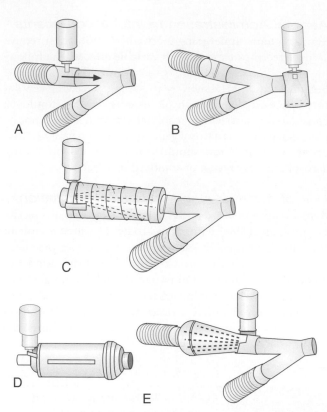

FIGURE 4-51 Devices for adapting a pressurized metered-dose inhaler to a ventilator circuit. A, Inline. B, Elbow. C, Collapsible chamber. D, Rigid chamber. E, Cone-shaped chamber in which aerosol is directed retrograde to gas flow to the patient. (Modified from Dhand R, Tobin MJ: Bronchodilator delivery with metered-dose inhalers in mechanically ventilated patients, *Eur Respir J* 9:585, 1996.)

through a simple elbow adapter typically results in the least pulmonary deposition, with most of the aerosol impacting in either the ventilator circuit or the tracheal airway. Higher aerosol delivery percentages occur only when a spacer is placed inline in the ventilator circuit (Figure 4-51). These spacers allow an aerosol "plume" to develop before the bulk of the particles impact on the surface of the circuit or endotracheal tube. The result is a more stable aerosol mass that can penetrate beyond the artificial airway and be deposited mainly in the lung. This leads to a better clinical response at lower dosages.[90] For medications delivered by pMDI, the amount of drug required to achieve the same therapeutic endpoint is similar for intubated patients (8%) and nonintubated patients (8% to 10%).[91] One study showed that 4 puffs produced maximum bronchodilation in stable patients with chronic obstructive pulmonary disease (COPD) receiving ventilatory support. Differences in response may be due to the level of airway obstruction and the techniques used for assessing response.

Techniques for assessing the response to a bronchodilator in intubated patients undergoing mechanical ventilation differ from those used in the care of spontaneously breathing patients because expiration is passive during mechanical ventilation, and forced expiratory values (PEFR, forced vital capacity [FVC], and forced expiratory volume in 1 second [FEV_1]) cannot normally be obtained. Additional techniques can be used for mechanically ventilated patients because (1) a change in the differences between peak and plateau pressures (the most reliable indicator of a change in airway resistance during continuous mechanical ventilation) can be measured, (2) auto-positive end-expiratory pressure (auto-PEEP) levels may decrease in response to bronchodilators, and (3) breath-to-breath variations make measurements more reliable when the patient is not actively breathing with the ventilator.[58] Box 4-14 outlines the optimum technique for drug delivery by pMDI to intubated patients undergoing mechanical ventilation.

Intrapulmonary Percussive Ventilation

Intrapulmonary percussive ventilation (IPV) provides high-frequency oscillation of the airway while administering aerosol using an integrated nebulizer (Percussionaire, Bird Technologies, Sandpoint, Idaho). Reychler et al.[84] compared aerosol administration during IPV with administration with a standard jet nebulizer. The MMAD was smaller with IPV than with the jet nebulizer (0.2 μm versus 1.89 μm), and the fine-particle fraction was also lower (16.2% versus 67.5%). However, the lung dose was similar (2.49% with IPV versus 4.2% with the jet nebulizer alone). The authors concluded that IPV was too variable and thus too unpredictable to recommend for drug delivery to the lung.

During high-frequency oscillatory ventilation (HFOV) with the Sensormedics 3100A and B ventilators (Viasys, cardinal Health, Dublin, OH), aerosol delivery can be difficult because of the high continuous flows (20 to 30 L/min) that pass through the ventilator circuit, diluting and scavenging aerosol. Demers et al.[85] reported placement of a VM mesh nebulizer (Aeroneb Pro) between the ventilator circuit and the endotracheal tube using a 15-mm pediatric T-adapter. They found that 10.25% (±6%) of the dose was delivered to a filter distal to the 3.0 endotracheal tube with infant settings. This was much greater than the 0.47% (±0.1%) deposition with the same nebulizer placed in the inspiratory limb. The authors noted that the ventilator alarm did not sound when the nebulizer was turned on or off or when the device was opened so that medication could be added.

Factors that Affect Aerosol Delivery during Mechanical Ventilation

In vitro testing has helped identify a number of factors that can optimize the efficiency of aerosol delivery during mechanical ventilation. These include the nebulizer type, the nebulizer's position in the ventilator circuit, continuous flow in the circuit, the inspiratory flow rate, the I:E ratio, humidity, and gas density.

Nebulizer Type and Position. Ari and others[86] studied SVNs, USNs, pMDIs, and VM nebulizers in an adult ventilator with no continuous or bias flow under both wet and dry conditions. Aerosol generators were placed either between the ventilator circuit and the patient's airway or in the inspiratory limb of the ventilator circuit at 6 inches from the Y, or 6 inches from the ventilator and before the heated humidifier under wet conditions. Jet nebulizers, operating continuously, delivered more aerosol particles when placed closer to the ventilator, where the aerosol tubing acts as a reservoir. In contrast, all the aerosol generators that do not add gas flow into the ventilator circuit appear to be most efficient when placed in the inspiratory limb, 6 inches from the Y. With the addition of continuous bias or trigger flow in the ventilator circuit, aerosol generators placed at the ventilator may be more efficient.

The inspiratory flow rate and I:E ratio can affect aerosol delivery. The lower the flow and the longer the inspiratory time, the greater the amount of aerosol delivered. Inspiratory flow has been shown to be the more important variable using pMDIs. Deposition increased twofold at 40 L/min

---

BOX 4-14	Technique for Using a Pressurized Metered-Dose Inhaler with a Ventilator Circuit

1. Assess the need for medication.
2. Establish the ventilator dose of 4 puffs (for bronchodilators with a standard dose of 2 to 4 puffs) with heated humidity for stable patients with chronic obstructive pulmonary disease (COPD). Higher doses may be required to treat an acute exacerbation.
3. Adjust the ventilator:
   · Leave the humidifier on (remove the heat and moisture exchanger [HME] from between the pressurized metered-dose inhaler [pMDI] and the patient).
   · To optimize delivery: Ensure a tidal volume of 400 ml or higher (for adults). Reduce the peak inspiratory flow rate as tolerated. Use ramp or sine wave flow patterns. Increase the TI/TTOT to 0.3 or greater. Turn off continuous flow through the circuit.
4. Shake the pMDI and warm it to hand temperature.
5. Place the pMDI in the chamber or other type of adapter in the ventilator circuit's inspiratory limb at the Y or between the elbow and the endotracheal tube. Use an adapter that has been shown in vitro to deliver greater than 10% of the dose.
6. Actuate the pMDI at the beginning of inspiration.
7. Wait 15 seconds or longer between actuations (the inhaler need not be shaken between puffs up to a total of 8 actuations).
8. If the patient can take a spontaneous breath equal to or greater than 500 ml, coordinate actuation with the beginning of a deep, spontaneous breath and encourage the patient to hold the breath for 4 to 10 seconds.
9. After administering the total dose, collapse or remove chamber from the circuit, replace the HME, and return all ventilator parameters to pretreatment settings. A small-volume adapter may be left inline as long as it does not create a leak or pool condensate.
10. Monitor the patient for an adverse response.
11. Assess the outcome of the treatment.

compared with 80 L/min, whereas a difference of less than 25% was seen in the I:E ratio (between 1:1 and 1:3) at either inspiratory flow. Flow patterns can make a significant but small difference, with descending ramp wave patterns providing higher efficiency than square wave patterns at the same peak flow.

Tidal volumes seem to be an issue only when the delivered volume is not sufficient to move the aerosol from the generator to the end of the patient airway in a single breath. A 6-foot adult circuit has an internal volume of 600 ml. Consequently, an aerosol generated at the ventilator would not reach the patient with a 500-ml tidal volume. Additional flow in the circuit could drive the aerosol down the inspiratory limb and improve efficiency.

Classic in vitro models of mechanical ventilation have demonstrated up to a 50% reduction in aerosol delivery with heated/humidified versus dry ventilator circuits. This difference may be partly due to a limitation of the model used. Adding a simulation of exhaled humidity has been shown to reduce the difference between wet and dry circuits. In general, it is not a good idea to subject a patient with a bypassed upper airway to dry, cold gas, which may precipitate bronchospasm and changes in the airways, just to increase aerosol deposition. It is far better to increase the dose than to turn off the humidifier.

Gas density has been demonstrated to make a substantial difference in aerosol delivery. Helium-oxygen mixtures in the ventilator circuit in concentrations greater than 50% have been demonstrated in vitro to increase aerosol delivery with SVNs, VM nebulizers, and pMDIs by up to 50%. It is easier to Controlling the helium-oxygen concentration is easier when a pMDI, USN, or VM aerosol generator is used.

Controlling Environmental Contamination

Nebulized drugs that escape from the nebulizer into the atmosphere or are exhaled by the patient can be inhaled by anyone in the vicinity of the treatment. The risk associated with this environmental exposure is clear, and it can arise with a variety of drugs. Pentamidine and ribavirin both have been associated with health risks to health care providers, even with the use of filters on the exhalation ports of nebulizers, containment and scavenger systems, high-efficiency particulate air (HEPA) filter hoods, and ventilation systems.

Continuous pneumatic nebulizers (standard SVNs) produce the greatest amount of secondhand aerosol, and most of the aerosol produced (up to 60%) passes directly into the environment. The Respirgard II nebulizer, which was developed for administration of pentamidine, added one-way valves and an expiratory filter to contain aerosol that is exhaled and not inhaled (Figure 4-52). Breath-actuated nebulizers and pMDIs offer another alternative, because these devices tend to generate less secondhand aerosol. A study that surveyed respiratory therapists found that they were more than twice as likely as physical thera-

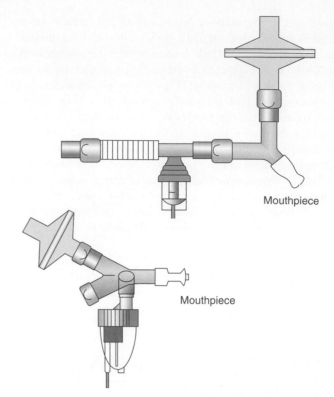

FIGURE 4-52 Nebulizers using a combination of one-way valves and filters collect exhaled aerosol and reduce secondhand aerosol exposure.

pists to develop asthma-like symptoms during the course of their careers. The authors associated this increased incidence of asthma-like symptoms with the administration of ribavirin and exposure to gluteraldehyde.[92] Over the years, there have been anecdotal reports of respiratory care clinicians who developed a sensitivity to secondhand aerosol from bronchodilators. Further research is required to provide a more thorough understanding of the hazards of secondhand exposure to aerosols in the clinical setting.

Patients with infectious diseases, such as tuberculosis (TB) or severe acute respiratory syndrome (SARS), require respiratory isolation. It is imperative that caregivers protect themselves and their patients when working with infected patients. A variety of techniques are available for protecting caregivers and patients from environmental exposure during aerosol drug therapy. As was already mentioned, the greatest occupational risk for exposure to secondhand aerosols has been associated with administration of ribavirin and pentamidine. Conjunctivitis, headaches, bronchospasm, shortness of breath, and rashes have been reported among those administering these drugs.[87] These problems can be reduced by treating patients receiving aerosolized ribavirin or pentamidine in a private room, booth, or tent or at a special station designed to minimize environmental contamination.

Negative-Pressure Rooms. When ribavirin or pentamidine is administered in a private room, the room should be equipped for negative-pressure ventilation with adequate air exchanges (at least six per hour) to clear the room of residual aerosols before the next treatment. HEPA filters should be used to filter room or tent exhaust, or the aerosol should be scavenged to the outside.

Booths and Stations. Booths or stations should be used for sputum induction and aerosolized medication treatments given in any area where more than one patient is treated. The area should be designed to provide adequate airflow to draw aerosol and droplet nuclei from the patient into an appropriate filtration system or an exhaust system directly to the outside. Booths and stations should be adequately cleaned between patients.

A variety of booths and specially designed stations are available for delivery of pentamidine or ribavirin. The Emerson containment booth (Figure 4-53) is an example of a system that completely isolates the patient during aerosol administration. All gas is drawn through a prefilter and a HEPA filter. In areas where proper air exchanges do not exist, devices such as the Enviracaire have been used to provide local exhaust ventilation through a HEPA filter medium. Few data exist to support the efficacy of these devices, although they are enjoying increasing popularity in the home environment.

The AeroStar Aerosol Protection Cart (Respiratory Safety Systems, San Diego, California) is a portable patient isolation station for administration of hazardous aerosol-

CLINICAL ROUNDS 4-6

The medical director of the respiratory care department asks you to design a protocol for administering aerosolized pentamidine. Describe the protective measure that should be taken to ensure safe delivery of this drug.

See Evolve Resources for the answer.

ized medication. It can be used during sputum induction and for pentamidine treatment. The patient compartment is collapsible and has a swing-out counter and three polycarbonate walls. Captured aerosols are removed with a HEPA filter. A prefilter is used to retain larger dust particles and to prevent early loading of the more expensive HEPA filter. (See Clinical Rounds 4-6.)

Filters and nebulizers used in treatments with pentamidine and ribavirin should be treated as hazardous wastes and disposed of accordingly. Goggles, gloves, and gowns should be used as splatter shields and to reduce exposure to medication residues and body substances. The staff should be screened for adverse effects of exposure to the aerosol medication. The risks and safety procedures should be reviewed regularly.

In addition to the risks associated with administration of aerosol medication, the risk of TB transmission has become a great concern because of an increase in case numbers and the development of multidrug resistant strains of the organism. TB is transmitted in the form of droplet nuclei (0.3 to 0.6 μm) that carry tuberculosis bacilli. Patients with known or suspected tuberculosis need private rooms with negative-pressure ventilation that exhausts to the outside. If environmental isolation is not possible or the health care worker must enter the patient's room, personal protective equipment should be used.

Personal Protective Equipment. Personal protective equipment is recommended when care is provided for any patient with a disease that can be spread by the airborne route.[88] The greatest risks that respiratory therapists encounter usually involve tuberculosis or chickenpox. Although environmental controls should be instituted in the care of these patients, standard and airborne precautions should also be implemented. A variety of masks and respirators have been recommended for use when caring for a patient with tuberculosis or other respiration-transmitted diseases. Traditional surgical masks, particulate respirators, disposable and reusable HEPA filters, and powered air-purifying respirators (PAPRs) have been used. No data are available determining the most effective and most clinically useful device to protect health care workers and others, although the U.S. Occupational Safety and Health Administration (OSHA) requires specific levels of protection (HEPA and PAPRs).

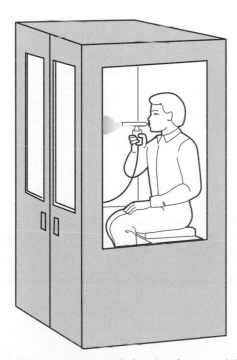

FIGURE 4-53 An environmental chamber for aerosol delivery to patients filters all exhaled gas through a high-efficiency particulate air (HEPA) filter.

KEY POINTS

- Conditioning of inhaled and exhaled gas is accomplished primarily by the nose and upper airway. Bypassing the upper airway without providing similar levels of heat and humidity to inhaled gas can cause damage to the respiratory tract.
- The primary goal of humidification is to maintain normal physiologic conditions in the lower airways.
- Gases delivered to the nose and mouth should be conditioned to 20° to 22° C with 10 mg/L of water vapor (50% relative humidity).
- When being delivered to the trachea, gases should be warmed and humidified to 32° to 40° C with 36 to 40 mg/L of water vapor (greater than 90% relative humidity).
- A humidifier is a device that adds invisible molecular water to gas.
- Temperature is an important factor affecting humidifier output. The higher the temperature, the greater the water vapor capacity of the delivered gas.
- Bubble, passover, wick, and, membrane humidifiers and HMEs are the major types of humidifiers. Active humidifiers incorporate heating devices, as well as a source of water with reservoir and/or feed systems.
- Most HMEs are passive, capturing both heat and moisture from expired gas and returning it to the patient at about 70% efficiency. HMEs are not recommended for use with infants because of issues related to increased mechanical dead space and use of uncuffed endotracheal tubes, which allow some exhaled gas to bypass the HME.
- Common problems with humidification systems include condensation, cross-contamination, and ensuring proper conditioning of the inspired gas.
- Bland aerosol therapy with sterile water or saline is used to (1) treat upper airway edema, (2) overcome heat and humidity deficits in patients with tracheal airways, and (3) help obtain sputum specimens.
- LVNs and USNs are used to generate bland aerosols. Delivery systems include a variety of direct airway appliances and mist tents.
- Common problems with bland aerosol therapy are cross-contamination and infection, environmental safety, inadequate mist production, overhydration, bronchospasm, and noise.
- An aerosol is a suspension of solid or liquid particles in gas. In the clinical setting, therapeutic aerosols are made with atomizers or nebulizers.
- The general aim of aerosol drug therapy is delivery of a therapeutic dose of the selected agent to the desired site of action.

- Where aerosol particles are deposited in the respiratory tract depends on their size, shape, and motion and on the physical characteristics of the airways. Key mechanisms causing aerosol deposition include inertial impaction, sedimentation, and brownian diffusion.
- For targeting aerosols for delivery to the upper airway (nose, larynx, and trachea), particles in the 5- to 50-μm MMAD range are used; 1- to 5-μm particles are used for the lower airways and lung parenchyma (alveolar region).
- The primary hazard of aerosol drug therapy is an adverse reaction to the medication being administered. Other hazards are related to infection control, airway reactivity, and systemic effects of bland aerosols.
- Drug aerosol delivery systems include pMDIs, DPIs, SVNs, LVNs, USNs, VM nebulizers, hand-bulb atomizers, and nasal spray pumps.
- Metered-dose inhalers and dry powder inhalers are the preferred method for maintenance delivery of bronchodilators and steroids to spontaneously breathing patients. The effectiveness of this therapy is highly technique dependent.
- Accessory devices, spacers, and holding chambers are used with pMDIs to reduce oropharyngeal deposition of a drug and to overcome problems with poor hand-breath coordination.
- LVNs and SVNs with continuous feed can be used to provide continuous aerosol delivery when traditional dosing strategies are ineffective in controlling severe bronchospasm.
- Small-volume USNs can be used to administer bronchodilators, anti-inflammatory agents, and antibiotics.
- Careful, ongoing patient assessment is the key to an effective bronchodilator therapy protocol. Components of the assessment include a patient interview, observation, tests of expiratory airflow, measurement of vital signs, auscultation, blood gas analysis, and oximetry.
- Standard SVNs are less efficient than pMDIs, USNs, or VM nebulizers for aerosol drug delivery during mechanical ventilation. Device selection, proper positioning of the device, and ventilator parameter selection are needed to optimize deposition and achieve the desired clinical outcome.
- A variety of techniques are available for protecting patients and caregivers from environmental exposure during aerosol drug therapy.

ASSESSMENT QUESTIONS

See Evolve Resources for answers.

1. A gas at body temperature and ambient pressure (BTPS) contains:
   a. 10 mg/L of water vapor
   b. 30 mg/L of water vapor
   c. 33.9 mg/L of water vapor
   d. 43.9 mg/L of water vapor

2. If the temperature of a saturated gas decreases, which of the following occurs?
   a. Condensation develops.
   b. Absolute humidity increases.
   c. Relative humidity decreases.
   d. Water vapor pressure increases.

3. If a patient has an artificial airway in place, what should be the minimum level of absolute humidity provided to the patient's airways?
   a. 10 mg/L
   b. 20 mg/L
   c. 30 mg/L
   d. 40 mg/L

4. A sample of room air gas contains 10 mg/L of humidity. What is the relative humidity (RH) of the gas if the room temperature is 77° F?
   a. 10%
   b. 22%
   c. 43%
   d. 98%

5. Based on the AARC Clinical Practice Guideline, the temperature of medical gas delivered through an artificial airway should be:
   a. 20° to 25° C
   b. 31° to 35° C
   c. 36° to 40° C
   d. Over 45° C

6. Which of the following are potential problems that may arise in patients with a tracheostomy who are breathing nonhumidified oxygen at a rate of 6 L/min?
   I. Atelectasis
   II. Destruction of the airway epithelium
   III. Inspissation of secretions
   IV. Mucociliary dysfunction
   a. I and III only
   b. II and IV only
   c. I, II, III only
   d. I, II, III, and IV

7. Which of the following is a contraindication to use of an HME?
   a. Minute volume greater than 10 L/min
   b. Minimal secretions
   c. Small tidal volumes
   d. Short-term mechanical ventilation

8. Which of the following is classified as a passive humidifier?
   a. Bubble humidifier
   b. Ultrasonic nebulizer
   c. Wick humidifier
   d. Heat and moisture exchanger

9. Name four types of heating devices that can be used to increase the humidity output of an active humidifier.

10. Which of the following results in increased aerosol deposition?
    a. Large tidal volume
    b. Slow inspiratory flow rate
    c. Decrease in the expiratory peak flow
    d. Short expiratory times

11. The optimum range of aerosol particle sizes that are to be inspired for general deposition through the upper and lower airways is:
    a. 0.1 to 1 µm
    b. 1 to 5 µm
    c. 3 to 10 µm
    d. 5 to 15 µm

12. What is the recommended gas flow rate to operate an SVN?
    a. 1 L/min
    b. 6 to 8 L/min
    c. 10 L/min
    d. 15 L/min or more

13. What is the most important factor influencing aerosol deposition from an MDI?
    a. Tidal volume
    b. Inspiratory flow rate
    c. Respiratory rate
    d. Breath-hold

14. The active drug component of a typical pMDI accounts for what percentage of the total content of the mixture in the device?
    a. Less than 1%
    b. 10%
    c. 25%
    d. 60%

15. List six factors that can affect the performance of a small-volume nebulizer (SVN).

References

1. Kapadia FN, Shelley MP: Normal mechanisms of humidification, *Probl Respir Care* 4:395, 1991.
2. Primiano FP Jr, Montague FW Jr, Saidel GM: Measurement system for water vapor and temperature dynamics, *J Appl Physiol* 56:1679, 1984.
3. Shelley MP, Lloyd GM, Park GR: A review of the mechanisms and the methods of humidification of inspired gas, *Intensive Care Med* 14:1, 1988.
4. Ingelstedt S: Studies on the conditioning of air in the respiratory tract, *Acta Otolaryngol* 131(Suppl):1, 1956.
5. Chalon J, Loew D, Malbranche J: Effects of dry air and subsequent humidification on tracheobronchial ciliated epithelium, *Anesthesiology* 37:338, 1972.
6. Marfatia S, Donahoe PK, Henderson WH: Effect of dry and humidified gases on the respiratory epithelium in rabbits, *J Pediatr Surg* 10:583, 1975.

7. American Association for Respiratory Care: Clinical practice guideline: humidification during mechanical ventilation, *Respir Care* 37:887, 1992.
8. Chatburn RL, Primiano FP: A rational basis for humidity therapy, *Respir Care* 32:249, 1987.
9. Anderson S, Herbring BG, Widman B: Accidental profound hypothermia, *Br J Anaesth* 42:653, 1970.
10. Weinberg AD: Hypothermia, *Ann Emerg Med* 22:370, 1993.
11. Chen TY, Chen KT, Chang DP, et al: The effect of heated humidifier in the prevention of intra-operative hypothermia, *Acta Anaesthesiol Sin* 32:27, 1994.
12. Giesbrecht GG, Younes M: Exercise and cold-induced asthma, *Can J Appl Physiol* 20:300, 1995.
13. American Society for Testing and Materials (ASTM): *Standard specification for humidifiers for medical use* (F1690), Conshohocken, Pa, 1996, The Society.
14. Gray HSJ: Humidifiers, *Probl Respir Care* 4:423, 1991.
15. Klein EF et al: Performance characteristics of conventional prototype humidifiers and nebulizers, *Chest* 64:690, 1973.
16. Darin J, Broadwell J, MacDonell R: An evaluation of water-vapor output from four brands of unheated, prefilled bubble humidifiers, *Respir Care* 27:41, 1982.
17. Kallstron TJ: American Association for Respiratory Care: Clinical practice guideline: bland aerosol administration—2003 revision and update, *Respir Care* 48:529, 2003.
18. Mercer TT, Goddard RF, Flores RL: Output characteristics of several commercial nebulizers, *Ann Allergy* 23:314, 1965.
19. Hill TV, Sorbello JG: Humidity outputs of large-reservoir nebulizers, *Respir Care* 32:225, 1987.
20. Khajotia RR et al: Induced sputum and cytological diagnosis of lung cancer, *Lancet* 338:976, 1991.
21. Gershman NH, Wong HH, Liu JT et al: Comparison of two methods of collecting induced sputum in asthmatic subjects, *Eur Respir J* 9:2448, 1996.
22. Craven DE, Goularte TA, Make BJ: Contaminated condensate in mechanical ventilator circuits: a risk factor for nosocomial pneumonia, *Am Rev Respir Dis* 129:625, 1984.
23. International Organization for Standardization: *Heat and moisture exchangers for use in humidifying respired gases in humans* (ISO 9360), Geneva, 1992, The Organization.
24. Shelly MP: Inspired gas conditioning, *Respir Care* 37:1070, 1992.
25. Branson RD, Davis K: Evaluation of 21 passive humidifiers according to the ISO 9360 standard: moisture output, dead space, and flow resistance, *Respir Care* 41:736, 1996.
26. Ploysongsang Y et al: Effect of flow rate and duration of use on the pressure drop across six artificial noses, *Respir Care* 34:902, 1989.
27. Inui D, Oto J, Nishimura M: Effect of heat and moisture exchanger (HME) positioning on inspiratory gas humidification. Available at www.biomedcentral.com/1471-2466/6/19. Retrieved June 2007.
28. Jean-Claude L, Marc A, Charles C et al: Impact of humidification systems on ventilator-associated pneumonia, *Am J Respir Crit Care Med* 17:1276, 2005.
29. Prasad KK, Chen L: Complications related to the use of heat and moisture exchangers. *Anesthesiology* 72:958, 1990.
30. Nishida T et al: Performance of heated humidifiers with a heated wire according to ventilatory settings, *J Aerosol Med* 14:43, 2001.
31. Williams R et al: Relationship between the humidity and temperature of inspired gas and the function of the airway mucosa, *Crit Care Med* 24:1920, 1996.
32. Gilmour IJ, Boyle MJ, Streifel A: Humidifiers kill bacteria, *Anesthesiology* 75:A498, 1991.
33. Fink JB et al: Extending ventilator circuit change interval beyond two days reduces the likelihood of ventilator associated pneumonia (VAP), *Chest* 113:405, 1998.
34. Kollef MH et al: Mechanical ventilation with or without 7-day circuit changes: a randomized controlled study, *Ann Intern Med* 123:168, 1995.
35. Beydon L et al: Correlation between simple clinical parameters and the in vitro humidification characteristics of filter heat and moisture exchangers, *Chest* 112:739, 1997.
36. American College of Chest Physicians and National Heart, Lung and Blood Institute (NHLBI): National conference on oxygen therapy, *Respir Care* 29:922, 1984.
37. Branson RD, Chatburn RL: Humidification during mechanical ventilation, *Respir Care* 38:461, 1993 (editorial).
38. Dolovich MA et al: Consensus statement: aerosols and delivery devices, *Respir Care* 45:589, 2000.
39. Kim CS: Methods of calculating lung delivery and deposition of aerosal particles, *Respir Care* 45:695, 2000.
40. Dolovich MD: Assessing nebulizer performance, *Respir Care* 47:1290, 2002.
41. Newhouse MT, Dolovich M: Aerosol therapy in children. In Chernick V, Mellins RB, editors: *Basic mechanisms of pediatric respiratory disease: cellular and integrative,* Toronto, 1991, BC Decker.
42. Pierce AK, Sanford JP, Thomas GD et al: Long-term evaluation of inhalation therapy equipment and the occurrence of necrotizing pneumonia, *N Engl J Med* 282:528, 1970.
43. Wojnarowski C et al: Comparison of bronchial challenge with ultrasonic nebulized distilled water and hypertonic saline in children with mild to moderate asthma, *Eur Respir J* 9:1896, 1996.
44. American Association for Respiratory Care: Clinical practice guideline: selection of aerosol delivery device, *Respir Care* 37:891, 1992.
45. Glick RV: Drug reconcentration in aerosol generators, *Inhal Ther* 15:179, 1970.
46. American Association for Respiratory Care: Aerosol consensus conference statement—1991, *Respir Care* 36:916, 1991.
47. Dolovich M, Ruffin R, Corr D et al: Clinical evaluation of a simple demand inhalation MDI aerosol delivery device, *Chest* 84:36, 1983.
48. Fink JB: Metered-dose inhalers, dry powder inhalers and transitions, *Respir Care* 45:623, 2000.
49. Newman SP: Aerosol generators and delivery systems, *Respir Care* 36:939, 1991.
50. Fink JB, Rubin BK: Problems with inhaler use: a call for improved clinician and patient education, *Respir Care* 50:1360, 2005.
51. Chhabra SK: A comparison of "closed" and "open" mouth techniques of inhalation of a salbutamol metered-dose inhaler, *J Asthma* 31:123, 1994.
52. Hampson NB, Mueller MP: Reduction in patient timing errors using a breath-activated metered dose inhaler, *Chest* 106:462, 1994.
53. Wildhaber JH, Janssens HM, Pierart F, et al: High percentage lung delivery in children from detergent-treated spacers, *Pediatr Pulmonol* 29:389, 2000.
54. Dhand R, Fink JB: Dry powder inhalers, *Respir Care* 44:940, 1999.
55. Nerbrink O, Dahlback M, Hansson HC: Why do medical nebulizers differ in their output and particle characteristics? *J Aerosol Med* 7:259, 1994.
56. Dennis JH, Hendrick DJ: Design characteristics for drug nebulizers, *J Med Eng Technol* 16:63, 1992.
57. Hess D, Fisher D, Williams P et al: Medication nebulizer performance: effects of diluent volume, nebulizer flow, and nebulizer brand, *Chest* 110:498, 1996.
58. Goode ML et al: Improvement in aerosol delivery with helium-oxygen mixtures during mechanical ventilation, *Am J Respir Crit Care Med* 163:109, 2001.

59. Hess DR, Fink JB, Venkataraman ST et al: The history and physics of heliox, *Respir Care* 51:608, 2006.

60. Phipps PR, Gonda I: Droplets produced by medical nebulisers: effects on particle size and solute concentration, *Chest* 97:1327, 1990.

61. Rau JL, Ari A, Restrepo RD: Performance comparison of nebulizer designs: constant-output, breath-enhanced, and dosimetric, *Respir Care* 49:174, 2004.

62. Denyer J, Nikander K, Smith NJ: Adaptive aerosol delivery (AAD) technology, *Expert Opin Drug Deliv* 1:165, 2004.

63. Dolovich MB: Assessing nebulizer performance, *Respir Care* 47:1290, 2002.

64. Rubin BK, Fink JB: Aerosol therapy for children, *Respir Care Clin N Am* 7:175, 2001.

65. Janssens HM, Tiddens HA: Aerosol therapy: the special needs of young children, *Paediatr Respir Rev* 7(Suppl 1):S83, 2006.

66. Bhashyam AR, Wolf MT, Marcinkowski AK et al: Aerosol delivery through nasal cannulas: an in vitro study, *J Aerosol Med* 21(2):181-188, 2008.

67. Kendrick AH, Smith EC, Wilson RSE: Selecting and using nebuliser equipment, *Thorax* 52(Suppl 2):S92, 1997.

68. Alvine GF, Rodgers P, Fitzsimmons KM et al: Disposable jet nebulizers: how reliable are they? *Chest* 101:316, 1992.

69. Zainuddin BM, Tolfree SEJ, Short M et al: Influence of breathing pattern on lung deposition and bronchodilator response to nebulized salbutamol in patients with stable asthma, *Thorax* 43:987, 1988.

70. Oie S, Kamiya A: Bacterial contamination of aerosol solutions containing antibiotics, *Microbios* 82:109, 1995.

71. Kacmarek RM, Kratohvil J: Evaluation of a double-enclosure double-vacuum unit scavenging system for ribavirin administration, *Respir Care* 37:37, 1992.

72. Phillips GD, Millard FJL: The therapeutic use of ultrasonic nebulizers in acute asthma, *Respir Med* 88:387, 1994.

73. Thomas SH, O'Doherty MJ, Page CJ et al: Delivery of ultrasonic nebulized aerosols to a lung model during mechanical ventilation, *Am Rev Respir Dis* 148:872, 1993.

74. American Association for Respiratory Care: Clinical practice guideline: delivery of aerosols to the upper airway, *Respir Care* 39:803, 1994.

75. Dhand R: Nebulizers that use a vibrating mesh or plate with multiple apertures to generate aerosol, *Respir Care* 47:1406, 2002.

76. Vecellio L: The mesh nebulizer: a recent technical innovation for aerosol delivery, *Breathe* 2:253, 2006.

77. Dolovich MB, Fink JB: Aerosols and devices, *Respir Care Clin N Am* 7:131, 2001.

78. Dolovich MB, Ahrens RC, Hess DR et al: Device selection and outcomes of aerosol therapy: evidence-based guidelines: American College of Chest Physicians/American College of Asthma, Allergy, and Immunology, *Chest* 127:335, 2005.

79. American Association for Respiratory Care: Clinical practice guideline: selection of a device for delivery of aerosol to the lung parenchyma, *Respir Care* 41:647, 1996.

80. American Association for Respiratory Care: Clinical practice guideline: selection of an aerosol delivery device for neonatal and pediatric patients, *Respir Care* 40:1325, 1995.

81. National Asthma Education and Prevention Program: *Expert panel report II: guidelines for the diagnosis and management of asthma*, Bethesda, Md, 1997, National Institutes of Health.

82. Fink J, Dhand R: Bronchodilator resuscitation in the emergency department. Part 2. Dosing, *Respir Care* 45:497, 2000.

83. Duarte A, Fink J, Dhand R: Inhalation therapy during mechanical ventilation, *Respir Care Clin N Am* 7:233, 2001.

84. Reychler G, Wallemacq P, Rodenstein DO et al: Comparison of lung deposition of Amikacin by intrapulmonary ventilation and jet nebulization by urinary monitoring, *J Aerosol Med* 19:199, 2006.

85. Demers B, Gilley D, Fink JB: *Nebulizer position impacts aerosol deposition during high-frequency oscillatory ventilation (HFOV)*, San Diego, Calif, 1995, American Thoracic Society.

86. Ari A: Evaluation of position of aerosol devices in two different ventilator circuits during mechanical ventilation, http://www.rejournal.com/abstracts/2007/index.cfm.

87. Harrison R: Reproductive risk assessment with occupational exposure to ribavirin aerosol, *Pediatr Infect Dis J* 9(Suppl):S1025, 1990.

88. Garner JS: Guideline for isolation precautions in hospitals, *Infect Control Hosp Epidemiol* 17:53, 1996.

89. Dhand R: Aerosal therapy with metered-dose inhalers during mechanical ventilation: the need for in vitro tests. *Resp Care* 43:699-702, 1998.

90. Dhand R, Tobin MJ: Bronchodilator delivery with metered-dose inhaler in mechanically-ventilated patients. *Eur Respir J* 9:585, 1996.

91. Fink JB, Dhand R, Duarte AG, et al: Aerosal delivery from a metered-dose inhaler during mechanical ventilation. *Am J Respir Care Med* 154:381-387, 1996.

92. Christiani DC, Kern DG: Asthma Risk and Occupation as a Respiratory Therapist. *Am Rev Respir Dis* 148(3):671-674, 1993.

INTERNET RESOURCES

Humidity

American College of Chest Physicians: Patient Instruction for Inhaled Devices: http://www.chestnet.org/patients/guides/inhaledDevices.php

Humidity and Humidification Lecture: http://www.usyd.edu.au/anaes/lectures/humidity_clt/humidity.html

Infoplease.com: http://www.infoplease.com/ce6/weather/A0824520.html

Humidity calculator: http://www.bom.gov.au/lam/humiditycalc.shtml

Relative humidity: http://en.wikipedia.org/wiki/Relative_humidity

Relative humidity: http://www.fphcare.com/humidification/relative_humidity.asp

Virtual Hospital: http://www.vh.org

Aerosol

The Aerosol Society: http://www.aerosol-soc.org.uk/index.asp

American Association of Aerosol Research: www.aaar.org

Guide to Aerosol Delivery Devices: http://www.aarc.org/education/aerosol_devices/aerosol_delivery_guide.pdf

American Association for Respiratory Care (AARC) Clinical Practice Guideline for aerosol therapy: http://www.rcjournal.com/cpgs/Journal of Aerosol Medicine: http://www.liebertonline.com/loi/jam

American College of Chest Physicians: Patient Instruction for Inhaled Devices: http://www.chestnet.org/patients/guides/inhaledDevices.php

American College of Chest Physicians (ACCP) Patient Education Guides: http://www.chestnet.org/patients/guides/

International Society of Aerosol in Medicine: http://www.isam.org/

RDD Online: http://www.rddonline.com/education/index.asp

Total Ozone Mapping Spectrometer: http://toms.gsfc.nasa.gov/aerosols/aerosols.html

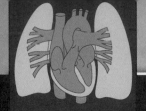

Principles of Infection Control

J.M. CAIRO

OBJECTIVES

Upon completion of this chapter, you will be able to:
- Identify the major groups of microorganisms associated with nosocomial pneumonia.
- List four factors that can influence the effectiveness of a germicide.
- Define the terms *high-level disinfection*, *intermediate-level disinfection*, and *low-level disinfection*.
- Describe the process of pasteurization and its application to the disinfection of respiratory care equipment.
- Explain how quaternary ammonium compounds, alcohols, acetic acid, phenols, glutaraldehyde, hydrogen peroxide, and iodophors and other halogenated compounds are used as disinfectants.
- Name the four physical methods commonly used to sterilize medical devices.
- Discuss the principle of ethylene oxide sterilization.
- Identify infection risk devices used in respiratory care.
- Describe three components of an effective infection surveillance program.
- Compare standard precautions with transmission-based precautions.
- List the most common agents associated with febrile respiratory illnesses that are potential causes of mass casualty events.

KEY TERMS

acid-fast bacillus	disinfecting	low-level disinfection
acid-fast stain	droplet precautions	normal flora
aerobes	eukaryotic	nosocomial
airborne	facultative	pasteurization
airborne precautions	fomites	pathogenic
anaerobes	fungicide	prokaryotic
autoclave	germicide	spirochetes
autotroph	gram stain	standard precautions
bacilli	gram-negative	staphylococci
bactericide	gram-positive	sterilizing
chemical sterilant	health care–associated	streptobacilli
cleaning	infections (HAIs)	streptococci
cocci	heterotroph	transmission-based precautions
contact precautions	high-level disinfection	universal precautions
decontamination	indirect contact	vectors
diplobacilli	infection surveillance	vehicles
diplococci	intermediate-level disinfection	virucide
direct contact	isolation techniques	

Preventing **health care–associated infections (HAIs)** is a formidable task for respiratory therapists. It is particularly challenging because devices used for respiratory care are potential reservoirs and **vehicles** for the transmission of infectious microorganisms. Additionally, many patients receiving respiratory care, especially those of extreme age or who are recovering from thoracoabdominal surgery, have an increased risk of developing **nosocomial** pneumonia. Underlying diseases, depressed sensorium, and immunosuppression can also add to the risk of acquiring a nosocomial infection.[1]

This chapter is a review of the aspects of microbiology and infection control that respiratory care practitioners must understand to prevent health care–associated infections. Specifically, the following are described here: (1) the microorganisms most often associated with nosocomial pneumonia; (2) the accepted methods for **cleaning, disinfecting,** and **sterilizing** reusable respiratory care equipment; (3) effective methods of **infection surveillance;** and (4) the proper use of **isolation techniques** to prevent person-to-person transmission of microorganisms.

PRINCIPLES OF CLINICAL MICROBIOLOGY

Microbiology is the study of microorganisms such as bacteria, viruses, protozoa, fungi, and algae. All these organisms, with the possible exception of algae, are **pathogenic** and therefore can produce infectious diseases in susceptible hosts.[1] Clinical microbiology is primarily concerned with the isolation, identification, and control of these pathogenic, or disease-producing, organisms.

The active participation of clinical microbiologists in infection control is essential for the identification and treatment of nosocomial infections, as well as for the prevention of these diseases. The process of identifying the infectious agent responsible for the nosocomial infection is fairly straightforward. Diagnosis of an infectious disease requires isolation of the suspected pathogen from the site of infection. The specimen then is inoculated onto agar or into a broth containing vital nutrients and incubated for a specified period. In many cases the organism is allowed to grow at body temperature in a specially designed incubator. It is important that those performing the collection process use aseptic techniques to prevent microbial contamination from adjacent tissue and **normal flora.** Although normal microbial flora, which are microorganisms normally found in or on a particular body site, do not usually cause infectious disease, these organisms can present problems, because they can overgrow the pathogen and produce erroneous results.

Identification of microorganisms is most often accomplished by direct examination of the specimen through microscopy with the aid of biologic staining techniques. Metabolic and immunologic tests may also help clinical microbiologists discern the nature of the invading microbe, especially with regard to its susceptibility to antibiotics.

Control of pathogenic microorganisms is based on the elimination of infections and prevention of the spread of infectious diseases through infection control techniques. Infections that overwhelm a person's immune system usually are eradicated by enhancing the host's innate immunity with antibiotics and immunizations. Decontamination of diagnostic and therapeutic medical equipment, furniture, and commonly used items and surfaces, as well as the use of barrier precautions (i.e., isolation precautions), are examples of infection control techniques.

A variety of microorganisms can be isolated from the hospital environment. A brief description of the major groups of pathogenic organisms associated with nosocomial pneumonia follows. More detailed information about the science of microbiology can be found in the references listed at the end of the chapter.[1-3]

Survey of Microorganisms

Bacteria

Bacteria are **prokaryotic,** unicellular organisms that range in size from 0.5 to 50 μm. Bacteria generally are classified according to their morphology (shape) and their staining and metabolic characteristics. Certain bacteria also can produce endospores, which are intermediate bacterial forms that develop in response to adverse condition. As is discussed later in this chapter, bacterial endospores can regenerate to vegetative cells when conditions improve.

As Figure 5-1 shows, the primary bacterial shapes are **cocci** (spherical), **bacilli** (rodlike), and **spirochetes** (spiral). Cocci that occur in irregular clusters are called *staphylococci.* Cocci and bacilli that occur in pairs are called *diplococci* and *diplobacilli,* respectively; chains of cocci and bacilli are called *streptococci* and *streptobacilli,* respectively.

The classification of bacteria according to their staining characteristics usually is accomplished with simple staining techniques, such as the **gram stain** and the **acid-fast stain.** A gram stain separates bacteria into two general classes: those that retain an initial gentian violet stain after an alcohol wash **(gram positive)** and those that do

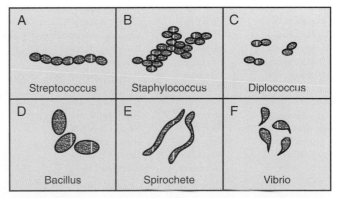

FIGURE 5-1 The morphology of bacteria. **A,** Streptococcus. **B,** Staphylococcus. **C,** Diplococcus. **D,** Bacillus. **E,** Spirochete. **F,** Vibrio.

not retain the initial violet stain **(gram negative).** Gram-positive organisms appear blue or violet; gram-negative organisms have a red appearance that results from a counterstain of the red dye safranin. Notable gram-positive pathogens are *Bacillus anthracis, Streptococcus pneumoniae, Staphylococcus aureus, Corynebacterium diphtheriae,* and *Clostridium* sp. (e.g., *C. botulinum, C. perfringens, C. tetani*). Gram-negative pathogens include *Pseudomonas aeruginosa, Escherichia coli, Klebsiella pneumoniae, Haemophilus influenzae, Serratia marcescens, Bordetella pertussis, Neisseria meningitidis,* and *Legionella pneumophila*.[2] Clinical Rounds 5-1 provides a clinical scenario that shows how gram stains can be used in the differential diagnosis of lower respiratory tract infections.

Acid-fast stains (also called *Ziehl-Neelsen stains*) are used to identify bacteria that belong to the genus *Mycobacterium*. These microbes retain a red (carbol-fuchsin) dye after an acid wash, thus *acid-fast bacillus* is used synonymously with *Mycobacterium*. *Mycobacterium tuberculosis* organisms are responsible for pulmonary, spinal, and miliary tuberculosis. The incidence of tuberculosis has increased considerably during the past decade, especially in patients infected with the human immunodeficiency virus (HIV; see the following discussion of viruses).

Metabolic characterization of bacteria usually involves identifying the substrate requirements for growth or the production of specific enzymes by the microbe. For example, bacteria require moisture and a source of nutrients for optimum growth. Organisms that require simple inorganic nutrients to sustain themselves are called **autotrophs,** whereas bacteria that require complex organic nutrients are referred to as **heterotrophs.** Atmospheric requirements can vary considerably among bacteria. Bacteria that require oxygen for growth are called *aerobes,* and those that can grow without oxygen are called *anaerobes.* **Facultative** anaerobes are bacteria that have limited oxygen tolerance. Although bacteria can be found in environments with temperatures ranging from $-5°$ to $80°$ C, pathogenic organisms typically grow at temperatures between $20°$ and $40°$ C.[4] Metabolic characterization may also involve the identification of various enzymes required for optimum growth of the organism. Examples of enzyme markers commonly quantified include catalase and coagulase.

As mentioned previously, certain bacteria form endospores under adverse conditions. Endospores are metabolically active life forms that can maintain their viability in the presence of dryness, heat, and poor nutrition. Their robust nature makes them especially resistant to disinfectants and a constant source of concern for infection control personnel. The most notable sources of bacterial endospores are from the aerobic *Bacillus* sp. and the anaerobic *Clostridium* sp.

Table 5-1 lists some commonly encountered bacterial genera, along with a summary of their morphologic, staining, and metabolic characteristics.

CLINICAL ROUNDS 5-1

Laboratory examination of a sputum sample from a febrile patient with a productive cough (purulent, blood-streaked sputum) reveals the presence of gram-positive diplococci and many segmented neutrophils. Suggest a possible diagnosis based on these findings.

See Evolve Resources for the answer.

TABLE 5-1

Commonly Encountered Bacteria Along with Morphologic, Staining, and Metabolic Characteristics

Genera	Gram Stain	Shape/Configuration	Aerobic/Anaerobic	Species
Bacillus	Positive	Rod, chain	Aerobic	*B. anthracis*
Bordetella	Negative	Rod	Aerobic	*B. pertussis*
Clostridium	Positive	Rod, separate, chain, pairs, palisade	Anaerobic	*C. tetani, C. botulinum, C. perfringens*
Corynebacterium	Positive	Rod, palisade	Aerobic	*C. diphtheriae*
Diplococcus	Positive	Coccus, encapsulated pairs	Aerobic	*D. pneumoniae*
Staphylococcus	Positive	Coccus, clusters	Aerobic	*S. aureus*
Streptococcus	Positive	Coccus, chain	Aerobic	Groups A, B, C, and D
Mycobacterium	Positive	Rod, separate, or "cords"	Aerobic	*M. tuberculosis, M. leprae*
Neisseria	Positive	Coccus, pairs	Aerobic	*N. meningitidis*
Proteus	Negative	Rod, separate	Aerobic	*N. mirabilis, N. vulgaris*
Pseudomonas	Negative	Rod, separate	Aerobic	*P. aeruginosa*
Serratia	Negative	Rod, separate	Aerobic	*S. marcescens*
Escherichia	Negative	Rod, separate	Aerobic, facultatively anaerobic	*E. coli*
Klebsiella	Negative	Rod, separate	Aerobic	*K. pneumoniae*
Haemophilus	Negative	Rod, separate	Aerobic	*H. influenzae, H. haemolyticus, H. parainfluenzae*
Salmonella	Negative	Rod, separate	Aerobic, facultatively anaerobic	*S. typhi, S. enteritidis*

From Kacmarek RM, Mack CW, Dimas S: *The essentials of respiratory care,* ed 3, St Louis, 1990, Mosby.

Viruses

Viruses are submicroscopic parasites that consist of a nucleic acid core surrounded by a protein sheath. They range in size from 20 to 200 nm. Viruses typically are described as nonliving because they must invade a living organism to replicate. Viruses generally are classified according to their structure (i.e., icosahedral, helical, or complex) and nucleic acid content (i.e., deoxyribonucleic acid [DNA] or ribonucleic acid [RNA]). They also can be differentiated by the type of host they invade (i.e., animal, plant, or bacteria).

The most commonly encountered pathogenic viruses are listed in Table 5-2. They include the influenza viruses, paramyxoviruses, adenoviruses, coronaviruses, rhinoviruses, enteroviruses, herpes viruses, rubella viruses, hepatitis virus, and human immunodeficiency viruses. Viruses are responsible for a number of respiratory illnesses, including the common cold, croup, tracheobronchitis, bronchiolitis, and pneumonia. The hepatitis viruses and HIV are particularly important pathogens because they are spread by direct contact (i.e., through sexual contact or blood and serum). Universal isolation precautions were

TABLE 5-2

Commonly Encountered Pathogenic Viruses

Virus	Transmission Route	Diseases
Influenza	Respiratory tract	Tracheobronchitis Pneumonia Susceptibility to bacterial pneumonia
Paramyxoviruses		
Mumps	Respiratory tract	Parotitis Orchitis Pancreatitis Encephalitis
Measles (rubeola)	Respiratory tract	Rash, systemic illness Pneumonia Encephalomyelitis
Parainfluenza	Respiratory tract	Upper respiratory disease Croup, pneumonia
Respiratory syncytial virus	Respiratory tract	Bronchitis Bronchiolitis Pneumonia
Adenoviruses	Respiratory tract Conjunctivae	Tracheobronchitis Pharyngitis Conjunctivitis
Coronavirus	Respiratory tract Gastrointestinal tract	Severe acute respiratory syndrome (SARS)
Rhinoviruses	Respiratory tract	Rhinitis Pharyngitis
Enteroviruses		
Coxsackie	Respiratory tract Gut	Systemic infections Meningitis Tracheobronchitis Myocarditis
Polio	Gut	Central nervous system damage (including anterior horn cells, paralysis)
Herpesviruses		
Herpes simplex	Oral Genital Eye	Blisters, latent infection Keratoconjunctivitis
Varicella Herpes zoster	Respiratory tract	Vesicles—all ectodermal tissues (skin, mouth, respiratory tract)
Cytomegalovirus	Not known	Usually disseminated disease in newborns and immunodeficient individuals
Rubella	Respiratory tract	Systemic mild illness, rash, congenital anomalies in embryo
Hepatitis	Blood, body fluids	Hepatitis Systemic disease
Rabies	Bites or saliva on cut	Fatal nervous system damage
Human Immunodeficiency Virus (HIV)	Blood, body fluids	Acquired immunodeficiency syndrome (AIDS)

From Scanlan CL, Spearman CB, Sheldon RL: *Egan's fundamentals of respiratory care,* ed 6, St Louis, 1995, Mosby.

designed to prevent the transmission of these types of infections. Isolation precautions for blood-borne pathogens are discussed in detail later in this chapter.

Rickettsiae *and* Chlamydiae *Spp.*

Rickettsiae and *Chlamydiae* spp. are unusual microorganisms that are intracellular parasites. Organisms of both species are less than 1 μm in diameter. Their complex structures resemble that of bacteria, but they act like viruses because they require a living host to replicate.[4] *Rickettsiae* sp. are transmitted by insects (e.g., lice, fleas, ticks), and *Chlamydiae* sp. are transmitted by contact or the **airborne** route. Common rickettsial diseases include typhus, Rocky Mountain spotted fever, and Q fever. (Note that Q fever is spread by the aerosol route rather than by insect vectors.) Chlamydial infections are also associated with pneumonia, sinusitis, pharyngitis, and bronchiolitis.[4]

Protozoa

Protozoa are unicellular eukaryotes that occur singly or in colonies. Protozoan infections are common in tropical climates, especially where sanitation is poor or lacking. Common examples of protozoan infections include amebiasis, malaria, and trypanosomiasis.[4] The most important protozoan that can invade the lung and cause pneumonia is *Pneumocystis carinii*. *Pneumocystis carinii* pneumonia (PCP) is common in immunocompromised patients, particularly those infected with HIV. It is worth noting that although *Pneumocystis* spp. are classified as protozoans, they are more closely related to fungi.[5]

Fungi

Fungi are **eukaryotic** organisms that include molds and yeast. Molds consist of chains of cells or filaments called *hyphae* and reproduce asexually by forming spores. Yeasts are unicellular fungi that reproduce sexually or asexually by budding. Fungal infections or mycoses can occur in normal healthy individuals, but they are more prevalent in patients with compromised immune function (i.e., opportunistic infections). Fungal infections in otherwise healthy individuals usually are caused by *Histoplasma capsulatum*, *Coccidioides immitis,* and *Blastomyces dermatitidis.* Opportunistic fungal infections typically are caused by *Candida albicans* and *Aspergillus fumigatus*.[3,4]

Transmission of Infectious Diseases

The public's awareness of infectious diseases has increased dramatically during the last two decades with the emergence of HIV and acquired immunodeficiency syndrome (AIDS), the Ebola and severe acute respiratory syndrome (SARS) viruses, and the threat of bioterrorism. It is important to recognize that the transmission of infectious diseases requires three elements for the spread of infectious materials: (1) a source of pathogens, (2) a mode of transmission for the infectious agent, and (3) a susceptible host. Nosocomial pneumonia is most often caused by bacteria;

BOX 5-1	Bacteria Commonly Associated with Ventilator-Associated Pneumonia (VAP)

- *Pseudomonas aeruginosa*
- *Staphylococcus aureus*
- Enterobacteriaceae
- *Haemophilus influenzae*
- *Streptococcus* spp.

From Chastre J, Fagon J-V: Ventilator-associated pneumonia, *Am J Resp Crit Care Med* 165:872, 2002.

TABLE 5-3
Routes of Infectious Disease Transmission

Mode	Type	Examples
Contact	Direct	Hepatitis A
		Venereal disease
		Human immunodeficiency virus (HIV)
		Staphylococcus spp.
		Enteric bacteria
	Indirect	*Pseudomonas* spp.
		Enteric bacteria
		Hepatitis B and C
		HIV
	Droplet	Measles
		Streptococcus spp.
Vehicle	Water-borne	Shigellosis
		Cholera
	Food-borne	Salmonellosis
		Hepatitis A
Airborne	Aerosols	Legionellosis
	Droplet nuclei	Tuberculosis
		Diphtheria
	Dust	Histoplasmosis
Vector-borne	Ticks and mites	Rickettsia, Lyme disease
	Mosquitoes	Malaria
	Fleas	Bubonic plague

From Wilkins RL, Stoller JK, Scanlan CL: *Egan's fundamentals of respiratory care,* ed 8, St Louis, 2003, Mosby.

viruses and fungi contribute to a lesser extent. Box 5-1 provides a list of bacteria typically associated with ventilator-associated pneumonia (VAP).[5] It is worth noting that the most common source of pathogenic microorganisms is infected patients, but contaminated water, food, and medications are also sources of infectious material.

Infectious particles can be transmitted by four routes: contact, vehicles, airborne, and vectors (Table 5-3). **Direct contact** occurs when the infectious organism is physically transferred from a contaminated person to a susceptible host through touching or sexual contact. **Indirect contact** involves transfer of the infectious agent to a susceptible host via a fomite (e.g., clothing, surgical bandages, instruments, equipment).[2] Transfer of infectious materials by vehicles most often occurs through contaminated water and food, although intravenous fluids, blood and blood products, and medications can also occasionally harbor infectious particles.[6] Airborne, or respiratory transmission involves the transfer of infectious particles through aerosol droplets and dust particles. Infectious agents are transferred by the vector route when an insect transfers the infectious particle from a host to susceptible individual.[4] Transmission of infections by vectors is rarely associated with nosocomial infections. Clinical Rounds 5-2 presents an exercise to test your understanding of infection transmission.

A variety of mechanical and immunologic factors usually protect the host from becoming infected with pathogenic organisms.[6] Alterations in mechanical barriers that occur when the skin and mucous membranes are breached during surgery, endotracheal intubation, or placement of indwelling catheters can significantly increase an individual's risk of developing a nosocomial infection. Defects in immune function that occur because of an underlying disease or as a result of therapeutic interventions (e.g., radiation therapy, pharmacologic therapies) can also increase the risk for infection. Table 5-4 lists several conditions, possible precipitating causes, and common pathogens associated with hospitalized patients at risk for developing nosocomial infections.

INFECTION CONTROL METHODS

The purpose of any hospital infection control program is to prevent the spread of nosocomial infections. The two most important concepts to understand about infection control are decontamination of patient care items and isolation precautions.

Decontamination, or the removal of pathogenic microorganisms from medical equipment, is accomplished by cleaning, disinfection, and sterilization with an appropriate **germicide** (i.e., an agent that destroys pathogenic microorganisms). *Cleaning* is the removal of all foreign material, particularly organic matter (e.g., blood, serum, pus, fecal matter) from objects with hot water, soap, detergent, and enzymatic products. *Disinfection* is the removal of most pathogenic microorganisms except bacterial endospores. Liquid chemicals and **pasteurization** are the most common disinfection methods used. *Sterilization* is the elimination of all forms of microbial life. It can be accomplished by either physical or chemical processes.

CLINICAL ROUNDS 5-2

As previously discussed, infectious agents can be transmitted by a variety of means, including contact, vehicle, airborne, and vector routes. Identify the most probable means of transmission for the following infectious particles:

· *Pseudomonas aeruginosa* organisms
· HIV
· *Mycobacterium tuberculosis* organisms
· *Rickettsiae* sp.

See Evolve Resources for the answer.

TABLE 5-4

Medical Conditions and Common Pathogens in Hospitalized Patients with Increased Susceptibility to Nosocomial Infections

Condition	Possible Cause	Common Pathogens
Skin and mucosal barrier disruption	Burns	*Staphylococcus* aureus
	Foley catheter	*Pseudomonas* aeruginosa
	Intravenous catheter	Enterobacteriaceae
	Surgical wound	*Candida* spp.
	Endotracheal tube	
Neutropenia	Oncochemotherapy	*P. aeruginosa*
	Drug reactions	Enterobacteriaceae
	Autoimmune process	*Staphylococcus epidermidis*
	Leukemia	*S. aureus, Aspergillus* sp.
Disruption of normal flora	Antibiotic therapy	*Clostridium difficile*
	Oncochemotherapy	*Candida* spp.
Altered T cells	Cushing's syndrome	*Mycoplasma tuberculosis*
	Corticosteroid therapy	Fungal infections
	Hodgkin's disease	Herpes viruses
	Acquired immunodeficiency syndrome (AIDS)	*Pneumocystis carinii*
	Organ transplantation	Toxoplasmosis
Hypogammaglobulinemia	Nephrotic syndrome	*Streptococcus pneumoniae*
	Multiple myeloma	*Haemophilus influenzae*
		Enterobacteriaceae
Hypocomplementemia	Systemic lupus erythematosus	*Neisseria meningitidis*
	Liver failure	*S. pneumoniae*
	Vasculitis	Enterobacteriaceae

From Chatburn RL: Decontamination of respiratory care equipment: what can be done, what should be done, *Respir Care* 34:98, 1989.

Factors Influencing the Effectiveness of Germicides

As was previously stated, germicides are agents used to destroy pathogenic microorganisms. They destroy these microorganisms by damaging their cell membranes, denaturing their proteins, or disrupting their cellular processes.[2] **Bactericides** destroy all pathogenic bacteria, **virucides** destroy viruses, and **fungicides** kill fungi. *Germicide* is a general term used to describe an agent that destroys pathogenic microorganisms on living tissue and inanimate objects; *disinfectant* is used to describe agents that destroy pathogenic microorganisms on inanimate objects only.[7]

A number of factors can affect disinfection and sterilization, including the number, location, and innate resistance of the microorganisms; the concentration and potency of the germicide; the duration of exposure to the germicide; and the physical and chemical environment in which the germicide is used.[8] A brief discussion of several key points to remember when using germicides follows.

Number and Location of Microorganisms

The amount of time required to kill microorganisms is roughly proportional to the number of microorganisms present. Cleaning helps reduce the number of microbes to a manageable number. The location of the microorganisms can also influence the effectiveness of a germicide, because physical barriers can prevent contact of the germicide and the microbe. Therefore, it is imperative that the germicidal agent have direct contact with any part of the device that is exposed to potential pathogens. Consequently, proper disassembly (and assembly) of equipment during the decontamination process can be a limiting factor when the effectiveness of a physical or chemical agent is assessed.

Microbial Resistance

The presence of microbial capsules can increase a microorganism's resistance to disinfection and sterilization. This resistance generally is overcome by increasing the exposure time of the microbe to the germicide. Bacterial spores are the most resistant microbes, followed by mycobacteria, nonlipid or small viruses, fungi, lipid or medium viruses, and vegetative bacteria (e.g., *Staphylococcus* and *Pseudomonas* spp.). The resistance of gram-positive and gram-negative microorganisms to disinfection and sterilization is similar, except for *Pseudomonas aeruginosa*, which shows greater resistance to some disinfectants.[9,10]

Concentration and Potency of the Germicide

In general, a disinfectant's potency increases as its concentration increases. (Iodophors are an exception.) It is important to remember, however, that germicides are affected differently by concentration adjustments; that is, diluting a germicide influences the amount of time required for disinfection or sterilization.

Physical and Chemical Factors

The effectiveness of a germicide depends on the temperature, pH, and relative humidity of the environment in which it is used. Generally, the activity of most germicides increases as the temperature increases. Increasing the pH improves the antimicrobial activity of some disinfectants (e.g., glutaraldehyde and quaternary ammonium compounds); increasing the alkalinity of other agents reduces their effectiveness (e.g., phenols, hypochlorites, iodine). Relative humidity is an important determinant of the activity of gaseous disinfectants (e.g., ethylene oxide, formaldehyde).

Cleaning

Cleaning is the first step in the decontamination process. Figure 5-2 is a schematic of a typical cleaning area for respiratory care equipment. Note that the space is divided into dirty and clean areas, which have separate entries and exits. This design helps ensure that clean equipment is not mixed in with or contaminated by soiled items.

The cleaning process usually begins with disassembly of the equipment to help ensure that dirt and organic matter are removed from surfaces that are not necessarily visible when the device is assembled. Ultrasonic systems sometimes are used for cleaning equipment with crevices that are difficult to clean. These ultrasonic devices create small bubbles that can penetrate and dislodge dirt and organic material, particularly in hard to reach crevices.

As stated, cleaning usually is done with soaps, detergents, and enzymatic products. Soaps and detergents contain amphipathic molecules that help dissolve fat and grease by reducing surface tension so that water can penetrate the organic matter. The amphipathic nature of these agents relates to their ability to dissolve both polar and nonpolar molecules; that is, they can dissolve polar, or water-soluble (hydrophilic), substances and nonpolar, or water-insoluble (hydrophobic), substances. Soaps are not bactericidal but may be combined with a disinfectant. Detergents are weakly bacteriocidal against gram-positive organisms, but they are not effective against tubercle bacilli and viruses.[4]

Cleaning can be done by hand with a scrub brush or with an automatic system. These automatic systems are similar to the dishwasher found in the home. Dirty equipment goes through a series of wash and rinse cycles before automatically undergoing pasteurization or cold disinfection.

After the equipment is cleaned, it should be dried to remove residual water, because moisture can alter the effectiveness of disinfectants and sterilizing agents. For example, water can dilute the disinfectant or change its pH.[7] Residual moisture can also combine with ethylene oxide to form ethylene glycol, a toxic chemical that is difficult to remove.[4] To prevent recontamination, equipment should be reassembled in a clean area separate from the area for processing soiled equipment. Clean equipment should never be allowed to sit on open counters for a prolonged time.

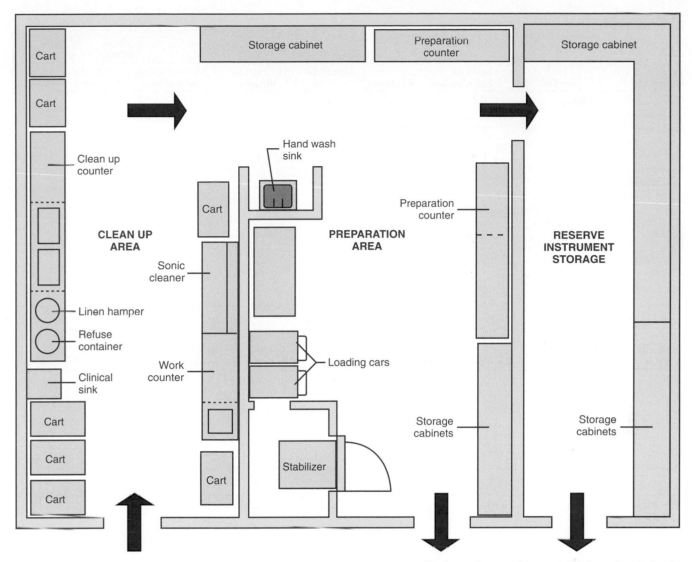

FIGURE 5-2 Schematic of a typical cleaning area for respiratory care equipment. (Redrawn from Perkins JJ: *Principles and methods of sterilization in health sciences,* Springfield, Ill, 1978, Charles C Thomas.)

Disinfection

By definition, disinfection differs from sterilization because it lacks sporicidal properties.[8] Disinfection can be accomplished by physical and chemical methods. Pasteurization is the most common physical method of disinfection. Quaternary ammonium compounds, alcohols, acetic acid, phenols, iodophors, sodium hypochlorite, glutaraldehyde, and hydrogen peroxide are examples of chemical disinfectants. Table 5-5 lists some commonly used disinfectants and their germicidal properties.

It is important to note that certain disinfectants (e.g., hydrogen peroxide, peracetic acid, glutaraldehyde) can eliminate spores with sufficient exposure time (i.e., 6 to 10 hours). Disinfectants that can eliminate spores are called **chemical sterilants. High-level disinfection** occurs when chemical sterilants are used at reduced exposure times (less than 45 minutes). High-level disinfectants kill bacteria, fungi, and viruses but do not kill bacterial spores unless the spores are exposed to the disinfectant for an extended time. **Intermediate-level disinfectants** remove vegetative bacteria, tubercle bacteria, some viruses, and fungi but do not necessarily kill spores. **Low-level disinfectants** kill most vegetative bacteria, some fungi, and some viruses. Box 5-2 summarizes the properties of an ideal disinfectant.

Pasteurization

Pasteurization uses moist heat to coagulate cell proteins. The exposure time required to kill vegetative bacteria depends on the temperature. Two techniques are commonly used: the flash process and the batch process. In the flash process, the material to be disinfected is exposed to moist heat at 72° C for 15 seconds. With the batch process, equipment is immersed in a water bath heated to 63° C for 30 minutes. The batch process can kill all vegetative bacteria and some viruses, including HIV. The flash process is used to pasteurize milk and other heat-labile liquids. Most

TABLE 5-5

Germicidal Properties of Disinfectants and Sterilization Agents

Level of Germicide	Use Dilution	Level of Disinfection	Bacteria	Lipophilic Viruses	Hydrophilic Viruses	INACTIVES		
						Mycobacterium tuberculosis	Mycotic Agents	Bacterial Spores
Isopropyl alcohol	60% to 95%	Int	+	+	−	+	+	+
Hydrogen peroxide	3% to 25%	CS/High	+	+	+	+	+	±
Formaldehyde	3% to 8%	High/Int	+	+	+	+	+	±
Quaternary ammonium compounds	0.4% to 1.6% aqueous	Low	+	+	−	−	±	
Phenolic	0.4% to 5% aqueous	Int/Low	+	+	±	+	±	
Chlorine	100-1000 ppm free chlorine	High/Low	+	+	+	+	+	±
Iodophors	30-50 ppm free iodine	Int	+	+	+	±	±	
Glutaraldehyde	2%	CS/High	+	+	+	+	+	±

	IMPORTANT CHARACTERISTICS							
Shelf Life > 1 Week	Corrosive/ Deleterious Effects	Residue	Inactivated by Organic Matter	Skin Irritant	Eye Irritant	Respiratory Irritant	Toxic	Easily Obtainable
+	±	−	+	±	+	−	+	+
+	−	−	±	+	+	−	+	+
+	−	+	−	+	+	+	+	+
+	−	−	+	+	+	−	+	+
+	−	+	±	+	+	−	+	+
+	+	+	+	+	+	+	+	+
+	±	+	+	±	+	−	+	+
+	−	+	−	+	+	+	+	+

From Rutala WA: Disinfection, sterilization, and waste disposal. In Wenzel RP, editor: *Prevention and control of nosocomial infections,* Baltimore, 1997, Williams & Wilkins.

Int, Intermediate; *CS,* chemical sterilant; +, yes; −, no; ±, variable results.

*Inactivates all indicated microorganisms with a contact time of 30 minutes or less, except bacterial spores, which require a 6- to 10-hour contact time.

respiratory care equipment can withstand the conditions of the batch process.

Quaternary Ammonium Compounds

Quaternary ammonium compounds (Quats) are organically substituted ammonium compounds that are cationic detergents containing four alkyl or heterocyclic radicals and a halide ion. The halide may be substituted by a sulfate radical. They are thought to interfere with the bacteria's energy-producing enzymes, denature its essential cell proteins, and disrupt the bacterial cell membrane.[8,11,12] Quats are bactericidal, fungicidal, and virucidal against lipophilic viruses. They are not sporicidal or tuberculocidal or virucidal against hydrophilic viruses. They are inactivated by organic material, and their effectiveness is reduced by cotton and gauze pads, which may absorb some of their active ingredients.[8] Quats are routinely used to sanitize noncritical surfaces (e.g., floors, walls, furniture) and can generally retain their activity for as long as 2 weeks if they are kept free of organic material.[7]

Alcohols

Ethyl and isopropyl alcohol are the two most common alcohols used for disinfection. Both are bactericidal, fungicidal, and virucidal, but they do not kill bacterial spores. The optimum concentrations of both alcohols range from 60% to 90%. Their ability to disinfect decreases significantly at concentrations below 50%.[8]

Alcohols are thought to kill microorganisms by denaturing proteins. This is a reasonable hypothesis considering that absolute ethyl alcohol, a dehydrating agent, is less bactericidal than an ethyl alcohol and water mixture, because proteins are denatured more quickly in the presence of water.[13] Although alcohols have been shown to be effective in fairly short periods (less than 5 minutes), the Centers for Disease Control and Prevention (CDC) recommends that exposure times of 15 minutes be required for 70% ethanol.[7]

Alcohols are used to disinfect rubber stoppers of multiple-use medication vials, oral and rectal thermometers, stethoscopes, and fiberoptic endoscopes. They also can be used to clean the surfaces of mechanical ventilators and areas used for medication preparation.[8] Alcohols are good solvents and can remove shellac from equipment surfaces. They can cause swelling and hardening of rubber and plastic tubes after prolonged and repeated use.

Acetic Acid
Acetic acid (white household vinegar) is used extensively as a means of decontaminating home care respiratory equipment. It also is used in hospitals but on a limited basis. Because of its acidic nature (pH ~2), its presumed mechanism of bactericidal action involves lowering a microbe's intracellular pH, thus inactivating its energy-producing enzymes.

The optimum concentration of acetic acid is 1.25%, which is the equivalent of one part 5% white household vinegar and three parts water. It has been shown to be an effective bactericidal agent (particularly against *P. aeruginosa*), but its sporicidal and virucidal activity has not been documented.[14]

Peracetic acid, or peroxyacetic acid, is acetic acid to which an oxygen atom has been added. It has been shown to be an excellent disinfectant with sterilization capabilities.[4] Peracetic acid is a strong oxidizing agent that kills microbes by denaturing proteins, disrupting cell wall permeability, and oxidizing cellular metabolites.[15] However, its strong oxidizing action is also a shortcoming, because it can corrode brass, iron, copper, and steel.[8]

Phenols
Carbolic acid, the prototype of the six-carbon aromatic compounds known as phenols, was first used as a germicide by Lister in his pioneering work on antiseptic surgery.[8] Although carbolic acid is no longer used as a disinfectant, chemical manufacturers have synthesized numerous phenol derivatives that have been shown to be effective bactericidal, fungicidal, virucidal, and tuberculocidal agents. (Note that these derivatives are not sporicidal.) Phenol derivatives contain an alkyl, phenyl, benzyl, or halogen substituted for one of the hydrogen atoms attached to the aromatic ring. Commonly used phenols include orthophenylphenol and orthobenzylparachlorophenol.

Phenols kill microbes by denaturing proteins and injuring the cell wall. They are used primarily as surface disinfectants for floors, walls, and countertops. Phenols are readily absorbed by porous material, and residual disinfectant can cause skin irritation. They have been associated with hyperbilirubinemia in neonates when used as disinfectants in nurseries.[16]

Iodophors and Other Halogenated Compounds
An iodophor is a solution that contains iodine and a solubilizing agent or carrier. This combination results in a chemical that provides a sustained release of free iodine in an aqueous solution.[8] The best known iodophor is povidone-iodine, which is used as an antiseptic and disinfectant.

Iodophors penetrate the cell wall of microorganisms, and their mode of action is thought to be disruption of protein and nucleic metabolisms. They are bactericidal, tuberculocidal, fungicidal, and virucidal, but they are not effective against bacterial spores. Note that solutions formulated for antiseptic use are not suitable for disinfectant use because antiseptic solutions contain significantly less free iodine than those formulated as disinfectants.

Sodium hypochlorite contains free available chlorine in an aqueous solution. Three forms of chlorine are present in the sodium hypochlorite mixture: free chlorine (Cl_2), hypochlorite anion (OCl^-), and hypochlorous acid ($HOCl$). It has been suggested that these forms of chlorine kill microbes by interfering with cellular metabolism, denaturing proteins, and inactivating nucleic acids.[8,17,18] Sodium hypochlorite (household bleach) demonstrates a range of "-cidal" activities. A 1:100 dilution is bactericidal, tuberculocidal, and virucidal in 10 minutes and fungicidal in 1 hour. The CDC recommends that a 1:10 dilution be used to clean blood spills.[4,19] However, it is not sporicidal. Although sodium hypochlorite is inexpensive and relatively fast acting, it is corrosive to metals. It forms bischloromethyl ether (a carcinogen) when it comes in contact with formaldehyde and trihalomethane when hot water is hyperchlorinated. It has a limited shelf life and is inactivated by organic matter.

Glutaraldehyde

Glutaraldehyde solutions have been some of the most common disinfectants used in respiratory care departments. As stated, these solutions can be used as chemical sterilants if exposure time is extended. They kill microbes by alkylating hydroxyl, sulfhydryl, carboxy, and amino groups of microorganisms, which ultimately interfere with protein synthesis.[8] Alkaline and acid glutaraldehyde solutions are commercially available.

Alkaline glutaraldehyde is packaged as a mildly acidic solution (2% glutaraldehyde) that is activated with a bicarbonate solution, yielding a solution with a pH of 7.5 to 8.5. It is bactericidal, fungicidal, tuberculocidal, and virucidal with an exposure time of 10 minutes. It is sporicidal with an exposure time of 6 to 10 hours. The average shelf life of alkaline glutaraldehyde is 14 days to 1 month. It is irritating to skin and mucous membranes (particularly the eyes). For this reason, the Occupational Safety and Health Administration (OSHA) limits exposure of workers to 0.2 ppm airborne alkaline glutaraldehyde. Union Carbide, a manufacturer of glutaraldehyde, recently suggested that the threshold for exposure be lowered to 0.1 ppm. Individuals working with glutaraldehyde should wear protective eyewear, masks, gloves, and splash gowns or aprons.[20,21] Ideally, glutaraldehyde should be used under a fume hood or in a room that is under negative pressure.

Acid glutaraldehyde, which has a pH of 2.7 to 3.7, is available as a 2% solution that does not require activation and comes ready to use. Acid glutaraldehyde is similar to alkaline glutaraldehyde in effect—it is bactericidal, tuberculocidal, and fungicidal; however, the exposure time must be extended to 20 minutes for acid glutaraldehyde to be tuberculocidal. The activity of an acid glutaraldehyde solution can be enhanced by warming it to 60° C. At this temperature, acid glutaraldehyde is bactericidal, fungicidal, and virucidal in 5 minutes, tuberculocidal in 20 minutes, and sporicidal in 60 minutes.[4] Acid glutaraldehyde is not irritating to the skin and mucous membranes as is alkaline glutaraldehyde. Its shelf life is approximately 30 days.

Hydrogen Peroxide

Commercially available 3% solutions of hydrogen peroxide are effective disinfectants of bacteria (including *Mycobacterium* sp.), fungi, and viruses and are active within 10 minutes at room temperature. Higher concentrations (6% to 25%) and prolonged exposure are required for sterilization. Hydrogen peroxide is sporicidal in 6 hours at 20° C; it is effective against spores in 20 minutes at 50° C.[8]

Hydrogen peroxide kills microorganisms by forming hydroxyl radicals that can attack membrane lipids, nucleic acids, and other essential compounds. Note that catalase-positive aerobes and facultative anaerobic bacteria can inactivate metabolically produced hydrogen peroxide by degrading it into water and oxygen.

Sterilization

As with disinfection, sterilization techniques generally are divided into physical and chemical methods. Physical methods most often rely on heat, specifically dry heat, boiling water, steam under pressure (autoclave), and incineration. Ionizing radiation (i.e., γ-rays and x-rays) also has been shown to be an effective method of sterilization; however, this method is used on a limited basis in hospitals. The most commonly used chemical for sterilization is ethylene oxide. (See Table 5-5 for a comparison of the advantages and disadvantages of various sterilization methods.)

Heat

Probably the simplest and surest means of destroying microorganisms is burning or incineration. This method is reserved for items that are disposable or are so contaminated that reuse is prohibited.[4] It should be recognized that, besides destroying the material being sterilized, incineration creates air pollution.

Dry heat is another effective method of heat sterilization. Its use is limited to items that are not heat sensitive. Temperatures must be maintained between 160° and 180° C for 1 to 2 hours to accomplish sterilization. Dry heat is routinely used to sterilize laboratory glassware and surgical instruments, but it cannot be used for heat-sensitive items made of rubber or plastic.

Boiling water kills vegetative bacteria and most viruses in 30 minutes; however, its effectiveness against spores, especially those of thermophilic organisms, is somewhat questionable. Boiling water is commonly used to sterilize metal surgical instruments. As with dry heat, it cannot be used for heat-sensitive equipment. Because water boils at a lower temperature at high altitudes, exposure time must be prolonged when this form of sterilization is used at high elevations.[4,6]

Steam under pressure, or autoclaving, is a highly effective and inexpensive method of sterilization. Of the aforementioned techniques, autoclaving is probably the most versatile. It is routinely used on laboratory glassware, surgical instruments, liquids, linens, and other heat- and moisture-resistant materials. The technique of autoclaving is fairly simple. Items to be autoclaved are cleaned and wrapped in linen, gauze, or paper. They are placed in a chamber like that shown in Figure 5-3, and the chamber is closed and secured. The chamber is evacuated of air, moisture is added (100% humidity), and the pressure inside is raised to 15 to 20 psig. Air is evacuated from the chamber, because residual air prolongs the penetration time of steam, thus increasing the total autoclave cycle

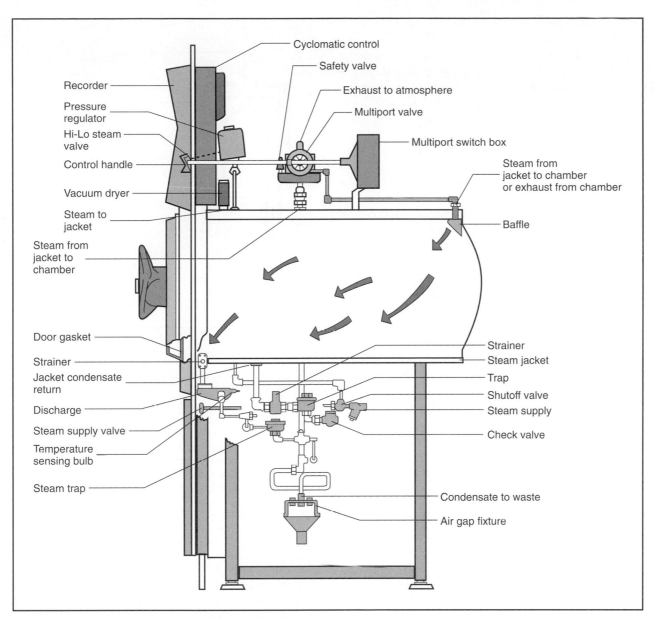

FIGURE 5-3 Components of an autoclave. (From Perkins JJ: *Principles and methods of sterilization in health sciences,* Springfield, Ill, 1978, Charles C Thomas.)

time. Pressure is used to raise the temperature of the steam, which is critical because the amount of time required to achieve sterilization depends on the temperature inside the autoclave. For example, at atmospheric pressure, steam has a temperature of 100° C. At 15 psig, it has a temperature of 121° C, and at 20 psig it has a temperature of 132° C. At 121° C, all microbes and spores are killed within 15 minutes; at 132° C, killing occurs in 10 minutes.

Because the process of autoclaving depends on several factors, heat-sensitive and biologic indicators are routinely used to ensure quality control during the process. Heat-sensitive tape used to package materials for autoclaving changes color when exposed to a given temperature for a prescribed amount of time. The most common biologic

indicators for autoclaving are strips of paper impregnated with *Bacillus stearothermophilus* spores. These strips should be used weekly (at a minimum) to ensure that the autoclave is working properly.

Ethylene Oxide

Ethylene oxide (ETO) is a sterilant that has been used since the 1950s. It is a colorless gas that is flammable and explosive. It kills microorganisms by alkylating proteins, DNA, and RNA, thus interfering with cellular metabolism.[11] ETO originally was combined with chlorofluorocarbons (CFCs), which acted as a stabilizing agent. Under provisions of the Clean Air Act of 1993, CFCs were phased out in 1995 because of their detrimental effect on the ozone layer. Currently, ETO is used alone or in combination with different stabilizing agents, such as carbon dioxide or hydrochlorofluorocarbons.

ETO kills all microorganisms and spores; bacterial spores are more resistant than vegetative microbes. The effectiveness of ETO depends on the gas concentration (450 to 1200 mg/L), the temperature (29° to 65° C), the humidity (45% to 85% relative humidity), and the exposure time (2 to 5 hours).[8] Generally, increases in the ETO concentration and temperature shorten the sterilization time.

All equipment to be sterilized with ETO must be free of water, because water interferes with the sterilization process. Additionally, equipment must be packaged in ETO-permeable materials, such as paper, muslin, or plastic bags made of polyethylene or polypropylene. The actual process of automated ETO sterilization consists of several stages: a preconditioning phase and a gas injection phase, exposure of the item to the ETO, evacuation of gas from the chamber, and an air-washing period.[8] After sterilization, all equipment exposed to ETO must be aerated before use. Note that the aeration time usually is not considered part of the sterilization time and usually is accomplished by mechanical aeration for 8 to 12 hours at 50° to 60° C. Aeration at room temperature is considered dangerous because of ETO's toxicity.

Biologic indicators, similar to those used for autoclaving, must be used to monitor the effectiveness of ETO. *Bacillus subtilis* spores generally are used for this purpose. Figure 5-4 shows a typical device for monitoring sterilization. *B. subtilis* organisms imbedded in a paper strip are housed within a plastic capsule inside a glass ampule containing a growth medium (e.g., tryptic soy broth).[8] The ampule is placed among the materials to be sterilized. After the sterilization cycle, the ampule is crushed and the paper strip is immersed in the liquid. The strip then is incubated according to the manufacturer's directions. Microbe growth is indicated by changes in the turbidity of the growth medium after incubation.[2]

Inhalation of ETO has been associated with nose and eye irritation, dyspnea, headache, nausea, vomiting, dizziness, and convulsions.[22] Direct contact with ETO causes skin irritation and burns. OSHA and The Joint Commission (TJC) provide general guidelines for the safe use of ETO. The current OSHA standard for ETO exposure is 1 ppm in 8 hours, with a maximum short-term exposure of 5 to 10 ppm for 15 minutes.[23]

Identifying Infection-Risk Devices

Not all reusable patient care items must be sterilized. Whether a medical device should be cleaned and disinfected or sterilized depends on its intended use. In 1968, E. H. Spaulding devised a classification scheme that could be used by infection control professionals in the planning of disinfection and sterilization methods for patient care items and equipment.[24,25] Spaulding's classification system placed devices into three categories based on the degree of

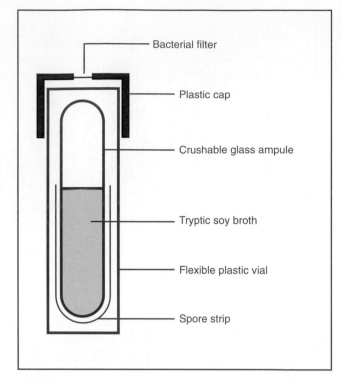

FIGURE 5-4 Biologic sterilization indicators: the capsule contains a strip impregnated with bacterial spores, a pH indicator, and a culture medium (e.g., tryptic soy broth). After sterilization, the ampule is crushed, releasing the culture medium onto the strip containing the spores. Incomplete sterilization is indicated if the capsule turns yellow. (Redrawn from Boyd RF, Hoerl BG: *Basic medical microbiology*, ed 3, Boston, 1986, Little, Brown.)

risk of infection involved in their use. The categories are critical, semicritical, and noncritical.

Critical items must be sterilized, because they are introduced into sterile tissue or the vascular system (e.g., surgical instruments, implants, cardiac and urinary catheters, heart-lung and hemodialysis equipment, needles). Because semicritical items (e.g., ventilator tubing) come in contact with intact mucous membranes, a minimum of high-level disinfection is recommended. Respiratory care and anesthesia equipment, endoscopes, and thermometers are semicritical items. High-level disinfection is effective against blood-borne pathogens (i.e., HIV, hepatitis B virus) and *Mycobacteria tuberculosis*. Noncritical items come in contact with intact skin but not mucous membranes. Intact skin acts as an effective barrier to most microorganisms, therefore sterility is not critical. Common examples of noncritical items are face masks, ventilators, stethoscopes, and blood pressure cuffs. Table 5-6 lists examples of medical devices and how they are classified according to Spaulding's system. Box 5-3 contains a summary of the guidelines for processing reusable respiratory care equipment.

Box 5-4 describes several strategies for preventing the spread of pathogenic organisms by in-use respiratory care

TABLE 5-6

Infection Risk Categories for Medical Equipment

Category	Description	Examples	Processing
Critical	Devices introduced into the bloodstream or other parts of the body	Surgical devices Cardiac catheters Implants Heart-lung and hemodialysis components	Sterilization
Semicritical	Devices that contact intact mucous membranes	Endoscopes Trachea tubes Ventilator tubing Face masks Blood pressure cuffs	High-level disinfection
Noncritical	Devices that touch only intact skin or do not contact patient	Face masks Blood pressure cuffs Ventilators	Detergent washing Low- to intermediate-level disinfection

Modified from Chatburn RL: Decontamination of respiratory care equipment: what can be done, what should be done. In Scanlan CL, Spearman CB, Sheldon RL: *Egan's fundamentals of respiratory care,* ed 6, St Louis, 1995, Mosby.

BOX 5-3   Guidelines for Processing Reusable Respiratory Care Equipment

- All reusable respiratory care equipment should undergo low- or intermediate-level disinfection as part of the initial cleaning.
- All reusable breathing circuit components (including tubing and exhalation valves, medication nebulizers and their reservoirs, large-volume jet nebulizers and their reservoirs) should be considered semicritical items.
- Semicritical items should be sterilized between patient use; heat-stable items should be autoclaved, and heat-labile items should undergo ethylene oxide (ETO) sterilization.
- If sterilization is not feasible, semicritical items should undergo high-level disinfection or pasteurization.
- The internal machinery of ventilators and breathing machines need not be routinely sterilized or disinfected between patients.
- Respirometers and other equipment used to monitor multiple patients should not directly touch any part of a ventilator circuit or a patient's mucus membranes. Rather, disposable extension pieces and low-resistance high-efficiency particulate air (HEPA) filters should be used to isolate the device. If the device cannot be isolated from the patient or circuit, it must be sterilized or receive high-level disinfection before use on other patients.
- After use on one patient, nondisposable resuscitation bags should be sterilized or should receive high-level disinfection before use on other patients.
- External surfaces, ports, and internal channels of bronchoscopes should be cleaned with water and a detergent before being immersed in a high-level disinfectant. All channels of the bronchoscope should be perfused for at least 20 minutes and then rinsed with sterile water, followed by an alcohol rinse, and then dried using filtered air. Forceps and specimen brushes should be sterilized separately from the bronchoscope.

Modified from Wilkins RL, Stoller JK, Scanlan, CL: *Egan's fundamentals of respiratory care,* ed 8, St Louis, 2003, Mosby. Data from Chatburn RL: Decontamination of respiratory care equipment: what can be done, what should be done, *Respir Care* 34:98, 1989; AARC Technical Standards and Safety Committee: Recommendations for respiratory therapy equipment: processing, handling, and surveillance, *Respir Care* 22:928, 1977.

BOX 5-4   Strategies for Preventing the Spread of Pathogenic Organisms by In-Use Respiratory Care Equipment[2,6,36]

- Large-volume reusable nebulizers and humidifiers should always be filled with sterile distilled water before initial use. When fluid is replenished, any fluid remaining in these devices should be emptied and the reservoir filled completely. Prefilled, sterile disposable humidifiers should be used whenever possible.
- Large-volume room air humidifiers that create aerosols should not be used unless they can be sterilized or subjected to high-level disinfection at least daily and filled only with sterile water.
- Large-volume jet nebulizers and medication nebulizers and their reservoirs and tubing should be changed or replaced every 24 hours with equipment that has undergone high-level disinfection.
- Prefilled, sterile, disposable humidifiers that are used with oxygen-delivery devices do not need to be changed between patients in high-use area, such as the recovery room; they can be used safely for up to 30 days. The tubing and oxygen-delivery device should be changed between patients.
- In-use ventilator circuits, including their humidifiers and nebulizers, should be changed every second or third day (48 to 72 hours). If a heat and moisture exchanger bacterial filter (i.e., artificial nose) is used instead of a water humidifier, changing the circuit between patients may be satisfactory.
- Water condensate in the ventilator and nebulizer tubing should be discarded and not drained back into the reservoir.

equipment (e.g., nebulizers, ventilator circuits, manual resuscitators, oxygen therapy apparatuses). Of particular note is the frequency of ventilator circuit changes. A number of studies have tried to address this issue by looking at the incidence of ventilator-associated pneumonia (VAP) as a function of the time interval between ventilator circuit changes. Historically, circuits were changed daily. In 1986 Craven et al.[26] found that the incidence of VAP was significantly reduced if the circuits were changed at 48-hour intervals compared with every 24 hours. Subsequent studies have suggested that the interval between ventilator circuit changes can be extended for even longer periods.[27] Although extending the time between circuit changes clearly does not increase the incidence of VAP, the optimum interval remains unclear.[28,29]

SURVEILLANCE

Ongoing surveillance is required to ensure that an infection control program is providing adequate protection for patients and health care providers. Surveillance typically consists of three components: monitoring of equipment processing procedures, routine sampling of in-use equipment, and identifying suspected pathogens microbiologically.[4] Equipment processing is monitored using the aforementioned chemical and biologic indicators. In-use equipment can be routinely sampled with sterile cotton swabs, liquid broth, and aerosol impaction. Swabs can be used to obtain samples from easily accessible surfaces of respiratory care equipment. Liquid broth can be used to obtain samples when cotton swabs cannot reach many parts of the equipment (e.g., inside tubing). Aerosol impaction is used to sample the particulate output of nebulizers.

Microbiologic identification requires the hospital's clinical laboratory staff to work with clinicians to identify infectious organisms. Clinical microbiologists can provide information about nosocomial infections from direct smears and stains, cultures, serologic tests, and antibiotic susceptibility testing. Identification of the cause of a nosocomial infection is essential for preventing and minimizing hospital epidemics.[4] Clinical Rounds 5-3 provides a

---

CLINICAL ROUNDS 5-3

The hospital infection control committee notifies your department that the incidence of nosocomial pneumonia in the recovery room increases significantly during the month of December. It has been suggested that the source of the pneumonia could be reusable, large-volume jet nebulizers. How would you determine whether in-use, large-volume jet nebulizers are responsible for this outbreak of pneumonia? How could you monitor the effectiveness of the sterilization of these devices?

See Evolve Resources for the answer.

---

test of your understanding of the principles of infection control techniques.

ISOLATION PRECAUTIONS

In 2007 the CDC, in cooperation with the federal Healthcare Infection Control Practices Advisory Committee (HICPAC; formerly the Hospital Infection Control Practices Advisory Committee), revised its guideline for isolation precautions in the health care setting.[1] The revised guideline contains information on the history of isolation practices, along with recommendations for isolation precautions in a variety of health care settings. The revised recommendations are intended for acute care hospitals and for subacute and extended care facilities.

Like the 1996 recommendations, the revised recommendations establish two levels of precautions: **standard precautions** and **transmission-based precautions.** Standard precautions are to be used with all patients, regardless of their diagnosis or presumed infection status. Standard precautions represent a combination of **universal precautions** and body substance isolation precautions; they apply to blood, all body fluids (secretions and excretions [except sweat]), nonintact skin, and mucous membranes. Standard precautions involve the use of personal protective equipment (PPE), as well as the proper handling of potentially contaminated equipment and items in the patient's environment. Standard precautions, therefore, are designed to reduce the risk of transmission of microorganisms from both recognized and unrecognized sources of infection in the health care setting.[1]

Transmission-based precautions are designed to interrupt transmission of known or suspected pathogens that can be transmitted by airborne or droplet routes or by direct contact with skin and contaminated surfaces. Transmission-based precautions are for the care of patients with highly transmissible or epidemiologically important pathogens that necessitate additional precautions to stop their transmission. Box 5-5 gives a synopsis of the various types of isolation precautions and a list of conditions that require each type of precaution. Table 5-7 lists clinical syndromes and conditions that warrant additional precautions to prevent the transmission of epidemiologically important pathogens upon confirmation of diagnosis.

Fundamentals of Isolation Protection

Hand washing is the most important prevention strategy for protecting health care workers from becoming infected through contact with infected patients. It also reduces the risk of health care workers transmitting infectious microorganisms from one patient to another or from a contaminated site to a clean site on the same patient.[30-33] Health care workers should wash their hands before caring for any patient; however, it is particularly important that they

BOX 5-5	Infection Control Precautions and Patients Who Require Them

STANDARD PRECAUTIONS

Use standard precautions for the care of all patients.

AIRBORNE PRECAUTIONS

In addition to standard precautions, use airborne precautions for patients known to have or suspected of having serious illnesses transmitted by airborne droplet nuclei. Examples of such illnesses include:

- Measles
- Varicella (including disseminated zoster)*
- Tuberculosis[†]

DROPLET PRECAUTIONS

In addition to standard precautions, use droplet precautions for patients known to have or suspected of having serious illnesses transmitted by large-particle droplets. Examples of such illnesses include:

- Invasive *Haemophilus influenzae* type b disease (meningitis, pneumonia, epiglottis, and sepsis)
- Invasive *Neisseria meningitidis* disease (meningitis, pneumonia, and sepsis)
- Other serious bacterial respiratory infections spread by droplet transmission, including:
  - Diphtheria (pharyngeal)
  - *Mycoplasma* pneumonia
  - Pertussis
  - Pneumonic plague
  - Streptococcal pharyngitis, pneumonia, or scarlet fever in infants and young children
- Serious viral infections spread by droplet transmission, including:
  - Adenovirus*
  - Influenza
  - Mumps
  - Parvovirus B19
  - Rubella

CONTACT PRECAUTIONS

In addition to standard precautions, use contact precautions for patients known to have or suspected of having serious illnesses easily transmitted by direct patient contact or by contact with items in the patient's environment. Examples of such illnesses include:

- Gastrointestinal, respiratory, skin, or wound infections or colonization with multidrug-resistant bacteria (judged by the infection control program to be of special clinical and epidemiologic significance based on current state, regional, or national recommendations).
- Enteric infections with a low infectious dose or prolonged environmental survival, including *Clostridium difficile* organisms.
- For diapered or incontinent patients: Enterohemorrhagic *Escherichia coli*, *Shigella* sp., hepatitis A, or rotavirus.
- Respiratory syncytial virus, parainfluenza virus, or enteroviral infections in infants and young children.
- Skin infections that are highly contagious or that may occur on dry skin, including:
  - Diphtheria (cutaneous)
  - Herpes simplex virus (neonatal or mucocutaneous)
  - Impetigo
  - Noncontained abscesses, cellulitis, or decubiti
  - Pediculosis
  - Scabies
  - Staphylococcal furunculosis in infants and young children
  - Zoster (disseminated or in an immunocompromised host)*
- Viral/hemorrhagic conjunctivitis
- Viral hemorrhagic infections (Ebola, Lassa, or Marburg)

Modified from Garner JS: Guideline for isolation precautions in hospitals, *Infect Control Hosp Epidemiol* 17:53, 1996.

*Certain infections require more than one type of precaution.

[†]See the CDC guidelines for environmental infection control in health-care facilities.[48]

wash them before and after performing invasive procedures or touching wounds or patients at high risk of infection.

Routine hand washing should involve a soap and water wash with a rubbing action to create a lather over both hands for at least 15 seconds. Hands should be rinsed thoroughly and dried with disposable or single-use towels or an air drier.[30] The CDC updated its recommendations for hand washing technique on October 25, 2002.[31] These updated guidelines specify that alcohol-based hand rubs should be used in conjunction with traditional soap and water to protect patients in health care settings. Alcohol-based hand rubs typically are applied to the hands after the hands have been dried following the soap and water wash. In many cases these alcohol-based handrubs can be substituted for the traditional hand washing with soap and water. As effective as these agents can be as an adjunct to infection control, it is important to recognize that frequent use of alcohol-based formulations for hand antisepsis can cause drying of the skin unless skin conditioning

agents are added to the formulations. In addition, alcohol-based hand rubs are flammable and have flash points in the range of 21° to 24° C, depending on the type and concentration of alcohol. Therefore, alcohol-based hand rubs should be stored away from high temperatures and flames, in accordance with the recommendations of the National Fire Protection Agency.[31]

Gloves are worn for several reasons: (1) to protect the health care worker from contact with blood and body fluids (i.e., blood-borne pathogens); (2) to provide a barrier so that resident and transient microorganisms on the hands of health care workers are not transferred to patients during patient care or medical or surgical procedures; and (3) to prevent health care workers from indirectly transmitting pathogens from an infected patient to another patient.[30,34] It is important to remember that hand washing is essential after removing gloves after each patient contact because hands can be contaminated during glove removal. Defects or tears in gloves also can allow contamination of the hands.[35,36]

TABLE 5-7

Clinical Syndromes and Conditions Warranting Additional Empiric Precautions to Prevent the Transmission of Infectious Disease*

Clinical Syndrome or Condition[†]	Clinical Syndrome or Condition[‡]	Empiric Precautions
Diarrhea		
Acute diarrhea with a likely infectious cause in an incontinent or diapered patient	Enteric pathogens[§]	Contact
Diarrhea in an adult with a history of recent antibiotic use	*Clostridium difficile*	Contact
Meningitis	*Neisseria meningitidis*	Droplet
Rash or exanthems, generalized, etiology unknown	*Neisseria meningitidis*	Droplet
Petechial/ecchymotic with fever	Varicella	Airborne contact
Vesicular Condition		
Maculopapular with coryza fever	Rubeola (measles)	Airborne
Respiratory Infections		
Cough/fever/upper lobe pulmonary infiltrate in a human immunodeficiency virus (HIV)–negative patient or a patient at low risk for HIV infection	*Mycobacterium tuberculosis*	Airborne
Cough/fever/pulmonary infiltrate in an HIV-negative patient or a patient at high risk for HIV infection	*Mycobacterium tuberculosis*	Airborne
Paroxysmal or severe persistent cough during periods of pertussis activity	*Bordetella pertussis*	Droplet
Respiratory infections, particularly bronchiolitis and croup, in infants and young children	Respiratory syncytial or parainfluenza virus	Contact
Risk of multidrug-resistant microorganisms	Resistant bacteria[‖]	Contact
History of infection or colonization with multidrug-resistant organisms		
Skin, wound, urinary tract infection in a patient with a recent hospital or nursing home stay in a facility where multidrug-resistant organisms are prevalent	Resistant bacteria[‖]	Contact
Skin or wound infection	*Staphylococcus aureus*	Contact
Abscess or draining wound that cannot be covered	Group A streptococcus	

Modified from Garner JS: Guideline for isolation precautions in hospitals, *Infect Control Hosp Epidemiol* 17:52, 1996.

*Infection control professionals are encouraged to modify or adapt this table according to local conditions. To ensure that appropriate empiric precautions are always implemented, hospitals must have systems in place for evaluating patients routinely according to these criteria as part of their preadmission and admission care.

[†]Patients with the syndromes or conditions listed may present with atypical signs or symptoms (e.g., pertussis in neonates and adults may not cause a paroxysmal or severe cough). The clinician's index of suspicion should be guided by the prevalence of specific conditions in the community and by clinical judgment.

[‡]The organisms listed are not intended to represent the complete, or even the most likely, diagnosis, but rather are possible etiologic agents that require additional precautions until they can be ruled out.

[§]These pathogens include enterohemorrhagic *Escherichia coli*, *Shigella sp.*, hepatitis A, and rotavirus.

[‖]Resistant bacteria as judged by the infection control program to be of special clinical or epidemiologic significance, based on current state, regional, or national recommendations.

Gowns and other protective apparel (e.g., shoe covers) are worn to prevent contamination of clothing and to protect the skin from blood and body fluid exposure.[29] This protective apparel should be impermeable to liquids and worn only once, then discarded. OSHA's final rule on blood-borne pathogens requires gowns and protective apparel to be worn.[37]

Face shields or masks with protective eyewear should be worn whenever splashing or spraying of blood or body fluid is possible (e.g., when obtaining arterial blood gas samples and inserting intravascular catheters). They may also be mandated in special circumstances stated in OSHA's final rule on blood-borne pathogens.[37] Face masks are used to prevent the spread of large-particle droplets transmitted by close contact (e.g., when working with patients who are coughing or sneezing). Note that the efficacy of wearing a mask to prevent the transmission of *Mycobacterium tuberculosis* organisms is questionable. The most recent guidelines established by the National Institute of Occupational Safety and Health (NIOSH) require that health care workers use respiratory protective devices, such as the N-95 respirator, to prevent the inhalation of airborne droplet nuclei, particularly when caring for patients with severe acute respiratory syndrome (SARS), tuberculosis (TB), or smallpox.[1] A wide range of respirators that meet NIOSH standards are available to prevent the inhalation of droplet nuclei. (Clinical Rounds 5-4 presents a brief discussion of the several types of protective respirators currently available.)

CLINICAL ROUNDS 5-4

Personal protective respirators that are used in hospital infection control programs must be certified by the National Institute of Occupational Safety and Health (NIOSH) and the U.S. Food and Drug Administration (FDA). Each type of mask typically is identified with a letter and a number code. The letter specifies whether the mask is not resistant (N), somewhat resistant (R), or strongly resistant (P) to oil degradation; the number following the letter refers to its particulate filtering efficiency. For example, an N-95 mask is not oil resistant, and it filters out 95% of the particles that attempt to flow through it. More information about personal protective respirators can be found at the NIOSH Personal Protective Technology Laboratory Web site: http://www.cdc.gov/niosh/npptl/default.html.

Patient care equipment and articles that may serve as **fomites** for the transmission of infectious particles (e.g., needles, scalpels, and other sharp objects) should be disposed of in specially designated containers. Disposable medical gas therapy devices, such as nebulizers and tubing, should be discarded in a sturdy bag or container. Reusable items should be sterilized or disinfected by standard procedures to prevent the transmission of infectious microorganisms from patient to patient. Disposable items should be disposed of according to hospital and applicable government regulations. Care must be taken not to contaminate the outside of the bag when it is handled and transported.

Fluids and medications used to treat patients should be sterile, therefore only sterile water should be used to fill nebulizers and humidifiers. Unused portions of large bottles of sterile water should be discarded within 24 hours. Single-dose ampules of sterile water and normal saline are ideal for small-volume nebulizers. Multidose vials should be stored according to manufacturer's specifications (e.g., refrigerated after opening). Single-dose and multidose vials should not be used beyond the date on the label.[2]

Standard Precautions

As was stated previously, standard precautions are a synthesis of previous CDC guidelines for universal precautions and body substance isolation techniques. Hands should be washed between patients and between tasks and procedures on the same patient to prevent cross-contamination of different body sites.[1,26] Gloves, masks, protective eyewear, and splash-proof gowns should be worn when there is a chance of splashing blood, body fluids, secretions, and excretions or contact with contaminated items. Needles and other sharp objects should be handled with care to prevent injuries. Needles should not be recapped; when recapping a syringe is necessary, both hands should never be used, instead, the one-hand "scoop" technique or a mechanical device to recap syringe needles safely.[30]

Three new elements have been added to standard precautions to reinforce existing infection control recommendations[38]: respiratory hygiene/cough etiquette, safe injection practices, and the use of masks by clinicians performing catheter insertion or injection of materials into spinal or epidural spaces via lumbar puncture procedures. Note that these recommendations focus on protection of the patient, whereas the other recommendations evolved from the original universal precautions, which were designed to protect health care personnel.

Respiratory hygiene/cough etiquette has five components: (1) education of health care staff, patients, and visitors; (2) signage that provides instructions about isolation procedures for family members and visitors accompanying the patient; (3) source control measures, such as using a surgical mask on a coughing patient when tolerated; (4) hand hygiene after contact with respiratory secretions; and (5) spacial separation of patients with respiratory infections in common waiting areas.[1]

Safe injection practices focus on reinforcing the importance of using proper aseptic techniques. Specifically, safe injection practices involve the use of a sterile, single-use, disposable needle and syringe for each injection. Additionally, single-dose medication vials should be used whenever possible to avoid contamination of injection equipment and medication.

Finally, recent evidence suggests that the use of face masks by health care providers participating in procedures involving lumbar puncture, spinal and epidural anesthesia, and the insertion of central venous lines can significantly limit the dispersal of oropharyngeal droplets and thus protect the patient from droplet-borne infectious materials.[39]

Airborne Precautions

Airborne precautions have two major components: (1) placement of the infected patient in an area with appropriate air handling and ventilation and (2) use of respiratory protective equipment by health care workers and visitors entering the patient's room.[29,30] When an infected patient must be transported, the patient should wear a surgical mask to minimize dispersal of droplet nuclei. Current standards require that infected patients be placed in a private, negative-pressure isolation room. Negative air pressures in the room should be monitored relative to other areas of the hospital. SARS, measles, chickenpox (primary varicella zoster), and tuberculosis are illnesses that require airborne precautions. Because varicella zoster organisms can also be transmitted by direct contact, infected patients may also require contact isolation.

Droplet Precautions

Droplet precautions are designed to prevent the transmission of microorganisms contained in droplets generated by sneezing, coughing, or talking or during procedures such as bronchoscopy and suctioning.[29] Precautions include gloves, masks, and protective eyewear. Special air handling and ventilation are not required. *Haemophilus influenzae* type b organisms and *Neisseria meningitidis* organisms are transmitted by this route. Other serious infections are adenovirus, influenza, parvovirus B19, pertussis, streptococcal pharyngitis, pneumonia, and scarlet fever.[30] As with airborne precautions, infected patients should wear a surgical mask to minimize transmission of droplet nuclei.

Contact Precautions

Contact precautions are recommended for patients infected with pathogenic organisms that can be spread by direct patient contact or through contact with items in the patient's environment.[26] Contact precautions require the patient to be isolated in a private room with a bath. Health care workers should wear masks, gloves, and gowns when caring for these patients. Illnesses that require contact isolation include gastrointestinal, respiratory, and skin infections. Some organisms responsible for these illnesses are *Clostridium difficile*, *Shigella* sp., hepatitis A, respiratory syn-

cytial virus, and the parainfluenza virus. Patients colonized with multidrug-resistant organisms of special clinical and epidemiologic significance also require contact isolation. Table 5-8 summarizes the HICPAC infection control guidelines for standard and transmission-based precautions. Clinical Rounds 5-5 provides a problem-solving exercise on isolation precautions typically required in the clinical setting.

CLINICAL ROUNDS 5-5

You are on call in the emergency department when one adult and two children are admitted after a house fire. The children incurred only minor cuts and bruises, but the adult sustained third-degree burns over 60% of his body. What precautions should you take when treating a burn patient?

See Evolve Resources for the answer.

TABLE 5-8

HICPAC Guidelines for Standard and Transmission-Based Precautions

Precautions	Scenario	Hand Hygiene	Gowns/Gloves	Mask and Eye Protection	Environmental Controls
Standard	Use for all patients, regardless of confirmed or suspected presence of an infectious agent.	Should be performed before patient contact, after touching blood, body fluids, and contaminated items, immediately after removing gloves, and between patient contacts.	Gowns should be worn when contact of clothing or exposed skin with blood or body fluids is anticipated. Gloves should be worn for touching blood, body fluids, contaminated items, mucous membranes or nonintact skin.	A surgical mask and eye protection should be worn during procedures and patient care activities likely to generate splashes or sprays of blood or body fluids, especially suctioning and endotracheal intubation.	Routine care, cleaning, and disinfection of environmental surfaces.
Contact*	Use for infectious agents spread by direct or indirect contact with patients or their environment (e.g., vancomycin-resistant enterococcus, *Clostridium difficile*, respiratory syncytial virus).	As above	Gowns and gloves should be worn for all interactions that involve contact with the patient or contaminated areas of the patient's environment. Gown and gloves should be donned on room entry for pathogens known to be transmitted through environmental contamination.	As above	Single-patient room is preferred. When a single-patient room is not available, consultation with infection control practitioners is recommended to assess other options, such as cohorting.

TABLE 5-8

HICPAC Guidelines for Standard and Transmission-Based Precautions—cont'd

Precautions	Scenario	Hand Hygiene	Gowns/Gloves	Mask and Eye Protection	Environmental Controls
Droplet*	Use for infectious agents that are spread through close respiratory or mucous membrane contact with respiratory secretions (e.g., *Bordetella pertussis*, influenza, *Neisseria meningitidis*).	As above	As per standard precautions	A mask should be donned on room entry. Eye protection should be used per standard precautions.	As above. Curtains should be drawn between beds in shared patient rooms, and the patient should wear a mask when transported out of the hospital room.
Airborne*	Use for infections agents that remain infectious over long distances when suspended in air (e.g., *Mycobacterium tuberculosis* and varicella and rubeola viruses).	As above	Per standard precautions	A fit-tested N-95 respirator or a powered air-purifying respirator should be worn whenever the patient's room is entered.	Patients should be placed in a monitored, airborne infection isolation room, maintained with six to 12 air exchanges per hour and negative pressure relative to surrounding areas.

From Daugherty EL. Health care worker protection in mass casualty respiratory failure: infection control, decontamination, and personal protective equipment. *Respir Care* 2008;53(2):201-214. Adapted from Siegel JD, Rhinehart E, Jackson M, et al. The healthcare infection control practices advisory committee. 2007 Guideline for isolation precautions: preventing transmission of infectious agents in healthcare settings. June, 2007. http://www.cdc.gov/ncidod/dhqp/pdf/guidelines/isolation2007.pdf.
*Transmission-based precautions (always used in addition to standard precautions).

INFECTION CONTROL ISSUES IN MASS CASUALTY SITUATIONS

Considerable time and effort have been devoted to the development of an effective rapid response plan for a mass casualty event, such as a severe influenza pandemic. Federal, state, and local governments, as well as many health-related organizations and professional societies, have presented documents to guide clinicians on the epidemiology and treatment of community-acquired severe respiratory illnesses.[40,41]

Febrile respiratory illness (FRI) caused by community-acquired pneumonia is a common reason for admission to the intensive care unit (ICU). Although bacterial and viral organisms are most often cited in the etiology of FRI, a relatively small group of agents have the potential to cause widespread epidemics that can severely affect our health care system.[42] Box 5-6 provides a list of naturally occurring or intentional causes of febrile respiratory illnesses that can lead to a sustained mass casualty event. Although it is beyond the scope of this text to discuss every aspect of infection control in an FRI mass casualty event, it should be apparent that early detection and isolation of infected patients are the cornerstones of an effective disaster infection control plan. It is imperative that all potentially involved health care workers be knowledgeable about the plan and receive education in the proper use of personal protective equipment (PPE). Table 5-9 provides a summary of isolation precautions for five specific infectious biologic agents associated with mass casualty respiratory failure. More detailed information about emergency preparedness can be found on the Evolve Resources site that accompanies this text.

BOX 5-6 | **Naturally Occurring or Intentional Causes of Febrile Respiratory Illness that Can Lead to a Mass Casualty Event**

Influenza*
Viral hemorrhagic fevers*
Severe acute respiratory syndrome (SARS) coronavirus*
Smallpox*
Plague*
Tularemia
Anthrax

From Sandrock CE: Severe febrile respiratory illnesses as a cause of mass critical care, *Respir Care* 53:40, 2008.
*Contagious condition.

TABLE 5-9

Recommended Precautions for Biologic Agents Associated with Mass Casualty Respiratory Failure

Agent	Mode of Transmission	Patient Placement	Type and Duration of Precautions
Smallpox	Inhalation of droplets or aerosols	Patients should be placed in airborne isolation whenever possible. In a mass exposure situation, cohorting may be appropriate.	Standard, contact, and airborne precautions should be used until all scabs have separated (3-4 weeks). Only immune health care workers should care for infected patients. Nonimmune individuals who are exposed should receive postexposure vaccination within 4 days.
Anthrax	Person-to-person transmission does not occur with respiratory or gastrointestinal tract anthrax. Person-to-person transmission of cutaneous anthrax is extremely rare.	No restrictions	Standard precautions. If presence of aerosolized powder or environmental exposure is suspected, airborne precautions should be used, and exposed persons should be decontaminated.
Pneumonic plague	Inhalation of respiratory droplets. Risk of transmission is low during the first 20-24 hours of illness.	Patients should be placed in private rooms whenever possible, and cohorted if private rooms are unavailable.	Use standard precautions. Droplet precautions should be used until the patient has received at least 48 hours of appropriate therapy.
SARS*	Droplet and contact transmission. Opportunistic airborne transmission is possible.	Airborne infection isolation	Standard, droplet, and airborne precautions with eye protection should be continued for the duration of potential infectivity.
Pandemic influenza	Presumed transmission is primarily via large respiratory droplets, but opportunistic airborne transmission also is possible.	Airborne infection isolation	Standard, droplet, and airborne precautions with eye protection should be continued for 14 days after the onset of symptoms or until an alternative diagnosis is made.

From Daugherty EL. Health care worker protection in mass casualty respiratory failure: infection control, decontamination, and personal protective equipment. *Respir Care* 2008;53(2):201-214. Adapted from Siegel JD, Rhinehart E, Jackson M, et al. The healthcare infection control practices advisory committee. 2007 Guideline for isolation precautions: preventing transmission of infectious agents in healthcare settings. June, 2007. http://www.cdc.gov/ncidod/dhqp/pdf/guidelines/isolation2007.pdf. and Centers for Disease Control and Prevention. Public health guidance for community-level preparedness and response to severe acute respiratory syndrome (SARS), version 2; supplement I: Infection control in healthcare, home, and community settings; III: infection control in healthcare facilities. January 8, 2004. http://www.cdc.gov/ncidod/sars/guidance/i/pdf/healthcare.pdf.
*SARS, Severe acute respiratory syndrome.

KEY POINTS

▶ Three elements are required for spread of an infectious disease: a source of pathogens, a mode of transmission of the infectious agent, and a susceptible host.

▶ Nosocomial pneumonia is most often caused by bacteria, but viruses, protozoa, and fungi contribute to a lesser extent. Most nosocomial bacterial pneumonias are described as polymicrobial, and gram-negative bacilli are the predominant microbes identified.

▶ The four routes of transmission of health care–associated infections are the contact route, vehicle route, airborne route, and vector route.

▶ A number of factors can affect disinfection and sterilization, including the number, location, and innate resistance of the microorganism. The effectiveness of a germicide depends on its concentration and potency, the duration of exposure to the germicide, and the physical and chemical environment in which the germicide is used.

▶ Three levels of disinfection are possible: high-level disinfection kills bacteria, fungi, and viruses. Spores can also be destroyed with high-level disinfection, but an extended exposure time is required. Intermediate-level disinfection removes vegetative bacteria, tubercle bacteria, some viruses, and fungi but does not kill spores.

Low-level disinfection kills most vegetative bacteria, some fungi, and some viruses.

▶ Quaternary ammonium compounds (QACs or Quats), alcohols, acetic acid, phenols glutaraldehyde, hydrogen peroxide, and halogenated compounds are highly effective chemicals used to disinfect floors, countertops, and the outer surface of respiratory care equipment.

▶ Four methods are commonly used to sterilize medical devices: (1) dry heat; (2) boiling water and steam under pressure (autoclave); (3) ionizing radiation; and (4) ethylene oxide.

▶ Reusable medical equipment can be categorized as critical, semicritical, or noncritical, depending on the degree of risk of infection involved in their use.

▶ The effectiveness of an infection control program should be monitored routinely with mechanical, chemical, and biologic indicators.

▶ Standard precautions are a synthesis of previous guidelines for universal precautions and body substance isolation techniques. Transmission-based precautions involve specific requirements for dealing with possible contaminants that can be spread by airborne, droplet, and contact routes.

ASSESSMENT QUESTIONS

See Evolve Resources for the answers.

1. Which of the following organisms are gram-negative bacteria often associated with nosocomial pneumonia?
   a. *Pseudomonas aeruginosa*
   b. *Diplococcus pneumoniae*
   c. *Clostridium botulinum*
   d. *Staphylococcus aureus*

2. *Mycobacterium tuberculosis* organisms are:
   a. Gram-negative bacilli
   b. An anaerobic infection
   c. Acid-fast bacteria
   d. Spore-producing bacteria

3. All of the following are transmitted through the respiratory route *except:*
   a. Rubella
   b. Rhinoviruses
   c. Varicella
   d. HIV

4. Briefly describe the most recent CDC guidelines for proper hand hygiene.

5. Which of the following disinfectants can be used as a chemical sterilant?
   a. Povidone-iodine
   b. Acetic acid
   c. Glutaraldehyde
   d. Isopropyl alcohol

6. Indicate whether each of the following presents a critical, semicritical, or noncritical risk of infection.
   a. Ventilator tubing
   b. Swan-Ganz catheter
   c. Blood pressure cuff
   d. Endoscope (bronchoscope)
   e. Endotracheal tubes

7. Which of these clinical conditions warrants additional precautions to prevent the spread of epidemiologically significant pathogens?
   a. Meningitis
   b. Pertussis
   c. Measles
   d. Diarrhea in an adult with a history of recent antibiotic use

8. The best method of sterilizing a bronchoscope is:
   a. Ethylene oxide
   b. Soaking in 2% glutaraldehyde for 10 hours
   c. Soaking in 70% isopropyl alcohol for 20 minutes
   d. Steam autoclave

9. Which of the following methods should *not* be used to sterilize plastic oxygen masks?
   a. Ethylene oxide
   b. Steam autoclave
   c. 70% Isopropyl alcohol
   d. 2% Alkaline glutaraldehyde

10. Which of the following conditions requires the application of contact precautions?
    a. Legionellosis
    b. Diphtheria
    c. Hepatitis
    d. Rubella

11. Which of the following are potential causes of skin and mucosal barrier disruption?
    I. Foley catheters
    II. Intravenous catheters
    III. Endotracheal tubes
    IV. Burns
       a. I and II only
       b. II and III only
       c. I, II, and IV only
       d. I, II, III, and IV

12. *Bacillus anthracis* is a(n):
    a. Gram-negative bacterium
    b. Anaerobic infection
    c. Acid-fast bacterium
    d. Spore-producing bacterium

13. Name three elements that must be present for the spread of infectious materials.

14. Describe various techniques that are routinely used to determine the effectiveness of sterilization.

15. Which of the following precautions should be taken with a patient under respiratory isolation?
    I. The patient should have a private room.
    II. Gowns should be worn by all those entering the room.
    III. Articles contaminated with secretions must be disinfected or discarded.
    IV. Masks must be worn by all individuals who will be in close contact with the patient.
       a. II and III only
       b. III and IV only
       c. I, II, and III only
       d. I, III, and IV only

16. Define *standard precautions*.

17. Match the following:
    1. _____ HIV   a. Bronchitis, bronchiolitis
    2. _____ Respiratory syncytial virus   b. Fungal infection
    3. _____ Parainfluenza   c. Croup, pneumonia
    4. _____ Influenza   d. Tracheobronchitis
    5. _____ Histoplasmosis   e. AIDS

18. Give an example of a disease that is transmitted by each of the following routes of transmission:
    a. Contact (direct)
    b. Vehicle (food-borne)
    c. Airborne (droplet nuclei)
    d. Vector-borne (fleas)

References

1. Siegel JD, Rhinehart E, Jackson M et al: *Guideline for isolation precautions: preventing transmission of infectious agents in health-care settings,* Atlanta, 2007, Centers for Disease Control and Prevention.
2. Wilkins RL, Stoller JK, Scanlan CL: *Egan's fundamentals of respiratory care,* ed 8, St Louis, 2003, Mosby.
3. Niederman MS, Sarosi GA, Glassroth J: *Respiratory infections: a scientific basis for management,* Philadelphia, 2001, WB Saunders.
4. Kacmarek RM, Mack CW, Dimas S, editors: *The essentials of respiratory care,* ed 4, St Louis, 2005, Elsevier-Mosby.
5. Chastre J, Fagon J-V: Ventilator-associated pneumonia, *Am J Resp Crit Care Med* 165:872, 2002.
6. Schaberg DR: How infections spread in the hospital, *Respir Care* 34:81, 1989.
7. Chatburn RL: Decontamination of respiratory care equipment: what can be done, what should be done, *Respir Care* 34:8, 1989.
8. Rutala WA: Disinfection, sterilization, and waste disposal. In Wenzel RP, editor: *Prevention and control of nosocomial infections,* Baltimore, 1997, Williams & Wilkins.
9. Favero MS et al: Gram-negative water bacteria in hemodialysis systems, *Health Lab Sci* 12:321, 1987.
10. Rutala WA, Cole EC: Ineffectiveness of hospital disinfectants against bacteria: a collaborative study, *Infect Control* 8:501, 1987.
11. Sykes G: *Disinfection and sterilization,* ed 2, London, 1965, E & FN Spon.
12. Petrocci AN: Surface active agents: quaternary ammonium compounds. In Block SS, editor: *Disinfection, sterilization, and preservation,* ed 3, Philadelphia, 1983, Lea & Febiger.
13. Morton HE: Alcohols. In Block SS, editor: *Disinfection, sterilization, and preservation,* ed 3, Philadelphia, 1983, Lea & Febiger.
14. Chatburn RE, Kallstrom TJ, Bajaksouzian MS: A comparison of acetic acid with a quaternary ammonium compound for the disinfection of hand-held nebulizers, *Respir Care* 33:179, 1988.
15. Block SS: Peroxygen compounds. In Block SS, editor: *Disinfection, sterilization, and preservation,* ed 3, Philadelphia, 1983, Lea & Febiger.
16. Rutala WA: APIC guideline for selection and use of disinfectants, *Am J Infect Control* 18:99, 1990.
17. Bloomfield SF, Uso EE: The antibacterial properties of sodium hypochlorite and sodium dichloroisocyanurate as hospital disinfectants, *J Hosp Infect* 6:20, 1985.
18. Favero MS, Bond WW: Chemical disinfection of medical and surgical materials. In Block SS, editor: *Disinfection, sterilization, and preservation,* ed 3, Philadelphia, 1983, Lea & Febiger.
19. U.S. Department of Labor: Bloodborne pathogens and acute care facilities, *OSHA* 3128, 1992.
20. Gorman SP, Scott EM, Russell AD: A review: antimicrobial activity, uses, and mechanisms of action of glutaraldehyde, *J Appl Bacteriol* 48:161, 1980.
21. Association for the Advancement of Medical Instrumentation: American National Standard—safe use and handling of glutaraldehyde-based products in health care settings, ANSI/AAMI ST58, 1996.
22. Gross JA, Haas MI, Swift TR: Ethylene oxide neurotoxicity: report of four cases and review of the literature, *Neurology* 29:978, 1979.
23. Occupational Safety and Health Administration: Occupational exposure to ethylene oxide—OSHA, final standard, *Fed Regist* 49:25734, 1984.
24. Garner JS: Guideline for isolation precautions in hospitals, *Infect Control Hosp Epidemiol* 17:53, 1996.
25. Spaulding EH: Chemical disinfection of medical and surgical materials. In Lawrence CA, Block SS, editors: *Disinfection, sterilization, and preservation,* ed 3, Philadelphia, 1968, Lea & Febiger.
26. Craven DE, Connolly MG, Lichtenbery DA et al: Risk factors for pneumonia and fatality in patients receiving continuous mechanical ventilation, *Am Rev Respir Dis* 133:792, 1986.
27. Fink JB, Krasue SA, Barrett L et al: Extending ventilator circuit change interval beyond 2 days reduces the likelihood of ventilator-associated pneumonia, *Chest* 113:405, 1998.
28. Hess DR, Kallstrom TJ, Mottram CD et al: American Association for Respiratory Care: care of the ventilator circuit and its relation to ventilator associated pneumonia, *Respir Care* 48:869, 2003.
29. Branson RD: The ventilator circuit and ventilatory-associated pneumonia, *Respir Care* 50:774, 2005.
30. Larson E: APIC guideline for handwashing and hand antisepsis in health care settings, *Am J Infect Control* 23:251, 1995.
31. Centers for Disease Control and Prevention: Guideline for hand hygiene in health-care settings, *MMWR* 51(RR16):1, 2002.
32. Rorberts E: *Infection control in respiratory care: strategies for JCAHO compliance,* Marblehead, Mass, 2005, HCPro.
33. Garner JS, Favero MS: Guideline for handwashing and hospital environmental control, *Infect Control* 7:231, 1986.
34. Olsen R et al: Examination gloves as barriers to hand contamination and clinical practice, *JAMA* 350, 1993.
35. Doebbeling B et al: Removal of nosocomial pathogens from the contaminated glove: implications for glove reuse and handwashing, *Ann Intern Med* 109:394, 1988.
36. Cadwallader HL, Bradley CR, Ayliffe GA: Bacterial contamination and frequency of changing ventilator circuits, *J Hosp Infect* 5:65, 1990.
37. U.S. Department of Labor, Occupational Safety and Health Administration: Occupational exposure to bloodborne pathogens: final rule, *Fed Regist* 56:64175, 1991.
38. Centers for Disease Control and Prevention: Guidelines for environmental infection control in health-care facilities, *MMWR* 52(RR-10):1, 2003.
39. Centers for Disease Control and Prevention: Guidelines for the prevention of intravascular catheter-related infections, *MMWR* 51(RR10):1, 2002.
40. Branson RD, Rubinson L: Mechanical ventilation in mass casualty scenarios. I, *Respir Care* 53:41, 2008.
41. Branson RD, Rubinson L: Mechanical ventilation in mass casualty scenarios. II, *Respir Care* 53:130, 2008.
42. Sandrock CE: Severe febrile respiratory illnesses as a cause of mass critical care, *Respir Care* 53:40, 2008.

Bibliography

Bartlett JG et al: Bacteriology of hospital-acquired pneumonia, *Arch Intern Med* 146:868, 1986.
Boucher RM: Cidex and sonacide compared, *Respir Care* 22:790, 1977.
Centers for Disease Control and Prevention: Guideline for hand hygiene in health-care settings, *MMWR* 51(RR16):1, 2002.
Centers for Disease Control and Prevention: Guidelines for preventing the transmission of tuberculosis in health-care settings, with special focus on HIV-related issues, *MMWR* 39(RR-17):1, 1990.
Hierholzer WJ: Guideline for prevention of nosocomial pneumonia, *Respir Care* 39:1191, 1994.

Internet Resources

American Association for Respiratory Care: http://www.aarc.org
National Center for Infectious Disease: http://www.cdc.gov/ncidod

Centers for Disease Control and Prevention: http://www.cdc.gov

Guidelines for Hand Hygiene in the Healthcare Setting: http://www.cdc.gov/mmwr/preview/mmwrhtml/rr5116a1.htm

The Joint Commission: http://www.jointcommission.org

Health Resources and Services Administration (HRSA): http://www.hrsa.gov

Infectious disease search engine: www.infectiousdiseases.about.com

Federation of American Scientists: http://www.fas.org/promed

Office of the United States Surgeon General: http://www.surgeongeneral.gov

AIDS Clinical Trials Information Service: http://www.actis.org

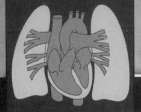

Chapter 6

Airway Management Devices

ASHLEY SHILLING
CHARLES G. DURBIN, JR.

OUTLINE

OBJECTIVES

Upon completion of this chapter, you will be able to:

- Recognize normal airway anatomy.
- Describe a complete airway examination.
- Describe ways to displace the tongue to improve gas exchange in unconscious patients.
- List patient characteristics that may contribute to difficult mask ventilation or intubation.
- List several complications associated with improper placement of oral and nasopharyngeal airways.
- Explain how to place the laryngeal mask airway and the Combitube in unconscious patients.
- Describe the appropriate sequence of steps for inserting an endotracheal tube to provide a secure airway.
- Identify at least three ways to confirm proper placement of an endotracheal tube.
- Name three airway devices that can facilitate the placement of an endotracheal tube in the event of difficult laryngoscopy.
- Discuss the most common problems facing intubated patients and identify strategies to avoid and equipment used to treat these complications.
- Identify the equipment necessary to perform invasive ventilation (transtracheal or surgical airway) and describe a procedure for airway entry.
- Review the equipment and steps used to obtain sputum samples from patients with endotracheal and tracheostomy tubes.
- Describe three ways to wean patients from tracheostomy tubes.
- List three methods that allow patients with a tracheostomy tube to speak.
- Identify various types of manual resuscitators and discuss the common hazards associated with use of these devices.

KEY TERMS

Berman airway	fiberoptic bronchoscope	nasotracheal intubation
cardiopulmonary resuscitation (CPR)	French sizes	nonrebreathing valve
Combitube	Guedel airway	oropharyngeal airway
double-lumen endotracheal tube (DLET)	laryngeal mask airway (LMA)	percutaneous dilatory tracheostomy (PDT)
duckbill valve	laryngoscope	retrograde wire intubation
endotracheal tube (ETT)	leaf valve	sniffing position
face mask ventilation (FMV)	Lukens sputum trap	spring-loaded valve
Fastrach®	Macintosh blade	tracheostomy tube (TT)
	Miller blade	translaryngeal intubation
	nasopharyngeal airway	

One of the most dramatic and rapidly fatal medical emergencies occurs when a person loses the ability to breathe spontaneously. This can be caused by upper airway obstruction, as with foreign body aspiration; lower airway obstruction, as with severe bronchospasm or a tension pneumothorax; or altered respiratory drive, as with depressant drugs or secondary to a neurologic insult. Failure to restore adequate respiratory gas exchange can result in hypoxic brain injury or death within 3 minutes. These serious consequences have led to universal acceptance of the ABCs of resuscitation (*airway, breathing,* and *circulation*), with establishment of an adequate airway as the highest priority.

This chapter reviews the normal anatomy of the airway, as well as the devices and means used to establish and maintain a patent upper airway and respiratory gas exchange. The discussion includes minimally invasive techniques, such as bag-mask-valve ventilation (or face mask ventilation) and supraglottic airway devices, as well as infraglottic devices such as the **endotracheal tube (ETT)** and **tracheostomy tube (TT).** Table 6-1 briefly describes some of these devices and techniques and separates them into supraglottic and infraglottic airways. Additional equipment used for patients with artificial airways, and some of the risks and problems encountered in their use, are described in this chapter.

Many airway devices and tools for airway management have been developed over the years, and some fit only a small clinical niche. Although scientific evidence substantiates the use and safety of some of these devices, others have yet to prove their practicality. With the ever-evolving alternatives to laryngoscopy and the traditional endotracheal tube, we have improved our ability to manage the airway on multiple levels and have reduced the need for emergency surgical airway intervention. Because it would be impractical to cover all the new and changing artificial airways and their adjuncts, the chapter focuses on selected equipment that is commonly used and that can serve as models for other equipment. Additional material can be found on the Evolve Resources.

AIRWAY ANATOMY

To understand airway management, one must have an appreciation of normal airway anatomy. Figure 6-1 shows the normal upper airway and tracheal anatomy in an adult. The airway has two natural access routes, the nasopharynx and the oropharynx, both of which lead to the pharynx, the larynx, and ultimately the trachea. The larynx consists of three large cartilaginous structures: the thyroid and cricoid cartilages and the epiglottis. It is essential to identify the true vocal cords and the glottic opening, but one also should understand the spatial relationships of the surrounding structures, including the vestibular folds (the false cords), the arytenoid cartilages, and the vallecula, as well as the relationship of the epiglottis to these structures.

The glottic opening, formed by the thyroarytenoid ligaments, or vocal cords, is the narrowest portion of the adult airway and usually the limiting factor that determines the size of the tube that can be placed into the trachea. The cricoid cartilage, which is the only complete tracheal ring, is usually found at the sixth cervical vertebra level (C6) in the adult and at the C4 level in the infant and young child. Unlike in the adult, the cricoid cartilage is the narrowest portion in the pediatric airway until approximately age 6. The cricoid cartilage is an important landmark for cricothyroidotomy (discussed later in the chapter). In the adult, the trachea divides at the carina into the mainstem bronchi, typically at the level of the fifth thoracic vertebral body (T5).

The sensory innervation of the oropharynx and the trachea is shown in Figure 6-2. The anterior part of the tongue is innervated by the fifth cranial nerve (CN V), the trigeminal nerve. The posterior one third of the tongue, extending to the superior surface of the epiglottis, is supplied by CN IX, the glossopharyngeal nerve. Understanding this innervation pattern is important, because it is responsible for an active gag reflex. The inferior surfaces of the epiglottis and the vocal cords are innervated by a branch of the vagus nerve (CN X), the internal branch of

TABLE 6-1

Devices and Techniques Used to Establish and Maintain a Patent Upper Airway and Respiratory Gas Exchange

Device or Maneuver	Description	Concerns and Contraindications
Supraglottic Airway Maneuver or Device		
Extreme extension (sniffer's position)	Extension of the occiput with the head extended	Unstable cervical spine
Jaw thrust or chin lift	Anterior displacement of the mandible with or without dislocation of the temporomandibular joints	Temporomandibular joint disease, fractured mandible, or unstable cervical spine
Anesthesia face mask	Assisted or controlled ventilation using a rubber or plastic mask contoured to fit the patient's face	Trauma to the face, presence of a beard, or abnormal anatomy, with resultant poor mask fit
Oropharyngeal airways	Rigid, curved device with an air passage that is placed through the mouth with the end resting distal to the tongue above the glottic opening	Gagging or vomiting, improper size, incorrect placement
Nasopharyngeal airways	Soft or semirigid, hollow tube placed through the nares, the tip lying distal to the tongue above the glottic opening	Gagging or vomiting (usually better tolerated in patients who are not comatose); posterior pharyngeal wall dissection; severe bleeding
Laryngeal mask airways	Custom-formed, soft mask with a hollow tube fitting into the pyriform sinuses directly above the larynx	Placement may be difficult, mask may fold, epiglottis may obstruct laryngeal opening, trachea is not protected from aspiration, positive pressure ventilation more difficult to generate
Combitube	Double-lumen device inserted blindly with one lumen providing ventilation and the other commonly in the esophagus	Not considered a secure airway device; should not be used in patients with intact gag or esophageal disease; may cause injury to the esophagus, trachea, or surrounding soft tissue
Infraglottic Airway Device		
Endotracheal tubes (ETTs)	Semirigid, hollow tube placed into the trachea with or without an inflatable cuff	Usually requires special devices (e.g., laryngoscopy) and technical skill for consistent correct placement; tracheal placement must be objectively confirmed and esophageal placement and ETT displacement avoided
Intubating laryngeal mask airways (LMAs)	Laryngeal mask airway designed to align the glottis with the LMA and allow blind endotracheal intubation through the hollow channel of the LMA	Requires training and practice; placement may be difficult
Lightwand	Rigid, light stylet that relies on transillumination of the trachea to confirm ETT placement	Ambient lights must be turned off during placement; difficult to use in patients with thick, short neck; blunt trauma
Indirect laryngoscope	Uses mirrors, lenses, or fiberoptic technology to view the glottis and allow insertion of the ETT under direct visualization	Often expensive and requires extensive training and experience
Flexible fiberoptic bronchoscopy	Flexible fiberoptic bronchoscope that allows visualization of the airway with minimal neck extension; procedure can be done with the patient awake or asleep	Expensive and requires practice to master technique
Transtracheal invasive airway	Emergent, direct entry into the trachea below the larynx with a large-bore needle, or surgical incision with insertion of an ETT	Hypoxia, bleeding, nerve or esophageal injury; failure to establish an airway; gas dissection or pneumothorax
Tracheostomy tubes	Hollow tube, with or without a cuff, that is electively inserted directly into the trachea through a surgical incision or with a wire-guided progressive dilation technique	Hypoxia, bleeding, nerve or esophageal injury; failure to establish the airway due to nontracheal placement; displacement

the *superior laryngeal nerve*. The region of the trachea below the cords is supplied by another branch of the vagus nerve, the *recurrent laryngeal nerve*. All the muscles of the larynx are innervated by the recurrent laryngeal nerves except for the cricothyroid muscles, which are controlled by the external branch of the superior laryngeal nerves.

Understanding the innervation of the airway allows the practitioner to block the sensory nerves, which is crucial when performing an awake intubation. Thorough anesthesia of the airway is needed to prevent coughing and gagging, which can cause discomfort, increased risk of aspiration and can prevent successful intubation.

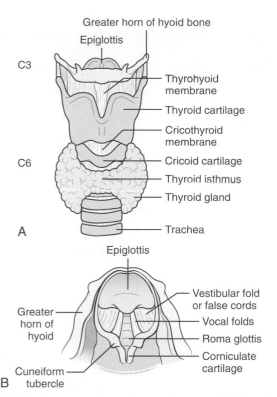

FIGURE 6-1 A, Anterior view of the adult larynx. **B,** View from above the vocal cords as would be seen during laryngoscopy.

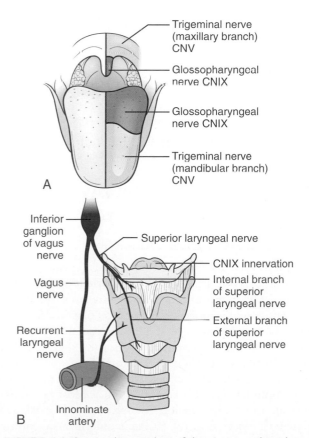

FIGURE 6-2 Sensory innervation of the airway and trachea.

AIRWAY EXAMINATION

The risks of airway management in the critically ill are greater than for patients undergoing elective procedures.[1] The incidences of both difficult airway management and inadvertent esophageal intubation are significantly higher than with airway management in the controlled environment of the operating room.[2] During elective surgery, the incidence of failed intubation is quite low (0.05 to 0.35%), and the incidence of failed intubation and inability to mask is even lower (0.01% to 0.03%).[3-7] Because difficulties with airway management occur even under ideal conditions, reliable methods of predicting these problems have been sought. Specialized equipment can improve success and prevent a catastrophe with an unanticipated difficult airway.

It is imperative to obtain an airway history from the patient or from a review of past medical records before attempting to establish an artificial airway. Important points that indicate a problem may exist include (1) a known history of difficult intubation, (2) the presence of obstructive sleep apnea, (3) temporomandibular joint disease, (4) previous airway surgery, and (5) anatomic abnormalities of the head, neck, or airway. Although a complete airway examination might be impossible in an emergency or on a comatose or uncooperative patient, a cursory examination of the airway for various characteristics and gross abnormalities proves beneficial in many instances. Table 6-2 lists important points of the airway examination and findings that are cause for concern.[8]

Patient mouth opening, a dental examination, cervical range of motion, and the thyromental distance are all common components of the airway examination. Several classification systems have been developed to help predict the ease or difficulty of providing **face mask ventilation (FMV)** or intubating patients. One of the most commonly used systems was described by Mallampati et al.[9] and later modified by Samsoon and Young.[4] This system (Table 6-3) attempts to predict the difficulty of visualizing the glottic structures during laryngoscopy. The examination should be performed with the patient sitting upright, and the individual should not be asked to phonate, as this may elevate the palate and improve the view improved while the airway is examined. Despite the use of this classification system and other components of the airway examination, a difficult intubation often is unanticipated. A number of prospective and retrospective studies have attempted to correlate the airway examination and patient characteristics with the ease of FMV and intubation.

At times, intubation may be difficult or impossible, and predicting the patients at high risk can help the practitioner assemble back-up devices and prepare to use advanced techniques. Predictors of difficult intubation include (1) a Mallampati airway class III or IV, (2) a thyromental distance of less than 6 cm, (3) mouth opening of less than 4 cm, (4) reduced atlanto-occipital neck extension,

TABLE 6-2

Suggested Components of the Preoperative Airway Physical Examination

Airway Examination Component	Concerning Findings
1. Length of upper incisors	Relatively long
2. Relation of maxillary and mandibular incisors during normal jaw closure	Prominent "overbite" (maxillary incisors extend anterior to mandibular incisors)
3. Relation of maxillary and mandibular incisors during voluntary protrusion	Mandibular incisors unable to be placed anterior to (mandible in front of) maxillary incisors
4. Interincisor distance	Less than 3 cm with maximum voluntary mouth opening
5. Visibility of uvula	Not visible when tongue is protruded with patient in sitting position (e.g., Mallampati class higher than II)
6. Shape of palate	Highly arched or very narrow
7. Compliance of mandibular space	Stiff, indurated, occupied by mass, or nonresilient
8. Thyromental distance	Less than three ordinary finger breadths
9. Neck length	Short
10. Neck bulk	Thick
11. Range of motion of head and neck	Patient cannot touch tip of chin to chest or cannot extend head on neck

TABLE 6-3

Mallampati Classification with Samsoon and Young Modifications to Airway Classes

Class	View with Patient Sitting, without Phonation
I	Faucal pillars, soft palate, and uvula visible
II	Uvula masked by base of tongue
III	Only base of uvula and soft palate visible
IV	No visualization of uvula or soft palate; only hard palate visible

From Mallampati SR, Gatt SP, Gugino LD et al: A clinical sign to predict difficult tracheal intubation: a prospective study, *Can Anaesth Soc J* 32:429, 1985; and Samsoon GL, Young JR: Difficult tracheal intubation: a retrospective study, *Anaesthesia* 42:487, 1987.

(5) increased body mass index (BMI), and (6) a large neck circumference.[10-12]

When difficult intubation is anticipated, additional personnel should be available and plans should be established beforehand. The American Society of Anesthesiologists (ASA) has proposed a difficult airway algorithm (Figure 6-3) to help direct airway management and improve patient outcome in the event of a difficult airway.[8] If difficult mask ventilation or intubation is encountered, it is essential to document the reason for this for future caregivers. For example, a patient who has a bloodied airway secondary to trauma may not present with the same challenges during a future intubation, whereas a patient with a small mouth opening and anterior larynx is unlikely to show improvements in the ease of future intubations. *It is essential to document the characteristics that make an airway challenging.* Making patients aware that they experienced a difficult intubation is essential as well. Patients should be told to inform future caregivers of their history of a difficult airway, just as they would tell a physician of a known drug allergy. In addition, a Medi-Alert bracelet may be advisable, especially in a patient with a high likelihood of needing invasive airway management in the future.

ESTABLISHING A PATENT AIRWAY

Displacing the Tongue

Simple maneuvers often can restore breathing in patients with upper airway obstruction. In the supine position and when the pharyngeal and tongue muscles lose tone, the tongue falls backward and may occlude the pharynx. Elevating the head and extending the neck advance the jaw and move the tongue forward, helping to open an obstructed or closed airway. This so-called **sniffing position** (Figure 6-4) opens the upper airway and places the long axes of the mouth, pharynx, and larynx in alignment. This head position provides for a tighter fit for a bag-mask-valve manual resuscitator and is also optimal for endotracheal intubation under direct vision. By forcing the jaw anteriorly with a jaw thrust or a chin lift maneuver, the tongue is moved farther from the hard and soft palates, and a patent upper airway that allows air exchange may be achieved. Figures 6-5 and 6-6 demonstrate these techniques.

SUPRAGLOTTIC AIRWAY DEVICES

Anesthesia Face Mask

The anesthesia face mask is a noninvasive means of ventilating and oxygenating an apneic patient. Traditionally made of rubber, most modern masks are latex free, disposable, and usually made of silicone or plastic. Clear face masks have the advantage of allowing visualization of the patient's face for condensation (indicating successful Face Mask Ventilation (FMV)) or cyanosis, vomit, or blood in the mask. In addition, patients find the clear plastic less claustrophobic than the opaque rubber. Most face masks have an inflatable cushion to optimize the mask seal, allowing a better fit to the patient's unique facial configuration and contour (Figure 6-7). Most adult masks come

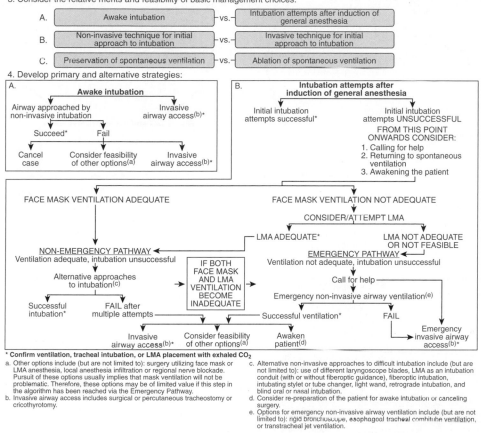

AMERICAN SOCIETY
OF ANESTHESIOLOGISTS

DIFFICULT AIRWAY ALGORITHM

1. Assess the likelihood and clinical impact of basic management problems:
   A. Difficult ventilation
   B. Difficult intubation
   C. Difficulty with patient cooperation or consent
   D. Difficult tracheostomy
2. Actively pursue opportunities to deliver supplemental oxygen throughout the process of difficult airway management
3. Consider the relative merits and feasibility of basic management choices:

A.   Awake intubation   -vs.-   Intubation attempts after induction of general anesthesia

B.   Non-invasive technique for initial approach to intubation   -vs.-   Invasive technique for initial approach to intubation

C.   Preservation of spontaneous ventilation   -vs.-   Ablation of spontaneous ventilation

4. Develop primary and alternative strategies:

A.   Awake intubation

Airway approached by non-invasive intubation   Invasive airway access(b)*

Succeed*   Fail

Cancel case   Consider feasibility of other options(a)   Invasive airway access(b)*

B.   Intubation attempts after induction of general anesthesia

Initial intubation attempts successful*   Initial intubation attempts UNSUCCESSFUL

FROM THIS POINT ONWARDS CONSIDER:
1. Calling for help
2. Returning to spontaneous ventilation
3. Awakening the patient

FACE MASK VENTILATION ADEQUATE   FACE MASK VENTILATION NOT ADEQUATE

CONSIDER/ATTEMPT LMA

LMA ADEQUATE*   LMA NOT ADEQUATE OR NOT FEASIBLE

NON-EMERGENCY PATHWAY
Ventilation adequate, intubation unsuccessful

EMERGENCY PATHWAY
Ventilation not adequate, intubation unsuccessful

Alternative approaches to intubation(c)

IF BOTH FACE MASK AND LMA VENTILATION BECOME INADEQUATE

Call for help

Emergency non-invasive airway ventilation(e)

Successful intubation*   FAIL after multiple attempts

Successful ventilation*   FAIL

Invasive airway access(b)*   Consider feasibility of other options(a)   Awaken patient(d)

Emergency invasive airway access(b)*

* Confirm ventilation, tracheal intubation, or LMA placement with exhaled CO₂

a. Other options include (but are not limited to): surgery utilizing face mask or LMA anesthesia, local anesthesia infiltration or regional nerve blockade. Pursuit of these options usually implies that mask ventilation will not be problematic. Therefore, these options may be of limited value if this step in the algorithm has been reached via the Emergency Pathway.
b. Invasive airway access includes surgical or percutaneous tracheostomy or cricothyrotomy.

c. Alternative non-invasive approaches to difficult intubation include (but are not limited to): use of different laryngoscope blades, LMA as an intubation conduit (with or without fiberoptic guidance), fiberoptic intubation, intubating stylet or tube changer, light wand, retrograde intubation, and blind oral or nasal intubation.
d. Consider re-preparation of the patient for awake intubation or canceling surgery.
e. Options for emergency non-invasive airway ventilation include (but are not limited to): rigid bronchoscope, esophageal tracheal combitube ventilation, or transtracheal jet ventilation.

FIGURE 6-3 Difficult airway algorithm established by the American Society of Anesthesiologists. (From the American Society of Anesthesiologists Task Force: Practice guidelines for management of the difficult airway, *Anesthesiology* 98:1269, 2003.)

with a device for attaching a mask strap to improve the success and reduce the work of providing FMV, as well as a standard 15-mm attachment for the ventilator tubing or a manual resuscitator. Most mask manufacturers provide six to eight numbered sizes to fit patients ranging from the neonate to the adult. Sizes 3, 4, and 5 typically are used for adults.

To provide FMV, the E and C configuration is used; the fingers of the left hand rest on and elevate the mandible to prevent bruising of the soft tissue and obstruction of the oropharynx with submandibular soft tissue pressure (Figure 6-8). The mask should fit over the bridge of the nose and form a tight seal. The mask should not be pushed onto the face, because this obstructs the airway; rather, the patient's mandible should be pulled up into the mask. Two-handed bag-mask-valve techniques may be needed for obese or bearded patients or patients with a difficult mask fit. Ventilatory pressures less than 20 cm H₂O should be used to prevent the forcing of gas into the patient's stomach. Jaw thrust, maximized sniffing positioning, two-

handed mask technique, and oral or nasal airways, as discussed later, help facilitate successful face mask ventilation. Signs of effective mask ventilation include the presence of carbon dioxide (CO₂) on capnography, condensation in the mask, a taut and refilling (non–self-inflating or anesthesia) bag, adequate bilateral breath sounds, and symmetric chest rise.

The skills needed to provide adequate ventilation by a bag-mask-valve device are of paramount importance and must be acquired by all who want to manage an airway successfully. Practitioners must always remember that even if a patient cannot be intubated, providing FMV allows for adequate oxygenation and partial CO₂ removal and buys time until a definitive airway can be established.

Although manual resuscitation ventilation with a bag-mask-valve device is one of the mainstays of airway management, it is not without complications. Common problems include injury to the surrounding soft tissues and nerves, such as the mandibular branch of the facial nerve and the mental nerves; injury to the eyes, including

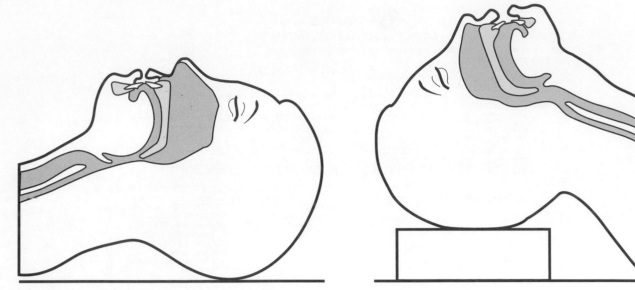

FIGURE 6-4 Sniffing position, the optimum position for opening the upper airway, can be achieved by supporting the occiput on a solid surface and extending the head. This is also the optimum position for oral intubation with a curved laryngoscope blade.

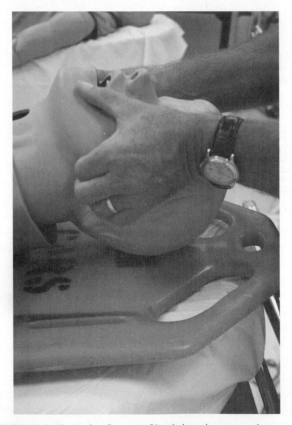

FIGURE 6-5 The index fingers of both hands are used to perform a jaw thrust maneuver, which displaces the temporomandibular joints anteriorly, achieving a patent airway without neck extension. This is particularly useful for patients with cervical spine injuries.

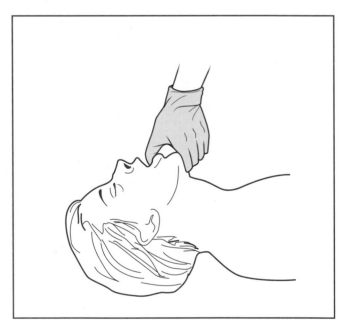

FIGURE 6-6 The chin lift is another maneuver for opening the upper airway by moving the tongue anteriorly, and it can be performed successfully without extending the cervical spine.

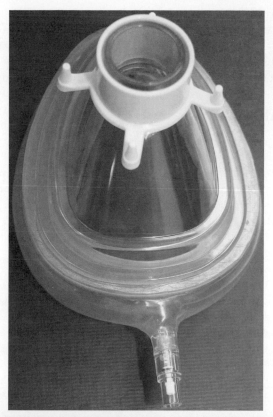

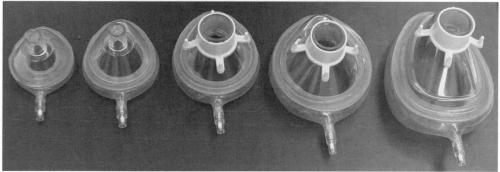

FIGURE 6-7 The anesthesia face mask is made of plastic and contains an inflatable rim to form a tight seal with the face.

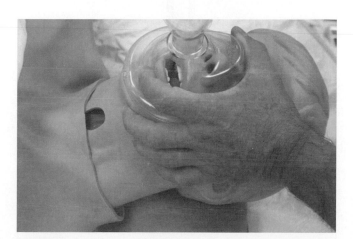

FIGURE 6-8 Note the E and C formation of the hands during mask ventilation.

raceon eyes

corneal abrasions; insufflation of the stomach, leading to gastric distention and regurgitation; and inability to ventilate a patient.

Difficulty in providing mask ventilation is indicated by a poor mask seal despite proper technique, excessive gas leakage, and difficulty initiating ingress or egress of respiratory gases. The incidence of difficult mask ventilation ranges from 1% to 5%, with impossible mask ventilation ranging from 0.1% to 0.2%.[12,13] Patient characteristics shown to reduce the success of mask ventilation include obesity (BMI greater than 26 or 30), Mallampati airway class III or IV, age greater than 55 years, poor mandible protrusion, lack of teeth, and history of snoring.[12,13] A beard is the only acutely modifiable risk factor. Troubleshooting for a bearded patient includes placing an occlusive adhesive dressing over a beard to improve the mask seal or using a water-soluble lubricant on the beard to smooth down the facial hair and form a better seal. In addition, the mask may be removed and the patient can be ventilated by placing the end of the airway circuitry in the patient's mouth and occluding the patient's nose. In extreme situations, the beard can be shaved.

OROPHARYNGEAL AIRWAYS

In some patients, providing FMV can be difficult and simple manual maneuvers are ineffective at opening an air passage past an obstructing tongue. A number of devices have been developed to displace the tongue and create a passage for air during FMV. The most common device for this purpose is the **oropharyngeal airway** (Figure 6-9).

A **Guedel airway** (Figure 6-10) consists of a hollow, central channel for air passage, a buccal flange, a bite block portion, and a curved part that follows the contour of the hard palate. Most are single-use, plastic devices with color-coded inserts based on size. The airway must extend past the posterior part of the tongue to allow air to pass. Variants of these airways are available, such as the Cath-guide, which includes three internal channels, the middle channel

being a dedicated suction port. Oral airways are available in six sizes and cost roughly $1 each.

The **Berman airway** (Figure 6-11) is similar in shape to the Guedel airway but has a different cross-sectional profile, and it does not have a protected central channel.

Oral airways are available in a variety of lengths. The standard for oral airways established by the American National Standards Institute (ANSI) is that the size is the "nominal" length in millimeters. This measurement convention is shown in Figure 6-12. Because jaw sizes differ markedly among individuals, the correct-size oropharyngeal airway can be estimated to be the one that reaches from the angle of the jaw or the meatus of the ear to the lips. Choosing an airway that is too large is safer than

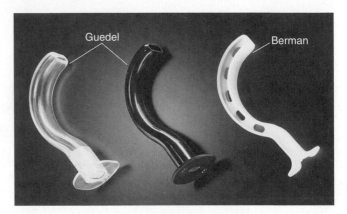

FIGURE 6-11 The Guedel and Berman airways are upper airway devices used to provide air passage distal to an obstructing tongue. (Courtesy Cardinal Health Respiratory Care Products and Services, McGaw Park, Ill.)

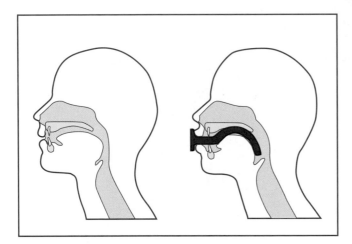

FIGURE 6-9 Anatomic insertion of an oral airway.

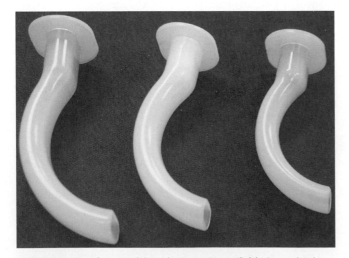

FIGURE 6-10 The Guedel oral airway is available in multiple sizes to fit patients ranging from neonates to adults.

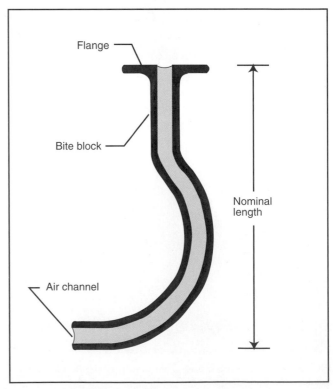

FIGURE 6-12 Oral airway components.

choosing one that is even slightly too small, because the tongue will not be bypassed by an airway that is too short, and therefore the obstruction will not be relieved. If the airway is too long, the excess length protrudes from the mouth, but the airway may be adequate.

An oropharyngeal airway may be inserted into an unconscious person in several ways. Using a tongue blade or gloved fingers, the practitioner can open the mouth and then insert the airway, following the curve of the hard palate and seated with the tip past the back of the tongue. Getting the tip past the flaccid tongue is sometimes difficult, but it is essential for success. To reduce the likelihood of the airway tip getting hung up on the back of the tongue, the practitioner can insert the airway upside down, with the tip riding along the hard palate until it is past the tongue, and then rotate the airway 180 degrees. A modification of this technique that may be less traumatic to the palate is to insert the airway rotated 90 degrees from the side of the mouth, using it like a tongue blade to move the tongue out of the way, and then rotate it back 90 degrees to seat it. These three insertion techniques are illustrated in Figure 6-13.

The correct size of airway and proper seating are essential for creating an open air passage with an oropharyngeal airway. An important sign that the distal airway tip may not have passed the back of the tongue is protrusion of the flange from the patient's mouth. If attempts to push the airway farther in just bounce it back out, it probably is catching on the back of the tongue and should be removed and replaced immediately using one of the previously described methods of insertion. An alternative technique for seating an airway that has failed to pass the tongue is to perform a jaw thrust and use the thumbs to push the airway in past the anteriorly displaced tongue (Figure 6-14).

Care must be taken when placing an oropharyngeal airway in awake patients. Oropharyngeal airways are contraindicated in patients who retain protective airway reflexes because gagging, vomiting, or laryngospasm may result. Dental damage can occur if the patient forcibly bites the hard plastic or metal airway. If the patient struggles to expel the airway, attempts at insertion should be abandoned and an improved head position or a **nasopharyngeal airway** should be used to open the upper airway.

Specialized oral airways have been developed to allow blind and fiberoptic-directed endotracheal intubation. The simplest of these is an Ovassapian airway, a hollow bite block that protects the endoscope from damage if the patient reflexively bites down during the procedure (Figure 6-15). Airways that facilitate intubation either have open channels or are split devices that can be removed, leaving the ETT in place.

NASOPHARYNGEAL AIRWAYS

Nasopharyngeal airways, which are also called *nasal trumpets* or *nasal airways,* are better tolerated than are oral airways by semiawake patients who retain some protective airway reflexes.

Nasopharyngeal airways resemble shortened, uncuffed endotracheal tubes. Most are for single use and are made of soft latex or polyethylene. The end is flared to prevent the tube from falling back into the airway and being lost in the patient. The ANSI sizing system requires that the internal diameter (ID) be given in millimeters, although **French sizes** (i.e., the external circumference in millimeters) are also frequently used. The critical size for these airways is the airway length, which must be long enough to pass beyond the tongue base but not enter the esophagus. Each manufacturer uses a different length to diameter ratio, therefore determining the proper airway for a specific patient may be a matter of trial and error. The correct length of the nasopharyngeal airway can be estimated by positioning the airway along the side of the head. For proper function, the tip should extend past the angle of the jaw. An airway that is too long may enter the esophagus and not provide an air passage. Unlike oropharyngeal airways, nasopharyngeal airways that are too short will not make a bad airway worse, they just will not improve the problem.

Nasal bleeding can complicate insertion of the nasopharyngeal airway. Caution should be used with patients who are coagulopathic. The correct insertion technique, generous lubrication, and vasoconstrictive agents can reduce the frequency of nasal bleeding. A mixture of a local anesthetic solution (i.e., 4% lidocaine) and phenylephrine (Neo-Synephrine) or oxymetazoline (Afrin) is effective in this regard. In emergency situations, the airway should only be well lubricated to avoid the delay involved in waiting for drugs to take effect.

The airway is inserted parallel to the floor of the nasal pharynx and slightly medially with constant, gentle pressure (Figure 6-16). Clinicians often make the mistake of attempting to insert the airway "up the nose" (i.e., parallel to the long axis of the nose), which increases the likelihood of bleeding and fails to secure placement. If undue resistance is met on one side of the nose, insertion should be attempted on the other side, or a smaller diameter airway may be needed. Softer airways are less likely to cause bleeding and conform to a distorted passageway as they pass through a narrow nasal channel. However, they also are more likely to obstruct and prevent passage of a suction catheter. If only a small airway can be passed through the external nasal passage, it may not function because of its concomitant short length.

Uncuffed ETTs can be used as nasopharyngeal airways (Figure 6-17). The tube length can be customized to fit the individual patient's anatomy. A long, thin tube can be created by trimming the tube to the proper length. The tube connector can be used to prevent the tube from disappearing into the nose; however, the friction fit may be inadequate to prevent accidental separation. Also, the connector's internal diameter is smaller than that of the tube and may prevent passage of a suction catheter and limit gas flow during ventilation. Leaving extra length so that the tube can be taped at the correct distance is another solution, but it may reduce the efficiency of ventilation.

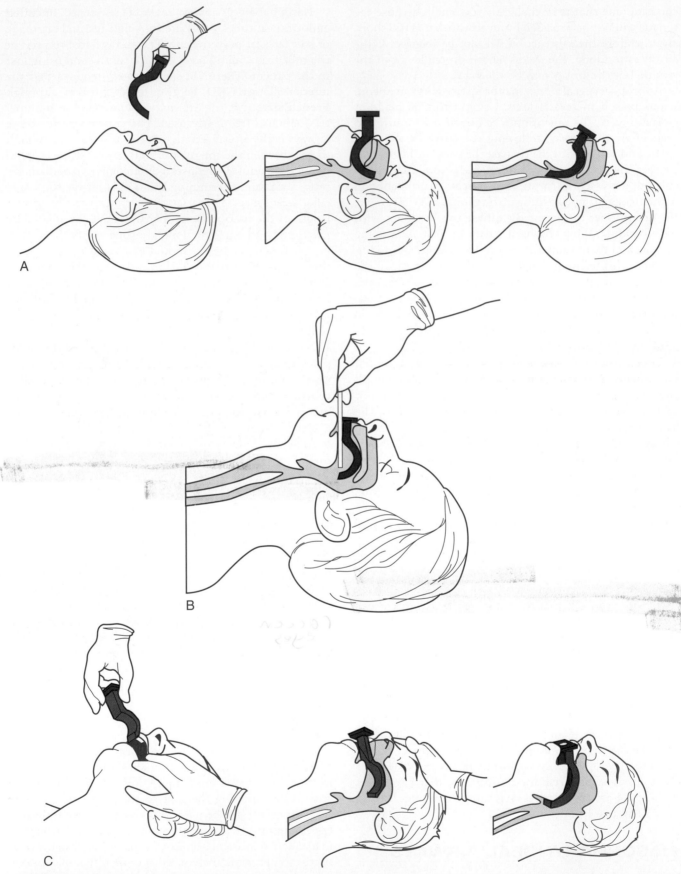

FIGURE 6-13 A, Antianatomic insertion of an oral airway. **B,** Anatomic insertion of an oral airway with a tongue blade. **C,** Insertion of an oral airway from the side of the mouth. The airway itself can be used as a tongue blade to displace the tongue while the airway is inserted.

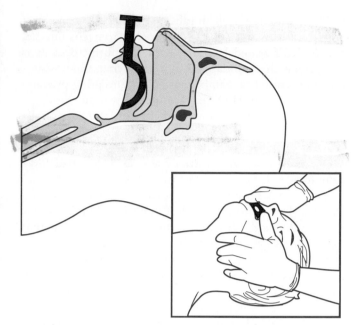

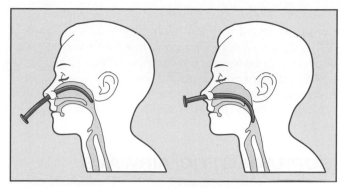

FIGURE 6-16 Placement of a nasopharyngeal airway. For correct insertion of the device, the tip is advanced directly posteriorly—not upward—because the nasopharynx lies directly behind the external nares.

FIGURE 6-14 A jaw thrust is performed to seat the oropharyngeal airway, which has become blocked by the tongue. If the correct-size oropharyngeal airway fails to seat properly and protrudes from the mouth, performing a jaw thrust and using the thumbs to insert the airway provides proper placement.

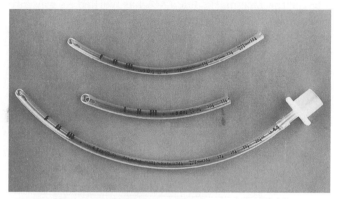

FIGURE 6-17 Uncuffed endotracheal tubes can be used as nasopharyngeal airways.

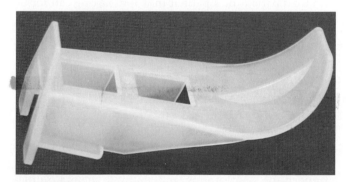

FIGURE 6-15 Intubating airways can be used to support and direct a fiberoptic bronchoscope and endotracheal tube into the trachea with direct vision. The incomplete channel allows separation of the scope from the airway after tracheal intubation.

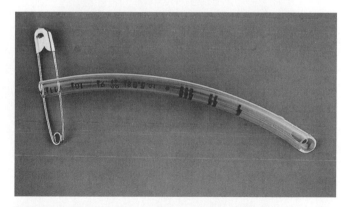

FIGURE 6-18 Inserting a safety pin just through the tube wall helps secure a custom-cut endotracheal tube used as a nasopharyngeal airway.

Cut-down endotracheal tubes are often used for nasopharyngeal airways in infants and children. Accidental movement can be prevented by placing a safety pin through the side of the tube, avoiding compromise of the center lumen with the tube with tape (Figure 6-18).

As mentioned previously, nasal bleeding is a concern, therefore nasopharyngeal airways should be used with caution in patients prone to uncontrollable bleeding. If bleeding occurs, topical vasoconstrictors can be applied, and the bleeding source can be directly tamponaded by leaving the device in place. Significant hemorrhage may necessitate a transfusion. A relative contraindication for

use of a nasopharyngeal airway is a Le Fort II or III facial fracture or a basilar skull fracture. Entry into the maxillary antrum, orbit, or base of the skull or penetration of the brain by the airway is possible, although unlikely, therefore this risk must be weighed against the urgency of the need for the airway and the failure of other techniques. Sinus infection is a long-term risk of nasopharyngeal tube placement.

As with oral airways, fiberoptic or blind tracheal entry can be facilitated with a nasopharyngeal airway. Removal of the device after intubation is more difficult, however, because split devices are not commercially available. Nasopharyngeal airways are useful for protecting the nose from trauma during blind nasotracheal suctioning. Once securely in place, they are usually well tolerated, even by awake individuals.

SUPRAGLOTTIC AIRWAYS

Laryngeal Mask Airway

The **laryngeal mask airway (LMA)** was invented by Dr. Archie Brain in the 1980s and was approved by the U.S. Food and Drug Administration (FDA) in 1991 as a substitute for the face mask. The LMA has worked its way into the difficult airway algorithm, as seen previously, as well as into the operating room and the toolboxes of emergency medical technicians (EMTs) and respiratory therapists.

The LMA consists of a plastic tube attached to a silicone laryngeal mask (Figure 6-19). It is designed to form a low-pressure seal in the laryngeal inlet by means of an inflated cuff. Note that the cuff pressures should not exceed 60 cm

H_2O. The LMA is placed blindly, with the tip resting against the upper esophageal sphincter (cricopharyngeus muscle) and the cuff seated laterally in the pyriform fossa. It is equipped with a standard 15-mm slip fitting, and positive-pressure ventilation can be delivered. Ventilating pressure exceeding 20 cm H_2O may result in volume loss, gas leakage, and ventilation around the cuff and potentially into the stomach. This device does not replace endotracheal intubation, because the lung is not protected from aspiration; the LMA essentially acts as a modified FMV technique.

The LMA is a useful emergency airway device for several reasons: (1) insertion is simple, can be done blindly, and is easy to teach and learn; (2) it provides a patent airway that usually is superior to that obtained with an oral or nasopharyngeal device; (3) it does not require airway manipulation or extreme head positioning and minimizes flexion and extension of the cervical spine; (4) it eliminates the need to place a foreign body in the patient's trachea and causes less bronchospasm and coughing in patients with asthma and irritable airways; and (5) once the LMA is in place, the user's hands are free for other tasks. A major drawback of the LMA is aspiration from gastroesophageal reflux disease (GERD) or a full stomach, because the LMA does not reliably seal the tracheal inlet.

Contraindications to elective use of the LMA include a nonfasted patient or a patient in whom fasting cannot be confirmed; retained gastric contents; and decreased pulmonary compliance. Box 6-1 lists the major contraindications to use of an LMA. Sizes are based on weight and range from 1 (neonates) to 6 (adults who weigh more than 100 kg) (Table 6-4). Normal adult females usually tolerate a size 4, and adult males tolerate a size 5. Use of a larger size with less air in the cuff often improves the ability to ventilate and may reduce the risk of mucosal damage and a sore throat.

Before the LMA is inserted, the cuff is inflated and examined for discoloration and ability to maintain inflation; it then is deflated completely and everted. A water-soluble lubricant is used on the back side of the cuff to help it slide past the hard and soft palates. The insertion

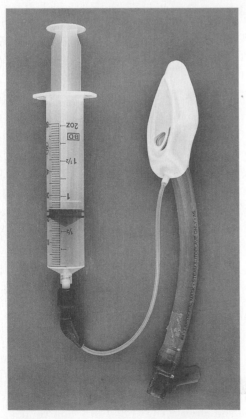

FIGURE 6-19 For correct insertion of a laryngeal mask airway (LMA), the cuff should be deflated completely with the mask forming an upward, open bowl configuration. This minimizes the risk of oral damage and helps prevent the mask from folding over during insertion.

BOX 6-1	Contraindications to Use of a Laryngeal Mask Airway

CONTRAINDICATIONS TO ELECTIVE USE OF A LARYNGEAL MASK AIRWAY
· Full stomach or inability to confirm fasting status
· Retained gastric contents
· Severe gastroesophageal reflux
· Decreased pulmonary compliance that necessitates high ventilation pressures

CONTRAINDICATIONS TO EMERGENT USE OF A LARYNGEAL MASK AIRWAY
· Patient conscious and/or resisting placement of the laryngeal mask airway

TABLE 6-4		
Sizing of Laryngeal Mask Airways		
Mask Size	Age Group	Patient Weight
1	Neonates/infants	Up to 5 kg
1½	Infants	5-10 kg
2	Infants/children	10-20 kg
2½	Children	20-30 kg
3	Children	30-50 kg
4	Adults	50-70 kg
5	Adults	70-100 kg
6	Large adults	>100 kg

technique is shown in Figure 6-20. A black line along the length of the tube marks the center of the device and is used to prevent and detect rotation after placement. The head may be extended and a finger used to guide the deflated cuff past the tongue and pharynx. The tube is held in place with the other hand while the guiding fingers are withdrawn. The tube then is advanced until it is fully seated and resistance to further insertion is felt. With the tube free in the mouth, the cuff is inflated. If it is seated correctly in the pyriform sinuses, the tube will move about 1 to 2 cm out of the mouth. This should be done "hands free" and without any ventilation equipment attached to the tube. If the mask is too small, it may pass down the esophagus, and no backward movement will occur on cuff inflation.

The final test of correct placement is the presence of adequate breath sounds over both lung fields and not over the stomach with manual ventilation. End tidal CO_2 ($ETCO_2$) should also be present. If ventilation fails, the head position may be altered (further extension usually is helpful), or the LMA can be inserted further or removed and reinserted. If the patient has a significant air leak and peak inspiratory pressures less than 20 cm H_2O, a larger LMA may be needed.

After the device has been properly placed and a patent airway obtained, the tube is secured with tape. Either spontaneous or positive-pressure ventilation can be used. Tidal volumes of 8 ml/kg are recommended for manual ventilation. Close attention still must be paid to the airway when it is secured with the LMA because loss of airway patency can occur, caused by dislodgement or twisting of the device, foreign body aspiration, obstruction of the LMA, or laryngospasm.

Blind (or fiberoptic) intubation with a cuffed endotracheal tube can be performed through an LMA to establish a definitive or secure airway (Figure 6-21). (A modification specifically designed for this purpose, the intubating LMA, is described later.) Occasionally the epiglottis is trapped in the LMA (it usually lies on top of the mask cuff), but this seems to have little effect on its function. The LMA is particularly beneficial in patients known or expected to have a difficult airway. Pregnant and obese patients predictably have improved ventilation with an LMA compared with

mask techniques. The LMA is potentially lifesaving when intubation and other ventilation devices have failed.

Use of LMAs is becoming widespread outside the operating room because mastering the necessary LMA skills is easier that mastering those needed for effective mask ventilation or endotracheal intubation. Emergency personnel are reporting excellent results in field use. Increased use of these devices in infants and pediatric patients is especially encouraging, because the skills necessary for other airway techniques in these patients are difficult to learn and maintain. The American Heart Association recommends instruction in the use of the LMA in basic lifesaving (BLS) training as an alternative to bag-mask ventilation. In ACLS, use of the LMA is considered as a IIa (acceptable to use) recommendation.

After use, reusable LMAs should be mechanically washed with a mild soap solution and autoclaved at a temperature of 134° C or less. The cuff must be evacuated completely or it will rupture during the sterilization process. Glutaraldehyde should not be used, because it is absorbed into the silicone and is quite toxic to the laryngeal mucosa. LMAs may be resterilized 100 to 200 times; marked discoloration and failure of the pilot tube and cuff to hold pressure are indications that the tube should be discarded. Disposable, single-use LMAs in adult sizes have been produced by several manufacturers and are now more commonly used than multiuse devices. Although reusable silicone rubber LMAs can cost as much as $200, the disposable models cost around $10. It is important to emphasize that these latter devices *should not* be reused. In addition to the LMA Classic (multiuse) and LMA Unique (single use), the LMA Flexible and LMA Proseal are available to meet specific needs. The LMA Flexible has a wire-reinforced tubing that allows greater flexion and greater adaptability for attaching the LMA to an airway circuit or during surgery. The LMA Proseal has an additional lateral tube that ends at the tip of the LMA and allows venting of the stomach (Figure 6-22). A gastric tube can be placed through this additional channel and may reduce gastric distention and the risk of pulmonary aspiration.[14] It is worth mentioning that the Proseal is touted as capable of generating 50% higher seal pressures. In addition to the aforementioned supraglottic airway devices, the LMA has been modified to act as a conduit to intubation (see later discussion).

LMA North America (San Diego, CA) manufactured the first supra-glottic airway device. Since then, a multitude of extraglottic airway devices have arrived on the market, including the Cobra (Engineered Medical Systems, Indiapolis, IN); King Laryngeal Tubes (King Systems, Noblesville, IN), which have a gastric access port; the Aura laryngeal mask (Ambu, Inc.); and the Portex Soft-Seal Laryngeal Mask (Smith Medical). Each device has its unique features, including single use to reduce cross-contamination, clear tubes with built-in bite blocks, reinforced tips to prevent folding during insertion, and various characteristics relating to the angle and composition of the tube portion (Figures 6-23 and 6-24).

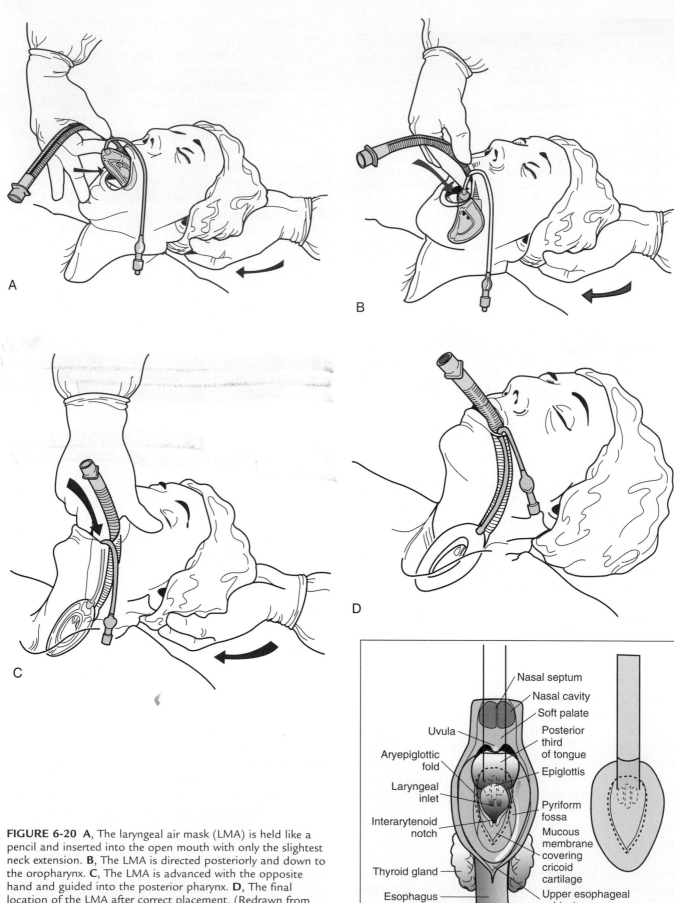

FIGURE 6-20 A, The laryngeal air mask (LMA) is held like a pencil and inserted into the open mouth with only the slightest neck extension. **B**, The LMA is directed posteriorly and down to the oropharynx. **C**, The LMA is advanced with the opposite hand and guided into the posterior pharynx. **D**, The final location of the LMA after correct placement. (Redrawn from Gensia Automedics, San Diego, Calif.)

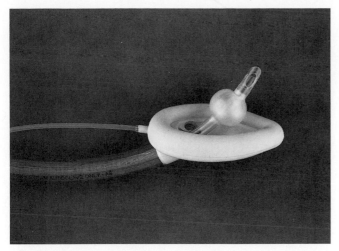

FIGURE 6-21 The laryngeal air mask can be used as a conduit for intubation.

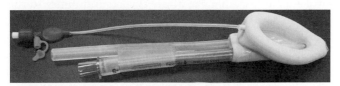

FIGURE 6-22 The LMA Proseal contains a port for gastric suction and venting of the stomach.

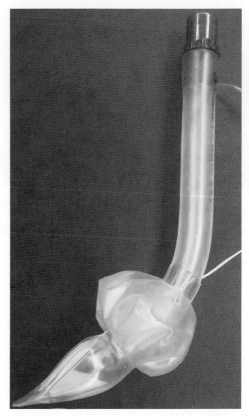

FIGURE 6-24 The Cobra is another supraglottic airway device.

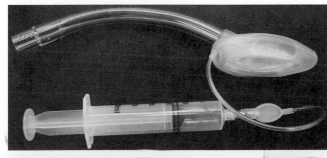

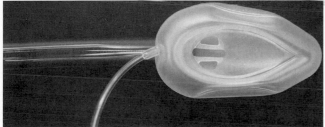

FIGURE 6-23 The LMA Unique is disposable to reduce the risk of cross-contamination.

Fastrach Laryngeal Mask Airway

As mentioned previously, a modification of the LMA has been developed to facilitate blind intubation in patients needing a secure airway. This modified version takes advantage of the fact that the LMA is simple to place and rests

directly above the larynx. The prototype of this intubating LMA, the **Fastrach**® (LMA North America), is shown in Figure 6-25. It consists of an LMA cuff mounted on a curved, hollow metal shaft, preformed to fit into an average airway. Initially, the Fastrach was a nondisposable, metal-containing device covered with silicone and packaged with a wire-reinforced ETT and an ETT stabilizer. Newer, disposable versions made of polyvinyl chloride are now available. The Fastrach has a flexible epiglottic elevating flap and a handle that allows control and manipulation of the mask orientation, which improves the chances of successful blind intubation. After intubation, the Fastrach is removed using the ETT stabilizer or stylet to prevent the endotracheal tube from becoming dislodged during removal of the LMA portion.

Benefits of the Fastrach include the fact that it can be used with minimal mouth opening (3 cm) and can ventilate the patient during the various steps of placement of the LMA and finally the ETT. Placement is blind, therefore this is a useful technique for a bloodied airway in which fiberoptic visualization would prove difficult. In addition, minimal cervical neck motion is involved, compared with direct laryngoscopy. Major disadvantages of the Fastrach are the cost ($500 for the reusable model and $90 for the disposable device) and the fact that it is available only in adult sizes. Despite these drawbacks, the Fastrach has become an important part of emergency and difficult airway equipment carts.

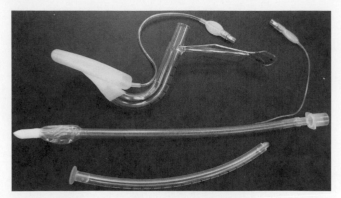

FIGURE 6-25 The Fastrach laryngeal mask airway allows intubation through the LMA. The intubating LMA is shown with its special Silastic endotracheal tube and tube pusher, which is used to help remove the LMA and leave the endotracheal tube in place.

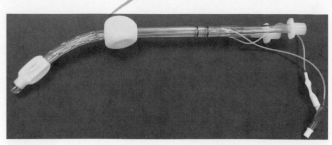

FIGURE 6-26 The Combitube is a supraglottic airway device that is useful for saving patients from failed intubations.

Combitube

The esophageal tracheal **Combitube** is a double-lumen device designed to provide a patent upper airway when inserted blindly in comatose patients with airway difficulty or after failed intubation. The two cuffs, proximal and distal, are designed to seal the esophagus and the pharynx (Figure 6-26). The tube can be placed blindly or during a failed laryngoscopy procedure. With blind insertion, the tube should be lubricated and inserted through the mouth, following the contour to the pharynx. Insertion continues until the depth mark reaches the lips or significant resistance is encountered. The distal cuff should be inflated with 12 to 15 ml of air, and the chest and abdomen should be auscultated for breath sounds or gurgling in the epigastrium. The small distal lumen usually advances into the esophagus, but in the case of a tracheal entry of the distal lumen, the Combitube can be used as a conventional endotracheal tube (Figure 6-27). If the distal tip enters the esophagus, both cuffs need to be inflated (the proximal cuff with 85 to 100 ml of air and the distal with 15 ml of air) to prevent air from escaping through the esophagus. Ventilation is then provided through the proximal lumen, which opens in a series of holes into the hypopharynx.

The benefits of the Combitube are that it allows a blind technique, it is easy to learn, and it allows the patient's head to remain in the neutral position. The esophageal cuff affords some protection from regurgitation, but as with the LMA, the Combitube is not considered a secure airway device. A nasogastric tube can be inserted through the esophageal lumen into the stomach for decompression. The Combitube is made in two sizes, 37 and 41 Fr; 41 Fr is recommended for patients over 60 inches in height. As of now, the Combitube is not suitable for pediatric use. The device is contraindicated for patients with a vigorous gag, in the presence of esophageal disease, or after ingestion of a caustic substance. Complications from the Combitube include dysphagia; a sore throat; and injury to the pyriform sinus and esophageal wall, which can result in subcutaneous emphysema, pneumomediastinum, pneumoperitoneum, or esophageal rupture.

SUBGLOTTIC AIRWAY DEVICES

Endotracheal Tubes

The endotracheal tube was first described in the 1800s and has since become the gold standard of airway management. ETTs allow ventilation with high levels of positive pressure, provide direct access to the lower airway for secretion removal and drug delivery, prevent aspiration of foreign material into the lung, and permit bronchoscopic examination of the peripheral airways. Placement of an ETT requires a high degree of skill and specialized equipment (i.e., laryngoscopes); risks during placement attempts include hypoxia, hypercarbia, and attendant cardiovascular changes. Before an ETT can be placed, adequate gas exchange must be established with another airway device or maneuver. Intubation may be an urgent procedure, but it should rarely be performed in a patient without a previously established patent airway and some evidence of reasonable gas exchange. *If a patent airway and gas exchange cannot be established by simple means, an invasive airway (needle or surgical cricothyrotomy)—not insertion of an ETT through the mouth or nose—should be performed without delay.*

As shown in Figure 6-28, the conventional, or Murphy-type, ETT consists of a round, plastic tube with a beveled tip, a sidehole (Murphy eye) opposite the bevel, a cuff attached to a pilot balloon with a **spring-loaded valve,** and a 15-mm standard connector. The tube has distance markers and a radiopaque marker imbedded along its length. The Murphy eye allows gas flow if the bevel tip becomes occluded. ETTs that lack a Murphy eye are called Magill-type tubes. ETTs are sized by internal diameter (in millimeters), although occasionally French sizes are

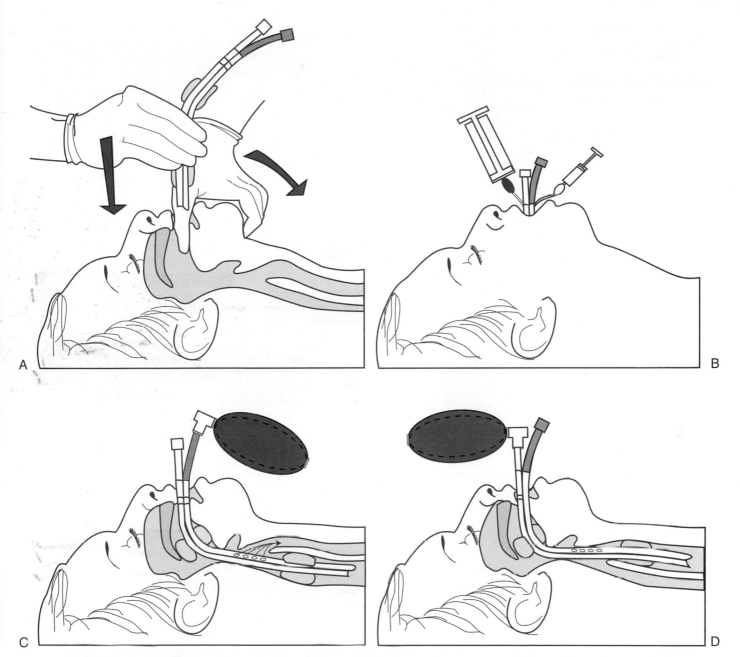

FIGURE 6-27 The Combitube is inserted with the head in the neutral position **(A)** and both cuffs inflated **(B)**. The two possible locations of the distal lumen are the usual esophageal location **(C)** and, in rare cases, the trachea **(D)**.

reported. Uncuffed tubes generally are used for children, because the smaller lumen necessary to accommodate a cuff would further compromise an airway that is already small in diameter. Also, the narrowest part of an infant's airway is below the larynx at the cricoid ring, and a snug fit at this level permits positive-pressure ventilation. The correct size of tube for an infant or a child can be determined only during actual intubation; a tube that will not pass easily down the trachea should be changed for a smaller diameter tube. To prevent postintubation croup or subglottic stenosis, an air leak of about 20 cm H_2O should be obtained in children intubated with an uncuffed ETT.

Many variants of the basic ETT design have been developed to solve clinical problems. The plastic tube tends to collapse and obstruct when bent at an acute angle, which frequently occurs in the posterior pharynx with a nasally placed ETT. A spiral wire–imbedded tube (Figure 6-29) helps prevent this problem, but these tubes are flimsy and do not hold a preformed arch shape, which makes them difficult to place in the trachea. Another solution to the bending and kinking problem is the RAE tube (Ring-Adair-Elwin), which has a preformed bend for oral or nasal intubation. Illustrations of these tubes can be seen on the Evolve Web site.

AIDS TO ENDOTRACHEAL INTUBATION

Laryngoscopes

The ETT is placed through the mouth or nose into the trachea, and the cuff forms a seal against the tracheal wall. Placement of the ETT usually is performed using a **laryngoscope,** which allows direct visualization of the larynx and control of the supraglottic structures. The first glottiscope was invented in the 1800s (Historical Note 6-1).[15-17] The modern laryngoscope was not invented until the 1940s and consisted of a handle containing a battery and a detachable blade with a light bulb. Figure 6-30 shows the two basic types of laryngoscope blades: a straight blade **(Miller blade)** and a curved blade **(Macintosh blade).** Note that direct laryngoscopy is performed slightly differently with the two types of blades. With either blade attached, the handle is held like a hammer in the left, usually nondominant hand (although "left-handed" models have been made, which are made to be held in the right hand) with the blade below the hand and the long axis directed forward (Figure 6-31). The mouth is opened, and the blade is inserted along the right side of the tongue. After the blade is past the base of the tongue, it is brought back to the midline of the oral cavity, moving the tongue completely to the left. With the straight blade, the epiglottis is identified and lifted with the tip of the blade, the jaw and epiglottis are lifted forward and upward (not rocked backward, which would cause trauma to the upper teeth), and the light then shines on the larynx and down the trachea. With a curved blade, the epiglottis is identified and the tip inserted above it into the vallecula, the space between the tongue base and the epiglottis. Using the same forward and upward lift, the larynx is illuminated, and the ETT can be passed into the trachea. The light is located farther down toward the blade tip on straight blades and brightly illuminates the larynx, whereas the light on curved blades is about midway down the blade and illuminates the pharynx and supraglottic area. The broad flange of the curved blade (Figure 6-32) gives better tongue control and more working room for tube insertion than does the straight blade. In children, the epiglottis is less rigid and longer than in adults and often a straight-blade technique (i.e., lifting the epiglottis) is necessary, even if a curved blade is used. Table 6-5 shows the standard Cormack-Lehane classification of the glottic view with laryngoscopy.[18]

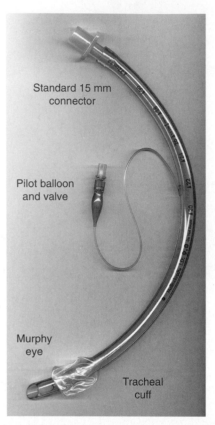

Standard 15 mm connector

Pilot balloon and valve

Murphy eye

Tracheal cuff

FIGURE 6-28 The components of a cuffed endotracheal tube.

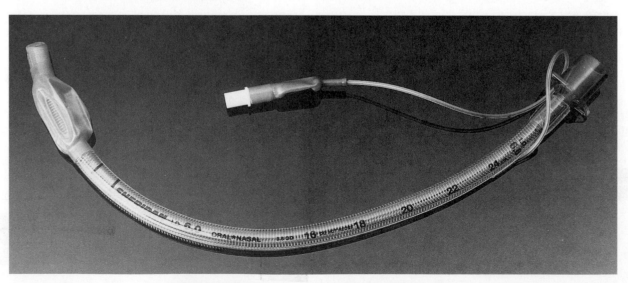

FIGURE 6-29 Spiral wire–reinforced endotracheal tube.

The basic laryngoscope blades have been modified over the years to deal with an anterior larynx, small mouth opening, cervical spine immobility, and a small sternal space. The size and shape of the flange and the location of the light on the curved blade are common features for innovation. Ports for suction or oxygen insufflation have been added. Straight blades have been modified in their cross-sectional shape to give better tongue control or working room during insertion of an ETT. No standardized size equivalency is represented in blade numbers, but a #0 or #1 blade generally is correct for infants, and a #3 blade usually is appropriate for average adults. The angle at which the blade leaves the handle is another area of modification. An acute angle may improve visualization, and an obtuse or offset angle may allow insertion of the blade when pendulous breasts or an orthopedic apparatus is in the way. An angled blade tip, a mirror, or a prism may allow the clinician to see "around the corner" into the larynx. In addition, short handles have been made to help with blade insertion in patients with a small sternal space. These specialized devices are often expensive and require considerable practice to master. Some of these devices are illustrated on the Evolve Web site.

Disposable laryngoscope blades (Figure 6-33) made of plastic or stainless steel have gained popularity because of the reduced risk of cross-contamination. Both the straight and curved blades come in sterile packaging and in the traditional sizes of the reusable blades. Other benefits of disposables are the elimination of sterilization and maintenance. Some evidence indicates that blades still contain protein matter even after sterilization.[19] In some cases, the disposable plastic blades have been reported to bend or snap. Other studies have shown that disposable blades lead to increased intubation times, greater peak force generated during intubation, and increased failed intubations during rapid sequence intubations.[20]

Although the ability to see the laryngeal structures is useful, a good view does not guarantee easy ETT insertion. Manipulation of the ETT into the trachea can be

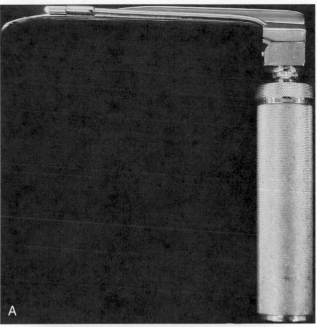

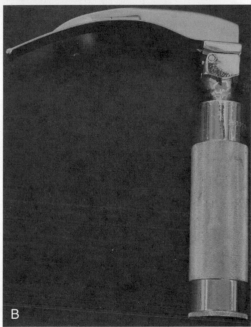

FIGURE 6-30 A, The Miller blade is a common version of the straight blade and **B,** the Macintosh blade is a type of curved blade.

TABLE 6-5

Cormack-Lehane Grades of Glottic Exposure during Direct Laryngoscopy

Grade	Description
I	Full vocal cords exposure
II	Only posterior commissure of glottis visible
III	Only epiglottis visible
IV	No exposure of glottis or epiglottis

From Cormack RS, Lehane J: Difficult tracheal intubation in obstetrics. *Anaesthesia* 39:1105, 1984.

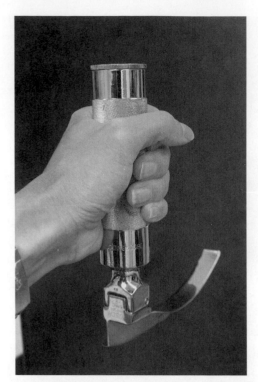

FIGURE 6-31 The laryngoscope is held like a hammer in the left hand.

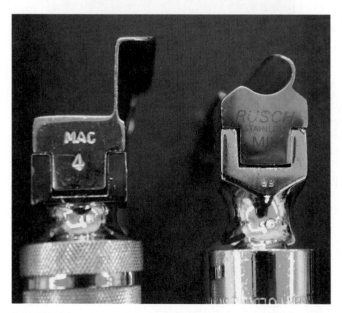

FIGURE 6-32 Cross section of straight and curved blades. The broad flange of the curved blade gives better tongue control and working room during intubation.

facilitated in several ways. The first consideration is proper head position. The sniffing position is ideal for opening the upper airway and aligning the trachea for intubation. The next consideration is the position of the intubator's head. The intubator's head should be far enough away from the patient's mouth to allow binocular vision (Figure 6-34A). If the intubator is too close to the airway (Figure 6-34B), depth perception is compromised. In general, if the

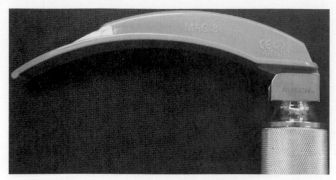

FIGURE 6-33 Disposable laryngoscope blade comes in a variety of materials, including plastic (pictured) and stainless steel.

arm holding the laryngoscope is 90 degrees or more at the elbow, the eye distance is correct. In difficult intubations, the larynx often is described as "anterior"; this means that the laryngeal opening is above the field of vision with the laryngoscope inserted. A malleable stylet can be inserted into the ETT to provide stiffness and can be bent to give the tube an upward hook at its end. This "hockey stick curve" is very useful if the problem is an anterior location of the larynx. Intubation often can be accomplished with this curved tip, even if a direct laryngeal view is not possible. The stylet should be lubricated before it is placed into the ETT so that it can be easily withdrawn. Another solution to controlling the ETT tip is the Endotrol Tube (Wellcor Boulder, CO). With this device, an implanted string with a pull-ring directs the tip anterior when pulled (Figure 6-35). This device is particularly well suited for blind **nasotracheal intubation.**

Endotracheal Tube Guide/Intubating Stylet

Even when the larynx cannot be seen during laryngoscopy, it may be possible to pass a rigid stylet blindly into the trachea. Called the Eschmann stylet, gum elastic bougie, or intubating introducer catheter, this device is useful with an anterior larynx or when the epiglottis can be seen but little or no glottic opening can be visualized. Ranging from 35 cm (pediatric) to 100 cm (depending on the manufacturer) and averaging 5 mm in diameter, the endotracheal tube guide has a 35-degree angle several centimeters from the tip (Figure 6-36). This allows for the washboard feeling or tracheal clicks when the device is advancing down the trachea over the tracheal rings. An ETT can be threaded over the stylet to achieve intubation. Variations include hollow centers that allow oxygenation and ventilation, and a channel for a fiberoptic scope to allow visual guidance through the glottic opening (Clinical Rounds 6-1).

Blind Intubation

Another approach to tracheal intubation is through the nasal passage. Blind nasotracheal intubation usually is performed in spontaneously breathing, semiconscious individuals. As with a nasopharyngeal airway, a well-

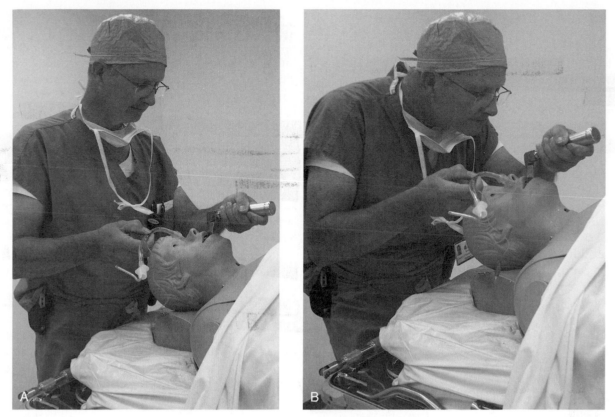

FIGURE 6-34 A, The correct head to trachea distance during intubation allows depth perception to be maintained. **B,** If the intubator is too close to the airway, the proper distance for depth perception is not present, and intubation becomes more difficult.

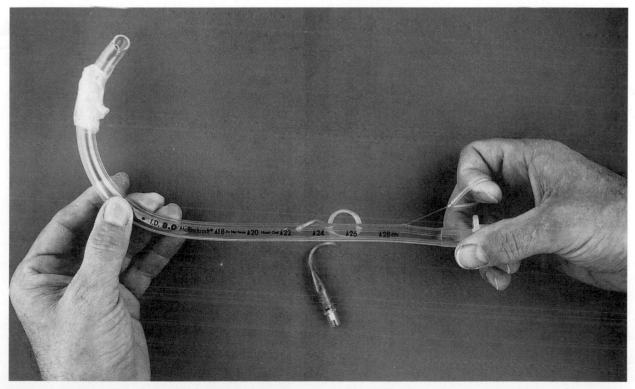

FIGURE 6-35 The Endotrol Tube has a string that when pulled directs the tip of the endotracheal tube anteriorly during intubation attempts.

lubricated ETT is inserted posteriorly, directly through the nares into the nasopharynx. Topical local anesthetics and vasoconstrictors should reduce patient discomfort and bleeding. Instead of the sniffing position, a neutral or slightly flexed head position is optimal for blind nasal intubation. Breath sounds or moisture in the tube is used to identify the tip location and the timing of tube advancement. Breath sounds or moisture disappears when the tube enters the esophagus. The ETT is placed just above the larynx and rapidly advanced 1 to 2 cm during inspiration, when the cords are maximally abducted. If tracheal topical anesthesia is not used, a vigorous cough follows successful tracheal intubation. Turning the head to one side or the other, flexing the neck further, or pushing the thyroid cartilage posteriorly may lead to success. Use of a fiberoptic bronchoscope may be necessary to complete nasotracheal intubation in some difficult circumstances. A nasally inserted ETT can be directed anteriorly into the trachea using a laryngoscope in the mouth and Magill forceps on an anesthetized patient, although care must be taken not to rip the cuff with the sharp teeth of the Magill forceps.

Blind oral ETT insertion techniques have been described. Proper placement can be achieved by using two fingers to retract the epiglottis and direct the tube tip anteriorly. The Berman intubating airway (Berman II) is an oropharyngeal airway with a hooked end and an open channel for an ETT. The ETT is placed through the channel while the tip is used to lift the vallecula. The tube can be passed into the trachea blindly and then separated from the open channel of the airway. The effectiveness of these blind techniques depends on the experience and skill of the individual; they are unlikely to be successful in the hands of a novice.

COMPLICATIONS OF INTUBATION

Intubating patients is not a benign procedure, and the incidence of complications during intubation has been reported to be as high as 30%.[1] Complications from intubation can be conveniently grouped into traumatic and cardiorespiratory complications. Traumatic problems include damage to the teeth and soft tissues of the lips and mouth, vocal cord injury, laryngeal cartilage dislocation, and perforation or rupture of the pharynx, larynx, trachea, or esophagus. In addition, corneal abrasions or injuries to the face, eyes, or cervical spine may occur during attempted laryngoscopy. Cardiorespiratory complications include the hemodynamic consequences of intubation or placement of a foreign body in the trachea, such as hypertension, tachycardia, vagal reactions (bradycardia and fainting), and ventricular arrhythmias. Respiratory complications include hypoxia, hypercarbia, aspiration, laryngospasm, and bronchospasm. Increased intracranial and intraocular pressure may also occur during intubation. Long-term intubation can lead to granuloma formation, mucosal ulceration or necrosis from high ETT cuff pressures, and vocal cord paralysis. Subglottic stenosis is another potential consequence of long-term intubation.

CONFIRMATION OF TRACHEAL INTUBATION

Objective confirmation of tracheal placement, rather than esophageal intubation, is imperative. This is especially true after intubation using a blind technique. The most sensitive way to confirm correct placement is to detect expired carbon dioxide with a capnograph or a color-change capnometry device like the one shown in Figure 6-37. Even

---

CLINICAL ROUNDS 6-1

You are called to the lobby of the hospital, where an elderly man is lying unresponsive on the floor. A cursory examination reveals a patent airway, no respiratory efforts, and no pulse. How do you prioritize resuscitation? How do you plan to intubate this patient on the floor?

See Evolve Resources for the answer.

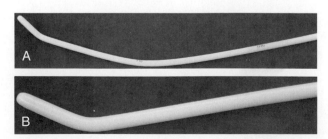

FIGURE 6-36 An intubating stylet or gum elastic bougie can be useful when a patient has an anterior larynx.

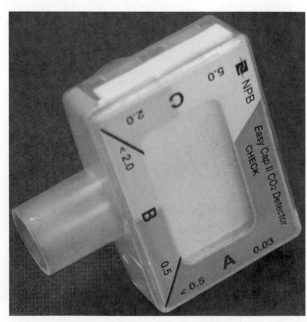

FIGURE 6-37 Calorimetric capnometer.

during an esophageal intubation, carbon dioxide may be detected for the first several breaths. CO_2 detection devices also are not as useful when cardiac output is profoundly depressed (e.g., during chest compressions for cardiac arrest). In addition, once a traditional color change device or capnogram is wet, it stops changing color. Newer products include 24-hour capnogram devices and moisture-repellant devices that maintain function despite 100% humidity.

A syringe or bulb can also be used to detect esophageal versus tracheal intubation. With this technique, because of negative pressure, the syringe or rubber bulb expands if the ETT is in the trachea but remains collapsed if it is in the esophagus (Figure 6-38). The primary advantage of this technique is that it does not depend on cardiac function or CO_2 delivery to the lungs to confirm correct tube placement. False-positive and false-negative results have been reported with this device in obese and pregnant patients. Auscultation should be performed in at least three areas after intubation. This examination should reveal bilateral thoracic breath sounds but no audible sounds over the gastric area. Sounds from esophageal and gastric ventilation can be heard transmitted to the chest and may be misleading.

Directly viewing the trachea with a bronchoscope passed through the ETT is another way to confirm correct placement. After exiting the distal end of the ETT, the broncho-scope should be above the carina (Figure 6-39). Although chest radiography (anteroposterior view) is useful for determining the tube depth in the chest relative to the carina, it does not provide information about the appropriate location in the trachea. A lateral film can identify tracheal rather than esophageal placement, but the other techniques described give rapid feedback on incorrect placement in enough time to prevent disaster (Clinical Rounds 6-2). Other indications that the ETT is in the trachea are seeing the chest rise and condensation in the tube with each breath, as well as palpating the ETT cuff in the trachea during rapid inflation.

After the ETT is in place in the trachea, the cuff can be used to form a seal with the tracheal wall. Usually air is inflated through the one-way valve in the pilot balloon until a seal forms or high pressure develops. Most ETT cuffs are large-volume, low-pressure devices meant to contact a large portion of the tracheal wall with a low pressure. Because of tracheal mucosal blood pressure flow characteristics, the cuff pressure should be below 25 mm Hg to prevent tracheal ischemic damage. A manometer for determining and regulating cuff pressure is shown in Figure 6-40. If a manometer is not available, a "just seal" or "minimal seal" technique can be used to minimize the lateral tracheal wall pressure from the inflated cuff. For some patients who require high airway pressure for mechanical ventilation, the cuff pressure cannot be kept below 25 mm Hg without significant volume loss. The amount of pressure used should be enough to guarantee adequate ventilation and protection from aspiration. An alternative to an inflatable cuff is a self-inflating cuff that is filled with foam. Before insertion, this type of cuff must be actively deflated and clamped; the clamp then

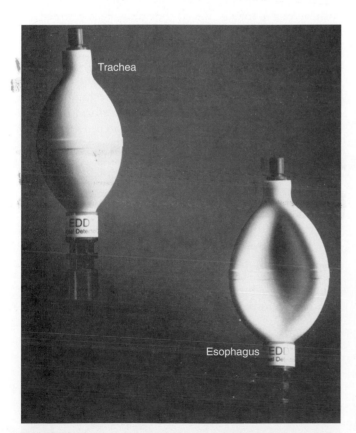

FIGURE 6-38 An esophageal detection device is another means of detecting tracheal or esophageal intubation. (Courtesy ARC Medical.)

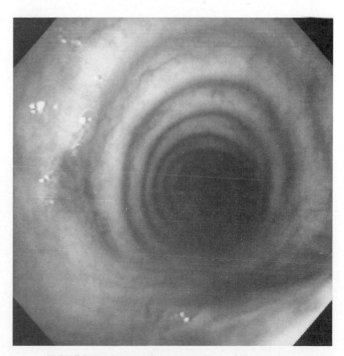

FIGURE 6-39 Bronchoscopic view of the trachea.

is removed, and the cuff is allowed to expand to form a seal. The pilot port of foam-filled cuffs does not have a valve.

A common problem with ETTs is, if they are inserted or migrate too far into the trachea, the cuff may obstruct a bronchus, or only one lung may be ventilated. Right mainstem intubation is most common, because the angle of take-off of the right main bronchus is less than that of the left. This is especially common in children because the distance between the glottis and the carina is so small.

ADJUNCTS TO ENDOTRACHEAL INTUBATION

Lighted Stylets or Lightwand

Lighted stylets or the Lightwand can be used to blindly place ETTs (Figure 6-41). This technique relies on pharyngeal and tracheal transillumination to identify the correct location of the stylet. The stylet should be lubricated before it is inserted into the ETT. The stylet can be molded into roughly a 90-degree bend to achieve entry into the anterior trachea. The patient's neck should be in the neutral position, although a jaw thrust can help with movement of the stylet and tube. The room lights should be turned off or dimmed, and the stylet should be placed blindly into the patient's oropharynx or nasopharynx. A dim, diffuse glow is characteristic of esophageal entry, whereas a bright, V-shaped light can be seen with tracheal entry. A lateral transillumination often indicates entry into the pyriform fossae. Once the characteristic pattern of light is seen on the neck, the ETT should be advanced off of the stylet and the stylet withdrawn. As with any form of intubation, the position of the tube in the trachea must be confirmed.

The lighted stylet technique is used when direct laryngoscopy is not possible because of cervical neck extension. A mouth opening of only 6 to 8 mm is required, and this can be useful in patients with an anterior larynx or a bloody airway. One drawback of this intubating technique is the need to turn the ambient lights off to perform transillumination. Furthermore, this procedure can prove challenging, if not impossible, in a patient with a short or excessively large, thick neck or darkly pigmented skin. It can prove equally difficult in a patient with a thin neck, because esophageal entry can look bright on transillumination and can be misleading. Although generally safe, this technique may cause blunt trauma to the airway and, less frequently, heat damage from the light source.

Indirect Laryngoscopy

Another procedure that has gained popularity among clinicians is indirect laryngoscopy. Indirect laryngoscopy

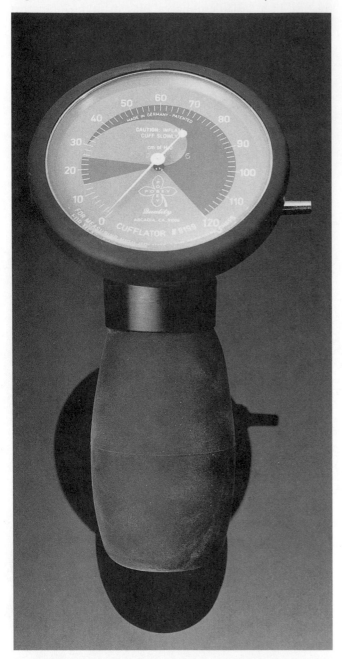

FIGURE 6-40 A manometer is a device used for measuring ETT cuff pressure.

CLINICAL ROUNDS 6-2

A 56-year-old man who has experienced cardiopulmonary arrest is admitted to the emergency department. Several attempts to insert an ETT have not established a definitive and secure airway. What alternative methods could be used to establish a secure airway for this patient?

See Evolve Resources for the answer.

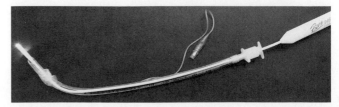

FIGURE 6-41 The Lightwand can be useful in patients with cervical immobility or instability.

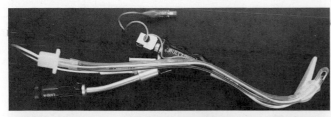

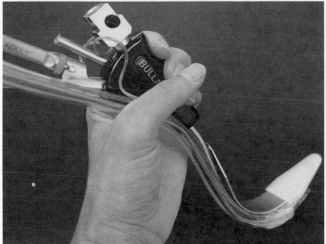

FIGURE 6-42 The Bullard scope is used for indirect laryngoscopy.

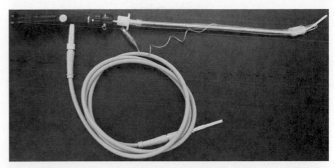

FIGURE 6-43 The optical stylet is another example of a device used for indirect laryngoscopy.

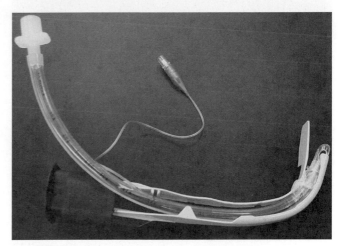

FIGURE 6-44 The Airtraq is a battery-operated, disposable device for indirect laryngoscopy.

devices rely on lenses, mirrors, or fiberoptic technology to obtain a clear view of the glottic opening and cords. Many of these devices have an optional attached video camera, which can be a useful aid for teaching airway anatomy and intubation skills. One of the first indirect, rigid fiberoptic laryngoscopes was the Bullard scope, an anatomically shaped device with a curved blade on the end and a fiberoptic bundle that allows visualization of the glottis without alignment of the oropharynx with the larynx (Figure 6-42). The Bullard scope has a built-in adjustable focusing system, suction port, and an introducing stylet. The fiberoptic bundle allows visualization of the cords and placement of the ETT under visualization. This device has proved useful for patients with temporomandibular immobility, micrognathia, and an anterior larynx. Because it requires less neck movement than direct laryngoscopy, it also has been helpful in patients with cervical spine instability.[21] Other rigid fiberoptic laryngoscopes include the WuScope and Upsherscope, which are variations of the Bullard scope.

A simpler rigid fiberoptic stylet, often called the optical stylet, consists of an anatomically shaped tube with a light on the distal end and an adjustable eyepiece proximally (Figure 6-43). An ETT can be mounted on the tube and advanced into the airway under fiberoptic guidance once the stylet has been advanced into the airway. Like the Bullard scope, the optical stylet allows visualization of the larynx without requiring alignment of the various axes of the airway.

A myriad of optical indirect laryngoscopes allow visualization of the airway but do not rely on fiberoptics for vis-

ibility. The Airtraq (King Systems) (Figure 6-44) is an example of a battery-operated, disposable device that provides an angular, mirrored, magnified view during the laryngoscopic procedure. It consists of one optical channel and a guiding channel for ETT placement. As with the Bullard scope, this device is beneficial in patients with minimal mouth opening (18 mm is necessary), an unstable cervical spine, and an anterior larynx. This and similar devices can be used with mounted video cameras; they include the GlideScope (Verathon Medical, Bothel, WA) and the DCI Video Laryngoscope System (Karl Storz Endoscopy, Tuttlingen, Germany). Maintaining a clear view with all these devices is mandatory, and blood and excessive secretions reduce their success rates. Experience is a primary determinant of success, and the devices with cameras may offer better opportunities for vicarious experience in a teaching situation.

Flexible Fiberoptic Bronchoscopy

Flexible fiberoptic bronchoscopy generally is considered the gold standard for intubation of a patient known to have a difficult airway or an unstable neck. Laryngoscopy with a flexible **fiberoptic bronchoscope** allows ETT insertion under laryngeal visualization using the scope as a guide for the endotracheal tube (Figure 6-45). The ETT is threaded over the scope before endoscopy and need only

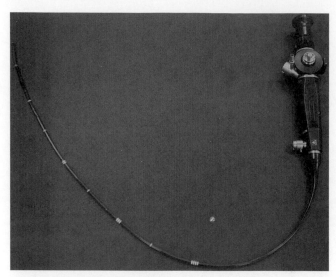

FIGURE 6-45 A flexible fiberoptic bronchoscope is useful for intubation in an awake patient known to have a difficult airway.

CLINICAL ROUNDS 6-3

After an emergency intubation of a patient in the surgical intensive care unit, a capnometer is attached to the ETT to confirm its placement. The indicator shows a carbon dioxide level of zero. How would you interpret this finding?

See Evolve Resources for the answer.

be advanced off the scope once the bronchoscope enters the airway. After airway entry with the scope is confirmed visually, the tube can be advanced over the scope and into the trachea. Because the scope is smaller than the ETT, the tube may need to be rotated gently to allow passage between the cords and into the trachea. This technique can be used for either oral or nasal intubation. Indications include a history or suspicion of difficult intubation, an unstable cervical spine or inability to move the cervical spine, anatomic abnormalities, and also ETT placement conformation and assessment. Contraindications to the use of this device include lack of skill or training in its use, inability to maintain oxygenation in the patient during the procedure, and significant bleeding or upper airway debris that blocks visualization. In addition, the fiberoptic bronchoscope is expensive and prone to damage without careful handling. Skill in fiberoptic examination of an unintubated patient is a prerequisite for use of this technique (Clinical Rounds 6-3). Fiberoptic intubation can be performed in awake or comatose patients. During an awake intubation, complete topical anesthesia is needed to prevent hemodynamic consequences, coughing, bronchospasm, and laryngospasm.

Retrograde Wire Intubation

The **retrograde wire intubation** technique is yet another means of placing an ETT with the added benefit of not requiring manipulation of the cervical spine. Because this technique takes several minutes or longer, it should not be performed on a patient who is acutely hypoxic. The retrograde wire technique requires an Angiocath or a needle, a guide wire, and forceps. The Angiocath (or needle) should be placed through the cricothyroid membrane in a cephalad direction and the needle withdrawn, leaving the Angiocath in the trachea. The guide wire then is advanced through the Angiocath in a cephalad direction until it can be retrieved through the nose or mouth. The wire should be pulled taut, and the ETT should be passed over the guide wire either orally or nasally and advanced into the trachea. Once the ETT is in the trachea, the guide wire should be removed and ETT placement should be confirmed (Figure 6-46).

Complications of the retrograde wire technique include failure to establish an airway, bleeding or hematoma at the needle puncture site, subcutaneous emphysema at the needle puncture site, laryngospasm, pneumothorax, and cord damage. Although this is a viable technique in a controlled situation, it is slow and requires practice to perform quickly and successfully. A kit with all the required components is available commercially and includes a wire stiffener to help advance the ETT.

SPECIALIZED ENDOTRACHEAL TUBES

Occasionally the need arises to provide selective ventilation to a single lung or a different kind of ventilatory support to each lung. Specialized ETTs that allow independent lung ventilation are available. These tubes were developed for bronchoalveolar lavage (to treat alveolar proteinosis) and for performing differential lung function tests before a pneumonectomy. They have been refined and frequently are used to improve surgical exposure and reduce risks during anesthesia for lung surgery or resection. Sometimes a **double-lumen endotracheal tube (DLET)** is used outside the operating room to protect the "good," or healthy, lung from blood contamination in patients with massive hemoptysis or infection from an empyema (Figure 6-47). They may also be useful in patients with a bronchopleural fistula. Probably the most common use of these devices outside the operating room is after single-lung transplant, when the compliance of the native lung and that of the transplanted lung are very different. Two ventilator systems can be used to titrate the appropriate support for each lung independently. More detail about DLETs is available on the Evolve Web site.

Other specialized ETTs may have distal airway channels. One is the Hi-Lo Jet endotracheal tube (Mallinckrodt Medical), in which the additional lumen can be used for distal airway pressure monitoring during jet ventilation (Figure 6-48). Another specialized ETT has a lumen designed for tracheal drug delivery (Figure 6-49). Recognition that aspiration of small amounts of infective oral secretions into the lung around the ETT cuff plays a role

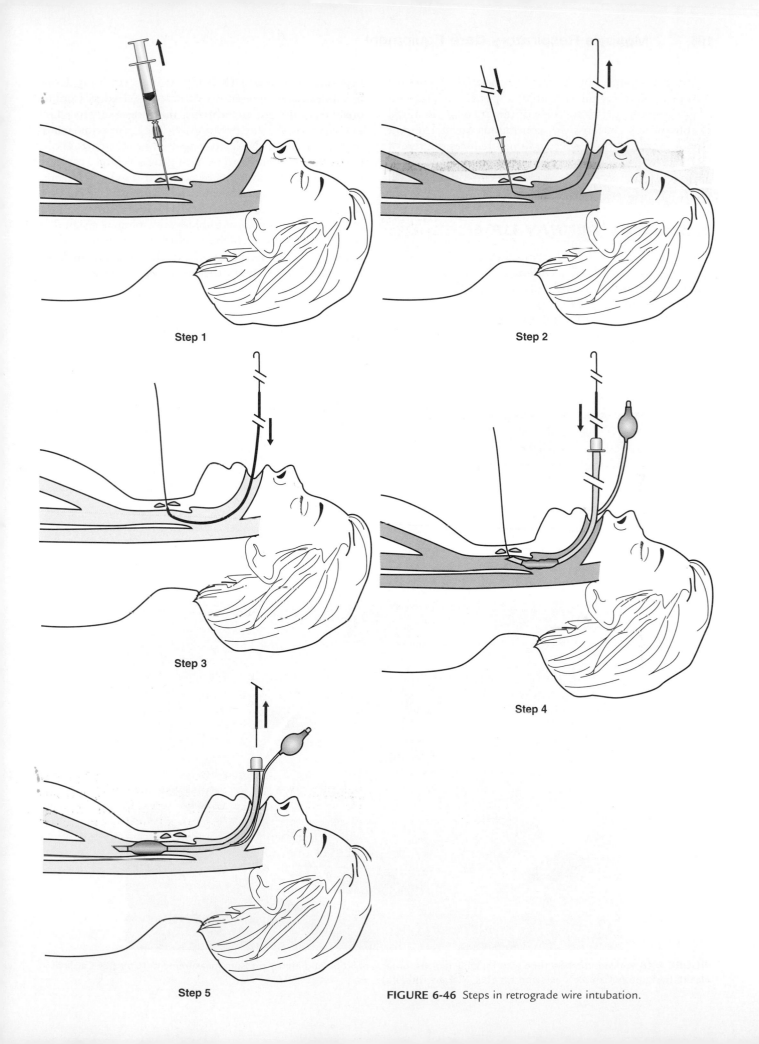

Step 1

Step 2

Step 3

Step 4

Step 5

FIGURE 6-46 Steps in retrograde wire intubation.

in the development of ventilator-associated pneumonia (VAP) has led to the production of a specialized ETT with a large suction port above the cuff (Figure 6-50). Removal of subglottic secretions with continuous or intermittent aspiration through the suction lumen reduces the risk of VAP. Use of this specialized ETT is recommended to help reduce nosocomial pneumonia in patients requiring prolonged infraglottic intubation.

SURGICAL AIRWAY DEVICES

On rare occasions, establishment of a patent airway with the previously described techniques (i.e., head position, oral and nasal airways, LMA, and Combitube) is unsuccessful. If the patient cannot be ventilated at all with a mask and an airway cannot be secured, invasive airway access should be established quickly to prevent hypoxia and its cardiovascular sequelae, as well as anoxic brain or organ injury. (Historical Note 6-2 presents a description of the

first surgical airways.) The simplest invasive airway device is a large-bore intravenous catheter inserted percutaneously through the cricothyroid membrane (a procedure known as a *needle cricothyroidotomy*). The cricothyroid membrane is an easily identified space between the thyroid cartilage and the cricoid ring. A 14-gauge or larger catheter over a needle intravenous device is attached to a syringe and inserted through the cricothyroid membrane at a slightly caudad direction. Continuous aspiration is applied to the syringe until air or bubbles are aspirated, a sign that the needle has entered the trachea. The catheter then is advanced off the needle into the trachea in a caudad direction. Figure 6-51 shows the position of the catheter. To

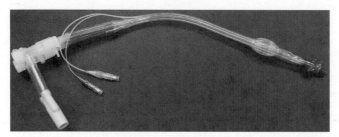

FIGURE 6-47 Double-lumen endotracheal tube used for lung isolation.

HISTORICAL NOTE 6-2

History of Tracheostomy[22]

· As early as 2000 BC, the Rgveda described a healed tracheostomy incision.
· Around 400 BC, Hippocrates condemned tracheostomy because of the risk to the carotid arteries.
· In 1546, Brasavola becomes the first person known to perform a tracheostomy for tonsillar obstruction.
· In the seventeenth century, tracheostomy becomes lifesaving and honored as a procedure to be performed in patients with severe diphtheria.
· Lorenz Heister coined the term **tracheotomy** in 1718 as a substitute for laryngotomy or bronchotomy.

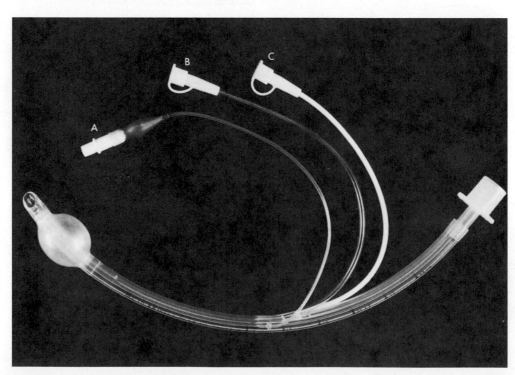

FIGURE 6-48 An endotracheal tube with multiple lumens for jet ventilation and airway pressure measurement. (Courtesy Cardinal Health Respiratory Care Products and Services, McGaw Park, Ill.)

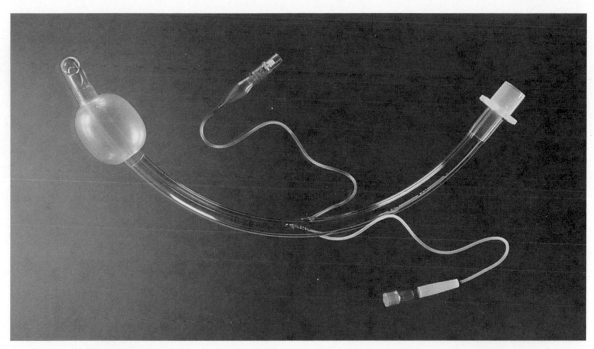

FIGURE 6-49 An endotracheal tube with an additional port to be used for the instillation of medications. (Courtesy Cardinal Health Respiratory Care Products and Services, McGaw Park, Ill.)

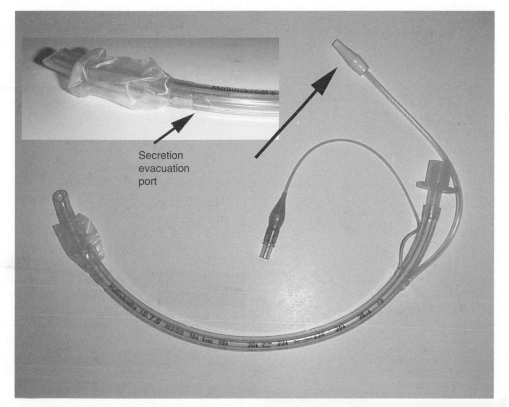

Secretion
evacuation
port

FIGURE 6-50 The Hi-Low Evac tube has a portal for suctioning subglottic secretions and is used as part of a program to reduce the incidence of ventilator-associated pneumonia in intubated patients.

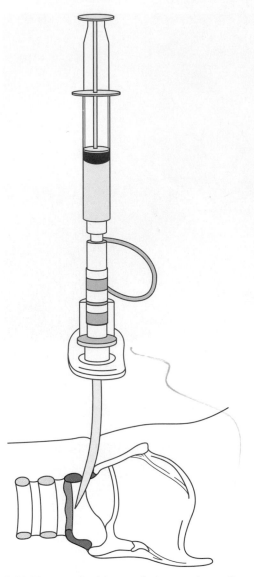

FIGURE 6-51 Transtracheal jet ventilation can be performed through a large-bore intravenous catheter or a special tracheal entry device placed through the cricothyroid membrane or trachea.

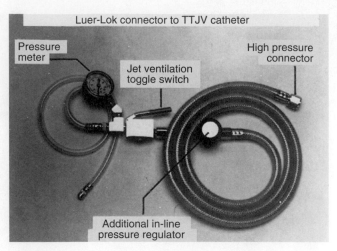

FIGURE 6-52 High-pressure jet ventilator system. (From Benumof JL: *Airway management: principles and practice,* St Louis, 1996, Mosby.)

provide adequate gas delivery through a tracheal needle, a high-pressure gas source (50 psi) must be used. A pressure interrupter or Saunders valve (Figure 6-52) is attached to the catheter with a Luer-Lok system to prevent disconnection from the catheter during ventilation. Expiration is passive and occurs through the upper airway. With brief jets of gas and intermittent pauses to allow for passive exhalation, normal ventilation and oxygenation can be maintained with this technique. It must be kept in mind, however, that the patient will become hypercarbic with time, and a needle cricothyroidotomy is merely a temporizing measure. With complete apnea, CO_2 rises approximately 2 to 3 mm Hg every minute.

It is important to use caution with the bursts of high-pressure gas to minimize the risk of barotrauma. The amount of pressure delivered should be enough to cause the chest to rise and to maintain oxygenation. If a high-

pressure system is unavailable, the catheter can be connected to a plungerless 3-ml syringe, which can then be adapted to fit with the tube connector of a size 7 ETT. This can be used in an emergency, and the patient can be hand ventilated for a short time while an alternative ventilation method is secured. For successful emergency use, the appropriate equipment must be assembled and ready for use ahead of time. Complications of needle–jet ventilation consist of formation of a false passage into subcutaneous tissue, development of subcutaneous emphysema, creation of a pneumothorax, bleeding, failure to ventilate, and damage to neck structures.

A cricothyroidotomy is a surgical incision into the trachea that passes through the cricothyroid membrane. A conventional ETT or tracheostomy tube (TT) can be placed through the incision. Routine airway equipment can be used to provide ventilation and oxygen delivery with the tube in place. A single horizontal slash incision through the skin to the trachea is performed. A small ETT (size 5) should be placed through the hole into the trachea to allow for the smallest incision to minimize bleeding and potential damage from scarring or stenosis. A significant gas leak around the tube through the cricothyroid incision can be occluded with sterile gauze. Bleeding usually is minimal because no large vascular structures lie in the area of the incision. Complications include false placement and failure to provide adequate gas exchange, bleeding, infection, and damage to other neck structures. Subglottic or laryngeal stenosis may be a long-term problem after cricothyroidotomy. Most authorities suggest elective conversion of an emergency cricothyroidotomy to a formal tracheostomy within 24 hours to reduce the likelihood of these severe problems.

Although not considered an emergency technique, **percutaneous dilatory tracheostomy (PDT)** has become a common means of providing direct tracheal access for long-term airway management. Because of its effectiveness, simplicity, and relatively low incidence of complications, this technique for placement of a TT often is performed in the intensive care unit (ICU) and recently was suggested as an alternative means of securing an emergency airway.

PDT can be performed by several different methods. The most common is the Ciaglia method, in which a guide wire is placed between the first and second or second and third tracheal rings and a series of stiff, plastic, tapered dilators is pushed through the soft tissues and the tracheal wall over the guide wire until an opening of sufficient size to accommodate the desired tracheostomy tube is created. PDT usually is performed on an anesthetized or a comatose patient and is done in the ICU or the operating room. It is worth mentioning that the PDT requires some neck extension and a sterile field.

Although some clinicians continue to perform PDT with a blind entry into the trachea, most have adopted a technique of observing and directing needle and wire placement using fiberoptic bronchoscopy.[23] This may help prevent inadvertent injury of the membranous tracheal (posterior) wall or too lateral a location of the tracheostomy.[24] A respiratory therapist often is requested to assist with the bronchoscopy and occasionally to administer sedative medications (in jurisdictions where the scope of practice laws and demonstrated competence allow). To allow visualization of the upper rings of the trachea with the bronchoscope, the ETT must be withdrawn until the tip rests in the larynx. This creates a significant gas leak during ventilation, because the ETT cuff is no longer in the trachea. Patients experiencing severe hypoxic respiratory failure may deteriorate during this time and may benefit from conversion to open surgical tracheostomy rather than persistence with attempting PDT.

In patients who require a tracheostomy only for airway access or protection, an LMA often can replace the endotracheal tube to provide the route for bronchoscopic visualization. The view of the larynx is unhampered when bronchoscopy is performed this way, which allows accurate identification of the tracheal anatomy. The bronchoscopic view of wire placement shown in Figure 6-53 was obtained this way.

Griggs et al.[25] developed an alternative to the sequential dilator technique. Their technique uses a tracheal spreader modified to thread over the wire and a cutting forceps to create the skin path and tracheal stoma. As with the Ciaglia technique, the trachea is entered between the appropriate tracheal rings with an intravenous catheter. Aspiration of air confirms tracheal entry. Bronchoscopy can also be used to prevent incorrect placement. Note that tracheal injury may be higher with this technique than with the other PDT techniques, especially if the procedure is performed without bronchoscopy.

The Blue Rhino dilator is a single, tapered dilator that is used instead of the sequential dilators of the Ciaglia method (Figure 6-54).[26] It has a lubricated coating that makes insertion very easy. It is softer and therefore may be less likely to damage the membranous tracheal wall.

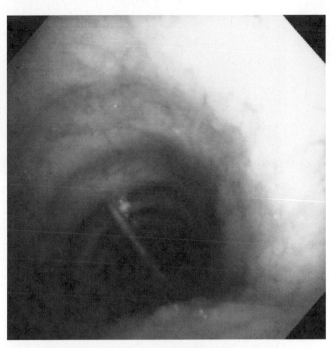

FIGURE 6-53 Wire is placed in the trachea in preparation for percutaneous dilatory tracheostomy.

Because only a single dilator must be passed, insertion of the tracheal tube is accomplished more quickly.[27] A significant amount of downward force is required to advance the stomal dilators and tracheostomy tube. This pressure often collapses the trachea and occasionally fractures a tracheal ring. The long-term significance of ring fracture is not known, but occasionally it has caused airway obstruction after decannulation.

PDT has been used as a technique for establishing an emergency airway. Divatia et al.[28] reported a patient who self-extubated but who could not be intubated or ventilated. They used a needle cricothyroidotomy to maintain oxygenation. After tracheal entry with a needle and high-pressure oxygen insufflation, a second needle was placed, followed by the guide wire, stomal dilator, and tracheostomy tube. With appropriate experience, PDT is likely to be more rapidly successful than a surgical tracheostomy in patients such as these.[29]

TRACHEOSTOMY TUBES

Similar to an ETT, a tracheostomy tube consists of a round, plastic tube—with or without a cuff, pilot balloon, and valve—with a standard 15-mm connector. Metal TTs (Jackson tubes) occasionally are used to maintain a patent stoma, allow for suctioning, or gradually reduce the size of a stoma. These tubes are rarely equipped with a cuff and need adapters to be mated with standard airway equipment. TTs are bent at about a 90-degree angle to fit flat against the skin and lie parallel to the axis of the trachea. As with ETTs, TT sizes are assigned as the internal diameter in millimeters, although the use of French sizes is still popular. TTs generally are more rigid than ETTs, although

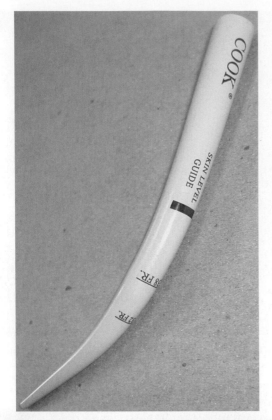

some are flexible. TTs are now available that are less likely to kink and must be carefully selected to fit the patient correctly. TTs typically have a collar that is used to secure the tube. The distance from the collar to the bend, the length of the tube distal to the bend (Figure 6-55), and the size and shape of the cuff vary by manufacturer and may be quite different. Some tubes have movable collars that accommodate different skin to trachea distances. The standard adaptor may be part of a removable connector or inner cannula.

TTs usually are placed occluded with a blunt, solid obturator that makes passage through the tissues less traumatic. The obturator is removed after the tube is in place but should remain with the patient and should be conveniently available for reinsertion in the TT if it is accidentally dislodged. Some surgeons place strong tagging sutures at the corners of the tracheal incision that can be grasped and pulled forward to expose the tract and facilitate reinsertion of a displaced TT. If ventilation is difficult after urgent replacement of a dislodged TT, the problem may be that the TT is not in the trachea, and manual ventilation through the upper airway should be initiated without

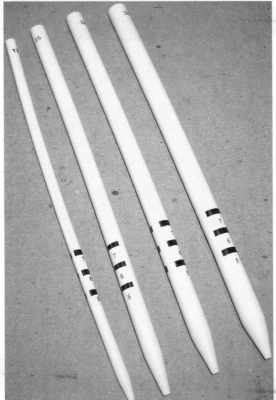

FIGURE 6-54 The Blue Rhino dilator is a single tapered dilator used for percutaneous dilation (top figure) in place of the sequential dilator described by Ciaglia.

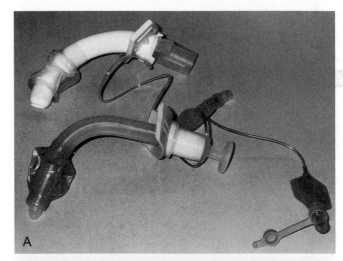

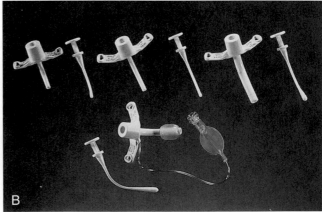

FIGURE 6-55 A, Tracheostomy tubes (TTs) come in preformed shapes with lengths that are not standardized. **B,** A conventional cuffed TT and general uncuffed TTs. Obstructors are used to occlude the TT end during replacement or tube changes. (**B** courtesy Shiley, Mallinckrodt, St Louis, Mo.)

delay. TT cuffs come in various sizes and, as with ETT cuffs, can cause mucosal ischemia if overpressurized (i.e., cuff pressure should not exceed 25 cm H_2O). Cuff pressure monitoring and pressure reduction are methods of reducing complications associated with the maintenance of TTs.

Although modern materials are less toxic than the hard rubber from which ETTs and TTs originally were made, these artificial airways can damage the structures through which they pass. TTs and ETTs can damage the larynx, as well as the trachea, from cuff pressure and tip trauma. TTs can cause damage at cuff and tip locations and at the tracheal stoma. Severe vocal cord damage and laryngeal stenosis are dreaded complications of **translaryngeal intubation.** These complications typically are difficult to treat and may permanently disable the patient. They increase with the duration of intubation and the larger diameter of the tube. If the need for tracheal intubation is predicted to exceed 2 weeks (in adults), a tracheostomy is often performed to reduce laryngeal complications. Trauma to the trachea from the tube cuff or tip can result in ulcers, cartilage loss, tracheomalacia, or rupture, which are complications of both TTs and ETTs. Granulation tissue may form at the TT stoma; also, after removal of the TT, stenosis at the stomal site may occur in up to 10% of patients. Treatment of these complications is difficult and often requires resection of tracheal segments or placement of a stent.

Tracheotomy Tube Adjuvants

With intubation, the patient's ability to speak is lost because the TT bypasses the vocal cords. This loss of communication and control can lead to psychological stress. Several methods for allowing seminormal speech with a tracheostomy have been developed. A fenestrated TT has a hole in the curved portion of the tube above the cuff that can be used to allow air to pass into the upper airway through the larynx so that normal speech is possible. When positive-pressure ventilation is needed, an inner, nonfenestrated cannula can be inserted. A one-way valve attached to the TT allows inspiration from the TT and exhalation upward through the larynx.

Two available devices to aid speaking are the Passy-Muir valve and the Olympic Trach-Talk (Figure 6-56). These devices can be used only in patients capable of initiating and maintaining spontaneous ventilation. Obviously, without an open upper airway, unobstructed fenestration, or a deflated TT cuff, a lethal, closed system with no portal for exhalation would exist. When one-way valves are attached to patients with artificial airways, careful observation for immediate problems with exhalation is essential (Clinical Rounds 6-4). In patients unable to sustain unaided ventilation, an extra port on the TT can be used to provide gas flow through the larynx. The Vocalaid (Portex) Smith Medical TT (Figure 6-57) was designed for this purpose, although speech with it usually is only a whisper. Vibrating devices can be used in the mouth or on the neck to produce audible

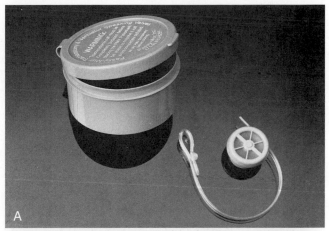

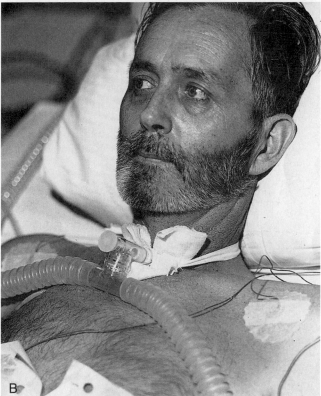

FIGURE 6-56 A, Passy-Muir speaking valve. **B,** Olympic Trach-Talk speaking device.

speech when mouthing words. Restoration of the ability to speak in patients with artificial airways can improve the patient's mood, increase cooperation with caregivers, and accelerate recovery.

When the need for a TT no longer exists, the patient should be weaned from the tracheostomy. If the tube is simply removed and the stoma covered with an occlusive dressing, the stoma will close in several days. Some clinicians prefer to gradually reduce the size of the TT every few days until only a small tube is in place. If direct tracheal access but not ventilation is needed for a longer time, several devices can be used to keep a stoma patent. A 4-mm, uncuffed metal or Silastic TT allows tracheal suctioning and causes very little airway obstruction in most adult patients. If rein-

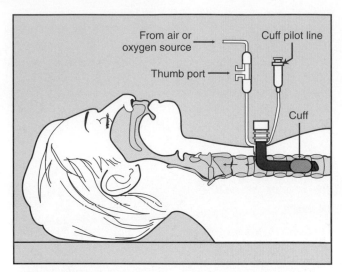

FIGURE 6-57 Vocalaid speaking tracheostomy tube (not available in U.S).

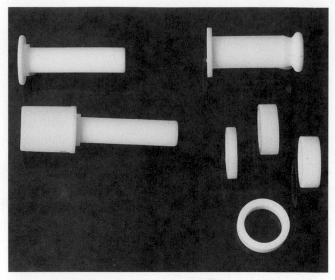

FIGURE 6-58 Olympic tracheostomy button.

CLINICAL ROUNDS 6-4

A patient has a fenestrated TT in place. To evaluate the patient's ability to move air around the tube and into the upper airway, what procedure should the respiratory therapist perform?

See Evolve Resources for the answer.

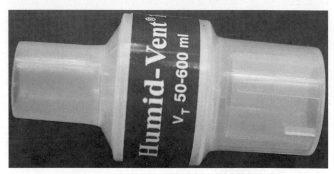

FIGURE 6-59 The Humidivent is a passive humidification system.

sertion of a larger, cuffed tube is later needed, the tract can be easily dilated to accommodate the larger tube.

Another device used to maintain a tracheostomy stoma is the tracheal button (Figure 6-58). It protrudes slightly into the airway but usually is less obstructive than a small TT. It usually is kept capped or plugged unless airway access is needed; it cannot be effectively used to provide positive-pressure ventilation, but it can be exchanged for a cuffed TT if necessary.

EQUIPMENT USED TO MANAGE ARTIFICIAL AIRWAYS

Patients who have been intubated or those with tracheostomy tubes bypass the nasopharynx and oropharynx during respirations. Humidifying and warming of inspired gases are primary functions of the upper airway. Active or passive humidification systems should be used in patients with ETTs or TTs for a prolonged period. Figure 6-59 shows a passive humidification system. (Chapter 4 presents a more detailed description of humidification systems available for patients with artificial airways.) Even with these devices, airway secretions may be increased because of tracheal irritation and thickened as a result of inadequate humidification or infection. In addition to the lack of humidification, the ability to cough is severely compromised because the glottis cannot be closed when the patient is intubated. Secretions must be aspirated from the lung in most intubated patients. Suction catheters are illus-

trated in Figure 6-60A. Suction catheters are available in a variety of sizes and designs; however, the general recommendation is that the catheter diameter should be no more than half the internal diameter of the artificial airway. It is important to recognize that suction catheters are sized according to the tube's circumference (i.e., French size). The tube's inner diameter can be converted to the catheter's circumference, or French size, by multiplying the internal diameter by 3 (actually 3.14, or Pi). The appropriate catheter size for the tube can then be determined by dividing the product by 2. For example, a size 8 (inner diameter) TT requires a 12 French catheter.

$$(8 \times 3) \div 2 = 12\,Fr$$

Preoxygenation, sterile preparation, and standard infection precautions should be used during endotracheal suctioning. Inline closed-system suction devices (Figure 6-60B) may reduce the caregiver's and patient's risk of exposure to infectious disease, lower costs, and compromise ventilation less during suctioning. Sterile sputum samples can be obtained using a **Lukens sputum trap** (Figure 6-61). Box 6-2 (see Evolve) provides a sample protocol for the suctioning of patients with artificial airways. Care must be taken during suctioning to prevent mucosal trauma and injury.

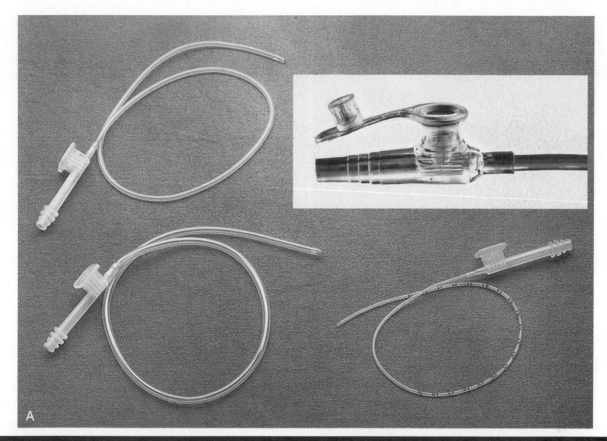

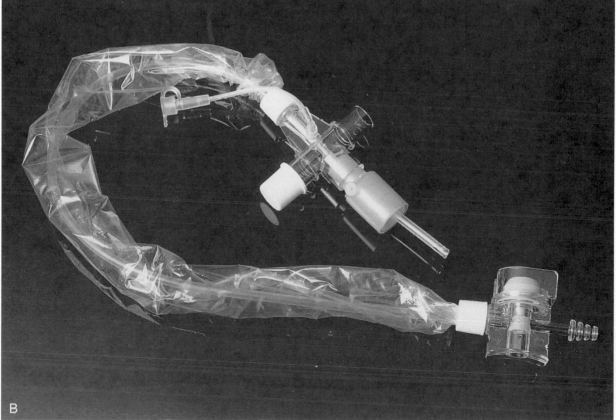

FIGURE 6-60 A, Types of suction catheters. **B,** Closed-system suction catheter. (**A** courtesy Cardinal Health Respiratory Care Products and Services, McGaw Park, Ill.)

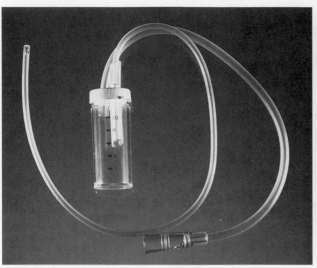

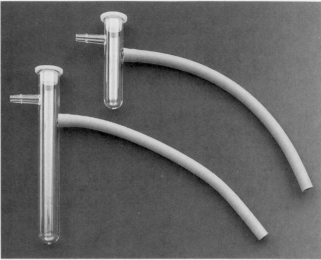

FIGURE 6-61 Uncontaminated sputum samples can be collected with a Lukens sputum trap. (Courtesy Cardinal Health Respiratory Care Products and Services, McGaw Park, Ill.)

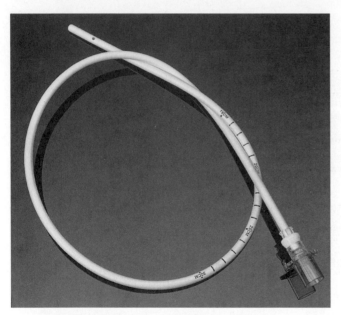

FIGURE 6-62 An endotracheal tube changer.

Many devices have been developed to help secure ETTs and TTs. Effective methods of securing these tubes are especially important in children. In addition to tube holders and securing devices, judicious use of sedation and physical restraints is important for the comfort and safety of the intubated patient and to prevent inadvertent extubation.

Changing an ETT may pose significant risk to critically ill patients. A tube exchanger designed specifically for this purpose is shown in Figure 6-62. The tube exchanger is inserted through the ETT, and the tube is withdrawn and removed. Oxygen can be insufflated through the tube changer during the procedure. A new ETT can be slipped over the tube changer and threaded down it into the trachea. Occasionally the new tube may catch on the vocal cords or larynx and may need to be gently rotated into

position; however, this method is not always successful, therefore equipment for primary reintubation must be at hand.

A common indication of the need to change a tube is failure of the cuff to hold pressure. If the pilot balloon remains inflated and the tube transiently seals when more air is added but quickly develops a leak again, the cuff probably has herniated through the vocal cords. This can be remedied by deflating the cuff completely, advancing the ETT 2 to 3 cm, and reinflating the cuff. If the pilot balloon holds pressure while the syringe is attached but deflates when it is disconnected, the pilot tube valve probably is defective. This can be overcome by inserting a stopcock into the valve, inflating the cuff, and turning the stopcock off toward the cuff. The pilot balloon and valve can be replaced with a blunt needle, and the stopcock inserted into the pilot tube after the balloon has been cut off (Figure 6-63). These methods of valve and pilot balloon repair may save patients the risk and trauma of reintubation.

MANUAL RESUSCITATORS

Manual resuscitators (or resuscitator bags) are portable, handheld devices that provide a means of delivering positive-pressure ventilation to a patient's airway. These devices incorporate a self-inflating bag, an air intake valve, a **nonrebreathing valve** mechanism, an oxygen inlet nipple, and an oxygen reservoir, which may be an attached tube or bag.[30,31] Manual resuscitators can deliver room air, oxygen, or air/oxygen mixtures via a mask or through an adaptor that attaches directly to a patient's ETT.

As their name implies, manual resuscitators originally were designed to ventilate patients during **cardiopulmonary resuscitation (CPR),** but they have become an indispensable part of the management of mechanically ventilated patients. They can be used to hyperinflate patients with enriched oxygen mixtures before and after

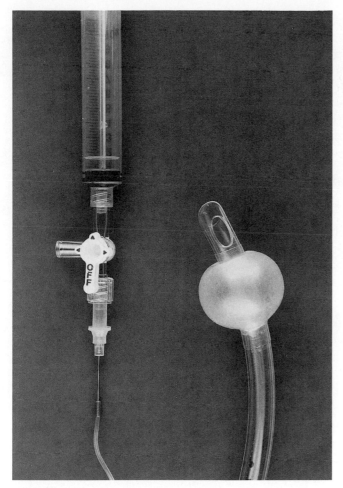

FIGURE 6-63 If the pilot balloon or pilot balloon valve fails to hold air, the entire assembly may be temporarily replaced by inserting a cut-off 19-gauge needle with a stopcock into the pilot tubing.

suctioning procedures, to generate airway pressures and large tidal volumes to expand atelectatic lung segments, and to ventilate bradypneic or apneic (ventilator dependent) patients while they are transported from one area of the hospital to another. Resuscitators differ in the type of valve used (see the following sections), the stroke and tidal volume potential, the amount of dead space, and the type of oxygen reservoir.

Types of Manual Resuscitators (Bag-Valve Units)

Manual resuscitators can be classified by the type of non-rebreathing valve used.[32] Therefore, two classes of resuscitators usually are described: those that use a spring-loaded mechanism and those that rely on pressure to affect diaphragm valves. Diaphragm valves can be subdivided into two types: a duckbill valve, and a leaf valve.

Spring-Loaded Valves

Spring-loaded devices use a nonrebreathing valve that consists of a disk or ball supported or attached to a spring.

When the operator compresses the self-inflating bag, the spring-loaded disk or ball is pushed against the exhalation port, occluding it, and gas is directed to the patient's airway. After the flow from the bag stops, the spring returns the disk or ball to the open position, and gas exhaled by the patient is vented to the atmosphere. Simultaneously, as gas enters the self-inflating bag through the one-way air inlet valve (which is attached to a reservoir), the bag inflates. The air inlet valve can be attached directly to the nonrebreathing valve or located separately at the bottom of the bag.

The most common examples of this type of manual resuscitator are the early Ambu (air-mask-bag unit) system, the Ohio Hope II bag, the Air Viva, and the Vital Signs Stat Blue Resuscitator. Early versions of the Ambu system used a spring-loaded, disk-type nonrebreathing valve that is no longer produced. The Hope II (Figure 6-64) and the Vital Signs Stat Blue (Figure 6-65) resuscitators both rely on the spring–disk-type nonrebreathing valve. Notice that the reservoir of the Hope II resuscitator, which allows for oxygen accumulation and potential delivery of 100% oxygen, is located on the bottom of the self-inflating bag. This reservoir is designed so that the angle of the oxygen inlet valve allows oxygen flows in excess of 30 L/min to be used without interrupting normal function. The Vital Signs Stat Blue Resuscitator differs from the Ohio Hope II bag because oxygen is drawn in through the neck, where a reservoir is attached.

Diaphragm Valves

Duckbill Valves. A **duckbill valve** incorporates a diaphragm-type nonrebreathing valve in place of spring-loaded mechanisms. The Laerdal Silicone Resuscitator, the Laerdal Adult Resuscitator, the Laerdal Infant and Child Resuscitators (Figure 6-66), the Hudson Life Saver II resuscitator, and the Life Design Systems disposable resuscitators are examples of devices that use the duckbill-type diaphragm valve.

The operating principle of these devices is comparable to that of spring-loaded resuscitators. Compression of the bag pushes a diaphragm against the exhalation ports. At the same time, the duckbill valve opens and gas flows to the patient. After the flow from the bag ceases, the duckbill valve closes, and the diaphragm is pushed away from the exhalation port. Exhaled gas can then exit through the exhalation ports. During reexpansion of the bag, the bag inlet valve allows air or oxygen from the reservoir to enter the self-inflating bag. Notice that the inlet valve is a simple one-way leaf valve that closes when the bag is compressed to prevent gas leakage. The one-way valve opens when the bag reexpands as a result of subatmospheric pressure inside the bag.

Leaf Valves. Resuscitators that use a **leaf valve** operate similarly to duckbill resuscitators. As shown in Figure 6-67, when the bag is compressed, a diaphragm swells and occludes the exhalation ports. The leaf valve in the middle of the diaphragm is pushed open, and gas is directed to the

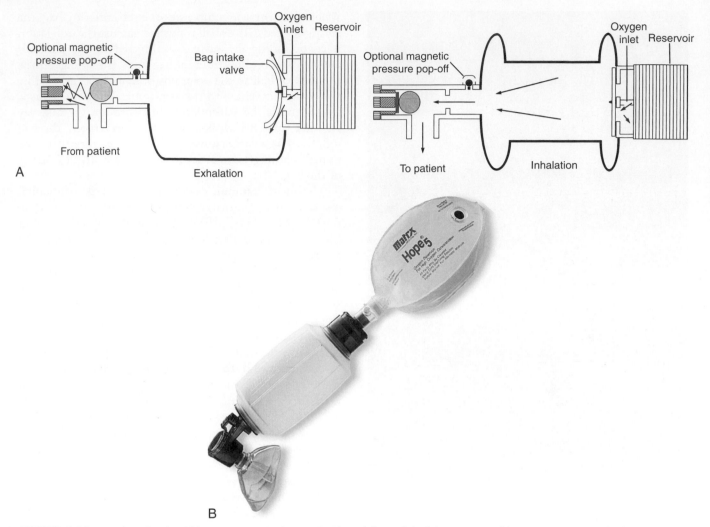

FIGURE 6-64 A, Valves for the Ohio Hope II resuscitator. **B**, The adult model of the Hope II with an oxygen reservoir. (**B** courtesy MDS Matrix, Orchard Park, N.Y.)

patient. During exhalation, the bag reexpands, creating a negative pressure that causes the diaphragm to move away from the exhalation ports. The leaf then closes and prevents exhaled gas from leaking into the bag. The bag inlet valve is opened, and the bag reinflates. The Respironics disposable resuscitator, the Hudson Lifesaver, and Robertshaw resuscitators are examples of devices that use leaf valves.

Standards for Manual Resuscitators

Standards for the design, construction, and use of manual resuscitators are published by the American Society for Testing and Materials (ASTM) and the International Standards Organization (ISO).[33,34] The ECRI (formerly Emergency Care Research Institute) and the American Heart Association (AHA) also provide standards for the use and evaluation of manual resuscitators, specifically relating to the level and timing of ventilation during CPR.[35] (Box 6-2 summarizes these standards.)

Table 6-6 compares the performance patterns equired by the ASTM, ISO, and AHA standards; however, delivery of a tidal volume of 800 mL (as specified by the AHA) may not be possible unless a patient is intubated. Figure 6-68 shows the results of several studies in which investigators measured the average tidal volumes delivered by one-handed compression of the bag.[36-41] It has been suggested that the lower tidal volumes could have resulted either from an inability to maintain an adequate mask seal while ensuring a patent airway or from gastric expansion. Another consideration is that the operator may be unable to deliver an appropriate tidal volume unless the bag is compressed with both hands.

Although manual resuscitators may differ in design, it generally is agreed that the ideal manual resuscitator should have certain characteristics.[42-44] Box 6-3 lists the characteristics of the ideal manual resuscitator.

Oxygen-Powered Resuscitators

Oxygen-powered resuscitators are pressure-limited devices that work similarly to reducing valves. A typical oxygen-powered resuscitator consists of a demand valve that can be manually operated or patient triggered. Oxygen-powered resuscitators can deliver 100% oxygen at flows of less than 40 L/min. Inspiratory pressures generally are limited to 60 cm H_2O, but the pressure-relief valve may be set to 80 cm H_2O if necessary.

Figure 6-69 shows an example of an oxygen-powered resuscitator. When the manual control actuator is depressed, oxygen enters the device from a 50-psig gas source and flows to the patient through a standard 15:22-mm (ID:OD) connector. The connector can be coupled to a mask, an ETT, a TT, or an esophageal obturator airway.

All types of manual resuscitators have various features that allow for adaptation to specific situations. These include syringe ports for administration of medication, metered-dose inhaler (MDI) connections, and specialized coverings to allow use in toxic environments. In addition, resuscitators allow for the addition of positive end-expiratory pressure (PEEP) valves, which have resistance characteristics that allow the addition of 1 to 20 mm Hg of positive end-expiratory pressure.

Hazards Associated with Manual Resuscitators

The most common hazards encountered with manual resuscitators are delivery of excessively high airway pressures, a defective or malfunctioning nonrebreathing valve, and faulty pressure-relief valves.[45] Excessively high airway pressures are more likely in patients who are intubated than in patients ventilated with a bag-mask-valve device. A nonrebreathing valve that is stuck in the inspiratory position because of improper assembly, inadvertent squeezing of the bag while the patient exhales, or obstruction of the exhalation port (e.g., by a mucous plug) all can produce dramatic increases in airway pressure. Defective nonrebreathing valves may cause an inspiratory leak, resulting in part of the tidal volume escaping through the exhalation port and not being delivered to the patient. Low tidal volumes also can occur with use of an inappropriately sized mask or failure to maintain an adequate seal between the mask and the patient's face. Improper setting of the pressure-relief valve can cause gas delivery at excessively high pressures and increase the risk of barotrauma.

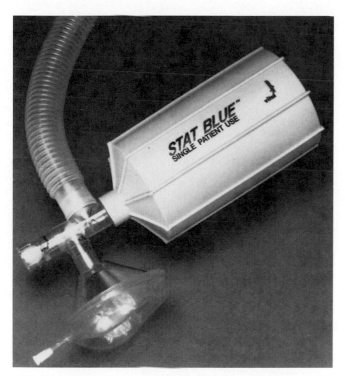

FIGURE 6-65 Vital Signs Stat Blue Resuscitator. (Courtesy Vital Signs, Totowa, N.J.)

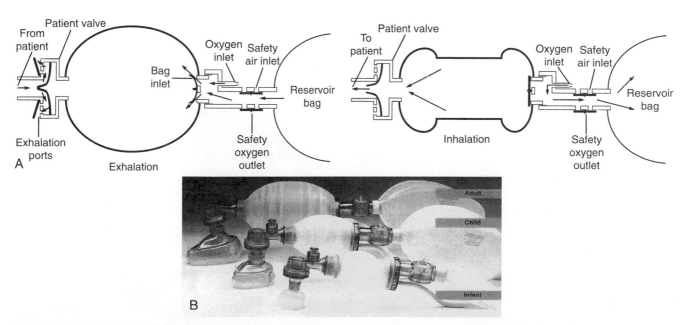

FIGURE 6-66 A, Valves for the adult and child with an oxygen reservoir system for adults. **B,** The Laerdal adult and infant resuscitators with oxygen reservoir systems. (**B** courtesy Laerdal Medical, Wappingers Falls, N.Y.)

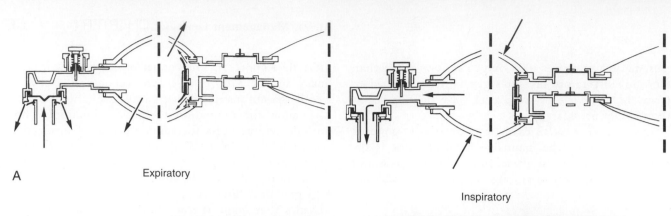

A   Expiratory

Inspiratory

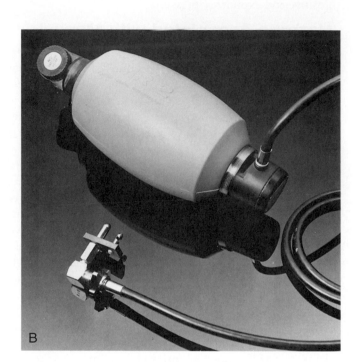

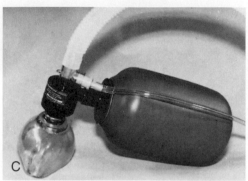

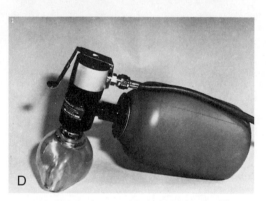

FIGURE 6-67 **A,** Operation of the leaf diaphragm valve for a Hudson Manual Resuscitator (as well as for a Robertshaw Bag Resuscitator). **B,** Hudson Lifesaver Manual Resuscitator with a manufacturer-supplied reservoir system attached. **C,** A modified reservoir system with 22-mm T-connection used for attaching the oxygen inlet at a right angle to the bag-inlet valve. **D,** Robertshaw Demand Valve attached to the bag inlet for providing 100% oxygen or other source gas to the bag. (**A** courtesy Hudson Oxygen Therapy Sales, Temecula, Calif.)

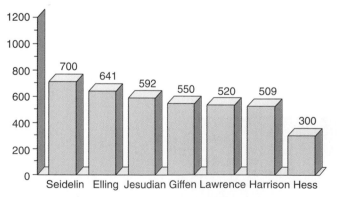

FIGURE 6-68 Tidal volumes produced by bag-valve-mask devices. (From Barnes TA: *Core textbook of respiratory care practice,* ed 2, St Louis, 1994, Mosby.)

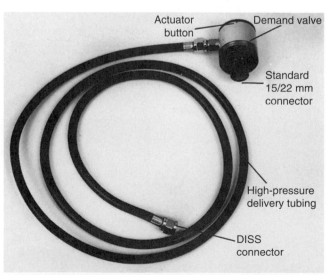

FIGURE 6-69 Oxygen-powered resuscitator. (From Scanlan CL, Wilkins RL, Stoller JK: *Egan's fundamentals of respiratory care,* ed 7, St Louis, 1998, Mosby.)

BOX 6-2	Standards for the Design and Construction of Manual Resuscitators

1. The American Society for Testing and Materials (ASTM) and the International Organization for Standardization (ISO) recommend that manual resuscitators be capable of delivering a fractional inspired oxygen (F_IO_2) of 0.85 with an oxygen flow of 15 L/min. Recognize that these are minimum requirements and may not be optimal for treating patients during cardiopulmonary resuscitation. It therefore is prudent to choose a device that can deliver an $F_IO_2 \geq 0.95$.
2. Manual resuscitators must be able to operate at extreme temperatures ($-180°$ to $600° C$) and at a relative humidity of 40% to 96%.
3. Adult resuscitators should deliver a tidal volume of at least 600 ml into a test lung set at a compliance of 0.02 L/cm H_2O and a resistance of 20 cm H_2O/L/sec.
4. The resuscitator's nonrebreathing valve must be designed so that the valve will not jam at oxygen flow rates up to 30 L/min.
5. If the resuscitator valve malfunctions because of a foreign obstruction (e.g., vomitus), the valve must be restored to proper function within 20 seconds.
6. Patient connectors of the resuscitator valve must have a 15:22-mm (internal diameter to outside diameter [ID:OD]) fitting.
7. Resuscitators used for adults should not have a pressure-limiting system. Bag-valve devices used for children must incorporate a pressure-release valve that limits peak inspiratory pressure to 40 ± 10 cm H_2O; devices used for infants may incorporate a pressure-release valve that limits peak inspiratory pressure to 40 ± 5 cm H_2O.
8. When a pressure-limiting system is incorporated into a resuscitator, an override capability must exist that is readily apparent to the operator (i.e., it should be easily visible that the valve is on or off), and an audible signal should indicate that the gas is being vented. The override mechanism should be provided for times when lung impedance is high and the patient has an endotracheal tube in place.
9. The resuscitator must be able to operate after being dropped from a height of 1 m onto a concrete floor.

BOX 6-3	Features of an Ideal Manual Resuscitator

1. The resuscitator should be lightweight and easily held in one hand.
2. It should have standard 15:22-mm (internal diameter to outside diameter [ID:OD]) patient adaptors.
3. The bag-valve device should be easy to disassemble, clean, and reassemble.
4. It should be constructed of durable materials (e.g., rubber, silicone, polyvinyl chloride).
5. The nonrebreathing valve should prevent back leaking of patient-exhaled gases into the bag. It should have a low resistance to inspiratory and expiratory airflow and a small dead space volume (<30 ml for adult models). The nonrebreathing valve should be transparent to allow detection of vomitus or any other obstruction.
6. A manual resuscitator should be able to deliver oxygen concentrations of 0.4 when oxygen is available.
7. The bag construction should allow rapid refill so that faster respiratory rates can be achieved as necessary.
8. The volume of the self-inflating bag should be at least twice the volume to be delivered, because not all of the bag volume is delivered when the bag is compressed. For example, adult resuscitators should have a volume of 1600 mL or more to be able to deliver a tidal volume of 800 mL. Resuscitation bags used for children should have a volume of at least 500 mL, and infant bags should hold at least 240 mL.
9. The bag-valve device should allow a positive end-expiratory pressure valve or spirometer attachments to measure exhaled volumes. It should be equipped with a tap for monitoring airway pressure with an aneroid manometer.
10. Every manual resuscitator should be supplied with a face mask that attaches to the standard patient connector of the resuscitator. The mask should provide an effective seal when applied to the patient's face.

TABLE 6-6

Ventilation Patterns Specified by Standards for Fractional Delivered Oxygen (F_DO_2) and Ventilation for Bag-Valve Devices

Specification	Ventilation Pattern (ml × cycles/min) ASTM[4]	ISO[5]	AHA[6]	O₂ Flow (L/min)	Compliance L/cm H_2O	Resistance cm H_2O/L/sec
Fractional Delivered Oxygen (F_DO_2)						
Adult	600 × 12	600 × 12	800 × 12	15	0.020	20
Child	300 × 20	15/kg × 20	N/A	15	0.010	200
Infant	20 × 60	20 × 60	6-8 kg × 40	15	0.001	400
Ventilation						
Adult	600 × 20	600 × 20	800 × 12		0.020	20
Child 1	300 × 20	15/kg × 20	N/A		0.010	20
Child 2	70 × 30	150 × 25	N/A		0.010	20
Infant 1	70 × 30	20 × 60	6-8/kg × 40		0.010	*20
Infant 2	20 × 60	N/A	N/A		0.010	400

From Barnes TA: *Core textbook of respiratory care practice*, ed 2, St Louis, 1994, Mosby.
ASTM, American Society for Testing and Materials; *ISO*, International Organization for Standardization; *AHA*, American Heart Association; *F_DO_2*, fraction of delivered oxygen; *N/A*, not available.

KEY POINTS

▶ Inadequate gas exchange is an acute emergency. Failure to restore adequate respiratory gas exchange can result in hypoxic brain injury or death within minutes.

▶ An understanding of the normal airway anatomy is essential for effective airway maintenance.

▶ The incidence of difficult airway management and inadvertent esophageal intubation is significantly higher in the critical care setting than when intubation is performed in the operating room.

▶ Various devices, such as oral and nasopharyngeal airways, laryngeal mask airways, and other supraglottic airway devices, can be used in emergency situations to improve the patency of the upper airway and permit manual ventilation.

▶ ETTs and TTs are definitive devices for airway management, allowing for ventilation with high levels of positive pressure as well as directing access to the lower airways for secretion removal and drug delivery.

▶ Correct sizing, proper placement, and securing of ETTs and TTs are essential for creating and maintaining an open airway.

▶ Objective confirmation of tracheal tube placement rather than esophageal intubation is imperative.

▶ Complications from endotracheal intubation typically are divided into traumatic and cardiorespiratory complications. Traumatic problems include damage to the teeth and soft tissues. Cardiorespiratory complications included hemodynamic compromise and hypoxia, hypercapnia, and aspiration.

▶ An adjunct to endotracheal intubation, such as lighted stylets, indirect laryngoscopy, and rigid fiberoptic stylets, can significantly improve the probability of successful ETT placement.

▶ Providing adequate, routine bronchial hygiene should be a primary concern of respiratory therapists caring for patients with ETTs or TTs.

▶ Manual resuscitators can be classified according to the type of nonrebreathing valve used. Two types of devices typically are described: those that rely on a spring-loaded mechanism and those that rely on pressure to affect diaphragm valves.

▶ The most common hazards encountered with manual resuscitators include delivery of excessively high airway pressures, a defective or malfunctioning nonrebreathing valve, and faulty pressure-relief valves.

ASSESSMENT QUESTIONS

See Evolve Resources for the answers.

1. The most important concern in an unconscious person is:
   a. Establishing a patent airway
   b. Calling for help
   c. Administering oxygen by mask
   d. Preventing aspiration

2. A finding on the physical examination that may indicate a difficult intubation is:
   a. A large mouth opening
   b. A thyromental distance of 8 cm
   c. Prominent incisors
   d. A long neck

3. The laryngeal mask airway:
   a. Is a definitive, secure airway
   b. Can be easily inserted in a conscious patient
   c. Bypasses upper airway obstructions
   d. Can be used to provide positive-pressure ventilation in patients with reduced pulmonary compliance

4. Benefits of the laryngeal mask airway include all of the following *except:*
   a. Requires less cervical range of motion during placement than direct laryngoscopy
   b. Requires less training to insert than an endotracheal tube
   c. Can be a conduit to fiberoptic intubation
   d. Prevents pressure injuries and damage to pharyngeal tissues

5. ETT placement can be confirmed by all of the following *except:*
   a. Capnogram color change
   b. Breath sounds over the epigastrium
   c. Fiberoptic bronchoscopy through the ETT to visualize the carina
   d. Easy expansion of the syringe of an esophageal detection device

6. Which of the following is the preferred artificial airway for a patient with liver failure who is vomiting blood?
   a. Nasotracheal intubation with a cuffed tube
   b. Oral intubation with a cuffed tube
   c. Laryngeal mask airway
   d. Cricothyroidotomy with a cuffed tube

7. A Combitube is placed in an unconscious patient. If breath sounds are clearly heard when ventilating through the pharyngeal lumen with both cuffs inflated, which of the following is true?
   a. A gastric tube should not be passed through the esophageal lumen.
   b. The lung is not protected from aspiration.
   c. Oxygen should be added to the esophageal lumen.
   d. More air should be placed in the pharyngeal cuff.

8. During placement of an appropriately sized oropharyngeal airway, the flange protrudes from the mouth. Attempts to insert it result in the device popping back out. This could be caused by:
   a. The airway catching on the back of the tongue
   b. The use of an airway that is too small
   c. A foreign body in the pharynx
   d. False teeth

ASSESSMENT QUESTIONS—cont'd

9. Which of the following is a complication of performing a cricothyroidotomy?
   a. Gas embolism syndrome
   b. Cervical spinal cord injury
   c. Stroke
   d. Subcutaneous emphysema

10. The most important concern with blind nasal intubation is:
    a. Failure to recognize esophageal intubation
    b. Nasal hemorrhage
    c. Sinusitis
    d. Loss of the ability to speak

11. After oral intubation, no carbon dioxide is detected during exhalation. This could be due to:
    a. Esophageal intubation
    b. Cardiac arrest
    c. Low cardiac output
    d. All of the above

12. A patient has a 7 (inner diameter) TT in the trachea. What size suction tube should be used?
    a. 10 F
    b. 12 F
    c. 14 F
    d. 16 F

13. List three important points in an airway examination.

14. Which size of laryngoscope blade should be used to attempt intubation of an average adult?
    a. #0
    b. #1
    c. #3
    d. #6

15. Which of the following are complications associated with TT placement?
    I. Hypoxia
    II. Hemorrhage
    III. Nerve injury
    IV. Gas dissection of the tissues surrounding the tracheotomy site
    a. I and II only
    b. II and III only
    c. I, II, and IV only
    d. I, II, III, and IV

16. Trauma from overinflation of an endotracheal tube cuff can result in:
    I. tracheal ulcers
    II. tracheal cartilage loss
    III. tracheal malacia
    IV. tracheal rupture
    a. I only
    b. I and II only
    c. II, III, and IV only
    d. I, II, III, and IV

17. The proper ETT size for a premature infant is:
    a. 2-mm inner diameter
    b. 3-mm inner diameter
    c. 4-mm inner diameter
    d. 4.5-mm inner diameter

18. A large, adult male patient has a 7-mm (inner diameter) ETT in place and is being mechanically ventilated. Cuff pressures of 35 cm H_2O are required to maintain an adequate cuff seal. Which of the following strategies would you suggest to correct this problem?
    a. Lower cuff pressures to no more than 25 cm H_2O
    b. Change the ETT to an 8.5-mm (inner diameter) tube
    c. Request placement of a TT
    d. Periodically deflate and inflate the cuff

19. A patient who has undergone a single-lung transplant is to be ventilated with two ventilators connected in tandem. What is the most appropriate type of airway to use?
    a. Magill-type ET
    b. Murphy-type ET
    c. DLET
    d. Combination of TT and oral ETT

20. What is the minimum F_IO_2 that a manual resuscitator with a reservoir should deliver according to ASTM and ISO recommendations?
    a. 0.4 with an oxygen flow of 8 L/min
    b. 0.7 with an oxygen flow of 10 L/min
    c. 0.85 with an oxygen flow of 15 L/min
    d. 1 with an oxygen flow of 6 L/min

21. Which of the following are standards recommended for the design and construction of manual resuscitators?
    I. Manual resuscitators must be able to operate at a relative humidity of 40% to 96%.
    II. Adult resuscitators must deliver a tidal volume of at least 600 mL into a test lung set at a compliance of 0.02 L/cm H_2O.
    III. The resuscitator's nonrebreathing valve must be designed so that the valve will not jam at oxygen flows up to 40 L/min.
    IV. Resuscitators that are used for adults should have a pressure-limiting system.
    a. I only
    b. I and II only
    c. I, II, and III only
    d. I, II, III, and IV

References

1. Jaber S, Amraoui J, Lefrant JY et al: Clinical practice and risk factors for immediate complications of endotracheal intubation in the intensive care unit: a prospective, multiple-center study, *Crit Care Med* 34:2355, 2006.

2. Walz J, Zayaruzny M, Heard S: Airway management in critical illness, *Chest* 131:608, 2007.

3. Hawthorne L, Wilson R, Lyons G et al: Failed intubation revisited: 17-year experience in a teaching maternity unit, *Br J Anaesthes* 76:680, 1996.

4. Samsoon GL, Young JR: Difficult tracheal intubation: a retrospective study, *Anaesthesia* 42:487, 1987.

5. Rocke DA, Murry WB, Route CC et al: Relative risk analysis factors associated with difficult intubation in obstetric anesthesia, *Anesthesiology* 77:597, 1993.

6. Lyons G: Failed intubation, *Anaesthesia* 40:759, 1985.

7. Adnet F, Racine SX, Borron SW et al: A survey of tracheal intubation difficulty in the operating room: a prospective observational study, *Acta Anaesthesiol Scand* 45:327, 2001.

8. American Society of Anesthesiologists Task Force: Practice guidelines for management of the difficult airway, *Anesthesiology* 98:1269, 2003.

9. Mallampati SR, Gatt SP, Gugino LD et al: A clinical sign to predict difficult tracheal intubation: a prospective study, *Can Anaesth Soc J* 32:429, 1985.

10. Iohom G, Ronayne M, Cunningham AJ: Prediction of difficult tracheal intubation, *Eur J Anaesthes* 20:31, 2003.

11. el-Ganzouri AR, McCarthy RJ, Tuman KJ et al: Preoperative airway assessment: predictive value of a multivariate risk index, *Anesthes Analg* 91:1197, 1996.

12. Kherterpal S, Han R, Tremper K et al: Incidence and predictors of difficult and impossible mask ventilation, *Anesthesiology* 105:885, 2006.

13. Langeron O, Huraux C, Guggiari M et al: Prediction of difficult mask ventilation, *Anesthesiology* 92:1229, 2000.

14. Brain AL, Verghese C, Strube PJ: The LMA "ProSeal": a laryngeal mask with an oesophageal vent, *Br J Anaesth* 84:650, 200.

15. Bailey B: Laryngoscopy and laryngoscopes: who's the first?—the forefathers/four fathers of laryngology, *Laryngoscope* 106:939, 1996.

16. Bailey BJ: What's all the fuss about?: the laryngoscope pages cause an international incident, *Laryngoscope* 106:925, 1996.

17. Cooper R: Laryngoscope: its past and future, *Can J Anesth* 51:R6, 2004.

18. Cormarck RS, Lehane J: Difficult tracheal intubation obstetrics, *Anaesthesia* 39:1105, 1984.

19. Miller DM, Youkhana I, Karunaratne WU et al: Presence of protein deposits on "cleaned" re-usable anaesthetic equipment, *Anaesthesia* 56:1069, 2001.

20. Evans A, Vaughan RS, Hall JE et al: A comparison of the forces exerted during laryngoscopy using disposable and non-disposable laryngoscope blades, *Anaesthesia* 58:869, 2003.

21. Hastings RH, Vigin AC, Yand BY et al: Cervical spine movement during laryngoscopy with the Bullard, Macintosh, and Miller laryngoscopes, *Anesthesiology* 82:859, 1995.

22. Lindman JP, Morgan CE, Dixon S: Tracheostomy, eMedicine, 2006.

23. Oberwalder M, Weis H, Nehoda H et al: Videobronchoscopic guidance makes percutaneous dilational tracheostomy safer, *Surg Endosc* 18:839, 2004.

24. Fernandez L, Norwood S, Roettger R et al: Bedside percutaneous tracheostomy with bronchoscopic guidance in critically ill patients, *Arch Surg* 131:129, 1996.

25. Griggs W, Worthley L, Gilligan J et al: A simple percutaneous technique, *Surg Gynecol Obstet* 170:543, 1990.

26. Bewsher M, Adams A, Clarke C et al: Evaluation of a new percutaneous dilational tracheostomy set apparatus, *Anaesthesia* 56:859, 2001.

27. Byhahn C, Wilke H, Habig S et al: Percutaneous tracheostomy: Ciaglia Blue Rhino versus the basic Ciaglia technique of percutaneous dilational tracheostomy, *Anesth Analg* 91:882, 2000.

28. Divatia J et al: Failed intubation managed with subcricoid transtracheal jet ventilation followed by percutaneous tracheostomy, *Anesthesiology* 96:1519, 2002.

29. Dult M, Ault B, Ng P: Percutaneous dilational tracheostomy for emergent airway access, *J Intensive Care Med* 18:222, 2003.

30. Fink JB: Volume expansion therapy. In Burton GC, Hodgkin JE, Ward JJ, editors: *Respiratory care: a guide to clinical practice*, ed 4, Philadelphia, 1997, JB Lippincott.

31. McPherson SP: *Respiratory care equipment*, ed 5, St Louis, 1995, Mosby.

32. Barnes TA, Watson ME: Cardiopulmonary resuscitation and emergency cardiac care. In Barnes TA, editor: *Core textbook of respiratory care practice*, ed 2, St Louis, 1994, Mosby.

33. American Society for Testing and Materials: *Standard specification for performance and safety requirements for resuscitators intended for use with humans*, Designation F-920-985, Philadelphia, 1988, The Society.

34. ISO Technical Committee ISO/TC 121: Anesthetic and respiratory equipment: International Standard ISO 8382: resuscitators intended for use with humans, Geneva Switzerland, 1988, The Organization.

35. Emergency Cardiac Care Committee, American Heart Association: *Textbook on advanced cardiac care*, ed 4, Dallas, 1996, The Association.

36. Eiling R, Plitis J: An evaluation of emergency medical technicians' ability to use manual ventilation devices, *Ann Emerg Med* 12:765, 1983.

37. Giffen PR, Hope CE: Preliminary evaluation of a prototype tube-valve-mask ventilator for emergency artificial ventilation, *Ann Emerg Med* 20:262, 1991.

38. Harrison RR et al: Mouth-to-mask ventilation: a superior method of rescue breathing, *Ann Emerg Med* 11:74, 1982.

39. Hess D, Baran C: Ventilatory volumes using mouth-to-mouth, mouth-to-mask, and bag-valve-mask techniques at various resistances and compliances, *Respir Care* 32:1025, 1987.

40. Jesudian MC et al: Bag-valve-mask ventilation: two rescuers are better than one—preliminary report, *Crit Care Med* 13:122, 1985.

41. Seidelin PH, Stolarek IH, Littlewood DG: Comparison of six methods of emergency ventilation, *Lancet* 2:1274, 1986.

42. Hess D, Goff G, Johnson K: The effects of hand size, resuscitator brand, and the use of two hands on volume delivered during adult bag-valve ventilation, *Respir Care* 34:805, 1989.

43. Barnes TA: Emergency ventilation techniques and related equipment, *Respir Care* 37:673, 1992.

44. Melker RJ, Banner MJ: Ventilation during CPR: two rescuer standards reappraised, *Ann Emerg Med* 14:397, 1985.

45. Dorsch JA, Dorsch SE: *Understanding anesthesia equipment*, ed 4, Philadelphia, 1998, Lippincott, Williams & Wilkins.

Internet Resources

Airway images from the University of Miami: http://umdas.med.miami.edu

American Association for Respiratory Care: www.aarc.org

American Society of Anesthesiologists: www.asahq.org

Healthcare Professionals Resources: www.healthanswers.com

The Internet Journal of Anesthesiology: www.ispub.com/journals/ija.htm

The Internet Journal of Emergency and Intensive Care Medicine: www.ispub.com/journals/ijeicm.htm

Mallinckrodt Corporation: www.mallinckrodt.com

National Library of Medicine (Medline/Grateful Med Services): http://www.nlm.nih.gov/portals/healthcare.htm   accessed 9/14/2008

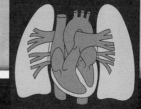

Chapter 7

Lung Expansion Devices

J.M. CAIRO

OUTLINE

Incentive Spirometers
    Volume-Displacement Devices
    Flow-Dependent Devices
Intermittent Positive-Pressure Breathing (IPPB)
    Devices
    Puritan Bennett Devices
    Bird Devices
    Vortran (IPPB) Device
Positive Airway Pressure (PAP) Devices
    Continuous Positive Airway Pressure
    Expiratory Positive Airway Pressure
    Positive Expiratory Pressure

Chest Physiotherapy Devices
    Manual Percussors
    Pneumatically Powered Devices
    Electrically Powered Percussors
High-Frequency Oscillation Devices
    Intrapulmonary Percussive Ventilation
    Flutter Valve Therapy
    High-Frequency Chest Wall Oscillation
      Devices
Mechanical Insufflation-Exsufflation

OBJECTIVES

Upon completion of this chapter, you will be able to:
· Compare volume-displacement and flow-dependent incentive spirometers.
· Describe two types of machines used to administer intermittent positive-pressure therapy.
· Discuss how expiratory positive airway pressure (EPAP), continuous positive airway pressure (CPAP), and positive expiratory pressure (PEP) therapies are used to mobilize secretions and treat atelectasis.
· Identify the major components of pneumatically and electrically powered percussors.
· Describe the theory of operation of four devices that enhance clearance of airway secretions by producing high-frequency oscillations to the lungs and chest wall.
· Discuss how mechanical insufflator-exsufflator devices can enhance airway secretions in patients with respiratory muscle weakness or paralysis.

KEY TERMS

Bennett valve
diluter regulator
flow-dependent incentive
    spirometer
Flutter valve
gas collector exhalation valve
high-frequency percussive
    breaths

magnetic valve resistors
mainstream nebulizers
mechanical
    insufflator-exsufflator
negative end-expiratory
    pressure (NEEP)
PEP therapy
Phasitron

sidestream nebulizers
spring-loaded valve resistors
sustained maximum inspiration
    (SMI)
underwater seal resistors
volume-displacement incentive
    spirometer
weighted-ball resistors

Bronchial hygiene therapy is an integral part of respiratory care. Various strategies and devices are used to help patients achieve and maintain optimum lung function, including lung expansion or hyperinflation therapy and airway secretion clearance techniques. The most common strategies involve deep-breathing exercises, directed coughing, postural drainage, endotracheal suctioning, and medical aerosol therapy.

The primary indication for lung expansion therapy is to prevent atelectasis. If left untreated, atelectasis can result in pulmonary shunting, hypoxemia, hypercapnia and, ultimately, respiratory failure. Factors that contribute to the development of atelectasis include retained secretions, altered breathing patterns, pain associated with surgery and trauma, chronic obstructive and restrictive pulmonary diseases, prolonged immobilization in a supine position, and increased intra-abdominal pressure.

The most common devices used by respiratory care practitioners in this type of therapy include incentive spirometers, intermittent positive-pressure breathing (IPPB) devices, chest wall percussors, and high-frequency oscillation devices. Selection of the appropriate device should be based on the patient's ability to perform the assigned therapy. Continuation of or changes in therapeutic goals should be determined by frequent assessment of the patient's status through physical assessment and review of laboratory test values.

INCENTIVE SPIROMETERS

Incentive spirometry (IS) is a lung expansion technique designed to mimic natural sighing or yawning by encouraging the patient to take slow, deep breaths.[1,2] It is a simple and relatively safe method of preventing atelectasis in alert patients who are predisposed to shallow breathing (e.g., patients recovering from thoracic or upper abdominal surgery; patients with chronic obstructive pulmonary disease [COPD] who are recovering from surgery; and patients who are immobilized or confined to bed).[3] The only contraindication to IS is a patient who is confused, uncooperative, or unable to deep breathe effectively (i.e., the vital capacity is less than 10 ml/kg, or the inspiratory capacity is less than one third of the predicted value).[2,3]

Although commercially produced incentive spirometers have been available for about 2 decades, the concept of **sustained maximum inspiration (SMI)** has been used since the latter part of the nineteenth century. Before the introduction of incentive spirometers, clinicians used devices and techniques such as blow-bottles, blow-gloves, and carbon dioxide–induced hyperventilation to accomplish the goal of having the patient take deep breaths to prevent atelectasis.

The principle of IS is based on the idea that the patient is encouraged to achieve a preset volume or flow, which is determined from predicted values or baseline measurements. Commercially available incentive spirometers are classified as either *volume-displacement* or *flow-dependent* devices. With volume-displacement devices, the volume of air the patient inspires during an SMI is measured and displayed. In contrast, flow-dependent devices measure the inspiratory flow the patient achieves during a maximum sustained inspiratory effort. Volume displacement can be derived with these latter devices by multiplying the flow achieved by the amount of time the flow is maintained.

No prospective studies as yet have demonstrated that IS is superior to other hyperexpansion methods that rely on natural deep-breathing exercises. Indeed, evidence suggests that deep breathing alone—without an incentive spirometer—can be beneficial for preventing or reversing pulmonary complications in some postoperative patients.[4-6] The advantage of using an incentive spirometer may be related to the fact that patients receive immediate visual feedback about whether they are achieving the prescribed goal (Clinical Rounds 7-1). Furthermore, patients can perform the treatment regimen without the direct supervision of a respiratory therapist after they have demonstrated mastery of the technique, which allows a cost-effective approach to lung expansion therapy. Clinical Practice Guideline 7-1 summarizes the Clinical Practice Guideline for Incentive Spirometry established by the American Association for Respiratory Care (AARC).[2]

Volume-Displacement Devices

Figure 7-1 is a schematic of a prototype of the **volume-displacement incentive spirometer.** The operational principle is simple: the patient inhales air through a mouthpiece and corrugated tubing attached to a flexible

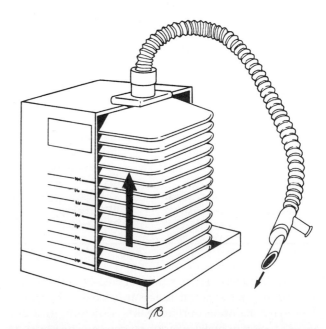

FIGURE 7-1 Volume-displacement incentive breathing exerciser. (From Eubanks DH, Bone RC: *Comprehensive respiratory care: a learning system,* ed 2, St Louis, 1990, Mosby.)

Incentive Spirometry (IS)

Clinical Practice Guideline 7-1

■ **INDICATIONS**
1. Conditions predisposed to the development of pulmonary atelectasis, such as upper abdominal surgery, thoracic surgery, and surgery in patients with chronic obstructive pulmonary disease (COPD)
2. Pulmonary atelectasis
3. Restrictive lung defects associated with quadriplegia or dysfunctional diaphragm

■ **CONTRAINDICATIONS**
1. Patient cannot be instructed or supervised to ensure appropriate use of the device.
2. Patient is unable to deep breathe effectively (e.g., vital capacity is less than 10 mL/kg, or inspiratory capacity is less than one third of that predicted).

■ **COMPLICATIONS**
1. Patient must be closely supervised, or therapy must be performed exactly as ordered.
2. Therapy is inappropriate as the only treatment for major lung collapse or consolidation.
3. Hyperventilation
4. Barotrauma (emphysematous lungs)
5. Discomfort secondary to inadequate pain control
6. Hypoxia secondary to interruption of oxygen therapy if face mask or shield is used
7. Exacerbation of bronchospasm
8. Fatigue

■ **ASSESSMENT OF OUTCOME**
Absence of or improvement in signs of atelectasis:
1. Decreased respiratory rate
2. Resolution of fever
3. Normal pulse rate
4. No crackles on auscultation, or improvement in previously absent or diminished breath sounds
5. Normal chest radiograph
6. Improved arterial oxygenation
7. Increased vital capacity and peak expiratory flows
8. Return of functional residual capacity or vital capacity to preoperative values without lung resection
9. Improved inspiratory muscle performance

■ **MONITORING**
Direct patient supervision is not necessary once the patient has demonstrated mastery of the technique; however, preoperative instruction, volume goals, and feedback are essential to optimum performance.

Modified from the American Association for Respiratory Care: AARC clinical practice guideline: incentive spirometry, Respir Care 36:1402, 1991.

plastic bellows. The volume of air displaced is indicated on a scale located on the device enclosure. After the patient has achieved the maximum volume, the individual is instructed to hold this volume constant for 3 to 5 seconds. The patient then can remove the mouthpiece and exhale, while the bellows expands to the starting position. Some authors have suggested that patients should perform a minimum of 5 to 10 breaths per session every hour while awake.[2] Note that the respiratory therapist does not have to be present for each performance, and patients should be encouraged to perform this therapy independently.

Incentive spirometers for adults typically have a total volume capacity of about 4 L, and those for children have a volume capacity of about 2 L. The Volurex incentive spirometer (DHD Medical Products, Wampsville, New York)

(Figure 7-2A) is a disposable device that operates similarly to the prototype unit described previously. It is slightly more sophisticated, however, in that after the patient inhales, the plastic bellows must be released by the push of a button before it returns to its starting position. The Voldyne 5000 Volumetric Exerciser (Hudson RCI, Temecula, California) (Figure 7-2B) and the Airlife Incentive Spirometer (Allegiance, McGaw Park, Illinois) (Figure 7-2C) consist of a movable piston in a clear cylinder. As the patient inhales, the piston rises and the inspired volume is indicated on a scale engraved on the side of the cylinder. A flow indicator is included as a visual aid to encourage the patient to take slow, deep breaths.

Most incentive spirometers are designed for single-patient use; multiple-use devices are available, but they are

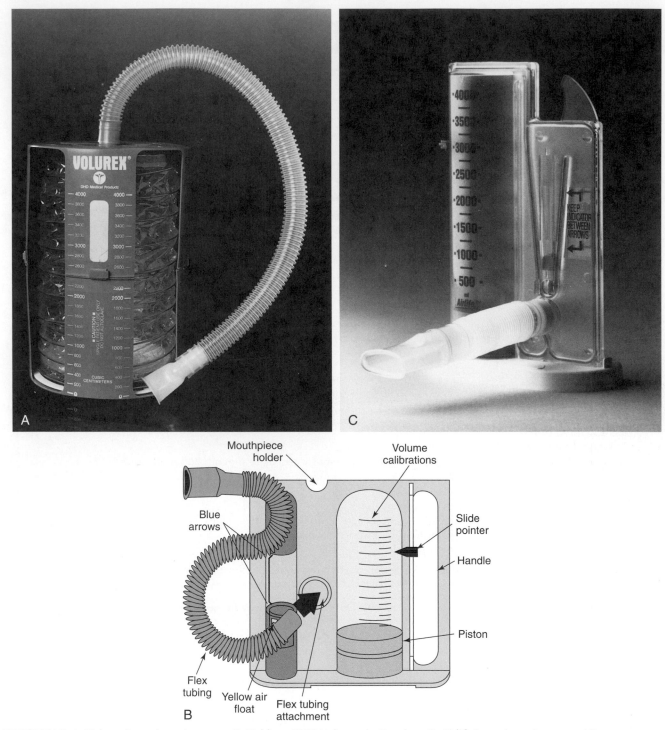

FIGURE 7-2 A, Volurex incentive spirometer. **B**, Voldyne 5000 Volumetric Exerciser. **C**, Airlife incentive spirometer. (**C** courtesy Allegiance, McGaw Park, Ill.)

rarely used anymore. Single-patient devices usually are made of plastic and can be discarded after the patient has completed the course of therapy. (Actually, patients should be encouraged to keep these devices and use them if similar respiratory illnesses develop.) Multiple-use incentive spirometers usually are electrically powered devices that use disposable mouthpieces and flow tubes and typically require that a respiratory therapist be available during the treatment.

Flow-Dependent Devices

Figure 7-3 shows an example of a **flow-dependent incentive spirometer,** which consists of a mouthpiece and corrugated tubing connected to a manifold composed of three flow tubes containing lightweight plastic balls. As the patient inhales through the mouthpiece, negative pressure is created within the tubes, causing them to rise. The device is designed so that the number of balls and the level to which they rise depend on the flow achieved. At lower flows, the first ball rises to a level that depends on the magnitude of the flow. As the inspiratory flow increases, the second ball rises, followed by the third ball. The flow achieved by the patient can be estimated based on the manufacturer's specifications. For example, with the Hudson RCI TriFlo II incentive spirometer, the patient must achieve a flow of 600 ml/sec to raise the first ball. A flow of 900 ml/sec is required to raise the second ball, and a flow of 1200 ml/sec must be generated to raise the third ball. As with volume-displacement incentive spirometers, it is important that the patient perform a maximum sustained inspiration.

The CliniFlo incentive spirometer (DHD Medical Products) (Figure 7-4) consists of a single plastic tube containing an indicator that rises as the patient makes an inspiratory effort. An adjustable volume selector can be used to vary the patient effort necessary to attain the desired inspiratory capacity. The CliniFlo contains an oxygen port that allows the clinician to provide supplemental oxygen if necessary. The Inspirx (Intertech Resources, INC., Keene, NH) incentive spirometer uses a similar design but can also display the number of successful efforts and the maximum flow achieved.[3] The LVE (lung volume exerciser) (Hudson RCI) (Figure 7-5) uses a different type of design: the patient inhales through a mouthpiece and corrugated tubing connected to a dual-chamber device. The two chambers of this device are arranged in series. The ball in the inner chamber rises when the patient achieves a flow that equals the inspiratory flow selected by the operator. Inspiratory flows vary from 200 ml/sec to 1200 ml/sec.

INTERMITTENT POSITIVE-PRESSURE BREATHING (IPPB) DEVICES

Intermittent positive-pressure breathing is a short-term therapeutic modality that involves the delivery of inspiratory positive pressure to spontaneously breathing patients. Since its introduction in 1947, IPPB has been used for a variety of purposes, including short-term ventilatory support and lung expansion therapy and as an aid in the delivery of aerosolized medications.[7,8] Over the past 2 decades, the effectiveness of IPPB as a therapeutic modality has been questioned rigorously, resulting in a reassessment of the indications for its prescription. The AARC produced a Clinical Practice Guideline in 1993 and a revised version in 2003 to provide a rational basis for prescribing and administering IPPB treatments (Clinical Practice Guideline 7-2 presents a summary of this guideline).[8,9] Although it has been suggested that negative positive-pressure

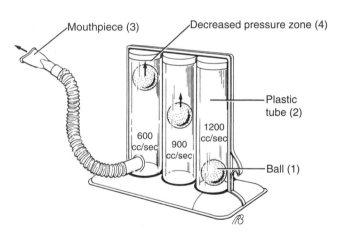

FIGURE 7-3 Flow-dependent incentive spirometer. (From Eubanks DH, Bone RC: *Comprehensive respiratory care,* St Louis, 1985, Mosby.)

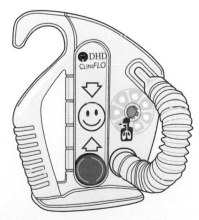

FIGURE 7-4 CliniFlo Low-Flow Breathing Exerciser incentive spirometer.

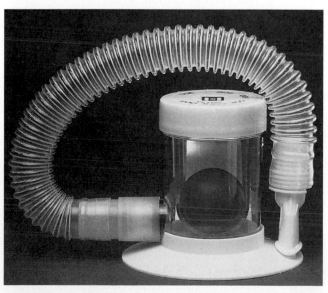

FIGURE 7-5 LVE (lung volume exerciser) incentive spirometer. (Courtesy Hudson RCI, Temecula, Calif.)

Intermittent Positive Pressure Breathing (IPPB)

Clinical Practice Guideline 7-2

■ INDICATIONS

1. The need to improve lung expansion, particularly for patients who demonstrate clinically important atelectasis when other forms of therapy, such as incentive spirometry, chest physiotherapy (CPT), deep-breathing exercises, and positive airway pressure (PAP), are unsuccessful. It may also be useful for patients who cannot cooperate with standard lung expansion techniques.
2. Inability to clear secretions adequately because of pathosis that severely limits the patient's ability to ventilate or cough effectively.
3. As an alternative to endotracheal intubation and continuous ventilatory support for patients requiring short-term ventilatory support. Devices specifically designed to deliver noninvasive positive-pressure ventilation (NPPV) should also be considered.
4. To deliver aerosolized medications to patients fatigued as a result of respiratory muscle weakness. Note that this guideline does not address aerosol delivery for patients on long-term mechanical ventilation. It may also be used to deliver aerosolized medications to patients unable to use a metered-dose inhaler (MDI).
5. IPPB may reduce the sensation of dyspnea and its associated discomfort during nebulizer therapy in patients with severe hyperinflation.

■ CONTRAINDICATIONS

1. Untreated tension pneumothorax
2. Elevated intracranial pressure (>15 mm Hg)
3. Hemodynamic instability
4. Recent facial, oral, or skull surgery
5. Tracheoesophageal fistula
6. Recent esophageal surgery
7. Active hemoptysis
8. Nausea
9. Air swallowing
10. Active, untreated tuberculosis
11. Radiographic evidence of a bleb
12. Hiccups

■ HAZARDS

1. Increased airway resistance and work of breathing
2. Barotrauma, pneumothorax
3. Nosocomial infection
4. Hypocarbia (hypocapnia)
5. Hemoptysis
6. Hyperoxia when oxygen is the gas source
7. Gastric distention
8. Impaction of secretions associated with inadequately humidified gas mixture
9. Psychological dependence
10. Impeded venous return
11. Exacerbation of hypoxemia
12. Hypoventilation or hyperventilation
13. Increased mismatch of ventilation and perfusion
14. Air trapping, auto-PEEP, overdistended alveoli

■ ASSESSMENT OF NEED

1. Presence of clinically significant atelectasis.
2. Reduced pulmonary function: forced vital capacity (FVC) <70% of predicted; maximum voluntary ventilation (MVV) <50% of predicted; or vital capacity (VC) <10 ml/kg of predicted, precluding an effective cough.
3. Neuromuscular disorders or kyphoscoliosis associated with reduced lung volumes.
4. Fatigue or respiratory muscle weakness with impending respiratory failure.
5. Based on proven therapeutic efficacy, variety of medications, and cost-effectiveness, the metered-dose inhaler (MDI) with a spacing device or holding chamber should be the first method considered for administration of aerosol therapy.

Intermittent Positive Pressure Breathing (IPPB)—cont'd

6. If effective, the patient's preference for a positive-pressure device should be honored.
7. IPPB may be indicated for patients who are at risk for the development of atelectasis and are unable or unwilling to perform deep-breathing exercises without assistance.

■ ASSESSMENT OF OUTCOMES

1. A minimum delivered tidal volume of at least one third of the predicted inspiratory capacity ($1/3 \times 50$ ml/kg) has been suggested (e.g., 1200 ml for a 70-kg individual).
2. Increase in forced expiratory volume in one second (FEV_1) or peak expiratory flow (PEF).
3. Improved cough with treatment, leading to better clearance of secretions.
4. Improvements in chest radiographs
5. Improved breath sounds
6. Favorable patient response

■ MONITORING

1. Machine performance: trigger sensitivity, peak pressure, flow setting, fractional inspired oxygen (F_IO_2), inspiratory time, expiratory time, plateau pressure, positive end-expiratory pressure (PEEP)
2. Respiratory rate
3. Delivered tidal volume
4. Patient's subjective response to therapy
5. Sputum production (quantity, color, consistency)
6. Skin color
7. Breath sounds
8. Blood pressure
9. Arterial hemoglobin saturation by pulse oximetry if hypoxemia is suspected
10. Intracranial pressure (ICP) in patients for whom it is of critical importance
11. Chest radiograph

Modified from the American Association for Respiratory Care: AARC clinical practice guideline: intermittent positive pressure breathing—2003 revisions and update, Respir Care 438:540, 2003.

ventilation (NPPV) may be considered a form of IPPB, the current clinical practice guideline does not provide guidance on this therapeutic modality.[9]

In the critical care setting, IPPB can be used every 1 to 6 hours as tolerated. In these cases, the IPPB order should be reevaluated at least daily. Continuation or discontinuation of the order should be based on the assessment outcomes for the patient obtained during each treatment session. When it is prescribed in the general care setting, IPPB typically is ordered 2 to 4 times daily and usually is determined by the patient's response to therapy. In these cases, therapy should be reevaluated at least every 72 hours or with any change in the patient's health status. Similarly, patients receiving IPPB therapy in the home should be reevaluated periodically and with any change in health status.[9]

It should be recognized that although IPPB is not the therapy of choice when other modalities can be used for aerosol delivery or lung expansion in spontaneously breathing patients, it can be potentially beneficial when IS, chest physiotherapy, deep-breathing exercises, and positive airway pressure (PAP) techniques have been unsuccessful (Clinical Rounds 7-2).

IPPB can be administered with any device that can deliver intermittent positive pressure to the airway (e.g.,

CLINICAL ROUNDS 7-2

A 38-year-old man is admitted to the hospital from a rehabilitation center with a diagnosis of pneumonia. He has quadriplegia and permanent brain damage as a result of a motor vehicle accident. He also has a permanent tracheostomy but does not require ventilatory support. Current evaluation reveals the following: temperature 103° F; respiratory rate = 28 breaths/min; heart rate = 100 beats/min; pulse oximetry oxygen saturation (SpO_2) on 30% heated tracheostomy collar is 93%. Copious amounts of thick, green secretions are present, and the patient coughs only when stimulated with suctioning. Crackles are present in both bases. Based on these findings, what form of respiratory care would you recommend?

See Evolve Resources for the answer.

conventional mechanical ventilators or manual resuscitators), but it most often is performed with specially designed electrically and pneumatically powered ventilators. These IPPB machines usually are categorized as patient-triggered, pressure- and time-limited, and pressure- or flow-cycled mechanical ventilators. Regardless of the manufacturer, all

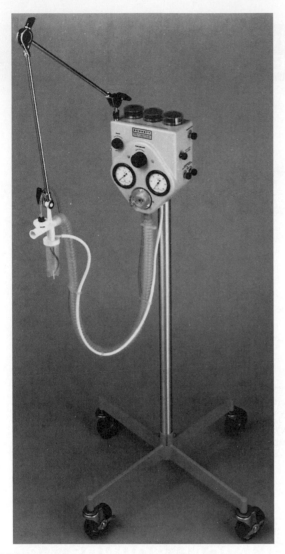

FIGURE 7-6 Bennett PR-1 ventilator. (Courtesy Tyco Healthcare, Puritan Bennett, Pleasanton, Calif.)

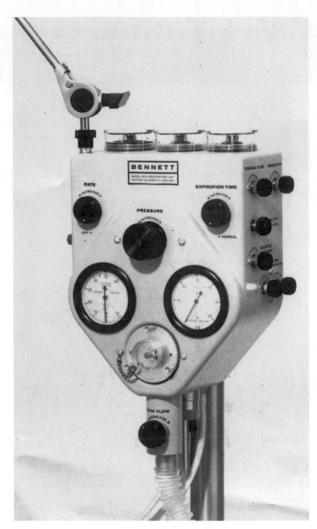

FIGURE 7-7 Bennett PR-2 ventilator. (Courtesy Tyco Healthcare, Puritan Bennett, Pleasanton, Calif.)

IPPB machines require a 45- to 55-psig gas source, such as a compressed-gas cylinder, a bulk air or oxygen system, or an air compressor. Furthermore, they all incorporate control valves that begin inspiration when a negative pressure is generated by the patient and terminate it when a preset pressure or flow is achieved. The amount of negative pressure (i.e., patient effort) required to initiate inspiration depends on the sensitivity of the device, which may be fixed or adjustable. The pressure that must be achieved to end inspiration, and thus initiate exhalation, typically can be adjusted to as high as 60 cm H_2O.[8,9]

Machines manufactured by Puritan Bennett (Tyco Healthcare, Pleasanton, California) and Bird Products (Viasys Healthcare, Palm Springs, California) still are the most widely used devices for IPPB therapy. A relatively recent advance in IPPB equipment is the introduction of a single-use, disposable device by Vortran Medical Technology (Sacramento, California). A brief description of these devices follows.

Puritan Bennett Devices

Puritan Bennett manufactures pneumatically and electrically powered IPPB machines. The tank ventilator (TV), pedestal ventilator (PV), and pedestal respirator (PR) series are pneumatically powered IPPB machines; the air-powered (AP) series of ventilators are electrically powered. The PR-1 and PR-2 models are the most commonly used pneumatically powered IPPB devices. The AP-4 and AP-5 models are the most commonly used electrically powered IPPB machines.

Puritan Bennett PR Series

The PR-1 (Figure 7-6) and PR-2 (Figure 7-7) ventilators are pneumatically powered devices that can be time or pressure triggered, but both are flow cycled and pressure limited. (Note that time cycling allows these devices to provide controlled, short-term ventilatory support.) They can deliver either 100% source gas or air-diluted source gas.

The PR-2 has adjustable controls for setting the pressure limit and the sensitivity or level of negative pressure

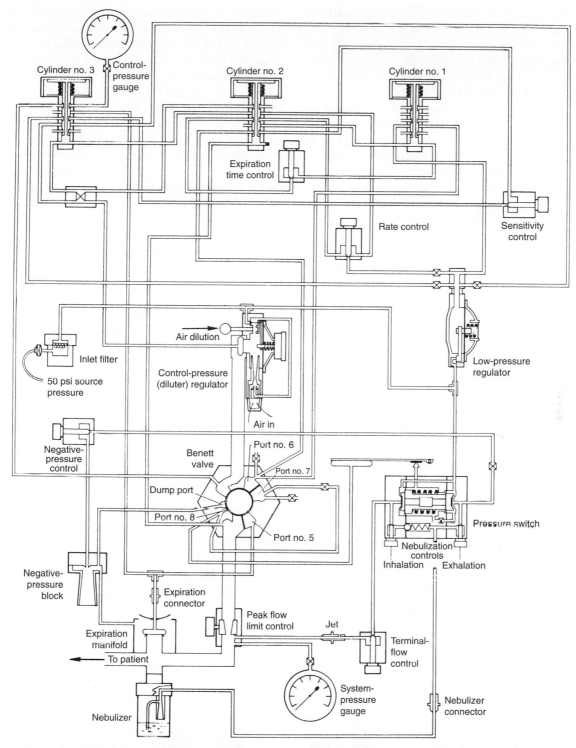

FIGURE 7-8 Flow schematic of the Bennett PR-2 ventilator as shown from behind the device. (Courtesy Tyco Healthcare, Puritan Bennett, Pleasanton, Calif.)

that must be achieved to initiate inspiration. It also has controls for adjusting the peak flow, inspiratory and expiratory nebulizer gas flows, and **negative end-expiratory pressure (NEEP).** A terminal flow control is provided for minor leak compensation. In contrast, the PR-1 does not have a peak flow control or the capability of providing NEEP. The PR-1 does not have separate controls for inspi-

ratory and expiratory nebulization; instead, inspiratory nebulization is a composite of continuous nebulization and the inspiratory nebulizer flow. The PR-1 does not have an expiratory time control.

Gas flow through the PR-2 ventilator is shown in Figure 7-8. (Note that gas flow through the PR-1 is comparable.) Compressed gas from a 50-psig gas source enters the ventilator through a brass filter. It is directed to a **diluter regulator,** to the nebulizer pressure switch, and to a low-pressure regulator. The diluter regulator (Figure 7-9) is an adjustable reducing valve that regulates the gas pressure delivered to the patient. It can be set from 0 to 30 cm H_2O using a control knob on the front panel of the machine. Gas flow to a nebulizer switch controls the flow of gas to the nebulizer during inspiration and expiration. Nebulizer flow can be adjusted with two knobs on the lower part of the machine's side panel. (Note that the nebulizer is powered by 100% source gas; therefore, use of the nebulizer affects the delivered fractionated inspired oxygen [F_1O_2] when the PR-2 is set to air dilution mode.) Gas flow to the nebulizer also controls a Venturi that allows the application of NEEP from 0 to −6 cm H_2O. The NEEP level can be adjusted with a knob just above the inspiratory nebulizer control on the side panel. NEEP originally was proposed as a means of reducing the level of air trapping experienced by some patients during IPPB. Because it subsequently was found that applying NEEP actually increased the level of air trapping, this therapeutic mode is no longer used.

From the diluter regulator, gas flows to the **Bennett valve,** which consists of a counterweighted, hollow drum with attached vanes (Figure 7-10). (It is called a Bennett valve for Dr. Ray Bennett, who invented it in 1945 for use in high-altitude aircraft breathing apparatuses. After World War II, the valve was adapted for medical applications.[10]) The drum rotates in a special housing on the front and rear jeweled bearings.* As Figure 7-10A shows, the drum vane creates a barrier between atmospheric and circuit pressures. Inspiration is triggered when the patient removes enough volume from the tubing to create a pressure gradient of 0.5 cm H_2O across the valve, thus causing it to rotate counterclockwise (B). (Note that the manufacturer presets the sensitivity of the machine at 0.5 cm H_2O, but the sensitivity [or amount of patient effort] that must be exerted to trigger inspiration can be changed by rotating the sensitivity knob counterclockwise.) The sensitivity of this valve is ultimately controlled by gas that flows to the low-pressure regulator mentioned previously. Gas flow from the low-pressure regulator is directed to the Bennett valve via a port located just above the upper drum vane. As the sensitivity is increased, the gas flow through the port rotates the drum counterclockwise toward inspiration, making it easier for the patient to trigger the ventilator (i.e., the patient can trigger inspiration with less effort). A small flow of gas from the valve travels out of the exhalation valve line and inflates an exhalation diaphragm, preventing gas from escaping through the exhalation port during the inspiratory phase. Gas, which is directed into the breathing circuit and to the patient, flows through the valve, holding it open. As the pressure proximal to the valve is kept constant, the pressure gradient decreases, allowing gravity to cause a counterweight to slowly rotate the valve clockwise, back toward the closed position (C). When the flow through the valve decreases to 1 to 3 L/min, the force of gravity is sufficient to swing the valve completely closed, thus terminating inspiration (D). After the valve is closed, gas flow to the exhalation diaphragm is halted and the diaphragm deflates, allowing gas from the patient circuit to flow into the room.

*It is important to recognize that the bearing and housing have serial numbers that must match. These components are specially machined, and mismatching of the serial numbers or damage to the bearing will impair the function of the valve.[9]

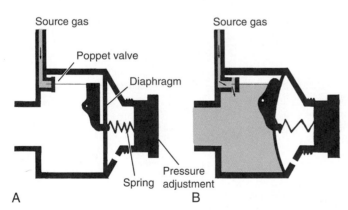

FIGURE 7-9 Bennett diluter regulator. **A,** Pressure equals spring tension. **B,** Pressure is below spring tension.

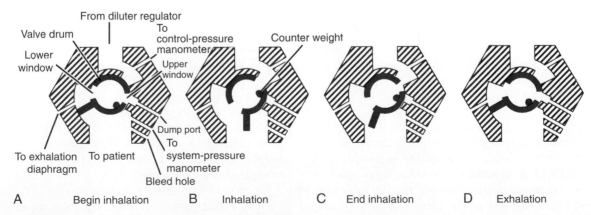

FIGURE 7-10 Functional diagram of the Bennett valve. (Courtesy Tyco Healthcare, Puritan Bennett, Pleasanton, Calif.)

Notice that the Bennett valve also includes a port (which releases gas from within the drum to atmospheric pressure [exhalation]), a bleed hole (which allows a small leak when the valve opens to prevent it from recoiling or fluttering), and two manometer ports (see Figure 7-10A). One of these manometer ports is for controlling pressure from the diluter regulator, and the other monitors pressure in the patient circuit.

Puritan Bennett AP Series

The AP-4 and AP-5 units (Figure 7-11) are electrically powered, pressure-limited ventilators. Unlike the PR series, these devices are only patient triggered, therefore they can be used for IPPB therapy but not for providing short-term ventilatory support of apneic patients. As shown in Figure 7-12, air from the unit's compressor passes through a filter and flows to the Venturi jet in the pressure control and then to a needle valve that controls the level of nebuliza-tion. The Venturi jet entrains additional air through an intake filter, and the AP machines have a spring-disk release valve instead of the diluter regulator of the PR series. When the pressure in the system control unit exceeds that of the spring tension, the pressure pushes the disk to the left, allowing the excess pressure to vent to ambient pressure. Note that the spring tension on the disk, and thus the peak pressure, can be adjusted to values of 0 to 30 cm H_2O. With all gas venting through the release valve, the Bennett valve rotates shut, starting exhalation. When the Bennett valve opens, gas flows from the control unit to the patient.

Puritan Bennett Circuits

The basic components of the Puritan Bennett breathing circuit comprise large-bore corrugated tubing, a nebulizer, and an exhalation valve. Two types of nebulizers are available: **mainstream nebulizers** (Bennett slip/stream) and **sidestream nebulizers** (Bennett Twin) (Figure 7-13).

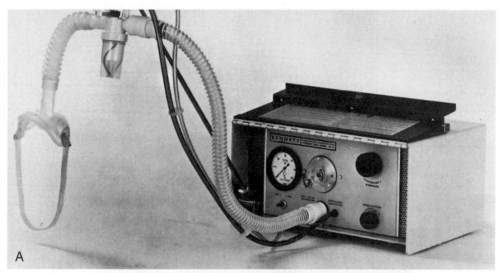

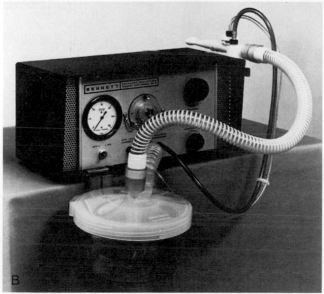

FIGURE 7-11 A, Bennett AP-4. **B**, Bennett AP-5. Both units are air compressor–driven ventilators. (Courtesy Tyco Healthcare, Puritan Bennett, Pleasanton, Calif.)

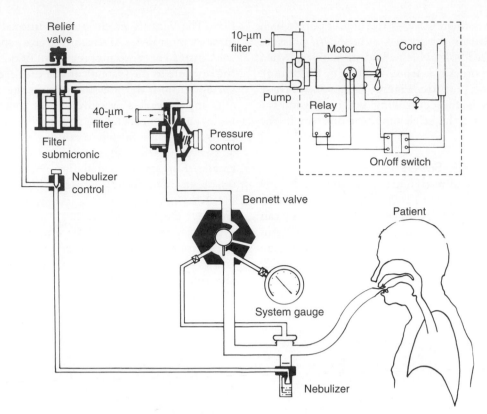

FIGURE 7-12 Functional diagram of the Bennett AP series ventilators. (Courtesy Tyco Healthcare, Puritan Bennett, Pleasanton, Calif.)

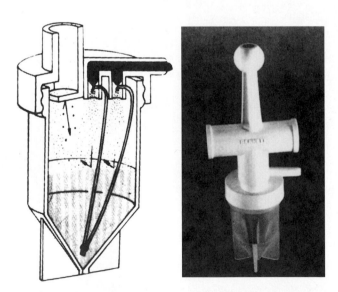

FIGURE 7-13 Bennett Twin jet nebulizer. (Courtesy Tyco Healthcare, Puritan Bennett, Pleasanton, Calif.)

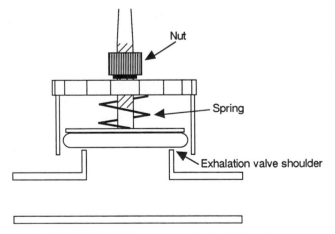

FIGURE 7-14 Bennett retard exhalation valve.

The Bennett retard exhalation valve (Figure 7-14) consists of a spring that is compressed as the diaphragm nut is tightened. When the nut is loosened, the spring pushes the diaphragm closer to the shoulder of the exhalation valve, causing a resistance to expiratory gas flow. The **gas collector exhalation valve** (Figure 7-15) allows expired gases to be measured through one directional port.

Bird Devices

The prototype Bird ventilator is the Mark 7, which was designed and developed by Forrest M. Bird, founder of the Bird Corporation. Bird subsequently introduced the Mark 8, which functions similarly to the Mark 7 but can provide a flow of source gas during the expiratory phase, thus allowing the operator to apply a negative expiratory pressure. A second generation of Bird ventilators was introduced in the late 1970s and provided additional capabilities. These latter units, however, also used the same ceramic control valve and ambient and pressure compartments as the first generation of Bird ventilators.

Before the components of the various Bird IPPB ventilators are described, their basic operational principle should be discussed. This principle has been referred to as magnetism versus gas pressure and can be described using the schematic in Figure 7-16. Notice that the schematic includes a series of boxes. Each box is divided into two compartments by a diaphragm, which has metal clutch plates attached to either side. Permanent magnets, which are aligned with the clutch plates, are located in each compartment. The left compartment is exposed to atmospheric pressure through a port in the lower left corner of box. The pressure on the right side of each box can be varied by moving gas into and out of a port in the lower right corner of the box.

If the two compartments are subjected to atmospheric pressure (Figure 7-16A), there is no pressure difference between them and the diaphragm remains straight. When a pressure gradient is created between the right and left compartments, the diaphragm flexes. In Figure 7-16B, as gas volume is removed from the right compartment, the pressure inside the compartment drops to below atmospheric pressure, causing the diaphragm and the attached metal plates to flex to the right. The clutch plate on the right is now close to the magnet on the right, and the plate and magnet are attracted to each other. Although the pressure on the right may return to atmospheric pressure (Figure 7-16C), the diaphragm remains attracted to the right magnet until sufficient gas volume and pressure are added to the right side to overcome the magnetic attraction (Figure 7-16D). When sufficient positive pressure

exists to overcome the magnetic attraction, the diaphragm is pushed to the left, where it will remain.

Bird Mark 7 Series

The Mark 7 is a pneumatically powered ventilator that can be time, pressure, or manually triggered and time or pressure cycled. Similar to the Puritan Bennett PR series, the Mark 7 can be used to provide short-term ventilatory support, but it is primarily used as a means of delivering IPPB therapy.

Figure 7-17 shows the major components of the Bird Mark 7 ventilator. Gas flow through the Mark 7 is shown in Figure 7-18. During inspiration (Figure 7-18A), negative pressure generated by the patient (along with atmospheric pressure in the left compartment) causes the diaphragm to move toward the right, away from the left compartment. Gas flow is allowed to pass through the ceramic control switch and then splits, traveling in the left side to the Venturi jet and passing to the line powering the nebulizer and exhalation valve. The Venturi jet then entrains air, and gas moves through the Venturi gate to the patient. This gas enters the patient's lungs, and the pressure begins to build in the right compartment. Thus at the beginning of inspiration, gas flow into the circuit comes from three sources: (1) the Venturi jet, (2) the air the Venturi entrains, and (3) the nebulizer jet. As end-inspiration is approached, the pressure in the right compartment equals the forward pressure through the Venturi jet, and the Venturi gate closes. The gas from the Venturi jet is then forced into the left side of the machine, flushing that compartment with source gas. After the Venturi gate closes, the only gas flowing into the patient's system during the remainder of inspiration comes from source gas through the nebulizer jet. Eventually this jet adds enough gas to make the pressure exceed the magnetic attraction of the right (pressure-controlled) magnet. The diaphragm, clutch plate, and ceramic switch are then forced to the left, occluding gas flow into the respirator and starting exhalation. The amount of pressure needed to end inspiration depends on the magnetic attraction between the right clutch plate and the corresponding magnet. As with the left clutch plate and magnet, the amount of attraction is related to the distance between the right plate and its magnet. The

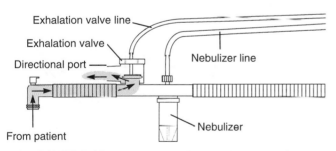

FIGURE 7-15 Bennett gas collector exhalation valve.

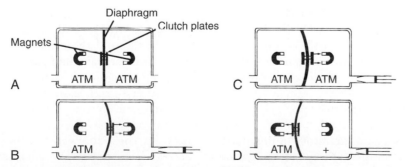

FIGURE 7-16 Pressure changes across the diaphragm with magnetic force. See text for explanation. *ATM,* Atmospheric pressure. (Modified from Viasys Healthcare, Critical Care Division, Palm Springs, Calif.)

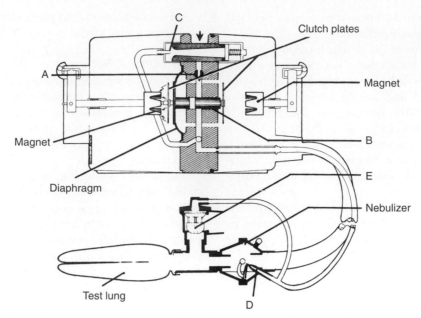

FIGURE 7-17 Structure of the Bird Mark 7 ventilator. (Modified from Viasys Healthcare, Critical Care Division, Palm Springs, Calif.)

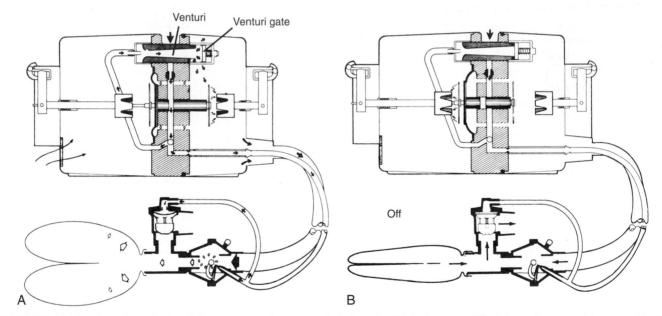

FIGURE 7-18 Gas flow through the Bird Mark 7 ventilator. **A,** Inhalation. **B,** Exhalation. (Modified from Viasys Healthcare, Critical Care Division, Palm Springs, Calif.)

distance, and thus the peak inspiratory pressure, can be set with the pressure adjustment lever on the right side of the machine. Because gas is no longer flowing into the flow control valve, the gas in the lines below the ceramic switch exits through the jets. The diaphragm and exhalation valve are now uncharged, and the existing positive pressure in the patient circuit simply pushes the exhalation valve gate open, allowing the patient to exhale passively (Figure 7-18B).

The Mark 7 has a pneumatic expiratory timing device that can be used to provide pressure-cycled ventilation. The timer is a pneumatic cartridge with an adjustable leak (Figure 7-19). On inspiration, the cartridge is charged by source gas, which enters via a one-way valve. The gas pushes the diaphragm to the left, depressing the spring and moving the plunger and arm to the left. The leak from the cartridge around the needle valve control is small compared with the incoming gas flow. Thus after inspiration has begun, the unit is completely charged until inhalation ends. At end-inspiration, no source gas is supplied to the cartridge, and the one-way entrance valve closes. The only way for gas to leave the cartridge is the leak past the needle valve on the outflow track. As gas leaks out, pressure decreases, and the diaphragm is pushed to the right by the spring. Concurrently, the plunger and its attached arm are moved slowly to the right. After the arm touches the clutch

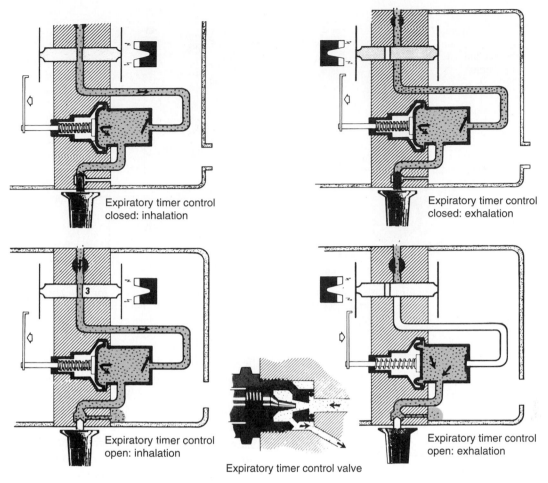

Expiratory timer control
closed: inhalation

Expiratory timer control
closed: exhalation

Expiratory timer control
open: inhalation

Expiratory timer control
open: exhalation

Expiratory timer control valve

FIGURE 7-19 Exhalation timer and control. (Modified from Viasys Healthcare, Critical Care Division, Palm Springs, Calif.)

plate, the clutch plate is pushed away from the magnet, and the ceramic switch is moved into the "on" position. Thus the length of expiratory time is controlled by the needle valve; the greater the leak past the needle valve, the faster the cartridge discharges and the shorter the exhalation time.

Notice that directly below the ceramic switch is the Air-Mix control. As shown in Figure 7-19, it is a two-position switch that allows for delivery of either an air-mixed gas (varying F_IO_2) or a gas with an F_IO_2 of 1. When this switch is pushed in, the O-rings seal the incoming source gas and direct it out the reed-covered bleed hole in the center body, providing a constant flow during the inspiratory phase. When the Air-Mix control switch is pulled out, the top O-ring blocks the bleed hole, and gas is directed to the jet of the Air-Mix Venturi. The decompression port above the bleed hole allows the plunger to be pushed in without compressing the gas behind it, therefore functionally it plays no part in the Air-Mix control. In the Air-Mix (switch pulled out) setting (Figure 7-20A), source gas comes from (1) the Venturi jet, (2) the air entrained by the Venturi system, and (3) the nebulizer jet. In the Air-Mix position, the Venturi is activated, producing a descending flow pattern and an irregular pressure waveform that ranges

from ascending to rectangular, depending on the compliance and resistance of the patient's respiratory system. In the 100% setting (i.e., switch pushed in; Figure 7-20B), two sources provide gas flow throughout inspiration, producing a square wave or constant flow pattern and an ascending pressure waveform.

The Mark 7A respirator is an updated version of the Mark 7 respirator. It features apneustic flowtime, a mechanical means of simulating a dynamic (time-cycled) postinspiratory breath hold for increased distribution and retention of inspired aerosols. In addition to the apneustic flowtime device, the Mark 7A has an independent flow control that permits precise regulation of gas flow.

Bird Mark 8 Series

The Bird Mark 8 ventilator (Figure 7-21) is functionally similar to the Mark 7, but it can provide a constant flow of source gas during the expiratory phase. The knob for adjusting the level of flow is on top of the machine, connected to a needle valve and a flow interrupter switch. The switch is a pneumatic cartridge containing a plunger, spring, and diaphragm. During inspiration, gas flows through the ceramic switch, which charges the cartridge and blocks the flow of 50-psig source gas to the Venturi.

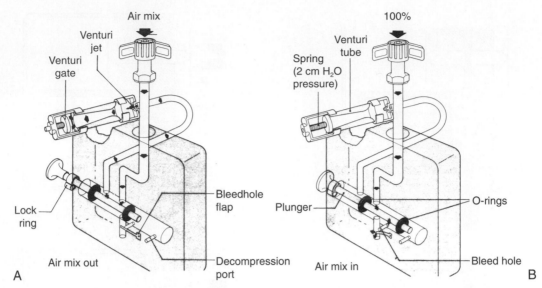

FIGURE 7-20 Air-Mix control for the Bird Mark 7 ventilator. The schematics show typical patterns for flow and pressure during Air-Mix *(left)* and 100% oxygen *(right)*. (Modified from Viasys Healthcare, Critical Care Division, Palm Springs, Calif.)

During expiration, gas flowing through the Venturi entrains expired gases from the circuit and the patient and directs them out the exhalation valve.

The Bird Mark 8 originally was designed to allow for the application of NEEP. As previously stated, NEEP has been shown to be ineffective in reducing air trapping and is no longer used.

Bird Mark 10 and 14 Series

The Mark 10 and Mark 14 ventilators are similar to the Mark 7 series, except that they do not have an Air-Mix control, which means that they can operate only in the air dilution mode. In addition, they have a control for providing inspiratory flow acceleration, which can be used to compensate for leaks in the system. The primary difference between the Mark 14 series and the Mark 10 series is that Mark 14 ventilators can produce pressures as high as 200 cm H_2O.[10]

Vortran Intermittent Positive-Pressure Breathing Device

The Vortran IPPB device provides short-term, pressure-triggered, pressure-cycled, constant-flow ventilatory support in combination with aerosol delivery.[11] The primary advantage of this device is that it is relatively compact and inexpensive compared with conventional IPPB devices. Also, Vortran IPPB units are single-patient, multiple-use devices, which reduces the incidence of nosocomial infections from cross-contamination.

The major components of the Vortran IPPB device include a pressure modulator coupled with a nebulizer (Figure 7-22). The unit runs on a continuous flow of gas of up to 40 L/min. (Flows of 40 L/min are automatically achieved when the unit is connected to a 50-psig source gas; flows of 15 to 40 L/min can be achieved by connecting the system to a 50-psig source gas using a standard hospital flowmeter.) Peak inspiratory pressures can be adjusted between 20 and 50 cm H_2O, and the device can produce a positive-end expiratory pressure (PEEP) of 2 to 5 cm H_2O (the manufacturer reports that the set PEEP typically is one tenth of the peak pressure). The inspiratory time and rate can be adjusted over a wide range (i.e., 8 to 20 breaths per minute). As Table 7-1 shows, the estimated delivered tidal volume depends on the flow and the inspiratory time.

The device's nebulizer, which provides the continuous flow of gas and a patient demand valve, can hold 20 ml of solution for nebulization. The nebulizer is also equipped with an air entrainment valve, which allows the patient to entrain additional air through the nebulizer. (Note that the F_IO_2 will vary with the amount of room air entrained by the patient through the nebulizer.)

Recent studies have demonstrated that the Vortran IPPB device can achieve inspiratory flows and tidal volumes comparable to those produced by conventional IPPB units. Furthermore, this device offers an alternative for the delivery of IPPB to hospitalized and home care patients. It is important to recognize that the Vortran IPPB device's modulator is similar to that of a pop-off valve. The device is *not* equipped with a redundant pop-off valve and should not be used with patients with endotracheal or tracheostomy tubes. It should be used cautiously when IPPB is administered with a mask.

POSITIVE AIRWAY PRESSURE (PAP) DEVICES

Positive airway pressure techniques, which include continuous positive airway pressure (CPAP), expiratory positive airway pressure (EPAP), and positive expiratory

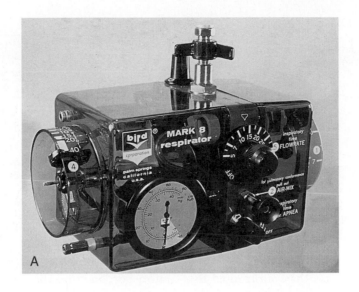

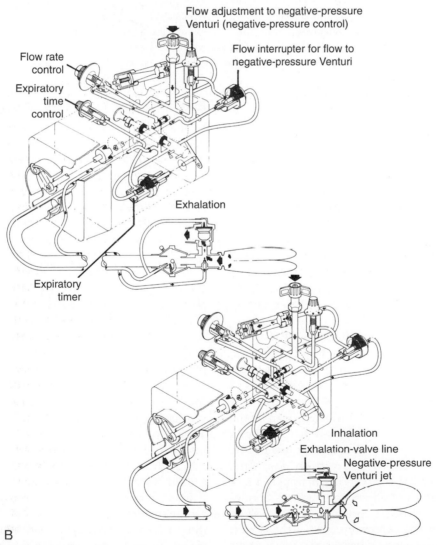

FIGURE 7-21 A, Bird Mark 8 ventilator. **B**, Bird Mark 8 flow diagram. (Modified from Viasys Healthcare, Critical Care Division, Palm Springs, Calif.)

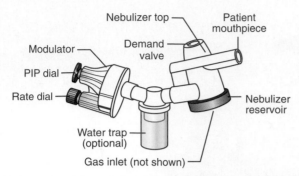

FIGURE 7-22 Major components of the Vortran intermittent positive-pressure breathing device. (Redrawn from Vortran Medical Technology: *Vortran IPPB user's guide*, Sacramento, Calif, 2005, Vortran.)

TABLE 7-1

Estimated Tidal Volume (mL) delivered at Various Flow (LPM) and Inspiratory Time (seconds)

Flow (LPM)	Inspiratory Time (seconds)					
	0.5	1	1.5	2	2.5	3
15	125	250	375	500	625	750
20	167	333	500	667	833	1000
25	208	417	625	833	1042	1250
30	250	500	750	1000	1250	1500
35	292	583	875	1167	1458	1750
40	333	667	1000	1333	1667	2000

From Vortran Medical Technology: *Vortran IPPB user's guide*, Sacramento, Calif, 2005, Votran.

pressure (PEP), are airway adjuncts that can be used to enhance bronchial hygiene therapy by reducing air trapping in susceptible patients.[1] As such, these techniques have been shown to be quite effective in mobilizing retained secretions, preventing or reversing atelectasis, and optimizing the delivery of bronchodilators to patients with cystic fibrosis and chronic bronchitis. The AARC has produced a Clinical Practice Guideline for PAP adjuncts to bronchial hygiene therapy, which should be read before PAP therapy is performed on patients.[12] Clinical Practice Guideline 7-3 summarizes several important points from this guideline.

Continuous Positive Airway Pressure

Continuous positive airway pressure therapy involves the application of positive pressure to a patient's airways throughout the respiratory cycle (i.e., the airway pressure is consistently maintained between 5 and 20 cm H_2O during both inspiration and expiration). It is accomplished by having the patient breathe from a pressurized circuit that incorporates a threshold resistor in the expiratory limb.

Figure 7-23 shows four types of threshold resistors: **underwater seal resistors, weighted-ball resistors, spring-loaded valve resistors,** and **magnetic valve resistors.**[13] With underwater seal resistors, tubing attached to the expiratory port of the circuit is submerged under a column of water. The level of CPAP is determined by the height of the column. Weighted-ball resistors consist of a specially milled steel ball placed over a calibrated orifice, which is attached directly above the expiratory port of the circuit. It is important that the balls are maintained in a vertical position to ensure consistent pressure.[1] Spring-loaded valve resistors rely on a spring to hold a disk or diaphragm down over the expiratory port of the circuit. Magnetic valve resistors contain a bar magnet that attracts a ferromagnetic disk seated on the expiratory port of the circuit. The amount of pressure required to separate the disk from the magnet is determined by the distance between them (i.e., the greater the distance between the magnet and

the disk, the lower the pressure required to open the expiratory port and thus the lower the level of CPAP).

All these valves operate on the principle that the level of PAP generated within the circuit depends on the amount of resistance that must be overcome to allow gas to exit the exhalation valve. The main advantage of threshold resistors is that they provide predictable, quantifiable, and constant force during expiration that is independent of the flow achieved by the patient during exhalation.[1,13]

Expiratory Positive Airway Pressure

Expiratory positive airway pressure is another method of delivering PAP to spontaneously breathing patients. EPAP differs from CPAP because it involves the creation of PAP only during expiration. With EPAP, the patient generates a subatmospheric pressure on inspiration and then exhales against a threshold expiratory resistance similar to that described for CPAP devices. Airway pressures during EPAP can be set at 10 to 20 cm H_2O.

Positive Expiratory Pressure

Positive expiratory pressure (PEP) has received considerable attention during the past 10 years, especially in the management of patients with cystic fibrosis. The rationale for performing **PEP therapy** is similar to that for the use of CPAP and EPAP, except that PEP seems to be less cumbersome and more manageable for patients.

Figure 7-24A shows a prototype device that can be used for PEP therapy. The device includes a mouthpiece (or ventilation mask), a T-piece assembly with a one-way valve, a series of fixed orifice resistors (or an adjustable orifice resistor), and a pressure manometer. The theory of operation of these PEP devices is that the patient exhales against a fixed resistance, creating a back pressure that in turn helps maintain airway patency in patients who experience airway closure (e.g., bronchiectasis). The Thera-PEP device (Smith Medical, Carlsbad, California) (Figure 7-24B) provides a series of fixed orifices that can be used to accommodate patients over a wide range of lung capacities. The amount of PAP generated with the fixed-orifice resistor varies with the size of the orifice and the level of expiratory flow produced by the patient. For example, for any given

Use of Positive Airway Pressure Adjuncts to Bronchial Hygiene Therapy

Clinical Practice Guideline 7-3

■ INDICATIONS
1. To reduce air trapping in patients with asthma or chronic obstructive pulmonary disease (COPD)
2. To help mobilize retained secretions in patients with cystic fibrosis or chronic bronchitis
3. To prevent or reverse atelectasis
4. To optimize bronchodilator delivery in patients receiving bronchial hygiene therapy

■ CONTRAINDICATIONS
1. Patients unable to tolerate the increased work of breathing (acute asthma, COPD)
2. Intracranial pressure >20 mm Hg
3. Hemodynamic instability
4. Recent facial, oral, or skull surgery
5. Acute sinusitis
6. Epistaxis
7. Esophageal surgery
8. Active hemoptysis
9. Nausea
10. Known or suspected tympanic membrane rupture or other middle ear pathologic condition
11. Untreated pneumothorax

■ ASSESSMENT OF OUTCOME
1. Increased sputum production in a patient producing more than 30 mL/day of sputum without positive expiratory pressure suggests that therapy should be continued.
2. Improved breath sounds (i.e., diminished breath sounds change to adventitious breath sounds) that can be auscultated over the larger airways, demonstrating that therapy is indicated.
3. Patient's response to therapy.
4. Changes in vital signs: moderate changes in respiratory rate or pulse rate are expected, but bradycardia, tachycardia, an increasingly irregular pulse, or a drop or dramatic increase in blood pressure are indications to stop therapy.
5. Changes in arterial blood gases or oxygen saturation should improve as atelectasis resolves.

■ MONITORING
1. Patient's response to pain, discomfort, dyspnea, and therapy in general
2. Pulse rate and cardiac rhythm (if electrocardiogram is available)
3. Breathing pattern and rate
4. Sputum production (quantity, color, consistency, and odor)
5. Mental function
6. Cyanosis or pallor
7. Breath sounds
8. Blood pressure
9. Pulse oximetry (if hypoxemia with the procedure has been previously demonstrated or is suspected)
10. Blood gas analysis (if indicated)
11. Intracranial pressure in patients for whom this value is of critical importance

Modified from the American Association for Respiratory Care: AARC Clinical practice guideline: use of positive airway pressure adjuncts to bronchial hygiene therapy, Respir Care 38:516, 1993.

expiratory flow, the smaller the resistor's orifice, the greater the expiratory pressure generated. Conversely, for a given orifice size, the higher the expiratory flow, the greater the expiratory pressure generated.[1] For this reason, the patient must be encouraged to achieve a flow high enough to maintain expiratory pressure at 10 to 20 cm H_2O. Notice that bronchodilator therapy with a metered-dose inhaler (MDI) or small-volume nebulizer (SVN) can be performed simultaneously by attaching these devices to the inspiratory port of the mask or mouthpiece. The AeroPEP (Monaghan Medical, Plattsburg, New York) is a specially designed device with a pressurized MDI, a valved holding chamber, and a fixed-orifice resistor for simultaneously administering aerosol therapy and PEP.

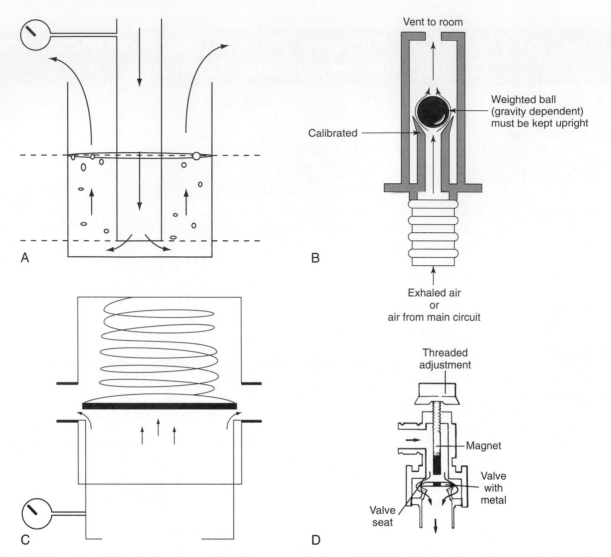

FIGURE 7-23 Four types of threshold resistors. **A,** Underwater seal resistor. **B,** Weighted-ball resistor. **C,** Spring-loaded valve resistor. **D,** Magnetic valve resistor. (**A** and **C** redrawn from Burton GG, Hodkin JE, Ward JJ: *Respiratory care: a guide to clinical practice,* ed 4, Philadelphia, 1997, JB Lippincott; **B** redrawn from Pilbeam SP: *Mechanical ventilation: physiological and clinical applications,* ed 2, St Louis, 1992, Mosby; **D** from Spearman CB, Sanders GH: Physical principles and functional designs of ventilators. In Kirby RR, Smith RA, Desautels DA, editors: *Mechanical ventilation,* New York, 1985, Churchill Livingstone.)

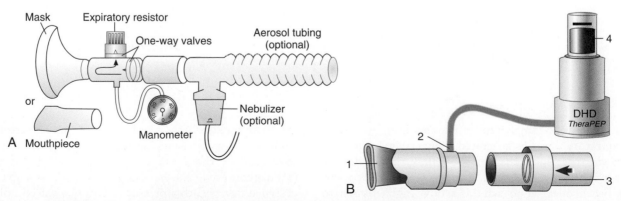

FIGURE 7-24 A, Prototype PEP device. **B,** Thera-PEP device. (Courtesy Smith Medical, Carlsbad, Calif.)

1. The mask is applied tightly but comfortably over the patient's nose and mouth. When a mouthpiece is used, the patient is instructed to form a tight seal around the mouthpiece.
2. The patient is instructed to inspire through the one-way valve to a volume that is greater than the normal tidal volume, but not to the total lung capacity.
3. At the end of inspiration, the patient is encouraged to actively but not forcefully exhale to functional residual capacity (FRC) to achieve an airway pressure of 10 to 20 cm H_2O.
4. The patient should perform 10 to 20 breaths through the device, then perform a series of 2 or 3 huff coughs to clear loosened secretions.
5. This cycle should be repeated 5 to 10 times during a 15- to 20-minute session.

The procedure for performing PEP therapy is presented in Box 7-1. Several factors should be considered when a therapeutic regimen is created using these devices. The level of resistance chosen should allow the patient to achieve the therapeutic goal of generating PEP of 10 to 20 cm H_2O with an inspiratory to expiratory ratio (I:E) of 1:3 or 1:4. The patient should perform 10 to 20 breaths through the device, then perform a series of 2 or 3 huff coughs to clear loosened secretions. This cycle should be repeated 5 to 10 times during a 15- to 20-minute session. Finally, the patient should be encouraged to learn to self-administer this therapy, although more than one session may be required to ensure patient proficiency in the use of these devices.

CHEST PHYSIOTHERAPY DEVICES

Chest physiotherapy (CPT) is a collection of techniques to help clear airway secretions and improve the distribution of ventilation. Historically these techniques have included breathing exercises, directed coughing, postural drainage, and chest percussion. Newer techniques involving the delivery of high-frequency oscillations to the lungs and chest wall are receiving increased interest as alternative methods for clearance of airway secretions.

Percussion and vibration, both of which involve the application of mechanical energy to the chest wall and lungs, provide a means of loosening retained secretions from the walls of the tracheobronchial tract. After they are loosened, the secretions can be coughed up and expectorated, or they can be removed by suctioning.

Percussion can be accomplished using either the hands or various mechanical or electrical devices. For this discussion, chest percussors have been divided into three categories: manual percussors, pneumatically powered devices, and electrically powered devices. Devices that produce vibrations to the lungs and chest wall are discussed separately in the section on high-frequency oscillation devices.

Manual Percussors

The traditional method of administering CPT involves cupping the hand (as if scooping water from a basin) and clapping on the patient's chest wall. Although this technique is quite effective in most cases, it can be tiring for the person administering the therapy and somewhat painful for the patient (if performed by someone inexperienced in CPT). As a result of these potential problems, several companies have produced some simple manual percussors that are fairly inexpensive and easy to use. Figure 7-25 shows a typical manual percussor made by DHD Medical Products. This device is made of soft vinyl and is formed to the shape of the palm. It is available in neonatal, pediatric, and adult sizes.

Pneumatically Powered Devices

Pneumatically powered percussors are driven by a compressed-air or oxygen source that operates at 45 to 55 psig. Although devices may differ in the number of accessories provided, each device usually comprises a high-pressure

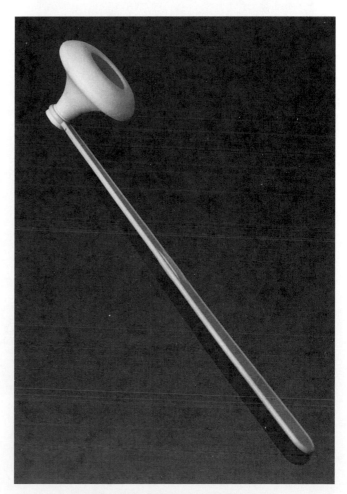

FIGURE 7-25 DHD's manual percussor.

hose, a body with controls for varying the frequency and force of percussive strokes, and a remote head with a concave applicator. Several common examples of pneumatically powered percussors are the Fluid Flo (Med Systems, San Diego, California) (Figure 7-26), the Hudson Pediatric, Temecula, California, the Mercury MJ, MJ Instrument Co. Sialkot, PK and the Fluid Flo percussors. The Strom PPS3, the Mercury MJ, and the Fluid Flo are designed for pediatric and adult patients. The Fluid Flo is only for adult patients.

Electrically Powered Percussors

Most electrically powered percussors are powered by electrical outputs of 110 V of alternating current, although some units are battery powered. Several of the more common units available in the United States are produced by General Physiotherapy (St. Louis, Missouri) (the Vibramatic/Multimatic, the Flimm Fighter, and the Neo-Cussor), Strom, and Nellcor Puritan Bennett (Vibrator/Percussor Boulder, Colorado). Most units typically have a variable control switch for setting the frequency of percussions and can be used for both adult and pediatric patients.

Each system, however, has unique features. The Vibramatic/Multimatic (Figure 7-27) produces two directional forces: one produces a stroking action that operates perpendicular to the chest wall to loosen mucus attached to the tracheobronchial tubes, and the other operates parallel to the chest wall and moves the mucus toward the central airways. The Flimm Fighter is designed primarily for home use. It comes with a foam pad and a Velcro belt to allow self-application of the device. The Neo-Cussor is a battery-operated device that uses a disposable applicator and is specifically designed for use with neonates and pediatric patients. The Vibrator/Percussor allows for independent control of frequency and stroke intensity.

HIGH-FREQUENCY OSCILLATION DEVICES

Administration of high-frequency oscillations to the lungs via the airway opening or through the chest wall has been shown to be quite effective in mobilizing secretions in

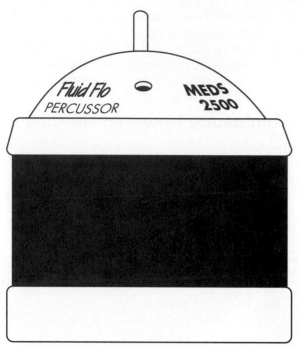

FIGURE 7-26 Fluid Flo pneumatic percussor. (Courtesy Med Systems, San Diego, Calif.)

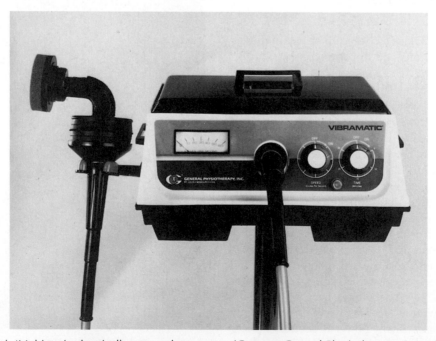

FIGURE 7-27 Vibramatic/Multimatic electrically powered percussor. (Courtesy General Physiotherapy, St Louis, Mo.)

select patient groups. Although the mechanism of action of these devices is uncertain, several factors are thought to enhance clearance of airway secretions. Some of these factors may include reducing the viscoelasticity of sputum through sheering forces generated during the oscillations, transient changes in airflow that occur during the inspiratory and expiratory phases of each oscillation, and redistribution of lung volume to airways partially obstructed by mucus.[14]

The most commonly used devices for delivering high-frequency oscillation therapy include the Percussionaire intrapulmonary percussive ventilation (IPV) device (Percussionaire, Sandpoint, Idaho), the Flutter valve, the Vest (Advanced Respiratory, St. Paul, Minnesota), and the Hayek Oscillator (Breasy Medical Equipment, London, England). IPV devices and Flutter valves transmit high-frequency oscillation via the airway opening, whereas the Vest and the Hayek Oscillator produce vibration of the chest wall by delivering high-frequency oscillations to the external chest wall.

Intrapulmonary Percussive Ventilation

IPV, a form of oscillator therapy, was introduced by Forrest Bird in 1979 as an adjunct technique for mobilizing airway secretions.[15] It involves the delivery of **high-frequency percussive breaths** into the patient's airways instead of applying percussions to the outside of the chest wall, as in standard CPT techniques (Clinical Rounds 7-3).

The Percussionaire Intrapulmonary Percussive Ventilator (IPV-1) is the prototype IPV device (Figure 7-28). It is manually cycled and can provide pressure- or flow-targeted breaths. Inspiration can be triggered manually by selecting a push-button control on the nebulizer (i.e., the patient typically is instructed to trigger inspiration by depressing the button for 5 to 10 seconds). Alternately, the therapist can trigger the percussive cycle by pressing the inspiration button on the control panel. Expiration is manually cycled by releasing the inspiratory control button.

The Percussionaire is powered by a 25- to 50-psi compressed-gas source. Figure 7-29 shows gas flow through the IPV-1 unit.[15] Gas enters the unit and passes through a filter before flowing into a pressure regulator, which reduces the pressure to a value preset by the operator. From there, gas flows to (1) an oscillator cartridge and a **Phasitron,** which increases and decreases air pressures; (2) a nebulizer; and (3) a remote control. Gas travels from the Phasitron outlet through small-bore tubing to the Phasitron unit, which contains a sliding Venturi (Figure 7-30). The Venturi slides forward during the impact phase, and a burst of air travels into the Venturi orifice, which in turn entrains room air (i.e., for each unit of gas that passes through the Venturi, 4 units of air are entrained). This enhanced burst of gas then passes through the mouthpiece to the patient. After the injection phase, the Venturi slides back, and the expiratory valve simultaneously opens, allowing the patient to passively exhale.

The nebulizer receives high-pressure gas from the internal regulator via the small-bore tubing connected to the front of the unit. Air flows through the jet, past the nebulizer, creating an area of reduced pressure that draws medication from the reservoir. A high-pressure gas at the top of the jet meets the stream of medication, creating a mist that is delivered to the circuit. Note that the entrainment post of the Venturi is connected to the nebulizer by large-bore aerosol tubing, allowing the patient to receive the mist during the percussive phase of operation.

The Percussionaire can deliver percussive pressures of 25 to 40 cm H_2O at about 100 to 300 cycles per minute, or 1.7 to 5 Hz (Figure 7-31). The effectiveness of IPV therapy,

CLINICAL ROUNDS 7-3

A 22-year-old man previously diagnosed with cystic fibrosis is admitted to the emergency department after a recent history of upper respiratory infection. A physical examination reveals that the patient is alert and cooperative; his respiratory rate is 40 breaths/min. Coarse, wet breath sounds are heard over all lung fields. He reports producing copious amounts of purulent, foul-smelling sputum for the past 3 days. His heart rate is 110 beats/min, and his oral temperature is 102° F. The arterial blood pressure is 150/100; the maximum inspiratory pressure (MIP) is −50 cm H_2O; and the pulse oximetry oxygen saturation (SpO_2) is 90%. Chest radiographs show bilateral pneumonia.

The pulmonology resident suggests using IPPB treatments. Do you agree with this suggestion?

See Evolve Resources for the answer.

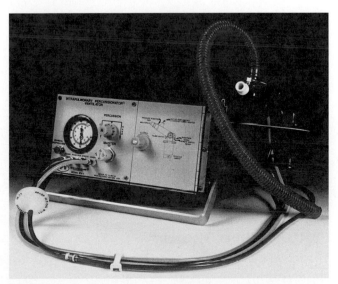

FIGURE 7-28 Percussionaire Intrapulmonary Percussive Ventilator (IPV-1). (Courtesy Percussionaire, Sandpoint, Idaho.)

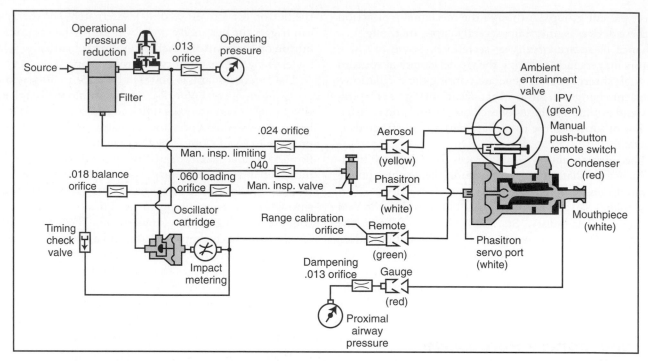

FIGURE 7-29 Gas flow through the IPV-1. (Courtesy Percussionaire, Sandpoint, Idaho.)

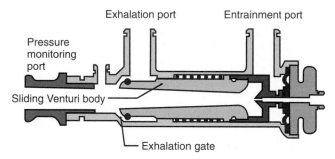

FIGURE 7-30 Phasitron unit used in the IPV-1. (Courtesy Percussionaire, Sandpoint, Idaho.)

compared with traditional CPT techniques, is still under investigation. It has been suggested that IPV may provide another potentially useful method of improving sputum mobilization in certain patients (e.g., those with cystic fibrosis or chronic bronchitis). Although a study by Deakins and Chatburn[16] provided encouraging results for this type of therapy for the treatment of atelectasis in pediatric patients compared with conventional CPT techniques, additional studies are needed to more clearly define the appropriate indications and contraindications for IPV therapy.

Flutter Valve Therapy

The concept of "flutter" mucus clearance therapy was first introduced by Freitag et al.[17] The appeal for this device undoubtedly is influenced by it simplicity of design and by the fact that it is relatively easy for patients to use. The

Flutter valve (Scandipharm, Birmingham, Alabama) consists of a pipe-shaped apparatus with a steel ball in a bowl covered by a perforated cap (Figure 7-32).[17] The steel ball creates a positive expiratory pressure (similar to a PEP device) that helps prevent early airway closure, and the internal dimensions of the pipe allow the steel ball to "flutter," resulting in the creation of a series of high-frequency oscillations that are transmitted to the lung through the airway opening. The Acapella (Smith Medical, Carlsbad, California) (Figure 7-33) uses a counterweighted plug and magnet to create the expiratory resistance. Unlike the Flutter valve, which the patient must use while seated upright or standing, the Acapella can be used in the upright or supine position, according to the manufacturer.

Box 7-2 summarizes the protocol for administering Flutter valve therapy.[14] A number of studies have demonstrated that this therapy is a viable alternative to standard CPT techniques in select patient groups. Further in vivo studies involving greater numbers and more diverse patient groups are required to better determine the effectiveness of Flutter valve therapy devices compared with other airway clearance techniques involving positive airway pressure.

High-Frequency Chest Wall Oscillation Devices

The Vest and the Hayek Oscillator can be used to deliver high-frequency external chest wall oscillations. The Vest was developed by Warwick and colleagues. As Figure 7-34 shows, it consists of a nonstretchable, inflatable vest that extends over the entire torso area down to the iliac crest.[14] Chest wall vibrations are delivered to the vest through a

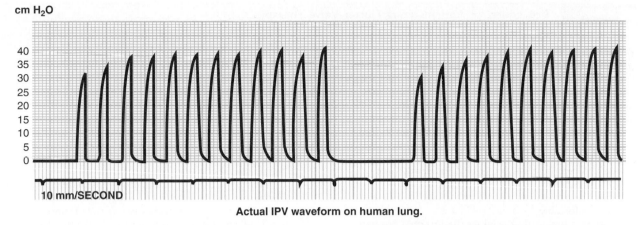

cm H₂O

10 mm/SECOND

Actual IPV waveform on human lung.

FIGURE 7-31 Pressure waveform generated during operation of the IPV-1. (Courtesy Percussionaire, Sandpoint, Idaho.)

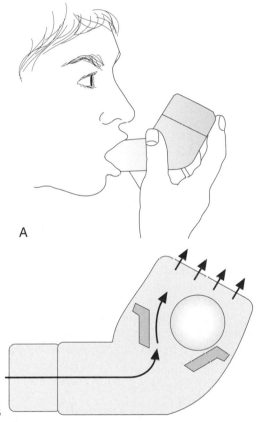

A

B

FIGURE 7-32 **A**, Position of the Flutter valve in the patient's mouth. **B**, During exhalation, the position of the steel ball is the result of an equilibrium between the pressure of the exhaled gas, the force of gravity on the ball, and the angle of the cone where the contact with the ball occurs. As the steel ball rolls and bounces up and down, it creates oscillation in the airway. (From Hess DR, MacIntyre NR, Mishoe SC, et al: *Respiratory care: principles and practice,* St Louis, 2002, WB Saunders.)

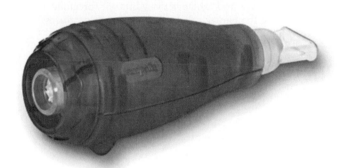

FIGURE 7-33 Acapella. (Courtesy Smith Medical, Carlsbad, Calif.)

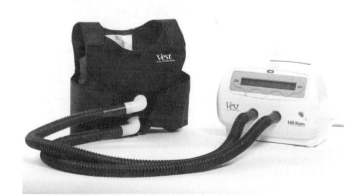

FIGURE 7-34 The Vest airway clearance system. (Courtesy Advanced Respiratory, St Paul, Minn.)

series of pressure pulses produced by an air compressor connected to the vest by a vacuum hose. A remote control switch also is available to start and stop the device. The patient can adjust the intensity and frequency of the pressure pulses to achieve pressures ranging from approxi-mately 25 to 40 mm Hg over a frequency range of 5 to 25 Hz, respectively.

The Hayek Oscillator (Figure 7-35), which is technically classified as an electrically powered noninvasive ventilator, consists of a flexible chest cuirass that is applied over the

BOX 7-2	Procedure for Administering Flutter Valve Therapy

1. Assess whether Flutter valve therapy is indicated and design a treatment program.
   a. Bring the equipment to the bedside and provide initial therapy, adjusting the pressure settings to meet the patient's needs.
   b. After the initial treatment or patient training, communicate the treatment plan to the patient's physician and nurse and provide instruction to the nursing staff, if required.
2. Explain that Flutter therapy is used to reexpand lung tissue and help mobilize secretions. Patients should be taught to huff.
3. Instruct the patient to:
   a. Sit comfortably.
   b. Take in a breath that is larger than normal but that does not fill the lungs completely.
   c. Seal the lips firmly around the Flutter device mouthpiece and exhale actively but not forcefully, holding the Flutter valve at an angle that produces maximum oscillation.
   d. Perform 10 to 20 breaths.
   e. Remove the Flutter mouthpiece and perform 2 or 3 huffs and then rest as needed.

   f. Repeat this cycle 4 to 8 times, not to exceed 20 minutes.
4. Evaluate the patient for ability to self-administer the therapy.
5. When appropriate, teach the patient to self-administer Flutter therapy. Observe the patient conduct the self-administration on several occasions to ensure proper uncoached Flutter technique before allowing the patient to self-administer without supervision.
6. When patients are also receiving bronchodilator aerosol, administer in conjunction with Flutter therapy by administering the bronchodilator immediately before the Flutter breaths.
7. If the Flutter device becomes visibly soiled, rinse it with sterile water and shake and air-dry. Leave the device within reach at the patient's bedside.
8. Send the Flutter device home with the patient.
9. In the patient's medical record, document the procedures performed (including the device, number of breaths per treatment, and frequency), the patient's response to therapy, the patient teaching provided, and the patient's ability to self-administer the treatment.

From Fink JB: High-frequency oscillation of the airway and chest wall, *Respir Care* 47:799, 2002.

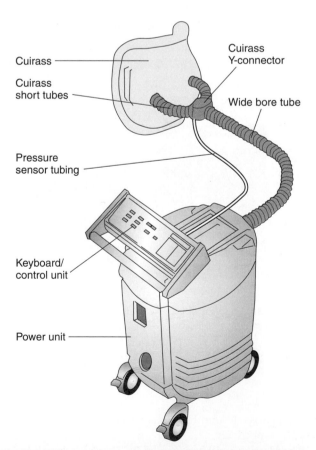

Cuirass

Cuirass short tubes

Cuirass Y-connector

Wide bore tube

Pressure sensor tubing

Keyboard/ control unit

Power unit

FIGURE 7-35 Schematic of the Hayek Oscillator. (From Hess DR, MacIntyre NR, Mishoe SC, et al: *Respiratory care: principles and practice,* St Louis, 2002, WB Saunders.)

chest wall. Its unique design characteristics allow for delivery of both negative and positive pressures to the chest wall during the respiratory cycle. Thus negative pressure is delivered during the inspiratory portion of the cycle, causing the chest wall and lungs to expand, and positive pressure is delivered while the patient exhales to produce a forced expiration. The frequency of oscillations, the I:E ratio, and the inspiratory pressure are controlled by a microprocessor, which can be programmed by the respiratory therapist according to the patient's needs. The frequency of oscillations can range from 8 to 999 oscillations per minute, and the I:E ratio can be varied from 6:1 to 1:6. Inspiratory and expiratory pressures of −70 to 70 cm H_2O can be achieved.[13]

Several therapeutic regimens have been suggested to improve the efficacy of high-frequency oscillations for clearing airway secretions. However, more studies are required to determine the best method of using these devices.[1,18]

MECHANICAL INSUFFLATION-EXSUFFLATION

The purpose of the **mechanical insufflation-exsufflation device** is to replace or augment cough clearance in individuals with respiratory muscle weakness or paralysis (e.g., neuromuscular disease).[19] The original device, which was produced during the polio epidemic in the 1950s, consisted of a vacuum cleaner motor that was designed to produce either a positive or negative pressure across the airway opening. The popularity of these devices declined in the years after the polio epidemic, and it was not until the early 1990s that the J.H. Emerson Co. (Cambridge, Massachusetts) decided to redesign the device (originally called the In-Exsufflator) and market it as the *CoughAssist*. The redesigned device can generate positive pressures of 30 to 50 cm H_2O on inspiration for 1 to 3 seconds. The pressure is then reversed to −10 to −50 cm H_2O during exhalation, generating a mean expiratory flow of 7.5 L/sec (Figure 7-36).[3] Treatments can be administered via face mask or tracheal airway. Use of the device has increased considerably since the redesign, but its use is directed primarily to individuals with Duchenne's muscular dystrophy and spinal muscular atrophy.

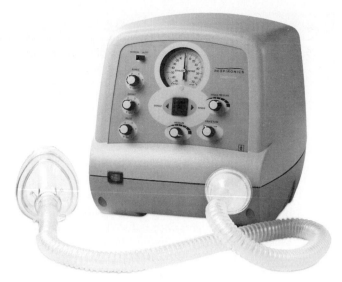

FIGURE 7-36 Cough Assisted (registered). (Courtesy Philips Respironics, Murrysville, PA.)

KEY POINTS

▶ The primary indications for lung expansion therapy are to prevent and treat atelectasis. One of the most important ways to accomplish this goal is to maintain effective clearance of airway secretions with lung inflation therapy.

▶ Various strategies and devices are available to accomplish airway clearance. Incentive spirometry, IPPB, PAP techniques, and CPT all have proved to be effective lung hyperexpansion methods.

▶ Newer devices that provide high-frequency oscillations to the lungs and chest wall are receiving considerable attention as viable alternatives to traditional bronchial hygiene techniques.

▶ Selection of the appropriate device and therapeutic modality should be based on the patient's ability to perform the procedure and on the therapeutic goals. Evaluation of the effectiveness of therapy should be based on the history and physical findings, chest radiographs, and a review of laboratory test results (i.e., arterial blood gas values).

ASSESSMENT QUESTIONS

See Evolve Resources for the answers.

1. What is the primary indication for lung inflation therapy?
   I. To prevent atelectasis
   II. To prevent hypoxemia
   III. To reverse hypercapnia
   IV. To reduce pulmonary shunting
      a. I only
      b. I and II only
      c. II and III only
      d. I, II, III, and IV

2. Incentive spirometry is indicated for patients who are predisposed to develop atelectasis. List four medical conditions for which incentive spirometry is indicated.

3. You are asked to show an adult patient how to properly use a TriFlo incentive spirometer. Although the patient appears to be following your instructions, she is unable to achieve the prescribed goal that you have established for her. Briefly describe several factors that could cause this problem.

4. Which of the following parameters is used to set the therapeutic goal for a patient using a volume-displacement incentive spirometer?
   a. Total lung capacity
   b. Inspiratory capacity
   c. Inspiratory reserve volume
   d. Expiratory reserve volume

5. You are asked to suggest a lung inflation therapy for a 55-year-old man who is 72 inches tall and weighs 85 kg. He has just undergone a cholecystectomy, and his chest radiograph shows right middle lobe atelectasis. He has a 10 pack-per-year history of smoking cigarettes, and his preoperative pulmonary function studies showed that his vital capacity was 20 mL/kg. He is alert and cooperative but complains of some upper abdominal pain when taking a deep breath. What modality would you suggest?

ASSESSMENT QUESTIONS—cont'd

6. Which of the following are contraindications to the administration of IPPB?
   I. Active hemoptysis
   II. Nausea
   III. Intracranial pressure >15 mm Hg
   IV. Recent esophageal surgery
   a. I and III only
   b. II and III only
   c. I, II, and III only
   d. I, II, III, and IV

7. The AARC Clinical Practice Guideline for IPPB states that this form of therapy is a viable lung expansion technique for patients with reduced lung function. Which of the following findings from a patient suggest that IPPB is warranted?
   I. FVC = 50% predicted
   II. FEV_1 = 70% predicted
   III. MVV < 50% predicted
   IV. VC = 15 mL/kg
   a. I only
   b. IV only
   c. II and III only
   d. I and III only

8. You can adjust the tidal volume delivered by a Bennett PR-2 ventilator by manipulating which of the following parameters?
   a. Inspiratory time
   b. Inspiratory flow
   c. Peak inspiratory pressure
   d. Trigger sensitivity

9. According to the manufacturer, the flow of gas from a Vortran IPPB device connected directly to a 50-psig gas source is:
   a. 10 L/min
   b. 25 L/min
   c. 40 L/min
   d. The flow will vary with the amount of gas entrained by the patient.

10. What types of percussive pressure does the Percussionaire IPV device deliver?
    a. 10 to 20 cm H_2O
    b. 25 to 40 cm H_2O
    c. 50 to 100 cm H_2O
    d. >200 cm H_2O

11. Name four types of threshold resistors used to administer CPAP.

12. Which of the following are considered positive outcomes to PEP therapy?
    I. Increased sputum production
    II. Increased respiratory rate
    III. Resolution of hypoxemia
    IV. Diminished breath sounds become adventitious sounds that can be auscultated over the larger airways.
    a. I only
    b. I and III only
    c. II and III only
    d. I, III, and IV only

13. The function of the steel ball in the Flutter device is to:
    a. Help prevent early airway closure
    b. Provide high-frequency oscillation
    c. Create a positive expiratory pressure
    d. All of the above

14. The Vest is used to:
    a. Provide positive pressure on exhalation
    b. Keep infants' core temperature stable
    c. Oscillate the chest wall to promote secretion clearance
    d. Provide biofeedback in the teaching of diaphragmatic breathing

15. Mechanical insufflation-exsufflation therapy has been shown to be most effective in patients with:
    a. Croup
    b. Duchenne's muscular dystrophy
    c. Asthma
    d. Acute respiratory distress syndrome

References

1. Fink JB, Hess DR: Secretion clearance techniques. In Hess DR, MacIntyre NR, Mishoe SC et al, editors: *Respiratory care: principles and practice,* Philadelphia, 2002, WB Saunders.
2. American Association for Respiratory Care: AARC clinical practice guideline: incentive spirometry, *Respir Care* 36:1402, 1991.
3. Wilkins RL, Stoller JK, Scanlan CL: *Egan's fundamentals of respiratory care,* ed 8, St Louis, 2003, Elsevier-Mosby.
4. Gooselink R, Schever K, Cops P et al: Incentive spirometry does not enhance recover after thoracic surgery, *Crit Care Med* 29:679, 2000.
5. Overend TJ, Anderson CM, Lucy SD et al: The effect of incentive spirometry on postoperative pulmonary complications: a systematic review, *Chest* 120:971, 2001.
6. Craven JL, Evans GA, Davenport PJ, et al: The evaluation of incentive spirometry in the management of postoperative pulmonary complications, *Br J Surg* 61:793, 1974.
7. Petz TJ: Physiologic effects of IPPB, blow bottles, and incentive spirometry, *Curr Rev Respir Ther* 1:107, 1979.
8. American Association for Respiratory Care: AARC clinical practice guideline: intermittent positive pressure breathing (IPPB), *Respir Care* 38:1189, 1993.
9. American Association for Respiratory Care: AARC clinical practice guideline: intermittent positive pressure breathing—2003 revisions and update, *Respir Care* 48:540, 2003.
10. McPherson SP: *Respiratory care equipment,* ed 5, St Louis, 1995, Mosby.
11. Vortran Medical Technology: *Vortran IPPB user's guide,* Sacramento, Calif, 2005, Vortran.
12. American Association for Respiratory Care: AARC clinical practice guideline: use of positive airway pressure adjuncts to bronchial hygiene therapy, *Respir Care* 38:516, 1993.
13. Pilbeam SP, Cairo JM: *Mechanical ventilation,* ed 4, St Louis, 2006, Elsevier-Mosby.
14. Fink JB, Mahlmeister MJ: High-frequency oscillation of the airway and chest wall, *Respir Care* 47:797, 2002.

15. Percussionaire: *Operator's manual for the Percussionaire intrapulmonary percussive ventilation (IPV-1) unit,* Sandpoint, Idaho, 1990, Percussionaire.

16. Deakins K, Chatburn R: A comparison of intrapulmonary percussive ventilation and conventional chest physiotherapy for the treatment of atelectasis in the pediatric patient, *Respir Care* 47:1162, 2002.

17. Freitag L, Long WM, Kim CS et al: Removal of excessive bronchial secretions by asymmetrical high-frequency oscillations, *J Appl Physiol* 67:614, 1989.

18. Scherer TA, Barandun J, Martinez E et al: Effect of high-frequency oral airway and chest wall oscillations and conventional chest physical therapy on expectoration in patients with stable cystic fibrosis, *Chest* 113:1019, 1998.

19. Finder J: Review of airway clearance technologies 2006, *RT Magazine,* July 2006, pp 23-26.

Internet Resources

American Association for Respiratory Care: http://www.aarc.org

American Society of Anesthesiologists: http://www.asahq.org

American College of Chest Physicians: http://www.chestnet.org

American Thoracic Society: http://www.thoracic.org

National Library of Medicine (free access to Medline): http://www.nlm.nih.gov/medlineplus/

History of Medicine Website: http://www.nlm.nih.gov/hmd/collections/digital/syllabi/index.html

Medline Plus Search Engine: http://medlineplus.gov/

Medscape: http://www.medscape.com

Medical Business Search Engine: http://www.infomedical.com

Medical Encyclopedia: http://www.nlm.nih.gov/medlineplus/encyclopedia.html

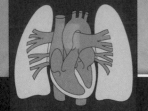

Assessment of Pulmonary Function

J.M. CAIRO

OBJECTIVES

Upon completion of this chapter, you will be able to:
·   Identify three types of volume-collecting spirometers.
·   Explain the operational theory of thermal flowmeters.
·   Name three types of pneumotachometers.
·   Describe three types of body plethysmographs.
·   Discuss the standards for lung function testing established by the American Thoracic Society and the European Respiratory Society.
·   Compare the nitrogen washout and the helium dilution techniques for measuring functional residual capacity and residual volume.
·   Explain the operational theories of strain gauge, variable inductance, and variable capacitance pressure transducers.
·   Describe various conditions that interfere with the operation of impedance pneumographs.
·   List and describe measured and derived variables commonly used to assess respiratory mechanics.
·   Compare the operational principles of the two types of oxygen analyzers used in the clinical setting.
·   Describe two techniques for monitoring nitrogen oxides in the clinical setting.
·   Identify the components of a normal capnogram.
·   Assess an abnormal capnogram and suggest possible pathophysiologic processes that could contribute to the contour of the carbon dioxide waveform.
·   Compare closed-circuit and open-circuit indirect calorimeters.
·   Calculate energy expenditure using measurements obtained during indirect calorimetry.
·   Explain how indirect calorimetry can be used to determine substrate utilization patterns in healthy individuals and in those with cardiopulmonary dysfunctions.

KEY TERMS

accuracy	energy expenditure (EE)	peak inspiratory pressure (PIP)
airway resistance (R_{aw})	Fleisch pneumotachograph	plateau pressure (P_{plat})
alveolar ventilation	functional residual capacity	pneumotachographs
ammonia	(FRC)	polarographic
anemometers	galvanic analyzer	precision
aneroid manometer	Haldane transformation	quenching
auto-positive end expiratory	indirect calorimetry	Raman effect
pressure (auto-PEEP)	inert gas techniques	repeatability
bell factor	kymograph	reproducibility
body plethysmography	lung and chest wall compliance	residual volume (RV)
capnogram	mainstream capnograph	respiratory system compliance
chemiluminescence monitoring	maximum voluntary ventilation	sidestream capnograph
closed-circuit method	(MVV)	spirogram
dead space ventilation	metabolic carts	Stead-Wells spirometer
Doppler effect	minute ventilation ($\dot{V}_E$)	thermal flowmeters
dry rolling seal spirometers	Monel screen	total lung capacity (TLC)
electrical impedance	open-circuit method	vital capacity (VC)
electrochemical	P_{100} ($P_{0.1}$)	Wheatstone bridge
electrochemical monitoring	paramagnetic	work of breathing
electromechanical transducer	peak flowmeters	

Respiration is the exchange of oxygen and carbon dioxide between an organism and its environment. Normal gas exchange in humans requires efficiently operating chest bellows and lungs, an alveolar-capillary network in which ventilation and blood flow are evenly matched, intact systemic circulation for transporting oxygen from the lungs to the tissues and carbon dioxide from the tissues to the lungs, and integrated neural and chemical control mechanisms that regulate pH, oxygen, and carbon dioxide levels in the blood.[1] If any of these processes fail, hypoxia, hypercapnia and, ultimately, respiratory and cardiovascular failure may result.

Advances in microprocessor technology have significantly improved our ability to evaluate patient respiratory function, both in the laboratory and at the bedside. This chapter discusses the devices and techniques commonly used by respiratory therapists to assess the respiratory system mechanics, gas exchange, and metabolic function of patients with cardiopulmonary disease.

RESPIRATORY SYSTEM MECHANICS

Ventilation can be defined as the movement of air between the atmosphere and the lungs. Gas flow into and out of the respiratory system is influenced by the pressure gradient between the airway opening and the alveoli and the impedance offered by the lungs and the chest wall. Respiratory muscular effort or the force generated by a mechanical ventilator establishes the pressure gradient between the atmosphere and the alveoli. The impedance to airflow results from the elastic and frictional forces offered by the lungs and thorax.[2]

The mechanics of breathing can be assessed by measuring the air volume exchanged during ventilation, the gas flow into and out of the lungs, and the pressure that must be generated to achieve a given volume or flow during breathing. Derived variables (e.g., **airway resistance [R_{aw}], lung and chest wall compliance,** and **work of breathing**) can be calculated using these three measurements.

The usefulness of respiratory mechanics measurements ultimately depends on the accuracy and precision of the equipment used. **Accuracy** can be explained as how closely a measured value is related to the true (correct) value of the quantity measured. The accuracy of any instrument depends on its linearity and frequency response, its sensitivity to environmental conditions, and how well it is calibrated.[3] The accuracy of mechanics measurements is also influenced by patient cooperation while the test is performed. In most cases, patient cooperation depends on a firm understanding of how the test is to be performed. If the technologist does not properly instruct patients in how to perform the test, the results can be severely affected. **Precision** is the expression of an instrument's ability to reproduce a measurement (i.e., **repeatability**). The precision of a measuring device can be quantified by calculating the standard deviation of repeated measurements made by the device.[3]

Volume and Flow Measurements

A spirometer is a device for measuring volume or flow changes at the airway opening. Therefore spirometers generally are classified by whether they measure lung volume changes or airflow. Volume-displacement devices measure lung volume changes by collecting exhaled gas into an expandable container and noting the amount of displace-

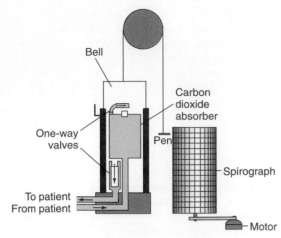

FIGURE 8-1 Water-sealed spirometer. (Modified from materials provided by Collins Medical, Braintree, Mass.)

ment that occurs. Typical examples of volume-collecting devices include water-sealed spirometers, bellows spirometers, and **dry rolling seal spirometers.** Flow-sensing devices measure airflow by using thermal, or "hot wire," **anemometers,** turbine flowmeters, and differential pressure **pneumotachographs.**

Water-Sealed Spirometers

As Figure 8-1 shows, a water-sealed spirometer consists of a bell that is sealed from the atmosphere by water. The patient is connected to the bell in rebreathing fashion by a breathing circuit, which consists of tubing with one-way valves and a carbon dioxide absorber. The bell, which is made of metal (usually aluminum), is suspended by a chain and pulley mechanism with a weight that counterbalances the weight of the bell.* A pen attached to the chain-and-pulley mechanism records bell movements on a separate, motor-driven rotating drum called a **kymograph.** As patients exhale into the system, the bell moves upward and the attached pen moves proportionately downward on graph paper, creating a **spirogram.** Inhalation causes the bell to move downward and the pen to move upward. The rotating drum can be set to move at a constant speed (32, 160, or 1920 mm/min), allowing the operator to measure volume changes relative to time. The slower speeds (32 and 160 mm/min) are used for measuring tidal volume, **minute ventilation ($\dot{V}_E$),** and **maximum voluntary ventilation (MVV).** The slower speeds are also used for specialized measurements (e.g., the diffusion capacity of carbon monoxide [$D_L CO$]). The fastest speed (1920 mm/min) is used for recording volume changes during forced vital capacity (FVC) maneuvers.

Two bell sizes are available: 9 L and 13.5 L. The volume of the bell determines how many millimeters the pen moves when a given volume is displaced. For example, a 9-L bell moves 1 mm for every 20.93 mL of gas displaced, and a 13.45-L bell moves 1 mm for every 41.73 mL of gas displaced. (Note that the number of milliliters of gas that must be displaced to cause the kymograph pen to move 1 mm is called the **bell factor.**) The total gas volume displaced during a breath is calculated by multiplying the number of millimeters the pen is displaced on the spirogram by the bell factor for the spirometer.

The **Stead-Wells spirometer** (Figure 8-2) is similar in design to the original Collins water-sealed spirometer except that a plastic bell is used instead of the metal one; this eliminates the need for a counterweight, because the bell weighs less. Stead-Wells spirometers show excellent frequency response characteristics, especially when recording rapid-breathing maneuvers such as FVC, timed expiratory volume measurements (e.g., forced expiratory volume in 1 second, or FEV_1), and MVV. Stead-Wells spirometers are available in 7-, 10-, and 14-L bell sizes. The pen recorder for the Stead-Wells spirometer is attached directly to the bell, therefore as the bell moves upward during exhalation, the pen inscribes on the spirogram in an upward motion. Conversely, the bell and pen move downward during inhalation.

Bellows Spirometers

With bellows spirometers, exhaled gases are collected into an expandable bellows (Figure 8-3). Air entering the bellows causes the free wall of the bellows to move outward, and its displacement is directly related to the volume of air exhaled. Volume changes can be recorded by attaching a pen recorder or a potentiometer to the free wall of the bellows.

The bellows usually is constructed of silicone rubber or plastic, and several different designs are currently available. These designs differ in that the free wall can move horizontally, vertically, and/or diagonally. The frequency response of these devices is good, therefore they can be used to measure lung volume changes during rapid-breathing maneuvers (e.g., FVC, FEV_1, and MVV).

Dry Rolling Seal Spirometers

Dry rolling seal spirometers consist of a canister containing a piston that is sealed to it with a rolling, diaphragm-like seal. As Figure 8-4 shows, gas entering the cylinder displaces the piston. The large surface area of the piston minimizes the mechanical resistance to movement and gives these devices good frequency response characteristics. A pen recorder or potentiometer attached to the cylinder shaft detects the piston's movement and registers the signal on an output display (e.g., graph paper or an oscilloscope).

Thermal Flowmeters

Figure 8-5 is a schematic of a thermal, or hot wire, anemometer. These devices use sensors that are temperature-

---

*The counterweight minimizes the effects of gravity acting on the metal bell.

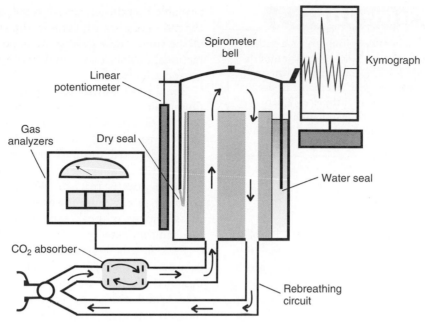

FIGURE 8-2 Stead-Wells spirometer. (From Ruppel G: *Manual of pulmonary function testing,* ed 9, St Louis, 2009, Mosby.)

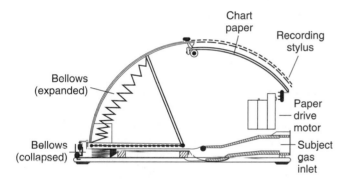

FIGURE 8-3 Wedge-bellows spirometer. (Modified from material provided by Vitalograph, Shawnee Mission, Kan.)

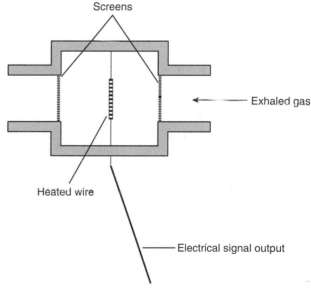

FIGURE 8-5 Thermal ("hot wire") anemometer.

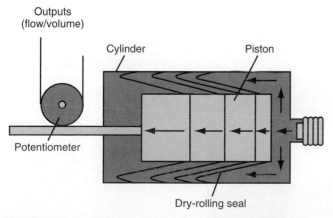

FIGURE 8-4 Dry rolling seal spirometer. (Courtesy Datex-Ohmeda, Madison, Wis.)

sensitive, resistive elements (e.g., thermistor beads or heated wires). **Thermal flowmeters** operate on the principle that as gas passes over the thermistor bead or the heated wire, the sensor cools and its resistance changes in proportion to the gas flow past it.* With thermistor beads, cooling increases resistance, whereas with a heated wire, cooling decreases resistance. The gas flow can be calculated, because the amount of power needed to maintain the temperature of the heating element above the ambient temperature is related to the velocity of the gas flow. Actu-

*The amount of cooling depends on the viscosity and the thermal conductivity of the gas measured.

CLINICAL ROUNDS 8-1

You are asked to perform bedside spirometry on a patient receiving bronchodilator therapy. You connect the mouthpiece to the measuring device (a heated wire [thermal] flowmeter) and instruct the patient to breathe in deeply and exhale forcefully into the mouthpiece. When the patient does this, you notice that the digital display fails to register a reading of estimated volume. What could cause this type of problem?

See Evolve Resources for the answer.

ally, the signal is related to the log of the velocity of gas flow and therefore must be linearized.[3] Thermal flowmeters are unidirectional devices and cannot be used for measuring bidirectional flows during breathing. Clinical Rounds 8-1 presents a decision-making problem involving a thermal flowmeter spirometer.

Turbine Flowmeters

Turbine flowmeters (Figure 8-6) use a rotating vane or turbine to measure gas flow. As gas flows through the device, the vane turns at a rate dependent on the flow rate of the gas. The flow rate can be measured by counting the number of times the vane turns, which can be done mechanically (by linking the vane to a needle attached to a calibrated display) or electronically (by using a light beam that is interrupted each time the vane turns).

Turbine flowmeters (e.g., handheld respirometers) usually are accurate for flows of 3 to 300 L/min. They are portable and easy to use, but they are slow to respond to flow changes because of inertia (low-frequency response). Some turbine devices, such as those found in commercially available **metabolic carts,** use a bias flow of gas to keep the turbine constantly turning, thereby reducing the inertia of the vane. These devices are good for measuring unidirectional flow, but they are inaccurate for measuring bidirectional flows.[2]

Some **peak flowmeters** operate by measuring the gas flow against a rotating vane. The operating mechanism consists of a pivoted vane with an attached needle indicator. The rotation of the vane is opposed by air resistance and a calibrated spring. During a forced exhalation, the vane and the indicator needle rotate until the maximum available flow is reached. Because the indicator needle attached to the vane is spring loaded, it maintains the measurement of peak expiratory flow (PEF) until it is mechanically reset.

Peak flowmeters typically are calibrated in liters per minute. The Wright Peak Flow Meter (Figure 8-7A), designed by B.M. Wright, can measure flows of 60 to 1000 L/min with an accuracy of ±10 L/min. Its reproducibility is within ±2 L/min. Because of its wide range, it can be used to measure peak flows for both pediatric and adult patients. Reusable and disposable mouthpieces are available in pediatric and adult sizes, so these devices can be used for multiple patients.[3]

Increased use of peak flowmeters in the management of asthmatics has prompted many medical device manufacturers to market inexpensive peak flowmeters that are durable and easy to use (Figure 8-7B). These expendable units are constructed of plastic and operate with a piston and spring mechanism. Exhaled air pushes against the piston, causing the needle to move on a calibrated scale. Although the accuracy and reproducibility of these devices are similar to nonexpendable peak flowmeters, they typically operate over a slightly narrower range of flows (80 to 800 L/min).

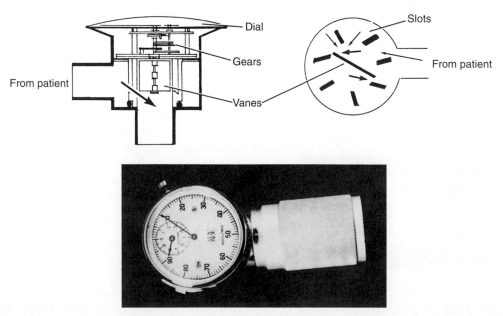

FIGURE 8-6 Turbine flowmeter.

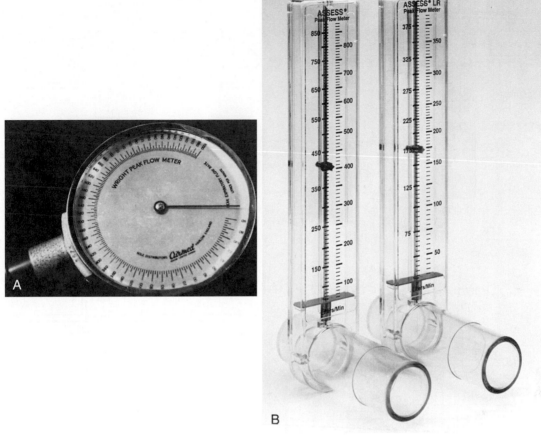

FIGURE 8-7 A, Wright peak flowmeter. **B,** Commercially available disposable peak flowmeter. (**B** courtesy Respironics/HealthScan, Cedar Grove, N.J.)

Pneumotachographs

Figure 8-8 shows several different types of pneumotachographs, including a Fleisch-type pneumotachograph, a screen pneumotachograph, a variable orifice pneumotachograph, and an ultrasonic pneumotachograph. All these devices, except the ultrasonic pneumotachograph, operate on the principle that gas flow through them is proportional to the pressure drop that occurs as the gas flows across a known resistance. Ultrasonic pneumotachographs rely on the **Doppler effect** to quantify the airflow velocity.

The **Fleisch pneumotachograph** (see Figure 8-8A) uses a bundle of brass capillary tubes arranged in a parallel manner to create the known resistance.[4] A differential pressure transducer monitors the pressures before and after the resistance and converts the difference into a flow signal. (With unidirectional flow, a single pressure measurement is required.) A heater is attached to raise the temperature of the entering gas and prevent moisture condensation on the capillary tubes.*

Fleisch pneumotachographs are most accurate when the gas flow is smooth, or laminar. Turbulent airflow, which occurs at high flows or with obstructions or bends in the breathing circuit, can adversely affect the accuracy of airflow measurements. Turbulent airflow can also be caused by increases in the gas viscosity. Therefore compensating for different viscosities is important, either mathematically or by calibrating the instrument with the gas mixture breathed during measurement. For example, room air has a viscosity of 184 poise (P), and 100% oxygen has a viscosity of 206P. A pneumotachograph calibrated with room air will show an error of 12% if it is used to measure airflow in a patient breathing 100% oxygen.[5]

Ceramic pneumotachographs are similar in design to Fleisch pneumotachographs, except that they use ceramic material containing a number of parallel channels to create the fixed resistance. The ceramic channels smooth the air flowing through them and provide a constant resistance to airflow. A heating element is incorporated into the design. The temperature of the gas mixture flowing through these devices tends to equilibrate with the temperature of the ceramic material because of the high heat capacity of the ceramic. In addition, moisture that condenses during

---

*The accumulation of moisture on the capillary tubes can change their resistance and this alters the accuracy of the device.

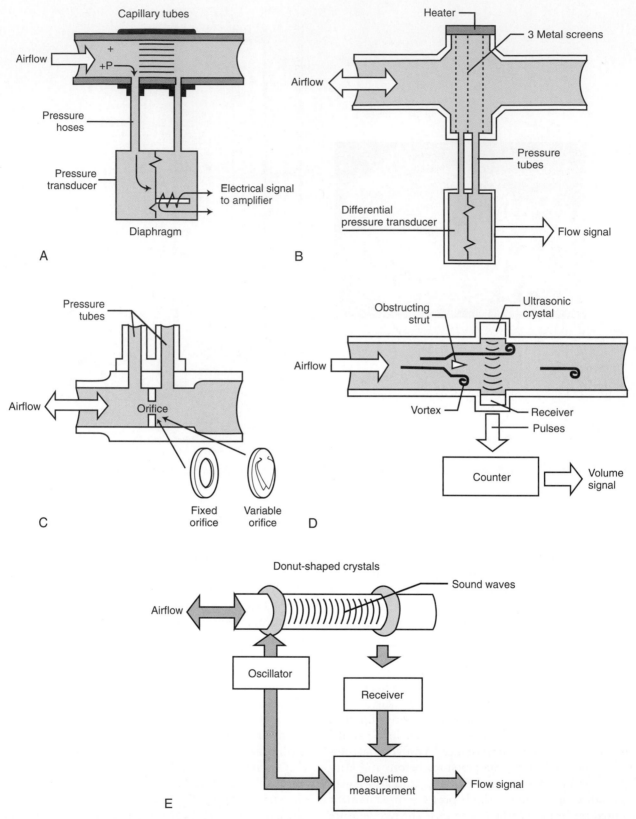

FIGURE 8-8 Pneumotachographs. **A,** Fleisch type device. **B,** Screen type device. **C,** Variable orifice device. **D,** Vortex ultrasonic device. **E,** Nonvortex device. (Redrawn from Sullivan WJ, Peters GM, Enright PL: Pneumotachography: theory and clinical application, *Respir Care* 29:736, 1984.)

breathing tends to be absorbed by the porous ceramic material rather than occluding the tubes.[5]

Screen pneumotachographs (Figure 8-8B) use a series of fine-mesh screens to create a fixed resistance. Most of these devices use a stainless steel **(Monel) screen** with a mesh size of 400 wires/inch.[5] When a triple screen configuration is used, the center screen acts as the main resistive element, and the two outer screens smooth the airflow and protect the inner screen from particulate matter.[5] Similar to Fleisch-type devices, a heating element is incorporated to prevent water condensation on the metal screens.

Some screen devices use fibrous material, which looks like a paper filter, instead of metal screens to create the known resistance. These devices operate at ambient temperature and therefore do not require a heating element. The main advantage of these devices is that they are inexpensive and disposable, which allows patients to have their own peak flowmeter, reducing the risk of cross-contamination. The disadvantages are that they are unidirectional devices, and accuracy varies by device.[5] Also, moisture absorbed by the paper filter can severely affect the device's accuracy.

Variable orifice pneumotachographs (Figure 8-8C) are disposable, bidirectional, flow-measuring devices that use a variable area, flexible obstruction for measuring flow as a function of the pressure differential generated by the obstruction. They contain minimum dead space (about 10 mL) and can measure flows from 1.2 to 180 L/min.[2] Although the flow-pressure characteristics of variable orifice pneumotachographs are nonlinear (i.e., nonproportional at very low and high flows), this discrepancy can be compensated for electronically.

Vortex ultrasonic flowmeters (Figure 8-8D) use struts to create a partial obstruction to gas flow. As gases flow past these struts, whirlpools, or vortices, are produced. The frequency at which these whirlpools are produced is related to gas flow through the struts. An ultrasonic transmitter perpendicular to the flow produces sound waves that are modulated by the frequency of the vortices. The extent of modulation related to actual flow is then determined.[6] Vortex ultrasonic flowmeters are not affected by the viscosity, density, or temperature of the gas being measured. They are unidirectional devices and therefore cannot measure inspiratory and expiratory flow simultaneously.[2]

Nonvortex ultrasonic flowmeters (Figure 8-8E) estimate airflow by projecting pulsed sound waves along the longitudinal axis of the flowmeter (i.e., parallel to the gas flow instead of across it). The theory is that the speed of the ultrasonic wave transmission is influenced by the rate of gas flow through the device.[4] Nonvortex ultrasonic flowmeters are not affected by moisture or the viscosity of the gas being breathed and can be used to measure bidirectional flows.

Measurement of Residual Volume

Vital capacity (VC) and its subdivisions can be measured in the pulmonary function laboratory with any of the aforementioned spirometers. Measurements of **residual volume (RV), functional residual capacity (FRC),** and **total lung capacity (TLC)** are obtained using **body plethysmography** and **inert gas techniques,** such as nitrogen washout and helium dilution.[6-8]

Body Plethysmography

A body plethysmograph (or "body box") is a rigidly walled, airtight enclosure (Figure 8-9). A number of variables can be measured with a body plethysmograph, but FRC and R_{aw} are by far the most common measurements obtained with this devices. Airway conductance (G_{aw}), which is the reciprocal of R_{aw}, and specific airway conductance (sG_{aw}; or, conductance per unit of lung volume) are calculated variables that also are routinely reported.

Two types of body plethysmographs are usually described: constant-volume chamber (variable pressure) devices and constant-pressure chamber (volume displacement) devices. Thoracic volume changes can be determined by measuring changes in pressure within a constant-volume chamber device or by measuring changes in volume within a constant-pressure chamber. Changes in a patient's thoracic volume can also be obtained by measuring changes in airflow into and out of a constant-pressure chamber.[8]

Constant-volume chamber (variable pressure) devices are the most common plethysmographs. With these

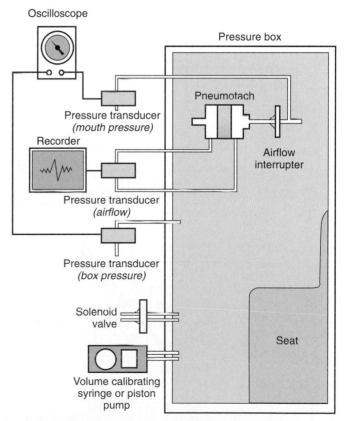

FIGURE 8-9 Schematic of a contrast volume (pressure) plethysmograph. (Redrawn from Miller WF, Scacci R, Gast LR: *Laboratory evaluation of pulmonary function,* Philadelphia, 1987, JB Lippincott.)

devices, the patient sits in the enclosure, which has a pressure transducer within the wall of the device, and breathes through a mouthpiece connected to an assembly containing an electronic shutter and a differential pressure pneumotachometer. Mouth pressure and box pressure changes measured during tidal breathing and panting maneuvers performed by the patient at the end of a quiet expiration are displayed on an oscilloscope and directed to a microprocessor unit that calculates the FRC from empirically derived pressure-volume relationships.[3,7,8] (Note that the reference pressure-volume relationships are empirically derived using an electronically driven piston to deliver known volumes into the enclosure. Pressure changes associated with a known volume change are recorded in the system's microprocessor and used to calculate the FRC.) The microprocessor corrects for variations in ambient temperature and pressure from data entered manually by the technologist.

The FRC is calculated using the following relationship:

$$V_{FRC} = \Delta V \div \Delta P \times P_B - P_{H2O}$$

where ΔV and ΔP are the box volume and alveolar pressure changes measured during the panting maneuver, P_B is the ambient barometric pressure, and P_{H2O} is the water vapor pressure (assume 47 mm Hg for 37° C). The V_{FRC} is then

corrected for the volume displaced from the box by the patient.[8]

Airway resistance is derived from two separate maneuvers. In the first maneuver, the patient pants while the mouth shutter is open so that flow changes ($\dot{V}$) can be measured. In the second part of the measurement, the mouth shutter is closed at the patient's end-expiratory or FRC level, and the patient is instructed to continue panting while maintaining an open glottis. This maneuver provides a measure of the driving pressure that is used to move air into the lungs (i.e., P_{mo}). It is important to recognize that airflow and mouth pressure measurements are recorded separately and therefore must be related to changes in the plethysmograph, or box pressure, to ensure accurate readings. The R_{aw} ultimately is derived using the following relationship:

$$R_{aw} = P_{mo} \div \dot{V}$$

Inert Gas Techniques

Nitrogen washout tests are performed with the equipment shown in Figure 8-10, including a spirometer with a rapidly responding nitrogen analyzer, a source of 100% oxygen, a nonrebreathing valve, and the appropriate tubing.[3,7,9] The FRC is determined by initiating the test at the end of a

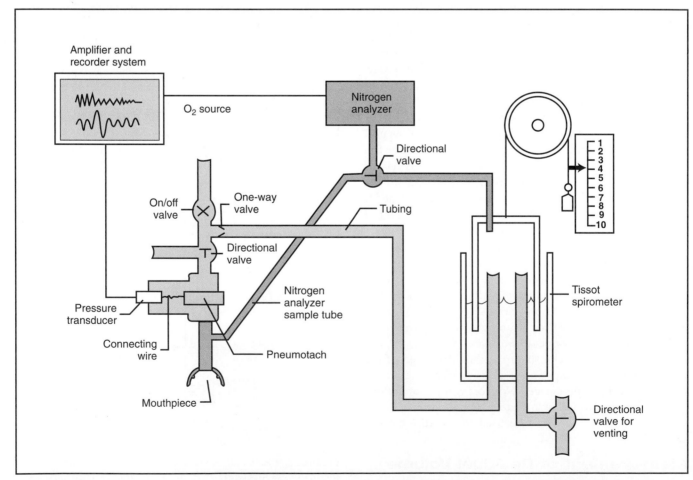

FIGURE 8-10 Breathing circuit for performing nitrogen washout test. (Redrawn from Miller WF, Scacci R, Gast LR: *Laboratory evaluation of pulmonary function*, Philadelphia, 1987, JB Lippincott.)

quiet expiration. The patient inspires 100% oxygen and exhales into the spirometer through the nonrebreathing valve. The patient continues to breathe the 100% oxygen until the exhaled nitrogen concentration is less than 1.5%. The nitrogen volume present in the lungs at the beginning of the test (i.e., FRC) can be determined by first measuring the total volume of exhaled gas and then multiplying this volume by the percentage of nitrogen in the mixed expired air, which is measured with the nitrogen analyzer.[8,10] The resultant volume represents the nitrogen volume in the lungs at the beginning of the test. Multiplying this volume by 1.25 allows the lung volume at the beginning of the test to be determined.* Remember that the resultant volume is measured under ambient conditions (ambient temperature and pressure, saturated [ATPS]) and must be converted to BTPS (body temperature, ambient pressure and saturated with water vapor).

Helium dilution tests can be performed using an apparatus such as the one shown in Figure 8-11. Note that this type of device contains a spirometer with a thermal conductivity analyzer (for measuring helium), a mixing fan, a source of helium and oxygen, and the appropriate tubing for a rebreathing breathing circuit.[3,8] The FRC is measured while the patient breathes into and out of a reservoir containing known concentrations of helium and

oxygen. As the patient breathes into and out of the system, the added volume of air from the patient's lungs dilutes the helium concentration. The end point of the test is reached when the helium percentage remains steady for 2 minutes, indicating that the helium is equilibrated between the spirometer and the patient's lungs. The FRC volume is calculated as

$$FRC = (He_{mL} \div He_{final}) - (He_{mL} \div He_{initial}) - Vrb - Vcorr$$

where He_{mL} is the number of milliliters of helium added to the system, $He_{initial}$ is the helium concentration at the beginning of the test, He_{final} is the helium concentration at the end of the test, Vrb is the apparatus dead space, and $Vcorr$ is a correction volume for the amount of helium theoretically absorbed by the body, respiratory quotient (RQ) changes, and changes in nitrogen in the circuit.[3,8]

It is important to recognize that inert gas techniques can measure gas volumes only in communicating airways (i.e., airways that are open between the mouth and the alveoli), whereas body plethysmography measures all the volume in the thorax (i.e., thoracic lung volume). Therefore inert gas measurements of FRC for patients with chronic obstructive pulmonary distress and severe air trapping are lower than FRC measurements from body plethysmography.

Lung Function Testing Standards

Since 1979, the American Thoracic Society (ATS) has provided a series of standardization documents on

---

*The correction factor of 1.25 is used because the room air that filled the patients lungs before the test began contains approximately 80% nitrogen.

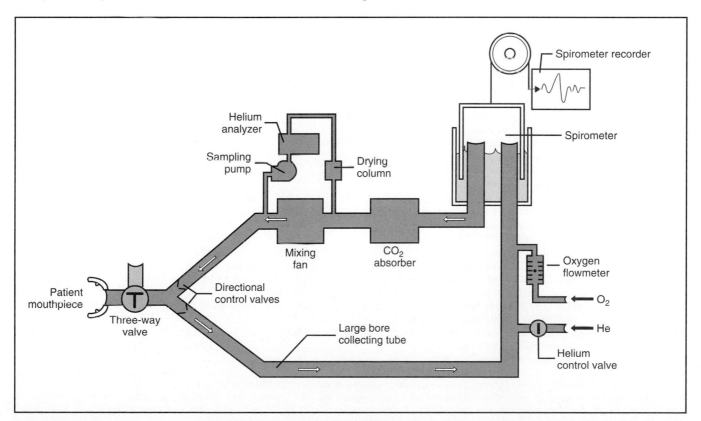

FIGURE 8-11 Breathing circuit for performing helium dilution tests. (Redrawn from Miller WF, Scacci R, Gast LR: *Laboratory evaluation of pulmonary function,* Philadelphia, 1987, JB Lippincott.)

instruments and techniques used during spirometric testing. The initial goal of these recommendations was to improve the performance characteristics of spirometers and reduce the variability of laboratory testing.[11,12] During the 1990s, the ATS widened the scope of its recommendations to include guidelines for the selection of reference values, the performance of spirometry, and the quality control of spirometers, as well as minimal recommendations for monitoring devices.[13,14]

Comparable documents have been released by the European Respiratory Society (ERS) during the past 25 years, beginning with the European Community for Coal and Steel document on standardized lung function testing.[15] The European documents were similar to those released by the ATS except that the ERS standards provided guidance for measuring lung volumes and did not include separate recommendations for monitoring devices.

In 2000, the ATS and the ERS came together in a millennium project to issue a set of unified standards for lung function tests.[16] The result of this collaborative effort was a series of documents published in 2005 that provides guidance on measurement and interpretation of spirometry, diffusing capacity, and lung volume tests.[8,10,17,18] The most notable items addressed in these updated standards relate to terminology, infection control, and reporting of data. Although the standards for spirometry and lung volume measurements are comparable to those in earlier published statements, some noteworthy changes were made. For example, the repeatability standard for FEV_1

was changed from 200 mL to 150 mL.[10] Note that the term *repeatability* is now used in place of **reproducibility.** Repeatability is a measure of the closeness of agreement for a series of successive measurements of the same variable when they are recorded under identical conditions over a period of time (i.e., methodology, instrument, location).[10] Reproducibility describes the closeness of agreement of successive measurements of a variable when the conditions have changed (e.g., measurement of the FEV_1 before and after administration of a bronchodilator).

It is important to recognize that the updated standards do not include separate recommendations for monitoring devices. Table 8-1 presents a summary of the updated standards for equipment used in spirometry. The complete set of standards has been published in the *European Respiratory Journal,* and they also can be downloaded from the ATS website (www.thoracic.org).

Quality Control

Attention to quality control for laboratory equipment is essential for assuring the accuracy of pulmonary function measurements. An effective quality control program includes documentation of daily and quarterly calibrations checks, repairs and other alterations that may be required to return malfunctioning equipment to acceptable operation, and dates of computer software and hardware updates.[17] Table 8-2 provides a summary of the components of a typical quality control program.

TABLE 8-1

Range and Accuracy Recommendations Specified for Forced Expiratory Maneuvers

Test	Range/Accuracy (BTPS)	Flow Range $L \cdot s^{-1}$	Time(s)	Resistance and Back Pressure	Test Signal
VC	0.5-8 L, ±3% of reading or ±0.050 L, whichever is greater	0-14	30		3-L Calibration syringe
FVC	0.5-8 L, ±3% of reading or ±0.050 L, whichever is greater	0-14	15	<1.5 $cmH_2O \cdot L^{-1} \cdot s^{-1}$ (0.15 $kPa \cdot L^{-1} \cdot s^{-1}$)	24 ATS waveforms, 3-L Cal Syringe
FEV_1	0.5-8 L, ±3% of reading or ±0.050 L, whichever is greater	0-14	1	<1.5 $cmH_2O \cdot L^{-1} \cdot s^{-1}$ (0.15 $kPa \cdot L^{-1} \cdot s^{-1}$)	24 ATS waveforms
Time zero	The time point from which all FEV_t measurements are taken			Back extrapolation	
PEF	Accuracy ±10% of reading or ±0.30 $L \cdot s^{-1}$ (20 $L \cdot min^{-1}$), whichever is greater, repeatability: ±5% of reading or ±0.15 $L \cdot s^{-1}$ (10 $L \cdot min^{-1}$), whichever is greater	0-14		Mean resistance at 200, 400, 600 $L \cdot min^{-1}$ (3.3, 6.7, 10 $L \cdot s^{-1}$) must be <2.5 $cmH_2O \cdot L^{-1} \cdot s^{-1}$ (0.25 $kPa \cdot L^{-1} \cdot s^{-1}$)	26 ATS flow waveforms
Instantaneous flows (except PEF)	Accuracy, ±5% of reading or ±0.200 $L \cdot s^{-1}$, whichever is greater	0-14		<1.5 $cmH_2O \cdot L^{-1} \cdot s^{-1}$ (0.15 $kPa \cdot L^{-1} \cdot s^{-1}$)	Data from manufacturers
$FEF_{25-75\%}$	7.0 $L \cdot s^{-1}$, ±5% of reading or ±0.200 $L \cdot s^{-1}$, whichever is greater	±14	15	Same as FEV_1	24 ATS waveforms
MVV	250 $L \cdot min^{-1}$ at V_T of 2 L within ±10% of reading or ±15 $L \cdot min^{-1}$, whichever is greater	±14 (±3%)	12-15	<1.5 $cmH_2O \cdot L^{-1} \cdot s^{-1}$ (0.15 $kPa \cdot L^{-1} \cdot s^{-1}$)	Sine wave pump

From Miller MR, Hankinson J, Brusasco V et al: Standardisation of spirometry, *Eur Resp J* 26:319-338, 2005.
BTPS: body temperature and ambient pressure saturated with water vapour; VC: vital capacity; FVC: forced vital capacity; ATS: American Thoracic Society; FEV_1: forced expiratory volume in one second; FEV_t: forced expiratory volume in t seconds; PEF: peak expiratory flow; $FEF_{25-75\%}$: mean forced expiratory flow between 25% and 75% of FVC; MVV, maximum voluntary ventilation; V_T: tidal volume.
Reproduced with the permission of the European Respiratory Society. This content has not been reviewed by the European Respiratory Society prior to release, therefore the European Respiratory Society may not be responsible for any errors, omissions or inaccuracies, or for any consequences arising there from, in the content.

TABLE 8-2		
Key Aspects of Quality Control for Pulmonary Function Testing Equipment		
Test	**Minimum Interval**	**Action**
Volume	Daily	Calibration check with a 3-L syringe
Leak	Daily	3 cm H_2O (0.3 kPa) constant pressure for 1 minute
Volume linearity	Quarterly	1-L increments with a calibrating syringe measured over entire volume range
Flow linearity	Weekly	Test at least three different flow ranges
Time	Quarterly	Mechanical recorder check with stopwatch
Software	New versions	Log installation date and perform test using "known" subject

From Miller MR, Hankinson J, Brusasco V et al: Standardisation of spirometry, *Eur Resp J* 26:319-338, 2005.
Reproduced with the permission of the European Respiratory Society. This content has not been reviewed by the European Respiratory Society prior to release, therefore the European Respiratory Society may not be responsible for any errors, omissions or inaccuracies, or for any consequences arising there from, in the content.

Calibration checks of a spirometer can be accomplished with a 3-L calibrated syringe. Notice that calibration involves establishing a relationship between sensor-determined values of flow and volume with the actual flow and volume; calibration checks are used to validate that the device is within the calibration limits.[17] Daily calibration checks of the volume-measuring capability and the presence of leaks usually involve a single discharge of a 3-L syringe into the device. More extensive calibration checks over the entire volume range of the spirometer should be conducted intermittently (e.g., every 3 months). The linearity of a volume-measuring device can be determined by injecting a series of consecutive 1-L samples of air and comparing the observed volume with the corresponding accumulative volume.[17] Daily calibration checks of flow-measuring spirometers should include injecting 3-L discharges from the calibration syringe using flows varying from 0.5 to 12 L/sec. Weekly volume calibration checks of flow measuring spirometers should be performed to verify the linearity of these devices. This can be accomplished by injecting 3-L discharges of air into the device at low, medium, and high flows.

It is important to recognize that daily calibration checks help define the day-to-day laboratory variability.[17,18] More frequent checks are required when the equipment is used for industrial surveys or other circumstances in which large numbers of individuals are being tested.

Pressure Measurements

In Chapter 1, several simple devices that can be used to measure pressure (e.g., U-shaped tubes and mercury barometers) were described. These devices are effective in measuring constant or slowly changing pressures (e.g., atmospheric pressure) but limited in their ability to measure dynamic pressures. Pressure changes such as those that occur during breathing can be measured with an **aneroid manometer** or an **electromechanical transducer.**

An aneroid manometer (Figure 8-12) consists of a vacuum chamber with a flexible cover or diaphragm that flexes when pressure is applied to it. This flexing motion is translated into a pressure measurement via a lever system attached to a calibrated scale. The Bourdon gauge, which consists of a coiled tube with a needle attached to a calibrated scale by a gear mechanism (see Chapter 1), is a variation of this concept. As the pressure in the Bourdon

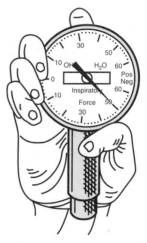

FIGURE 8-12 Aneroid manometer. (From Pilbeam SP: *Mechanical ventilation: physiological and clinical applications*, ed 3, St Louis, Mosby 1998.)

tube increases, its force tends to straighten the tube, causing the attached needle to become displaced. The amount of displacement is measured on the calibrated scale.

Aneroid manometers are used extensively in mechanical ventilators and as independent units for instantaneous pressure measurements, such as maximum inspiratory and expiratory pressures. The pressure is displayed relative to atmospheric pressure or as gauge pressure (psig). Thus a gauge pressure of 5 mm Hg measured at sea level (1 atm = 760 mm Hg) corresponds to an absolute pressure of 765 mm Hg. Although aneroid manometers can measure a wide range of pressures, their frequency response is low.

Electromechanical transducers generally are classified as strain gauge devices, variable inductance devices, or variable capacitance devices.[3] Strain gauge pressure transducers (Figure 8-13A) use sensors consisting of a metal wire or semiconductor incorporated into a **Wheatstone bridge** circuit. When pressure is applied to the sensor, the wire or semiconductor elongates, causing its electrical resistance to increase. The increased resistance reduces the output voltage by an amount that is proportional to the applied pressure.

The variable inductance transducer (Figure 8-13B) consists of a stainless steel diaphragm positioned between two coils. When the diaphragm is not flexed, the inductance of

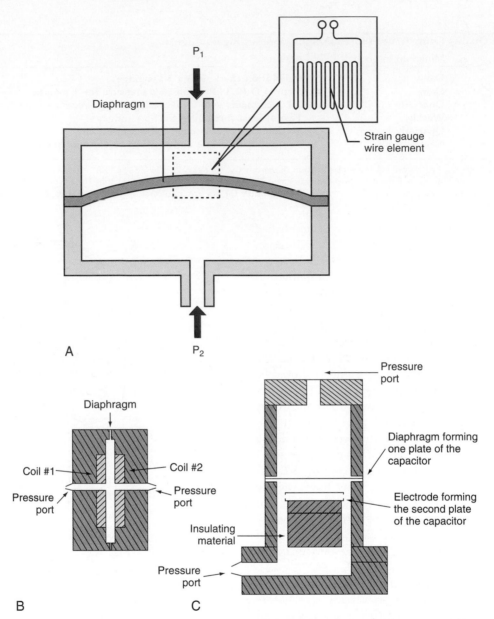

FIGURE 8-13 Electromechanical transducers. **A,** Strain gauge device. **B,** Variable inductance device. **C,** Variable capacitance device. (**B** and **C** courtesy Snow M: Instrumentation. In Clause JL, editor: *Pulmonary function testing guidelines and controversies,* New York, 1992, Academic Press.)

the two coils is equal. The diaphragm flexes when pressure is applied, changing the inductance between the two coils by an amount proportional to the applied pressure.

The variable capacitance transducer (Figure 8-13C) operates similarly to the variable inductance device except that the diaphragm of the capacitance device constitutes one plate of a capacitor. The other half of the plate is a stationary electrode. Displacement of the diaphragm alters the capacitance of the device and changes the output voltage in a manner that is proportional to the applied pressure.[3]

Strain gauge and variable inductance pressure transducers are commonly used for measuring respiratory and cardiovascular pressures. These devices respond quickly to pressure changes and thus have good frequency response

characteristics over a wide range of pressures. They usually are quite stable, being relatively insensitive to vibration and shock.[3] Variable capacitance transducers are large, bulky, very sensitive to vibration, and have poor frequency response compared with strain gauge and variable inductance types of transducers.

Bedside Measurement of Respiratory Mechanics

A number of commercial systems are now available for measuring bedside respiratory mechanics, especially during mechanical ventilation. These include "stand alone" units, such as the BICORE CP-100 Pulmonary Monitoring System (Cardinal Health, San Diego, California), as well as microprocessor units incorporated into

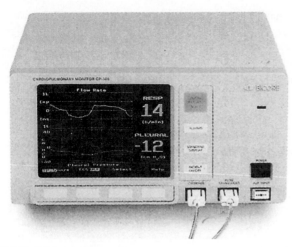

FIGURE 8-14 BICORE pulmonary monitor. (Courtesy Cardinal Health, San Diego, California.)

some ventilators (e.g., Siemens Servo 300 and Drager E4 ventilators).

The BICORE CP-100 pulmonary monitor (Figure 8-14) uses variable orifice pneumotachographs to measure airflow and airway pressures and an electronic transducer attached to a triple-lumen esophageal catheter to measure esophageal pressures (i.e., esophageal pressure is about equal to intrapleural pressure). These catheters are multifunctional and may be used for gastric suctioning and feeding. The catheter can be positioned by noting the pressure recorded as the catheter is inserted. Its ideal position is in the lower third of the esophagus; this position is easily detected, because when the catheter enters the stomach, a positive pressure is recorded. Therefore, after the pressure becomes positive, the catheter can be positioned correctly by retracting it until the pressure returns to a negative value. The catheter then can be anchored to the nose with surgical tape.

Airflow and pressure measurements are relayed to the system's microprocessor and displayed on a cathode ray tube (CRT). The system can display real-time tracings of airway pressure, tidal volume, and airflow measured at the mouth (Figure 8-15). The microprocessor unit can also provide flow-volume, pressure-volume, and pressure-flow plots, along with calculations of R_{aw}; patient-ventilator compliance; intrinsic, or **auto-PEEP; P_{100} ($P_{0.1}$);** and work of breathing. Although both the BICORE CP-100 and Ventrak systems can be used with spontaneously breathing patients, they are almost exclusively used by clinicians to monitor the respiratory system mechanics of mechanically ventilated patients.

As previously mentioned, many of the new ventilators can also provide measurements of respiratory mechanics. These ventilators have pressure and airflow transducers for measuring airway pressures and airflow, which can be displayed in real time. A microprocessor incorporated into the system's hardware provides calculations of R_{aw}, lung

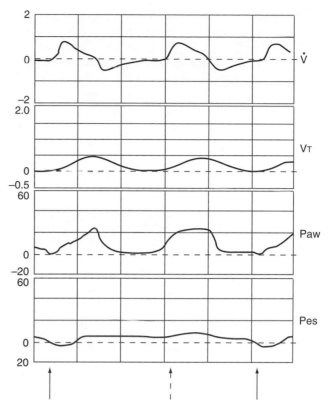

FIGURE 8-15 Real-time tracings of airway pressure, tidal volume, and airflow at the mouth recorded during mechanical ventilation. (From MacIntyre NR, Gropper C: Monitoring ventilatory function. II. Respiratory system mechanics and muscle function. In Levine RL, Fromm RE, editors: *Critical care monitoring: from prehospital to ICU,* St Louis, 1995, Mosby.)

compliance, and auto-PEEP. (See Chapter 11 for a discussion of intrinsic PEEP, or auto-PEEP.)

Impedance Plethysmography

Impedance plethysmographs estimate lung volume changes by measuring the changes in electrical impedance between two electrodes placed on the chest wall. **Electrical impedance,** which is opposition to the flow of an alternating current, is determined by the resistance and capacitance of the circuit through which the current must pass. In the case of lung volume measurements, changes in chest wall impedance are caused by variations in the amount of blood, bone, and tissue present. Therefore, as the chest wall expands during inspiration, the thoracic blood volume increases. Conversely, as the lungs deflate during expiration, the thoracic blood volume decreases, and its electrical impedance decreases. Note that the contributions of air to electrical impedance are minimal.

The electrodes used in impedance plethysmography are similar to the standard electrocardiograph electrodes and are placed in the midclavicular line at the level of the manubrium. A constant high-frequency (100 kHz), low-amplitude electrical current is passed between the two electrodes, and the return voltage is used to calculate the impedance. Variations in impedance measured during the respiratory cycle are demodulated and displayed as a waveform. The respiratory rate is extrapolated from a 4- to 6-breath average.[19]

Impedance pneumography is most often used in home apnea monitoring units (Figure 8-16). Each unit contains adjustable low and high respiratory rate alarms. The sensitivity of the monitor can be adjusted by the operator to prevent false alarms because of changes in impedance caused by movement instead of by changes in respiration.

It has been suggested that bradycardia and upper airway obstruction may cause these monitors to fail to recognize apnea.[20,21] In the case of bradycardia, cardiac oscillations and intrathoracic blood volume changes cause an increase in impedance, which is sensed as part of the respiratory cycle. Continued respiratory efforts in the presence of upper airway obstruction are sensed as normal respiratory efforts.

Respiratory Inductive Plethysmography

Respiratory inductive plethysmography is based on the principle developed by Konno and Mead[22] that the respiratory system moves with 2 degrees of freedom; that is, it consists of two moving parts: the rib cage and the abdomen. During inspiration, the rib cage moves outward as the lungs expand in the thorax. Simultaneously, the abdomen is displaced outward by the downward movement of the diaphragm. Because the two compartments are arranged in a series, the sum of the two displacements can be used to calculate the volume of air inspired (Figure 8-17).

The respiratory inductive plethysmograph consists of two elastic cloth bands into which insulated polytetrafluo-

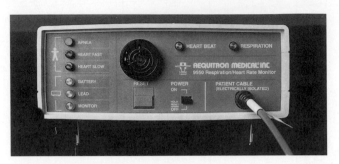

FIGURE 8-16 Apnea monitor.

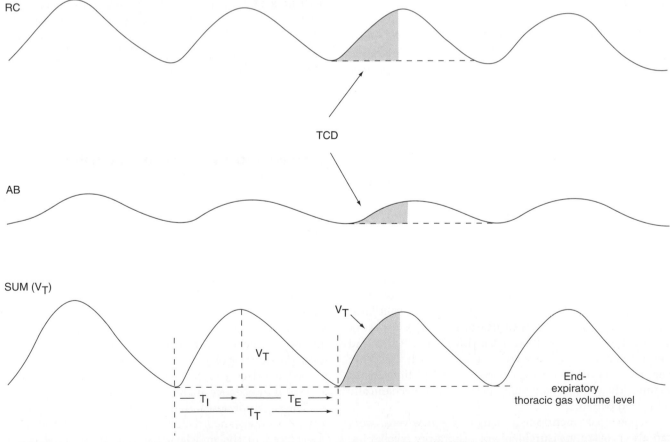

FIGURE 8-17 Idealized respiratory inductive plethysmography tracing showing rib cage *(RC)*, abdominal *(AB)*, and total compartment displacement *(TCD)*. Note that RC and AB motions are in synchrony. TCD equals the sum of RC and AB. Inspiratory time *(T_I)*, expiratory time *(T_E)*, and total respiratory time *(T_T)* are marked on the TCD tracing. (From Branson R, Campbell RS: Impedance pneumography, apnea monitoring, and respiratory inductive plethysmography. In Kacmarek RM, Hess D, Stoller JK: *Monitoring in respiratory care*, St Louis, 1993, Mosby.)

roethylene wire has been sewn in a sinusoidal pattern.[23] One band is placed around the rib cage, and the other is placed around the abdomen. The wires of the two bands are connected to an oscillator, which provides a 20-mV alternating current voltage at a frequency of 300 kHz. Changes in the cross-sectional diameter of the wire caused by changes in the rib cage or abdominal diameter alter the oscillatory frequencies as a function of changes in self-inductance.[20] The frequency alterations are processed and converted to analog voltages, which are displayed on an oscilloscope or with a pen recorder.

The clinical indices most often reported from respiratory inductive plethysmography are the tidal volume (V_T) and respiratory rate. The total compartmental displacement (TCD; or, the sum of rib cage plus abdominal movements) can be expressed as TCD/V_T. The percentage of the total displacement (i.e., tidal volume) contributed by rib cage (RC) movement is expressed as % RC/V_T.

Respiratory inductive plethysmography has been used extensively in research on respiratory muscle function. It has also been used clinically as a means of monitoring the breathing patterns of patients in sleep laboratories, in pulmonary function laboratories, and in intensive care units (ICUs). In the ICU, it has been used primarily to identify the uncoordinated thoracoabdominal movements associated with respiratory muscle fatigue or failure.

Clinical Applications of Respiratory Mechanics Measurements

Respiratory mechanics data can provide valuable information about the ventilatory capacity of a patient with cardiopulmonary disease. These data generally are divided into two categories: measured and derived variables. Measured variables include lung volumes and capacities, airflow, and airway and intrapleural pressures. R_{aw}, **respiratory system compliance,** and work of breathing are derived variables that can be calculated from volume, flow, and pressure measurements.[23]

Box 8-1 lists some of the more common respiratory mechanics measurements used by clinicians.

Lung Volumes and Airflow

Laboratory measurements of lung volumes focus on the standard subdivisions shown in Figure 8-18. As previously stated, simple spirometers can measure three of the four standard lung volumes (i.e., [V_T], inspiratory reserve volume [IRV], and expiratory reserve volume [ERV]) and therefore the VC and inspiratory capacity (IC). They also can measure all the dynamic lung volumes, including FVC, FEV_1, forced expiratory flow from 25% to 75% of the vital capacity (FEF_{25-75}), and peak flows. The residual volume (RV), functional residual capacity (FRC), and total lung capacity (TLC) cannot be measured with simple spirometry; they require specialized equipment and procedures, such as body plethysmography and inert gas techniques. Simple spirometry routinely is used to diagnose individuals suspected of having a pulmonary dys-

---

BOX 8-1	Respiratory Mechanics Measurements

STANDARD LUNG VOLUMES AND CAPACITIES
- Tidal volume (V_T or TV)
- Inspiratory reserve volume (IRV)
- Residual volume (RV)
- Total lung capacity (TLC)
- Vital capacity (VC)
- Functional residual capacity (FRC)
- Inspiratory capacity (IC)

DYNAMIC LUNG VOLUMES (FLOWS)
- Forced vital capacity (FVC)
- Forced expiratory volume in 1 second (FEV_1)
- Forced expiratory flow from 25% to 75% of the vital capacity (FEF_{25-75})
- Peak expiratory flow (PEF)

MINUTE VENTILATION
- Minute volume ($\dot{V}_E$, $\dot{V}_I$, or MV)
- Breathing frequency (f_B)

RESPIRATORY PRESSURES
- Maximum inspiratory pressure (MIP)
- Maximum expiratory pressure (MEP)
- Peak airway inspiratory pressure (PIP)
- Plateau pressure (P_{plat})

Reproduced with the permission of the European Respiratory Society. This content has not been reviewed by the European Respiratory Society prior to release, therefore the European Respiratory Society may not be responsible for any errors, omissions or inaccuracies, or for any consequences arising there from, in the content.

CLINICAL ROUNDS 8-2

The following lung volume measurements were obtained from a 65-year-old man whose chief complaint is shortness of breath on exertion, which has increased significantly during the past year. He has a 40 pack-per-year history of cigarette smoking (i.e., he smoked two packs of cigarettes per day for 20 years). FVC is 60% of predicted, FEV_1 is 50% of predicted, FEF_{25-75} is 40% of predicted, FEV_1/VC is 60% of predicted, RV is 140% of predicted, and FRC is 150% of predicted. Interpret these results.

See Evolve Resources for the answer.

---

function, to monitor the effectiveness of therapeutic interventions used to treat patients with pulmonary disease, for disability evaluations, and for public health screenings. (Box 8-2 lists the indications for spirometry.) Full lung volume tests usually are reserved for patients who have abnormal spirometric results.[10] Table 8-3 describes the characteristic lung volume changes associated with obstructive and restrictive pulmonary disorders, and Clinical Rounds 8-2 presents a case related to lung volume measurements in a patient with chronic obstructive pulmonary disease (COPD).

At the bedside, the most commonly measured lung volume is the expired minute volume. In spontaneously breathing patients, the minute volume usually is measured with a handheld respirometer. For mechanically ventilated patients, the minute volume can be measured by attaching

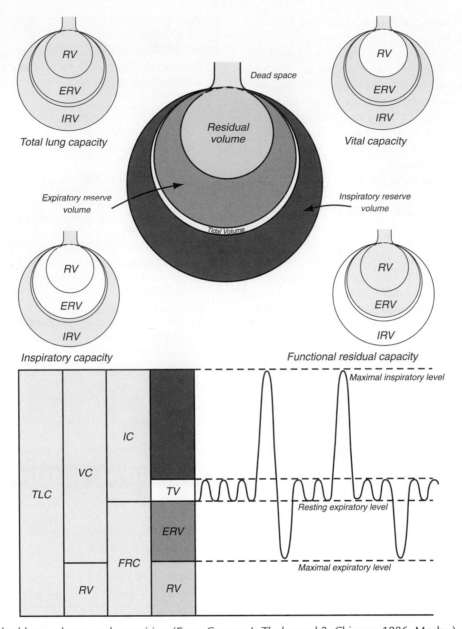

FIGURE 8-18 Standard lung volumes and capacities. (From Comroe J: *The lung,* ed 3, Chicago, 1986, Mosby.)

a spirometer to the exhalation valve of the ventilator. In most newer ventilators, a flow transducer is incorporated into the system design to give continual updates of the V_T and the minute volume. (Note that the minute volume can be calculated based on 5 to 10 breaths and extrapolated to a minute volume value.)

Minute ventilation expresses the patient's ventilatory needs in liters per minute. It is influenced by the metabolic demands of the tissues and the level of **alveolar ventilation.** For example, elevated minute volumes are associated with increased metabolic rates and/or reductions in effective ventilation (decreased alveolar ventilation or increased **dead space ventilation**).

Monitoring of dynamic lung volumes can also alert the clinician to significant changes in a patient's R_{aw}. Peak expiratory flow (PEF) measurements are routinely moni-

tored at the bedside to assess the effectiveness of bronchodilator therapy. The same devices can be used at home by asthmatic patients to monitor daily variations in airway resistance and thus guide therapeutic interventions.[14] (Clinical Practice Guideline 8-1 summarizes the American Association for Respiratory Care [AARC] Clinical Practice Guideline for assessing the response to a bronchodilator at the point of care.)

Airflow measurements during mechanical ventilation can signal changes in the resistance and compliance of the patient-ventilator system. For example, high-frequency ripples on the inspiratory flow tracing can indicate turbulent flow caused by secretions in the airway or water in the ventilator circuit.[24] Expiratory flow limitations should be suspected if the decay in expiratory flow is linear rather than exponential.[7]

DIAGNOSTIC PURPOSES

· To evaluate symptoms, signs, or abnormal laboratory test results
· To measure the effect of disease on pulmonary function
· To screen individuals at risk of having pulmonary disease
· To assess preoperative risk
· To assess prognosis
· To assess health status before beginning strenuous physical activity programs

MONITORING

· To assess therapeutic intervention
· To describe the course of diseases that affect lung function
· To monitor individuals exposed to injurious agents
· To monitor for adverse reactions to drugs with known pulmonary toxicity

DISABILITY/IMPAIRMENT EVALUATIONS

· To assess patients as part of a rehabilitation program
· To assess risks as part of an insurance evaluation
· To assess individuals for legal reasons

PUBLIC HEALTH

· Epidemiologic surveys
· Derivation of reference equations
· Clinical research

Modified from Miller MR, Hankinson J, Brusasco V et al: Standardisation of spirometry, *Eur Resp J* 26:319-338, 2005.

TABLE 8-3	

Static and Dynamic Lung Volume Changes Associated with Obstructive and Restrictive Pulmonary Disease

	Obstructive Pulmonary Disease	Restrictive Pulmonary Disease
TLC	Increased	Decreased
FRC	Increased	Normal or decreased
VC	Normal or decreased	Decreased
FEV₁	Decreased	Decreased
FEV₁/VC	Decreased	Normal
FEF₂₅₋₇₅	Decreased	Normal
MVV	Decreased	Decreased in severe disease

FEF₂₅₋₇₅, Forced expiratory flow from 25% to 75% of the vital capacity; *FEV₁*, forced expiratory volume in 1 second; *FEV₁/VC*, ratio of forced expiratory volume in 1 second to vital capacity; *FRC*, functional residual capacity; *MVV*, maximum voluntary ventilation; *TLC*, total lung capacity; *VC*, vital capacity.

Airway Pressures

The most common airway pressure measurements made on spontaneously breathing patients are the maximum inspiratory pressure (MIP) and maximum expiratory pressure (MEP), **peak inspiratory pressure (PIP),** and static pressure, or **plateau pressure (P_plat).**

The MIP is obtained by measuring the maximum sustained pressure patients achieve while making a forceful inspiration starting at the residual volume. The MEP is recorded while the patient makes a forceful effort starting at the TLC. The MIP and MEP are easily obtained from spontaneously breathing patients with an aneroid manometer such as that shown in Figure 8-12. The MIP normally is −60 to −100 cm H_2O, and the MEP is 80 to 100 cm H_2O.

The PIP and P_{plat} are measured during mechanical ventilation. Instantaneous PIP is the peak inspiratory pressure generated during a tidal breath. It can be measured with an aneroid manometer that is incorporated into the ventilator (see Chapter 11). The PIP can be derived from continuous recordings of airway pressure, which can be made during the breathing cycle using a strain gauge transducer. The P_{plat} represents the amount of pressure needed to maintain the tidal volume in the patient's lungs during a period when gas flow is absent. It is determined by the compliance of the lungs and the chest wall. The P_{plat} is measured during mechanical ventilation by temporarily occluding the expiratory valve of the ventilator at the end of a tidal inspiration and noting the new pressure level. In most newer ventilators, a manual control is incorporated into the ventilator circuit to operate an inflation-hold shutter valve, which closes at the end of inspiration.[24,25]

Figure 8-19 shows a tracing of the measurement of the PIP and P_{plat}. Note that the PIP is greater than the P_{plat}; however, remember that the PIP is a dynamic measurement, and the P_{plat} is measured under static conditions. The PIP represents the total force that must be applied to overcome the elastic and frictional forces offered by the patient-ventilator system, whereas the P_{plat} represents that portion of the total pressure required to overcome only elastic forces.

Increases in the elastance of the respiratory system (i.e., decreases in compliance of the lung or chest wall) increase both the PIP and P_{plat}. Elevated R_{aw} increases the peak airway pressure but does not affect the P_{plat}.

Airway Resistance

Airway resistance is the opposition to airflow from non-elastic forces of the lung. It can be calculated by subtracting the P_{plat} from the PIP and dividing the resultant pressure

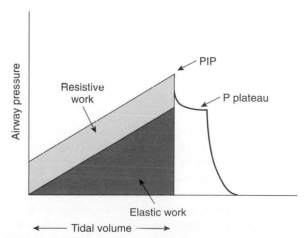

FIGURE 8-19 Airway pressure tracing showing peak airway pressure and plateau pressure. (From Pilbeam SP: *Mechanical ventilation,* ed 3, St Louis, 1998, Mosby.)

Assessing the Response to Bronchodilator Therapy at the Point of Care

Clinical Practice Guideline 8-1

■ **INDICATIONS**
1. To confirm appropriateness of therapy
2. To individualize patient's dose per treatment or frequency of administration
3. To help determine the patient's status during acute and long-term pharmacologic therapy
4. To determine the need for change of therapy

■ **CONTRAINDICATIONS**
In cases of acute severe distress, some assessment maneuvers may be contraindicated or should be postponed until therapy and supportive measures have been instituted.

■ **HAZARDS/COMPLICATIONS**
Forced exhalations may be associated with bronchoconstriction, airway collapse, and paroxysmal coughing with or without syncope.

■ **LIMITATIONS OF METHODOLOGY**
1. Cost and accessibility.
2. Patient inability to perform forced vital capacity (FVC) or peak expiratory flow (PEF) maneuvers.
3. Accuracy and reproducibility of peak flowmeters vary among models and units, therefore results from the same device should be compared for consistency and accuracy.
4. The measurement of peak flows is an effort-dependent test. The patient should be encouraged to perform the maneuver vigorously. Three trials are desirable; report the best of the three peak flows measured.
5. An artificial airway increases resistance and may limit inspiratory and expiratory flows.

■ **RESOURCES**
1. Equipment may include portable laboratory spirometer, peak flowmeter, stethoscope, and pulse oximeter. Spirometers and peak flowmeters should meet ATS standards.
2. Personnel performing the tests should be licensed or credentialed respiratory care practitioners or individuals with equivalent knowledge.
3. The patient or family caregiver providing maintenance therapy must demonstrate an ability to monitor and measure the response to the bronchodilator, use proper technique for administering medication and using the devices, modify doses and frequency as prescribed and instructed in response to adverse reactions or increased severity of symptoms, and appropriately communicate the severity of symptoms to the physician.

■ **MONITORING**
The following observations can assist the clinician in assessing the patient's response to bronchodilator therapy:
1. Patient's general appearance, use of accessory muscles, and sputum volume and consistency
2. Patient's vital signs and FVC, FEV_1, PEF, and pulse oximetry measurements
3. In ventilator patients, PIP, P_{plat}, increased inspiratory/expiratory flows (F-V loops), and decreased auto-PEEP

Modified from the American Association for Respiratory Care: AARC clinical practice guideline: capnography, Respir Care 40:1300, 1995.

by the airflow. R_{aw} resistance averages 2 to 5 cm H_2O/L/sec. It is determined primarily by the caliber of the airway (according to Poiseuille's law, a twofold decrease in the airway diameter results in a 16-fold increase in R_{aw}). Thus retention of secretions, peribronchiolar edema, and bronchoconstriction associated with asthma result in increased airway resistance. Smoke inhalation can also cause severe bronchoconstriction. Conversely, bronchodilation causes a reduction in R_{aw}, such as occurs after administration of a bronchodilator (see Clinical Practice Guideline 8-1).

Respiratory System Compliance

Respiratory system compliance can be defined simply as the distensibility of the lungs and the chest wall. Lung-thorax compliance can be determined by dividing the tidal volume by the P_{plat}. The normal compliance of the respiratory system averages 0.1 L/cm H_2O.

Pathologic conditions (e.g., pulmonary interstitial fibrosis, atelectasis, and pulmonary vascular engorgement) reduce the compliance of the pulmonary parenchyma, resulting in increases in both the P_{plat} and PIP (i.e., decreasing lung compliance). Conditions such as kyphoscoliosis and myasthenia gravis increase the PIP and P_{plat} by reducing chest wall compliance.[22]

Work of Breathing

In normal, healthy individuals, the work of breathing constitutes only about 2% to 5% of total oxygen consumption; however, this value can rise sharply with a pathologic pulmonary condition. Therefore increases in airway resistance or decreases in respiratory system compliance can lead to considerable increases in work of breathing and thus oxygen consumption.

Although considerable interest has arisen in using work of breathing measurements in clinical practice, the technique is somewhat difficult to master and limited in use. Its most practical uses have been in establishing optimum levels of pressure-support ventilation and determining the work of breathing for various forms of ventilatory support.

Table 8-4 summarizes the lung mechanics measurements used to assess patients receiving ventilatory support.

MEASUREMENT OF INSPIRED OXYGEN

Oxygen Analyzers

Two types of analyzers generally are used for measuring the oxygen concentration in inspired gases: **electrochemical** analyzers (including **polarographic** and galvanic devices) and electrical analyzers. A brief discussion of **paramagnetic** analyzers is included for historical purposes (Historical Note 8-1).

TABLE 8-4

Measurements of Lung Mechanics Used to Assess Ventilatory Function in Mechanically Ventilated Patients with Obstructive and Restrictive Pulmonary Diseases

Variable	Description	Measuring Technique
Effective compliance (C_{eff})	The reciprocal of the elastic property of the patient-ventilator system (in mL/cm H_2O)	Mandatory (i.e., passive inspiration expiration) breath (V_T); end-inspiratory pause of at least 1 second (P_{plat}); corrected for tubing compression. Calculation: $C_{eff} = V_T/(P_{plat} - \text{Total PEEP})$
Inspiratory resistance	Inspiratory resistive component of patient-ventilator system impedance (cm $H_2O \times sec \times L^{-1}$)	Mandatory (i.e., passive inspiration and expiration) breath (V_T) with fixed constant flow over fixed time (T_i); end-inspiratory pause as described for C_{eff}. Calculation: $R_1 = \dfrac{P_{peak} - P_{plat}}{V_T/T_i}$
Expiratory resistance	Expiratory resistive component of the patient-ventilator system (cm $H_2O \times sec \times L^{-1}$)	Mandatory (i.e., passive inspiration and expiration) breath (VT); end-inspiratory pause as described for C_{eff}. Calculation: $R_E = \dfrac{P_{plat} - \text{Total PEEP}}{\text{Flow at onset of exhalation}}$
Mean airway pressure	Average airway pressure over a respiratory cycle	Mean airway pressure should be reported over a time period that includes a representative number of machine- and patient-cycled breaths.
Negative inspiratory force (NIF)	Maximum negative inspiratory pressure generated by patient against closed circuit	One-way valve allowing expiration; 15 to 20 seconds.
Intrinsic positive end-expiratory pressure (auto-PEEP)	Positive end-expiratory alveolar pressure resulting from inadequate expiratory time, dynamic airway collapse, or both	Auto-PEEP measurement is clinically important but may be difficult during spontaneous or assisted breathing. It is recommended that the ventilator be equipped with an expiratory hold control to facilitate manual determination of auto-PEEP by airway occlusion as close to the proximal airway as possible; circuit pressures should stabilize during the expiratory hold. Measurement reflects total PEEP but tends to underestimate the intrinsic component because of pressure equilibration in compliant circuitry.

From MacIntyre NR, Gropper C: Monitoring ventilatory function. II. Respiratory system mechanics and muscle function. In Levine RL, Fromm RE, editors: *Critical care monitoring: from prehospital to ICU,* St Louis, 1995, Mosby.

Electrochemical Analyzers

Electrochemical analyzers are the most commonly used oxygen analyzers. They generally are classified as galvanic or polarographic devices.

A **galvanic analyzer** uses an oxygen-mediated chemical reaction to generate an electrical current. A gold cathode and a lead anode are immersed in a potassium hydroxide bath (Figure 8-20A). The gas sample is separated from the bath by a semipermeable membrane that usually is made of polytetrafluoroethylene (Teflon). As oxygen diffuses across the membrane into the hydroxide solution, it reacts with water and free electrons from the gold cathode to form hydroxyl ions (OH^-). The OH^- ions diffuse toward the lead (Pb) anode, forming lead oxide (PbO_2), water, and free electrons. The flow of the electrons produces a current that can be measured with an ammeter, and the amount of current flow detected is directly related to the oxygen concentration. (Note that galvanic oxygen analyzers do not have to be "turned on." They continually read 21% oxygen when the sensor is exposed to room air, therefore it is important to keep the sensor capped to prolong its life.)

Polarographic analyzers also use an oxygen-mediated chemical reaction to create current flow, but they differ slightly in design from galvanic devices (Figure 8-20B). Polarographic analyzers contain a platinum cathode and a silver anode immersed in a potassium hydroxide bath. Also, they typically use a 9-V battery to polarize the silver

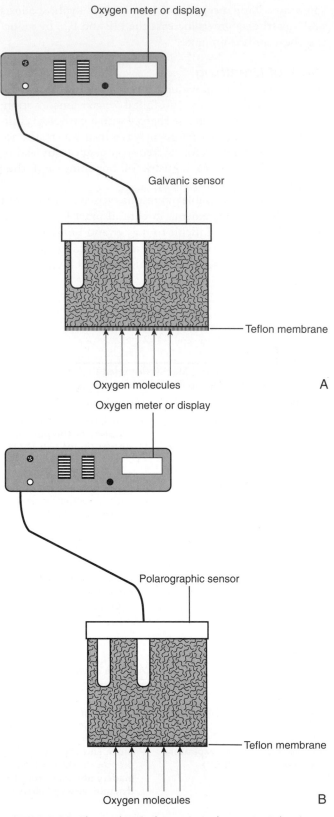

FIGURE 8-20 Electrochemical oxygen analyzers. **A,** Galvanic device. **B,** Polarographic device.

anode, resulting in an improved response time because the OH^- ions are attracted to the difference in electrical charge. The reaction formula basically is similar to that of galvanic analyzers, but the reaction time is faster.

Galvanic and polarographic analyzers can be used for intermittent or continuous monitoring of the fractional inspired oxygen (F_IO_2) and can be used with flammable gases during anesthesia. Because they respond to changes in partial pressure, readings can be affected by changes in ambient pressure, as may occur during mechanical ventilation or at high altitudes. Although galvanic analyzers have a slower response time than polarographic analyzers, they do not require an external power supply, and their electrodes may last longer.

Commercially available galvanic analyzers are made by Teledyne, Hudson, Biomarine, and Ohmeda. Polarographic oxygen analyzers are available from SensorMedics/Viasys Healthcare, Hudson-Ventronics, IL, IMI, Teledyne, and Critikon.

Electrical Analyzers

Electrical analyzers operate on the principle of thermal conductivity and use an electronic device called a *Wheatstone bridge* (Figure 8-21). Two parallel wires receive current flow from an external power source, usually a battery. One of these wires, which serves as the reference, is exposed to room air. The other wire is located in the sample chamber and is exposed to the gas being analyzed. If the sample gas contains a higher oxygen to nitrogen ratio than room air, the sample wire cools, and its resistance decreases because oxygen is a better conductor of heat than nitrogen. Consequently, current flow increases through the sample wire compared with the reference wire. An ammeter detects the change in current flow and relates it to the oxygen concentration.

The primary advantage of an electrical analyzer is that it compares the oxygen concentration of an unknown gas with ambient air. Therefore it is responsive to changes in the percentage of oxygen instead of partial pressure, and it is unaffected by changes in pressure (e.g., those that occur with altitude changes). However, several problems can occur with these devices. For example, the Wheatstone bridge can generate significant amounts of heat and therefore is dangerous to use in the presence of flammable gases. Also, contaminant gases can dissipate heat at rates different from those of oxygen and nitrogen; therefore, if gases other than oxygen and nitrogen are present, the F_IO_2 levels may be erroneous.

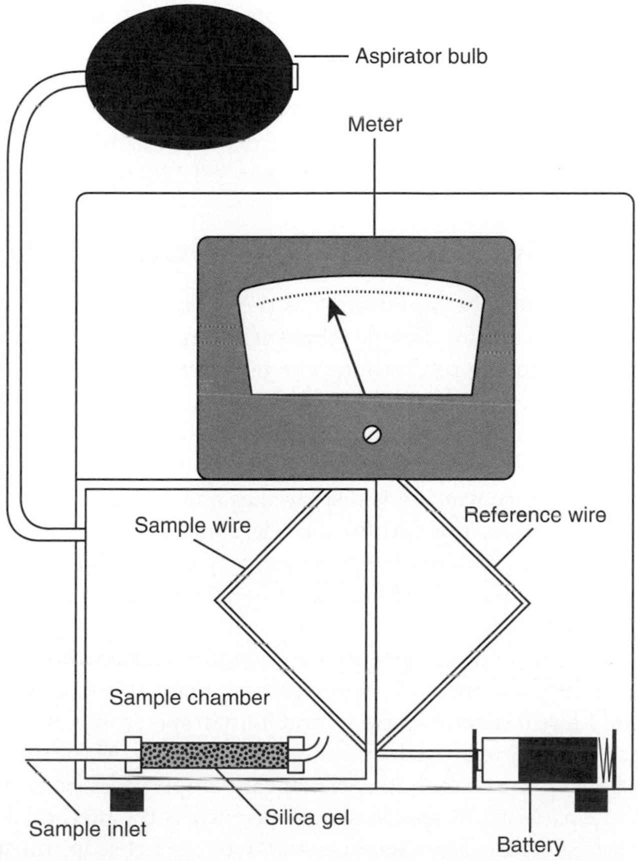

FIGURE 8-21 Electrical oxygen analyzer showing Wheatstone bridge circuit.

MEASUREMENT OF NITROGEN OXIDES

As was discussed in Chapter 3, nitric oxide (NO) is a simple, diatomic molecule that can cause vasodilation, macrophage cytotoxicity, and platelet adhesion.[27] NO has been used to successfully treat pulmonary hypertension in neonates and to improve gas exchange in critically ill patients.[28,29]

Because of the potential for pulmonary toxicity induced by high levels of NO and nitrogen dioxide (NO_2), it is important to monitor the concentration of these molecules when nitric oxide is used clinically. Body and Hartigan[29] provided an excellent review of NO measurement. Two types of monitoring systems are routinely used when nitric oxide is administered: chemiluminescence monitoring and electrochemical monitoring.

Chemiluminescence Monitoring

Chemiluminescence monitoring involves the quantification of gas-specific photoemission.[27] Gases sampled by the chemiluminescence monitor react with ozone (O_3) to produce nitrogen dioxide with an electron in an unstable, excited state (NO_2^*). Because this unstable molecule decays to its lower energy (ground) state, photons are emitted with energies in the wavelength range of 600 to 3000 nanometers (nm).[27] Photon emissions are measured by photomultiplier tubes and electronically converted into a displayable signal.

Nitrogen dioxide levels can be measured indirectly by converting NO_2 to NO with a catalytic or chemical converter and then measuring the NO concentration as described previously.[29] Thermal catalytic converters, which are made of stainless steel, operate at temperatures of 600° to 800° C.[24] Chemical converters rely on molybdenum and carbon to convert NO_2 to NO. Although chemical converters must be replenished periodically, they can be used at lower temperatures and are more stable than catalytic converters. They are also less affected by interference from other gases.

The NO_2 concentration is determined by measuring the total concentration of nitrogen oxides and subtracting the NO concentration. Figure 8-22 shows the schematics of two types of commercially available chemiluminescence nitrogen oxide monitors. A single–reaction chamber model (Figure 8-22A) is used to measure NO and NO_2. This system operates on the principle that the NO_2 converter is switched into the sample line at 10- to 30-second intervals. A dual–reaction chamber device (Figure 8-22B) uses two separate chambers to measure NO and NO_2, and a single photomultiplier tube measures the outputs of both chambers.

The accuracy of a chemiluminescence monitor can be altered either by variations in the sample gas composition or by interference with the operation of the photomultiplier tubes. Variations in the composition of the sample gas can result from **quenching** of excited states of nitrogen dioxide, false identification of contaminant gases (e.g., NO_2), and alterations in the viscosity of the sample gas by background gases. Quenching occurs when NO_2 is converted to ground state NO_2 by inadvertent collisions of the former gases with other background gases, such as oxygen, carbon dioxide, and water.[27] **Ammonia** (NH_2) and nitrous oxide (N_2O) are two gases that can be falsely identified as NO_2. Increases in the viscosity of the sample gas (such as can occur with high percentages of oxygen) reduce the gas flow into the reaction chamber, thus reducing the number of NO molecules entering the chamber. Inaccuracies caused by photomultiplier tube interference generally are associated with photon emissions from contaminating gases in the sample reaction chamber and with thermal fluctuations.

Electrochemical Monitoring

Electrochemical monitoring is based on a principle similar to that used with polarographic (Clark) electrodes; that is, gases diffusing across a semipermeable membrane react with an electrolyte solution, generating a current flow between two polarized electrodes as electrons are liberated or consumed.[27]

An electrochemical NO analyzer (Figure 8-23) consists of three electrodes (a sensing electrode, a counter electrode, and a reference electrode) immersed in an electrolyte solution that contains a highly conductive concentrated acid or alkali solution. The electrodes are separated from the gas sample to be analyzed by a semipermeable membrane. NO and NO_2 from the unknown gas sample diffuse across a semipermeable membrane and react with the electrolyte solution near the sensing electrode, generating electrons in the following oxidation reaction:

$$NO + 2H_2O \rightarrow HNO_3 + 3H^+ + 3e^-$$

The electrons generated are consumed at the counterelectrode through the reduction of oxygen, or

$$O_2 + 4H^+ + 4e^- \rightarrow 2H_2O$$

Balancing the equations at both electrodes yields the following equation:

$$4NO + 2H_2O + 3O_2 \rightarrow 4HNO_3$$

NO_2 can be measured by electrochemical analysis using a similar principle. In this series of reactions, NO_2 is reduced to NO at the sensing electrode, and H_2O is oxidized at the counterelectrode, or

$$NO_2 + 2H^+ + 2e^- \rightarrow NO + H_2O$$
$$2H_2O \rightarrow 4H^+ + 4e^- + O_2$$

The accuracy of NO/NO_2 electrochemical monitors can be altered by increases in ambient pressure (as occur with positive-pressure ventilation) and also by the presence of background gases (e.g., carbon dioxide [CO_2], carbon monoxide [CO], and [NH_2]) that have lower oxidation potentials than the sensor potential. The accuracy of these electrochemical monitors is also limited in the clinical setting for NO concentrations less than 0.1 ppm.[30]

Box 8-3 lists the standards set by the U.S. Food and Drug Administration (FDA) for NO and NO_2 monitoring devices. Table 8-5 shows a comparison of chemiluminescence and electrochemical nitrogen oxide analyzers.

CAPNOGRAPHY (CAPNOMETRY)

Capnography, or capnometry, is the continuous measurement of carbon dioxide concentrations at the airway opening during respiration. The term *capnography* is used to describe the technique in which the carbon dioxide concentration is displayed as a graphic waveform called a **capnogram;** *capnometry* is the technique in which the carbon dioxide concentration is displayed as a numeric reading.[28] In both cases, the carbon dioxide concentration can be displayed in millimeters of mercury (i.e., mm Hg), representing the partial pressure, or as a percentage of carbon dioxide.[31]

Several methods are used to measure carbon dioxide, including infrared (IR) spectroscopy, mass spectroscopy, and Raman spectroscopy. IR and Raman spectrometers are portable devices used by individual patients. Mass spectrometers are shared devices that can sample gases from 10 to 12 patients. IR spectroscopy currently is the method of choice in critical care settings, and mass spectroscopy most often is used in surgical suites. The use of Raman spectroscopy for capnography is limited.

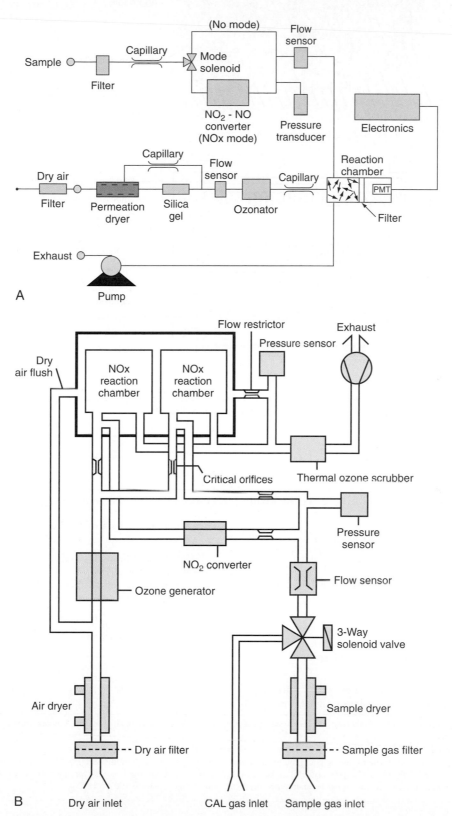

FIGURE 8-22 Schematic illustrating two types of chemiluminescence nitrogen oxide monitors. **A,** Single–reaction chamber chemiluminescence device. **B,** Dual–reaction chamber chemiluminescence device. (From Body S, Hartigan PM, Shernan SK, et al: Nitric oxide: delivery, measurement, and clinical application, *J Cardiothorac Vasc Anesth* 9:748, 1995.)

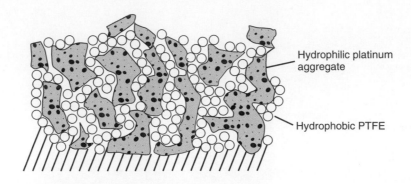

A   PTFE backing tape membrane

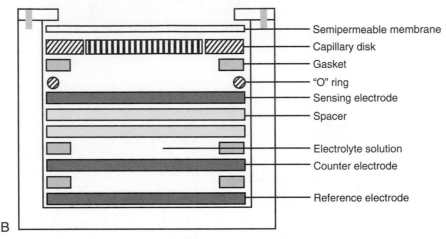

B

FIGURE 8-23 Schematic of an electrochemical nitrogen oxide monitor. (From Body S, Hartigan PM, Shernan SK, et al: Nitric oxide: delivery, measurement, and clinical application, *J Cardiothorac Vasc Anesth* 9:748, 1995.)

BOX 8-3	Proposed Standards for Nitric Oxide (NO) and Nitrogen Dioxide (NO_2) Monitoring Devices*

MONITORING RANGE
1 ppm NO lower limit. No upper limit specified
1 to 5 ppm NO_2

ACCURACY[†]
≤20 ppm NO; ± 20% of NO concentration, or 0.5 ppm, whichever is greater.
>20 ppm NO; ± 10% of NO concentration
± 20% of NO_2 concentration

RESPONSE TIME
10% to 90% of full signal response time <30 seconds

ALARMS
Audible and visual alarms: for NO, an upper level alarm able to be sent from 2 ppm NO to maximum signal; for NO_2, an upper level alarm able to be sent from 2 ppm NO_2 to maximum signal.

OTHER CONSIDERATIONS
Electrical safety (IEC601-1)
Electromagnetic compatibility and immunity (IEC601-1-2)
Environmental protection (temperature, humidity, and spill resistance)
Environmental pollution
Software safety (IEC601-1-4)

Modified from Body SC, Hartigan PM: Manufacture and measurement of nitrogen oxides. In Hess D, Hurford WE, editors: Inhaled nitric oxide I, *Respir Care Clin N Am* 3:414, 1997.
*These standards have been proposed by the U.S. Food and Drug Administration (FDA).
[†]The stated accuracy must be present in the following background gases: 0 and 5 ppm NO_2 (for NO monitoring); 0, 10, and 40 ppm NO (for NO_2 monitoring); 21%, 60%, and 95% oxygen and 0%, 50%, and 100% relative humidity. If the monitoring device is placed within the ventilator circuit and subject to lung inflation pressures, the accuracy must be maintained over a pressure range of −15 to 100 cm H_2O.

TABLE 8-5		
Comparison of Chemiluminescence and Electrochemical Monitoring Devices		
Factor	Electrochemical Device	Chemiluminescence Device
Cost	$2,500 to $5,800	$11,00 to $23,000
Ease of use	+++	+
Ease of servicing	+++	+
Ease of setup	+++	+
Accuracy	+	+++
Response time	10 to 30 seconds	0.15 to 20 seconds
Measurement range	++	+++
Size	+++	+
O$_2$% correction required	No	Yes
Ozone production	No	Yes

Modified from Body S, Hartigan PM, Shernan SK, et al: Nitric oxide: delivery, measurement, and clinical application, *J Cardiothorac Vasc Anesth* 9:748, 1995.

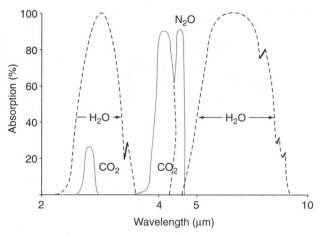

FIGURE 8-24 Infrared absorption spectra for carbon dioxide, nitrous oxide, and water. (From Hess D: Capnometry and capnography: technical aspects, physiologic aspects, and clinical applications, *Respir Care* 35:558, 1990.)

Infrared Spectroscopy

IR spectroscopy is based on the principle that molecules containing more than one element absorb IR light in a characteristic manner.[32] Normally, carbon dioxide maximally absorbs infrared radiation at 4.26 μm. The carbon dioxide concentration of a gas sample can be estimated because the amount of carbon dioxide in a gas sample is directly related to the amount of infrared light absorbed.[33]

The peak carbon dioxide absorption is very close to the absorption peaks for water and nitrous oxide (Figure 8-24). Therefore, if water or nitrous oxide is present, the carbon dioxide readings during IR monitoring can be erroneous. The effects of water vapor can be eliminated by passing the gas sample through an absorbent (i.e., drying the sample) before it is analyzed. Nitrous oxide artifacts can be removed with filters or by using correction factors.[34]

The two types of infrared capnographs are a single-beam, negative filter device (Figure 8-25A) and a double-beam, positive filter capnograph (Figure 8-25B). With the single-beam device, the sample gas is directed to a sample chamber that lies between the IR radiation source and a detection chamber. A chopper blade with two transparent cells (one containing carbon dioxide and the other containing nitrogen) is positioned between the sample chamber and the detector. Gas passing through the sample must pass through the circulating chopper cells before reaching the detection chamber. As the blade turns, two signals are generated, the ratio of which is detected and used to calculate the carbon dioxide concentration.

In the double-beam analyzer, gas is drawn into a sample chamber that contains a cuvette made of sodium chloride and sodium bromide.[32] IR radiation is beamed through the cuvette containing the sample of gas to be analyzed and through a reference chamber containing gas free of carbon dioxide. The carbon dioxide in the sample chamber absorbs

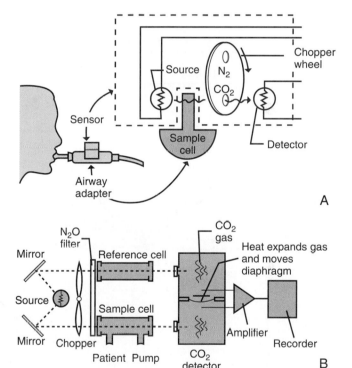

FIGURE 8-25 A, Single-beam nondispersive infrared capnograph. **B,** Double-beam nondispersive infrared capnograph. (Redrawn from Gravenstein JS, Paulus DA, Hayes TJ: *Capnography in clinical practice,* Boston, 1989, Butterworth.)

some of the radiation, thereby reducing the amount of radiation reaching the detector. The difference between the radiation transmitted through the sample cell and the radiation transmitted through the reference causes a diaphragm within the detector chamber to move. This movement is converted into an electrical signal, which is amplified and displayed in millimeters of mercury (representing the partial pressure) or a percentage of carbon dioxide.[35]

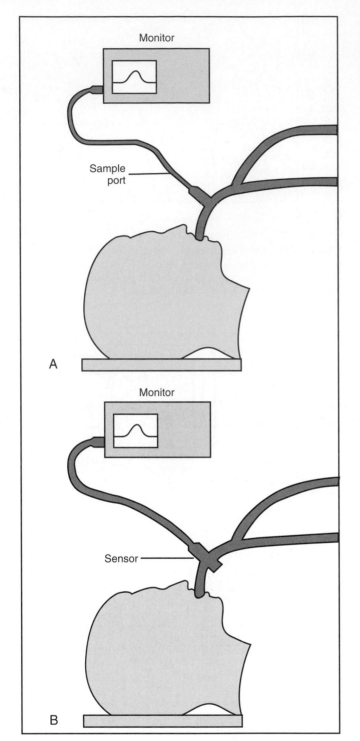

FIGURE 8-26 Classification of capnographs by sampling technique. **A,** Sidestream capnograph: exhaled gas is extracted through small-bore tubing and transported to a console containing the infrared sensor. **B,** Mainstream capnograph: exhaled gas is measured at the airway.

500 mL/min through a narrow-bore polyethylene tube and transferred to the sample chamber, which is located in a separate console. With a **mainstream capnograph** (Figure 8-26B), analysis is performed at the airway, and gas passes into the sampling chamber, which is attached directly to the endotracheal tube (ETT).

Although sidestream devices are quite reliable, they have a slight delay between sampling and reporting times because of the time required to transport the sample from the airway to the sample chamber. Consequently, these devices may not be appropriate for patients breathing at high rates (e.g., neonates). The plastic tube that transports sample gas from the airway to the analyzer is prone to plugging by water and secretions and therefore can lead to erroneous readings. Contamination with ambient air from leaks in the sample line also is a concern. Clinical Rounds 8-3 illustrates a common problem that occurs with a sidestream capnograph.

A mainstream capnograph does not have a delay between sampling and reporting times because the analyzer is attached directly to the ETT. However, these devices add dead space to the airway, which must be quantified to prevent erroneous readings of the partial pressure of carbon dioxide. The additional weight placed on the artificial airway by this type of analyzer increases the possibility of dislodgment or complete extubation. It should also be recognized that because this type of analyzer is directly attached to the airway, it is subject to damage from mishandling (i.e., dropping the device on the floor).

Mass Spectroscopy

Mass spectroscopy is based on the principle that gas molecules can be identified by their mass to charge ratio when they are passed through a magnetic field (Figure 8-27). The gas to be analyzed is aspirated into a chamber and ionized by a stream of electrons emitted from a filament. The ionized gas molecules are accelerated and deflected by a magnetic field onto a collector plate. The amount of deflection depends on their mass to charge ratio. The gas molecules are then separated according to their mass to charge ratio, and as they reach the collector plate, they generate a signal that is picked up by a detector. The strength of the signal, which depends on the number of particles detected, can then be amplified and displayed.[36]

Clinicians generally classify infrared analyzers as sidestream or mainstream devices, depending on the method used to sample gases at the airway. With a **sidestream capnograph** (Figure 8-26A), the gas to be analyzed is aspirated from the airway at a flow rate of approximately

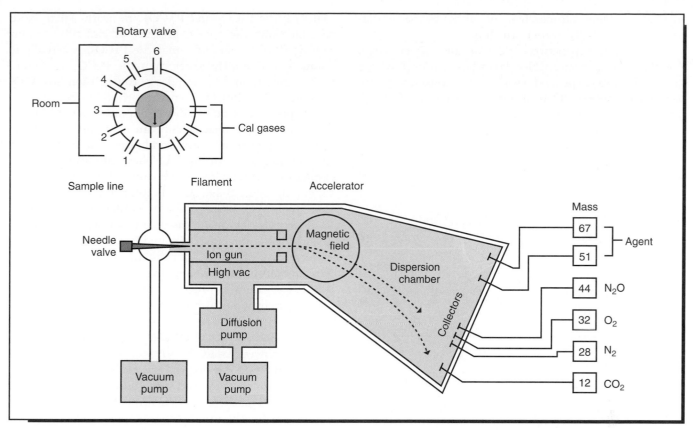

FIGURE 8-27 Schematic of a mass spectrometer. (Redrawn from Gravenstein JS, Paulus DA, Hayes TJ: *Capnography in clinical practice,* Boston, 1989, Butterworth.)

Although mass spectrometers are expensive, they can be used for several patients (i.e., multiplexing in the surgical suite) and can be used to measure gases other than carbon dioxide, including oxygen, nitrogen, and nitrous oxide. This added capacity does have drawbacks, however, because carbon dioxide and nitrous oxide have the same molecular weight. Therefore separation on the basis of weight alone can lead to erroneous readings. This problem is overcome by ionizing N_2O to N_2O^+ and CO_2 to C^+.[33,36]

Raman Spectroscopy

Raman spectroscopy relies on the **Raman effect,** which occurs when light interacts with gas molecules to cause rotational or vibrational energy changes in the gas molecules. The light that is emitted from a gas molecule as it relaxes to its original state results in a shift in the wavelength that is characteristic of the molecule being analyzed. For example, monochromatic radiation passed through a gas mixture demonstrates a spectral change that depends on the structure of the individual molecules present in the gas mixture.[36]

Although Raman spectroscopy has been available for some time, its use in clinical medicine is still somewhat limited. Because the accuracy of these devices has been shown to be similar to that of mass spectroscopy, future use of this technology is promising.

Physiologic Basis of Capnography

Under normal circumstances, inspired air contains very little carbon dioxide (about 0.3%). Expired air, on the other hand, contains about 4% to 6% carbon dioxide. Figure 8-28 shows an idealized capnogram of a resting individual who is quietly breathing room air. This waveform, which is divided into four phases, reflects the elimination of carbon dioxide from the lungs during respiration. During phase 1, gas is exhaled from the large conducting airways, which contain essentially no carbon dioxide. In phase 2, some alveolar gas containing carbon dioxide mixes with gas from the smaller conducting airways, and the carbon dioxide concentration rises. During phase 3, the carbon dioxide concentration curve remains relatively constant, as primarily alveolar gas is exhaled (alveolar plateau).* On inspiration (phase 4), the concentration falls to zero.

The amount of carbon dioxide in exhaled air depends on the balance between carbon dioxide production and the elimination. Production is determined primarily by the metabolic rate, whereas elimination depends on alveolar

---

*The concentration of carbon dioxide at the end of the alveolar phase (just before the inspiration begins) is called the end-tidal PCO_2 ($P_{ET}CO_2$).

ventilation, which ultimately is influenced by the ventilation/perfusion ($\dot{V}/\dot{Q}$) ratio of the lungs.

The relationship between the $\dot{V}/\dot{Q}$ and gas exchange (i.e., the partial pressure of alveolar carbon dioxide [PACO$_2$]) therefore can be expressed with $\dot{V}/\dot{Q}$ relationships. Figure 8-29 shows three $\dot{V}/\dot{Q}$ relationships that can affect the partial pressure of arterial carbon dioxide (PaCO$_2$). In Figure 8-29A, ventilation and perfusion are equally matched; the PaCO$_2$ and PACO$_2$ are nearly equal. Note that although the partial pressure of end tidal carbon dioxide (P$_{ET}$CO$_2$) should equal the PaCO$_2$, it actually is about 4 to 6 mm Hg lower than the PaCO$_2$. In Figure 8-29B, ventilation declines relative to perfusion (low $\dot{V}/\dot{Q}$, or shunt). The PACO$_2$ eventually equilibrates with the partial pressure of carbon dioxide in mixed venous blood. This type of $\dot{V}/\dot{Q}$ relationship can exist throughout the lung in a number of clinical conditions, leading to higher than normal levels of P$_{ET}$CO$_2$. These conditions include respiratory center depression, muscular paralysis, and COPD. In Figure 8-29C, ventilation is higher than perfusion (high $\dot{V}/\dot{Q}$, or dead space ventilation). Physiologic dead space ventilation increases, and the PACO$_2$ approaches inspired air (0 mm Hg). Decreased P$_{ET}$CO$_2$ levels are found with this type of $\dot{V}/\dot{Q}$ relationship in patients with pulmonary embolism, excessive positive end-expiratory pressure (PEEP; mechanical or intrinsic), and any disorder involving pulmonary hypoperfusion.

Clinical Applications of Capnography

Capnography can be used both for spontaneously breathing patients and for those who are mechanically ventilated. Because capnography has been used primarily with mechanically ventilated patients, the AARC has prepared a guideline for the use of capnography to monitor such patients.[31] Clinical Practice Guideline 8-2 summarizes the key points of this guideline.

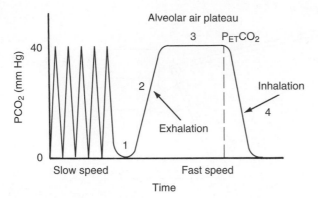

FIGURE 8-28 Idealized capnogram of a resting individual breathing room air. *1,* Exhaled gas from conducting airways; *2,* mixture of conducting airways and alveolar air; *3,* alveolar plateau; *4,* inspired air (0.3% CO$_2$). (From Pilbeam SP, Cairo JM: *Mechanical ventilation: physiological and clinical applications,* ed 4, St Louis, 2006, Mosby.)

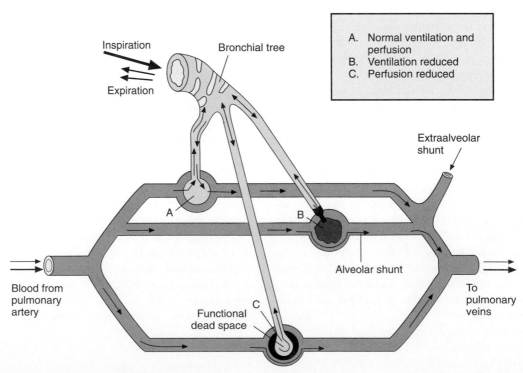

FIGURE 8-29 Ventilation/perfusion relationships. **A,** Normal. **B,** Low $\dot{V}/\dot{Q}$ (Modified from Despopoulos A, Sibernagl S: *Color atlas of physiology,* ed 4, New York, 1991, Thieme.)

Capnography/Capnometry during Mechanical Ventilation

Clinical Practice Guideline 8-2

■ INDICATIONS

Based on current evidence, capnography is useful for:

1. Monitoring the severity of pulmonary disease and evaluating the response to therapy, especially therapy intended to improve the dead space to tidal volume ratio (V_D/V_T) and ventilation/perfusion ($\dot{V}/\dot{Q}$) relationships. It may also provide valuable information about therapy for improving coronary blood flow.
2. Determining that tracheal rather than esophageal intubation has been achieved.
3. Monitoring the integrity of the mechanical ventilatory circuit and artificial airway.
4. Evaluating the efficiency of mechanical ventilatory support.
5. Monitoring the adequacy of pulmonary and coronary blood flow.
6. Monitoring carbon dioxide production.

■ CONTRAINDICATIONS

No absolute contraindications to capnography in mechanical ventilated adult patients have been established.

■ MONITORING

During capnography, the following should be recorded:

1. Ventilatory variables, including tidal volume, respiratory rate, positive end-expiratory pressure, inspiratory to expiratory (I : E) ratio, peak airway pressure, and respiratory gas concentrations.
2. Hemodynamic variables, including systemic and pulmonary pressures, cardiac output, shunt, and $\dot{V}/\dot{Q}$ imbalances.

Modified from the American Association for Respiratory Care: AARC clinical practice guideline: capnography, Respir Care 40:1321, 1995.

Capnogram Contours. In mechanically ventilated patients, capnography can be used to detect increases in dead space ventilation, hyperventilation and hypoventilation, apnea (periodic breathing), inadequate neuromuscular blockade in pharmacologically paralyzed patients, and carbon dioxide rebreathing. It also can be used to monitor gas exchange during cardiopulmonary resuscitation (CPR). Figure 8-30 shows various capnogram contours characteristic of several common situations.

When physiologic dead space increases, as in COPD, phase 3 becomes indistinguishable (Figure 8-30A). Hyperventilation is characterized by a reduction in the $PaCO_2$ and therefore in the $P_{ET}CO_2$ (Figure 8-30B). Conversely, hypoventilation is associated with elevated levels of $PaCO_2$ and $P_{ET}CO_2$ (Figure 8-30B). Figure 8-30C shows a capnogram from a patient demonstrating Cheyne-Stokes breathing. During bradypnea, phase 3 typically shows cardiac oscillations that result from the transferal of the beating heart motion to the conducting airways (Figure 8-30D). Rebreathing of exhaled gas is recognized because the capnogram does not return to baseline (Figure 8-30E). Figure 8-30F shows a capnogram demonstrating the characteristic phase 3 "curare cleft" that can occur when a patient is receiving insufficient neuromuscular blockade.[33,35]

Capnography also can be used to detect cessation of pulmonary blood flow, as occurs with pulmonary embolism and during cardiac arrest.[28,30,32] A number of investigators have advocated the use of capnography as an adjunct

to CPR. Laboratory studies suggest that capnography can be used as an indication of the progress and success of CPR. These studies demonstrated that the $P_{ET}CO_2$ increases as $\dot{V}/\dot{Q}$ is restored to normal.[32,33]

In addition, capnography can be used during CPR to detect accidental esophageal intubation.[31,35] The gastric partial pressure of carbon dioxide (PCO_2) generally is equal to room air. Therefore failure to detect the characteristic changes in the CO_2 concentration during ventilation may indicate esophageal intubation. However, low perfusion of the lungs is also associated with a low $P_{ET}CO_2$ and should not be confused with esophageal intubation. Also, the gastric PCO_2 may be elevated after mouth-to-mouth breathing or ingestion of a carbonated beverage.

Arterial to Maximum End-Expiratory PCO_2 Difference. The arterial to end-tidal partial pressure of carbon dioxide (a-et PCO_2) for tidal breathing should be negligible (essentially zero). It becomes elevated in patients with COPD, left heart failure, and pulmonary embolism because of an increase in physiologic dead space.[31-33,35]

Another technique that can be used to further evaluate the severity of disease is to compare the $PaCO_2$ measurements with the maximum expired PCO_2 measurements (the arterial to maximum expiratory PCO_2 gradient).[36,37] With this technique, the expired PCO_2 recorded at the end of a maximum exhalation to residual volume is compared with the $PaCO_2$. Normally, the difference between these two values is minimal. Interestingly, patients with COPD

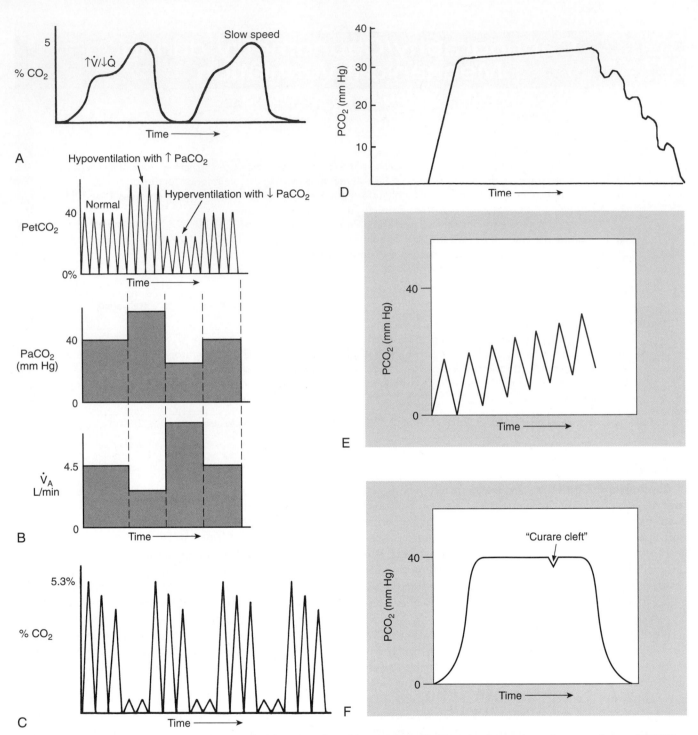

FIGURE 8-30 Capnogram contours associated with various breathing patterns. **A,** Chronic obstructive pulmonary disease (COPD). **B,** Hyperventilation and hypoventilation. **C,** Cheyne-Stokes breathing. **D,** Cardiac oscillations. **E,** Rebreathing of exhaled gases. **F,** Curare cleft. (From Pilbeam SP, Cairo JM: *Mechanical ventilation: physiological and clinical applications,* ed 4, St Louis, 2006, Mosby.)

and left heart failure do not show an arterial to maximum expiration PCO_2 difference, whereas patients with pulmonary embolism do show an increased gradient (Figure 8-31).

Volumetric Capnography. End-tidal CO_2 monitoring tracks exhaled CO_2 plotted over time; volumetric capnometry tracks exhaled CO_2 plotted relative to exhaled volume.

The NICO (Respironics, Murryville, Pennsylvania) is an example of a capnometer that can provide this type of monitoring (Figure 8-32).

Single-Breath Carbon Dioxide Curve. The single-breath CO_2 curve ($SBCO_2$) is produced by the integration of airway flow and CO_2 concentration and is presented on a breath-to-breath basis. As shown in Figure 8-33, this type

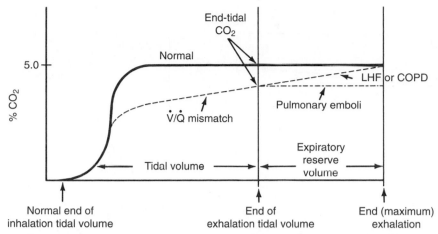

FIGURE 8-31 Capnogram illustrating exhaled carbon dioxide at the end of a quiet expiration and after a maximum expiration. The difference between these two values can be used to assess $\dot{V}/\dot{Q}$ relationships. A patient with COPD typically has an end-tidal carbon dioxide value that is less than that measured after a maximum expiration. In patients suspected of having a pulmonary embolus, the end-tidal and maximum expiratory carbon dioxide measurements are nearly equal. (From Darin J: *Curr Rev Respir Ther* 1:146, 1981; Erickson L, Wollmer P, Olsson CG et al: *Chest* 96:357, 1989; Hatle CJ, Rokseth R: *Chest* 66:352, 1974.)

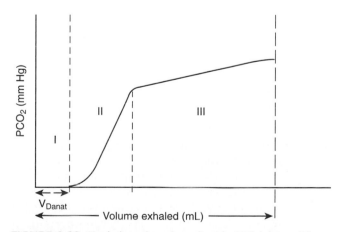

FIGURE 8-32 NICO monitor capnograph. (Courtesy Respironics, Murryville, Pa.)

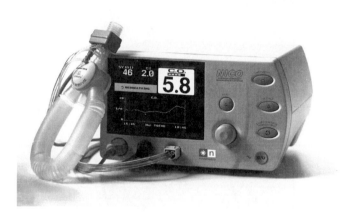

FIGURE 8-33 Single-breath carbon dioxide (CO_2) curve. The horizontal axis of the graph represents the expiratory/inspiratory volume; the vertical axis is the partial pressure of CO in mm Hg. See text for description of the graph. (From Pilbeam SP, Cairo JM: *Mechanical ventilation: physiological and clinical applications,* ed 4, St Louis, 2006, Mosby.)

of graph can provide information on anatomic dead space, alveolar dead space (when the $PaCO_2$ is known), and CO_2 elimination ($\dot{V}CO_2$) for each breath.

The $SBCO_2$ curve is divided into three phases:

· *Phase I:* The first part of the curve represents the volume exhaled from the anatomic dead space that is free of CO_2 (i.e., $FECO_2 = 0$).

· *Phase II:* The second part of the curve shows a rapid rise in $FECO_2$, which represents the transition between airway and alveolar exhaled gas.

· *Phase III:* The third phase is referred to as the *alveolar plateau,* which typically has a positive slope. The slope represents a rising $PACO_2$; the alveoli empty at different rates because of the anatomy of the lung and the various time constants of different units. (NOTE: Perfusion from the pulmonary artery maintains a relatively constant rate of flow past the alveoli. Although the blood is constantly delivering CO_2 to the alveoli, the alveoli get smaller during exhalation. Consequently, the CO_2 level increases in relation to a shrinking volume.)

If a horizontal line is drawn at the top of the curve to represent the percentage of carbon dioxide (% CO_2) in arterial blood, four distinct regions of the curve are established (Figure 8-34).

Area X represents the actual amount of CO_2 exhaled in the breath, assuming that no exhaled air is rebreathed. In other words, the area under the $SBCO_2$ curve is the volume of CO_2 in a single breath. Adding all the single breaths in a minute gives the $\dot{V}CO_2$; the same results that would occur if exhaled gas were collected using a Douglas bag. Area Y represents the amount of CO_2 that is *not* eliminated because of alveolar dead space (i.e., ventilated alveoli that are poorly perfused or receive no perfusion at all). Area Z represents the amount of CO_2 that was *not* eliminated because of anatomic dead space.

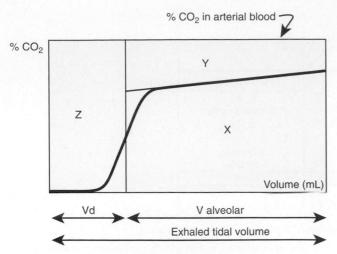

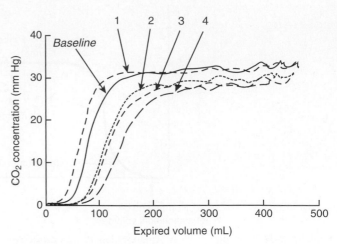

FIGURE 8-34 Graph of exhaled volume (x axis) versus % CO_2 (y axis). A horizontal line drawn at the top of the curve represents the % CO_2 in arterial blood. Three distinct regions are illustrated: Area X represents actual CO_2 exhaled in one breath; area Y is the amount of CO_2 not eliminated because of alveolar dead space; and area Z is the amount of CO_2 not eliminated because of anatomic dead space. V_d, Dead space volume; $V_{anatomic}$, alveolar volume. (Redrawn from material from Respironics, Murryvillle, Pa.)

FIGURE 8-35 Changes in volumetric CO_2 tracing in an experimental model when pulmonary artery blood flow was progressively restricted. Note that phase II shifts to the right as perfusion decreases. (From Pilbeam SP, Cairo JM: *Mechanical ventilation: physiological and clinical applications*, ed 4, St Louis, 2006, Mosby; Adapted from Thompson JE, Jaffe MB: Capnographic waveforms in the mechanically ventilated patient. *Respir Care* 50(1):100-109, 2005.)

This type of graphic analysis, along with direct measurement of the $PaCO_2$, can provide insight to some important physiologic parameters. The ratios of the areas created in the $SBCO_2$ curve can provide the same result as the relationship seen in the Enghoff-modified Bohr equation:

$$[PaCO_2 - P\bar{E}CO_2]/PaCO_2 = (Y+Z)/(X+Y+Z)$$

where $PaCO_2$ is the arterial partial pressure of carbon dioxide and $P\bar{E}CO_2$ is the mixed expired partial pressure for CO_2. (NOTE: X, Y, and Z are defined above.)

Four major factors influence the $PACO_2$: CO_2 production, perfusion of the lungs, diffusion, and ventilation. The balance of these four components represents the total transport and elimination of CO_2. It should be apparent that altering any one of the four without a compensatory change in the other three factors results in changes in the $PaCO_2$ and the volume of CO_2 eliminated through the lungs.[38] For example, $\dot{V}CO_2$ increases in patients with sepsis, fever, severe burns, trauma, and during increased work of breathing, in which the respiratory muscles produce additional CO_2 (i.e., conditions that can increase the volume of CO_2 produced are related to increases in metabolism). Therefore, if the metabolism increases and ventilation does not, the $PaCO_2$ rises and the amount of CO_2 exhaled during the $SBCO_2$ increases.

Figure 8-35 shows changes in volumetric CO_2 tracing that occur in an experimental model in which the pulmonary artery blood flow was progressively restricted. Volume and metabolism remain constant, and overall CO_2 production ($\dot{V}CO_2$) remains stable. As perfusion to the lung is progressively reduced (represented by curves 1 to 4), the phase II curve shifts to the right, showing increased dead space in the system. In this case, physiologic dead space

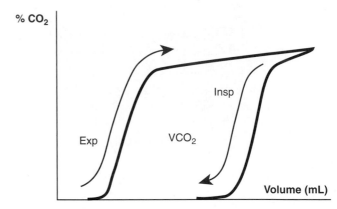

FIGURE 8-36 Single-breath CO_2 curve recorded during inspiration and expiration. % CO_2, Percentage of carbon dioxide; $\dot{V}CO_2$, carbon dioxide elimination; *exp*, expiration; *insp*, inspiration. (Courtesy Teb Tabor, Paris, France.)

increased. Notice that the area under the curves progressively decreases because less CO_2 is exhaled per breath. This is a simple explanation for a complex series of events. As the clinician becomes more familiar with the monitoring technique and applies physiologic principles, the two parameters provide a valuable assessment tool.[39]

$SBCO_2$ Loop of Inspiration and Exhalation. When the $SBCO_2$ graph includes both inspiration and exhalation, a loop is produced (Figure 8-36). The net volume of CO_2 exhaled in one breath is the area between the exhaled and inhaled CO_2 of this loop. Often the inspiratory portion of the curve is negligible. The net CO_2 in one breath is the difference between the amount of CO_2 inhaled and the amount exhaled.

Trending CO_2 Production and Alveolar Minute Ventilation over Time. As mentioned earlier, the NICO

CLINICAL ROUNDS 8-4

Volumetric capnography tracings for a patient being mechanically ventilated with 5 cm H_2O of PEEP have demonstrated a progressive decrease in phase II after the PEEP was increased to 10 cm H_2O. Describe the significance of this finding.

See Evolve Resources for the answer.

BOX 8-4	Formulae Used during Indirect Calorimetry

ENERGY EXPENDITURE

Weir Equation[44]

$$EE = [3.941\,(\dot{V}O_2) + 1.106\,(\dot{V}CO_2)]\,1.44 - 12.17\,(UN)$$

Modified Weir Equation

$$EE = [3.9\,(\dot{V}O_2) + 1.1\,(\dot{V}CO_2)] \times 1.44$$

SUBSTRATE UTILIZATION[45]

Carbohydrates

$$dS = 4.115\,(\dot{V}CO_2) - 2.909\,(\dot{V}O_2) - 2.539\,(UN)$$

Fats

$$dF = 1.689\,(\dot{V}O_2 - \dot{V}CO_2) - 1.943\,(UN)$$

Proteins

$$dP = 6.25\,(UN)$$

dS, *dF*, and *dP* represent grams of carbohydrate, fat, and protein, respectively, for a fasting individual.

---

monitor can trend data over time. The display for this purpose reports the CO_2 produced each minute ($\dot{V}CO_2$) rather than SBCO$_2$ curves. Trended data can be used for monitoring a variety of clinical procedures. For example, during a recruitment maneuver in a patient with acute respiratory distress syndrome (ARDS), trended CO_2 data will reveal a transient rise in CO_2 when previously closed alveoli are reopened. This tool can also be used in weaning patients. For example, if the patient's respiratory rate increases during a spontaneous breathing trial (SBT), monitoring of the $\dot{V}CO_2$ can help determine whether the patient's metabolic rate is increasing, thus working the respiratory muscles, or a change in dead space is affecting the patient's ability to wean.

Trending of CO_2 can also be useful for noting the time lag that can occur in CO_2 removal as a result of CO_2 stores (CO_2 bound in the cells or through bicarbonate or bound in the blood). With large stores, the time lag is long, whereas when stores are small, the time lag is short. For example, suppose the alveolar ventilation increases. As a result, $PaCO_2$ decreases, and the stores of CO_2 also start to decrease; however, this second part takes time. In this situation, if alveolar ventilator ($\dot{V}_A$), increases, the SBCO$_2$ increases and the $PaCO_2$ goes down initially. After a slight delay, because the production of CO_2 remains constant, the $PaCO_2$ remains low and the monitored exhaled $\dot{V}CO_2$ returns to baseline, indicating that a balance has returned (Clinical Rounds 8-4).[36]

INDIRECT CALORIMETRY AND METABOLIC MONITORING

Most clinicians rely on equations derived by Harris and Benedict[40] in 1919 to estimate patient energy requirements. These formulae can be quite appropriate for normal individuals and patients who are not critically ill, but their usefulness may be limited for some critically ill patients. Kinney[41] derived correction factors to compensate for the increased energy demands in critically ill patients (e.g., those with burns or bone fractures), but these factors are of limited help when a patient has multiple conditions simultaneously (e.g., sepsis and adult respiratory distress syndrome).

Advances in microprocessor technology have made it relatively easy for respiratory therapists to measure accurately the energy needs and substrate utilization patterns

of hospitalized patients. The technique used to accomplish this task is called indirect calorimetry.

Indirect Calorimetry

Indirect calorimetry is based on the theory that all of a person's energy is derived from the oxidation of carbohydrates, fats, and proteins and that the ratio of carbon dioxide produced to oxygen consumed (i.e., the respiratory quotient, or $\dot{V}CO_2/\dot{V}O_2$) is characteristic of the fuel burned.[42] **Energy expenditure (EE)** is calculated from $\dot{V}O_2$ and $\dot{V}CO_2$ measurements using the Weir equation, and substrate utilization patterns can be determined using equations such as those derived by Burszein et al.[43] and Consolazio et al.[44] Box 8-4 summarizes these equations.

Indirect calorimeters generally are classified according to their method of determining the $\dot{V}O_2$. Therefore two methods usually are described: the closed-circuit method and the open-circuit method. With the **closed-circuit method,** the patient breathes into and out of a container prefilled with oxygen. Oxygen consumption is determined by measuring the oxygen volume used by the patient. With the **open-circuit method,** the volumes of inspired and expired gases are measured, as well as the fractional concentrations of oxygen in each. The $\dot{V}O_2$ is then determined by calculating the difference between the amount of oxygen in inspired gas ($\dot{V}_I \times F_IO_2$) and the amount of oxygen in expired gas ($\dot{V}_E \times F_EO_2$).

Closed-Circuit Calorimeters

With closed-circuit devices, oxygen consumption can be determined by measuring either the oxygen volume removed from the device or the oxygen volume that must be added to the system to maintain the original oxygen volume.

Figure 8-37 illustrates a closed-circuit system in which the $\dot{V}O_2$ is determined by measuring the amount of oxygen removed from a reservoir over time. The system consists of

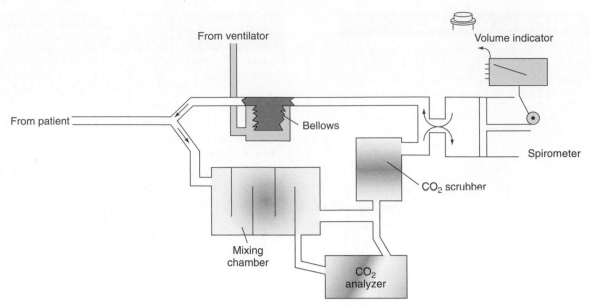

FIGURE 8-37 Closed-circuit indirect calorimeters. Oxygen consumption is estimated by measuring the amount of oxygen used from a reservoir. (From Branson RD: The measurement of energy expenditure: instrumentation, practical considerations, and clinical applications, *Respir Care* 35:640, 1990.)

a breathing circuit connected to a spirometer that is pre-filled with oxygen. The patient's exhaled gases are directed to a mixing chamber, then through a carbon dioxide absorber, and back to the spirometer. Carbon dioxide production ($\dot{V}CO_2$) can be measured by incorporating the carbon dioxide analyzer positioned between the mixing chamber and the carbon dioxide absorber. Closed-circuit calorimeters can be used both for spontaneously breathing and for mechanically ventilated patients.

Oxygen consumption is determined by measuring the oxygen volume removed from the spirometer. The volume of oxygen removed can be determined by measuring the change in the end-expiratory level. (Oxygen consumption is expressed in milliliters per minute.) The fractional concentration of mixed expired carbon dioxide ($FECO_2$) is determined by aspirating a sample of the mixed expired gas (from the mixing chamber) into the carbon dioxide analyzer between the mixing chamber and the spirometer. Carbon dioxide production is calculated by multiplying the fractional concentration of mixed expired carbon dioxide by the minute ventilation and is expressed in milliliters per minute.

Another variation of the closed-circuit technique for estimating oxygen consumption involves measuring the oxygen volume that must be replenished while the patient removes oxygen from the reservoir. This system consists of a breathing circuit, a bellows containing oxygen, a carbon dioxide absorber, and an ultrasonic transducer to monitor the bellows position. As the patient breathes into and out of the bellows, the oxygen used by the patient is replaced on demand by an external oxygen supply. The amount of oxygen that must be added to the system is a measure of oxygen consumption. These systems can be used for

spontaneously breathing and for mechanically ventilated patients.

Open-Circuit Calorimeters

Open-circuit calorimeters use mixing chambers, dilution techniques, and breath-by-breath measurements to determine oxygen consumption. With mixing chambers, expired gases are directed into a collecting chamber containing baffles to ensure adequate mixing of gases. A vacuum attached to the chamber aspirates a sample of the mixed expired gas and directs it into the oxygen and carbon dioxide analyzers. After they are analyzed, the gases are returned to the mixing chamber, and the entire volume of the mixing chamber is routed through a volume- or flow-sensing device.

Dilution systems also use a mixing chamber, but they use a bias flow of room air to dilute the gas sample and move it through the system. The amounts of oxygen and carbon dioxide exhaled are calculated by multiplying the fractional concentrations of oxygen and carbon dioxide by the total flow through the system, which usually is about 40 L/min.

Breath-by-breath devices measure the volume and fractional concentrations of oxygen and carbon dioxide in each breath. The amount of oxygen and carbon dioxide in inspired and mixed expired gases actually is determined by averaging the volumes and concentrations of several breaths. The number of breaths to be averaged can be preselected by the technologist or preset by the manufacturer.

Figure 8-38 is a schematic of an open-circuit indirect calorimeter. A flow- or volume-sensing device is used to measure the inspired and expired gas volumes, a polaro-

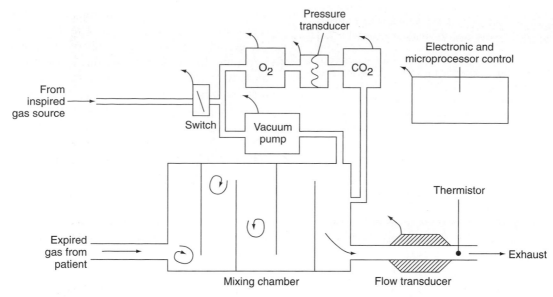

FIGURE 8-38 Open-circuit indirect calorimeter. Oxygen consumption and carbon dioxide production are estimated by multiplying the minute ventilation by the fractional concentration of oxygen and carbon dioxide during inspiration and expiration. (From Branson RD: The measurement of energy expenditure: instrumentation, practical considerations, and clinical applications, *Respir Care* 35:640, 1990.)

graphic analyzer is used to measure the fractional concentrations of oxygen, and a nondispersive infrared analyzer is used to measure the fractional concentration of carbon dioxide. Because changes in ambient temperature and pressure can affect gas concentrations, a sensor for measuring the ambient temperature and barometric pressure of the gases analyzed also is incorporated into the system.

Although open-circuit devices can be used for both spontaneously breathing and mechanically ventilated patients, special problems can arise when these systems are used with mechanically ventilated patients. Some of these problems include fluctuations in the F_IO_2 level, separation of the patient's inspired and expired gases from the continuous gas flow from the ventilator, and handling of water vapor.[45] Problems with fluctuations in the F_IO_2 level can be alleviated to some extent by using air/oxygen blenders or premixed gases.* Beyond F_IO_2 levels of 0.5 to 0.6, most systems are unreliable because of the **Haldane transformation** and should be viewed skeptically. Inspired and expired gases can be separated using isolation valves supplied by the manufacturer of the metabolic monitor. Water vapor is always a problem when continuous measurements are performed on ventilator patients, but the difficulty is accentuated when cascade humidifiers are used to supply humidity to the patient. Replacement of these humidifiers with artificial noses may help minimize the problem.

Practical Applications of Indirect Calorimetry

Spontaneously breathing patients breathing room air can be connected to an indirect calorimetry system by breathing through a mouthpiece or mask attached to a nonrebreathing valve. Specially designed canopies and hoods can also be used for spontaneously breathing patients who are not receiving ventilatory support.

Patients with ETTs or tracheostomy tubes (TTs) can be connected to the system if the nonrebreathing valve is placed directly onto the airway opening and expired gases are routed into the system. It is important to inflate the cuffs of ETTs and TTs when inspired and exhaled gases are to be measured, because failure to do so results in loss of expired air around the tube and erroneous measurements of $\dot{V}O_2$ and $\dot{V}CO_2$. For patients receiving a continuous flow of gas during ventilatory support, such as occurs when a bias flow is present, an isolation valve must be used to ensure that only the patient's exhaled gases are delivered to the system.

As previously stated, oxygen consumption and carbon dioxide production are calculated by comparing the fractional concentrations of oxygen and carbon dioxide of inspired and expired air. When the patient is breathing room air, however, it is reasonable to assume that the fractional concentration of inspired oxygen is 20.9%, and the fractional concentration of inspired carbon dioxide is 0.3%. For patients receiving enriched oxygen mixtures, the fractional concentration of inspired oxygen must be measured by the system. Fluctuations in the F_IO_2 can be caused by air leaks in the patient-ventilator/metabolic monitor system and by varying gas volumes and pressure demands, as occur during intermittent mandatory ventilation. Unstable air-oxygen blending systems in the ventilator

BOX 8-5	Conditions for Obtaining Indirect Calorimetry Measurements

1. The patient should be at rest and in a supine position for at least 30 minutes before the measurement is made.
2. The room temperature should be 20° to 25° C.
3. The patient should remain relaxed during the measurement (i.e., no voluntary physical activity).
4. Measurements should be recorded for 15 to 30 minutes or until the $\dot{V}O_2$ and $\dot{V}CO_2$ vary by less than 5%.

CLINICAL ROUNDS 8-5

While obtaining indirect calorimetric measurements from a mechanically ventilated patient receiving an F_1O_2 of 0.6, you notice that her $\dot{V}O_2$ continually varies from 250 to 800 ml/min over a 10-minute period. Briefly describe several possible causes for these erratic measurements.

See Evolve Resources for the answer.

circuit may also contribute to unstable F_1O_2 levels. In addition, clinical studies have demonstrated that currently available systems cannot provide accurate and reproducible $\dot{V}O_2$ measurements for patients breathing F_1O_2 at levels greater than 0.5. Box 8-5 contains a summary of conditions that should be observed when indirect calorimetry measurements are made (see Clinical Rounds 8-5).

Metabolic Monitoring

The main advantage of using indirect calorimetry instead of prediction equations (e.g., the Harris and Benedict equations) is that indirect calorimetry can provide actual measurements of a patient's caloric needs. Combined with nitrogen excretion measurements, indirect calorimetry can also provide information about substrate utilization, giving the clinician valuable insight into the types of substrates the patient is using to generate energy.

Energy Expenditure

Energy expenditure typically is expressed in kilocalories per day (kcal/day) or relative to an individual's body surface area (kcal/hr/m²). A normal, healthy adult uses 1500 to 3000 kcal/day, or about 30 to 40 kcal/hr/m².[42,43]

Many factors can influence the metabolic rate, including the type and rate of food ingested, the time of day of the measurement, the patient's activity level, and whether the patient is recovering from infection, surgery, or trauma.

Prolonged starvation is associated with a decreased metabolic rate. Eating raises the metabolic rate through a mechanism called *specific dynamic action*. Specific dynamic action is thought to be related to the digestion and absorption of food.[44] Energy expenditure shows diurnal variation (i.e., it is usually higher in the morning than in the evening), which may be related to the variations in hormone levels that naturally occur daily.[45] Changes in activity are a well-recognized factor that can alter the metabolic rate. Figure 8-39 shows how changes in physical activity can affect energy expenditure in a hospitalized patient. Note that sleep is associated with a reduction in the metabolic rate, and even the slightest exertion is associated with an increase in the metabolic rate. Fever, as can occur with bacterial and viral infection, also can have a profound effect on the metabolic rate. For example, an increase in body temperature of 1° F causes a 10% increase in the metabolic rate. Burns, long-bone fractures, and surgery can increase the metabolic rate by as much as 200%.[41]

Substrate Utilization Patterns

The substrate utilization pattern is the proportions of carbohydrates, fats, and proteins that contribute to the total energy metabolism. As was previously stated, the percentage of the total energy that a substrate contributes can be determined using the RQ. Remember that the RQ is the ratio of $\dot{V}CO_2$ to $\dot{V}O_2$. The RQs for various foods are shown in Table 8-6. When pure fat is burned, the RQ is 0.7. The RQ for pure carbohydrate is 1, and the RQ for protein is approximately 0.8. RQs greater than 1 are associated with lipogenesis (fat synthesis), metabolic acidosis, and hyperventilation. RQs less than 0.7 are associated with ketosis.

Healthy adults who consume a typical American diet derive 45% to 50% of their calories from carbohydrates, 35% to 40% from lipids, and 10% to 15% from proteins. The resultant RQ ranges from 0.8 to 0.85.[44] Under normal conditions, proteins normally contribute only minor amounts to energy metabolism. Note that the percentage of protein used represents the normal turnover rate for replenishing structural and functional proteins in the body. Proteins may contribute significantly to EE, however, in cases of starvation. For this reason, a nonprotein RQ usually is reported to indicate the contribution to RQ made by carbohydrates and lipids.

Substrate utilization is determined by the types of substrates ingested and an individual's ability to use various types of foods. For example, eating a large amount of

TABLE 8-6	
Variations in the Respiratory Quotient	
Substrate	**Respiratory Quotient**
Carbohydrate oxidation	1.0
Fat oxidation	0.7
Protein oxidation	0.8
Lipogenesis	>1.0

Metabolic Measurements Using Indirect Calorimetry during Mechanical Ventilation—2004 Revision and Update

Clinical Practice Guideline 8-3

■ INDICATIONS

1. In patients with known nutritional deficits or derangements. Multiple nutritional risk and stress factors that may considerably skew prediction by the Harris-Benedict equation include:
   a. Neurologic trauma
   b. Paralysis
   c. Chronic obstructive pulmonary disease (COPD)
   d. Acute pancreatitis
   e. Cancer with residual tumor burden
   f. Multiple trauma
   g. Amputations
   h. Patients in whom the height and weight cannot be accurately obtained
   i. Patients who fail to respond adequately to estimated nutritional needs
   j. Patients who require long-term acute care
   k. Severe sepsis
   l. Extremely obese patients
   m. Severely hypermetabolic or hypometabolic patients
2. When patients fail attempts at liberation from mechanical ventilation to measure the O_2 cost of breathing and the components of ventilation.
3. When the need exists to assess oxygen consumption ($\dot{V}O_2$) to evaluate the hemodynamic support of mechanically ventilated patients.
4. To measure cardiac output by the Fick methods.
5. To determine the cause or causes of increased ventilatory requirements.

■ CONTRAINDICATIONS

When a specific indication is present, no contraindications to performing a metabolic measurement using indirect calorimetry exist unless short-term disconnection of ventilatory support for connection of measurement lines results in hypoxemia, bradycardia, or other adverse effects.

■ HAZARDS/COMPLICATIONS

1. Closed-circuit calorimeters may cause a reduction in alveolar ventilation as a result of increased compressible volume of the breathing circuit.
2. Closed-circuit calorimeters may reduce the trigger sensitivity of the ventilator and result in increased work of breathing for the patient.
3. Short-term disconnection of the patient from the ventilator for connection of the indirect calorimetry apparatus may result in hypoxemia, bradycardia, and patient discomfort.
4. Inappropriate calibration or system setup may result in erroneous readings, causing incorrect patient management.
5. Isolation valves may increase circuit resistance and cause increased work of breathing and/or dynamic hyperinflation.
6. Inspiratory reservoirs may cause a reduction in alveolar ventilation as a result of increased compressible volume of the breathing circuit.
7. Manipulation of the ventilator circuit may cause leaks that may lower alveolar ventilation.

Modified from American Association for Respiratory Care: AARC Clinical practice guideline: metabolic measurements using indirect calorimetry during mechanical ventilation—2004 revision and update. Respir Care 49:107, 2004.

glucose raises the RQ to about 1, which suggests that carbohydrates are providing most of the energy expenditure. Prolonged starvation lowers the RQ to about 0.7, indicating that the individual is relying almost completely on fats for energy. Many systemic diseases adversely affect an individual's ability to use various types of substrates. For example, several studies have shown that patients with severe sepsis have RQs of approximately 0.7 because of their reliance on lipid metabolism for energy and an inability to use carbohydrates.[46]

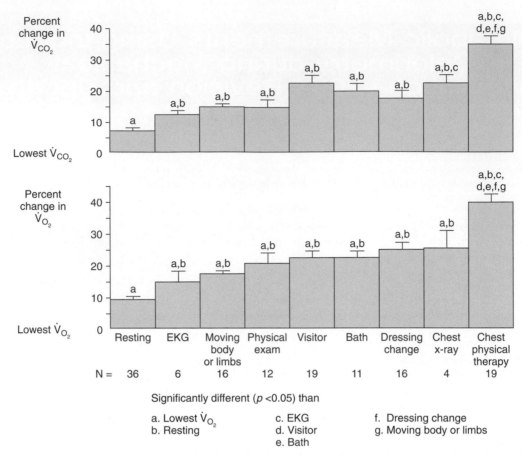

FIGURE 8-39 Variations in oxygen consumption and carbon dioxide production (expressed as percent change) associated with diagnostic and therapeutic interactions in a patient in the intensive care unit. (From Weismann C, Kemper MC, Damask M: The effects of routine interactions on metabolic rate, *Chest* 86:815, 1984.)

KEY POINTS

▶ Spirometers generally are classified as volume-collecting or flow-sensing devices. Common examples of volume-collecting devices include water-sealed spirometers, bellows spirometers, and dry rolling seal devices. The most commonly used flow-sensing devices include thermal and turbine flowmeters and pneumotachographs.

▶ Variable orifice pneumotachographs and vortex ultrasonic flowmeters are relatively low-cost pneumotachometers that can provide valuable bedside measurements of respiratory mechanics.

▶ The ATS/ERS unified standards for lung function testing provide guidance on the measurement and interpretation of spirometry, diffusing capacity, and lung volume tests.

▶ Respiratory inductive plethysmography is a noninvasive method of monitoring the breathing patterns of patients in sleep laboratories, pulmonary function laboratories, and intensive care units.

▶ Noninvasive measurements of respiratory system mechanics, such as vital capacity and its subdivisions, can be provide valuable information that can be used in the diagnosis and management of patients with cardiopulmonary dysfunctions.

▶ Measurements of FRC, RV, and TLC can provide valuable information for the management of patients with chronic obstructive and restrictive pulmonary diseases.

▶ Advances in microprocessor technology have significantly improved a respiratory therapist's ability to assess the ventilatory function of mechanically ventilated patients. Evaluation of airway resistance, respiratory system compliance, and work of breathing studies can provide information that can assist the management of these patients.

▶ Accurate measurements of the inspired oxygen concentration are essential for successful management of hypoxemic patients.

▶ Chemiluminescence and electrochemical monitoring are routinely used when nitric oxide is administered to prevent the potential toxic effects induced by high levels of NO and NO_2.

▶ Capnography is a simple, noninvasive method for monitoring the ventilatory status of spontaneously and mechanically ventilated patients. The contour of the

KEY POINTS—cont'd

capnograph can be evaluated to detect dead space ventilation, hyperventilation and hypoventilation, apnea, and periodic breathing.

▶ Volumetric capnography is a useful method for noninvasively assessing carbon dioxide elimination, which can be used to help wean patients from mechanical ventilatory support.

▶ Indirect calorimetry allows clinicians to obtain actual measurements of a patient's caloric needs rather than relying on prediction equations. Although prediction equations can provide useful estimates of metabolic requirements for normal, healthy individuals, they may underestimate the caloric and substrate needs of patients afflicted with multiple organ dysfunction.

ASSESSMENT QUESTIONS

See Evolve Resources for the answers.

1. Which of the following spirometers are classified as flow-sensing devices?
   I. Wright respirometers
   II. Hot wire anemometers
   III. Dry rolling seal spirometers
   IV. Stead-Wells spirometers
   a. I and II only
   b. II and III only
   c. II and IV only
   d. I, II, and III only

2. Which of the following can influence the accuracy of spirometer measurements?
   I. The linearity and frequency response of the device
   II. The device's sensitivity to environmental conditions
   III. The frequency of calibration
   IV. The presence of an obstructive or restrictive pulmonary disease
   a. I and II only
   b. II and III only
   c. I, II, and III only
   d. I, II, III, and IV

3. According to ATS/ERS standards, spirometers used to measure vital capacity should have an accuracy range (in BTPS) of:
   a. 5 L ± 10% of the reading, or 50 mL, whichever is greater
   b. 6 L ± 5% of the reading, or 50 mL, whichever is greater
   c. 7 L ± 3% of the reading, or 50 mL, whichever is greater
   d. 12 L ± 3% of the reading, or 50 mL, whichever is greater

4. Which of the following is considered the primary criterion for identifying the end of a successful nitrogen washout test?
   a. Patient becomes fatigued.
   b. Exhaled nitrogen concentration is less than 1.5%.
   c. Nitrogen percentage remains stable for 2 minutes.
   d. Exhaled volume equals the FRC.

5. Which of the following can cause erroneous measurements with impedance pneumography?
   I. Sinus tachycardia
   II. Upper airway obstruction
   III. Central apnea
   IV. Tachypnea
   a. I only
   b. II only
   c. II and III only
   d. I, II, and III only

6. Which of the following lung volumes cannot be measured by simple spirometry?
   I. VC
   II. RV
   III. TLC
   IV. IC
   a. I and II only
   b. II and III only
   c. III and IV only
   d. I, III, and IV only

7. Maximum inspiratory pressures normally are:
   a. −20 to −40 cm H_2O
   b. −50 to −80 cm H_2O
   c. −60 to −100 cm H_2O
   d. −150 to −200 cm H_2O

8. Which of the following measurements is considered a good indicator of a patient's effort during an FVC maneuver?
   a. FEV_1
   b. PEF
   c. FEV_1/FVC
   d. FEF_{25-75}

9. Lack of a definitive phase 3 on a capnogram most often is associated with:
   a. insufficient neuromuscular blockade
   b. cardiac oscillations
   c. $\dot{V}/\dot{Q}$ imbalances, such as occur with patients with emphysema or chronic bronchitis
   d. rebreathing of exhaled gases

ASSESSMENT QUESTIONS—cont'd

10. How many kilocalories of energy per day should a typical healthy adult ingest to maintain energy balance?
   a. 500 to 1000
   b. 900 to 1200
   c. 1200 to 1800
   d. 1500 to 3000

11. You notice that the FRC measured on a patient with COPD with the nitrogen washout technique is different from that measured with body plethysmography. In fact, the volume measured with the body box is approximately 500 mL greater than the FRC measured with nitrogen washout. Why might this difference exists?
   a. Trapped gas in the lungs
   b. Ventilation-perfusion mismatch
   c. Elevated carbon monoxide level in the patient's blood
   d. Severe hypercapnia

12. Which of the following analyzers can be used to measure nitric oxide?
   I. Chemiluminescence analyzer
   II. Polarographic analyzer
   III. Electrochemical analyzer
   IV. Capnography
   a. I only
   b. II only
   c. I and III only
   d. I, II, and III only

13. A patient receiving mechanical ventilatory support via an ETT is being monitored for oxygen consumption. Which of the following could lead to an erroneous measurement?
   I. The patient appears agitated.
   II. The measurement is performed immediately after the patient receives a physical therapy treatment.
   III. The F_IO_2 is 0.8.
   IV. The patient's ETT cuff is inflated to seal the airway.
   a. I and II only
   b. II and III only
   c. I, II, and III only
   d. I, II, III, and IV

14. The only source of nutrition administered to a patient is D_5W (i.e., 5% dextrose in water). What would you expect to find when measuring the RQ?
   a. 0.7 to 0.75
   b. 0.8 to 0.85
   c. 0.9 to 0.95
   d. 1

15. Which of the following patient conditions would you expect to be hypermetabolic (elevated $\dot{V}O_2$)?
   a. Starvation
   b. Fever
   c. Sedation
   d. Hypothermia

References

1. Wasserman K et al: *Principles of exercise testing and interpretation*, Philadelphia, 1994, Lea & Febiger.
2. East TD: What makes noninvasive monitoring tick?: a review of basic engineering principles, *Respir Care* 35:500, 1990.
3. Ruppel GL: *Manual of pulmonary function testing*, ed 9, St Louis, 2008, Elsevier-Mosby.
4. Fleisch A: Der pneumotachograph: ein apparacat zur beischwindig-kertregstrier der ateniluft, *Arch Ges Physiol* 209:713, 1925.
5. Sullivan WJ, Peters GM, Enright PL: Pneumotachography: theory and clinical application, *Respir Care* 29:736, 1984.
6. American Association for Respiratory Care: AARC clinical practice guideline: body plethysmography, *Respir Care* 46:506, 2001.
7. American Association for Respiratory Care: AARC clinical practice guideline: static lung volumes—2001 revision and update, *Respir Care* 46:531, 2001.
8. Wanger J, Clausen JL, Coates A et al: Standardization of the measurement of lung volumes, *Eur Respir J* 26:511, 2005.
9. Kacmarek RM, Hess D, Stoller JK: *Monitoring in respiratory care*, St Louis, 1993, Mosby.
10. Miller MR, Crapo R, Hankinson J et al: General considerations for lung function testing, *Eur Respir J* 26:153, 2005.
11. American Thoracic Society: Snowbird workshop on standardization of spirometry, *Am Rev Respir Dis* 119:831, 1979.
12. American Thoracic Society: Standardization of spirometry—1987 update, *Am Rev Respir Dis* 136:1285, 1987.
13. American Thoracic Society: Lung function testing: selection of reference values and interpretation, *Am Rev Respir Dis* 144:1202, 1991.
14. American Thoracic Society: Standardization of spirometry—1994 update, *Am Rev Respir Dis* 152:1107, 1995.
15. Quanjer PH, editor: Standardized lung function testing: report of the Working Party on Standardization of Lung Function Test, European Community of Coal and Steel, *Bull Eur Physiopathol Respir* 5:1, 1983.
16. Brusasco V, Crapo R, Viegi G: Coming together: the ATS/ERS consensus on clinical pulmonary function testing, *Eur Respir J* 26:1, 2005.
17. Miller MR, Hankinson J, Brusasco V et al: Standardization of spirometry, *Eur Respir J* 26:319, 2005.
18. MacIntyre N, Crapo RO, Viegi G et al: Standardization of the single-breath determination of carbon monoxide uptake in the lung, *Eur Respir J* 26:720, 2005.
19. Branson RD, Campbell RS: Impedance pneumography, apnea monitoring, and respiratory inductive plethysmography. In Kacmarek RM, Hess D, Stoller JK, editors: *Monitoring in respiratory care*, St Louis, 1993, Mosby.
20. Southhall DP et al: Undetected episodes of prolonged apnea and severe bradycardia in preterm infants, *Pediatrics* 72:541, 1983.
21. Wayburton D, Stork AR, Taeusch HW: Apnea monitoring in infants with upper airway obstruction, *Pediatrics* 60:742, 1967.
22. Konno K, Mead J: Measurement of the separate changes of rib cage and abdomen during breathing, *J Appl Physiol* 22:407, 1967.

23. Pellegrino R, Viegi G, Brusasco V et al: Interpretative strategies for lung function tests, *Eur Respir J* 26:948, 2005.

24. Marini JJ: Lung mechanics determination at the bedside: instrumentation and clinical application, *Respir Care* 35:669, 1990.

25. Osborne JJ, Wilson RM: Monitoring the mechanical properties of the lung. In Spence AA, editor: *Respiratory monitoring in the intensive care unit,* New York, 1980, Churchill Livingstone.

26. Pauling L, Wood RE, Sturdivant JH: Oxygen meter, *J Am Chem Soc* 68:795, 1946.

27. Etches PC et al: Clinical monitoring of inhaled nitric oxide: comparison of chemiluminescence and electrochemical sensors, *Biomed Instrum Technol* 29:134, 1995.

28. Miller CC: Chemiluminescence analysis and nitrogen dioxide measurement, *Lancet* 34:300, 1994.

29. Body S, Hartigan PM, Shernan SK, et al: Nitric oxide: delivery, measurement, and clinical application, *J Cardiothoracic Vasc Anesth* 9:748, 1995.

30. Purtz E, Hess D, Kacmarek R: Evaluation of electrochemical nitric oxide and nitrogen dioxide analyzers suitable for use during mechanical ventilation, *J Clin Monit* 13:25, 1997.

31. American Association for Respiratory Care: AARC clinical practice guideline: capnography, *Respir Care* 40:1321, 1995.

32. Stock MC: Capnography for adults, *Critical Care Clin* 11:219, 1995.

33. Hess D: Capnometry and capnography: technical aspects, physiologic aspects, and clinical applications, *Respir Care* 35:557, 1990.

34. Kennel EM, Andrews RW, Wollman H: Correction factors for nitrous oxide in the infrared analysis of carbon dioxide, *Anesthesiology* 39:441, 1973.

35. Gravenstein JS, Paulus DA, Hayes TJ: *Capnography in clinical practice,* Boston, 1989, Butterworth.

36. Pilbeam SP, Cairo JM: *Mechanical ventilation,* ed 4, St Louis, 2006, Mosby.

37. Davis PD, Parbrook GD, Kenny GNC: *Basic physics and measurement in anesthesia,* ed 4, Oxford, 1995, Butterworth-Heinemann.

38. Taskar V, Larsson A, Wetterberg T et al: Dynamics of carbon dioxide elimination following ventilator resetting, *Chest* 108:196, 1995.

39. Gravenstein JS, Jaffe MB, Paulus DA: *Capnography: clinical aspects—carbon dioxide over time and volume,* Cambridge, UK, 2004, Cambridge University Press.

40. Harris JA, Benedict F: *Standard basal metabolism constants for physiologists and clinicians: a biometric study of basal metabolism in man,* Philadelphia, 1919, JB Lippincott.

41. Kinney JM: The application of indirect calorimetry in clinical studies: assessment of energy metabolism in health and disease. In Kinney JM, editor: *Report of the first Ross conference on medical research,* Columbus, Ohio, 1980, Ross Laboratories.

42. Ferrannini E: The theoretical basis of indirect calorimetry: a review, *Metabolism* 37:287, 1987.

43. Burszein P et al: Utilization of protein, carbohydrate, and fat in fasting and postabsorptive subjects, *Am J Clin Nutr* 33:998, 1980.

44. Consolazio CJ, Johnson RE, Pecora LJ: *Physiological measurements of metabolic function in man,* New York, 1963, McGraw-Hill.

45. Weir JB: New method for calculating metabolic rate with special reference to protein metabolism, *J Physiology* 109:1, 1949.

46. Branson RD, Lacey J, Berry S: Indirect calorimetry and nutritional monitoring. In Levine RL, Fromm RE, editors: *Critical care monitoring,* St Louis, 1995, Mosby.

Internet Resources

American Association for Respiratory Care: http://www.aarc.org

Society of Critical Care Medicine: http://www.sccm.org

American Association of Cardiovascular and Pulmonary Rehabilitation: http://www.aacvpr.org

Canadian Journal of Respiratory Therapy: http://www.csrt.com

Virtual Hospital: http://www.vh.org

American Thoracic Society: http://www.thoracic.org/sections/publications/statements/index.html

Medline Search Engine: http://medline.cos.com

National Library of Medicine: http://www.nlm.nih.gov

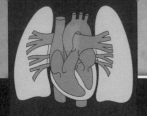

Chapter 9

Assessment of Cardiovascular Function

J.M. CAIRO

OUTLINE

Electrocardiography
  Electrophysiology of Cardiac Cells
Principles of Electrocardiography
  The Electrocardiograph
  The Normal Electrocardiogram
  Interpretation of Electrocardiograms

Hemodynamic Monitoring
  The Cardiac Cycle
  Pressure Measurements
  Cardiac Output Measurements
  Interpretation of Hemodynamic Profiles

OBJECTIVES

Upon completion of this chapter you will be able to:
· Discuss the electrophysiologic properties of the heart.
· Explain the principles of electrocardiography.
· Identify the major components of an electrocardiograph.
· Demonstrate the correct placement of electrodes on a patient to obtain a 12-lead electrocardiogram.
· Explain the various waves, complexes, and intervals that appear on a normal electrocardiogram.
· List and describe the most common dysrhythmias encountered in clinical electrocardiography.
· Describe the pressure, volume, and flow events that occur in the heart and major blood vessels during a typical cardiac cycle.
· Explain the principle of operation of various noninvasive and invasive devices routinely used to obtain blood pressure measurements.
· Describe various methods used to measure cardiac output.
· Interpret hemodynamic measurements obtained from patients in a critical care setting.

KEY TERMS

absolute refractory period
action potential
atrial diastole
atrial fibrillation
atrial flutter
atrial premature depolarizations
atrial systole
automaticity
cardiac cycle
cardiac work
conductivity
diastasis
diastolic depolarization
effective refractory period
excitability
floating electrodes
heart blocks

impedance cardiography
impedance plethysmography
incisura
isovolumetric contraction
isovolumetric relaxation
junctional escape rhythm
Korotkoff's sounds
murmurs
normal sinus rhythm
paroxysmal atrial tachycardia (PAT)
phonocardiogram
premature ventricular beats
premature ventricular depolarizations
pulmonary vascular resistance (PVR)

relative refractory period
rhythmicity
sinus arrhythmia
sinus bradycardia
sinus tachycardia
sphygmomanometer
systemic vascular resistance (SVR)
ventricular asystole
ventricular diastole
ventricular fibrillation
ventricular systole
ventricular tachycardia
volume conductor
Wolff-Parkinson-White (WPW) syndrome

Successful management of patients with cardiovascular and pulmonary dysfunctions requires a working knowledge of cardiovascular physiology. This knowledge can be applied clinically to quantify various aspects of cardiovascular function with techniques such as electrocardiography and hemodynamic monitoring. This chapter provides an overview of the most common devices and techniques used by respiratory therapists to assess cardiovascular function.

ELECTROCARDIOGRAPHY

Electrophysiology of Cardiac Cells

Contraction of cardiac muscle provides the energy required to propel blood through the circulation. Under normal circumstances, each heartbeat is initiated by specialized pacemaker cells of the heart, which have the property of rhythmic, spontaneous electrical activity. When these specialized pacemaker cells depolarize (i.e., become electrically activated), they cause other electrically excitable cells of the heart to depolarize, resulting in simultaneous activation of the right and left atria, followed by simultaneous activation of the right and left ventricles.[1,2]

To fully appreciate this ability of cardiac cells to initiate and conduct electrical impulses, we must consider three important aspects of the electrophysiology of the heart: **excitability, automaticity,** and **conductivity.** *Excitability* may be defined as the ability of a cell to respond to an electrical stimulus. *Automaticity* is the ability of certain specialized cells of the heart to depolarize spontaneously. These specialized cells, which are located at the sinoatrial (SA) and atrioventricular (AV) nodes, can initiate **action potentials** in the absence of nerve impulses from the central nervous system. *Conductivity* is the ability of cardiac tissue to propagate an action potential.

An understanding of the cellular events that occur during a heartbeat provides a foundation for the study of electrocardiography and for identifying abnormalities of the electrical activity of the heart. We therefore begin our discussion of electrocardiography with a brief description of the basic electrophysiologic properties of the heart.

Resting Membrane Potentials

Like other cells of the human body, cardiac cells are polarized; that is, the inside of a cardiac cell has a negative electrical charge relative to the outside of the cell. This property of polarization can be explained by the selective permeability of the cell membrane to various types of molecules and ions.[2] Large molecules, such as proteins, normally have a negative charge at physiologic pH. These negatively charged macromolecules are trapped within cells because they are too large to pass freely through pores in the membrane. Smaller ions, such as potassium, sodium, and calcium, are also influenced by the selective permeability characteristics of the cell membrane, although their movements across the membrane are governed primarily by chemical and

electrical gradients rather than particle size. For example, under normal resting conditions, the concentration of potassium ions is higher in the intracellular fluid than in the extracellular fluid. Conversely, the concentrations of sodium and calcium ions are higher in the extracellular fluid than in the intracellular fluid. If the membrane were freely permeable to all ions, it is reasonable to assume that an equal exchange of positive ions would occur across the membrane. In fact, the resting cell membrane is much more permeable to potassium ions than it is to sodium and calcium ions; therefore, more potassium ions leak from the cell than sodium or calcium ions leak into the cell. Thus, under resting conditions, the greater efflux of potassium out of the cell compared to the influx of sodium and calcium into the cell results in polarization of the cell membrane, with the intracellular charge being more negative than the extracellular charge. It is important to mention that electrical gradients also can influence the movement of these small ions across the cell membrane. In the situation described here, potassium movement out of the cell is promoted by the chemical concentration gradient and opposed by the electrical gradient between the inside and outside of the cell; sodium movement into the cell is promoted by both gradients. Table 9-1 shows the chemical composition of the intracellular and extracellular fluids.[1]

Another factor that must be considered in a discussion of the origin of the resting membrane potential is the sodium-potassium ATPase pump, an enzyme in the cell membrane. This pump functions to move out of the cell excess sodium that leaks into the cell and excess potassium that leaks out of the cell back into the intracellular compartment. It is important to recognize that the sodium-potassium pump moves more sodium out of the cell than it moves potassium back into the cell, thus adding to the potential difference across the cell membrane.[2] It also is worth noting that this pump represents an active (i.e., energy dependent) mechanism for moving ions across the cell membrane compared with the passive electrochemical forces previously discussed.

TABLE 9-1		
Chemical Composition of Intracellular and Extracellular Spaces		
	Extracellular Fluid	**Intracellular Fluid**
Na^+	142 mEq/L	10 mEq/L
K^+	4 mEq/L	140 mEq/L
Ca^{++}	2.4 mEq/L	0.0001 mEq/L
Mg^{++}	1.2 mEq/L	58 mEq/L
Cl^-	103 mEq/L	4 mEq/L
HCO_3^-	24 mEq/L	10 mEq/L
Phosphates	4 mEq/L	75 mEq/L
SO_4^-	1 mEq/L	2 mEq/L
Glucose	90 mg/dL	0-20 mg/dL
Proteins	2 gm/dL	5 gm/dL

Cardiac Action Potentials

As can other excitable tissue, cardiac cells can depolarize, rapidly initiating an action potential, and then repolarize. In muscle cells, action potentials are responsible for the initiation of muscle contraction. If an excitable cell is depolarized either by a propagated wave of excitation originally initiated by pacemaker cells or by artificial stimulation, it may reach a critical level, called its *threshold potential,* and an action potential occurs.[2]

Most of the excitable cardiac cells, including atrial and ventricular muscle cells, and the specialized conducting cells, such as Purkinje fibers, have action potentials like the one shown in Figure 9-1A. Pacemaker cells, including those of the SA node and AV node, have a slightly different type of action potential (Figure 9-1B). The latter type of action potentials is discussed in the section on pacemaker cell action potentials.

As Figure 9-1A shows, the action potential begins when the cell membrane of the excitable cell is exposed to a depolarizing current and eventually reaches its excitation threshold potential. The initial phase of this type of action potential (at the point where the cell reaches its threshold potential), referred to as *phase 0,* consists of a rapid upstroke or depolarization. This change in membrane potential to a more positive value occurs because of a rapid influx of sodium ions into the cell. (At the peak of phase 0, the inside of the cell actually becomes positive relative to the outside of the cell.) The increased conductance of sodium into the cell during this phase of the action potential is thought to occur as a result of activation of the so-called *fast* sodium channels in the cell membrane.[1,2] After several milliseconds, these sodium channels become inactivated and close. They remain closed until the cell reaches its resting membrane potential. As is discussed later in the chapter, when these fast sodium channels are closed, the cell is refractory to additional stimuli. During phase 1, the cell undergoes a partial repolarization, in which the membrane potential falls from a value of about 20 mV to a value of about 0 mV. It is thought that this partial repolarization results from a countercurrent flow of potassium out of the cell and to a decrease in sodium conductance into the cell with closure of the fast sodium gates. At this time, a series of slow calcium and sodium channels opens, and a plateau phase 2 is established. Phase 2 lasts approximately 200 to 300 msec. Phase 3 of the action potential begins when the myocardial cell starts to repolarize and return toward the negative resting membrane potential, or phase 4 of the action potential. This repolarization occurs because the membrane becomes more permeable to potassium ions, allowing a greater number of these charged ions to move outside of the cell, and inactivation of the slow channels for calcium and sodium. The increased efflux of positive potassium ions at the same time as the decreased influx of sodium and calcium ions results in restoration of the negative resting membrane potential.[1,2]

The period from the beginning of phase 0 to the middle of phase 3 is referred to as the **absolute** or **effective refrac-**

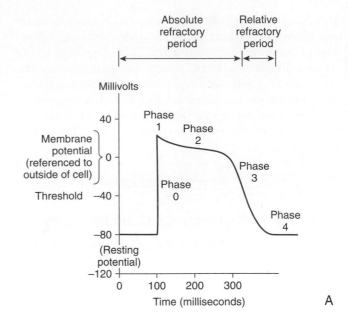

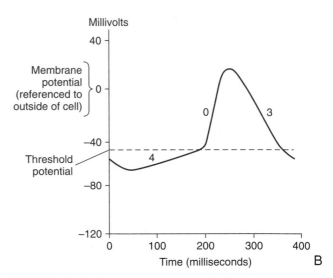

FIGURE 9-1 Cardiac action potentials. **A,** Fast-type action potentials, such as those seen in atrial and ventricular muscle and His-Purkinje fibers. **B,** Slow-type action potentials characteristic of nodal tissue, such as the SA node and AV node.

tory period, because regardless of the strength of the stimulus, the myocyte cannot be depolarized again. A **relative refractory period** follows immediately after the absolute refractory period (this period begins during the middle of phase 3 and lasts until the beginning of phase 4). During the relative refractory period, the myocyte can be depolarized again by a stronger than normal stimulus; however, the amplitude and duration of these action potentials are considerably reduced.

Pacemaker Action Potentials (Rhythmicity)

As was mentioned previously, pacemaker cells of the SA and AV nodes normally have action potentials that differ from those of other excitable cells of the heart. As shown in Figure 9-1B, the resting membrane potential and threshold potential of pacemaker cells are less negative than those of other excitable myocardial cells. Phase 0 of pacemaker cells is slower than the action potentials of atrial, ventricular, and Purkinje fiber myocardial cells. (Because the slope of phase 0 of the pacemaker cell's action potential is less than those of the atrial, ventricular, and Purkinje fiber action potentials, the former often are referred to as *slow* action potentials, whereas the latter are called *fast* action potentials.) In addition, pacemaker cells do not have a prolonged phase 2, or plateau (i.e., the action potential for these cells includes only phases 0, 3, and 4). The most important difference between the *slow* and *fast* action potentials is the rate at which pacemaker cells can elicit a spontaneous action potential during phase 4. It is thought that this ability of pacemaker cells to discharge automatically results from a progressive decrease in permeability of the cell membrane to potassium ions while the permeability of the membrane to sodium remains unchanged. As a result, the inside of the cell progressively depolarizes (i.e., phase 4 **diastolic depolarization**). When the threshold is reached, the action potential occurs. Although the frequency of discharge (i.e., the heart rate) is influenced primarily by the decrease in permeability of the membrane to potassium, the amplitude of the slow action potential is determined by the influx of calcium into the cell. Under normal conditions the SA node discharges approximately 60 to 100 times per minute, whereas the AV node discharges 40 to 60 times per minute. Although other myocardial cells, such as Purkinje fiber cells, can also discharge spontaneously, their discharge rate is so low (15 to 40 times per minute) that they do not normally act as pacemaker cells.

The heart rate can be increased by anything that increases the rate of spontaneous depolarization. That is, anything that increases the slope of the phase 4 diastolic depolarization raises the resting membrane potential (i.e., makes it less negative) or decreases the threshold potential. Conversely, the heart rate is decreased by anything that decreases the rate of spontaneous phase 4 depolarization, whether by decreasing the slope of phase 4, hyperpolarizing the resting membrane potential (making the resting membrane potential more negative), or raising the threshold potential.

Although it has been stated that the heart can initiate impulses in the absence of inputs from the central nervous system, it should be apparent that an individual's heart rate changes dramatically with alterations in the level of activation of the autonomic nervous system (i.e., sympathetic versus parasympathetic control). Norepinephrine and epinephrine, which mediate sympathetic control, can increase the heart rate by increasing the slope of the phase 4 diastolic depolarization, decreasing the threshold potential, or hypopolarizing the resting membrane potential; acetylcholine, which mediates parasympathetic control, can decrease the heart rate by decreasing the slope of the phase 4 depolarization, increasing the threshold potential,

or hyperpolarizing the resting membrane potential. It is important to understand that pacemaker cells receive continuous input from both divisions of the autonomic nervous system. Therefore the heart rate can be increased by an increase in sympathetic stimulation or by a decrease in parasympathetic activity. Conversely, it can be decreased by an increase in parasympathetic stimulation or by a decrease in sympathetic tone.

Conduction Pathways of the Heart

As was stated previously, conductivity is the ability of the heart to propagate impulses throughout the heart. This property of conductivity is remarkably consistent under normal circumstances. Depolarization of the SA node, which is located at the bifurcation of the superior vena cava and the right atrium, initiates the heartbeat by triggering a wave of excitation that spreads throughout the right and left atria as it moves toward the AV node. (NOTE: The SA node normally is considered the pacemaker of the heart because it has the highest rate of automatic discharge.) As shown in Figure 9-2, the movement of electrical impulses between the SA and AV nodes occurs through a series of high-speed internodal conduction pathways, referred to as the anterior, middle, and posterior *internodal pathways*. Impulses travel to the left atrium via a branch of the anterior internodal pathway, which is called *Bachmann's bundle.*[2]

As the impulse travels through the AV node, a 100-msec delay occurs in conduction. This important delay allows the atria to become fully depolarized and contract before ventricular excitation begins, thus allowing the atrial contraction and emptying (i.e., "atrial kick") to contribute optimally to ventricular filling. (The AV node is divided into three distinct regions: [1] an A-N region, which is a

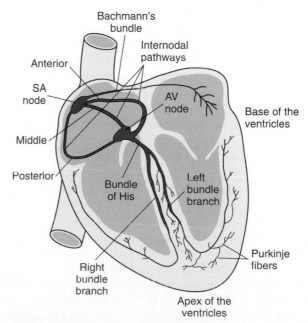

FIGURE 9-2 Electrical conduction system of the heart.

transitional zone between the atria and the AV nodal tissue; [2] an N region, which represents the middle of the AV node; and [3] an N-H region, in which nodal fibers gradually merge with the bundle of His and enter the Purkinje fiber system.) After the delay and depolarization of the AV node, the excitation wave spreads to the muscle cells of the ventricles via a specialized high-speed conduction system that starts at the *bundle of His* and then splits into the right and left bundle branches. The bundle branches ultimately divide into a complex network of specialized conducting fibers, the *Purkinje fibers,* located beneath the surface of the endocardium. Excitation of the ventricular muscle cells finally occurs as impulses travel cell to cell from the inner endocardial surface to the outer epicardial surface and from the apex to the base of the heart. Repolarization of the ventricles normally occurs from epicardium to endocardium; that is, in the opposite direction of depolarization. Repolarization of the ventricles also usually begins in the apex of the heart and travels toward the base.

PRINCIPLES OF ELECTROCARDIOGRAPHY

The electrocardiogram (ECG) is a graphic representation of electrical voltages generated by cardiac tissue. Because the heart can be considered an electrical generator within a **volume conductor,** electrical potentials measured at various points on the body surface can be related to electrical impulses traveling through the heart. (Although the term *volume conductor* sometimes is difficult to understand, it can best be explained in the following manner: The heart is surrounded by tissues that contain ions, which can conduct electrical impulses generated in the heart to the body surface, where these electrical signals can be detected by electrodes placed on the skin.) The electrical activity measured by the ECG is not directly comparable to the action potentials of any individual cell but rather represents *summed* information from many cells at any instant. Therefore the potential difference determined actually shows the resolved direction, or vector, with respect to a particular frame of reference, of the movement of a wave of depolarization as it travels within the heart.[2] The electrocardiograph is wired in such a way that a wave or vector of depolarization traveling toward the sensing or positive electrode results in an upward deflection on the recording paper or monitor. Conversely, a wave of depolarization moving away from the sensing electrode results in a downward deflection on the recording paper or monitor.

The contour of ECG waveforms remains relatively constant, although the heart rate may vary considerably.[2,3] For patients with heart disease, pathologic alterations in the excitability, **rhythmicity,** and conductivity of the heart can result in significant changes in the amplitude and duration of the ECG waveforms. In the following sections, several aspects of electrocardiography are considered, including standard methods for recording electrocardiograms and selective criteria that can be used to define a "normal" electrocardiogram. Finally, a clinically relevant approach to the analysis of ECGs is provided to facilitate recognition of abnormalities in cardiac electrical activity.

The Electrocardiograph

The major components of an electrocardiograph are shown in Figure 9-3. Electrodes placed on the patient's skin act as transducers to convert ionic potentials into electrical impulses. These electrical impulses are then transmitted to an amplifier before being registered on an output display, such as a graphic recorder or a cathode ray tube (CRT).

Electrodes

A variety of electrodes have been used in clinical electrocardiography, including plate electrodes, suction-cup electrodes, and **floating electrodes.** Plate and suction-cup electrodes are made of silver, nickel, or a similar alloy with high conductivity. A thin coat of conduction jelly or electrolyte paste, which reduces the impedance of the skin-electrode interface, is applied evenly to the electrode before it is attached to the body surface. Although both plate and suction-cup electrodes provide accurate and reliable results, their use in clinical electrocardiography has waned since the introduction of disposable floating electrodes. Floating electrodes consist of a silver–silver chloride electrode encased in a plastic housing. The surface of the electrode is covered with a conductive gel or paste. The entire electrode assembly can be attached to the skin with a double-sided ring, which adheres to the patient's skin and to the plastic housing of the electrode. These electrodes are referred to as "floating" electrodes because the only conductive path between the electrode and the patient's skin is the electrolyte gel or paste.

Lead Configurations

The standard electrocardiogram has 12 leads: three standard limb leads, three augmented limb leads, and six precordial or chest leads. The standard limb leads plus the augmented limb leads are oriented in a hexaxial arrangement that gives information about the frontal plane of the heart (i.e., the frontal plane of the heart is divided into six different angles). The chest leads provide information about electrical activity of the heart when it is observed in the horizontal plane. Figure 9-4 shows electrode placement for a standard 12-lead ECG.

The standard limb leads, which are designated leads I, II, and III, form an equilateral triangle, often referred to as *Einthoven's triangle* (Figure 9-5). These leads are bipolar, having one positive electrode and one negative electrode. In lead I, the right arm is negative and the left arm is positive. In lead II, the right arm is negative and the left leg is positive. In lead III, the left arm is negative and the left leg is positive. In all the standard limb leads, the right leg electrode serves as a ground. Notice that the limb electrodes may be attached to the torso rather than on the arms (i.e., *Mason-Liker* lead configurations).[4]

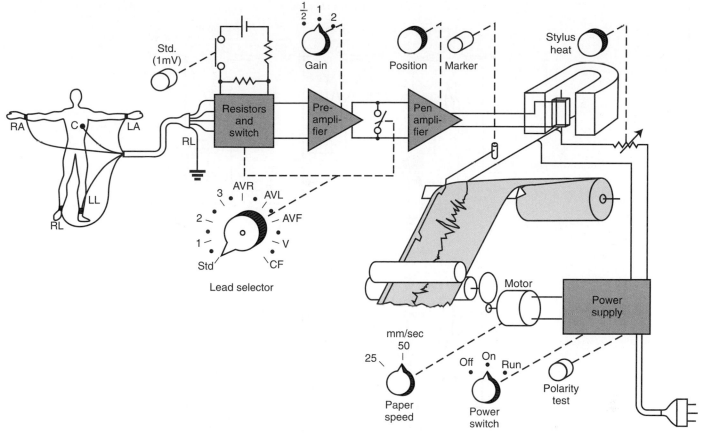

FIGURE 9-3 Major components of an electrocardiograph. (Modified from Cromwell L, Weibell FJ, Pfeiffer EA: *Biomedical instrumentation and measurements,* Englewood Cliffs, NJ, 1980, Prentice-Hall.)

The augmented leads, which are designated leads aVR, aVL, and aVF, are all unipolar; that is, each lead is arranged such that each one of the three limb electrodes is designated as the positive electrode, whereas the other two are taken together to be zero or the reference electrode. For example, in lead aVR, the right arm is the positive electrode and the left arm and left leg electrodes constitute the zero reference. In lead aVL, the left arm is positive and the right arm and left leg, taken together, are the zero reference. For lead aVF, the left leg is positive and the right arm and left arm, taken together, are the reference. The term *augmented* is applied to these electrodes because the waveforms generated with these lead configurations typically are electronically amplified one and one-half times the recorded amplitude before being displayed.[3]

The precordial or chest leads V_1 to V_6 are unipolar leads arranged around the chest. In these leads, the positive or exploring electrode is located at a standard position on the chest (Figure 9-4); the three limb electrodes are averaged together to create a reference, or the central terminal. In special cases, additional precordial leads may be used, including leads V_7, V_8, V_9, and V_3R, V_4R, V_5R, V_6R, V_7R, V_8R, and V_9R. Note that V_7 is located in the fifth intercostal space at the posterior axillary line.[4] Leads V_8 and V_9 are located at the angle of the scapula, over the spine at the level of V_3 and V_4. V_3R through V_9R are placed on the right side of the chest in a position oriented similarly to those of V_3 through V_9.[4]

During clinical exercise testing, modified chest leads (MCLs) often are used to monitor patients with suspected dysrhythmias. These leads include a positive electrode in the V_3 or V_5 position and a negative electrode placed on the left shoulder or forehead. For example, with the MCL3 lead, the positive electrode is at the V_3 position (Figure 9-6).[5]

Electrocardiographic Recorders

The typical ECG recorder includes a differential amplifier with filtering circuits and an output display, such as a strip chart recorder or a CRT (Figure 9-7). The differential amplifier and filtering circuits serve to increase the power output of the electrical signals detected by the surface electrodes and to remove extraneous electrical interference. Electrical interference, or "noise," can be caused by action potentials generated by skeletal muscle (electromyographic interference), fluorescent lights, and television and radio signals, as well as by other electrical monitoring devices attached to the patient. A special circuit that allows a 1-mV standardization voltage to be introduced into the system

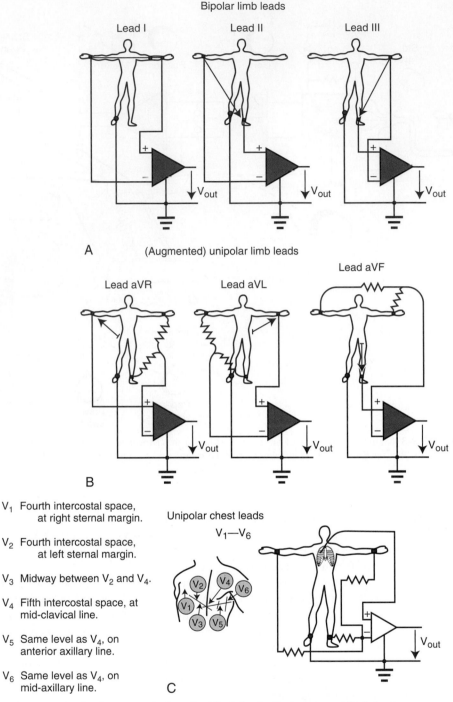

FIGURE 9-4 ECG lead systems. **A,** Standard limb leads. **B,** Augmented limb leads. **C,** Precordial or chest leads. (Modified from Cromwell L, Weibell FJ, Pfeiffer EA: *Biomedical instrumentation and measurements,* Englewood Cliffs, NJ, 1980, Prentice-Hall.)

also is included in the central processing unit so that the output display can be calibrated. In older ECG systems, a lead selector switch is used to access information from each of the 12 standard leads. Newer systems contain microprocessors that automatically access each of the standard 12 leads in sequence.

Most electrocardiographs have direct-writing recorders to provide permanent ECG records, as well as a CRT

for long-term monitoring. For direct-writing strip chart recorders, the ECG is inscribed on a moving sheet of heat-sensitive paper with an electrically heated stylus. The paper upon which the ECG is recorded is ruled in lines 1 mm apart, both vertically and horizontally. As discussed in the next section, when properly standardized, the amplitude and duration of waves, complexes, and intervals can be determined from the electrocardiogram.

Standard limb leads

Augmented leads

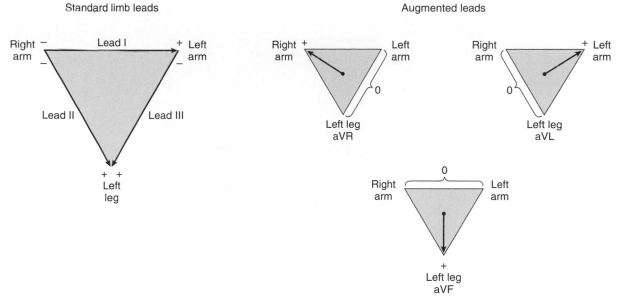

FIGURE 9-5 Einthoven's triangle.

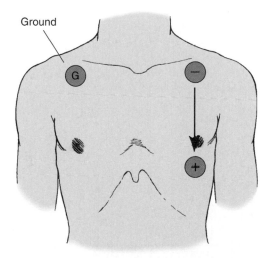

FIGURE 9-6 Electrode placement for modified chest leads (MCL3).

The Normal Electrocardiogram

Figure 9-8 shows the main waves, complexes, and intervals normally seen on an electrocardiogram.[2,6] (The ECG waveform shown in this figure is derived from lead II. Note that the amplitude of each of the waves varies, depending on the lead examined and the vectors of depolarization and repolarization.) It is important to understand that all ECGs are standardized; that is, ECGs are recorded on paper that is ruled in millimeters in the horizontal and vertical planes. Notice that the graph has heavy lines every fifth millimeter, both in the horizontal and vertical directions. When an ECG is recorded, the paper speed is set at 25 mm/sec, the equivalent of 1500 mm/min. As such, time is recorded on the *x* axis, with each millimeter representing

0.04 seconds and 0.2 seconds between each heavy vertical line. Marks often are seen at 75-mm intervals along the top of the strip, corresponding to 3-second intervals. ECGs also are calibrated so that each millimeter on the *y* axis is equal to 0.1 mV. Therefore, a 10-mm deflection vertically equals 1 mV.

Waves, Complexes, and Intervals

P Wave. The P wave represents depolarization of the atria. As was discussed previously, atrial depolarization normally begins at the SA node and travels from right to left and toward the AV node. The P wave is upward in leads I, II, aVF, and V_3 to V_6. It usually is inverted in leads aVR, V_1, and sometimes V_2. The P wave normally is 0.1 to 0.3 mV in amplitude and 0.06 to 0.1 second in duration. Atrial disease is associated with a prolongation of the P wave to greater than 0.1 second.

PR Interval. The PR interval, which is the time interval between the beginning of the P wave and the beginning of the QRS complex, represents the conduction time required for an impulse initiated in the atria to travel through the AV node. It normally ranges from 0.12 to 0.2 seconds in duration. The PR segment, which occurs between the end of the P wave and the beginning of the QRS complex, corresponds to the 0.1-second delay that occurs as the cardiac impulse travels through the AV node. Because the delay occurs after the atrial muscle mass has depolarized completely, the PR segment is on the line of zero potential, which is called the *isoelectric line*. Blocks in conduction through the AV node, which are discussed in greater detail later, may result in either prolonged PR intervals or P waves that are not followed by QRS complexes. These are called first-degree, second-degree, and third-degree AV blocks. Shortening of the PR interval is associated with pre-excitation syndrome (see Wolff-Parkinson-White syndrome later

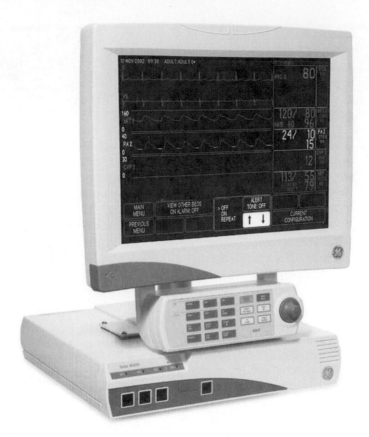

FIGURE 9-7 Typical electrocardiogram monitor used in a critical care unit. (Courtesy of GE Healthcare.)

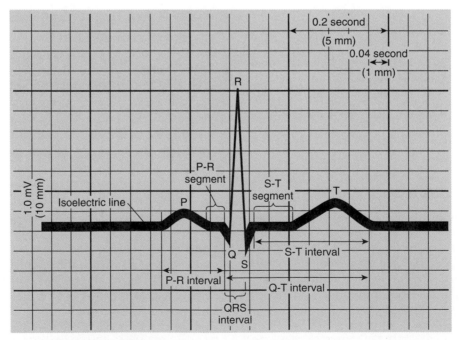

FIGURE 9-8 Normal electrocardiogram showing waves, complexes, and intervals.

in this chapter) and with atrial impulses initiated low in the atria near the AV node.

QRS Complexes. The QRS complex represents ventricular depolarization. A Q wave is a downward deflection that precedes the upward deflection of an R wave; an S wave is a downward deflection following an R wave. Figure 9-9 shows several types of QRS complexes that may be seen in ECGs. Under normal circumstances, the QRS duration is approximately 0.1 second because the high-speed conduction system of the bundle of His, left and right bundle branches, and the Purkinje fiber system allow rapid and complete depolarization of the ventricles. Prolonged QRS durations and abnormal-appearing QRS complexes indicate ventricular muscle cell–to–muscle cell conduction caused either by blocks in the high-speed conduction pathway or by initiation of ventricular depolarization by an ectopic focus. An ectopic beat typically is defined as electrical activation of the heart outside of the normal pacemaker cells (i.e., SA node). The QRS vector normally is upward in leads I, II, aVL, and V_5 and V_6. It usually is downward in leads aVR and V_1.

ST Segment. After the ventricles are completely depolarized, an ST segment appears on the ECG. The ventricles stay completely depolarized for a substantial interval, as noted in the discussion of the phase 2 plateau in the section on cardiac action potentials. The ST segment, which is measured from the end of the QRS complex to the begin-

ning of the T wave, falls on the isoelectric line. ST segments above and below the isoelectric line may be seen during myocardial injury as a result of "currents of injury" caused by ions moving into and out of injured cardiac cells. The *J point,* which is the junction between the QRS complex and ST segment, often is used as a reference for describing alterations in the ST segment.

T Wave. The T wave represents ventricular repolarization. It usually is upright in all leads except aVR. At first this may seem odd, because repolarization is the opposite of depolarization; however, as was noted previously, repolarization usually occurs in a direction opposite to that of depolarization. The T wave usually is rounded, and its amplitude is less than 0.5 mV in the limb leads and less than 1 mV in the precordial leads. It typically is 0.1 to 0.2 seconds in duration.

Repolarization is an energy-dependent phenomenon that is mainly a function of the movement of potassium ions. Any situation compromising the energy state, such as myocardial ischemia, injury, or infarction, therefore can affect this potassium balance of the heart, resulting in altered T waves. Tall T waves may suggest myocardial infarction, potassium excess, coronary ischemia, or ventricular overload. Inversion of T waves is related to coronary ischemia and injury. T wave inversion occurs in these situations if the T wave originally was upright. If the individual initially demonstrated inverted T waves, ischemia

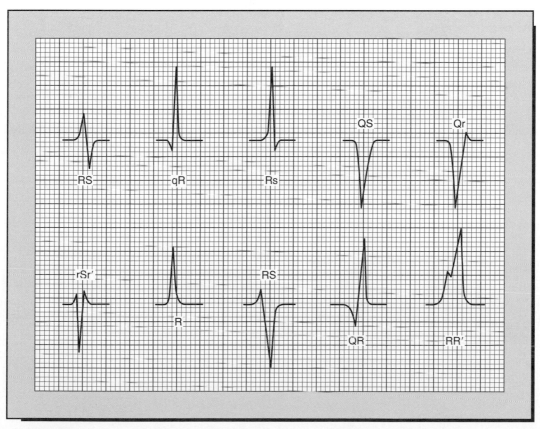

FIGURE 9-9 Types of QRS complexes. (Modified from Graver K: *A practical guide to ECG interpretation,* St Louis, 1991, Mosby.)

and injury produce an upright T wave. This sometimes is referred to as *pseudonormalization* of the T wave.[6]

Atrial repolarization is not usually visible in the ECG because it does not represent much electrical activity and it usually occurs during ventricular depolarization.

QT Interval. The QT interval is measured from the beginning of the QRS complex to the end of the T wave. It represents the time required for ventricular depolarization and repolarization to occur and also approximates the time of ventricular systole. For heart rates of 60 to 100 beats/min, the QT interval is approximately 0.4 seconds. Note that the QT interval varies inversely with the heart rate. Slowing the heart rate lengthens the QT interval, whereas increasing the heart rate shortens the QT interval. The QT interval can be prolonged in congestive heart failure, myocardial infarction, procainamide administration, hypocalcemia, and hypomagnesemia. The QT interval is shortened by digitalis, hypocalcemia, and hyperkalemia.[7]

U Wave. The U wave follows the T wave and precedes the succeeding P wave. It is thought to represent remnants of ventricular repolarization or repolarization of the papillary muscles. The amplitude and duration of U waves are considerably less than those of the T wave; however, the polarity of the U wave normally is in the same direction as the preceding T wave. When present, U wave amplitude is made more prominent by hypokalemia and bradycardia.[7]

Interpretation of Electrocardiograms

Alterations in the initiation and conduction of electrical impulses through the heart can result in abnormal cardiac rhythms or arrhythmias (also called *dysrhythmias*). A typical interpretation of an ECG contains information about the effective atrial and ventricular rates, an estimation of the mean ventricular electrical axis, and the presence of arrhythmias. The following sections of this chapter present basic techniques for interpreting ECGs.

Determination of the Heart Rate

Figure 9-10 shows a practical method for determining the heart rate from an ECG. To calculate the heart rate, count the number of cardiac cycles during a 6-second interval and multiply this number by 10. This can be easily accomplished because most ECG paper has vertical markings on the top of the paper corresponding to 3-second intervals when the paper speed is 25 mm/sec. Alternatively, if the patient's heart rate is fairly constant, you can calculate the effective ventricular rate by counting the number of millimeters between two successive R waves (i.e., the R-R interval) and dividing this number into 1500 (25 mm/sec = 1500 mm /min). The atrial rate can be calculated similarly by dividing the P-P interval or the number of millimeters between two successive P waves into 1500. Test your ability to calculate the heart rate using the ECG shown in Clinical Rounds 9-1.

Mean Electrical Axis. As was discussed previously, the mean ventricular axis of the heart represents the average direction and magnitude of the electrical activity of the heart. Figure 9-11 shows a method for determining the mean ventricular axis. Ordinarily, the frontal plane electrical axis is determined from the standard limb leads. In healthy subjects, the mean ventricular axis is between –30 and 105 degrees because of the anatomic position of the heart in the thorax and because the muscle mass of the left ventricle is approximately three times greater than that of the right ventricle. The axis rotates more to the left in normal subjects during expiration and when a subject lies down because the diaphragm rises. Rotation to the right occurs during inspiration and when a subject assumes an upright position. Chronic changes in the mean ventricular axis of the heart occur in pathologic conditions, such as left or right ventricular hypertrophy and myocardial

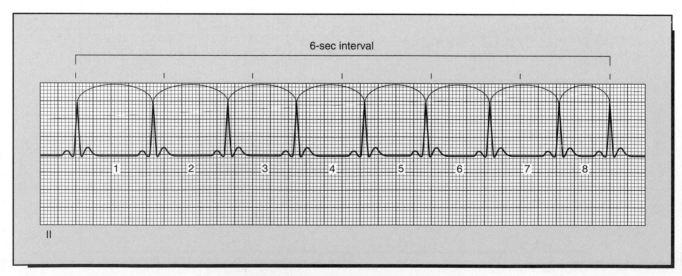

FIGURE 9-10 Determination of the heart rate.

CLINICAL ROUNDS 9-1

The electrocardiogram shown here was obtained from a healthy 20-year-old female during a maximum exercise effort. Calculate her effective ventricular heart rate.

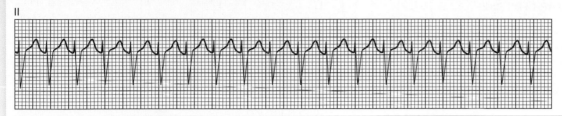

See Evolve Resources for the answer.

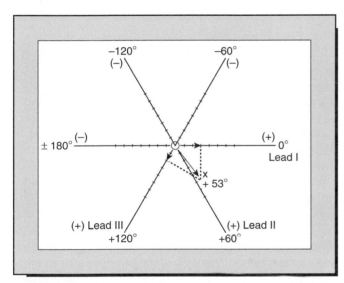

FIGURE 9-11 Simplified method of calculating the mean ventricular axis. The amplitude of the QRS complexes is plotted on the lead I and lead III axes, respectively. The axis is established by determining the resolved vector for these two values.

BOX 9-1	Interpretation of Electrocardiograms

I. Rate
   a. Atrial rate
   b. Ventricular rate
II. Rhythm (Supraventricular versus Ventricular Rhythm)
   a. Presence of P waves
   b. Measurement of the PR interval
   c. QRS duration
   d. QT duration
   e. Presence of premature atrial or ventricular beats
III. Conduction Disturbances
   a. AV blocks
   b. Intraventricular (bundle branch) blocks
IV. Mean Ventricular Electrical Axis
   a. Chamber enlargement (hypertrophy)
V. Ischemia and Infarction
   a. ST segment displacement
   b. T wave changes
   c. Abnormal Q waves
VI. Miscellaneous Findings
   a. Drug effects
   b. Electrolyte disturbances

infarction and during interventricular conduction delays or bundle branch blocks.

Pattern Regularity

To determine whether an abnormal rhythm is present, the examiner should ask the following questions while observing the ECG. First, are P waves present? Is each QRS complex preceded by a P wave (i.e., is there a 1:1 relationship between the number of P waves and the number of QRS complexes present)? Do the P waves have the same contour, or do they vary from beat to beat? Is the time interval between the initiation of the P wave and the QRS complex less than 0.2 seconds? Furthermore, does the PR interval have a repeatable value or does it continually vary? The contour of the QRS complexes should be noted. Is the QRS interval less than 0.1 seconds? If the QRS complexes are prolonged, do the QRS complexes show any abnormal

notching? Next, the examiner should look at the contour of the T wave. Is it peaked, depressed, or inverted? Finally, the position of the ST segment should be evaluated. Is it elevated or depressed below the isoelectric line by 2 mm for 0.08 seconds or greater? As the following section on identifying specific arrhythmias shows, the use of these criteria can reduce much of the difficulty associated with interpreting ECGs. Box 9-1 summarizes the various criteria that can be used to identify common arrhythmias encountered in clinical practice.

Box 9-2 lists the most common rhythms and dysrhythmias encountered in clinical medicine. They are described briefly in the following sections; examples of each may be found in Figures 9-12 through 9-20. Also note that unless stated otherwise, each of the arrhythmias shown is illustrated using lead II.

Sinus Rhythms. Remember that under normal circumstances, the heart rate is determined by the number of

BOX 9-2	Common Cardiac Rhythms and Arrhythmias Encountered in Clinical Practice

SUPRAVENTRICULAR RHYTHMS
Sinus rhythms
    Normal sinus rhythm
    Sinus tachycardia
    Sinus bradycardia
    Respiratory sinus arrhythmia

ATRIAL TACHYCARDIA
Atrial flutter
Atrial fibrillation
Junctional (nodal) rhythms

VENTRICULAR RHYTHMS
Ventricular tachycardia
Ventricular fibrillation
Wolff-Parkinson-White syndrome

HEART BLOCKS
Intraventricular (bundle branch) blocks
    Atrioventricular blocks
    First degree
    Second degree (Mobitz I and Mobitz II)
    Third degree (complete)

ABNORMAL BEATS
Premature atrial beats
Premature junctional beats
Premature ventricular beats

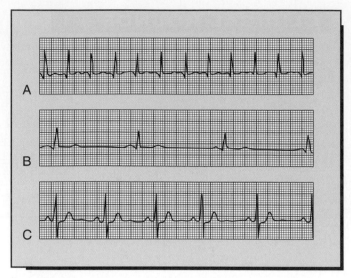

FIGURE 9-12 Sinus rhythms. **A,** Sinus tachycardia. **B,** Sinus bradycardia. **C,** Respiratory sinus arrhythmia.

times the SA node depolarizes per minute. In healthy subjects, if the resting heart rate is 60 to 100 beats/min and each QRS complex is preceded by a normally appearing P wave, the rhythm is referred to as a **normal sinus rhythm.**

In **sinus tachycardia** (Figure 9-12A), the SA node remains the source of cardiac excitation, but the ventricular rate exceeds 100 beats/min. Stimulation of the autonomic nervous system, as occurs with the administration of sympathomimetic amines (e.g., isoproterenol or epinephrine) or drugs that block parasympathetic impulses to the heart (e.g., atropine), cause considerable increases in the heart rate. Sinus tachycardia can also result from exertion, ingestion of large amounts of caffeine or nicotine, fever, anemia, hypoxemia, hypotension, myocardial ischemia, thyrotoxicosis, pulmonary emboli, and congestive heart failure.

Sinus bradycardia (Figure 9-12B) refers to a heart rate of less than 60 beats/min. Again, each QRS complex is preceded by a P wave. This rhythm is caused by increased vagal tone, as occurs during carotid sinus massage and after the administration of β-adrenergic blocking agents (e.g., propranolol). Clinically, sinus bradycardia most often is associated with hypothermia, eye surgery, increased intracranial pressure, cervical and mediastinal tumors, vomiting, myxedema, and vasovagal syncope. (Note that well-trained athletes may demonstrate sinus bradycardia because of an improved ventricular stroke volume. It is not

uncommon for these individuals to have resting heart rates as low as 40 beats/min.)

The term **sinus arrhythmia** (Figure 9-12C) is used to describe a regular acceleration of the heart rate during inspiration followed by a slowing of the heart rate during expiration. It should be noted that although these variations in the heart rate may be quite exaggerated, all QRS complexes have a normal duration and they are all preceded by P waves. Also, the PR interval is of normal duration. Sinus arrhythmias are common findings in children and young adults. (It has been suggested that sinus arrhythmias result from the lung inflation reflex or from activation of the Bainbridge reflex; inspiration causes a reduction in intrathoracic pressure, an increase in venous return, and a consequent stretching of the atria, which ultimately leads to an increase in the heart rate. Conversely, during expiration, intrathoracic pressure rises, atrial filling declines, and the heart rate slows.)

Supraventricular Arrhythmias. Supraventricular arrhythmias include atrial premature contraction, atrial flutter, atrial fibrillation (Figure 9-13), and junctional rhythm (Figure 9-14).

Atrial premature depolarizations are ectopic beats that can originate in any part of the atria. The terms *atrial premature contractions, premature atrial beats,* and *atrial extrasystole* are used synonymously in discussions of these arrhythmias. These beats are characterized by P waves that come before the next expected sinus depolarization. Because the atrial premature beat may cause depolarization of the SA node, the interval between the premature P wave and the next normal sinus P wave is equal to or slightly longer than the usual P-P interval. The configuration of the P wave of an atrial premature beat varies, depending on the site of the ectopy and the lead examined. For example, in lead II, if the impulse is generated high in the atria, the P wave has a normal upright appearance.

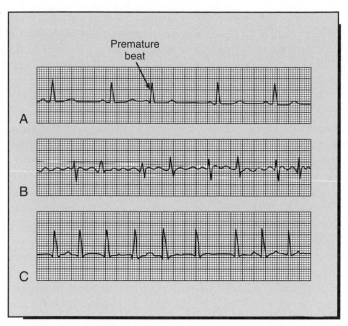

FIGURE 9-13 Supraventricular arrhythmias. **A,** Atrial premature depolarizations. **B,** Atrial flutter. **C,** Atrial fibrillation.

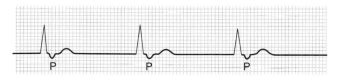

FIGURE 9-14 Junctional rhythm.

However, if the focus is low in the atria, the P wave appears inverted because its axis is directed superiorly.

Atrial tachycardia usually involves atrial rates of 150 to 250 beats/min. It can be caused by a number of agents, including stimulants such as caffeine, tobacco, and alcohol; sympathomimetic drugs; hypoxia; elevation of atrial pressure; and digitalis intoxication.

Paroxysmal atrial tachycardia (PAT) is a distinct clinical syndrome characterized by repeated episodes of atrial tachycardia that have an abrupt onset and last a few seconds to many hours. The genesis of this type of arrhythmia is a premature atrial depolarization with a prolonged AV conduction time.[1] The prolonged AV conduction time permits the impulse to be reflected back into the atrium (i.e., reentry), resulting in the production of this type of supraventricular tachycardia. Vagal stimulation, caused by gagging, carotid sinus massage, face immersion, or the Valsalva maneuver, often is helpful for determining the underlying rhythm because these maneuvers generally convert PAT to a normal sinus rhythm. Although PAT can be well tolerated in healthy young adults, it can cause serious problems in elderly patients with other forms of heart disease, such as coronary atherosclerosis and valvular stenosis. In the latter group of patients, PAT can lead to myocardial ischemia, infarction, or pulmonary edema.

In **atrial flutter,** the atrial rate is regular and ranges from 250 to 350 beats/min. The ventricular rate typically is about 125 to 150 beats/min, and it is regular if a constant degree of AV block is present. Atrial flutter waves (*F waves*) replace the normal P waves, giving the ECG a characteristic "sawtooth" or "picket fence" appearance.

As with atrial flutter, **atrial fibrillation** is characterized by gross irregularities in both atrial and ventricular depolarization. The atrial rate usually is 400 to 700 beats/min but generally cannot be quantified. P waves are replaced by fibrillatory waves. As shown in Figure 9-13, these fibrillatory waves vary in size and shape and are irregular in rhythm, causing an undulation of the baseline on the ECG. The ventricular rate is 120 to 200 beats/min. Note that this ventricular rate occurs because, as a result of the inherent refractoriness of the AV node, not every atrial depolarization that reaches the AV node is transmitted. Therefore only depolarizations that arrive at a period when the AV node is not refractory and that have sufficient strength are transmitted into the ventricles.

Atrial fibrillation may occur intermittently or as a chronic arrhythmia, in which case it is the result of some underlying form of heart disease, such as mitral stenosis, thyrotoxicosis, chronic pericarditis, and congestive heart failure. It also is a common finding in patients recovering from a myocardial infarction, particularly during exercise. However, it may occur paroxysmally in individuals with no apparent heart disease.

Junctional rhythms (see Figure 9-14) are impulses that originate in or near the AV node. The P wave may precede, coincide with, or follow the QRS, depending on the relative conduction times from the impulse's site of origin in the AV node to the atria and ventricles. Impulses generated high in the AV node are likely to be associated with a P wave that occurs before the QRS complex, whereas impulses generated low in the AV node result in a P wave that follows the QRS complex. Note that because of the retrograde transmission of the impulse into the atria, the P wave appears inverted in the ECG leads that face the left side of the heart (e.g., leads II, III, and aVF), whereas it appears upright in the leads that face the right side of the heart (e.g., leads aVR and V_1).

Junctional rates may vary from 40 to 60 beats/min to well over 100 beats/min. In the case of slower heart rates, the junctional rhythm may serve as an escape mechanism to protect ventricular function. This phenomenon occurs when the SA node either fails to depolarize or impulses generated by the SA node or atria fail to be conducted to the AV node. If the AV node is not depolarized within 1 to 1.5 seconds, it initiates an impulse called an *escape beat.* A series of these beats therefore is called a **junctional escape rhythm.** Junctional rates greater than 100 beats/min can occur because of an inherent instability in the AV node caused by ischemia or a toxin. This type of junctional rhythm is referred to as *junctional tachycardia.*

Ventricular Rhythms. Ventricular arrhythmias include **premature ventricular beats, ventricular tachycardia,**

and **ventricular fibrillation** (Figure 9-15). Premature ventricular beats (PVBs), which are often called *premature ventricular contractions (PVCs)*, occur when ectopic impulses originate in the ventricles before the normal sequence of depolarization beginning at the SA node. PVBs are characterized by the absence of P waves and the presence of wide QRS complexes (longer than 0.12 seconds in duration) that result from sequential activation of the two ventricles rather than the usual simultaneous activation. (Also, remember that the QRS duration is prolonged as a result of cell-to-cell conduction rather than through the normal high-speed conduction pathways in the His-Purkinje system.) Because this type of abnormal depolarization affects repolarization, T waves also are affected (i.e., inverted T waves).

In some instances, ectopic beats originating in the ventricles are conducted to the AV node and into the atria, resulting in inverted P waves. However, in most cases this does not occur, and the impulses generated in the ventricles are blocked from entering the atria; the SA node therefore is unaffected by the abnormal impulse. Consequently, the SA node continues to fire at its own inherent rate. Because the ventricles are refractory to any stimuli after activation, they typically show a "compensatory pause" between the generation of the PVB and the next normally conducted depolarization. This can be seen on an ECG by noting that the duration of two cardiac cycles (including the PVB) is the same as the duration of two normal cycles.

Premature ventricular depolarizations may occur alone or as multiples. *Ventricular bigeminy* refers to a rhythm in which every other beat is a premature ventricular beat. *Ventricular trigeminy* is the presence of a PVB on every third beat. Ventricular tachycardia exists when three or more PVBs occur in succession at a rate in excess of 100 beats/min. Usually during ventricular tachycardia, atrioventricular dissociation occurs; this simply means that the atria depolarize at a rate independent of the ventricular rate. P waves may be discernible between successive QRS complexes in ventricular tachycardia, but they generally are hard to find. Occasionally an impulse originating in the SA node reaches the AV node and ventricles during an interval when the ventricles are not in a refractory period. The SA node depolarization therefore is conducted into the ventricles, resulting in the production of a normal QRS complex or a "captured" beat.

PVBs can occur in normal, healthy subjects who ingest large amounts of caffeine, alcohol, or tobacco, or who are experiencing abnormally high levels of physical or mental stress. Ventricular tachycardia usually is associated with myocardial ischemia and infarction, excessive adrenergic stimulation, and digitalis toxicity. Premature ventricular depolarization that occurs during the T wave (i.e., during the ventricle's vulnerable period or supernormal period, which occurs immediately after the relative refractory period) may cause ventricular tachycardia and possibly even ventricular fibrillation.

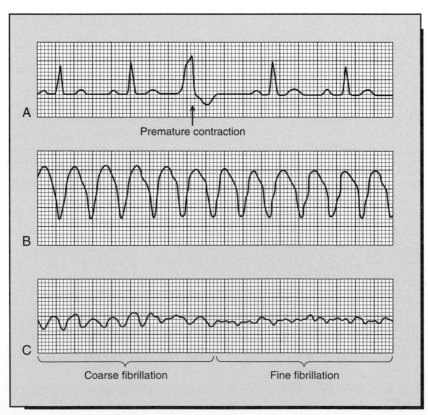

FIGURE 9-15 Ventricular arrhythmias. **A,** Premature ventricular beats. **B,** Ventricular tachycardia. **C,** Ventricular fibrillation.

In ventricular fibrillation, no effective ventricular contractions occur, and consequently there is no cardiac output. The ECG can show "coarse" or "fine" fibrillatory waves, which replace the normal PQRST waves. The terms *coarse* and *fine* refer to the amplitude of the fibrillatory waves. Ventricular fibrillation should be treated immediately with cardiopulmonary resuscitation (CPR), including the establishment of a patent airway so that the patient can be ventilated either by mouth-to-mouth methods or with a self-inflating (bag-valve-mask) resuscitator; external chest wall compressions; pharmacologic agents to maintain circulation; and electrical defibrillation. Coarse fibrillatory waves usually indicate that cardiovascular collapse has occurred recently and thus may respond to prompt defibrillation. Fine fibrillatory waves usually indicate that some time has elapsed since the onset of fibrillation and that the success rate for resuscitation may be significantly reduced.

Wolff-Parkinson-White (WPW) Syndrome is an unusual rhythm that results from the presence of an abnormal route of conduction that bypasses the AV nodes as the impulse travels from the atria to the ventricles.[6,8] In most cases, this abnormal route is attributed to a group of muscle fibers called the *bundle of Kent.* (It should be noted that other bypass tracts between the atria and the ventricles can also cause WPW preexcitation syndrome.) WPW syndrome is characterized by the presence of a P wave with an abnormally short PR interval. Probably the most ominous sign of WPW syndrome is the presence of an early, slurred upstroke of the QRS wave, often referred to as a *delta wave.* The QRS complex is prolonged, not because of a delay as the impulse travels through the ventricles, but because it started earlier than usual (preexcitation). Figure

9-16 shows a typical ECG tracing from a patient with WPW syndrome.

Ventricular Asystole is the complete absence of any ventricular electrical activity and thus the absence of ventricular contractions. Ventricular asystole typically occurs after ventricular fibrillation; however, it may occur as a primary event during cardiac arrest.

Heart Blocks. Heart Blocks, or abnormal conduction delays, may occur anywhere in the heart when the refractory period at a certain point in the conduction path is prolonged. Generally, heart blocks are divided into three categories: (1) SA blocks, (2) AV blocks, and (3) intraventricular (bundle branch) blocks.

Sinoatrial Blocks. SA blocks (Figure 9-17) occur when the impulse generated at the SA node is blocked before it can enter the atrial muscle. Typically, the ECG shows a sudden loss of P waves resulting from the absence of atrial depolarization. The contour of the QRS complex is normal, but the R-R intervals usually are prolonged, indicating the presence of a junctional escape rhythm. Transient sinoatrial blocks usually do not produce symptoms; prolonged SA blocks can cause dizziness and syncope, particularly if the escape rhythm is slow.

Atrioventricular Blocks. AV blocks occur when impulses generated at the SA node are abnormally prolonged or blocked in or near the AV node. Clinically, AV blocks are classified as first-degree, second-degree, or third-degree blocks. Figure 9-18 shows ECGs demonstrating each of these conduction delays.

A first-degree AV block is characterized by prolongation of the PR interval (i.e., longer than 0.2 seconds), although every impulse does result in ventricular depolarization. Patients with a first-degree AV block generally are asymptomatic if they do not demonstrate any other cardiovascular problems.

A second-degree AV block occurs when some of the impulses generated at the SA node fail to pass through the AV node into the ventricles. The ECG shows characteristic "dropped" beats (i.e., the P wave is not followed by a QRS complex), resulting from failure to conduct every impulse from the atria to the ventricles. A second-degree AV block

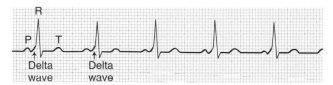

FIGURE 9-16 Electrocardiographic tracing from a patient with Wolff-Parkinson-White syndrome.

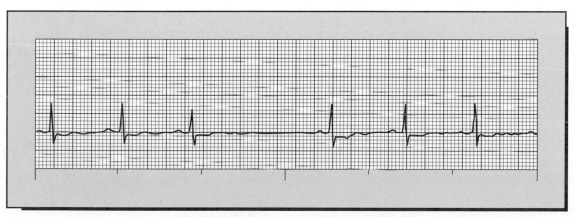

FIGURE 9-17 Sinoatrial (SA) conduction block.

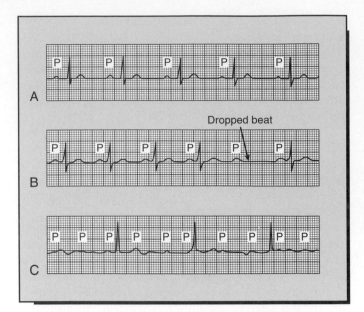

FIGURE 9-18 Atrioventricular (AV) blocks. **A,** First-degree block. **B,** Second-degree (Mobitz II) block. **C,** Third-degree block.

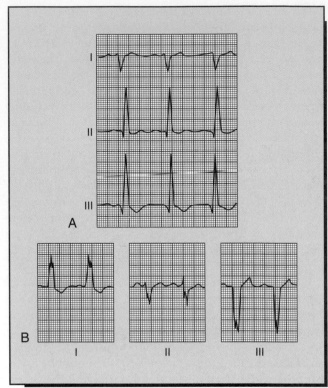

FIGURE 9-19 Intraventricular (bundle branch) blocks. **A,** Right bundle branch block. **B,** Left bundle branch block.

may be further described as a Mobitz type I (Wenckebach) block or a Mobitz type II (non-Wenckebach) block. In a Mobitz type I block, progressive prolongation of the PR interval occurs until at some point a QRS complex does not follow the P wave. In a Mobitz type II AV block, the PR interval does not show the progressive lengthening before the dropped beat.

Mobitz type I blocks usually are associated with blockage of the atrial impulses at the level of the atrial–AV node junction. They often are the result of increased parasympathetic tone or of the effects of drugs (e.g., digitalis or propranolol). Mobitz type II blocks typically occur below the level of the AV node, at the junction of the AV node and the bundle of His. Mobitz type II blocks are most often associated with an organic lesion in the conduction pathway. Mobitz type I blocks usually do not require treatment, whereas Mobitz type II blocks typically require the insertion of a permanent artificial pacemaker.

A third-degree AV block often is referred to as a *complete AV block,* because a complete dissociation of atrial and ventricular conduction occurs. The SA node continues to depolarize at a normal or elevated rate, but the ventricles "escape" to a slower rate. The ECG shows an atrial rate completely dissociated from the ventricular rate. Treatment of third-degree AV blocks usually requires the insertion of an artificial pacemaker if the ventricular rate is too low to permit normal activity.

Intraventricular Blocks. Intraventricular blocks, also called *bundle branch blocks,* occur when impulses are delayed or blocked in either the right or left branches of the Purkinje fiber system. The hallmark of this type of conduction delay is a prolongation of the QRS complex, because distal to the blockage, ventricular excitation must occur by cell-to-cell conduction.

In a right bundle branch block (Figure 9-19A), the QRS complex shows a characteristic rSR' pattern in the right precordial leads (i.e., leads V_1, V_2, and V_3) and a prolonged, deep S wave in the left precordial leads (leads V_4, V_5, and V_6). Vector analysis of ECGs from patients with a right bundle branch block shows that the mean ventricular axis is shifted to the right (greater than 90 degrees) as a result of the delayed cell-to-cell conduction through the right ventricle. Right bundle branch blocks are associated with hypertensive cardiac disease, cardiac tumors, rheumatic heart disease, pulmonary emboli, and congenital cardiac defects.

Left bundle branch blocks (Figure 9-19B) are characterized by the absence of Q waves in the left limb leads (i.e., leads I and aVL) and in the left precordial leads (i.e., leads V_4, V_5, and V_6). The QRS complexes in the left precordial leads show an rSR' configuration. The mean ventricular axis is shifted to the left in this type of block (less than 30 degrees). Although left bundle branch blocks are less common than right bundle branch blocks, they are almost always indicative of coronary artery disease or systemic hypertension. (Other possible etiologies include aortic stenosis, myocarditis, and congenital cardiac disease.)

Myocardial Ischemia and Infarction. If coronary blood flow is severely limited, as occurs with atherosclerosis or as a result of obstruction secondary to thromboembolism, the heart's oxygen demand exceeds its oxygen delivery and myocardial ischemia results. The inability of

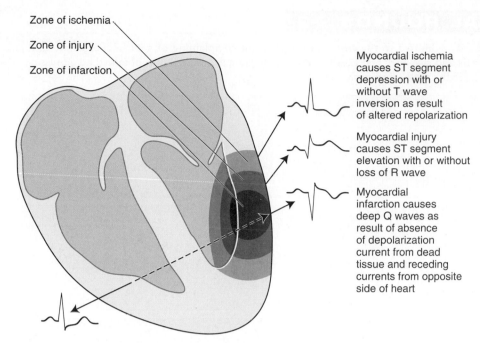

Zone of ischemia

Zone of injury

Zone of infarction

Myocardial ischemia causes ST segment depression with or without T wave inversion as result of altered repolarization

Myocardial injury causes ST segment elevation with or without loss of R wave

Myocardial infarction causes deep Q waves as result of absence of depolarization current from dead tissue and receding currents from opposite side of heart

FIGURE 9-20 Electrocardiogram changes associated with myocardial ischemia, injury, and infarction.

the coronary circulation to provide blood flow sufficient to meet the increased metabolic demands of the myocardium is manifested in the electrocardiogram.

As shown in Figure 9-20, three types of ECG changes are associated with myocardial ischemia, injury, and infarction: T wave inversion, ST segment elevation and depression, and abnormal Q waves. T wave inversion occurs during periods of transient ischemia. Transient ischemia affects repolarization waves before any other on the ECG because this period represents the most energy-sensitive activity of the heart.

ST segment alterations occur if ischemia progresses to injury. During myocardial injury, the cardiac cell membrane, or sarcolemma, is unable to maintain its integrity, and ions continue to stream into and out of the myocardial cells. These so-called currents of injury are responsible for depression or elevation of the ST segment.

If cardiac tissue is deprived of blood for a prolonged period, the tissue dies, leading to a myocardial infarction (MI). The most characteristic finding in myocardial infarction is the presence of abnormal Q waves. The abnormal Q waves are most notable on the left precordial leads in MIs that involve the left anterior descending and circumflex branches of the left coronary artery. These Q waves occur because of a lack of counterbalancing electrical forces on the affected side; as a result, the unaffected side demonstrates the predominant electrical forces. Consequently, a downward deflected (Q) wave, rather than an upright (R) wave, appears on the ECG.

Both clinical research and basic research have provided valuable information about localizing myocardial infarctions by electrocardiography. Table 9-2 lists the common

electrocardiographic changes associated with inadequate blood flow to various arteries supplying the heart.[6] A note of caution is appropriate concerning ECG findings associated with MI. Abnormal T waves, ST segment amplitude, and Q waves can occur with other serious cardiac disorders. For example, T wave changes and ST segment displacements (elevation or depression) are associated with pericarditis as well as myocardial ischemia, injury, and infarction (Clinical Rounds 9-2).

HEMODYNAMIC MONITORING

Electrocardiograms provide information about the electrical activity of the heart. Hemodynamic measurements provide valuable information about the mechanical function of the cardiovascular system. To fully appreciate the significance of these measurements, students must recognize that the cardiovascular system is essentially a hydraulic system, which consists of a pump that propels liquid (i.e., blood) through a series of branched tubes or blood vessels (i.e., arteries, capillaries, and veins) to supply the various organ systems of the body.

A functional description of any hydraulic system requires simultaneous evaluation of a variety of parameters, so that a reasonable estimate can be made of the system's performance characteristics.[9,10] Therefore the amount of force the heart must generate to propel the blood through the circulation depends on the impedance offered by the blood vessels. As such, measurements of intracardiac and intravascular pressures and cardiac output, along with computation of vascular resistance, can provide fundamental information about the mechanical

CLINICAL ROUNDS 9-2

A 45-year-old male is admitted to the emergency department complaining of shortness of breath and angina. The patient appears diaphoretic and cyanotic. The 12-lead electrocardiogram shown here was obtained on admission. What are the most significant electrocardiographic findings?

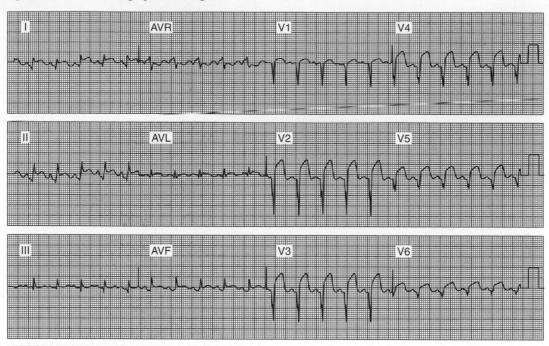

See Evolve Resources for the answer.

TABLE 9-2

Localization of Acute Myocardial Infarction

Anterior Infarcts

Anterolateral (occlusion of the anterior interventricular branch of the left coronary artery)	Deep Q waves in precordial leads V_3 to V_5 Loss of R waves in the left precordial leads (V_4 and V_5) ST segment elevation in lead I; ST segment depression in lead III
Anteroseptal (occlusion of the right division of the interventricular branch of the coronary artery)	Deep Q wave in precordial leads V_2 and V_3 Normal QRS complexes in limb leads I, II, and III S-T segment depression in limb lead II
Apical (occlusion of the terminal portions of the anterior interventricular branch of the left coronary artery)	Loss of R waves with deep Q waves in limb lead I and in precordial leads V_3 and V_4 ST segment elevation in lead I; S-T segment depression in lead III
Anterobasal (occlusion of a branch of the circumflex artery)	Small Q wave in limb lead I; large Q waves in precordial lead V_6 S-T segment elevation in leads I and V_6 T wave inversion in leads I and V_6

Posterior Infarcts

Posteroseptal (occlusion of the right coronary artery)	S-T segment depression in precordial leads V_3 and V_4
Posteroinferior (occlusion of the posterior interventricular branch of the right coronary artery)	Large Q waves in limb leads II and III and aVF S-T segment depression in leads I, V_3, and V_4; S-T segment elevation in lead aVF
Posterolateral (occlusion of the circumflex artery)	Q waves in leads aVL and V_6 S-T segment elevation and T wave inversion in limb leads II, III, and aVL

properties of the cardiovascular system and its ability to perform under varying conditions.

Technologic advances in the design of sensors, recording devices, and data analysis systems have greatly improved the ability to obtain accurate and reliable data that can be used in the diagnosis and treatment of patients with various types of cardiopulmonary dysfunction. Indeed, advances in solid-state electronics made during the past decade present possibilities for the future that were previously unimaginable.

Before the various devices routinely used to obtain hemodynamic measurements are described, a review of some basic physical principles as they apply to the heart and circulation is warranted.

The Cardiac Cycle

An appropriate place to begin the discussion of hemodynamics is to describe the pressure, volume, and flow events that occur in the heart and great vessels during a single heartbeat, or **cardiac cycle.** Figure 9-21 shows these events as they occur in the left heart chambers and the aorta.[10] The cardiac cycle typically is divided into two periods, a *systolic period,* during which the heart muscle is contracting and ejecting blood, and a *diastolic period,* during which the heart is relaxing and filling with blood. As shown in Figure 9-21, the cardiac cycle can be further divided into ventricular and atrial events.

Ventricular Events

Ventricular systole begins with a period of **isovolumetric contraction,** which follows the peak of the R wave on the ECG. During this period of contraction, ventricular muscle fibers shorten, but the volume of blood in the ventricle remains constant. The volume remains constant because the atrioventricular valves (i.e., mitral and tricuspid valves) and the semilunar valves (aortic and pulmonary valves) are closed. (Although the term *isometric contraction* often is used to describe this period, this is not a true isometric contraction, because some of the fibers shorten and others increase in length.[2]) During this period, the left ventricular pressure increases from 0 to about 80 mm Hg, and the right ventricular pressure increases from 0 to about 12 mm Hg.

As the ventricular muscle fibers continue to shorten and the left ventricle pressure exceeds the aortic diastolic pressure (about 80 mm Hg) and the right ventricle pressure exceeds the pulmonary artery diastolic pressure (about 12 mm Hg), a period of ejection occurs, and blood flows rapidly out of the ventricles as the semilunar valves open. At this point in the cycle, the pressures in the aorta and pulmonary artery increase from their diastolic values toward their peak systolic pressures (about 120 mm Hg and about 25 mm Hg, respectively). A longer phase, in which the ejection of blood is considerably reduced, immediately follows this period of rapid ejection and lasts until the pressures in the aorta and pulmonary artery decrease to about 80 mm Hg and about 15 mm Hg, respectively.

The rapid ejection period can be distinguished from the reduced ejection period by the contour of the aortic and pulmonary artery flow curves. During the rapid ejection period, the volume flow from the ventricle decreases sharply after the first third of the ejection. During the final two thirds of ejection, corresponding to the period of reduced ejection, the flow curve tapers. Thus blood flow into the aortic and pulmonary artery increases dramatically during the early period of ejection and gradually decreases during the latter stage of ejection. Notice that the pressures in the ventricles are higher than the pressures in the great vessels during the first third of ejection, whereas the reverse is true during the following two thirds of ventricular systole. Although it may not be apparent, the point of peak ejection occurs when the ventricular and aortic or pulmonary artery pressure tracings intersect.[1]

A period of **ventricular diastole** begins with closure of the aortic and pulmonary valve and can be identified by the presence of an **incisura** on the descending limb of the aortic or pulmonary artery pressure tracings. (This incisura, which is a small negative deflection on the aortic and pulmonary artery tracing, is thought to be associated with a transient reversal of flow that results from elastic recoil of these vessels after ventricular systole, which forces the blood to push against the respective semilunar valve.) The period between the closure of the semilunar valves and the opening of the atrioventricular valves is called **isovolumetric relaxation,** because the pressure in the ventricle falls dramatically, whereas the volume of the ventricle remains constant. As was described for isovolumetric contraction, the atrioventricular and semilunar valves are closed during isovolumetric relaxation. The aortic pressure gradually returns to its resting or diastolic value. This gradual decrease in pressure results from the inertia of blood flowing from the heart and to the elastic recoil of the aorta, which propels the blood through the systemic circulation even after ventricular systole has concluded. Upon opening of the atrioventricular valves, which occurs as the ventricular pressure drops below the atrial pressure, rapid ventricular filling begins. This rapid filling period typically occurs during the first third of ventricular filling, and it is followed by a longer period of reduced filling, or **diastasis.** Figure 9-22 shows another way to illustrate the pressure-volume changes that occur during each cardiac cycle. Although it may not be apparent, these changes are expressed independent of time and thus appear as a pressure-volume loop, with pressure and volume expressed on the abscissa, or *x* axis, and plotted on the ordinate, or *y* axis. Note that although the contours of the pressure, volume, and flow tracings for the left and right heart chambers, the aorta, and pulmonary artery are similar, there is a considerable difference in the magnitude of their values.

Atrial Events

Atrial systole begins immediately after the P wave which, as mentioned previously, is associated with atrial depolarization on the ECG. Atrial systole is indicated on the atrial

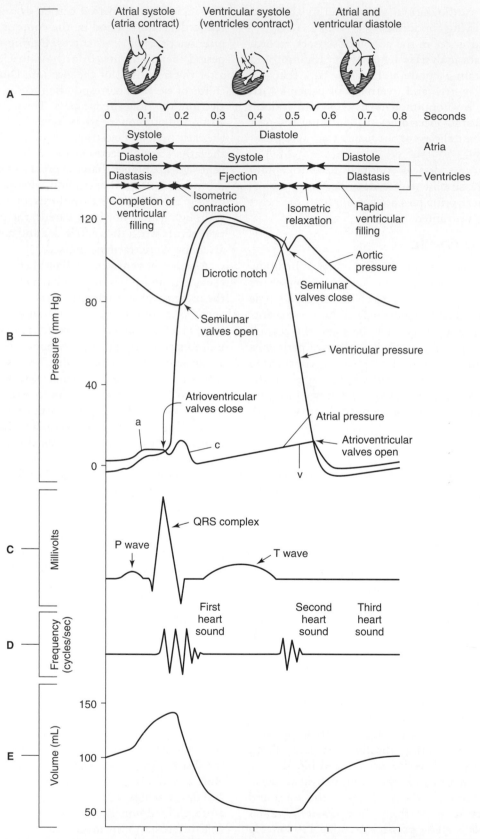

FIGURE 9-21 Pressure, volume, and flow changes that occur in the ventricles and great vessels during a typical cardiac cycle for a normal healthy individual. (From Pilbeam SP, Cairo JM: *Mechanical ventilation,* ed 4, St Louis, 2006, Mosby.)

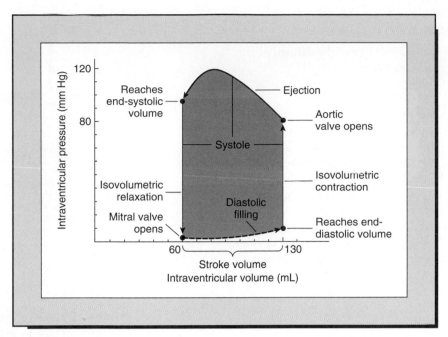

FIGURE 9-22 Pressure-volume graph illustrating changes during a normal cardiac cycle.

pressure tracing as an *"a" wave*. Under normal circumstances, ventricular filling occurs mainly during the period of **atrial diastole**, when the atrioventricular valves are open between the atria and ventricles. Atrial systole (i.e., the "atrial kick" mentioned previously) occurs just before the beginning of ventricular systole. Contraction of the atria normally contributes only a small amount of blood to ventricular filling. However, it can contribute a significant amount of blood to ventricular filling if the heart rate is increased and the period of diastasis is reduced. This occurs during ventricular tachycardia, because the higher heart rate results in a reduction in the volume of blood that passively enters the ventricle during atrial diastole.

The next important wave on the atrial pressure tracing is the *"c" wave*, which occurs at the beginning of atrial diastole. This wave coincides with the period of ventricular systole and is associated with a transient increase in atrial pressure as the pressure in the ventricle increases and forces the closed AV valves backward into the atrial chamber. It should be noted that the pressures in the two atria are normally only slightly higher than the ventricular pressures, indicating that minimal resistance exists between these two chambers when the valves are open. The atrial pressure wave shows a slight increase during atrial filling when the AV valves are closed and can be seen as a *"v" wave*. After the valves open, the pressure in the ventricle falls below the atrial pressure, and the atrial pressure tracing drops sharply as blood flows from the atria into the ventricles, initiating the period of ventricular filling.

Heart Sounds

Four heart sounds usually are associated with the various ventricular and atrial events of the cardiac cycle (see Figure 9-21). The first heart sound, typically designated S_1, occurs at the onset of ventricular contraction and is associated with closure of the atrioventricular valves and opening of the semilunar valves. It is a relatively low-pitched, high-intensity sound that is best heard over the apex of the heart. It has the longest duration of the four heart sounds. The second heart sound (S_2) occurs at the beginning of ventricular relaxation and is associated with closure of the semilunar valves and opening of the atrioventricular valves. It has a higher pitch and a lower intensity than the first heart sound. The third heart sound (S_3) occurs during early ventricular filling and normally is characterized as a low intensity, low-frequency sound. The fourth heart sound (S_4) occurs during atrial contraction. It also is a low-intensity, low-pitched sound. Under normal circumstances, only the first two heart sounds are audible through a stethoscope. The third and fourth heart sounds are not typically heard with a stethoscope but can be amplified and recorded graphically as a **phonocardiogram.**

The relationship between ventricular systole and diastole can be correlated with these various heart sounds by simply recognizing that ventricular systole occurs between S_1 and S_2 and ventricular diastole occurs during the period from S_2 to the next S_1. This division of the cardiac cycle based on heart sounds can be very useful when describing **murmurs** or abnormal heart sounds, which are associated with the generation of turbulent blood flow resulting from abnormal mechanical function of the heart, such as occurs when a valve fails to open or close properly. Clinicians typically describe a murmur as being a systolic murmur or a diastolic murmur, depending on when it is heard relative to S_1 and S_2. Test yourself on this principle by determining whether a stiff, calcified aortic valve causes a systolic or diastolic murmur.

Pressure Measurements

As stated in Chapter 1, pressure (P) may be defined as the force (F) exerted per unit area (A) or

$$P = F/A$$

where pressure can be measured in pounds per square inch (lb/in^2), dynes per square centimeter ($dynes/cm^2$), millimeters of mercury (mm Hg), centimeters of water (cm H_2O), or kilopascals (kPa). You might also remember that a variety of devices can be used to measure atmospheric pressures, most notably the mercury barometer and the aneroid barometer. This chapter focuses on the pressure-measuring devices routinely used to determine intracardiac and intravascular pressures. For purposes of continuity, devices routinely used to perform noninvasive measurements of arterial pressure are described first and then the devices used for invasive blood pressure measurements.

Noninvasive Devices

The simplest and most widely used technique for measuring arterial blood pressure involves the **sphygmomanometer** (Figure 9-23). This device consists of an aneroid manometer connected by rubber tubing to a cuff, which can be inflated with a hand bulb. Deflation of the cuff is accomplished with a pressure control valve, which is attached to the tubing that connects the hand bulb to the inflatable cuff.

For blood pressure measurement, the deflated cuff is wrapped snugly around the patient's arm so that the bottom edge of the cuff is approximately 2 to 3 cm above the antecubital fossa. Selecting the appropriate-size cuff is important, because using a cuff that is too big or too small can seriously affect the accuracy of the measurement. The width of the cuff should be approximately 40% to 50% of the circumference of the patient's arm. The length of the cuff should be approximately 80% to 100% of the patient's Humerus. For example, the standard blood pressure cuff used for adults is 5 inches wide and approximately 8 to 10 inches long. Pediatric cuffs are available for children younger than 5 years of age. These cuffs typically range from 1.5 to 3 inches wide and 3 to 6 inches long.[11,12] The measurements should be taken on an arm that is not being used for the infusion of fluids or drugs, because inflation of the cuff can obstruct the blood vessel and slow the infusion of the fluids.

While palpating the radial artery in the arm used for measurement, the examiner inflates the cuff to a pressure about 30 mm Hg above the pressure at which the radial pulse disappears. A stethoscope is placed over the brachial artery, and the cuff is gradually deflated at a rate of about 5 mm Hg/sec. The pressure at which a tapping sound is first heard as the cuff is deflated is the systolic pressure. The pressure at which these sounds become inaudible during cuff deflation is the diastolic pressure. The tapping sounds heard with the aid of the stethoscope are called **Korotkoff's sounds;** these are attributed to turbulent

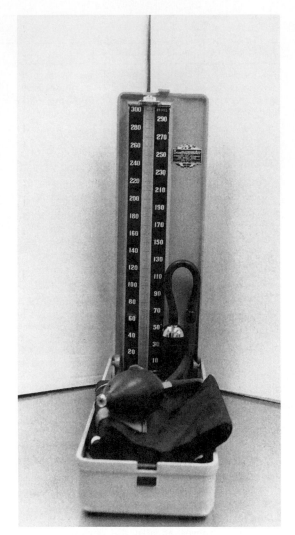

FIGURE 9-23 Sphygmomanometer. (Courtesy WA Braum, Copiague New York.)

blood flow that occurs when blood is forced through a partially occluded artery.[10] As the diameter of the vessel becomes larger with deflation of the compression cuff, blood flow becomes more laminar, and the turbulence that caused the tapping sound essentially disappears.

Automated blood pressure measurement systems (Figure 9-24) operate on similar principles. These systems are particularly convenient when frequent determinations of blood pressure are required, such as during surgical procedures or in the intensive care unit.[11] Automated blood pressure measurement systems use electricity in the form of either a 110-V, 60-Hz alternating current or a battery as the power source. As with the manual systems, the automated devices can be attached to different-size disposable cuffs. A microphone or ultrasound transducer attached to the cuff is used instead of the stethoscope to detect pressure pulsations that occur as the blood is forced through the partially occluded blood vessel during cuff deflation.

When the system is first activated, the cuff is inflated to a preset pressure and held constant for a period of pressure

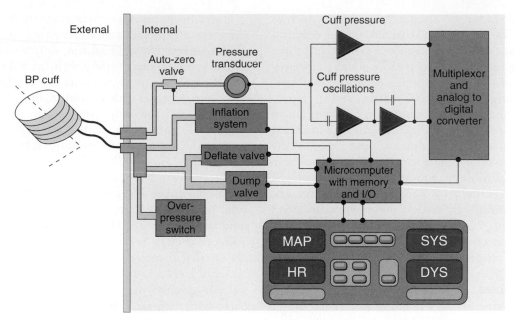

FIGURE 9-24 Automated blood pressure measurement system. (Courtesy of VIASYS, Pleasanton, Calif.)

stabilization (e.g., 160 mm Hg). The system then determines whether pressure oscillations are present and records the pressures as the cuff is deflated in a stepwise manner to atmospheric pressure (Figure 9-25). If oscillations are sensed during the period of pressure stabilization, indicating that the initial cuff pressure was less than the patient's peak systolic pressure, the system increases the inflation pressure on the next cycle. Conversely, the system decreases the inflation pressure on the next cycle if the inflation pressure was too high. The systolic and diastolic blood pressures, along with the mean arterial blood pressure, can be recorded graphically on an oscilloscope or registered on a light-emitting diode (LED) display. The system automatically zeros itself periodically by opening the transducer to the atmosphere.

Automated systems can automatically determine the maximum inflation pressure in the cuff, the cuff inflation time, and the cuff deflation rate by relying on a specially designed control circuit. These circuits are also designed to automatically reject oscillation artifacts that can interfere with the accuracy of the measurements. Audible and visual alarm systems are available on all systems. In many systems, the alarms are set at default values but can be manually adjusted by the operator.[12] In several commercially available systems, the alarms are automatically set around the initial readings of the patient's peak systolic, diastolic, and mean arterial pressures.

The most common errors in determining the arterial blood pressure with both manual sphygmomanometers and automated blood pressure monitoring systems are failure to use the proper size cuff, improper positioning of the cuff, improper deflation of the cuff, and motion artifacts. For example, an undersized cuff causes falsely elevated readings, whereas an oversized cuff results in

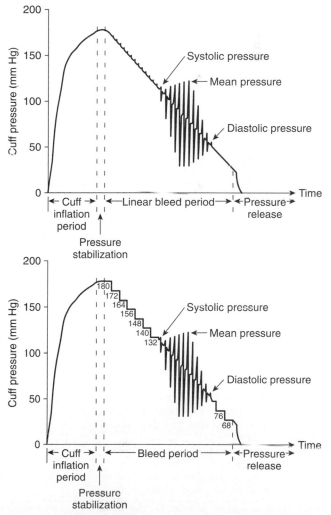

FIGURE 9-25 Pressure oscillation method for automated blood pressure measurement. (Courtesy Tyco Healthcare, Pleasanton, Calif.)

underestimated readings.[13] Mechanical problems, such as a defective pressure control valve or old, porous connecting tubing, also can lead to erroneous results. Improper cuff placement, such as moving it more peripherally away from the level of the heart, typically results in an abnormally high reading for the systolic pressure and an erroneously low diastolic pressure. The most common problem encountered with deflation of the cuff occurs in automated systems that fail to deflate because of obstruction of the cuff vent. This problem may also cause an erroneous zero setting, resulting in lower than actual pressure readings. Motion artifacts caused by patient shivering, tremors, convulsions, or simply by restless movements can affect the measurement. Although most automated systems can reject these extraneous signals, they occasionally fail to do so and therefore provide misleading information.

Invasive Devices

Invasive measurements, which allow determination of intravascular and intracardiac pressures, require insertion of fluid-filled catheters into the vascular space. For arterial blood pressure measurements, a catheter made of polyvinyl chloride is inserted into a peripheral artery, such as the radial, brachial, or dorsalis pedis artery. The insertion site should be chosen based on assessment of the integrity of the vessel and the presence of adequate collateral circulation. This can be accomplished using the modified Allen's test (see Chapter 10). Box 9-3 presents a summary of the technique for inserting and maintaining an indwelling arterial line catheter.[13]

BOX 9-3	**Technique for Insertion and Maintenance of an Indwelling Arterial Line Catheter**

1. Perform the Allen test before radial artery cannulation. Ischemic complications are lowest when the ulnar artery refill time is less than 5 seconds.
2. Use sterile technique for insertion (antiseptic preparation, gloves, drapes).
3. Choose percutaneous insertion over surgical cut-down when possible.
4. Use a 20-gauge catheter if the patient's wrist circumference is small.
5. Use a continuous flush system with a nondextrose solution (normal saline) containing heparin.
6. Use a transducer with a disposable dome.
7. Assess daily:
   a. Catheter site for evidence of inflammation
   b. Distal extremity for evidence of ischemia
8. Limit cannulation to 4 to 5 days at one site.
9. Remove catheter for:
   a. Distal ischemia
   b. Local infection
   c. Persistently damped pressure tracing
   d. Difficulty with blood withdrawal

Modified from Matthay RA, Wiedemann HP, Matthay MA: Cardiovascular function in the intensive care unit: invasive and noninvasive monitoring, *Respir Care* 30:432, 1985.

Right heart pressure measurements are obtained by inserting a catheter into a peripheral vein and slowly guiding it into the right atrium, right ventricle, and ultimately the pulmonary artery with the aid of fluoroscopy or real-time pressure measurements. A significant improvement in right heart catheterization, including fewer complications and the ability to perform this procedure at the bedside, came with the balloon-tipped, flow-directed pulmonary artery catheter introduced by Swan and Ganz in 1970.[14]

The standard balloon flotation catheter (Figure 9-26) is a multiple-lumen catheter constructed of polyvinyl chloride. Adult and pediatric catheters are available. The standard adult catheter is 110 cm long and comes in size 5 or 7 French (F) (the French number divided by 3.14, or π, is the external diameter of the catheter in millimeters).[2] Pediatric catheters are 60 cm long and available in either 4 or 5 F. All catheters are marked at 10-cm increments. The Swan-Ganz catheter, as it is commonly called, has an inflatable balloon attached to the tip of the catheter with multiple lumens that can be attached to pressure manometers or used for the injection of fluids.

In dual-lumen catheters, one lumen connects to a balloon at the tip of the catheter, and the other lumen runs the length of the catheter and terminates at a port at the distal end of the catheter. The second lumen's distal port can be used to monitor right ventricular pressure and pulmonary arterial (PA) pressure, or it can be used to obtain mixed venous blood samples when the catheter's distal end is positioned in the pulmonary artery. Triple-lumen catheters have an additional lumen that is connected to a proximal port 30 cm from the tip of the catheter. When the catheter is placed properly, the proximal port is located in the area of the right atrium and thus can be used to monitor the central venous pressure (CVP). Specially designed thermodilution catheters have a fourth lumen, which contains electrical wires that connect a thermistor located approximately 2 cm from the tip of the catheter to a cardiac output computer like the one shown in Figure 9-27. (Thermodilution cardiac output measurements are discussed in the section on cardiac output measurements.)

The catheter is introduced percutaneously into a peripheral vein, such as the antecubital, subclavian, internal or external jugular, or femoral vein. Surgical cut-down may be necessary if the antecubital route is used. The catheter is advanced using fluoroscopy or with the aid of continuous pressure monitoring and electrocardiography until the tip of the catheter enters the intrathoracic vessels. Alternatively, the distance required to enter the intrathoracic vessels can be ascertained by noting the 10-cm marks on the catheter. If the catheter is introduced through the antecubital route, this distance is approximately 40 to 50 cm. The distance for the femoral route is approximately 30 to 40 cm, and it is 10 to 15 cm if the internal jugular route is chosen.

After the catheter is positioned in the intrathoracic vessels, the balloon is inflated with a small volume of air

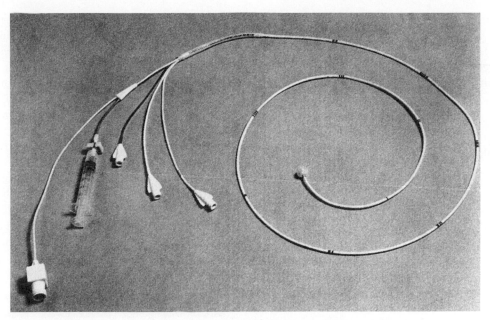

FIGURE 9-26 Balloon-tipped, flow-directed (Swan-Ganz) right heart catheter. (Courtesy Edwards-American Hospital Supply, Santa Ana, Calif.)

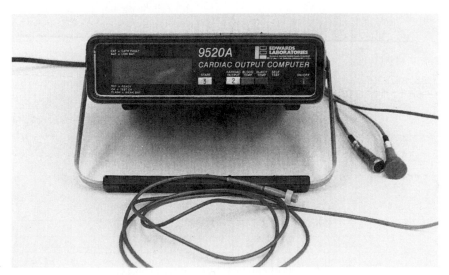

FIGURE 9-27 Cardiac output computer. (Courtesy Edwards-American Hospital Supply, Santa Ana, Calif.)

(about 0.8 mL). (Carbon dioxide [CO_2] sometimes is used to inflate the balloon, because if the balloon should rupture, the CO_2 is absorbed by the tissues rather than causing an air embolism.) The balloon on the tip of the catheter is carried by the blood (like a sail being pushed by the wind) into the ventricle and then to the pulmonary artery. It can be further advanced and wedged into a small pulmonary artery for measurement of the pulmonary artery occlusion pressure (PAOP; the term often is used interchangeably with *pulmonary artery wedge pressure* [PAWP]). The PAOP can be used as an estimate of the left atrial pressure and thus preload of the left ventricle (i.e., the left ventricular end-diastolic pressure [LVEDP], which is not easily measured in the critical care setting). Deflation

of the balloon after it is wedged in a small pulmonary artery typically causes the catheter to drift backward into the main pulmonary artery. Figure 9-28 shows a typical pressure tracing for a healthy adult during right heart catheterization with a Swan-Ganz catheter.

Box 9-4 provides a summary of the most common problems encountered during right heart catheterization. (Clinical Rounds 9-3 presents an exercise involving right heart catheterization.) It generally has been accepted that the number of critical incidences and problems associated with the use of balloon flotation catheters in critical care medicine has been relatively low in light of the number of catheterizations that have been performed during the past 30 years. However, recent editorials and articles appearing in the medical literature have raised questions regarding the risk-benefit ratio when this procedure is used in critically ill patients. A special commission established by the American College of Chest Physicians, the American Society of Anesthesiologists, and the American Thoracic Society was formed in 2001 to address these issues. A final report from the commission proposed and ultimately succeeded in implementing an educational program to better prepare clinicians using this technology. The program is administered through online education and can be easily accessed through the Web site of the Pulmonary Artery Catheter Education Project (www. PACEP.org).

Left heart catheterization, which involves placing a catheter into the aorta, left ventricle, and left atrium, requires a retrograde approach in which the catheter is inserted into a peripheral artery (usually the brachial or femoral artery) under fluoroscopic guidance.[15] A transseptal approach also can be used. In the transseptal technique, a specially designed catheter containing a retractable

---

BOX 9-4	Common Problems Encountered during Right Heart Catheterization

1. Arrhythmias
   a. Transient premature ventricular contractions (PVCs)
   b. Sustained ventricular tachycardia
   c. Ventricular fibrillation
   d. Atrial fibrillation
   e. Atrial flutter
2. Right bundle branch block
3. Pulmonary infarction
4. Pulmonary artery rupture
5. Catheter-related infections
6. Balloon rupture
7. Catheter knotting
8. Endocardial damage to:
   a. Valve cusps
   b. Chordae tendineae
   c. Papillary muscles
9. Complications at insertion site
   a. Pneumothorax
   b. Arterial puncture
   c. Venous thrombosis or phlebitis
   d. Air embolism

From Wiedermann HP, Matthay MA, Matthay RA: Cardiovascular-pulmonary monitoring in the intensive care unit, *Chest* 85:537, 656, 1984.

CLINICAL ROUNDS 9-3

A number of factors can lead to inaccurate pressure measurements during right heart catheterization with a balloon flotation catheter. Briefly describe how each of the following conditions would adversely affect these measurements:

1. Hypovolemic patient is ventilated with PEEP.
2. Therapist is unable to obtain a PAOP measurement.
3. Attending physician notes that the pressure tracings are erratic and difficult to decipher.

See Evolve Resources for the answer.

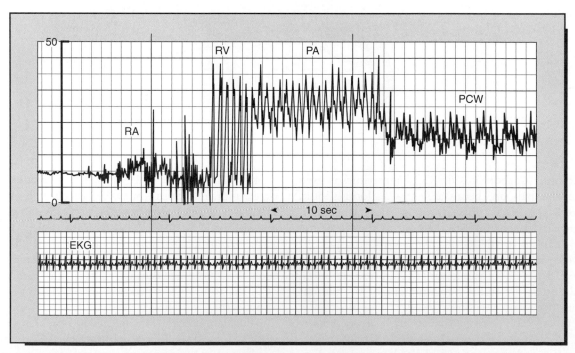

FIGURE 9-28 Pressure tracing obtained during a typical right heart catheterization in a healthy adult. (Redrawn from Grossman W: *Cardiac catheterization and angiography,* ed 3, Philadelphia, 1986, Lea & Febiger.)

needle is introduced into a peripheral vein and positioned in the right atrium.[15] The clinician then extends the needle and punctures the interatrial septum, establishing a communication between the distal tip of the catheter or needle, which lies within the left atrium, and the proximal opening of the catheter, which can be attached to a pressure transducer. Left heart catheterizations are performed in specially designed cardiac catheterization laboratories, whereas right heart catheterization can be performed either in a cardiac catheterization laboratory or at the bedside in the intensive care unit. Specific information on the procedures for left heart catheterization can be found in the references at the end of this chapter.

Pressure Transducers

A transducer can be defined simply as a sensor that converts one form of energy into another form. A pressure transducer is an electromechanical device that converts a pressure signal into an electrical signal, which can be recorded or displayed on some type of output device. The number and variety of pressure transducers available for clinical practice have increased during recent years. The principles upon which these devices are based are the electrical properties of resistance, capacitance, and inductance.

Figure 9-29 shows the three types of electromechanical transducers.[16] A resistance transducer (Figure 9-29A) consists of a thin metal diaphragm attached to four wires, forming a Wheatstone bridge. Remember from Chapter 1 that a Wheatstone bridge is an electronic circuit consisting of four resistors connected in parallel. One branch of the circuit contains two resistors (R1 + R2) that form a fixed resistance, and the second branch of the circuit is made up of two resistors (R3 + R4) that form a variable resistance.

As pressure is applied to the metal diaphragm, the attached wires are stretched, changing their length and diameter and their electrical resistance. This change in electrical resistance changes the output voltage by an amount that is proportional to the applied pressure.

The variable capacitance transducer (Figure 9-29B) also uses a flexible diaphragm to sense pressure changes. In this type of device, a thin metal diaphragm is linked to an electrode, forming a capacitor. Notice that when the diaphragm is not flexed, a small gap of air exists between the diaphragm and the electrode. As pressure is applied to the diaphragm, the gap narrows and ultimately causes the capacitor to discharge. As with the resistance transducer, the output voltage is directly proportional to the movement of the diaphragm and thus the pressure applied to it.

A variable inductance transducer (Figure 9-29C) consists of a stainless steel diaphragm attached to a soft iron core positioned between two coils. The application of pressure to the diaphragm results in downward displacement of the iron core, ultimately causing a change in the inductance of the two coils. The change in inductance caused by the movement of the iron core between the two coils is proportional to the applied pressure.

Strain gauge and variable inductance pressure transducers are the most frequently used devices because they can respond quickly to pressure changes. They both have good frequency response characteristics over a wide range of pressures. These devices are also quite stable and relatively insensitive to vibration and shock.[17] Variable capacitance transducers are usually large, bulky, and very sensitive to vibrations. They also have poor frequency response characteristics compared with strain gauge and variable inductance transducers.

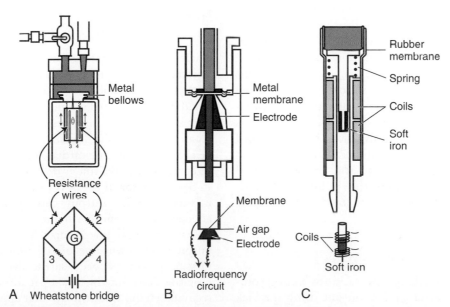

FIGURE 9-29 Electromechanical pressure transducers. **A,** Resistive transducer. **B,** Variable capacitance transducer. **C,** Variable inductance transducer.

Cardiac Output Measurements

Historically, invasive techniques involving right heart catheterization have been the preferred method of determining cardiac output in clinical medicine. The direct Fick method, which is based on a principle formulated by Adolph Fick, has served as the gold standard for cardiac output measurements for more than a century. The development of thermistors and the thermodilution technique for measuring cardiac output have largely supplanted the use of the Fick method in clinical medicine during the past 20 years. More recent advances in the development of noninvasive technologies, which are based on impedance plethysmography and the Doppler effect, may very well prove to be the methods of choice for measuring cardiac output in critically ill patients because of their accuracy and safety.

Noninvasive methods of measuring cardiac output, such as impedance plethysmography and the indirect Fick method, currently are available but are not routinely used by most critical care clinicians for cardiac output determinations. It is reasonable to assume, however, that clinicians will gain more confidence in these techniques and recognize their value in critical care medicine because they can provide another means of assessing the cardiopulmonary status of patients with minimal risk.[17]

Invasive Techniques

Direct Fick Method. The Fick principle states that the total uptake of a substance by an organ ($\dot{V}_x$) is directly related to the blood flow through the organ ($\dot{Q}$) and the arteriovenous concentration or content difference of the substance across the organ ($Ca_x - Cv_x$), or

Equation 9-1

$$\dot{V}O_2 = \dot{Q} \times (CaO_2 - C\overline{v}O_2)$$

We can determine the output of the right ventricle (i.e., pulmonary blood flow) by simultaneously measuring the total uptake of oxygen by the lungs, or oxygen consumption ($\dot{V}O_2$), and the arteriovenous oxygen content difference between arterial blood (CaO_2) and mixed venous blood ($C\overline{v}O_2$). Oxygen consumption is determined from measurements of the volumes and oxygen concentrations of a patient's inspired and expired gases, whereas the arteriovenous oxygen difference is determined by measuring the oxygen content of arterial blood obtained from a peripheral artery and that of a mixed venous sample obtained from the pulmonary artery. The cardiac output can by derived by simply applying Equation 9-1.

Equation 9-2

$$\dot{Q} = \dot{V}O_2 \div (CaO_2 - C\overline{v}O_2)$$

Clinical Rounds 9-4 presents a scenario for testing yourself on the calculation of cardiac output using the Fick method.

Indicator Dilution Methods. The indicator dilution method of determining cardiac output, also known as the *Stewart-Hamilton dye dilution technique*, is commonly used to measure cardiac output during cardiac catheterization because of its accuracy and simplicity.[15] A known amount of dye (e.g., indocyanine green or Evan's blue) is injected into a peripheral vein. The passage of dye through the pulmonary artery and its appearance and changing concentration in the arterial blood are recorded by continuously passing samples of arterial blood obtained from an indwelling radial, brachial, or femoral arterial line through a densitometer, which determines the concentrations of the dye in the blood. The results are recorded as time-concentration curves, which can be displayed on an oscilloscope and digitally processed to determine the cardiac output using the following relationship:

Equation 9-3

$$\dot{Q} = I/C_0$$

where $\dot{Q}$ is the cardiac output, I is the total amount of dye injected (measured in milligrams per minute), and C_o is the average concentration of dye in the first pass through the circulation (measured in milligrams per liter). As shown in Figure 9-30, if the first-pass curve is extrapolated with regard to time (dashed line), the effects of recirculation can be eliminated and the cardiac output can be calculated by integrating the area under the curve.

Several factors must be considered when this technique is used. Cardiac output determinations are adversely affected in patients with intracardiac shunts and also in patients with low cardiac output. With low cardiac output, the downslope of the time-concentration curve may be prolonged because the dye moves more slowly past the detector; this makes it difficult to differentiate recirculated dye from the dye that appears in the first-pass sample.

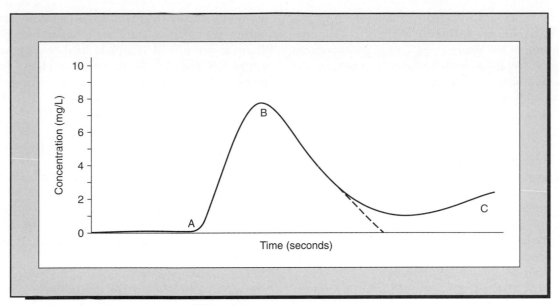

FIGURE 9-30 Indicator dilution curve.

The thermodilution technique of determining cardiac output is another variation of the indicator dilution method. For the thermodilution technique, approximately 10 mL of cold (or room temperature) sterile 0.9% saline or 5% dextrose is injected through the proximal port of an indwelling balloon-tipped, flow-directed catheter, and a small thermistor at the tip of the catheter senses changes in the temperature of the blood. A cardiac output computer, which is connected to the catheter through electrical contacts, calculates the cardiac output by relying on temperature relationships (similar to the time-concentration relationships mentioned with the dye dilution technique) that occur as the injected fluid changes the temperature of the blood sensed by the catheter's thermistor.

The thermodilution technique is widely used in the critical care setting. The advantage of this technique is that it does not require monitoring of arterial blood samples; measurements require only small volumes of injectate (e.g., cold normal saline), and therefore multiple determinations are possible and there is essentially no problem with recirculation. Inaccuracies can occur in patients with tricuspid valve insufficiency and intracardiac shunts. Measurements are also affected by a low cardiac output. When cardiac output is measured in mechanically ventilated patients, the normal saline should be injected during the end-expiration portion of the ventilatory cycle to ensure that consistent measurements are obtained.

Noninvasive Techniques

Impedance Plethysmography. Impedance plethysmography, as it is used in cardiac output measurements, is based on the principle that changes in blood volume associated with pulsations of blood as it passes through a

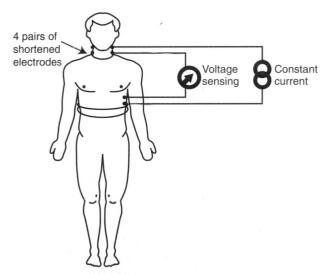

FIGURE 9-31 Impedance cardiograph.

blood vessel cause changes in the electrical impedance, or resistance, of the tissue surrounding the blood vessel.[17] This electrical impedance can be measured by passing a small amount of alternating current through the body segment in question. The amount of alternating electrical current is small enough that the patient does not feel it. An important application of this principle is the diagnosis of deep vein thrombosis.

Impedance Cardiography, a variation of impedance plethysmography, can be used to measure cardiac output. A series of two pairs of electrodes is placed on the thorax (Figure 9-31). The assumption is that changes in bioimpedance that occur with changes in the thoracic blood volume during ventricular systole and diastole can be used to calculate beat-to-beat changes in stroke volume and thus cardiac output. Electrical voltage signals sensed by the measuring electrodes are processed, along with a simultaneous recording of the patient's ECG, and an impedance cardiograph curve is derived. Different points on the impedance cardiograph curve can be labeled and used to calculate variables such as stroke volume and systolic time intervals.

Studies have demonstrated that cardiac output measurements made with thoracic electrical bioimpedance correlate with those obtained by thermodilution and the direct Fick method.[17] The potential uses for impedance cardiography include screening for cardiac disease, pacemaker adjustments, long-term continuous monitoring of cardiac output during surgery and in the intensive care unit, noninvasive hemodynamic measurements during cardiopulmonary stress testing, and monitoring of the effects of pharmacologic interventions.

Indirect Fick Method. As might be surmised from the name of this technique, the indirect Fick method is based on the Fick principle, which was described previously. In the indirect technique, however, cardiac output is determined through continuous measurements of CO_2 production rather than oxygen consumption. Arterial and mixed venous oxygen differences are replaced by noninvasive measurements of arterial CO_2 content and mixed venous CO_2 content, respectively.[18] CO_2 production is obtained from continuous measurements of the mixed expired CO_2 ($FECO_2$) and the expired minute ventilation ($\dot{V}_E$). The arterial CO_2 content is calculated from measurements of the partial pressure of the end-tidal CO_2 ($PETCO_2$) (to approximate the partial pressure of CO_2 in the arteries [$PaCO_2$]); the mixed venous CO_2 content is derived from measurements of the partial pressure of mixed expired CO_2 ($P\bar{v}CO_2$) when the patient intermittently rebreathes a 10% CO_2 mixture (at 10- to 15-second intervals). Cardiac output therefore is calculated as

Equation 9-4

$$\dot{Q} = \dot{V}CO_2/(P\bar{v}CO_2 - PETCO_2)$$

Results indicate that the indirect Fick technique may prove to be useful for measuring cardiac output in most patients; however, more studies are required to determine the accuracy of this technique in critically ill patients.

Interpretation of Hemodynamic Profiles

Interpreting hemodynamic data is a fairly straightforward task. However, using this information in the management of patients can be considerably more challenging for even the most skilled clinician. It is reasonable to state that the hemodynamic profile ultimately focuses on the factors that influence cardiac output, namely, the heart rate, preload, contractility, and afterload. Preload, which typically is defined as the filling pressure of the ventricle at the end of ventricular diastole, is estimated by measuring the end-diastolic pressures. As such, the right ventricular end-diastolic pressure (RVEDP) is used as an indicator of the right ventricular preload, and the left ventricular end-diastolic pressure (LVEDP) is used to estimate the left ventricular preload. Because both of these intracardiac pressures are difficult to measure in the critical care setting, clinicians rely on measurements of the CVP to estimate the RVEDP and measurements of the PAWP to estimate the LVEDP.

Contractility, which is related to the force the ventricle generates during each cardiac cycle, can be estimated using the ejection fraction or the ratio of the stroke volume to the ventricular end-diastolic volume. The ventricular afterload is the resistance the ventricle must overcome to eject blood and is estimated from calculations of systemic resistance and the pulmonary vascular resistance.

The information that follows in this section is meant to provide an overview of basic measurements obtained in a standard hemodynamic profile. It is not our purpose to provide an extensive analysis of the various factors and conditions that can influence a patient's hemodynamic status. A number of excellent references related to hemodynamic monitoring in clinical practice are listed at the end of this chapter for those readers interested in obtaining more detailed information about this area of clinical physiology.

Cardiac Output

Cardiac output is the volume of blood pumped by the heart each minute; it usually is expressed in liters or milliliters per minute. Cardiac output can be calculated by multiplying the heart rate by the stroke volume, which is the volume of blood pumped by the heart per beat (measured in liters or milliliters per beat). Alternatively, cardiac output can be measured using one of the techniques described in the previous section of this chapter on cardiac output determinations.

In many cases the cardiac output and the stroke volume may be expressed relative to the patient's body surface area (BSA), which can be easily obtained using a Dubois chart. This indexing technique allows the clinician to compare an individual's cardiac output or stroke output to that of normal healthy individuals of the same weight and height (the BSA is calculated using these two anthropometric values). The cardiac index is calculated by dividing the cardiac output by the BSA, or

Equation 9-5

$$\text{Cardiac Index} = \dot{Q}/\text{BSA}$$

Similarly, the stroke index is calculated by dividing the stroke volume by the BSA, or

Equation 9-6

$$\text{Stroke Index} = \text{SV}/\text{BSA}$$

The normal cardiac index for an adult is approximately 3.5 L/min/m^2. The stroke index normally ranges from

40 to 50 mL/beat/m^2. Cardiac output can be reduced by decreases in either the heart rate or stroke volume. Decreases in the effective ventricular rate usually are associated with an increase in parasympathetic tone or with various types of bradyarrhythmias. Decreases in stroke volume typically are associated with reductions in the preload or contractility of the heart or with an abnormally high afterload. Increases in cardiac output are associated with increases in the heart rate or stroke volume. Tachycardia associated with an increase in sympathetic tone or a decrease in parasympathetic tone increases cardiac output. Increases in stroke volume are associated with increases in preload and contractility and with reductions in afterload. Note that profound increases in the heart rate actually can reduce cardiac output by reducing the ventricular filling time and the resultant ventricular preload.

Vascular Resistance

Vascular resistance represents the impedance, or opposition to blood flow, offered by the systemic or pulmonary vascular beds. It influences the force the ventricular muscle must generate during cardiac contractions (remember that $\Delta P = \dot{Q} \times R$). It has been reported historically as dyne sec cm^{-5}; however, more recent publications have used the units of mm Hg/L/min. In this text, we use the units of dyne sec cm^{-5}.

Vascular resistance usually is described as **systemic vascular resistance (SVR)** or **pulmonary vascular resistance (PVR).** A simple way to think of these calculations is to understand that ΔP represents the pressure gradient across the vascular bed, and $\dot{Q}$ is the blood flow through the vascular bed. Thus the SVR can be calculated as follows:

Equation 9-7

$$SVR = (MAP - MRAP/SBF)80$$

where *MAP* is the mean arterial blood pressure (expressed in mm Hg); *MRAP* is the mean right atrial pressure (also expressed in mm Hg); and *SBF* is the systemic blood flow, or cardiac output. Clinicians routinely multiply the equation by 80 to convert the units of mm Hg/L/min to dyne sec cm^{-5}.

Similarly, the PVR is calculated as

Equation 9-8

$$PVR = (MPAP - MLAP/PBF)80$$

where *MPAP* is the mean pulmonary artery pressure, *MLAP* is the mean left atrial pressure (both measured in mm Hg), and *PBF* is the pulmonary blood flow, or cardiac output (expressed in L/min). Note that PAWP can be used in place of MLAP.

The normal SVR ranges from 900 to 1500 dyne sec cm^{-5}, and the PVR ranges from 100 to 250 dyne sec cm^{-5}. A variety of factors can influence vascular resistance, most importantly, the caliber of the blood vessels and the viscosity of the blood. Remember that $R = 8\eta l/\pi r^4$, where in

this case η is the viscosity of the blood, l is length, and r is the radius of the vessel. Thus the SVR can be increased in left ventricular failure and hypovolemia because of the vasoconstriction that results from stimulation of the baroreceptor reflex. The SVR may also be increased by an increase in blood viscosity, as occurs in polycythemia. The SVR is reduced by systemic vasodilation, such as occurs with moderate hypoxemia or after administration of pharmacologic agents such as nitroglycerin and hydralazine.

The PVR can increase significantly during periods of alveolar hypoxia or when high intraalveolar pressures are generated, such as during positive pressure ventilation. A low cardiac output can increase the PVR by causing derecruitment of pulmonary vessels. The PVR is reduced by administration of pulmonary vasodilator drugs, such as tolazoline and prostacyclin.

Cardiac Work

In Chapter 1, we defined *work* as the product of a force acting on an object to move it a certain distance. In calculations of **cardiac work,** the pressure generated by the heart during a ventricular contraction is used to quantify the amount of force developed, and the distance traveled is replaced with the volume of blood pumped by the heart, either as cardiac output or more often as stroke volume. The amount of work performed by each ventricle during the cardiac cycle can be quantified by applying the following formulae:

Equation 9-9

$$LSW = MAP \times SV \times 0.00136$$

Equation 9-10

$$RSW = MPAP \times SV \times 0.00136$$

where *LSW* is the left ventricular stroke work, *RSW* is the right ventricular stroke work, *MAP* is the mean arterial pressure, *MPAP* is the mean pulmonary artery pressure, *SV* is the stroke volume, and 0.00136 is a factor for converting mL-mm Hg to gram-meters. In most clinical situations, stroke work measurements are indexed to the BSA by dividing the LSW or RSW by the patient's body surface area. Therefore, the left ventricular stroke work index (LSWI) and right ventricular stroke work index (RSWI) are calculated as

Equation 9-11

$$LSWI = LSW/BSA$$

Equation 9-12

$$RSWI = RSW/BSA$$

The LSWI normally ranges from 0.5 to 0.6 kg-m/m^2, and the RSWI from 0.07 to 0.1 kg-m/m^2. It should be apparent from these equations that conditions that increase the stroke volume or mean pressure generated by the ventricles increase the amount of work the ventricle must perform.

KEY POINTS

▶ The assessment of cardiovascular function is an integral part of the management of patients with cardiopulmonary dysfunction.

▶ Conventional electrocardiography provides valuable information about the electrophysiologic properties of the heart: excitability, rhythmicity, and conductivity.

▶ The standard 12-lead ECG comprises three sets of leads: standard limb leads, augmented limb leads, and the precordial or chest leads. Analysis of these three sets of leads provides an electronic view of the heart both from a frontal and a horizontal perspective.

▶ A number of waves, complexes, and intervals should be quantified in the analysis of typical ECG waveforms. These include the P, QRS, and T waves, the PR interval, the QT interval, and the ST segment.

▶ Interpretation of the ECG should focus on three major factors: atrial and ventricular rates, the presence of abnormal rhythms or dysrhythmias, and calculation of the mean electrical axis.

▶ Hemodynamic monitoring provides valuable information about the mechanical function of the cardiovascular system. Noninvasive measurements of arterial blood pressure and heart sounds can give the clinician an overview of cardiovascular function. The most common invasive techniques use vascular and cardiac catheterization to assess pressure, volume, and flow events that occur during the cardiac cycle.

▶ Interpretation of the hemodynamic profile should focus on quantifying cardiac output, vascular resistance, and cardiac work.

ASSESSMENT QUESTIONS

See Evolve Resources for the answers.

1. Which of the following correctly describes the permeability characteristics of the resting membrane potential for a ventricular myocyte?
   a. $K^+ > Na^+$
   b. $Ca^{++} > Na^+$
   c. $Ca^{++} > K^+$
   d. $Na^+ = K^+$

2. Which of the following statements is true concerning nodal tissue action potentials?
   a. The action potential demonstrates five phases, like ventricular myocytes.
   b. The amplitude of this type of action potential is the same as an action potential for a ventricular myocyte.
   c. The threshold potential for this type of tissue is more negative than the threshold potentials for a ventricular myocyte.
   d. The slope of phase 4 of the SA node is greater than that of the ventricular myocyte.

3. For the lead aVF configuration, the positive electrode is placed on the:
   a. Right arm
   b. Left arm
   c. Right leg
   d. Left leg

4. A patient's ECG tracing shows an R-R interval of 15 mm. What is this patient's effective heart rate?
   a. 50 beats/min
   b. 75 beats/min
   c. 100 beats/min
   d. 150 beats/min

5. Which of the following electrocardiographic leads provides information related to the horizontal plane of the heart?
   a. Lead I
   b. Lead III
   c. Lead V_4
   d. Lead aVR

6. The last structure of the heart to depolarize is the:
   a. Left bundle branch
   b. Apex
   c. Endocardial surface of the right ventricle
   d. Epicardial surface of the base of the left ventricle

7. Which of the following is *not* characteristic of a respiratory sinus arrhythmia?
   a. The SA node is the pacemaker of the heart.
   b. The R-R interval is constant.
   c. A P wave precedes every QRS.
   d. The heart rate varies throughout the respiratory cycle.

8. The heart rate of an individual who demonstrates sinus tachycardia typically shows a ventricular rate of:
   a. Less than 60 beats/min
   b. 40 to 60 beats/min
   c. 60 to 100 beats/min
   d. Greater than 100 beats/min

9. For a person with a mean ventricular axis of 90 degrees, the amplitude of the QRS typically is greatest (upstroke) in which of the following leads?
   a. Lead I
   b. Lead III
   c. Lead aVF
   d. Lead V_3

10. Which of the following rhythms is characterized by the presence of delta waves on the ECG?
    a. First-degree AV block
    b. Bundle branch block
    c. Wolff-Parkinson-White syndrome
    d. Atrial fibrillation

11. Which of the following rhythms is characterized by a constant PR interval with intermittent loss of a QRS complex?
    a. Intraventricular conduction delay
    b. Second-degree (Mobitz I) AV block
    c. Second-degree (Mobitz II) AV block
    d. Respiratory sinus arrhythmia

ASSESSMENT QUESTIONS—cont'd

12. Which of the following statements is true concerning ventricular action potentials?
  a. The action potential demonstrates three phases (phases 0, 3, and 4).
  b. The amplitude of this type of action potential typically is about 60 mV.
  c. The threshold potential for this type of tissue is more negative that the threshold potentials for a nodal myocyte.
  d. The slope of phase 4 of the SA node is greater than that of the SA node myocyte.

13. During a normal cardiac cycle:
  I. the first heart sound is associated with atrial contraction
  II. the period of isovolumetric contraction follows closure of the semilunar valves
  III. the dicrotic notch of the aortic pressure tracing is associated with closure of the aortic and pulmonary valves
  IV. the pressure in the left ventricle is higher than aortic pressure during the period of maximum ejection
  a. I and II only
  b. III and IV only
  c. I, III, and IV only
  d. I, II, III, and IV

14. An increase in right ventricular preload can be estimated clinically by measuring:
  a. LVEDP
  b. RVEDP
  c. PAWP (PCWP)
  d. MPAP

15. A 30-year-old female has a stroke index of 50 mL/beat/m^2. If her body surface area is 2 m^2 and her heart rate is 60 beats/min, what is her cardiac output in liters per minute?
  a. 3.4 L/min
  b. 4 L/min
  c. 5.6 L/min
  d. 6 L/min

References

1. Berne RM, Levy MN: *Cardiovascular physiology*, ed 6, St Louis, 2001, Mosby.
2. Levitzky MG, Cairo JM, Hall SM: *Introduction to respiratory care*, Philadelphia, 1990, WB Saunders.
3. Scheidt S: *Basic electrocardiography*, West Caldwell, NJ, 1989, CIBA-GEIGY.
4. Cromwell L, Weibell FJ, Pfeiffer EA: *Biomedical instrumentation and measurements*, ed 2, Englewood Cliffs, NJ, 1980, Prentice-Hall.
5. Lipman BC, Cascio T: *ECG assessment and interpretation*, Philadelphia, 1994, FA Davis.
6. Scheidt S: *Interactive electrocardiography*, New York, 2000, Novartis.
7. Guyton AC, Hall JE: *Textbook of medical physiology*, ed 10, Philadelphia, 2000, WB Saunders.
8. Katz AM: *Physiology of the heart*, Philadelphia, 2001, Lippincott Williams & Wilkins.
9. Fishman AP, Richards DW: *Circulation of the blood*, Bethesda, Md, 1982, American Physiological Society.
10. Levine RL, Fromm RE: *Critical care monitoring*, St Louis, 1995, Mosby.
11. Parbrook GD, Kenny GNC, Davis PD: *Basic physics and measurement in anaesthesia*, New York, 1999, Butterworth-Heinemann.
12. Perloff D, Grim C, Flack J et al: Human blood pressure determination by sphygmomanometry, *Circulation* 88:2460, 1993.
13. Kascmarek RM, Hess D, Stoller JM: *Monitoring in respiratory care*, St Louis, 1993, Mosby.
14. Swan HJC, Ganz W, Forrester J et al: Catheterization of the heart in man with the use of a flow-directed balloon tipped catheter, *N Engl J Med* 75:83, 1975.
15. Baim DS, Grossman W: *Grossman's cardiac catheterization, angiography, and intervention*, ed 6, Philadelphia, 2000, Lippincott Williams & Wilkins.
16. Rushmer RF: *Structure and function of the cardiovascular system*, ed 2, Philadelphia, 1976, WB Saunders.
17. Weiss S, Calloway E, Cairo J et al: Comparison of cardiac output measurements by thermodilution and thoracic electrical impedance in critically ill versus non-critically ill patients, *Am J Emerg Med* 13:626, 1995.
18. Durbin CG: Noninvasive hemodynamic measurements, *Respir Care* 35:709, 1990.

Internet Resources

American Association for Respiratory Care Clinical Practice Guidelines: http://www.aarc.org
American College of Chest Physicians: http://www.chestnet.org
The Interactive Heart: http://library.thinkquest.org/C003758/home.htm
Heart Disease: http://www.pathguy.com/lectures/heart.htm
Introduction to Cardiothoracic Imaging: http://www.med.yale.edu/intmed/cardio/imaging/
The Merck Manual Online Resources: http://www.merckmedicus.com
The Visible Human Project: http://www.nlm.nih.gov/research/visible/visible_gallery.html
PA Catheter Insertion video: http://www.uth.tmc.edu/scriptorium/gallery/video/pa-catheter.htm

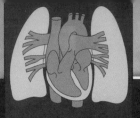

Blood Gas Monitoring

J.M. CAIRO

OBJECTIVES

Upon completion of this chapter you will be able to:

· Describe how to perform and evaluate the modified Allen test.
· Identify various sites used to obtain samples for blood gas analysis.
· Label the components of a modern, in vitro blood gas analyzer.
· Compare the operational principles of the pH, partial pressure of carbon dioxide (PCO_2), and partial pressure of oxygen (PO_2) electrodes.
· Apply values for the PO_2 at which 50% saturation of hemoglobin (P_{50}) occurs, bicarbonate, buffer base, and base excess in the interpretation of arterial blood gases.
· Explain the operational principle of CO-oximetry.
· Name the components of a quality assurance program for blood gas analysis.
· Compare the effects of hyperthermia and hypothermia on arterial blood gases.
· Describe physiologic and technical factors that can affect pulse oximeter readings.
· Identify various factors that can influence transcutaneous PO_2 and PCO_2 measurements.
· State criteria for identifying four types of acid-base disorders.

KEY TERMS

absorbance sensors
actual bicarbonate
Allen's test
amperometric
base excess/deficit
buffer base
capillary blood gas (CBG)
central processing unit (CPU)
Clark electrode
Clinical Laboratory
 Improvement Amendments
 of 1988 (CLIA-88)
electrochemical sensors
electrodes

fetal hemoglobin (HbF)
fluorescent sensors
fractional hemoglobin
 saturation
functional hemoglobin
 saturation
glucose oxidase
half-cells
Henderson-Hasselbalch
 equation
hyperbilirubinemia
in vitro
in vivo
invasive

Levy-Jennings charts
light-emitting diodes (LEDs)
microcuvette
Nernst equation
noninvasive
one-point calibration
optical plethysmography
optical shunting
oxygen content (O_2ct)
Partial pressure of carbon
 dioxide in arterial blood
 ($PaCO_2$)
Partial pressure of oxygen in
 arteries (PaO_2)

KEY TERMS—cont'd

palpebral conjunctiva	quality control (QC)	sulfhemoglobin (sulfHb)
pH	Sanz electrode	superior palpebral conjunctiva
photoplethysmography	servo-controlled	temperature correction
point of care (POC) testing	Siggaard-Andersen alignment	three-point calibration
potentiometric	nomogram	total hemoglobin (THb)
quality assurance (QA)	standard bicarbonate	two-point calibration

Measurements of arterial blood gases (ABGs) and **pH** are used extensively in the diagnosis and treatment of patients with acute and chronic illnesses. This is most evident in the management of critically ill patients, for whom ABG analysis can provide valuable information, such as acid-base status, ventilatory function, and oxygenation status.

Blood gas techniques generally are classified as **invasive** or **noninvasive.** Invasive blood gas analysis, which involves direct exposure of a sample of blood to a series of **electrochemical sensors** or **electrodes,** is considered the gold standard for measuring the hydrogen ion concentration (pH), partial pressure of carbon dioxide (PCO_2), and partial pressure of oxygen (PO_2) in the arterial blood. Until recently, invasive blood gas analysis could provide only intermittent **in vitro** measurements of a patient's blood gas and acid-base status; however, the development of fiberoptic catheters has extended the possibilities of **in vivo** blood gas monitoring by allowing for real-time determinations of the pH of arterial blood (pHa), **partial pressure of carbon dioxide in the arteries ($PaCO_2$), and partial pressure of oxygen in the arteries (PaO_2).**

Noninvasive techniques, which include pulse oximetry and transcutaneous monitoring, do not require blood samples and are performed with sensors placed on the surface of the body. Because pulse oximetry and transcutaneous monitoring can provide continuous estimates of blood gas levels with minimal risk to the patient, they are indispensable tools in the management of patients with unstable ventilatory and oxygenation status. Appropriate use of noninvasive monitoring can significantly reduce the need for more expensive invasive blood gas analysis.

This chapter describes the various devices and techniques commonly used to determine ABGs and pH. Some basic principles to ensure an understanding of how blood gas measurements can be used to assess a patient's acid-base and respiratory status are presented. You should remember, however, that ABGs must be interpreted in the context of other clinical indices, including other laboratory tests (e.g., hematology and electrolytes), chest radiographs, the patient's history, and the physical examination findings. Interpreting blood gas values without considering other clinical findings can lead to serious mistakes and ultimately can harm the patient.

INVASIVE BLOOD GAS ANALYSIS

Invasive blood gas analysis can be performed in a variety of settings, including hospitals, clinics, physicians' offices, and extended care facilities. The primary indications for invasive blood gas analysis are to quantify a patient's response to a diagnostic or therapeutic intervention and to monitor the severity and progression of a documented disease process.[1]

The American Association for Respiratory Care (AARC) has published a series of Clinical Practice Guidelines for ABG analysis to help ensure that these tests are performed in a safe and standardized manner.[1-3] Besides providing information on the equipment required to obtain blood samples, the guidelines also list the indications, contraindications, hazards, and complications of ABG analysis. The AARC Clinical Practice Guideline for blood gas analysis and hemoximetry[2] is summarized in Clinical Practice Guideline 10-1.

Health care professionals who perform blood gas analysis should understand patient assessment techniques and the relationship of the patient's history, physical findings, and various cardiopulmonary dysfunctions. Therefore individuals who perform blood gas analysis should be formally trained in respiratory care, cardiovascular technology, clinical laboratory sciences, nursing, medicine, or osteopathy.[1,2] Periodic reevaluation of these individuals should focus on all aspects of blood gas analysis, including the proper technique for obtaining blood samples, postsampling care of the puncture site, and safe handling of blood, needles, and syringes.[1,2]

COLLECTION DEVICES AND SAMPLING TECHNIQUES

Specimens for ABG analysis can be drawn from a peripheral artery by means of a percutaneous needle puncture or from an indwelling intravascular cannula. Mixed venous blood samples can be obtained with a flow-directed (Swan-Ganz) intracardiac catheter. For percutaneous sampling, blood most often is drawn from the radial, brachial, or femoral arteries or the dorsalis pedis artery of the foot.[3-5] Capillary blood samples from an earlobe or the side of the heel may

Blood Gas Analysis and Hemoximetry

Clinical Practice Guideline 10-1

■ SETTING
1. Hospital laboratories
2. Hospital emergency areas
3. Patient care areas
4. Clinical laboratories
5. Physicians' offices

■ INDICATIONS
1. Evaluate the adequacy of a patient's ventilatory, acid-base, or oxygenation status, oxygen-carrying capacity, and intrapulmonary shunt.
2. Quantify a patient's response to therapeutic intervention and/or diagnostic evaluation.
3. Monitor the severity and progression of documented disease processes.

■ CONTRAINDICATIONS
1. Improperly functioning analyzer or an analyzer that has not had its functional status validated by analysis of commercially prepared quality control products or tonometered whole blood, or participation in a proficiency testing program.
2. A specimen that has not been properly anticoagulated.
3. A sample that contains visible air bubbles.
4. A sample that has been stored in a plastic syringe at room temperature for longer than 30 minutes, stored at room temperature for longer than 5 minutes for a shunt study, or stored at room temperature in the presence of an elevated leukocyte or platelet count.
5. Sample is submitted without adequate background information, including patient's name or other unique identifier (e.g., medical record number, birth date or age, date and time of sampling), location of the patient, name and signature of the requesting physician or authorized individual, clinical indication and tests to be performed, sample source (arterial line, central venous catheter, peripheral artery), respiratory rate, fractional inspired oxygen (F_IO_2), ventilator settings (tidal volume, respiratory rate, mode, F_IO_2), body temperature, activity level, and working diagnosis. It is also imperative to have the signature of the person who obtained the sample.

■ HAZARDS/COMPLICATIONS
1. Infection of the specimen handler from blood containing human immunodeficiency virus (HIV), hepatitis B, or other blood-borne pathogens.
2. Inappropriate medical treatment of the patient based on improperly analyzed blood sample or from analysis of an unacceptable specimen, or from incorrect reporting of results.

■ LIMITATIONS OF PROCEDURE
1. Sample clotting as a result of improper anticoagulation or improper mixing.
2. Sample contaminated with air, improper anticoagulant or anticoagulant concentration, saline or other fluids, inadvertent sampling of systemic venous blood.
3. Delay in sample analysis.
4. Incomplete clearance of analyzer calibration gases and previous waste or flushing solution or solutions.
5. Hyperlipidemia (interference with electrode membranes).
6. Failure to obtain an adequate sample size.
7. Possible error in calculation of derived variables (e.g., hemoximetry oxygen saturation [SaO_2] may underestimate oxyhemoglobin [O_2Hb] because of the presence of carbon monoxide or methemoglobin).
8. Possible erroneous temperature-corrected results because of errors in measurement of the patient's temperature.

■ VALIDATION OF RESULTS
1. Analytic procedure conforms to recommended, established guidelines and follows the manufacturer's recommendations.
2. Results of pH–blood gas analysis fall within the calibration range of the analyzer and quality control product range.
3. Laboratory procedures and personnel are in compliance with quality control and recognized proficiency testing programs.
4. Questionable results should be reanalyzed (preferably on a separate analyzer), and an additional sample should be obtained if the discrepancy cannot be resolved. NOTE: The results of the analysis of the discarded sample should be documented, and the reason for discarding the sample should be given.

Blood Gas Analysis and Hemoximetry—cont'd

■ **ASSESSMENT OF NEED**

1. A valid indication in the patient to be tested supports the need for sampling and analysis.

■ **INFECTION CONTROL**

1. Staff, supervisors, and physician-directors associated with the pulmonary laboratory should be knowledgeable about the "Guidelines for Isolation Precautions in Hospitals," published by the Centers for Disease Control and Prevention (CDC) and the Hospital Infection Control Practices Advisory Committee (HICPAC).
2. The manager and medical director of the laboratory should maintain communication and cooperation with the institution's infection control service and the personnel health service to help ensure consistency and thoroughness in complying with the institution's policies related to immunization, postexposure prophylaxis, and community-related illnesses and exposures.

Modified from the American Association of Respiratory Care: Clinical practice guideline: Blood gas analysis and hemoximetry—2001 Revision and Update, Respir Care 46:498, 2001.

be substituted when arterial blood cannot be obtained. As is discussed later in the chapter, **capillary blood gas (CBG)** values may vary considerably from ABG values.

In the case of percutaneous puncture of the radial artery, a modified **Allen's test** should always be performed before the sample is obtained (Figure 10-1).[4,5] For this test, the patient clenches the fist to force blood from the hand. While the fist is formed, pressure is applied to the radial and ulnar arteries. The patient then is instructed to release the fist; the hand should appear blanched. When pressure on the ulnar artery is released, blood should return to the hand, causing the palm to blush and indicating that the ulnar artery is patent. If the palm does not blush, the ulnar artery is either absent or partially or totally occluded. Another sampling site, such as the brachial artery, should be chosen if the modified Allen's test is negative. Note that a similar test can be performed when blood is obtained from the dorsal artery of the foot. Pressure is applied directly over the artery to occlude it, and then pressure is applied to the nail of the big toe, causing it to blanch. When pressure on the big toe is released, color returns to the toe if the collateral circulation is sufficient from the posterior tibial and lateral plantar arteries.[6]

After tests have shown that sufficient collateral circulation is present, the site should be prepared for puncture. It should be cleaned with 70% isopropyl alcohol or another suitable antiseptic solution.[7] In some cases anesthetization of the puncture site may be necessary, which can be accomplished by injecting a local anesthetic such as 1% lidocaine HCl.[1,4,5] Proper administration of the anesthetic can alleviate some of the pain associated with the procedure and reduce the patient's anxiety.

Samples to be analyzed should be obtained with a small-gauge needle (23 to 25 gauge) attached to a glass or plastic syringe of low diffusibility containing an anticoagulant (sodium or lithium heparin, 1000 units/mL) (Figure 10-2).[1,2] For infants, 25- to 26-gauge scalp vein needles can be used to collect arterial samples. The blood should be

CLINICAL ROUNDS 10-1

How would a large air bubble affect the PCO_2 and PO_2 of an arterial blood sample taken from a normal healthy person breathing room air?

See Evolve resources for the answer.

drawn anaerobically to prevent contamination by room air. Room air that is inadvertently drawn into the syringe should be removed before analysis because contamination with room air can lead to erroneous results and ultimately compromise patient care. Clinical Rounds 10-1 gives an example of this type of problem in the clinical setting.

After blood has been withdrawn and the needle removed, direct pressure should be applied to the puncture site to prevent the formation of a hematoma. With adult patients with indwelling cannulas, 1 to 2 mL of blood should be removed and discarded before blood is removed for analysis. For infants, the discarded volume typically is only about 0.2 to 0.5 mL.* After the blood sample to be analyzed has been removed, the cannula should be flushed with several milliliters of normal saline to prevent blood coagulation in the cannula and loss of a functioning indwelling line.

As mentioned previously, CBG samples obtained from an earlobe or the side of the heel may be substituted for arterial blood samples in certain situations.[8] CBGs most often are used in pediatric patients, especially in the neonatal intensive care unit, to avoid multiple arterial sticks.[6,9,10] The site should be warmed before the sample is obtained to increase perfusion to the area (i.e., "arterializing"). "Arterialized" capillary samples actually contain a

---

*Remember that the volume of blood removed and discarded should be minimal; this is particularly important in neonates.

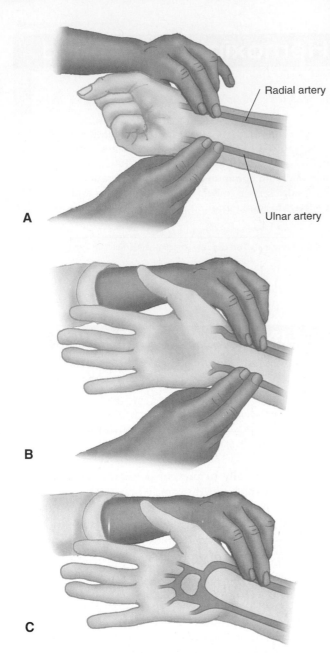

FIGURE 10-1 Modified Allen's test. **A,** The hand is clenched into a tight fist, and pressure is applied to the radial and ulnar arteries. **B,** The hand is opened (but not fully extended), and the palm and fingers are blanched. **C,** Pressure on the ulnar artery is removed, which should result in flushing of the entire hand. (From Wilkins RL, Stoller JK, Kacmarek RM: *Egan's fundamentals of respiratory care*, ed 9, St Louis, 2009, Mosby.)

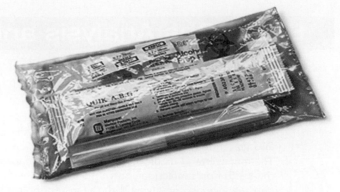

FIGURE 10-2 Commercially available blood gas kit. (Courtesy Marquest Medical Products, Vital Signs, Newark, N.J.)

TABLE 10-1	
Normal Blood Values for a Healthy Adult	
Parameter	**Value**
pH	7.40 ± 0.05
$PaCO_2$	40 ± 5 mm Hg
PaO_2	80-100 mm Hg
HCO_3^-	24 ± 2 mEq/L
Base excess	±2 mEq/L
O_2Hb	95% to 100%
HbCO	<1.5%
MetHb	<1.5%
THb	12-18 g/dL
Na^+	140 ± 5 mEq/L
K^+	4 ± 0.5 mEq/L
CL^-	101 ± 4 mEq/L
Ca^{++}	5 ± 0.5 mEq/L
Glucose	70-105 mg/dL
P_{50}	27 ± 2 mm Hg

CLINICAL ROUNDS 10-2

A CBG sample is obtained from a 2-day-old infant in apparent respiratory distress. The results indicate respiratory alkalosis (high pH, low PCO_2) and apparent hypoxemia (low PO_2). How would you interpret these findings?

See Evolve Resources for the answer.

combination of arterial and venous blood and therefore may not be equivalent to an arterial blood sample.[10,11] The correlation between capillary and arterial pH and PCO_2 measurements is better than the correlation between capillary and arterial PO_2 measurements. Consequently, CBGs more often are used to discern acid-base status rather than to assess a patient's oxygenation status. Table 10-1 presents accepted normal ABG values. Clinical Rounds 10-2 shows how CBGs can be used in clinical decision making.

Personnel responsible for performing blood gas analysis should understand that they are dealing with a potential biohazard and should take appropriate precautions when performing these tests.[12,13] Such precautions include wearing gloves, protective eyewear (goggles), and other barriers deemed necessary to prevent exposure. Needles used for blood sampling should be recapped with the one-handed "scoop" technique, or they can be removed after being inserted into a cork or similar device to shield the sharp end. Unused blood samples, needles, and other "sharps" should be discarded in appropriately marked containers. (See Chapter 5 for a full discussion of infection control principles in respiratory care.)

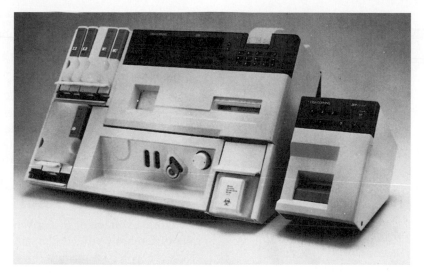

FIGURE 10-3 Modern in vitro blood gas analyzer. (Courtesy Corning Instruments, Chiron Diagnostics, Norwood, Mass.)

Specimens should be transported to the blood gas laboratory and analyzed as soon as possible after drawing because blood cells remain metabolically active in vitro; therefore a prolonged delay between obtaining and analyzing a specimen (longer than 5 minutes) can lead to erroneous results (i.e., a reduction in PO_2 and a rise in PCO_2). This problem is particularly evident in patients with high leukocyte counts.[4,5] Chilling the specimen to below 5° C by placing the syringe in ice water can reduce the metabolic rate of the white blood cells, minimizing this problematic effect.

MODERN IN VITRO BLOOD GAS ANALYZERS

Modern in vitro blood gas analyzers (Figure 10-3) have three electrodes for determining the pH, PCO_2, and PO_2 of a blood sample. They also have a **central processing unit (CPU)** for data management and outputs for displaying measured and derived variables. Many of these systems may also have sensors for providing hemoglobin (Hb), oxyhemoglobin, carboxyhemoglobin, and methemoglobin measurements, along with serum electrolyte and blood glucose measurements. Table 10-2 lists the normal values for the derived variables commonly recorded during blood gas analysis. Unlike early blood gas analyzers, which were cumbersome to operate and required large amounts of blood to make accurate measurements, modern analyzers are fully automated, self-calibrating devices that can analyze blood samples as small as 50 to 100 μL.

pH and Hydrogen Ion Concentration

S.P.L. Sorenson introduced the term *pH* as a shorthand way to express the hydrogen ion activity of solutions.[14,15] It is defined as the negative logarithm (base 10) of the hydrogen ion concentration, or

$$pH = -\log_{10}[H^+]$$

For example, a hydrogen ion concentration of 0.0000007 mol/L, or 1×10^{-7} mol/L, can be expressed as a pH of 7. Although scientific efforts have increased to express hydrogen ion concentrations in Système International (SI) units (i.e., nanomoles per liter [nmol/L]), the concept of pH is still recognized as a convenient and useful way of discussing a patient's clinical acid-base status.[15,16] Table 10-3 shows the relationship between hydrogen ion concentration and pH. Note that the pH decreases as the hydrogen ion concentration increases, and vice versa. Despite the fact that hydrogen ion activity is not exactly equal to the hydrogen ion concentration, these two terms are interchangeable for practical purposes in clinical situations.

In general chemistry textbooks, the pH scale is described as ranging from 1 to 14, with a pH of 7 representing universal neutrality. (Neutrality is defined as the pH of pure water, which contains 1×10^{-7} mol/L of hydrogen ions and 1×10^{-7} mol/L of hydroxyl ions.) A solution with a pH less than 7 is acidic, and a solution with a pH higher than 7 is alkaline. Although the pH of arterial blood can vary from

TABLE 10-2		
Normal Values for Derived Blood Gas Variables		
Variable	**Symbol**	**Normal Values**
Oxyhemoglobin	O_2Hb	≥95%
Carboxyhemoglobin	HbCO	<1.5%
Methemoglobin	metHb	<1.5%
Deoxygenated hemoglobin	HHb	<2%
Sulfhemoglobin	SulfHbs	<1%
Total hemoglobin	THb	Males: 15.8 ± 2 g/dL
		Females: 14 ± 2 g/dL
Partial pressure of oxygen at 50% saturation	P_{50}	27 ± 2 mm Hg

TABLE 10-3	
Hydrogen Ion–pH Relationships	
pH	**[H+]***
7.80	16
7.70	20
7.60	26
7.50	32
7.40	40
7.30	50
7.20	63
7.10	80
7.00	100
6.90	125
6.80	160

*Reported in nanomoles per liter.

6.9 to 7.8, it normally ranges (±2 standard deviations [SD]) from 7.35 to 7.45, with a mean pH of 7.4. For interpretative purposes, a blood pH less than 7.4 is considered acidic, and a blood pH higher than 7.4 is alkaline.

pH Electrode

The standard pH electrode, which sometimes is called the **Sanz electrode,** is composed of two **half-cells** connected by a potassium chloride (KCl) bridge (Figure 10-4).[17] One of the cells, the measurement half-cell, has a special glass membrane that is permeable to hydrogen ions (H^+). The measuring electrode is made of silver–silver chloride (Ag/AgCl) and immersed in a phosphate buffer solution with a pH of 6.84. The second cell, the reference half-cell, is composed of mercury–mercurous chloride (Hg/Hg_2Cl_2) (calomel) and is immersed in a solution of saturated KCl.

According to the **Nernst equation,** the electrical potential generated as H^+ ions pass through the glass membrane (EH^+) is a logarithmic function of the ratio of hydrogen ion concentration across the membrane, or

$$EH^+ = (RT/F) + \ln[(H_o^+)/(H_i^+)]$$

where R is the gas constant, F is Faraday's constant, T is the absolute temperature in Kelvin, H_o^+ is the hydrogen ion concentration outside the membrane, and H_i^+ is the hydrogen ion concentration inside the membrane. If you consider that at body temperature (37° C, or 310 K) the quantity (RT/F) is 61.5 mV, then the equation becomes

$$EH^+ = 0.0615 \times \log_{10}[H^+] \: or$$
$$EH^+ = 0.0615 \times pH$$

Therefore a voltage of 61.5 mV is developed for every pH unit difference between the sample and the measuring electrode, which is constant (6.84). Consider the following example: A voltage difference of 30.75 mV is measured when a sample is analyzed. This voltage difference equals 0.5 pH units (30.75 ÷ 61.5 = 0.5). The resultant pH can be calculated as 6.84 + 0.5 = 7.34.

It should be apparent that these devices are quite sensitive and therefore are adversely affected by changes in the permeability of the glass membrane, such as can occur when the electrode is damaged or coated with protein. As is discussed later in this chapter, an effective quality assurance program can prevent these types of problems.

Partial Pressures of Carbon Dioxide and Oxygen

As was discussed in Chapter 1, the partial pressure a gas exerts in a gas mixture is calculated by multiplying the fractional concentration of the gas by the total pressure of the gas mixture. For example, if oxygen makes up about 21% of the atmosphere and the barometric pressure is 760 mm Hg, the partial pressure of oxygen in room air is 0.21 × 760 mm Hg, or approximately 159 mm Hg.

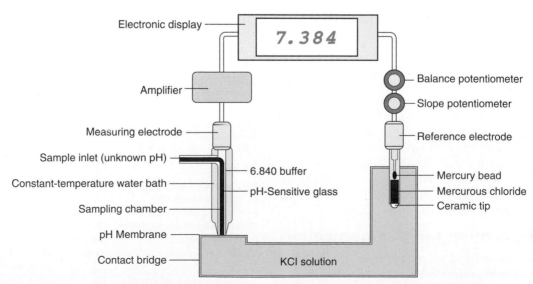

FIGURE 10-4 Schematic of the pH electrode. (From Hess DR, MacIntyre NR, Mishoe SC, et al: *Respiratory care: principles and practice,* St Louis, 2002, WB Saunders.)

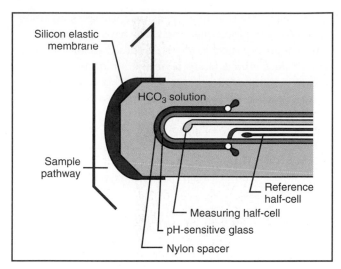

FIGURE 10-5 Stowe-Severinghaus PCO$_2$ electrode. (Redrawn from Shapiro BA, Peruzzi WT, Templin R: *Clinical application of blood gases*, ed 5, St Louis, 1994, Mosby.)

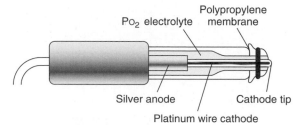

FIGURE 10-6 Clark PO$_2$ electrode. (From Hess DR, MacIntyre NR, Mishoe SC, et al: *Respiratory care: principles and practice,* St Louis, 2002, WB Saunders.)

The partial pressure of carbon dioxide in arterial blood (PaCO$_2$), which is regulated primarily by the respiratory system, can vary from 10 to 100 mm Hg. People breathing room air at sea level typically have a PaCO$_2$ of 35 to 45 mm Hg (the mean is 40 mm Hg; the range represents $\pm$2 SD). The partial pressure of oxygen in arterial blood (PaO$_2$) can range from 30 to 600 mm Hg, depending on the fractional concentration of inspired oxygen. For healthy people breathing room air at sea level, the PaO$_2$ usually is 80 to 100 mm Hg.

PCO$_2$ Electrode

The PCO$_2$ electrode was first described by Stowe in 1957 and later refined by Severinghaus and Bradley[18]; therefore the standard PCO$_2$ electrode is commonly called the *Stowe-Severinghaus electrode* (Figure 10-5). It is basically a pH electrode covered with a carbon dioxide–permeable Teflon or silicone (Silastic) membrane. A bicarbonate-buffered solution is held between the Teflon (or Silastic) membrane and the pH glass electrode by a nylon spacer. Carbon dioxide from the blood diffuses across the semipermeable Teflon (or Silastic) membrane and reacts with the water to form carbonic acid, which dissociates into hydrogen ions and bicarbonate. The reaction can be written as

$$CO_2 + H_2O \rightarrow H_2CO_3 \rightarrow H^+ + HCO_3^-$$

H$^+$ ions from the bicarbonate-buffered solution then diffuse across the glass electrode, and the pH of the solution is measured as described earlier. The pH is related to the PCO$_2$ by using the following modification of the **Henderson-Hasselbalch equation:**

$$pH = pK + \log(HCO_3^-/PCO_2)$$

Thus the PCO$_2$ is determined as a function of the change in pH of the bicarbonate solution (i.e., the pH changes by 0.1 unit for every 10–mm Hg increase in PCO$_2$).

The most common problems encountered with PCO$_2$ electrodes involve interference with the diffusion of CO$_2$ across the Teflon (or Silastic) membrane and the H$^+$ ions across the glass membrane (e.g., worn or cracked electrodes, protein deposits). If the bicarbonate solution dehydrates between the Teflon (or Silastic) membrane and the pH glass electrode, erroneous data can result. As with the pH electrode, these problems can be minimized by an effective quality assurance program.

PO$_2$ Electrode

The partial pressure of oxygen in blood is most commonly measured using the Clark electrode.[17] As Figure 10-6 shows, the **Clark electrode** consists of a negatively charged platinum electrode (cathode) and a positively charged Ag/AgCl reference electrode (anode) immersed in a phosphate-potassium chloride buffer, the pH of which can range from 7 to 10, depending on the manufacturer. The cathode and anode are connected by a KCl bridge. An external voltage is applied to the platinum electrode, creating a small potential difference of about 0.5 to 0.6 mV between it and the anode.* The active surface of the electrode is separated from the blood to be analyzed by a polyethylene or polypropylene membrane that is permeable to oxygen.

Figure 10-7 illustrates the principle of PO$_2$ measurement. Oxygen from the blood sample diffuses across the semipermeable plastic membrane into the KCl solution and reacts with the platinum cathode, altering the conductivity of the electrolyte solution. Specifically, the platinum cathode donates electrons, which reduce oxygen to produce hydroxyl ions:

$$O_2 + 2H_2O + 4e^- \rightarrow 4OH^-$$

The electrons donated by the cathode are derived from oxidation of Ag at the anode:

$$4Ag \rightarrow 4Ag^+ + 4e^-$$
$$Ag^+ + Cl^- \rightarrow AgCl$$

The volume of oxygen reduced at the cathode is directly proportional to the number of electrons used in the reac-

---

*Because an external polarizing voltage is applied to create this potential difference, the Clark electrode is called a *polarographic electrode.*

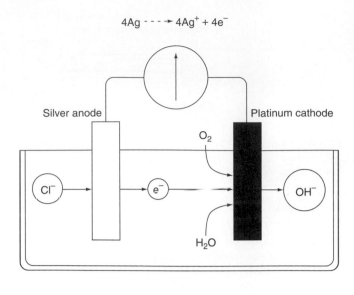

$$4Ag \dashrightarrow 4Ag^+ + 4e^-$$

Silver anode   Platinum cathode

O_2

Cl^- e^- OH^-

H_2O

☐ KCl solution

FIGURE 10-7 Principles of PO_2 measurements. See text for discussion. (From Shapiro BA, Peruzzi WT, Templin R: *Clinical application of blood gases*, ed 5, St Louis, 1994, Mosby.)

tion. Therefore the amount of oxygen diffusing across the membrane into the electrolyte solution can be determined by measuring the current change that occurs between the anode and the cathode when the electrode is exposed to a blood sample containing oxygen. Because the PO_2 is determined by measuring current changes that occur as oxygen is reduced, this technique is an example of an **amperometric** measurement; determinations of pH and PCO_2 as described above are examples of **potentiometric** measurements (i.e., they are based on voltage changes).

The electrical output of the Clark electrode, and thus its sensitivity for measuring PO_2, can be altered by several factors, including protein buildup, cracked electrodes, and loss of electrolyte. When blood samples are analyzed, the consumption of oxygen by the electrode leads to an underestimation of the partial pressure of oxygen in a blood sample by 2% to 6%. This phenomenon, which has been called the *blood gas factor*, is due to the slow rate of oxygen diffusion in fluids (i.e., oxygen consumed by the electrode is not replaced by oxygen from the blood).[19] The magnitude of the blood gas factor depends on the diameter of the cathode and the thickness of the membrane between the sample and the cathode. Exposure of the PO_2 electrode to nitrous oxide and halothane (gaseous anesthetic agents) may also alter its electronic output by increasing the production of peroxide ions.[16]

Derived Variables

Several variables can be calculated from the measurements of pH, $PaCO_2$, and PaO_2. The oxygen saturation of hemoglobin (SO_2), the partial pressure of oxygen at which Hb is 50% saturated (P_{50}), bicarbonate, buffer base, and base

excess/deficit are examples of derived variables. Although most modern blood gas analyzers have computer software that automatically calculates these variables, they can also be determined using formulae or nomograms that incorporate accepted constants. Note, however, that these derived variables are calculated and not measured. As such, they may be inaccurate compared with actual measurements because they may not necessarily account for all confounding factors. For example, calculations of oxygen saturation of hemoglobin do not account for the presence of dyshemoglobins, such as carboxyhemoglobin and methemoglobin.

Oxygen Saturation of Hemoglobin
The percentage of available hemoglobin that is saturated with oxygen can be calculated by using an equation empirically derived from the oxyhemoglobin saturation curve. These calculations do not account for all of the variables (e.g., the actual $PaCO_2$ or the presence of dyshemoglobins) that can affect this value and therefore can lead to erroneous conclusions about the level of oxyhemoglobin saturation. Direct measurement of oxyhemoglobin saturation is discussed along with oximetry later in this chapter. Directly measured values are more reliable and should be used instead of a derived oxygen saturation value when decisions are made about a patient's oxygenation status. Notice that although the calculated and the measured SO_2 are identical in many cases, this is not always true.

P_{50} Determinations
P_{50} is a convenient way of describing hemoglobin affinity for oxygen because it identifies the PO_2 in millimeters of mercury (mm Hg) when hemoglobin is 50% saturated with oxygen. It is determined by equilibrating a blood sample with various oxygen concentrations at 37° C, which can be accomplished with a tonometer connected to a series of certified gas mixtures.* As Figure 10-8 shows, alterations in hemoglobin affinity for oxygen are associated with shifting of the oxyhemoglobin dissociation curve. It is well established that the affinity of hemoglobin A (HbA, or normal adult hemoglobin) for oxygen (and thus the P_{50}) can be altered by changes in the pH, PCO_2, temperature, and concentration of 2,3-diphosphoglycerate (2,3-DPG) in arterial blood. The presence of **fetal hemoglobin (HbF)** and carboxyhemoglobin (HbCO) can also alter the oxyhemoglobin curve. P_{50} determinations are not routinely performed, but they can be helpful in diagnosing and managing hypoxemia associated with various types of hemoglobinopathies.

Bicarbonate, Buffer Base, and Base Excess
The **actual bicarbonate** is the concentration of HCO_3^- in the plasma of anaerobically drawn blood.[15] It is derived

---

*The P_{50} measurements are standardized for a pH of 7.4, a $PaCO_2$ of 40 mm Hg, and a temperature of 37° C.[17,19]

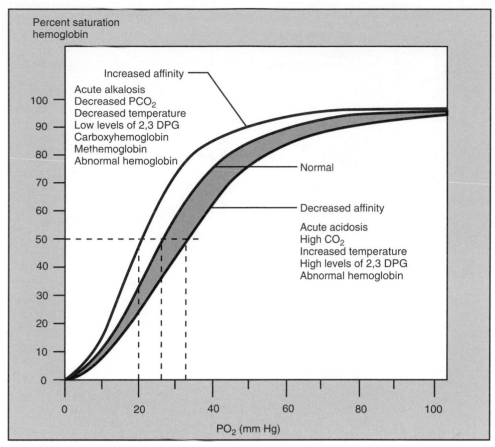

FIGURE 10-8 Effects of changes in pH, PCO_2, and 2,3-diphosphoglycerate (2,3-DPG) on the oxyhemoglobin dissociation curve. (Redrawn from Lane EE, Walker JF: *Clinical arterial blood gas analysis*, St Louis, 1987, Mosby.)

from measurements of pH and $PaCO_2$ using the Henderson-Hasselbalch equation. (Note that the **standard bicarbonate** is also derived from the Henderson-Hasselbalch equation, but it represents the bicarbonate concentration in a fully oxygenated plasma sample measured at a temperature of 37° C and a $PaCO_2$ of 40 mm Hg.) Plasma bicarbonate levels normally range from 22 to 26 mmol/L. The HCO_3^- becomes elevated in metabolic alkalosis and chronic respiratory acidosis and reduced in metabolic acidosis and chronic respiratory alkalosis.

The **buffer base** represents the sum of all the anion buffers in the blood, including bicarbonate, hemoglobin, inorganic phosphate, and negatively charged proteins.[17] The buffer base usually ranges from 44 to 48 mmol/L. The **base excess/deficit** is the number of millimoles of strong acid required to titrate a blood sample to a pH of 7.4 at a PCO_2 of 40 mm Hg. Theoretically, the buffer base and the base excess are not affected by changes in respiratory function; therefore they can be used to identify nonrespiratory disturbances in acid-base status. Figure 10-9 is a **Siggaard-Andersen alignment nomogram** for calculating the actual and standard bicarbonate, buffer base, and base excess concentrations.

Whole Blood Analysis: Electrolytes and Glucose

Many blood gas analyzers incorporate sensors for measuring electrolytes (e.g., Sodium (Na^+), Potassium (K^+), Chloride (Cl^-), Calcium (Ca^{++})) and metabolites (e.g., glucose). Table 10-4 presents the normal values for plasma electrolytes. The sensors used for electrolyte measurements are ion-selective electrodes, but those used to measure glucose are coated with an enzyme called **glucose oxidase.** Electrolytes are determined by potentiometric measurements, but metabolites are determined by amperometric measurements.

The typical electrolyte sensor is composed of a measuring half-cell and an external reference half-cell, which form a complete electrochemical cell. The measuring half-cell is made of a silver–silver chloride wire that is surrounded by an electrolyte-specific solution. For example, the electrolyte solution used in the sodium and chloride sensors contains a fixed concentration of sodium and chloride; the potassium sensor electrolyte contains a fixed concentration of potassium; and the calcium electrolyte contains a fixed concentration of calcium. The electrolyte solution is separated from the sample solution by an ion-selective

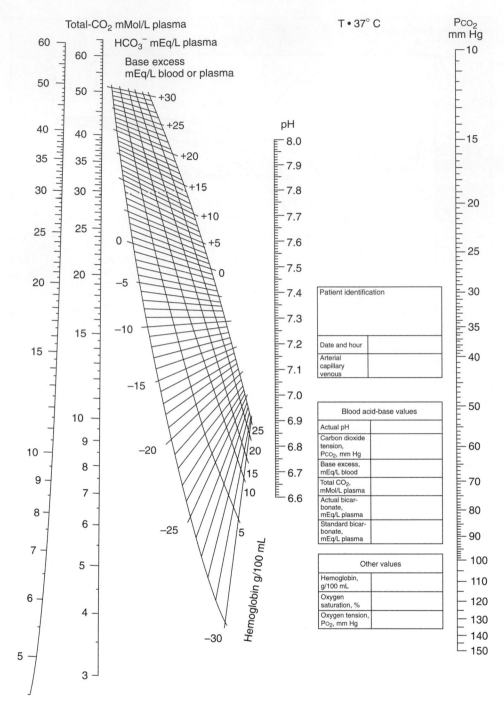

FIGURE 10-9 Siggaard-Andersen alignment nomogram. A line is drawn between the pH and PCO_2, and the actual bicarbonate is read directly at the intersection of this line. BE_b is hemoglobin dependent and can be read at the intersection of the constructed line and the patient's hemoglobin (Hb) value. Standard bicarbonate can be determined by constructing another line through the BE-Hb point and the PCO_2 of 40 mm Hg, and by reading the HCO_3^- scale. Buffer base can be computed from the equation BB = 41.7 + (0.42 × Hb) + BE. BE_{ECF} is calculated similarly to BE_b, but the BE_{ECF} is read off at the intersection of the constructed line and one third of the patient's Hb value. (Modified from Siggaard-Andersen O: Arterial blood gas analyzers. In Burton G, Hodgkin JE, Ward JJ, editors: *Respiratory care: a guide to clinical practice*, ed 4, Philadelphia, 1997, JB Lippincott.)

TABLE 10-4

Normal Values for Plasma Electrolytes

Parameter	Symbol	Normal Values
Sodium	Na^+	136-145 mEq/L
Potassium	K^+	3.5-5.0 mEq/L
Total calcium	Ca^{++}	9.9-11.0 mEq/L
Magnesium	Mg^{++}	1.5-2.5 mEq/L
Chloride	Cl^-	98-106 mEq/L
Glucose*	—	100 ± 20 mg/dL

*Although glucose is not classified as an electrolyte, it is included in this table for reference because many blood gas analyzers can now provide determinations of serum glucose concentrations.

membrane, and as the sample comes in contact with the membrane, a transmembrane potential develops across the membrane because of the exchange of ions across it. The potential developed across the membrane is compared with the constant potential of the external reference sensor, and the magnitude of the potential difference is proportional to the ion activity of the sample.

A glucose sensor consists of four electrodes:

- The measuring electrode, made of platinum and glucose oxidase, which is enclosed in a binder.
- A second reference electrode, which is composed of silver–silver chloride.
- A "counter" electrode, composed of platinum, which ensures that a constant polarizing voltage is applied to the sensor.
- A second "counter" electrode, which does not contain the enzyme glucose oxidase, to quantify interfering substances in the sample.

As the sample contacts the measuring electrode, glucose oxidase on the surface of the electrode converts the glucose in the sample to hydrogen peroxide and gluconic acid. The polarizing voltage applied to the electrode causes the hydrogen peroxide to oxidize, resulting in the loss of electrons. The loss of electrons causes current flow to be directly proportional to the glucose concentration of the sample.

Quality Assurance of Blood Gas Analyzers

The Joint Commission (TJC), the Centers for Medicare and Medicaid Services (formerly the Health Care Financing Administration), and the College of American Pathologists (CAP) have published standards that clinical blood gas laboratories must follow to ensure the accuracy and reliability of blood gas measurements. These standards, which are based on recommendations from the **Clinical Laboratory Improvement Amendments of 1988 (CLIA-88)**, require routine calibrations of instruments, as well as programs to assess **quality control (QC)** and **quality assurance (QA)**.[2,20,21]

Calibration standards for most blood gas analyzers are buffers for pH electrodes and specially prepared gases for the PCO_2 and PO_2 electrodes.[22] (Note that buffers and cali-

bration gases must be clearly labeled with reference values and defined confidence limits.) Verification of the instrument's calibration may vary according to the regulatory agency under which the laboratory is accredited or licensed (e.g., CAP, TJC).[2] Generally, every instrument in operation must undergo routine one- and two-point calibrations, which should include high and low pH, PCO_2, and PO_2 values. The **one-point calibration** involves adjusting the electronic output to a single, known standard. With two-point calibrations, the electrode's electronic output is adjusted to two known standards. A one-point calibration should be performed before an unknown sample is analyzed, unless the analyzer is programmed to perform a one-point calibration automatically at regular intervals (e.g., every 20 to 30 minutes). **Two-point calibrations** usually are performed at least three times daily, usually every 8 hours. In many cases, analyzers can be programmed to perform a two-point calibration at predetermined intervals. A **three-point calibration** should be performed every 6 months, or whenever an electrode is replaced. Three-point calibrations involve adding a third standard that is intermediate to the other standards to ensure linearity of the electrode response. A fourth level may be required if samples containing high O_2 levels are analyzed with the instrument.[2]

The National Institute of Standards and Technology (NIST) and the International Federation of Clinical Chemistry (IFCC) have established standards for the calibration of blood gas electrodes. A nearly normal pH buffer (pH = 7.384) is used for one-point calibrations; a second, lower pH buffer (pH = 6.84) is analyzed in the two-point calibration to ensure that the electronic output of the electrode is linear over a wide range of pH levels. The PCO_2 electrode is calibrated with two gas concentrations: a 5% CO_2 mixture for establishing the lower end of CO_2 levels encountered and a 10% CO_2 mixture for the high end of the range. The 5% mixture is used for one-point calibrations, but both mixtures are used in the two-point calibration to establish a linear slope for the electrode's electronic output. The PO_2 electrode is also calibrated with two gas mixtures, usually a gas mixture with 0% O_2 and another with 12% or 20% O_2.[17] The accuracy of oxygen electrodes may vary by as much as 20% for high PO_2 levels because of the lack of linearity between electronic output and oxygen tensions above 150 mm Hg. It has been suggested that this problem can be minimized by using additional calibration gases with higher concentrations of oxygen (i.e., greater than 20% O_2).

Quality control may be defined as a system that includes analysis of control samples (with a known pH, PCO_2, and PO_2), assessment of the measurements against defined limits, identification of problems, and specification of corrective actions. Internal quality control can be accomplished by periodic analysis of commercial products with known pH, PCO_2, and PO_2 values. Quality control materials include human or bovine whole blood samples that have been tonometered to exact gas tensions or commercially prepared aqueous buffers and perfluorocarbon emulsions that have been equilibrated with a series of known PCO_2 and PO_2 values by the manufacturer. Although tonometry remains the gold standard for quality control of PCO_2 and PO_2 electrodes, most laboratories use commercially prepared quality control systems for biosafety and convenience. It should be mentioned, however, that commercially prepared controls provide information on the instrument's precision—not the accuracy of the data. (Remember that *precision* refers to the reproducibility of repeat measurements, and *accuracy* relates to how close the measurement is to the correct value.) Also, commercial controls are susceptible to variations in room storage temperature and do not reflect temperature and protein errors in blood gas analyzers.[17]

Regardless of the type of quality control material used to assess an instrument's performance, the results should be recorded in a manner that allows the operator to detect changes in the operation of the blood gas analyzer. The most common method of recording quality control data involves the use of **Levy-Jennings charts** (Figure 10-10). These charts allow the operator to detect trends and shifts in electrode performance, which helps prevent problems associated with reporting of inaccurate data because of analyzer malfunction. For example, a trend (Figure 10-10A) typically is associated with protein buildup on an electrode membrane or an electrode that is nearing the end of its life expectancy. A shift (Figure 10-10B) can be due to a tear in the electrode membrane or loss of the electrolyte that bathes the electrode.

Quality assurance involves testing the proficiency of both personnel and equipment, providing a dynamic process of identification, evaluation, and resolution of problems that affect blood gas measurements.[22] CAP and the American Thoracic Society (ATS) currently offer two proficiency testing programs that provide a means of assessing blind samples (periodically) and the technical competence of laboratory personnel, and a means of reporting the variability of individual blood gas analyzers.

Proficiency testing materials usually include a series of unknown samples with target values that have been established by previously identified reference laboratories. At regular intervals throughout the year (i.e., a minimum of three times per year), all participating laboratories analyze unknown samples (typically three to five samples are used) and forward their results to the sponsoring organization collating the results from all laboratories. The criteria for acceptable results are defined, and the laboratory personnel are notified of their laboratory's performance. (Generally, an acceptable pH is within ±0.04 of the target value; PCO_2 values must be ±3 mm Hg or ±8% of the target value, whichever is greater; and PO_2 values must be within ±3 standard deviations.[17,19]) An unsatisfactory performance, which is failure to achieve any of the target values at a single event, necessitates that remedial action be taken and documented. Unsuccessful performance, which is associated with failure to achieve the target values for an analyte in two consecutive events or in two out of three consecutive events, can result in the placement of sanctions on the laboratory.[9-17,19,20] These sanctions can cause the laboratory to lose revenue because of suspension of Medicare and Medicaid reimbursement. The laboratory can be reinstated only through additional staff training, increased quality control procedures, and reapplication with evidence that the problems have been corrected.

Temperature Correction of Blood Gases

With most modern blood gas analyzers, the blood sample is heated and maintained at a constant temperature of 37° C during analysis. The term ***temperature correction*** refers to the application of mathematical formulae to adjust blood gas tensions to more accurately reflect the patient's core temperature (i.e., the temperature in the artery from which the blood sample was obtained). Whether these temperature corrections are necessary or even desirable is the subject of considerable debate. Those who favor temperature correction point out that corrected results are a true reflection of the individual's oxygenation and

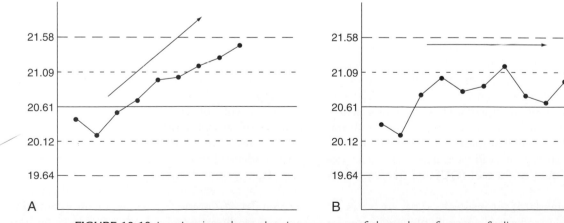

FIGURE 10-10 Levy-Jennings charts showing two types of electrode performance findings. **A,** Trend. **B,** Shift.

acid-base status. According to Mohler et al.,[23] the PaO_2 changes approximately 7% for each degree Celsius; the $PaCO_2$ changes about 4% per degree Celsius; and the pH changes by 0.0146 per degree Celsius. Proponents of reporting blood gases at 37° C believe that pH and $PaCO_2$ values standardized to a body temperature of 37° C reliably reflect the in vivo acid-base status of the patient and that correction of pH and $PaCO_2$ does not affect the calculated HCO_3.[17] Furthermore, most acid-base nomograms are calculated for 37° C, and considerable errors occur if temperature-corrected blood gas data are used with these nomograms. Although all commercial blood gas analyzers contain solid-state circuitry that can easily perform temperature corrections, most laboratories still report blood gases at 37° C because of the lack of consensus on the topic.

In Vivo Blood Gas Monitors

As was previously mentioned, recent advances in fiberoptic technology have made it possible to obtain continuous, in vivo ABG and pH measurements. A typical in vivo blood gas monitor has one or more optical sensors that are imbedded in a gas or ion-permeable polymer matrix. The sensors are connected to a central processing unit by a fiberoptic cable. The fiberoptic sensor is inserted into the intravascular space through an indwelling 20-gauge cannula. Light of a specific wavelength and intensity from the CPU is transmitted along the fiber to a **microcuvette** containing a fluorescent dye. The incident light striking the microcuvette is modified in proportion to the PO_2, PCO_2, or pH level of the blood, which is in contact with the microcuvette. The modified light is then transmitted back to the monitor through either the same optical path or a second fiber parallel to the fiber carrying the incident light.[24] Figure 10-11 shows an alternative extraarterial

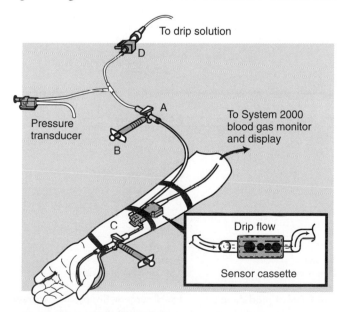

FIGURE 10-11 Fiberoptic blood gas monitor. (Redrawn from Shapiro BA, Peruzzi WT, Templin R, et al: Clinical performance of a blood gas monitor: a prospective, multicenter trial, *Crit Care Med* 21:487, 1993.)

blood gas monitor. In this case, the blood gas sensor is located in series with the arterial catheter.

Optical blood gas sensors generally are categorized by how they modify the initial optical signal; they are classified as either **absorbance** or **fluorescent sensors.**[17] With absorbance sensors, when light of a known wavelength and intensity is transmitted down the fiber and through the microcuvette, a fraction of the incident light is absorbed, and the remaining light is transmitted. The concentration of the analyte can be determined by measuring the intensity of the light striking the photodetector, because the amount of light transmitted is proportional to the concentration of the analyte in question (i.e., the pH, PCO_2, or PO_2).

Fluorescent sensors use dyes that fluoresce when they are struck by light in the ultraviolet or nearly ultraviolet visible range. Light from the monitor is transmitted to the microcuvette containing the dye. The dye absorbs the light energy of the optical excitation signal and emits a fluorescent signal that is returned to the monitor along the fiberoptic cable. The concentration of the analyte in question can be measured by determining the ratio of fluorescent light emitted to the original excitation light signal. The pH, PCO_2, or PO_2 of arterial blood can be determined by using sensing fibers containing dye systems that are analyte specific (i.e., most commercially available systems contain three analyte-specific sensing fibers).

Fluorescent sensors currently in use can measure pH values from 6.8 to 7.8, PCO_2 values from 10 to 100 mm Hg, and PO_2 values from 20 to 600 mm Hg. Compared with in vitro blood gas analysis, intraarterial blood gas monitoring systems are comparable for pH, but the correlation may not be as good for PCO_2 and PO_2 measurements.[24]

Calibration of Intraarterial Blood Gas Monitors

Intraarterial blood gas monitoring systems must be calibrated before insertion into a patient by immersion of the sensor in a buffer containing known pH, PCO_2, and PO_2 values. In vivo calibrations are complicated and subject to error, because adjustment must be made using single-point measurements from laboratory (in vitro) ABG analysis.

In many cases temperature corrections may be required because the sensor may be in a peripheral artery, where the measured temperature may not equal the patient's core temperature. Temperature corrections usually are accomplished by combining a temperature-measuring thermocouple with the analyte-specific sensor. By measuring the sensor's temperature, the pH or blood gas value may then be displayed as measured or corrected to 37° C (or some other user-entered patient temperature).

Point of Care (POC) Testing

Point of care testing is testing that is done outside the main hospital laboratory. POC testing typically involves the use of portable devices that can be located at or near the point of patient care. As such, these devices are not only portable but also lightweight (total weight is approximately 1 pound); this allows in vitro ABG and pH measurements to be made in the emergency department, intensive care unit, physician's office, or a transport vehicle.[25] Figure 10-12 shows a typical POC blood gas analyzer. POC devices usually are battery powered but can be powered by a standard AC electrical outlet. The system uses solid-state sensors, which rely on either fluorescence technology or thin-film electrodes that have been fabricated onto silicone chips. The microelectrodes are incorporated into a single-use disposable cartridge that also contains calibration reagents, a sampling stylus, and a waste container. In addition to the standard blood gas cartridges, several modules are available for the analysis of electrolytes (e.g., sodium, potassium, and chloride), lactates, blood urea nitrogen, glucose, and hematocrit. The results are shown on a liquid crystal display.

Measurements can be made on blood samples of less than 1 mL in 60 to 120 seconds. Manufacturers of POC devices state that these devices are accurate over a wide range of pH, $PaCO_2$, and PaO_2 values. For example, the manufacturer iSTAT (East Windsor, New Jersey) states that its device has a range of 6.8 to 8 for pH, 10 to 100 torr (mm Hg) for $PaCO_2$, and 5 to 800 (mm Hg) for PaO_2. The use of these devices is growing, especially as a replacement for "stat" laboratory services. Table 10-5 compares four commercial POC blood gas analyzers currently available.[25] Box 10-1 summarizes the potential advantages and disadvantages of POC testing.

CO-OXIMETRY

An oximeter is a device that can measure the oxyhemoglobin saturation of arterial, venous, mixed venous, or intracardiac blood. Two types of oximeters are routinely used in respiratory care: CO-oximeters and pulse oximeters. A CO-oximeter can provide simultaneous in vitro measurements of various hemoglobin gases, including oxyhemoglobin (O_2Hb), carboxyhemoglobin (HbCO), methemoglobin (metHb), **sulfhemoglobin (sulfHb),** and fetal hemoglobin (HbF), using whole blood samples. Pulse oximeters are noninvasive devices that provide only measurements of arterial oxyhemoglobin saturation. Pulse oximeters are discussed in detail in the section on noninvasive assessment of ABGs.

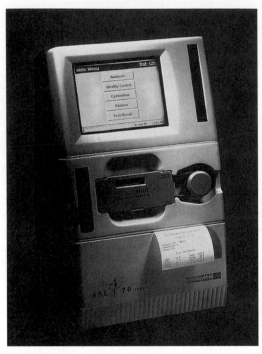

FIGURE 10-12 Point of care blood gas analyzer. (Courtesy Radiometer America, Cleveland, Ohio.)

TABLE 10-5				
Comparison of Four Point of Care Blood Gas Analyzers				
	StatPal II	**Gem 6**	**Gem Stat**	**Gem Premier**
Measured values	pH	pH	pH	pH
	PCO_2	PCO_2	PCO_2	PCO_2
	PO_2	PO_2	PO_2	PO_2
		Hct	Hct	Hct
		Ca^{++}	Ca^{++}	Ca^{++}
		K^+	K^+	K^+
			Na^+	Na^+
Calculated values	6	5	4	4
Sample volume	0.2 mL	2 mL	0.5 mL	0.2 mL
Analysis time	60 sec	130 sec	109 sec	92 sec
Samples/module	25	50 in 72 hr	50 in 72 hr	150 or 300 in 7 days
Interface	—	RS 232		
Data management	—	Hard copy of module in use	Hard copy of module in use	Hard copy or floppy disk storage of module in use

StatPal II (PPG Industries, Pittsburg, PA), Gem 6, Gem Stat, and Gem Premier (Mallinckrodt Sensor Systems, Ann Arbor, MI).
PCO_2, Partial pressure of carbon dioxide; PO_2, partial pressure of oxygen; *Hct*, hematocrit; *Ca*, calcium, *K*, Potassium; *Na*, Sodium.
From Levine RL, Fromm Jr RE: *Critical care monitoring: from pre-hospital to the ICU*, St Louis, 1995, Mosby.

Oximeters operate on the principle of spectrophotometry, which is based on the relative transmission or absorption of portions of the light spectrum.[26] The various forms of hemoglobin mentioned previously can be identified because each form has its own absorption spectrum. (Figure 10-13 shows the light spectra for each type of hemoglobin.) The concentration of a certain hemoglobin type can be determined using the Lambert-Beer law, which states that the transmission of a specific wavelength of light through a solution is a logarithmic function of the concentration of the absorbing species in the solution.[17,27]

The operating principle of a typical CO-oximeter is fairly straightforward. A blood sample is heated to 37° C and hemolyzed (either chemically or by high-frequency vibrations), creating a translucent solution. The solution is placed in a cuvette, which is positioned between a light source and a condenser and two photodetectors. A series of monochromatic light beams are simultaneously directed through the cuvette containing the sample of blood and through a blank solution (containing no hemoglobin).[17] The condenser lens system focuses the light passing through the sample cuvette onto a photodetector, which generates an electric current proportional to the intensity of the transmitted light and inversely proportional to the amount of light absorbed by the sample. The light passing through the blank solution is simultaneously focused onto

---

BOX 10-1	Advantages and Disadvantages of Point of Care Testing

POTENTIAL ADVANTAGES

· Decreased therapeutic turnaround time
· Rapid data availability
· Augmented clinical decision making
· Increased real-time patient management
· Shortened length of stay
· Decreased preanalytic error
· Decreased patient cost per episode
· Test clustering
· Decreased iatrogenic blood loss
· Increased patient throughput
· Fewer redundant blood tests
· Convenience for the clinician
· Improved clinician-patient interface
· Customized instrumentation
· Convenient when laboratory is inaccessible
· Rapid response to critical results
· Integration with performance maps, algorithms, and care paths

POTENTIAL DISADVANTAGES

· Lack of adequate documentation
· Quality control and proficiency testing issues
· Unauthorized testing
· Poor analytic performance
· Problems with training and competency
· Increased preanalytic error
· Data not recorded
· Sample handling error
· Limited test menu
· Decreased entry of results in patient record
· Postanalytic error (e.g., transcription error or communication failure)
· Need for separate license or licenses
· Failure to comply with regulations
· Increased costs
· Duplication of instruments and methods
· No critical values notification system and/or documentation

Modified from Kost GJ, Ehrmeyer SS, Chernow B: The laboratory-clinical interface: point of care testing, *Chest* 115:1142, 1999.

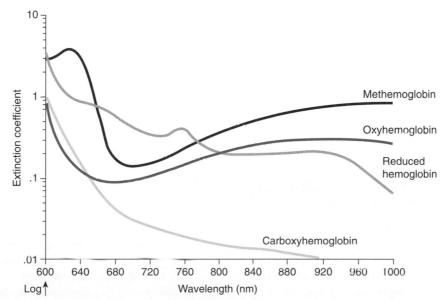

FIGURE 10-13 Absorption spectra for various species of hemoglobin. (From Pilbeam S: *Mechanical ventilation: physiological and clinical applications,* ed 3, St Louis, 1998, Mosby.)

a reference photodetector, which generates an electric current proportional to the light transmitted through the blank solution. The absorbance of the blank solution is then subtracted from the absorbances of the blood sample, and the resultant values are used to calculate the concentration of each type of hemoglobin in the blood sample. The normal concentrations of the various hemoglobin types are shown in Table 10-1.

Although blood can contain six different types of hemoglobin, most commercially available CO-oximeters provide measurements of only four types: O_2Hb, deoxyhemoglobin, metHb, and HbCO. Sulfhemoglobin and fetal hemoglobin are not usually determined by CO-oximetry, although the manufacturer Radiometer America (Westlake, Ohio) has introduced a CO-oximetry procedure to determine fetal hemoglobin. Although these results are different from reference methods, such as radioimmunoassay and chromatographic procedures, CO-oximeter analysis of fetal hemoglobin has been deemed clinically acceptable. Other reported values may include **total hemoglobin (THb)** and **oxygen content (O_2ct)**.

A number of factors can interfere with CO-oximetry measurements. Incompletely hemolyzed red blood cells, lipids, or air bubbles in the sample can scatter some of the incident light, producing erroneous measurements.[28,29] The presence of bilirubin (greater than 20 mg/dL of whole blood) or intravenous dyes (particularly methylene blue and indocyanine green) can also alter measurements because they absorb near-infrared (NIR) and infrared (IR) light. Absorbance of light by these substances lowers the actual oxyhemoglobin measured. The presence of fetal hemoglobin can also lead to false HbCO readings. Oxygenated fetal hemoglobin produces a 4% to 7% false carboxyhemoglobin level; reduced fetal hemoglobin yields a 0.2% to 1.5% false carboxyhemoglobin level.[17]

Calibration of CO-Oximeters

CO-oximeters should be routinely calibrated with solutions supplied by the manufacturer. These solutions typically are dye-based propylene glycol solutions that allow only for the calibration of total hemoglobin. Determination of the various forms of hemoglobin is accomplished by relating the relative absorbances recorded at the wavelengths tested. That is, the percentage of a particular hemoglobin type reported is derived from absorbance ratios at predetermined wavelengths.

NONINVASIVE ASSESSMENT OF ARTERIAL BLOOD GASES

Noninvasive blood gas monitoring has become a standard practice in respiratory care and anesthesiology. The importance of these devices in the management of patients with cardiopulmonary dysfunctions cannot be overstated. In just 30 years, pulse oximeters and transcutaneous pH, PCO_2, and PO_2 monitors have gone from expensive, bulky units to compact, affordable devices that can provide both continuous and intermittent pH, PCO_2, and PO_2 measurements that are reliable and accurate.

Pulse Oximetry

Pulse oximetry provides continuous, noninvasive measurements of the arterial oxygen saturation and pulse rate via a sensor placed over a digit, the earlobe, or the bridge of the nose. The sensor measures the absorption of selected wavelengths of light beamed through the tissue. Advances in microprocessor technology, coupled with improvements in the quality of **light-emitting diodes (LEDs)** and photoelectric sensors, have greatly improved the accuracy and reliability of these devices. Most clinicians now consider pulse oximetry an indispensable tool for monitoring the oxygenation status of patients at risk of hypoxemia.

Theory of Operation

Pulse oximetry is based on the principles of spectrophotometry and **photoplethysmography**.[30-32] As with CO-oximeters, pulse oximeters use spectrophotometry to determine the amount of hemoglobin (and deoxyhemoglobin) in a blood sample. Oxyhemoglobin and deoxygenated hemoglobin are differentiated by shining two wavelengths of light (660 and 940 nm) through the sampling site. As Figure 10-13 shows, at a wavelength of 660 nm (red light), deoxygenated hemoglobin absorbs more light than oxyhemoglobin. Conversely, oxyhemoglobin absorbs more light at 940 nm (IR light) than deoxygenated hemoglobin.

Photoplethysmography, or **optical plethysmography**, estimates the heart rate by measuring cyclic changes in light transmission through the sampling site during each cardiac cycle. That is, as the blood volume in the finger, toe, or earlobe increases during ventricular systole, light absorption increases and transmitted light decreases. Conversely, as blood volume decreases during diastole, absorbency decreases and transmitted light increases. The pulsatile and nonpulsatile components of a typical pulse oximetry signal are shown in Figure 10-14.

The percentage of oxyhemoglobin in a sample can be determined by first calculating the ratio of absorbencies for pulsatile and nonpulsatile flow at the two specified wavelengths, or

$$Red/Infrared = \frac{Pulsatile_{660nm}/Nonpulsatile_{660nm}}{Pulsatile_{940nm}/Nonpulsatile_{940nm}}$$

This ratio is then applied to an algorithm that relates the ratios of these two absorbencies to the oxyhemoglobin saturation.[32]

As mentioned previously, four types of hemoglobin can be measured by oximetry: reduced or deoxygenated hemoglobin (HHb), oxyhemoglobin, carboxyhemoglobin, and methemoglobin. Two terms often used to describe oxyhemoglobin saturation determinations are *fractional* and *functional saturations*. The **fractional hemoglobin saturation** is calculated by dividing the amount of oxyhemoglobin by the amount of all four types of hemoglobin present, or

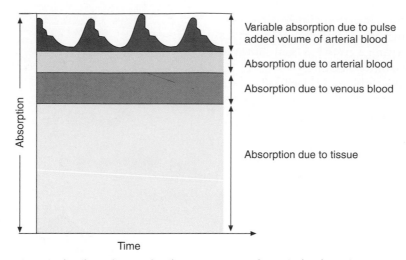

FIGURE 10-14 Pulsatile and nonpulsatile components of a typical pulse oximetry signal. (From McGough EK, Boysen PG: Benefits and limits of pulse oximetry in the ICU, *J Crit Ill* 4:23, 1989.)

$$\text{Fractional } O_2Hb = {}^-O_2Hb \div [HHb + O_2Hb + HbCO + metHb]$$

The **functional hemoglobin saturation** is calculated by dividing the oxyhemoglobin concentration by the concentration of hemoglobin capable of carrying oxygen. It may be written as

$$\text{Functional } O_2Hb = O_2Hb \div [HHb + O_2Hb]$$

Although laboratory CO-oximeters measure all four types of hemoglobin by using a series of wavelengths of light to identify each species, pulse oximeters use only two wavelengths to quantify the amount of O_2Hb and HHb present. Therefore laboratory CO-oximeters can report the fractional oxyhemoglobin saturation, and pulse oximeters can estimate the functional oxyhemoglobin saturation.

Physiologic and Technical Considerations

It is important to recognize that both physiologic and technical factors can influence the accuracy of pulse oximetry measurements.[33]

Low Perfusion States. The accuracy of a pulse oximetry reading depends on identification of an arterial pulse; therefore many conditions can interfere with proper pulse oximeter function. Hypovolemia, peripheral vasoconstriction from drugs or hypothermia, and heart-lung bypass (i.e., extracorporeal membrane oxygenation [ECMO]) are associated with a diminished pulsatile signal, resulting in an intermittent or absent oxygen saturation pulse oximetry (SpO$_2$) reading.[30] Some oximeters compensate for the weak signal associated with low perfusion states by increasing the signal output. The problem with this approach is that augmenting the signal also causes an increase in the signal-to-noise ratio, which can result in high levels of background noise that can contribute to erroneous results. A simpler approach is to reposition the oximeter sensor in an area of higher perfusion. For example, placing the oximeter probe on the ear instead of the finger may alleviate

some of the problems associated with reductions in peripheral perfusion.

Dysfunctional Hemoglobins. High levels of dysfunctional hemoglobins (i.e., HbCO and metHb) can adversely affect oxyhemoglobin measurement by pulse oximetry.[30] High HbCO levels can alter SpO$_2$ measurements because O_2Hb and HbCO have similar absorption coefficients for red light (660 nm); however, HbCO is relatively transparent to IR light (940 nm). Accordingly, significant levels of HbCO, as occur in carbon monoxide poisoning, lead to an overestimation of SpO$_2$.[30] (See Clinical Rounds 10-3 for a decision-making problem involving pulse oximetry.)

Methemoglobinemia, a complication associated with certain types of drugs (e.g., nitrites, benzocaine [a local anesthetic], and dapsone [an antibiotic used to treat malaria and *Pneumocystis carinii*]), can lead to erroneous SpO$_2$ values because metHb absorbs both red and IR light.[30] Methemoglobinemia is also associated with nitrate poisoning. If enough metHb is present to dominate all pulsatile absorption, the pulse oximeter will measure a red to IR ratio of 1:1, corresponding to an SpO$_2$ of about 85%. Consequently, the pulse oximeter reading will overestimate or underestimate the true oxyhemoglobin saturation.[30]

Dyes. Intravascular dyes can adversely affect SpO$_2$ values by absorbing a portion of the incident light emitted by the pulse oximeter diodes. Injection of methylene blue and indigo carmine during cardiac catheterization causes a false drop in SpO_2; indocyanine green has been shown to have little effect on pulse oximeter readings.[33]

Dark nail polish (particularly blue and black nail polish) can severely affect SpO_2 readings. Some have suggested that nail polish may affect pulse oximetry values by causing the shunting of light around the finger periphery.[34,35] In **optical shunting,** transmitted light never comes in contact with the vascular bed; therefore SpO_2 values can be erroneously high or low, depending on whether this light is pulsatile. This problem can be alleviated to a large extent by placing the device over the lateral aspects of the digit instead of over the nail. Theoretically, skin pigmentation should not affect pulse oximeter readings; however, in practice, SpO_2 readings are inconsistent for patients with dark pigmentation, possibly because of optical shunting.[36] **Hyperbilirubinemia,** a yellow discoloration of the skin associated with hepatic dysfunction, does not seem to affect pulse oximetry readings.[17]

Ambient Light. Fluorescent lights and other external light sources (e.g., heat lamps, fiberoptic light sources, and surgical lamps) have been shown to adversely affect heart rate and SpO_2 readings.[37] Most commercially available pulse oximeters attempt to compensate for this interference by continually cycling the transmitted red and infrared light on and off at a rate of about 480 cycles per second. In this process, the pulse oximeter cycles in three modes:

1. Red light on, IR off
2. IR on, red light off
3. Red light and IR off

By using this sequence, ambient light interference can be determined when both red and IR light sources are off. Subtracting any light measured during phase 3 from that measured during phases 1 and 2 provides a means of minimizing ambient light interference.

Calibration of Pulse Oximeters

Pulse oximeters are calibrated by manufacturers with data obtained from studies of healthy humans. Specifically, SpO_2 levels are compared with invasive hemoximetry oxygen saturations (SaO_2) measured simultaneously while each individual breathes several gas mixtures of different fractional inspired oxygen (F_IO_2). Therefore the accuracy and reliability of a pulse oximeter ultimately depend on the initial calibration algorithm programmed into the device by the manufacturer. Generally, pulse oximeters are accurate for oxygen saturations higher than 80%. Pulse oximeter saturations lower than 80% are questionable and should be confirmed with ABG analysis and hemoximetry.

Clinical Applications of Pulse Oximetry

Pulse oximetry probes are available in neonatal, pediatric, and adult sizes. Advances in LED and solid-state technology have led to the miniaturization of pulse oximeters and the manufacture of handheld devices (Figure 10-15). The response time of a pulse oximeter (i.e., how long it takes

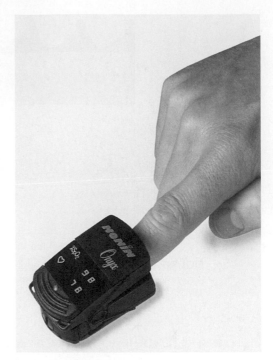

FIGURE 10-15 Handheld pulse oximeter. (Courtesy Nonin Medical, Plymouth, Minn.)

for a change in central circulation [left heart PO_2] to be detected by the pulse oximeter) depends on the location of the probe. Probes placed on fingers show a delay of 12 seconds or longer compared with a probe placed on the earlobe. Probes placed on the toe show an even greater lag time for detecting PO_2 changes.

Pulse oximetry is well recognized as an early warning system for detecting hypoxemia of patients with unstable oxygenation status. It can provide a continuous display of oxygen saturation, which can be used to monitor the oxygenation status of patients during surgery, mechanical ventilation, or bronchoscopy. It also can provide intermittent measurements of SpO_2, which can be useful, for example, in the management of home care patients.

Although pulse oximetry can be quite effective for adjusting oxygen therapy in hospitalized patients, its use in prescribing oxygen therapy for home care patients is questionable. Therefore caution should be exercised when pulse oximeter readings are used to prescribe oxygen therapy. Carlin et al.[38] demonstrated that the use of only pulse oximetry measurements could disqualify a significant number of patients applying for reimbursement for oxygen therapy. The guidelines established by the Centers for Medicare and Medicaid Services for qualifying for oxygen therapy require that the patient demonstrate a PaO_2 less than or equal to 55 torr (mm Hg) or a saturation less than or equal to 85%.[39] Because any of the physiologic or technical problems discussed previously can significantly affect pulse oximetry measurements, it is wise to use invasive ABG analysis to establish the need for oxygen therapy for chronically ill patients.

Clinical Practice Guideline 10-2 summarizes the AARC Clinical Practice Guideline for pulse oximetry, which provides valuable information to ensure that SpO_2 values are valid.

Transcutaneous Monitoring

Transcutaneous monitoring provides another method of indirect ABG assessment. Unlike pulse oximetry, which relies on spectrophotometric analysis, transcutaneous monitoring uses modified blood gas electrodes to measure the oxygen and carbon dioxide tension at the skin surface.[18,40,41] The conjunctival PO_2 electrode, a modification of the standard transcutaneous PO_2 electrode, measures the PO_2 of the **palpebral conjunctiva** surrounding the eyeball.

Transcutaneous PO₂

Figure 10-16A is a schematic of a transcutaneous PO_2 ($PtcO_2$) electrode, which consists of a **servo-controlled,** heated (Clark) polarographic electrode connected to a CPU.[40,41] The electrode is covered with a Teflon membrane, and the entire electrode assembly attaches to the skin surface with a double-sided adhesive ring. The electrode is heated to 42° to 45° C to produce capillary vasodilation below the surface of the electrode. Heating improves gas diffusion across the skin, because it increases local blood flow at the site of the electrode and alters the structure of the stratum corneum. The stratum corneum has been described as a mixture of fibrinous tissue within a lipid and protein matrix. It has been suggested that heating the skin to temperatures greater than 41° C melts the lipid layer, thus enhancing gas diffusion through the skin.[42]

The ratio of transcutaneous PO_2 to PaO_2 measured by hemoximetry (the $PtcO_2/PaO_2$ index) has been shown to be good for neonatal use, but it often is unreliable for critically ill adults.[43,44] Decreases in peripheral perfusion caused by reductions in cardiac output or increases in peripheral (cutaneous) resistance can significantly affect the accuracy of $PtcO_2$ measurements.[44,45] Current data indicate that when the cardiac index is greater than 2.2 L/min/m², the $PtcO_2/PaO_2$ index is 0.5, but when the cardiac index is less than 1.5 L/min/m², the $PtcO_2/PaO_2$ index is only 0.1.[46] Therefore hypoperfusion of the skin caused by pathologic states (e.g., septic shock, hemorrhage, or heart failure) or by increased vascular resistance (e.g., hypothermia or pharmacologic intervention) can lead to erroneous data.

Pulse Oximetry

Clinical Practice Guideline 10-2

■ INDICATIONS
Based on current evidence, pulse oximetry is useful for:
1. Monitoring arterial oxyhemoglobin saturation
2. Quantifying the arterial oxyhemoglobin saturation response to therapeutic intervention
3. Monitoring arterial oxyhemoglobin saturation during bronchoscopy

■ CONTRAINDICATIONS
Pulse oximetry may not be appropriate when ongoing measurements of pH, $PaCO_2$, and total hemoglobin are required. The presence of abnormal hemoglobins may be a relative contraindication.

■ LIMITATIONS
A number of factors, agents, and situations may affect readings and limit the precision and performance of pulse oximetry, including:
1. Motion artifacts
2. Abnormal hemoglobins (especially carboxyhemoglobin [HbCO] and methemoglobin [metHb])
3. Intravascular dyes
4. Exposure of the measuring sensor to ambient light sources
5. Low perfusion states
6. Skin pigmentation
7. Nail polish
8. Low oxyhemoglobin saturations (i.e., <83%)

■ MONITORING
The following information should be recorded during pulse oximetry:
1. Probe type; measurement site and date and time of measurement; and patient position and activity level.
2. Fractional inspired oxygen (F_IO_2) and mode of supplemental oxygen delivery.
3. Arterial blood gas (ABG) measurements and CO-oximetry results that may have been made simultaneously.
4. Clinical appearance of the patient (e.g., cyanotic, skin temperature).
5. Agreement between pulse oximeter heart rate and heart rate determined by palpation or electrocardiogram (ECG) recordings.

Modified from the American Association for Respiratory Care: Clinical practice guideline: pulse oximetry, Respir Care 36:1406, 1991.

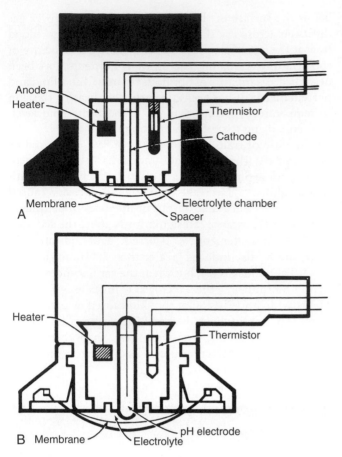

FIGURE 10-16 Transcutaneous electrodes. **A,** $PtcO_2$. **B,** $PtcCO_2$. (From Novametrix Medical Systems, Wallingford, Conn.)

Because the $PtcO_2$ is influenced by blood flow to the tissues, as well as by oxygen utilization by the tissues, changes in the $PtcO_2$ may be an early indicator of vascular compromise or shock. In fact, many $PtcO_2$ monitors display the power supplied to the electrode heater as a way of identifying perfusion problems at the site.

Transcutaneous PCO₂

The standard transcutaneous carbon dioxide ($PtcCO_2$) electrode is a modified Stowe-Severinghaus blood gas electrode composed of pH-sensitive glass with a Ag/AgCl electrode (Figure 10-16B). As with the $PtcO_2$ electrode, the $PtcCO_2$ electrode is heated to 42° to 45° C. $PtcCO_2$ values are slightly higher than the $PaCO_2$ value, primarily because of the higher metabolic rate at the site of the electrode caused by heating the skin. Most commercial instruments incorporate correction factors into their system's software to remove the discrepancy between the $PtcCO_2$ and $PaCO_2$.

Technical Considerations for Transcutaneous Monitoring

Clinical Practice Guideline 10-3 presents guidelines for transcutaneous monitoring of neonatal and pediatric patients that relate to the care, placement, and calibration of the electrodes.

Several points in the Clinical Practice Guideline deserve special attention:

1. Transcutaneous signals are adversely affected by dirt and hair; therefore before an electrode is placed on the patient's skin, the site should be cleaned with an alcohol swab. When hair is present, the site should be shaved to ensure good contact between the electrode and the skin. Before the electrode is attached to the patient, a drop of electrolyte gel or deionized water should be placed on the electrode's surface to enhances gas diffusion between the skin and the electrode.

2. Transcutaneous PO_2 monitors are calibrated with two-point calibration in which room air (PO_2 of about 150 mm Hg) is the high PO_2 of the calibration, and an electronic zeroing of the system is the low PO_2 of the calibration. The $PtcCO_2$ electrodes are also calibrated with a two-point calibration procedure. In this case, a 5% CO_2 calibration gas and a 10% CO_2 calibration gas are used for low and high calibration points, respectively. Electrodes should be calibrated before initial use on a patient. Manufacturers typically suggest calibration of an electrode each time it is repositioned.

3. Transcutaneous electrodes are bathed with a small amount of electrolyte solution, which can easily evaporate because heat is applied to the electrode. Loss of electrolyte either through evaporation or leakage from a torn membrane can adversely affect operation of the electrode. The electrolyte and the sensor's membrane should be checked regularly and changed weekly or whenever a signal drift during calibration is noticed. Because silver can deposit on the cathode, the electrode should be periodically cleaned according to the manufacturer's recommendations.

4. When transcutaneous PO_2 and PCO_2 readings are reported, the date and time of the measurement, the patient's activity level and body position, the site of electrode placement, and the electrode temperature should be noted. The inspired oxygen concentration and the type of equipment used to deliver supplemental oxygen should always be included. The clinical appearance of the patient, including assessment of peripheral perfusion (i.e., pallor, skin temperature), is important data to note. When invasive ABG measurements are available, they are recorded for comparison with $PtcO_2$ and $PtcCO_2$ readings.[45]

Burns are probably the most common problem that clinicians encounter during transcutaneous monitoring, because the site of measurement must be heated to 42° to 45° C. Repositioning the sensor every 4 to 6 hours can minimize this problem. For transcutaneous monitoring of neonates, the sensor should be repositioned more often.

INTERPRETATION OF BLOOD GAS RESULTS

As stated previously, ABG values can provide important information about a patient's acid-base, ventilatory, and

Transcutaneous Blood Gas Monitoring for Neonatal and Pediatric Patients— 2004 Revisions and Update

Clinical Practice Guideline 10-3

■ **INDICATIONS**
1. Monitoring the adequacy of arterial oxygenation or ventilation.
2. Quantifying a patient's response to diagnostic and therapeutic interventions.

■ **CONTRAINDICATIONS**
Relative contraindications to transcutaneous monitoring may be poor skin integrity and adhesive allergy.

■ **HAZARDS/COMPLICATIONS**
1. False-negative or false-positive results may lead to inappropriate treatment.
2. Tissue injury at the measurement site (e.g., blisters, burns, skin tears).

■ **LIMITATIONS**
The following factors may increase the discrepancy between arterial and transcutaneous values:
1. Hyperoxemia (partial pressure of arterial oxygen [PaO_2] > 100 mm Hg)
2. Hypoperfused state (e.g., shock)
3. Improper electrode placement
4. Vasoactive drugs
5. Skin factors (skinfold thickness or presence of edema)

■ **VALIDATION**
Arterial blood gas values should be compared with transcutaneous readings taken at the time of arterial sampling to validate the transcutaneous values. The validations should be performed when transcutaneous monitoring is initiated and periodically as dictated by the patient's clinical state.

■ **ASSURANCE OF CONSISTENCY OF CARE**
1. High- and low-limit alarms are set appropriately.
2. Appropriate electrode temperature is set.
3. Systematic electrode site change occurs.
4. Manufacturer's recommendations for maintenance, operation, and safety are followed.

■ **MONITORING**
The following information should be recorded at regular intervals (e.g., 1 to 4 hours):
1. Date and time of measurement.
2. Patient position, respiratory rate, activity level, fractional inspired oxygen (F_IO_2), mode of ventilatory support and settings.
3. Electrode placement site, electrode temperature, time of placement, results of simultaneously obtained in vitro arterial blood gas (ABG) analysis.
4. Clinical appearance of the patient, including perfusion, pallor, and skin temperature.

■ **INFECTION CONTROL**
Standard Precautions are recommended for all patients. The device probe should be cleaned between patient applications according to the manufacturer's recommendations. The external portion of the monitor should be cleaned according to the manufacturer's recommendations whenever the device remains in a patient's room for a prolonged period or if it becomes soiled or contaminated with potentially transmissible organisms.

Modified from the American Association for Respiratory Care: Clinical practice guideline: transcutaneous blood gas monitoring for neonatal and pediatric patients, Respir Care 49:1069, 2004.

oxygenation status. Blood gas analysis is also an integral part of more sophisticated procedures, such as cardiopulmonary and hemodynamic monitoring. It is beyond the scope of this book to discuss fully the interpretive value of blood gas measurements. Therefore a framework for ABG interpretation is provided here, but the titles of several texts and monographs on blood gas analysis are listed at the end of the chapter.

Acid-Base Status

Acid-base disorders can be categorized as either acidosis or alkalosis. Acidosis is associated with an increase in the plasma hydrogen ion concentration and a fall in the pH. Alkalosis is associated with a decrease in plasma hydrogen ion concentration and a rise in pH. The Henderson-Hasselbalch equation can be used to describe how changes in HCO_3 and $PaCO_2$ can be used to determine whether a metabolic, a respiratory, or a combined acid-base disorder is present. Consider these equations:

$$pH = pKa + \log(HCO_3^-)/(PaCO_2 \times 0.03) \; or$$
$$pH \sim (HCO_3^-)/(PaCO_2)$$

Acute decreases in HCO_3^- and increases in $PaCO_2$ are associated with decreases in pH and metabolic and respiratory acidosis, respectively. Conversely, acute increases in HCO_3^- and decreases in $PaCO_2$ are associated with increases in pH and metabolic and respiratory alkalosis, respectively. If only one of the parameters changes and the other stays within normal limits, the problem can be classified as an acute or uncompensated acid-base disorder. For example, a reduced pH with an increase in $PaCO_2$ and a normal HCO_3^- indicates an acute or uncompensated respiratory acidosis. If the reduced pH is associated with a decreased HCO_3^- and a normal $PaCO_2$, an acute or uncompensated metabolic acidosis is suggested. Note that a mixed acidosis or mixed alkalosis is also an uncompensated event. In the case of a mixed acidosis, the pH is less than 7.35 with the $PaCO_2$ greater than 45 mm Hg and the HCO_3^- less than 22 mEq/L. A mixed alkalosis is characterized by a pH greater than 7.45, a PCO_2 less than 35 mm Hg, and an HCO_3^- greater than 26 mEq/L. With compensated acid-base disorders, both the $PaCO_2$ and HCO_3 are out of their normal range of values. The interpretation of arterial blood gas values can therefore be an arduous task, particularly when one is trying to differentiate the source of the acid-base disturbance and the compensatory response. The following is offered as one method that can be used to interpret ABG measurements when compensation occurs. First, look at the pH and determine whether an acidosis or alkalosis is present. To determine the primary disorder, look at the $PaCO_2$ to decide whether a respiratory problem could have caused the altered pH. Next, look at the HCO_3^- to determine whether a metabolic disorder is responsible for the altered pH. After the origin of the acid-base disorder has been established, compensation can be discerned by examining whether the other variable has also changed. Consider the following situation: If a patient's pH is below 7.4, then the original problem could be caused by an increase in the $PaCO_2$ (i.e., respiratory acidosis) or a decrease in HCO_3^- (i.e., metabolic acidosis). The compensation for a respiratory acidosis would be a rise in HCO_3^-, whereas the compensation for a metabolic acidosis would be a reduction in the $PaCO_2$. The converse of this situation would follow the same line of logic. If the patient's pH is greater than 7.4, then the original problem could be caused by a reduction in the $PaCO_2$ (i.e., respiratory alkalosis) or an increase in HCO_3^- (i.e., metabolic alkalosis). The compensation for a respiratory alkalosis is loss of HCO_3^-, whereas the compensation for a metabolic alkalosis is CO_2 retention.

The level of compensation usually is described as partially compensated or fully compensated. If the pH is within the range of normal limits, the acid-base disorder is fully compensated. If not, it is partially compensated. For example, a respiratory acidosis is associated with a decreased pH and an increased $PaCO_2$. If HCO_3^- also has increased, there is evidence of metabolic compensation. If the pH is between 7.35 and 7.4, this is interpreted as a fully compensated respiratory acidosis. Table 10-6 summarizes the pH, $PaCO_2$, and HCO_3^- findings associated with various types of acid-base disturbances.

Ventilatory Status

A patient's ventilatory status can be assessed by looking at the $PaCO_2$. An increase in $PaCO_2$ is associated with hypoventilation and a respiratory acidosis. Conversely, a decrease in $PaCO_2$ is associated with hyperventilation and a respiratory alkalosis. As a general rule, a $PaCO_2$ greater than 50 mm Hg is classified as ventilatory failure and often is used as a criterion for initiating mechanical ventilatory support. Note that changes in the $PaCO_2$ must be interpreted relative to the patient's clinical condition. For example, patients with chronic obstructive pulmonary disease (COPD) often demonstrate chronic ventilatory failure (e.g., a $PaCO_2$ higher than 50 mm Hg with a pH within normal limits). Therefore acute ventilatory failure is said to exist in patients with COPD only if the $PaCO_2$ increases well above 50 mm Hg and the pH is below 7.3.

Oxygenation Status

A patient's oxygenation status can be evaluated by looking at the PaO_2 or the SaO_2. The relationship between these two values can then be illustrated graphically with an oxyhemoglobin dissociation curve (Figure 10-17). Note that a PaO_2 of 45 mm Hg is associated with an SaO_2 of approximately 80%; a PaO_2 of about 60 mm Hg corresponds to an SaO_2 of 90%; and a PaO_2 of 75 mm Hg is equivalent to an SaO_2 of 95%. For interpretative purposes, a PaO_2 of 60 to 80 mm Hg is classified as mild hypoxemia; a PaO_2 of 40

TABLE 10-6			
pH, PaCO$_2$, and HCO$_3^-$ Findings for Various Acid-Base Disturbances			
	pH	**PCO$_2$ (mm Hg)**	**HCO$_3^-$**
Respiratory Acidosis			
Acute	<7.35	>45	Normal
Partly compensated	<7.35	>45	>26
Compensated	>7.35 <7.40	>45	>26
Respiratory Alkalosis			
Acute	>7.45	<35	Normal
Partly compensated	>7.45	<35	<22
Compensated	<7.45 >7.40	<35	<22
Metabolic Acidosis			
Acute	<7.35	Normal	<22
Partly compensated	<7.35	<35	<22
Compensated	>7.35 <7.40	<35	<22
Metabolic Alkalosis			
Acute	>7.45	Normal	>26
Partly compensated	>7.45	>45	>26
Compensated	<7.45 >7.40	>45	>26

From Harwood R: *Exam review and study guide for perinatal/pediatric respiratory care*, Philadelphia, 1999, FA Davis.

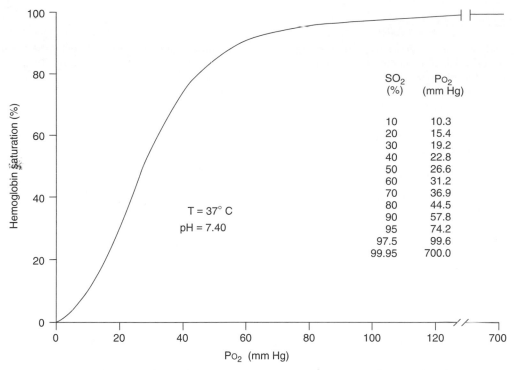

SO$_2$ (%)	Po$_2$ (mm Hg)
10	10.3
20	15.4
30	19.2
40	22.8
50	26.6
60	31.2
70	36.9
80	44.5
90	57.8
95	74.2
97.5	99.6
99.95	700.0

T = 37° C
pH = 7.40

FIGURE 10-17 Oxyhemoglobin dissociation curve. (From Lane EE, Walker JF: *Clinical arterial blood gas analysis,* St Louis, 1987, Mosby.)

TABLE 10-7

Criteria for Classifying Hypoxemia Using PaO$_2$ Measurements

Hypoxemia	PaO$_2$
Room Air Inspired; Patient Under 60 Years of Age	
Mild*	<80 mm Hg
Moderate	<60 mm Hg
Severe*	<40 mm Hg
Supplemental Oxygen Inspired; Patient Under 60 Years of Age	
Uncorrected	Less than room air acceptable limit
Corrected	Within the room air acceptable limit; <100 mm Hg
Excessively corrected	>100 mm Hg

*Subtract 1 mm Hg of oxygen to limits of mild and moderate hypoxemia for each year over age 60. A PaO$_2$ of 40 mm Hg indicates severe hypoxemia in any patient at any age.
Modified from Shapiro BA, Peruzzi WT, Templin R: *Clinical application of blood gases,* ed 4, Chicago, 1989, Mosby.

BOX 10-2	Examples of Disease States Associated with Various Types of Acid-Base Disorders

METABOLIC ACIDOSIS
Diabetes mellitus
Diarrhea
Methanol ingestion
Renal dysfunction
Salicylate intoxication

METABOLIC ALKALOSIS
Administration of excessive amounts of bicarbonate
Diuretic therapy
Ingestion of excessive amounts of antacids
Nasogastric suctioning
Vomiting

RESPIRATORY ACIDOSIS
Acute airway obstruction
Ingestion of excessive amounts of sedatives, opiates, and other respiratory depressants
Neuromuscular disorders
Pneumothorax
Restrictive pulmonary disease

RESPIRATORY ALKALOSIS
Anxiety
Encephalitis
Excessive mechanical ventilatory support
Progesterone

to 60 mm Hg is classified as moderate hypoxemia; and a PaO$_2$ less than 40 mm Hg is classified as severe hypoxemia. Table 10-7 provides PaO$_2$ and SaO$_2$ ranges for evaluating a patient's oxygenation status.

Box 10-2 lists examples of conditions and disease states associated with various acid-base disorders. As mentioned previously, blood gas measurements are meaningful only when they are interpreted in the context of other clinical findings. Interpretation of ABGs without other supporting clinical data can be misleading and lead to potentially harmful decisions in patient management.

KEY POINTS

- Blood gas analysis is an integral part of the management of patients with cardiopulmonary dysfunctions.
- Modern in vitro blood gas analyzers are fully automated systems that require only small amounts of blood for analysis and can provide intermittent measurements of pH, $PaCO_2$, and PaO_2, which give valuable information about a patient's acid-base, ventilatory, and oxygenation status.
- Many blood gas analyzers also allow for determinations of plasma electrolytes and metabolites, such as sodium, potassium, calcium, and glucose.
- Noninvasive devices, including pulse oximetry and transcutaneous monitoring, are an alternative to the standard in vitro blood gas analysis and allow for continuous blood gas surveillance.
- Pulse oximetry is based on the principles of spectrophotometry and photoplethysmography. Pulse oximeters use spectrophotometry to determine the amount of hemoglobin (and deoxyhemoglobin) in a blood sample, and photoplethysmography estimates the heart rate by measuring cyclic changes in light transmission through the sampling site during each cardiac cycle.

- A number of factors can influence the accuracy of pulse oximetry measurements, including the level of perfusion, the presence of dysfunctional hemoglobins, dyes, and interference from ambient light.
- Transcutaneous monitoring is a noninvasive method for estimating the arterial oxygen and carbon dioxide tensions. It uses modified blood gas electrodes to measure oxygen and carbon dioxide tensions at the skin surface.
- Point of care blood gas analyzers are cost-effective devices that can provide accurate and reliable blood gas analysis at the bedside.
- Blood gas measurements should be interpreted relative to other clinical indices, including the history and physical examination findings, chest radiographs, and other clinical laboratory tests.
- Blood gas abnormalities generally are classified as acidosis or alkalosis. Careful interpretation of blood gas findings can identify the etiology of the problem as being associated with a respiratory, metabolic, or mixed respiratory and metabolic condition.

ASSESSMENT QUESTIONS

See Evolve Resources for the answers.

1. Which of the following are current safety requirements for protection of the therapist during drawing of an ABG sample?
   I. Gloves
   II. Gown
   III. Protective eyewear (goggles)
   IV. Shoe covers
   a. I and III only
   b. II and III only
   c. II and IV only
   d. I, II, and III only

2. A positive Allen test indicates the presence of:
   a. An occluded radial artery
   b. A patent ulnar artery
   c. Inadequate arterial oxygenation to the hand
   d. Inadequate collateral circulation to the hand

3. The site most often used for sampling of arterial blood in adults is which of the following arteries?
   a. Brachial artery
   b. Dorsalis pedis artery
   c. Radial artery
   d. Femoral artery

4. Interpret the following ABG findings:
   pH = 7.5 PaO_2 = 60 mm Hg
   $PaCO_2$ = 30 mm Hg HCO_3^- = 24 mEq/L
   a. Acute metabolic alkalosis with mild hypoxemia
   b. Chronic metabolic acidosis with moderate hypoxemia
   c. Acute respiratory alkalosis with mild hypoxemia
   d. Chronic respiratory alkalosis with moderate hypoxemia

5. Which of the following conditions is associated with an acute respiratory acidosis?
   a. Barbiturate intoxication
   b. Excessive ingestion of antacids
   c. Emphysema
   d. Anxiety

6. A patient is admitted to the emergency department after a motor vehicle accident. In your initial assessment, you find that he is pale and his pulse is weak. You are unable to obtain a steady pulse oximeter reading. Which of the following is the most probable cause of the erratic pulse oximetry readings?
   I. Poor perfusion state
   II. Increased levels of carboxyhemoglobin
   III. Low PaO_2
   IV. Anemia
   a. I only
   b. I and II only
   c. I, II, and III only
   d. I, II, III, and IV

7. Which of the following can alter pulse oximetry readings?
   I. Low perfusion states, such as hypovolemic shock
   II. Dark blue nail polish
   III. Methemoglobinemia
   IV. Hyperbilirubinemia
   a. I and III only
   b. II and III only
   c. II and IV only
   d. I, II, and III only

ASSESSMENT QUESTIONS—cont'd

8. A patient's P_{50} is 37 mm Hg. Which of the following conditions could be responsible?
   I. Hypercarbia
   II. Decreased plasma levels of 2,3 diphosphoglycerate
   III. Acute acidosis
   IV. Carbon monoxide poisoning
   a. I and III only
   b. II and III only
   c. II and IV only
   d. I, II, and IV only

9. To function effectively, the reference pH electrode must be bathed in which of the following solutions?
   a. 1% Sodium bicarbonate
   b. Saturated potassium chloride
   c. 5% Hydrochloric acid
   d. 0.9% Sodium chloride

10. While assessing the Levy-Jennings graphs for PCO_2 values, you notice that the results for the last five quality assessment tests have increased progressively. Which of the following is the most likely cause of this finding?
   a. A leak in the electrode membrane
   b. Protein buildup on the electrode
   c. A damaged wire
   d. This is a normal membrane function.

11. Which of the following is *not* an anion buffer?
   a. Hemoglobin
   b. Inorganic phosphate
   c. Bicarbonate
   d. Organic calcium

12. According to CLIA standards, laboratory instruments used in the hospital for blood sample testing should undergo three-point calibrations at least:
   a. Daily
   b. Weekly
   c. Monthly
   d. Every 6 months

13. Compare the processes of quality control and quality assurance.

14. Arterial blood was obtained from a patient after open heart surgery. The patient's temperature is 35° C, and the measured PaO_2 is 80 mm Hg before temperature correction. The patient's actual PaO_2 is approximately:
   a. 70 mm Hg
   b. 80 mm Hg
   c. 90 mm Hg
   d. It cannot be determined from the information provided.

15. What are the consequences of maintaining the temperature of the transcutaneous PO_2 probe at 48° C?
   a. Thermal injury
   b. Low $PtcO_2$ readings
   c. Fire hazard
   d. Malignant hyperthermia

16. Which of the following tests is indicated for detecting carbon monoxide poisoning?
   a. Pulse oximetry
   b. ABGs
   c. CO-oximetry
   d. Transcutaneous $PtcO_2$

References

1. American Association of Respiratory Care: Clinical practice guideline: sampling for arterial blood gas analysis, *Respir Care* 37:913, 1992.
2. American Association of Respiratory Care: Clinical practice guideline: Blood gas analysis and hemoximetry—2001 Revision and Update, *Respir Care* 46:498, 2001.
3. Browning JA, Kaiser DL, Durbin CG: The effect of guidelines on the appropriate use of arterial blood gas analysis in the intensive care unit, *Respir Care* 34:269, 1989.
4. Bruck E et al: *Percutaneous collection of arterial blood for laboratory analysis*, National Committee for Clinical Laboratory Standards, H11A, 5:39, 1985.
5. National Committee for Clinical Laboratory Standards: *Procedures for the collection of diagnostic blood specimens by skin puncture*, ed 3, Villanova, Pa, 1992.
6. Koch G, Wendel H: Comparison of pH, carbon dioxide tension, standard bicarbonate, and oxygen tension in capillary blood and in arterial blood during the neonatal period, *Acta Paediatr Scand* 56:10, 1967.
7. Burritt MF, Fallon KD: *Blood gas preanalytical considerations: specimen collection, calibration, and controls*, National Committee for Clinical Laboratory Standards, C27-T 9:685, 1989.
8. Ehrmeyer S, Laessig RH: Measurement of the proficiency of pH and blood gas analyses by interlaboratory proficiency testing, *J Med Tech* 2:33, 1985.
9. Duc GV, Cumarasamy N: Digital arteriolar oxygen tension as a guide to oxygen therapy of the newborn, *Biol Neonate* 24:134, 1974.
10. McLain BI, Evans J, Dear PFR: Comparison of capillary and arterial blood gas measurements in neonates, *Arch Dis Child* 63:743, 1988.
11. Desai SD et al: A comparison between arterial and arterialized capillary blood in infants, *S Afr Med J* 41:13, 1967.
12. Centers for Disease Control: Update: universal precautions for prevention of transmission of human immunodeficiency virus, hepatitis B virus, and other blood-borne pathogens in health care settings, *MMWR* 37:377, 1988.
13. Department of Labor, Occupational Safety and Health Administration: Occupational exposure to bloodborne pathogens, 29 CFRR Part 1910.1030, *Fed Regist* Dec 6, 1991.
14. Moran RF et al: Oxygen content, hemoglobin oxygen, "saturation," and related quantities in blood: terminology, measurement, and reporting, National Committee for Clinical Laboratory Standards, C25-P 10:1, 1990.
15. Davenport HW: *The ABC of acid-base chemistry*, ed 3, Chicago, 1975, University of Chicago Press.
16. Brensilver JM, Goldberger E: *A primer of water and acid-base syndromes*, ed 8, Philadelphia, 1996, FA Davis.
17. Shapiro BA, Peruzzi WT, Kozlowski-Templin: *Clinical application of blood gases*, ed 5, St Louis, 1994, Mosby.
18. Severinghaus JS, Bradley FA: Electrodes for blood PO_2 and PCO_2 determination, *J Appl Physiol* 13:515, 1958.

19. National Committee for Clinical Laboratory Standards: *Clinical laboratory technical procedure manual*, ed 2, Pub GP2-A2, Illinois, 1992, Villanova.

20. Clinical Laboratory Improvement Amendments of 1988: Final rule, subpart H, *Fed Regist* Feb 1992.

21. Medicare, Medicaid, and CLIA Programs: CLIA-88 continuance of approval of the Joint Commission on Accreditation of Healthcare Organizations (JCAHO) as an accrediting organization, *Fed Regist* 67:65585, 2002.

22. Hansen JE et al: Assessing precision and accuracy in blood gas proficiency testing, *Am Rev Respir Dis* 141:1190, 1990.

23. Mohler JG et al: Blood gases. In Clausen JL, editor: *Pulmonary function testing: guidelines and controversies*, New York, 1982, Academic Press.

24. Barker SJ, Hyatt J: Continuous measurement of intraarterial pH, $PaCO_2$, and PaO_2 in the operating room, *Anesth Analg* 73:43, 1991.

25. MacIntyre NR et al: Accuracy and precision of a point-of-care blood gas analyzer incorporating optode, *Respir Care* 41:800, 1996.

26. Brown LJ: A new instrument for the simultaneous measurement of total hemoglobin, % oxyhemoglobin, % carboxyhemoglobin, % methemoglobin, and oxygen content in whole blood, *IEEE Trans Biomed Eng* 27:132, 1980.

27. Falholt W: Blood oxygen saturation determinations by spectrophotometry, *Scand J Clin Lab Invest* 15:67, 1963.

28. Severinghaus JW, Astrup PB: History of blood gas analysis. VI. Oximetry, *J Clin Monit* 2:270, 1986.

29. Nillson NJ: Oximetry, *Physiol Rev* 40:1, 1960.

30. Tremper KK, Barker SJ: Pulse oximetry, *Anesthesiology* 70:98, 1989.

31. Yang K, Brown SD, Gutierrez G: Noninvasive assessment of blood gases. In Levine RL, Fromm RE, editors: *Critical care monitoring: from pre-hospital to ICU*, St Louis, 1995, Mosby.

32. Pilbeam S: *Mechanical ventilation*, ed 3, St Louis, 1998, Mosby.

33. Scheller MS, Unger RJ, Kelner MJ: Effects of intravenously administered dyes on pulse oximetry readings, *Anesthesiology* 65:550, 1986.

34. Cote CJ et al: The effect of nail polish on pulse oximetry, *Anesth Analg* 67:685, 1988.

35. Rubin AS: Nail polish color can affect pulse oximeter saturation, *Anesthesiology* 68:825, 1988.

36. Emery JR: Skin pigmentation as an influence on the accuracy of pulse oximetry, *J Perinatol* 7:329, 1987.

37. Amar D et al: Fluorescent light interferes with pulse oximetry, *J Clin Monit* 5:135, 1989.

38. Carlin BW, Claussen JL, Ries AL: The use of cutaneous oximetry in the prescription of long-term oxygen therapy, *Chest* 94:239, 1988.

39. Kacmarek RM, Hess D, Stoller JK: *Monitoring in respiratory care*, St Louis, 1993, Mosby.

40. Lubbers DW: Theory and development of transcutaneous oxygen pressure measurement, *Int Anesthesiol Clin* 25:31, 1987.

41. Severinghaus JS, Stafford M, Bradley FA: Transcutaneous PO_2 electrode design, calibration, and temperature gradient problems, *Acta Anaesthesiol Scand* (Suppl) 68:118, 1978.

42. Baecjert P et al: Is pulse oximetry reliable in detecting hypoxemia in the neonate? *Adv Exp Med Biol* 220:165, 1987.

43. Reed RL et al: Correlation of hemodynamic variables with transcutaneous PO_2 measurements in critically ill patients, *J Trauma* 25:1045, 1985.

44. Lubbers DW: Theoretical basis of transcutaneous blood gas measurements, *Crit Care Med* 9:721, 1981.

45. American Association of Respiratory Care: Clinical practice guideline: transcutaneous blood gas monitoring for neonatal and pediatric patients, *Respir Care* 39:1176, 1994.

46. Wahr JA, Tremper KK: Non-invasive oxygen monitoring techniques, *Crit Care Clin* 11:199, 1995.

Internet Resources

AARC Clinical Practice Guidelines: http://www.aarc.org

Altitude Blood Gas Calculator: http://www.altitude.org/calculators/ABGcalculator.htm

College of American Pathologists: http://www.cap.org

The Joint Commission: http://www.jointcommission.org

The Virtual Hospital: http://www.vh.org

WebMD Arterial Blood Gases: http://www.webmd.com/a-to-z-guides/arterial-blood-gases

Lab Test Online: http://www.labtestsonline.org/understanding/analytes/blood_gases/test.html

Chapter 11

Introduction to Ventilators

SUSAN P. PILBEAM

OUTLINE

Part I: Physical Characteristics of Ventilators
Part II: Basic Components of Breath Delivery
Part III: Basic Modes of Ventilation

OBJECTIVES

Upon completion of this chapter you will be able to:

- List the two primary power sources used in mechanical ventilators.
- Compare and contrast negative-pressure and positive-pressure ventilation.
- Explain how a closed-loop ventilator system can perform self-adjustment.
- Define volume and pressure ventilation.
- Provide three additional names for pressure and volume ventilation.
- Name three volume-displacement designs and three flow-control valves.
- Compare the location of expiratory valves on current intensive care unit (ICU) ventilators with the location on older model ventilators.
- Draw the flow and pressure curves produced by linear drive and rotary drive piston ventilators.
- Explain the two fundamental principles of fluidics.
- Evaluate available positive end-expiratory pressure (PEEP) valves to determine whether a flow resistor or a threshold resistor is being used.
- Evaluate patient information to determine which expiratory maneuver is indicated: negative end-expiratory pressure (NEEP), continuous positive airway pressure (CPAP), PEEP, expiratory pause, or expiratory retard.
- Troubleshoot a freestanding CPAP system.
- Describe the four phases of a breath.
- Explain how pressure-, flow-, and volume-triggering mechanisms work to begin the inspiratory phase of a breath.
- Identify the graph of the flow-time, volume-time, and pressure-time curves for time-triggered, volume- or pressure-limited, time-cycled breaths.
- Identify a pressure-time curve showing patient triggering.
- Apply Chatburn's classification for ventilator modes.
- Explain the concept of having an adjustable flow drop-off feature for ending inspiration in pressure-support ventilation.
- Name at least one current use of CPAP.
- Define the modes of ventilation by their triggering, limiting (controlling), and cycling mechanisms.
- Compare the dual control mode of ventilation to adaptive ventilation.
- Contrast the three methods of achieving minimum minute ventilation as used by current-generation ventilators.
- Define each of the following modes of ventilation: APRV, PAV, NAVA, and ASV.
- List the five common methods of delivering high-frequency ventilation.

PART I PHYSICAL CHARACTERISTICS OF VENTILATORS

OUTLINE

Perspectives on Ventilator Classification
Introduction to Ventilators
Power Source—Input Power
    Pneumatically Powered Ventilators
    Electrically Powered Ventilators
    Combined Power: Pneumatically Powered and Electronically or Microprocessor-Controlled Ventilators
Pressure Delivery
    Positive-Pressure Ventilators
    Negative-Pressure Ventilators
    Combined-Pressure Devices
Control Systems and Circuits
    Open-Loop and Closed-Loop Systems
    Control Panel
    Pneumatic Circuit
Drive Mechanisms (Power Transmission and Conversion Systems)
    Compressors or Blowers
    Volume-Displacement Designs
    Flow-Control Valves
    Fluidic Elements in Power Transmission Design
    Contemporary Drive Mechanisms and Control Valves
Additional Devices Used During Patient Ventilation
    Expiratory Valves for Providing Positive End-Expiratory Pressure
    Continuous Positive Airway Pressure (CPAP) Devices

KEY TERMS

beam deflection	flow resistance	pneumatic circuit
chest cuirass	fluidic	pneumatically powered
closed-loop	high-frequency oscillator	positive-pressure ventilators
Coanda effect	high-frequency ventilation (HFV)	power transmission systems
combined-power	internal circuit	proportional solenoid valve
control panel	iron lung	rotary drive pistons
direct-drive pistons	linear-drive piston	separation bubble
electrically powered	microprocessor controlled	sinusoidal
external circuit	negative-pressure ventilators	threshold resistance
flip-flop component	open-loop	user interface
flow-control valves	patient circuit	

Advances in computer technology continue to be made at a rapid pace. Nowhere is the impact of modern technology more noticeable than in medical devices, particularly mechanical ventilators. A wide variety of mechanical ventilators is available for managing patients of different ages and in various settings. All of these share certain characteristics, as well as important functional properties. This chapter focuses on the classification of modes of ventilation, breath delivery, and the common physical characteristics of mechanical ventilators.

PERSPECTIVES ON VENTILATOR CLASSIFICATION

The use of ventilators in patient management is relatively young. In the United States, the earliest ventilators appeared in the 1950s and 1960s and were originally classified by a system used by Mushin et al.,[1] the purpose of which was to try to describe ventilator function. However, the technology of mechanical ventilation expanded so rapidly that the original classification system needed modification. Practitioners were becoming confused about terms used to describe ventilators and modes. In the late 1980s and early 1990s, Robert L. Chatburn tried to solve this problem by establishing a newer classification system.[2-5] Although a welcome change, this system was difficult for some practitioners to adopt.[6] As of this writing, Chatburn is continuing his efforts to bring uniformity to ventilator classification.[7-10]

Historically, classification systems attempted to describe the physical function of the ventilator. Chatburn's method attempts to do two things: First, it describes certain characteristics of the ventilator, such as its power source (e.g., electricity or compressed gases). Second, it describes the breath or breathing pattern delivered to the patient. For example, does the therapist want to target a specific volume to deliver to the patient, or is pressure the greater concern? Does gas flow start when the patient initiates a breath, or does the machine determine when flow starts? Does the ventilator measure a variable and change its function based on that measurement?

Although Chatburn's classification system seems appropriate, some respiratory therapists and physicians remain confused by the names applied to different modes and breath types. Part of this confusion exists because of the names manufacturers give to "new" modes. Typically, ventilator manufacturers give a recently designed mode a different name from any used in others' ventilators, even if the mode is the same as or very similar to one that exists on a competitor's ventilator. For example, Autoflow on the Dräger EvitaXL ventilator is similar in function to pressure-regulated volume control (PRVC) on the Servo[i]. This makes understanding ventilator nomenclature difficult.

In 2007 Chatburn revisited ventilator classification to provide an updated description of ventilators, how they are classified, and how they function to deliver a breath.[7] The reader is referred to his references for a complete description of this system.[7-10] This chapter includes and follows the key aspects of Chatburn's classification system.

INTRODUCTION TO VENTILATORS

A ventilator is basically a box connected to a power source that provides a breath or gas flow to a patient. The operator sets certain controls on the **control panel,** sometimes called the **user interface.** These settings determine the pattern of gas delivery the patient receives.

The classification of a ventilator begins with a description of the physical characteristics of the ventilator (Box 11-1).[11] It then proceeds to a description and classification of breath types and combinations of breaths, also referred to as *modes.*

POWER SOURCE—INPUT POWER

Power sources provide the machine with the energy to perform the work required to ventilate a patient. Ventilators fall into three categories of power sources: **pneumatically powered** ventilators, **electrically powered** ventilators, and **combined-power** ventilators.

Pneumatically Powered Ventilators

Pneumatically powered ventilators connect to high-pressure gas sources (35 to 100 psi) and use this pressure to power gas flow to the patient. In general, pneumatically powered ventilators used in an intensive care unit (ICU)

BOX 11-1	Components of a Ventilator

1. Ventilator power source or input power (electric or gas source)
   a. Electrically powered
   b. Pneumatically powered
   c. Combined power
   d. Manually powered
2. Positive- or negative-pressure ventilators
3. Control systems and circuits
   a. Open- and closed-loop systems to control ventilator function
   b. Control panel (user interface)
   c. Pneumatic circuit (internal and patient circuit)
4. Power transmission and conversion system
   a. Volume displacement, pneumatic designs
   b. Flow-control valves
5. Output (pressure, volume, and flow waveforms)

From Pilbeam SP, Cairo JM: *Mechanical ventilation: physiological and clinical applications,* ed 4, St Louis, 2006, Mosby/Elsevier.

---

use two 50-psi gas sources (oxygen and air) and have built-in reducing valves so that the operating pressure is lower than the source pressure. With pneumatically powered ventilators, gas flows down a pressure gradient from the wall, through the pressure-reducing valves, and to the patient without the need of a mechanical device such as a piston.

Two basic types of pneumatically powered ventilators are used: pneumatic ventilators and **fluidic** ventilators. Pneumatic ventilators may incorporate components such as Venturi devices or air entrainers, needle valves, flexible diaphragms, and spring-loaded valves to perform certain functions. For example, Venturi devices may be used to control an expiratory valve, and a needle valve may control the rate of gas flow during inspiration. Fluidic ventilators use fluidic components that are based on special pneumatic principles. Very few ventilators use the fluidic principle. (The section on fluidics later in this chapter presents a basic description of some fluidic components.)

Electrically Powered Ventilators

Electrically powered ventilators most often use standard electrical outlets (112 to 120 V alternating current [AC]) to power the internal components.* They also may have internal direct current (DC) batteries, which can provide electrical power during patient transport or in the event of a power failure. Some ventilators can also be connected to external DC batteries.

Electrically powered ventilators may use the electricity to power internal motors for operating air compressors, pistons, electrical solenoids, transducers, and microprocessors, all of which either provide gas flow to the patient or help control gas flow to the patient.

---

*In the United States, most standard electrical outlets use 112 V. Higher voltages (e.g., 220 V) are used in other countries.

Combined Power: Pneumatically Powered and Electronically or Microprocessor-Controlled Ventilators

One of the more common types of ventilators used in the ICU today is pneumatically powered and **microprocessor controlled.** Two 50-psi gas sources provide the pressure to deliver inspiratory gas flow. This gas flow usually is the same gas the patient receives during inspiration. Control of the inspiratory flow waveform is governed by a microprocessor. For example, the pattern of gas flow may be constant, producing a constant-flow waveform, or it may be rapid at the beginning of inspiration and gradually taper, producing a descending ramp waveform (see the section on inspiratory waveform and ventilator graphics later in this chapter). Programming of the microprocessor and its interaction with electrically operated flow valves or mechanical devices control this function. These ventilators require both electrical and pneumatic power sources.

PRESSURE DELIVERY

A ventilator does all or part of the work of breathing (WOB) for the patient. A ventilator can increase lung volume during inspiration by creating either negative- or positive-pressure gradients. The pressure gradient applied to the body results in gas flow to produce ventilation (Box 11-2).

Positive-Pressure Ventilators

A pressure gradient must exist for gas flow to occur. During normal spontaneous breathing, contraction of the inspiratory muscles initiates inspiration. During inspiration, the diaphragm contracts and descends, and the external intercostal muscles contract. The action of these muscles, especially the diaphragm, results in an increase in the intrathoracic volume. Intrapleural and intraalveolar pressures becomes subambient. This produces a pressure gradient from the mouth, which is at ambient pressure, to the alveoli, which are below ambient pressure. Consequently,

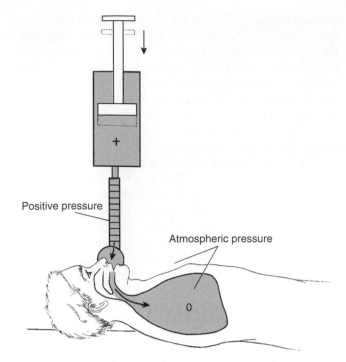

FIGURE 11-1 Application of positive pressure at the airway creates a pressure gradient between the mouth and the alveoli; as a result, gas flows into the lungs. (NOTE: This is a single-circuit ventilator, which is explained later in the chapter.)

air flows into the lungs. Expiration follows because passive relaxation of the respiratory muscles and chest wall recoil reduce the intrathoracic volume. Intraalveolar pressure becomes slightly positive (above ambient), and air flows out of the lungs.[11]

During positive-pressure ventilation, a supraatmospheric pressure is created at the mouth, and the intraalveolar pressure is ambient at the beginning of the breath. As a result, air flows into the lungs, expanding them and the chest wall (Figure 11-1). **Positive-pressure ventilators** are by far the most common method of ventilation used today. Expiration occurs the same way as in spontaneous ventilation.

Negative-Pressure Ventilators

Negative-pressure ventilators (NPVs) currently are rarely used in the ventilation of patients. A historical perspective on their function is presented in Historical Note 11-1 and Figure 11-2.

Combined-Pressure Devices

The most common example of a combined-pressure device is a **high-frequency oscillator.** This is a form of **high-frequency ventilation (HFV)** that produces oscillating gas pressure waveforms at the upper airway. The waveform is a **sinusoidal** pattern with positive- and negative-pressure oscillations produced at the upper airway by an oscillating device (Figure 11-3). The section in this chapter on high-frequency ventilation explains oscillator function.

BOX 11-2	Types and Examples of Pressure Ventilators

NEGATIVE-PRESSURE VENTILATORS
· Iron lung
· Chest cuirass

POSITIVE-PRESSURE VENTILATORS
· Most ventilators in use today are positive-pressure ventilators, such as the Puritan Bennett 840, the Servo[i], and the Hamilton G5 ventilators

POSITIVE/NEGATIVE PRESSURE VENTILATORS
· High-frequency oscillators

Negative-Pressure Ventilators

Negative-pressure ventilators (NPVs) generally enclose the thoracic area and create a subatmospheric pressure around the chest wall (see Figure 11-2). This negative pressure is transmitted across the chest wall, resulting in reduced intrapleural and intraalveolar pressures. The pressure at the mouth is atmospheric pressure, creating a pressure gradient between the mouth and the alveoli similar to the normal spontaneous pressure gradient. Air flows into the lungs. During exhalation, the negative pressure around the chest is returned to ambient, the intraalveolar pressure becomes slightly positive, and air flows out of the lungs. Examples of these types of devices are the **iron lung** *and the* **chest cuirass**.[11] *These ventilators currently are not widely used, but they occasionally are used in the home as an alternative form of ventilation for ventilator-dependent patients.*

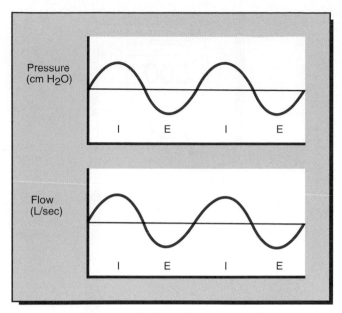

FIGURE 11-3 The sinusoidal waveform produced by an oscillator. *I,* Inspiration; *E,* expiration.

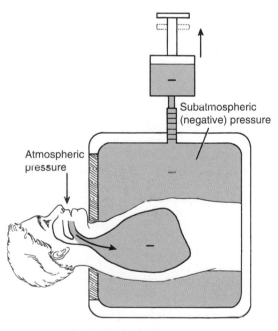

FIGURE 11-2 Application of subatmospheric pressure around the chest wall causes a pressure drop in the alveoli, and air flows into the lungs; this is referred to as *negative-pressure ventilation (NPV).*

Oscillators are used with neonatal, pediatric, and adult patients. The chapter on infant and pediatric ventilation provides an example of an oscillator, the Sensormedics 3100A.

CONTROL SYSTEMS AND CIRCUITS

A combination of mechanical, pneumatic, and electronic devices in the ventilator constitutes the control or decision-making functions of the unit. These control systems and circuits, which govern ventilator operation, can create an **open-loop** or a **closed-loop** system.

Open-Loop and Closed-Loop Systems

The terms *open loop* and *closed loop* describe the level of control within a ventilator. Unintelligent ventilators are called *open-loop systems.* When the operator establishes a setting, such as the tidal volume (V_T), the unit delivers the set amount of volume. In reality, this volume might leak into the room and never reach the patient. Unfortunately, an open-loop system cannot discern the difference between the volume actually delivered and the set volume and respond to this difference (Figure 11-4A).

Suppose a robot is pouring water from a 1-L beaker of water into a 0.75-L container. If not programmed otherwise, the robot pours the liter of water, filling the container but spilling the excess (0.25 L) on the ground. This is an example of open-loop programming. On the other hand, an intelligent robot that can see the container and determine when it is full can stop pouring, if programmed to do so. This example demonstrates closed-loop programming.

Closed-loop systems are intelligent systems that use a microprocessor to control function.[12] For example, the manufacturer programs a responsive system into the computer to deliver a specific quantity (e.g., V_T). This system measures the volume delivered by the ventilator and exhaled by the patient, makes a comparison, and adjusts the volume delivery based on this comparison to deliver the amount of volume set on the control panel. Figure 11-4B shows an algorithm for a closed-loop system.[11] This system is similar to cruise control on a car. You set the

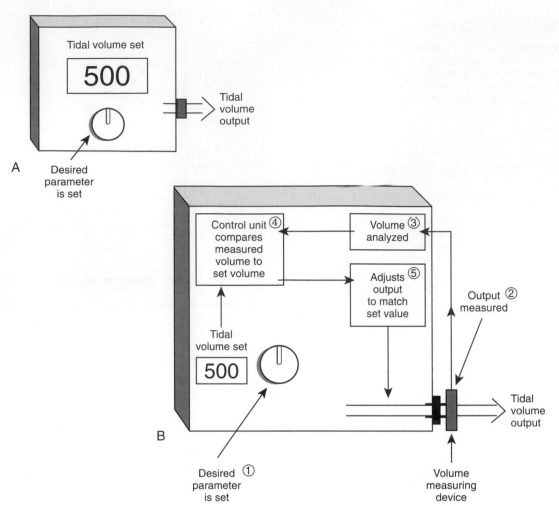

FIGURE 11-4 A, Open-loop system. The path through the device is straight from the control panel to the internal device and out to the patient. No feedback is provided to the ventilator about the output. **B,** The ventilator "closes the loop" by measuring the gas exhaled by the patient, comparing it to the set value, and feeding this information back to the machine. (See text for further explanation.) (From Pilbeam SP, Cairo JM: *Mechanical ventilation: physiological and clinical applications,* ed 4, St Louis, 2006, Mosby.)

cruise control at the speed you want the car to go. The car then compares the actual speed with how fast you want to go. If the car is going too slowly, the cruise control accelerates the car. You do not have to make any adjustments; the cruise control does it for you. This is a closed-loop system. It is closed because it compares the input to the output and "closes the loop" (Figure 11-4B). These systems are also called *feedback systems* and *servo-controlled systems.* An example of a closed-loop or intelligent system is an auto set point (Box 11-3).[5,7]

All new commercially available ventilators now have some form of closed-loop logic. However, they are not without problems. New modes of ventilation can be introduced on the market without any patient testing. The manufacturer has only to prove that the mode performs the intended function and that the software has been validated (Box 11-4).[13] Clinical Rounds 11-1 provides an exercise to test your understanding of closed- and open-loop systems.

BOX 11-3	Auto Set Point

With auto set point, the output of the ventilator is forced to follow or match an operator preset input based on several layers of conditional logic. The ventilator selects which operator-adjusted controls (set points) are enforced at the moment. For example, in the pressure augmentation mode of the BEAR 1000, inspiration starts out delivering a constant pressure. This action is modified by a series of "if-then" statements. If the set volume has not been met by the time flow decreases to the set value, the ventilator switches to volume ventilation and maintains the flow at the set flow value.

Control Panel

The control panel, or user interface, is located on the front of most ventilators. It contains the controls by which the operator can adjust such variables as the respiratory rate (f), V_T, set pressure (P_{set}), and inspiratory time (T_I) (Figure 11-5).

Pneumatic Circuit

The **pneumatic circuit** consists of a series of tubing that directs gas flow both within the ventilator (the **internal circuit**) and from the ventilator to the patient (the external or **patient circuit**).

Internal Circuit

The internal circuit conducts gas generated by the power source, passes it through various mechanical or pneumatic

---

BOX 11-4	Smart Modes, Handguns, and Tequila

Rob Chatburn reminds us with a quotation that applies very well to the use of closed-loop ventilation. "A computer lets you make more mistakes faster than any invention in human history . . . with the possible exception of handguns and tequila."

From Branson RD: Dual control modes, closed loop ventilation, handguns and tequila (editorial), *Respir Care* 46:232, 2001.

CLINICAL ROUNDS 11-1

Open-Loop and Closed-Loop Ventilator Systems

Part I

A respiratory therapist sets a ventilator tidal volume at 650 mL; the peak inspiratory pressure is 8 cm H_2O. The volume measured at the exhalation valve is 500 mL. These measurements occur over the next several breaths with no changes. Is this open-loop or closed-loop logic?

Part II

A respiratory therapist sets the tidal volume at 650 mL. After one breath, the exhaled volume measures 500 mL, and the peak pressure is 8 cm H_2O. After a second breath, the exhaled volume is 600 mL, and the peak pressure is 14 cm H_2O. After a third breath, the exhaled volume is 649 mL, and the peak pressure is 16 cm H_2O. What type of system is this?

See Evolve Resources for the answer.

---

mechanisms, and finally directs it to the **external circuit.** Internal circuits are either single or double circuits (Box 11-5).

In a single-circuit ventilator, the gas enters the ventilator and goes directly to the patient (Figure 11-6). This design is the most common one in currently used ventilators. A double-circuit ventilator consists of two gas sources. One gas source goes to the patient from a bag or bellows, and the other actively compresses the bag or bellows. A double circuit is also called a *bellows* or *"bag-in-a-chamber"* design. The double-circuit design has become nearly extinct. The most recent double-circuit ventilator on the market was the Cardiopulmonary Venturi ventilator (Figure 11-7).

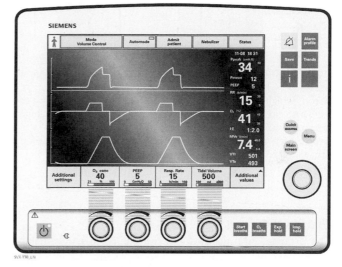

FIGURE 11-5 User interface of the Servo' ventilator. (Courtesy Maquet, Bridgewater, N.J.)

BOX 11-5	Types of Internal Circuits

- A single circuit is one in which the gas supply that powers the ventilator is the same gas that goes to the patient.
- A double circuit has a source gas that powers the unit by compressing a bag or bellows containing the gas that goes to the patient.

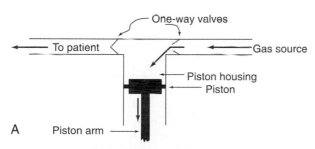

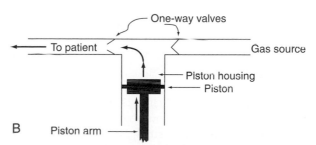

FIGURE 11-6 Single-circuit ventilator. **A,** Gases are drawn into the cylinder during the expiratory phase. **B,** During inspiration, the piston moves upward into the cylinder, sending gas directly to the patient circuit. (From Pilbeam SP: *Mechanical ventilation: physiological and clinical applications,* ed 3, St Louis, 1998, Mosby.)

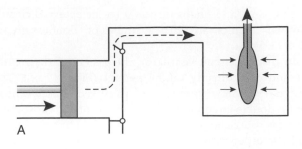

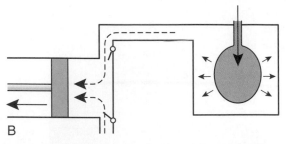

FIGURE 11-7 Simple diagram of a piston-driven, double-circuit system (i.e., bag-in-a-chamber). **A,** Forward stroke of the piston, which causes gas to flow to the chamber containing the bag (first circuit). The bag (second circuit) collapses, sending gas to the patient (inspiration). **B,** Backward stroke of the piston, with gas entering the piston cylinder. Gas also enters the bag, filling it for the next patient inspiration. (See text for description.)

External Circuit

The external circuit conducts the gas from the ventilator to the patient and from the patient through an expiratory valve to the room. The external circuit is commonly called the *ventilator circuit* or the *patient circuit* (Figure 11-8). Figure 11-8A shows a ventilator circuit with an externally mounted expiratory valve; Figure 11-8B shows a ventilator circuit with an internally mounted exhalation valve, the most common design used in critical care ventilators today.

With an external circuit, gas flows both through the main inspiratory line to the patient and to the expiratory valve line during inspiration. This line inflates a balloon or puts pressure on a diaphragm, closing a hole. The hole in the exhalation valve is where the patient's exhaled gases normally vent into the room. During inspiration the hole is covered by the balloon or diaphragm. During exhalation, no gas goes through the main inspiratory line or the expiratory valve line. The balloon deflates, and the patient's exhaled volume passes through the open hole (Figure 11-8A, enlarged portion).

Almost all new ventilator circuits use a patient circuit with the exhalation valve mounted inside the machine. These internal valves are usually low-resistance, large-diameter, flexible plastic diaphragms. They operate similar to the externally mounted expiratory valve. During inspiration either gas pressure or a mechanical device pushes the valve over the exhalation hole. Exhaled gas normally passes

through this hole. During exhalation the valve is opened and the patient's exhaled volume can pass through the hole.

DRIVE MECHANISMS (POWER TRANSMISSION AND CONVERSION SYSTEMS)

The power source, gas or electricity, provides the energy to power mechanical devices. This energy and the devices they control ultimately generate a pressure gradient. The pressure gradient provides all or part of the patient's work of breathing. These internal drive mechanisms are also called the **power transmission systems.** They transmit the original energy source (gas, electricity, or both) to direct gas flow to the patient.

From an engineering standpoint, two basic categories describe the power transmission systems in most conventional ventilators: those that control volume delivery and those that control flow delivery.[9,14,15] For electrically powered ventilators that control volume delivery, these systems might be compressors or blowers and volume-displacement devices. For pneumatically powered systems, the power transmission unit may consist of Venturi entrainers, flexible diaphragms, or specially designed pneumatic or fluidic elements. For pneumatically powered, microprocessor-controlled units, the power transmission devices might be **flow-control valves.**

In the past, respiratory therapy students spent a great deal of time studying ventilator systems because respiratory therapists often were called upon to repair the systems or at least to be able to answer questions about them. Now, less emphasis is placed on this information, and respiratory therapists no longer repair these devices. That function has been given to bioengineering departments and technical support personnel. The following section briefly reviews some examples of volume-displacement devices and flow-control valves.

Compressors or Blowers

Compressors can be driven by pistons, rotating blades (vanes), moving diaphragms, or bellows. Hospitals use large, piston-type, water-cooled compressors to supply high-pressure air for wall air outlets (see Chapter 2). Small, portable compressors are used to power small-volume nebulizers and similar devices. The most common type of compressor used for ventilators is the rotary compressor (Historical Note 11-2). The rotor acts as a fan, drawing air from the room, compressing it, and directing it through the ventilator's internal circuit. Examples of contemporary ventilators that use an internal rotary device are the LTV ventilator and the VIASYS AVEA ventilator (see Chapters 12 and 14).

Volume-Displacement Designs

Some ventilators use volume-displacement devices, including pistons, bellows, or similar "bag-in-a-chamber"

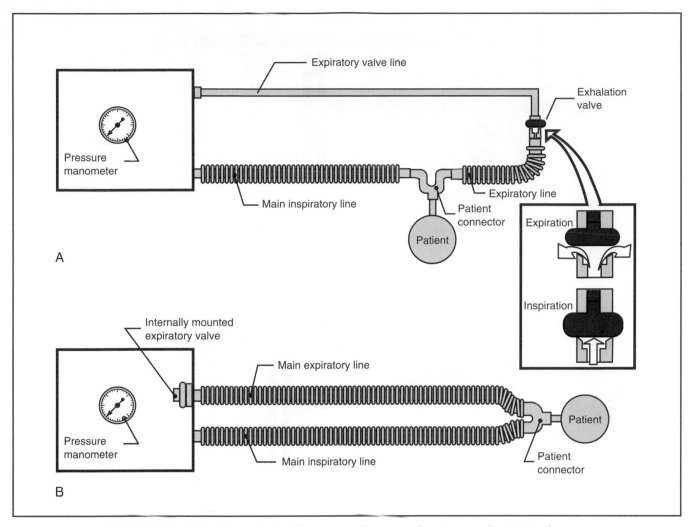

FIGURE 11-8 A, Ventilator circuit with an externally mounted expiratory valve. **B,** Ventilator circuit with an internally mounted exhalation valve. (See text for further explanation.)

HISTORICAL NOTE 11-2

Use of the Rotary Compressor
Some older ventilators developed in the 1950s and 1960s were never connected to wall air sources because at that time wall outlets for air were scarce. An internal compressor sometimes was used within the ventilator as the power source itself. For example, the rotating vane compressor in the MA-1 provided the pressure to power the drive mechanism. In this case, an electric motor powered a blower that held a series of blades, similar to a fan. The rotary blower forced air to flow into a canister containing a bellows. The forced air pushed up on the bellows, causing them to empty, and the gas inside the bellows flowed to the patient.

mechanisms to deliver a positive-pressure breath.[14] Some ventilators, such as the Cardiopulmonary Venturi, used the bag-in-a-chamber design (see Figure 11-7). Others, such as the Puritan Bennett 740 and 760 ventilators, use a piston design (see Chapter 12). Figure 11-9A shows an example of a single-circuit piston design. During the backward stroke of the piston, gas is drawn into the piston's cylinder. On the upward stroke of the piston, gas flows out of the cylinder, through the ventilator circuit, and to the patient. Some home care ventilators also use pistons.

Pistons

Two piston designs have been used for ventilators, direct drive and indirect drive. In a direct-drive piston, or **linear-drive piston,** special gearing connects an electrical motor to a piston rod or arm (see Figure 11-9A). The rod moves the piston forward linearly inside the cylinder housing at a constant rate. This movement normally produces a constant or rectangular waveform of gas flow to the patient, an ascending ramp volume waveform, and a relatively linear ascending ramp pressure waveform (Figure 11-10). Ventilators that incorporate linear-drive pistons are usually single-circuit units. Some high-frequency ventilators use **direct-drive pistons.**

Contemporary rolling seal or low-resistance materials have helped eliminate the friction of the early piston-

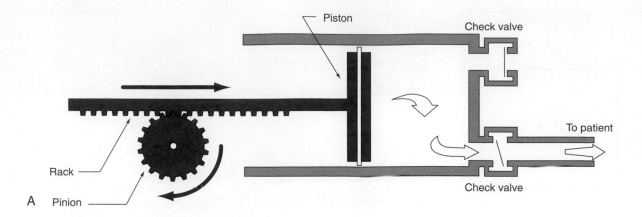

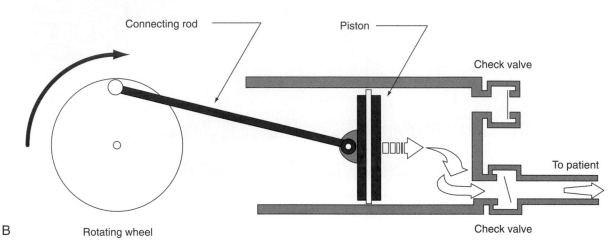

FIGURE 11-9 Linear **(A)** and rotary **(B)** piston-driven mechanisms for ventilators. (Redrawn from Dupuis Y: *Ventilators,* ed 2, St Louis, 1992, Mosby.)

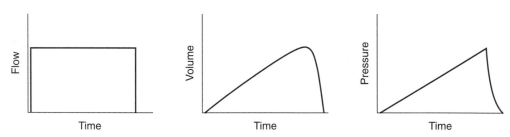

FIGURE 11-10 Flow-time, volume-time, and pressure-time curves generated by a linear-drive piston.

cylinder designs. For example, the Puritan Bennett 740 uses a low-resistance piston that provides all the gas flow to the patient and does not require an external high-pressure gas source to function (electrically powered). In addition, it can produce not only a constant flow but also a descending flow waveform.

Rotary, or nonlinear-drive, pistons are sometimes called *eccentric-drive pistons.* The nonlinear-drive piston is seldom used in ventilator design at this time, although the Lifecare PLV-100 and -102 and the Puritan Bennett Companion 2801 home care ventilator do use this design (see Chapter

14). Figure 11-9B illustrates the function of a nonlinear-drive piston. Historical Note 11-3 illustrates how this device works and the types of flow and pressure waveforms it produces.

Spring-Loaded Bellows

Another volume design unit uses a spring-loaded bellows as the force that delivers the breath (Figure 11-11).[16] A mixture of oxygen and air at the desired fractional inspired oxygen (F_IO_2) flows into the spring-loaded bellows. The operator can tighten the tension on the spring to increase

The Rotary Drive Piston
The first figure below shows a complete forward cycle of a rotary drive piston. The piston is connected to the outer edge of the rotary wheel. The piston's forward motion is short at the beginning of inspiration (A_1 to B_1), rapid at midinspiration (B_1 to C_1), and slow again at the end of inspiration (C_1 to D_1). This change in speed produces the sine wave–like flow curve shown by the second figure. Gas flow is slowest at the beginning and end of inspiration and fastest at midinspiration, producing a sine wave–like flow pattern. This type of waveform is characteristic of rotary drive pistons.

(NOTE: The rotary drive piston produces half of the sinusoidal wave during the inspiratory phase, but it is commonly referred to as a sine wave or a pattern similar to a sine wave.)

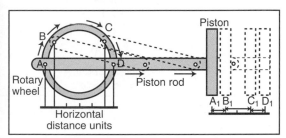

Diagram of a rotary-driven piston's movement. The times between points A and B, B and C, and C and D are equal. The piston travels different distances in the same amount of time and therefore moves at different speeds from A_1 to B_1, from B_1 to C_1, and from C_1 to D_1.

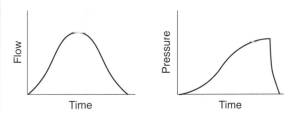

Flow-time and pressure-time curves created by a rotary-driven piston, positive-pressure ventilator during volume delivery.

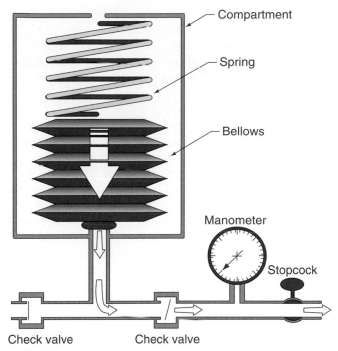

FIGURE 11-11 Spring-loaded bellows unit. (See text for description.) (Redrawn from Dupuis Y: *Ventilators,* ed 2, St Louis, 1992, Mosby.)

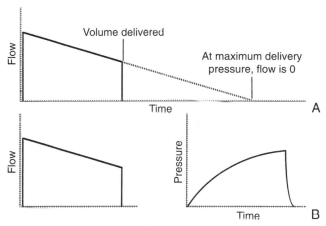

FIGURE 11-12 A, The primary flow-time curve from a spring-loaded bellows with a low working pressure and a high system resistance (i.e., high patient airway resistance and low lung compliance). **B,** Flow-time and pressure-time curves for this system when the breath is time cycled.

the force exerted against the bellows and the pressure delivered to the patient. The Servo 900C ventilator uses this type of power transmission system, which can be adjusted up to 120 cm H_2O. (NOTE: The Servo 900C is still used in some U.S. hospitals; however, it will no longer be serviced by the manufacturer after 2011. It will have been in service for 39 years upon its retirement.)

The flow and pressure curves produced by this system resemble those of a linear-drive piston when the working pressure is high and the system resistance (i.e., the patient's lung condition and the patient circuit) is low (see Figure 11-10). When the working pressure is low, especially when the system resistance is high, the flow curve descends during inspiration (Figure 11-12).

Flow-Control Valves

Most current ICU ventilators use valves that precisely control flow to the patient. In general, high-pressure sources of air and oxygen are mixed and delivered at the desired F_1O_2 to accumulator chambers. These chambers often are similar in shape to medical gas cylinders. They hold about 2 to 3 L of gas under pressure and act as reservoirs from which inspired gas for the patient can be withdrawn. The VIASYS AVEA is an example of a ventilator with an accumulator chamber.

Other ventilators, such as the Servo[i] (Maquet, Inc., Bridgewater, NJ), take the incoming gas sources individually, regulate their pressures to precise values, and then mix the gases directly without going through an accumulation chamber. This type of system tends to consume less gas during operation than one that uses an accumulator chamber.

Ultimately the gas is sent through one or more valves that control the inspiratory gas flow. These valves can be moved in small, precise increments and at varying rates because their activity is governed by a microprocessor. Because it responds so quickly, a flow-control valve can precisely control the exact pattern of gas and pressure. The more technology has advanced, the faster and more dependable flow valves have become. Three types of flow-controlling valves deserve further discussion: proportional solenoid valves, stepper motors with valves, and digital valves with on/off configurations.

Proportional Solenoid Valves

Proportional solenoid valves control flow by using an on/off switch (Figure 11-13). Commonly, this valve has a gate or plunger, a valve seat, an electromagnet, a diaphragm, a spring, two electrical contacts, and an adjustable electric current.

A proportional solenoid valve operates on a basic principle of physics concerning electricity and magnetism. When a current flows through a wire, it creates a magnetic field. Winding a wire into a coil increases the strength of the magnetic field around the wire. Adding an iron rod within the coiled wire further increases the magnetism and produces an electromagnet.

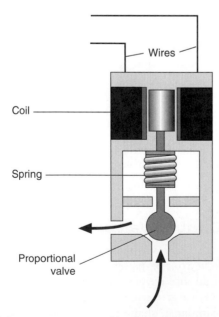

FIGURE 11-13 Proportional solenoid valve. Gas flows upward through the bottom of the valve and out through the side. (See text for description.) (Redrawn from Sanborn WG: Microprocessor-based mechanical ventilation, *Respir Care* 38:72, 1993.)

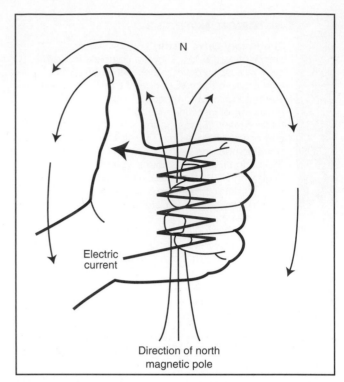

FIGURE 11-14 A solenoid uses a coil of wire. An electrical current is passed through the coil, generating a magnetic field. The direction of the magnetic field is indicated by the arrows. If you hold your left hand with your thumb pointed up and your fingers slightly curved, the curve of your fingers is the direction of the electrical current through the coil, and your thumb is pointed in the direction of magnetic north. (See text for further explanation.)

The polarity of an electromagnet can be determined using the left-hand rule (Figure 11-14). The curved fingers indicate the electric current, and the upward-directed thumb points to the north magnetic pole. When the rod is connected inline in the center of the coiled wire, it moves up and down, depending on the strength of the electric current and the magnetic field it creates. The action of this electromagnet basically describes how solenoid valves operate.[14]

The variation in the amount of current flowing through the coiled wire results in movement of the rod or plunger and causes the plunger to assume a specific position. Some solenoids are called *proportional solenoid valves* because the valves move in proportion to the current applied and open a hole or gate a proportional amount. Examples of ventilators with proportional solenoid valves are the Hamilton GALILEO, the Dräger EvitaXL, and the Maquet Servo[i].

In a proportional solenoid valve used to govern gas flow (see Figure 11-13), gas enters the bottom of the valve when the metal rod with the ball at the base moves upward. This movement opens a hole into the valve. The flow can then be directed out another hole and to the patient.

Stepper Motors with Valves

Stepper motors can move in very rapid, discrete steps to open or close a valve. Figure 11-15A shows an example of

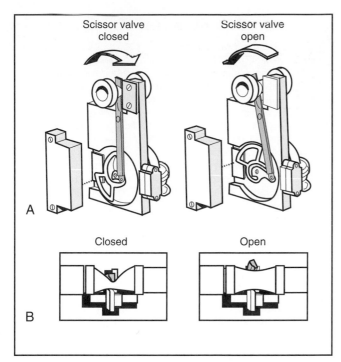

FIGURE 11-15 Stepper motor with a scissor valve in the Siemens Servo 900C ventilator. **A,** A cam on the motor controls the moving arm. On the left, the valve is shown in the closed position; on the right, it is completely open. **B,** Closing and opening of the internal circuit by the scissor valve. (**A** courtesy Maquet, Bridgewater, N.J.)

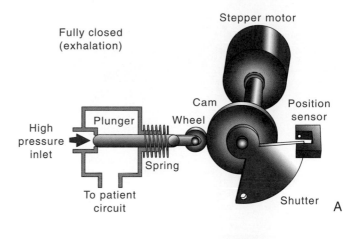

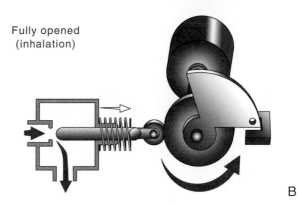

FIGURE 11-16 Schematic of a microprocessor-operated flow valve. (See text for description.) (Redrawn from Dupuis Y: *Ventilators,* ed 2, St Louis, 1992, Mosby.)

a stepper motor. Notice the lever arm. It is connected at its base to a rotating metal "wheel." The wheel moves in fixed steps, almost like the teeth on a gear. This movement is very rapid. As the wheel moves, the arm moves forward and back. The arm moves toward a fixed metal post to the right of the moving arm. The movement is like closing a pair of scissors. It closes a plastic tube, as shown on the lower left of Figure 11-15B. When the arm moves away from the metal post, the tube reopens, allowing gas to flow through it (right side of Figure 11-15B). Electricity is used to power the motor that controls the movement of the lever arm.

Figure 11-16 shows a microprocessor-controlled stepper motor, which consists of a cam connected to a stepper motor and a spring-loaded plunger attached to a wheel. The tension of the spring pushes the wheel against the perimeter of the cam. During exhalation, the plunger occludes the gas outlet and stops flow to the patient (Figure 11-16A). During inspiration, the motor turns the cam, and the spring tension relaxes, although contact is still maintained. Because of this action, the plunger moves to the right (Figure 11-16B), and gas flows to the patient. An optical sensor and a shutter (not shown) send information to the microprocessor about the position of the cam. With microprocessor control, the motor can rotate the cam in many specific steps and at different speeds, allowing the microprocessor to deliver gas flow in the pattern and amount the operator selects.[14,16,17]

Although some ventilators incorporate stepper motors as flow-control valves, several different motor and cam designs for controlling valve or poppet positions are used in each. The Bear 1000 and the Bird 8400 ventilators incorporate stepper motor–driven cam devices that actuate flow-control valves. Figure 11-17 shows an example of an externally actuated proportional valve.[14] Several different motor and cam designs are available for controlling valve or poppet position.

Digital Valve On/Off Configuration
With a digital valve on/off configuration, several valves operate simultaneously, assuming either an open or a closed position (Figure 11-18). An individual valve produces a specific flow by opening or closing an orifice of a particular size. Depending on which valves are open, the amount of flow can be varied. The Infant Star ventilator used this type of valve configuration.

Fluidic Elements in Power Transmission Design

Units that use fluidics, or fluid logic, to deliver gas flow to the patient do not require moving parts or electrical

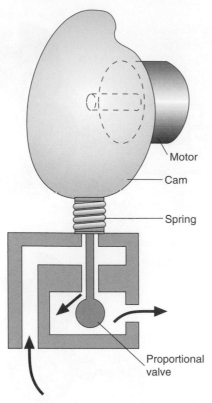

FIGURE 11-17 Example of an externally actuated proportional valve. (See text for description.) (Redrawn from Sanborn WG: Microprocessor-based mechanical ventilation, *Respir Care* 38:72, 1993.)

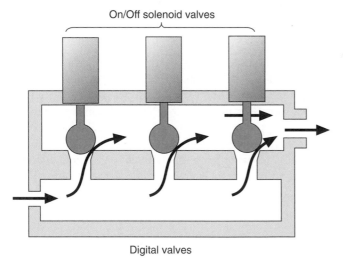

FIGURE 11-18 On/off digital valve design for flow control. Each valve controls a critical orifice and thus a specified flow. The number of discrete flow steps (from zero upward) becomes 2^n, where n is the number of valves. (Redrawn from Sanborn WG: Microprocessor-based mechanical ventilation, *Respir Care* 38:72, 1993.)

circuits to function. Control is provided solely through fluid dynamics. Fluidic units use air and oxygen as the operating media and have all the same basic functional controls as electrically operated ventilators.[18] The Bio-Med MPV 10 is an example of a fluidic ventilator (see Chapter 14).

Because some fluidic ventilators are not disrupted by electromagnetic interference, as is encountered in magnetic resonance imaging (MRI) suites, they can be used in this environment. Of course, they must be constructed of nonferrous metals, such as aluminum. Modifications can also be made to other ventilators to make them MRI compatible.[18]

Fluidic devices operate on two basic physical principles: wall attachment and **beam deflection.** The principle of wall attachment is commonly called the **Coanda effect,** a phenomenon that occurs when an air stream (jet stream) is forced through an opening (Historical Note 11-4 and Figure 11-19). The jet exits the opening, creating a localized drop in pressure adjacent to itself. Ambient air is drawn toward the jet stream on all sides as a result of the localized low pressure associated with the rapid movement of the jet through the air (Figure 11-19A).

When a wall is added to one side of the jet stream (Figure 11-19B), the entrained gas can enter only from the opposite side. However, a **separation bubble** (a low-pressure vortex) develops between the wall and the jet stream. The bubble attracts or bends the jet stream toward the wall. The pocket of turbulence forms an air foil, similar to that seen with an airplane wing.[16,17] When the gas entrained into the bubble from the jet stream equals the amount of air moving from the vortex flow of the bubble back to the jet stream, the attachment is stable.

The second important phenomenon of fluid logic is beam deflection. When a beam or jet of gas is moving through a fluidic device (Figure 11-20A, P_S to O_2), the direction of the beam can be changed by hitting the beam with another jet of gas (Figure 11-20B). The second gas jet usually comes from the side, at a right angle to the main jet stream (Figure 11-20B, C_1 to C_2). Note in Figure 11-20 how this changes the gas output in the device from O_2 to O_1.

The principles of wall attachment and beam deflection can be used to design a host of other devices, which in turn are used in the construction of fluidic ventilators. The nomenclature of fluidics originated in digital electronics, which is the reason many terms (e.g., **flip-flop component**

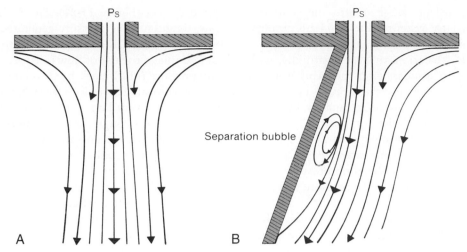

FIGURE 11-19 The Coanda effect (wall attachment phenomenon). **A,** Turbulent jet flow (P$_S$) causes a local drop in lateral pressure and draws air inward. **B,** A wall placed adjacent to the jet stream creates a low-pressure vortex or separation bubble. The gas stream tends to bend toward that wall. (From Dupuis Y: *Ventilators,* ed 2, St Louis, 1992, Mosby.)

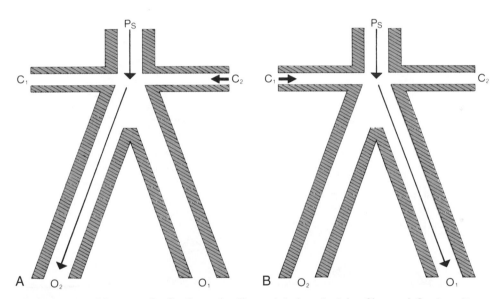

FIGURE 11-20 Diagram of a flip-flop valve illustrating the principle of beam deflection. (See text for explanation.) (From Dupuis Y: *Ventilators,* ed 2, St Louis, 1992, Mosby.)

and *OR/NOR gate*) seem unusual in relation to medical terminology. More details about fluidics are beyond the scope of this text.

Contemporary Drive Mechanisms and Control Valves

For more recently designed ventilators, such as the Servo^i and the Hamilton G5, little information is available from the manufacturer about the specific design of the internal components. This is primarily because technical support representatives are responsible for the repair of these units. Respiratory therapists have had less and less involvement with the repair and servicing of ventilators. Consequently, less emphasis is placed on discovering and learning the function of these newer machine designs.

ADDITIONAL DEVICES USED DURING PATIENT VENTILATION

In addition to the primary drive mechanism of a ventilator, other components are important to its operation. Such a component is the expiratory valve.

Expiratory Valves for Providing Positive End-Expiratory Pressure

Expiratory valves in a ventilator normally close during inspiration, directing gas flow into the patient's lungs, and open during exhalation, allowing the patient to exhale through a valve. Optimally designed expiratory valves allow unrestricted flow from the patient. Older valves often increased resistance to gas flow when expiratory flow was high or when the patient coughed into the ventilator circuit.[19] Newer ventilator systems try to avoid this problem by using very low-resistance, large-diameter valves.

Besides allowing exhalation to occur naturally, with pressures returning to atmospheric, the ventilator can apply positive pressure during exhalation to increase or restore the patient's functional residual capacity. In certain types of patients, the application of positive pressures during exhalation helps improve oxygenation; this technique is referred to as *positive end-expiratory pressure,* or *PEEP.* Use of PEEP elevates the baseline pressure above ambient (zero). Baseline pressure is the pressure sustained during expiration.

When PEEP is selected, it is the threshold-resistive characteristics of the expiratory valve that provide PEEP. The PEEP valve generally is located inside the ventilator housing. Pressure on exhalation is accomplished in one of two ways: **flow resistance** or **threshold resistance.**

Flow resistors direct expiratory flow through an orifice or resistor, such as a screw clamp, and act as expiratory retard devices (Figure 11-21). The higher the rate of gas flow, the higher the pressure generated. If the expiratory period is extended, the baseline pressure can return to zero. An example of the use of flow resistors is a positive expiratory pressure (PEP) mask used to combat atelectasis and aid the removal of secretions (see Chapter 7). It is used less commonly in ventilator circuits because the rapid flow from a patient's cough can cause pressure to be very high in the patient's lungs and airways.

Threshold resistors allow expiratory flow to continue unimpeded until the pressure in the circuit equals the threshold value set; that is, the desired PEEP level. A true threshold resistor is unaffected by the rate of flow (Figure 11-22). Most newer generation ventilators have PEEP capabilities built into their design and operate through the expiratory valves, which generally are located internally.

Spring-Loaded Valves

A spring-loaded valve may also be used to create PEEP (Figure 11-23). Changing the spring tension adjusts the

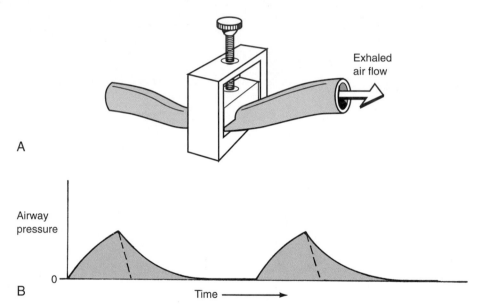

FIGURE 11-21 A, Screw clamp as an example of a flow resistor. **B,** Pressure-time curve for a normal breath with normal exhalation *(dashed line)* and with expiratory retard *(solid line).* (From Pilbeam SP: *Mechanical ventilation: physiological and clinical applications,* ed 3, St Louis, 1998, Mosby.)

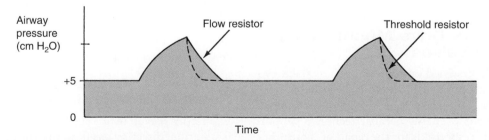

FIGURE 11-22 This airway pressure curve shows a mandatory breath plus positive end-expiratory pressure (PEEP) with two different expiratory flow curves. The solid line indicates pressure with a flow resistor; pressure can vary with flow. The dashed line represents a threshold resistor; flow leaves the lungs rapidly until the set baseline is reached. (From Pilbeam SP: *Mechanical ventilation: physiological and clinical applications,* ed 3, St Louis, 1998, Mosby.)

amount of pressure needed to move the valve off its seat and allows expiration to occur. When the circuit pressure equals the force applied on the valve by the spring, the valve closes. Some of these devices may have flow-resistor characteristics when expiratory flows are high. The Pulmonetics LTV 1000 is a currently used ventilator with an externally mounted PEEP valve (see Chapter 14). External PEEP valves also are commonly used on manual resuscitation bags.

Diaphragm Expiratory Valves

Diaphragm expiratory valves commonly incorporate a large-diameter diaphragm to control expiratory gas flow and PEEP. Figure 11-24 shows the diaphragm valve from a Servo[i] ventilator. Figure 11-25 uses a balloon to illustrate the function of the expiratory valve. During inspiration, the ventilator pressurizes the diaphragm (illustrated as a balloon) and closes an expiratory orifice (Figure 11-25A). During normal expiration, the pressure against the diaphragm (balloon) is released, and the patient's expiratory gas flow occurs unimpeded (Figure 11-25C). When PEEP is applied, a proportional pressure is held against the diaphragm (balloon) so that the pressure at the end of exhalation is equal to the PEEP value set by the operator (Figure 11-25B).

Magnetic and Electromagnetic Valves: PEEP Valves

Some PEEP valves use magnetic forces (Figure 11-26) or electromagnetic forces to oppose gas pressure.[20] A metallic valve is held on its seat by magnetic attraction supplied by an adjustable magnet. The threaded adjustment moves the

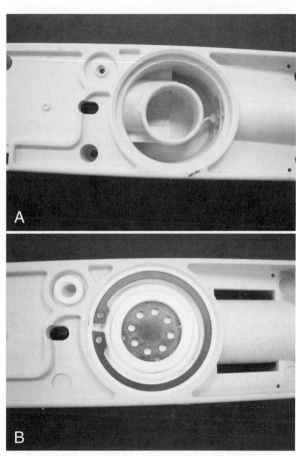

FIGURE 11-24 Diaphragm expiratory valve on the Servo[i] ventilator. **A,** Housing over which the expiratory diaphragm (valve) normally sits. The visible openings represent the channels through which expiratory gas is routed when the diaphragm is in position to allow exhalation. **B,** Diaphragm in position over the opening.

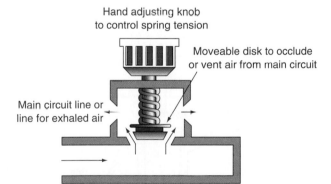

FIGURE 11-23 Spring-loaded positive end-expiratory pressure (PEEP) valve. (Modified from Pilbeam SP: *Mechanical ventilation: physiological and clinical applications,* ed 2, St Louis, 1992, Mosby.)

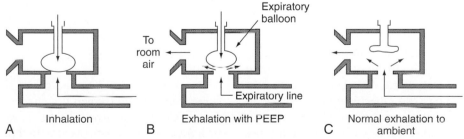

FIGURE 11-25 Functioning of a diaphragm expiratory valve. **A,** A balloon valve is used to illustrate inspiration; the balloon is fully inflated during inspiration, blocking the expiratory channel. Diaphragm valves function in the same way. **B,** The expiratory valve (balloon or diaphragm) remains partially pressured during exhalation and closes to keep positive pressure in the circuit at end-exhalation. **C,** The expiratory valve opens completely to allow unimpeded flow of the exhaled gas. (See text for description.) (From Pilbeam SP: *Mechanical ventilation: physiological and clinical applications,* ed 2, St Louis, 1992, Mosby.)

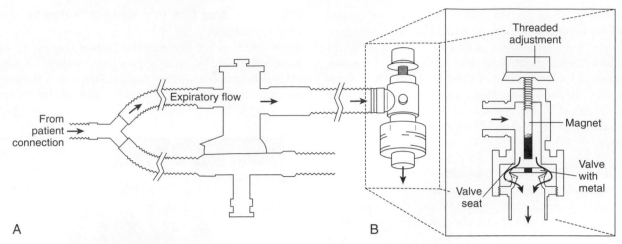

A

B

FIGURE 11-26 Magnetic positive end-expiratory pressure (PEEP) valve. **A,** The valve is connected to a typical ventilator circuit with the expiratory valve mounted inline. Arrows show the direction of expiratory flow. **B,** Detail of the magnetic valve. The threaded adjustment moves the magnet closer to or farther from the metal valve, which increases or decreases, respectively, the magnetic attraction. The greater the attraction, the greater the pressure needed to lift the valve from its seat.

magnet closer to or farther from the metal valve, causing an increase or decrease, respectively, in magnetic attraction. The greater the attraction, the greater the pressure needed to push the valve off its seat and allow gas flow from the circuit. If the cross-sectional area of the device is small or restricted, a magnetic PEEP valve can act as a flow resistor.

Electromagnetic valves are slightly different from magnetic valves, because solenoids are often used in their construction. In an electromagnetic valve, the amount of electric current that flows to the solenoid is regulated by a rheostat. The solenoid creates a downward force through an actuating shaft. The actuating shaft pushes against a diaphragm, which opposes expiratory gas flow. The stronger the current, the stronger the downward force and the higher the PEEP level. The Maquet Servo[i] and Hamilton Veolar ventilators use an electromagnetic device to control the expiratory diaphragm that controls the level of PEEP in the patient circuit (Figure 11-27).

Continuous Positive Airway Pressure (CPAP) Devices

Continuous positive airway pressure is very similar to PEEP. CPAP provides positive airway pressure, but it is restricted by definition to use in spontaneously breathing patients. Some CPAP devices are designed for home care to treat sleep apnea (these CPAP machines are described in Chapter 14). Some CPAP systems are used for neonates (see Chapter 13). CPAP also can be used for certain types of hospitalized patients who are able to breathe spontaneously but who need help with oxygenation. Examples of illnesses for which CPAP often is indicated include cardiogenic pulmonary edema and hypoxemic respiratory failure. In these cases, CPAP generally is provided by a ventilator or CPAP device.

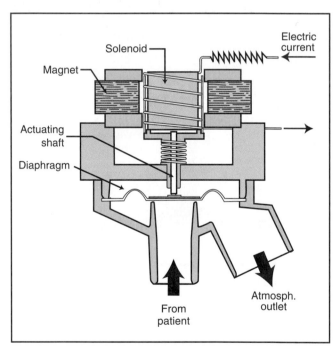

FIGURE 11-27 Electromagnetic threshold resistor of the Hamilton Veolar ventilator.

In a CPAP device, blended gas at the desired F_IO_2 can come from air and oxygen flowmeters, from a blender, or from a CPAP generator. The gas is warmed and humidified. A threshold resistor is attached to the expiratory end of the system. For example, the Downs CPAP generator (Figure 11-28) is connected to a gas source. A large-bore tube (22 mm) connects the generator with the patient's mask interface (Figure 11-29). The amount of CPAP is adjusted with a spring-loaded CPAP valve on the mask. Most valves are spring loaded with fixed pressures (e.g.,

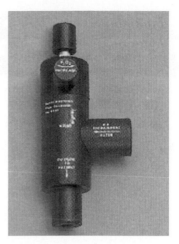

FIGURE 11-28 Downs continuous positive airway pressure (CPAP) generator. (Courtesy Vital Signs Corp., Totowa, N.J.)

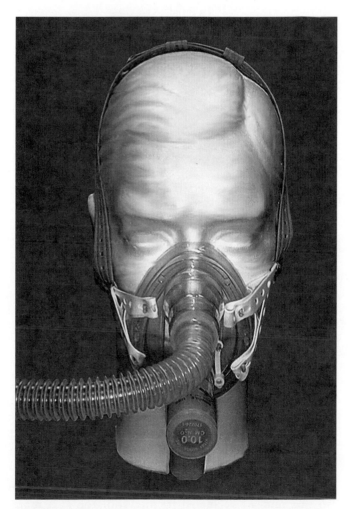

FIGURE 11-29 Model wearing a continuous positive airway pressure (CPAP) mask (spring-loaded valve) connected to a large-bore circuit, which connects to the Downs CPAP generator. Air flows into the large-bore tubing on the left to the patient. Air exits through the valve mounted on the mask (bottom of the mask). (Courtesy Vital Signs Corp., Totowa, N.J.)

5 cm H_2O, 7.5 cm H_2O), but other masks can be adjusted by tightening the spring. For monitoring purposes, a pressure manometer can be added to the circuit to monitor circuit pressure.

Sometimes a safety pressure-release valve is incorporated into a CPAP system. The safety pressure-release valve setting is slightly higher than the desired CPAP level. For example, if the CPAP is 10 cm H_2O, the safety pressure release might be set at 15 cm H_2O. If the normal threshold resistor (or, in this case, spring-loaded valve) jams, which would prevent gas flow from exiting the system, the safety pressure-release valve acts as a pop-off valve.

Including a safety pop-in valve is also important in case the source gas is turned off accidentally. A safety pop-in valve provides a source of ambient air for the patient in the event of loss of a source gas. Generally these pop-in valves open at a fairly low pressure (−1 to −2 cm H_2O).

A variety of problems can occur with a CPAP system; therefore the operator must make sure the safety systems (i.e., pop-off and pop-in valves) are in place and the patient is monitored. Some of these problems are:

· Inadequate flow to the patient
· Leaks in the system
· Loss of source gas flow
· Jamming or obstruction of the expiratory threshold resistor

Clinical Rounds 11-2 presents some exercises involving problems related to CPAP systems like the one previously described.

CLINICAL ROUNDS 11-2

Troubleshooting Freestanding CPAP Systems

Problem 1
A patient attached to a freestanding, continuous-flow CPAP system (e.g. the Down's CPAP generator) set at 10 cm H_2O appears to be in distress (e.g., supraclavicular retractions, accessory muscle use, pale and diaphoretic). The operator notices that the manometer drops to −1 cm H_2O during inspiration and rises to 10 cm H_2O during expiration. What do you think is the problem?

Problem 2
The low oxygen saturation alarm is sounding on a patient connected to a continuous-flow CPAP system. The operator notices that the manometer fluctuates around the zero point during both inspiration and expiration. What is the problem?

See Evolve Resources for the answers.

PART II BASIC COMPONENTS OF BREATH DELIVERY

OUTLINE

Model Description of Shared Work of Breathing
Type of Breath Delivery (Breath Classification)
Control Circuit
Control Variable
Phases of a Breath (Phase Variables)
Beginning of Inspiration: The Trigger Variable
Time Triggering
Patient Triggering
Other Triggering Mechanisms
Inspiratory Phase
Sloping or Ramping
Waveforms and Graphics
Limiting Factors during Inspiration
Maximum Safety Pressure
Termination of the Inspiratory Phase: Cycling Mechanism
Pressure Cycling
Time Cycling
Volume Cycling
Flow Cycling
Inspiratory Pause
Expiratory Phase: Baseline Variable
Baseline Pressure
Subambient Pressure (Negative End-Expiratory Pressure)
Continuous Gas Flow During Exhalation
Expiratory Hold: End-Expiratory Pause
Time-Limited Exhalation

KEY TERMS

assisted breath
auto-PEEP
baseline pressure
continuous positive airway
    pressure (CPAP)
control variable
control ventilation
cycle variable
end-expiratory pause
expiratory hold
flow triggering
high-frequency jet
    ventilation
high-frequency oscillation

inspiratory hold
inspiratory pause
limit variable
mandatory breath
negative end-expiratory pressure
    (NEEP)
neurally adjusted ventilatory assist
    (NAVA)
patient triggering
peak inspiratory pressure (PIP)
phase variables
plateau pressure (P_{plat})
positive end-expiratory pressure
    (PEEP)

pressure triggering
pressure ventilation (PV)
scalars
spontaneous breaths
static compliance
time triggering
total cycle time (TCT)
tubing compliance factor
tubing compressibility
trigger sensitivity
trigger variable
Y-connector

To accomplish breath delivery, the ventilator must be able to provide the four basic phases of a breath and assume all or part of the patient's work of breathing. The four phases, which are controlled by **phase variables,** are listed in Box 11-6. The following sections discuss these concepts in more detail.

MODEL DESCRIPTION OF SHARED WORK OF BREATHING

Two forces are available to perform work of breathing: the patient's muscles and the ventilator. The ventilator must also be adjustable so that the operator can balance the work between these two components. This balance is best described by the equation of motion (Box 11-7 and Figure 11-30). For a single breath, the compliance and resistance of the respiratory system do not change significantly, but the volume, pressure, flow, and time can vary and are regulated by the ventilator.[7,10] A more detailed description of the equation of motion is available elsewhere.[7]

Type of Breath Delivery (Breath Classification)

As mentioned previously, work of breathing can be provided by the ventilator and by the patient; therefore more

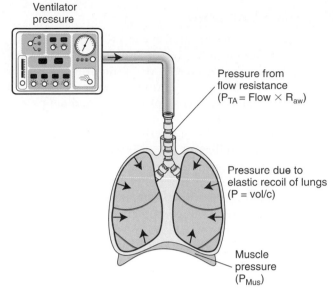

FIGURE 11-30 Model of the equation of motion: Muscle pressure + Ventilator pressure = Elastic recoil pressure + Flow resistance pressure. (See text for description.)

<table>
<tr><td>

BOX 11-6 **Four Phases of a Breath during Mechanical Ventilation and Phase Variables**

BREATH PHASES
1. End of expiration and beginning of inspiration
2. Delivery of inspiration
3. End of inspiration and beginning of expiration
4. Expiratory phase

PHASE VARIABLES
Phase variables are controlled by the ventilator and are responsible for each of the four parts of a breath. These variables are:
- Triggering: Begins inspiratory gas flow
- Limiting: Places a maximum value on a control variable (pressure, volume, flow, or time) during delivery of a breath
- Cycling: Ends inspiratory gas flow

</td></tr>
</table>

BOX 11-7 **Equation of Motion**

The equation of motion is a mathematical model that represents the interaction between the patient and the ventilator during inspiration (and expiration). The simplest version of this equation assumes that the complex respiratory system can be represented by a single resistance, R, representing the airways and the artificial airway (connected in series) and a single elastance, E, representing the lungs and chest wall.

There are two pressures to move gas into the lung, the pressure needed to move gas through the airway (flow resistance pressure) and the pressure to expand the lung and thorax (elastic recoil pressure). These two pressures are provided by the respiratory muscles (muscle pressure) and/or by a ventilator (ventilator pressure).

Equation 1
> Muscle pressure + Ventilator pressure = Elastic recoil pressure + Flow resistance pressure

Or, an abbreviated form can be used:

Equation 2
$$P_{mus} + P_{vent} = (V/C) + (R_{aw} \times Flow)$$

Where:
P_{mus} is the pressure generated by the muscles of ventilation (i.e., muscle pressure); if these muscles are not active, P_{mus} equals zero.
P_{vent} is the pressure generated by the ventilator at the upper airway.
V is the volume delivered.
C is the respiratory system compliance (recall that compliance is the inverse of elastance, $C = 1/E$).
V/C is the elastic recoil pressure.
R_{aw} is the respiratory system resistance.
$Flow$ is the gas flow during inspiration (i.e., $R_{aw} \times flow$, flow resistance).
Because $P_{vent} = R_{aw} \times Flow$, and alveolar pressure (P_A) = V/C, the following substitutions can be made in the equation above:
$$P_{mus} + P_{vent} = P_A + \text{Transairway pressure } (P_{TA})$$

---

than one type of breath delivery is possible. If the ventilator controls the timing and/or size of the breath, the breath is called a **mandatory breath;** in other words, the ventilator can start and end the breath, or it can simply end the breath.

An **assisted breath,** on the other hand, is one in which all or part of inspiration (or expiration) is performed by the ventilator doing work on the patient. If the pressure rises above the baseline pressure during inspiration, the breath is *assisted.* Note the baseline pressure is the pressure maintained during expiration.

Spontaneous breaths are those in which the patient controls the transition from inspiration to exhalation. For example, during CPAP the ventilator tries to maintain pressure at a constant value. The spontaneous breaths the patient takes during CPAP are unassisted, because the pressure remains at the baseline pressure.

Control Circuit

To use the drive mechanism and the gas delivery valves previously described, the ventilator must be programmed to manipulate pressure, volume, flow, and time to deliver a breath (inspiration) to the patient. A control circuit performs this function. A control circuit is part of the internal circuit and can consist of mechanical devices such as spring-loaded valves. It also can consist of pneumatic systems such as pressure regulators, entrainment devices, or fluidic components. The control circuits of earlier generation ventilators often were mechanical or pneumatic. Current ICU ventilators tend to use more sophisticated control circuits composed of programmed microprocessors and flow valves controlled by these microprocessors, as described earlier in this chapter. The control circuit is part of the ventilator classification.

Control Variable

The main parameter or variable controlled by the ventilator for any given breath is referred to as the **control variable.** This is the parameter the ventilator adjusts or manipulates to deliver inspiration. Pressure, volume, and flow are the three main control variables and are part of the breath classification.[7,9,10]

To help clarify which of the three control variables the ventilator is controlling to deliver inspiration, the following definitions can be used:

- If pressure delivery remains constant with changing patient lung characteristics (compliance [C] or airway resistance [R_{aw}]) but volume and flow vary, the breath's control variable is pressure.
- If pressure changes but the volume remains constant with changing patient lung characteristics, the breath's control variable is volume.

Flow can also be a control variable. When a ventilator is a flow controller, the volume and flow waveforms remain the same but the pressure varies. Most current ICU ventilators (e.g., the VIASYS AVEA and the GALILEO G5) function as flow controllers. These systems are very precise and can measure and adjust gas flow hundreds of times per second.

Figure 11-31 illustrates how a clinician can determine the control variable used to deliver any given breath.

In the clinical setting, the two control variables most commonly used are volume and pressure. Operators select either a volume they wish to deliver or a pressure they wish to deliver. Selection of a volume is called *volume-targeted ventilation,* which is also known as *volume ventilation, volume control,* and *volume-limited ventilation.* Selection of a pressure is called *pressure-targeted ventilation,* which is also known as *pressure ventilation, pressure-controlled ventilation,* or *pressure-limited ventilation* (Box 11-8). Confusion results from so many names having the same meaning.

PHASES OF A BREATH (PHASE VARIABLES)

When the term *breath* is used, it usually refers to inspiration. However, a breath really consists of a total respiratory cycle; that is, the time required for both inspiration (T_I)

BOX 11-8	Other Names for Volume and Pressure Ventilation

VOLUME VENTILATION
Volume-limited ventilation
Volume-controlled ventilation
Volume-targeted ventilation

PRESSURE VENTILATION
Pressure-limited ventilation
Pressure-controlled ventilation
Pressure-targeted ventilation

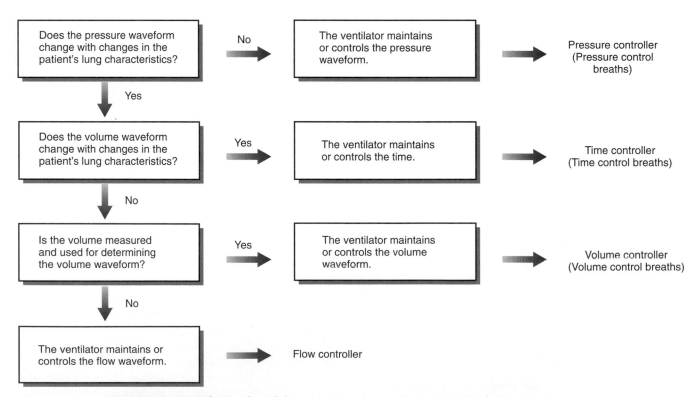

FIGURE 11-31 Defining a breath based on how the ventilator maintains the inspiratory waveform. (Criteria for determining the control variable during a ventilator-assisted inspiration.) (Modified from Chatburn RL, Volsko TA: Mechanical ventilators. In Wilkins RL, Stoller JK, Kacmarek RM: *Egan's fundamentals of respiratory care,* ed 9, St Louis, 2009, Mosby.)

and expiration (T_E) and the events that occur during that time. This time frame is also called the **total cycle time (TCT).** A ventilator must be capable of separating a breath into four parts, which proceed as follows (see Box 11-6):

1. The **trigger variable** begins inspiration.
2. Breath delivery (inspiration) is accomplished when the settings on the ventilator front panel (user interface) establish what will be controlled: pressure, volume, or flow. (As mentioned previously, these three are called *control variables*. The two most common are volume and pressure.)
3. The **cycle variable** ends the inspiratory phase and begins exhalation.
4. The **limit variable** limits the value for pressure, flow, volume, or time during delivery of inspiration, but it *does not end the breath*.

Pressures and flows can be controlled during exhalation; therefore the ventilator also can be involved in the expiratory phase.

BEGINNING OF INSPIRATION: THE TRIGGERING VARIABLE

The trigger variable begins the inspiratory phase. Ventilator breaths can be time, pressure, flow, or volume triggered. For example, when the trigger variable is time, the ventilator controls the beginning of inspiration based on the set rate. For example, if the rate is set at 12 breaths/min, a breath occurs every 5 seconds. Inspiratory flow starts 5 seconds after the last inspiration, thus providing **time triggering.**

When pressure, flow, or volume begins the breath, the patient controls the beginning of inspiration; this is called **patient triggering.**

The trigger variable must not be confused with the cycling variable. Triggering begins inspiration; cycling (discussed later) ends inspiration. This difference is mentioned because the term *cycle* historically meant the variable that began the breath, and some journal articles and technical manuals still occasionally misuse this terminology.

Time Triggering

As noted, with time triggering the ventilator controls the beginning of inspiration based on the set mandatory rate. The breath is mandatory.

Patient Triggering

Ventilators can be adjusted to sense the patient's inspiratory effort. The control set by the operator is commonly called the *sensitivity setting*, or **trigger sensitivity.** Pressure and flow are the most common variables used for patient triggering, but volume and neural triggering also can be used.

Pressure Triggering

Pressure triggering occurs when the ventilator senses a drop in pressure below baseline in the circuit. Pressure

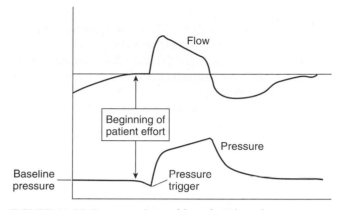

FIGURE 11-32 Pressure-triggered breath. When the pressure drops to the pressure trigger level, the inspiratory flow begins. (From Hess DR, MacIntyre NR, Mishoe SC, et al.: *Respiratory care: principles and practices*, Philadelphia, 2002, WB Saunders.)

CLINICAL ROUNDS 11-3

A patient has a baseline pressure of 10 cm H_2O during mechanical ventilation. The trigger sensitivity is set at -1 cm H_2O. At what pressure will the ventilator sense a patient effort and start inspiration?

See Evolve Resources for the answer.

triggering usually is set at -0.5 to -1.5 cm H_2O. In other words, the patient must make an inspiratory effort to reduce the pressure below baseline to begin inspiration (Figure 11-32). **Baseline pressure** is the pressure maintained at the airway during exhalation and the pressure from which inspiration begins. (See the discussion of the expiratory phase later in this section.)

Pressure generally is measured in three different places on ventilators because pressure transducers or sensors can be placed at three common locations:

- Within the internal ventilator circuit near the point where the main gas flow leaves the unit
- Where expired gas returns to the unit from the patient
- At the proximal airway (near the **Y-connector**)

In the third case, a small-bore plastic tubing extends from the front of the ventilator to the patient's Y-connector (Clinical Rounds 11-3). (See Chapter 8 for further information on pressure monitoring devices.)

Flow Triggering

Flow triggering occurs when a drop in flow is detected. In some ventilators a pneumotachograph (see Chapter 8) is located between the ventilator circuit and the patient to measure flow. In others, a background flow, also called a *base* or *bias flow,* is set either by the operator or by the ventilator itself. This flow is present during the expiratory phase. For example, the base flow may be set at approximately 5 to 10 L/min. A flow trigger is also set and can range from about 1 to 5 L/min, although this value varies with the type of ventilator used, the patient's size (baby or adult), and inspiratory effort. Most ventilator manufacturers recommend a value or have set values.

The ventilator measures the base flow during exhalation. When the flow drops by the amount set on the flow trigger, inspiration begins. For example, if the base flow is set at 7 L/min and the trigger is set at 3 L/min, the ventilator begins inspiration when the expiratory flow is measured at 4 L/min (7 L/min − 3 L/min = 4 L/min). Figures 11-33 and 11-34 show flow-trigger graphics and a flow-triggering device. Clinical Rounds 11-4 presents a practice problem in flow triggering.

Volume Triggering

Volume triggering occurs after the patient has inhaled a specific volume from the circuit. This type of triggering is used on the Dräger Babylog and Cardiopulmonary Venturi ventilator. By adjusting the trigger sensitivity (e.g., the range for the Venturi is 1 to 250 mL), the operator can change the effort required by the patient to begin inspiration. Just to give an example of how sensitive this can be, a tuberculin syringe has a volume of 1 mL. The operator can adjust the Venturi's sensitivity so that only 1 mL must be inhaled from the circuit to start inspiration.

Figure 11-35 shows how to determine the type of trigger variable used.

Other Triggering Mechanisms

Other methods of triggering include the following:
1. Manual triggering, in which the operator activates the "manual breath" or "start breath" control and delivers a mandatory breath based on the set variables.
2. Triggering from chest wall movement, as is available on the Star Sync module of the Infant Star ventilator (see Chapter 13).
3. Neural triggering from the electrical activity of the diaphragm, which is called **neurally adjusted ventilatory assist (NAVA)** and is available on the Maquet Servo[i].

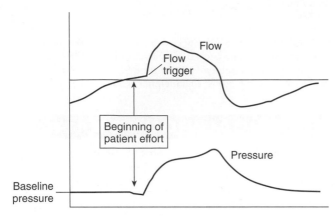

FIGURE 11-33 Flow-triggered breath. When the flow reaches the set flow-trigger level, the inspiratory flow begins. (From Hess DR, MacIntyre NR, Mishoe SC, et al.: *Respiratory care: principles and practices,* Philadelphia, 2002, WB Saunders.)

INSPIRATORY PHASE

One of the most important ventilator functions is delivery of inspiratory gas flow. The first positive-pressure volume ventilators were often classified by the strength of the force behind inspiratory delivery and by the evaluation of the

---

CLINICAL ROUNDS 11-4

The operator decides to use flow triggering for a patient and sets the base flow at 6 L/min and the trigger flow at 2 L/min. The base flow measurement must drop to what value before the ventilator will begin the inspiratory phase?

See Evolve Resources for the answer.

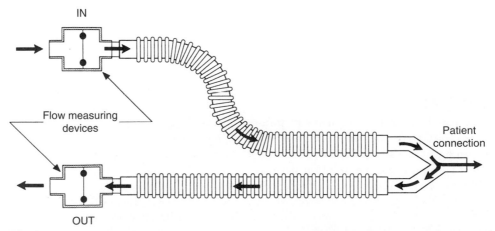

FIGURE 11-34 Schematic of flow triggering, which occurs when the patient makes an inspiratory effort and drops the flow through the patient circuit to the trigger level. (From Dupuis Y: *Ventilators,* ed 2, St Louis, 1992, Mosby.)

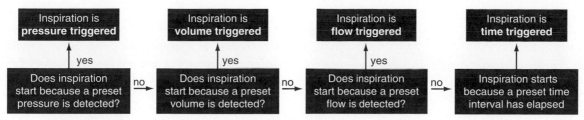

FIGURE 11-35 Criteria for determining the trigger variable during a breath on a mechanical ventilator. The determination is based on observation of the ventilator and ventilator graphics and on previous knowledge. (Modified from Chatburn RL, Volsko TA: Mechanical ventilators. In Wilkins RL, Stoller JK, Kacmarek RM: *Egan's fundamentals of respiratory care,* ed 9, St Louis, 2009, Mosby.)

HISTORICAL NOTE 11-5

Classification of Ventilators

The classification of ventilators previously was based on the power source. For example, the IMV Emerson ventilator was described as a high-pressure drive ventilator. A powerful electric motor was used to drive its rotary piston. Regardless of changes in a patient's lung characteristics, the ventilator could deliver the set volume, although pressure increased as the workload increased.

Ventilators also were classified according to the flow waveform they produced. For example, the IMV Emerson was also referred to as a non–constant-flow generator because the flow produced was not constant (in this case, it resembled a sine wave), and it produced the same sine pattern breath after breath, regardless of changes in the patient's lung characteristics.

From Mushin WW et al: *Automatic ventilation of the lungs,* Philadelphia, 1980, FA Davis; and Pilbeam SP, Cairo JM: *Mechanical ventilation: physiological and clinical applications,* ed 4, St Louis, 2006, Mosby/Elsevier.

BOX 11-9   A Flow-Controlled Breath

Any breath having a set flow waveform that does not change from one breath to the next—regardless of changes in lung characteristics—is a flow-controlled breath. If flow is controlled, the volume is also controlled. Therefore the breath is also a volume-controlled breath.

CLINICAL ROUNDS 11-5

Before inspiration, the pressure drops to −1 cm H_2O on the pressure manometer, and then inspiratory flow begins. During inspiration, the pressure rises to 20 cm H_2O and stays at 20 cm H_2O for 1.2 seconds. Then expiration begins. What are the trigger, limit, and cycle variables?

See Evolve Resources for the answer.

---

pressure, flow, and volume curves produced during inspiration (Historical Note 11-5). Current ICU ventilators are no longer classified by this method.

Delivery of inspiration is regulated primarily by a control variable. The three variables the ventilator can control are represented in the equation of motion described earlier—volume, flow, and pressure. The ventilator can control only one of these variables at a time.[7,10] (NOTE: It is intuitively understood that time is a part of the equation of motion. However, time generally is not the control variable selected to regulate inspiration.)

In theory, a ventilator that truly controls volume would directly measure volume by using a volume-measuring device such as a bellows or piston.[7] Current ventilators do not directly measure volume; however, volume can be controlled indirectly by controlling and measuring flow and time. A volume of gas is simply a flow of gas delivered within a certain time frame. If the flow and the time during which it is delivered are known, the volume can be determined (Volume = Flow × Time). Therefore a volume breath is one in which flow is also controlled (i.e., a flow-controlled breath) (Box 11-9). Flow-controller is probably a more accurate term than volume-controller.[*]

With **pressure ventilation (PV),** pressure is selected as the control variable. The pressure remains constant during inspiration, but the volume and flow delivered may change if the patient's lung characteristics change. See Clinical Rounds 11-5 for a problem related to breath variables.

Because time is not commonly used as a control variable, it was excluded from the previous discussion of these variables. However, when a ventilator delivers a time-controlled breath, pressure, volume, and flow may vary with changes in lung characteristics. Time is constant. Examples of timed breaths are those produced during **high-frequency jet ventilation** and **high-frequency oscillation.**

Sloping or Ramping

Most contemporary ICU ventilators allow the operator to adjust the slope of the pressure and flow curves at the beginning of inspiration. This feature, called *ramping,*

---

*In this text, the term *volume controlled* or *volume limited* also mean *flow controlled* or *flow limited.*

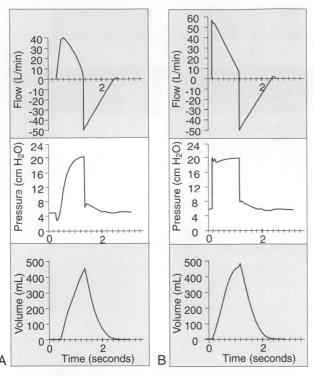

FIGURE 11-36 The effect of rise time, or sloping adjustment, during pressure-support ventilation. The top graph is flow-time, the middle graph is pressure-time, and the bottom graph is volume-time. Breath *A*, on the left, shows a slow rise time. Breath *B*, on the right, shows a more rapid rise time. Note how the pressure-time curve is visibly tapered in breath *A* compared to breath *B*. Flow is also tapered in breath *A* when the two are compared. (See text for further explanation.) (From Hess DR, MacIntyre NR, Mishoe SC, et al.: *Respiratory care: principles and practice*, Philadelphia, 2002, WB Saunders.)

inspiratory rise time adjustment, or *sloping,* allows the operator to change the rate of gas delivery at the very beginning of inspiration. When no sloping is selected, the ventilator delivers gas very rapidly at the beginning of inspiration. Flow and pressure rise to their set value as quickly as possible. On the other hand, when the operator uses the sloping or rise time control, pressure and flow delivery are tapered slightly until they reach their maximum value (Figure 11-36). Names for this feature vary from company to company. Some of these names are rise time, flow acceleration percent, inspiratory rise time percent, and slope adjustment.

In some ventilators, sloping can be used for either pressure-controlled (or targeted) breaths (PC) or volume-controlled (or targeted) breaths (VC). Other ventilators allow sloping only with pressure-targeted breaths. Additional information about sloping or ramping is available with each ventilator reviewed in Chapter 12.*

---

*Additional information about sloping, or rise time, is presented in reference 11.

Waveforms and Graphics

Monitoring and evaluation of graphic waveforms produced during ventilation are one method of determining the control variable for a breath. Although more detailed information about ventilator waveform graphics is available elsewhere,[11] a brief summary is provided here.

Pressure, volume, and flow graphed over time are called **scalars** (i.e., pressure-time, volume-time, and flow-time).[21] Six basic waveforms are produced for pressure, volume, and flow over time during ventilation (Figure 11-37). Figure 11-38 shows examples of the pressure, volume, and flow waveforms produced with several methods of pressure and volume ventilation.

Remember that during pressure ventilation, the delivered pressure pattern stays the same, regardless of changes in the patient's lung condition, but volume and flow delivery vary (Figure 11-39). During volume ventilation, the selected volume and flow wave patterns stay the same, but the pressure varies (Figure 11-40).

Limiting Factors during Inspiration

As reviewed previously, the ventilator controls one of the three primary control variables during inspiration and can also limit the variables. A limiting variable has a maximum value that cannot be exceeded during inspiration because the ventilator does not allow it; however, reaching the limit does not end inspiratory flow to the patient (Figure 11-41).

For example, in a bag-in-a-chamber ventilator (see Figure 11-7), the volume is limited to the gas volume in the bag. It cannot exceed that volume; however, delivery of the volume does not necessarily end the breath. The ventilator may continue to hold the bag in a collapsed state briefly before the bag is allowed to refill. This would add a brief period after volume delivery in which the ventilator pauses before beginning exhalation. In this example, inspiration is time cycling and volume limited (Clinical Rounds 11-6).

CLINICAL ROUNDS 11-6

For volume ventilation with the ventilators currently used in the intensive care unit (ICU), the operator sets a volume, flow, and mandatory rate. The ventilator does not measure volume. The ventilator calculates and sets the inspiratory time needed to achieve the set volume based on the set variables (volume, flow, and time [rate]). This technically makes them time cycled.

However, clinicians commonly consider them volume cycled, on the grounds that they achieve volume delivery by the time inspiratory flow ends but technically do not "measure" the volume using a volume-measuring device such as a bellows or bag.

Defend the argument that these ventilators are volume cycled rather than time cycled.

See Evolve Resources for the answer.

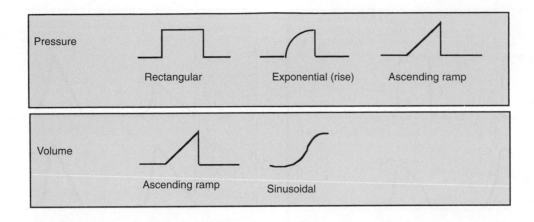

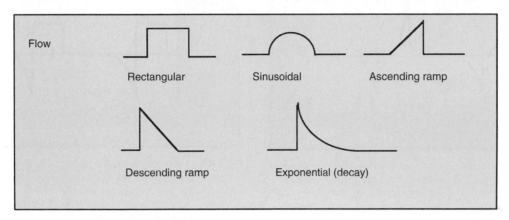

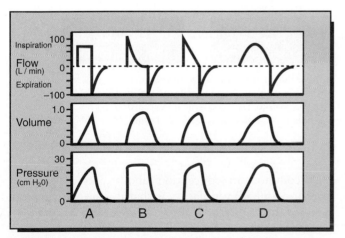

FIGURE 11-37 Examples of curves for pressure, volume, and flow. Pressure curves are usually constant, rising exponential, or ascending ramps. Volume curves are usually ascending ramps or sinusoidal (resembling a sine wave). Flow curves are commonly rectangular (constant), resemble sine waves, ramps (ascending or descending), and decaying exponential. (From Pilbeam SP: *Mechanical ventilation: physiological and clinical applications,* ed 3, St Louis, 1998, Mosby.)

FIGURE 11-38 Characteristic waveforms for flow *(top curve),* volume *(middle curve),* and pressure *(bottom curve)* in four forms of ventilation. **A,** Volume breath with constant flow. **B,** Pressure breath with a constant pressure delivery, a long inspiratory time (T_I) (flow returns to zero), and time cycling. **C,** Volume breath with a descending ramp flow pattern. **D,** Volume breath using a sinelike flow pattern. (From Pilbeam SP: *Mechanical ventilation: physiological and clinical applications,* ed 3, St Louis, 1998, Mosby.)

A ventilator is considered flow limited if the flow reaches a maximum value before the end of inspiration but does not exceed that value. For example, if the forward motion of a linear-drive piston is constant, the flow is constant and limited to the rate of forward motion and the volume in the piston housing (Flow = Volume ÷ Time).

Pressure limiting sets a maximum value for pressure, which is not exceeded during inspiration. After the pressure is reached, inspiration may continue, but no more pressure (and thus no more volume) is delivered to the patient (Figure 11-42). Excess pressure is vented through a pressure-release mechanism. Some ventilators have pressure-limited capabilities and use a mode called *time-cycled, pressure-limited ventilation* (Clinical Rounds 11-7) (see Chapter 12, VIASYS AVEA ventilator).

Maximum Safety Pressure

All ventilators have some type of feature that allows inspiratory pressure to reach but not exceed a maximum value during inspiration. This pressure usually is set by the operator at 10 cm H_2O above the peak pressure

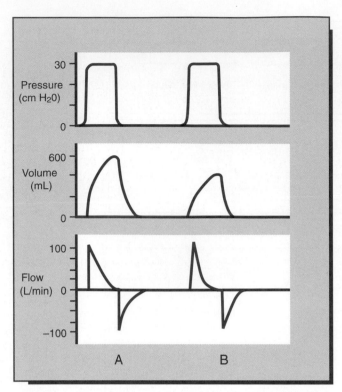

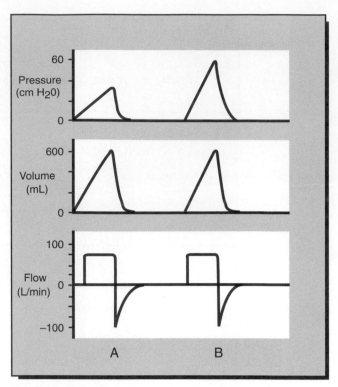

FIGURE 11-39 Examples of waveforms for pressure-targeted ventilation. The top waveform is pressure, the middle waveform is volume, and the bottom waveform is flow. **A,** Breath *A* waveforms show normal pressure, volume, and flow curves. **B,** Breath *B* waveforms indicate a patient with reduced lung compliance, showing reduced volume delivery. Note that for breath *B,* the flow curve returns to the zero baseline before exhalation begins. This is an example of a *pause* in pressure at the end of inspiration during pressure ventilation.

FIGURE 11-40 Example of a patient's lung condition becoming worse during volume-targeted ventilation. The top curve is pressure, the middle curve is volume, and the lower curve is flow. **A,** The waveforms show normal pressure, volume, and flow curves. **B,** The waveforms indicate that the patient's lungs have reduced compliance, showing increased pressure delivery while the volume and flow waveforms remain constant.

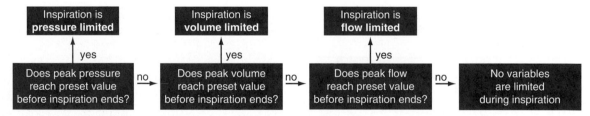

FIGURE 11-41 Criteria for determining the limit variable during a breath on a mechanical ventilator. The determination is based on observation of the ventilator and ventilator graphics and on previous knowledge. (Modified from Chatburn RL, Volsko TA: Mechanical ventilators. In Wilkins RL, Stoller JK, Kacmarek RM: *Egan's fundamentals of respiratory care,* ed 9, St Louis, 2009, Mosby.)

reached during inspiration. This particular setting on the control panel can have a variety of names (Box 11-10); the purpose of this feature is to prevent excessive pressure from damaging lung tissue. In most adult ventilators, inspiratory gas flow ends when this pressure is reached; thus the ventilator pressure cycles out of inspiration. Unfortunately, the labeling used on the control panel of most ventilators includes the term "pressure limit," which leads to a lot of confusion because this feature usually cycles the ventilator out of inspiration and does not just limit the pressure.

A common misconception about pressure-targeted (pressure-limited) ventilation is that if a specific pressure is set for the inspiratory control variable (e.g., 20 cm H_2O), the pressure cannot exceed that value. This is not true. If a patient coughs, the pressure can rise above the set value. It is important to set a safe upper pressure limit during pressure ventilation so that excessively high pressures do not occur. Again, a common upper pressure limit is about 10 cm H_2O above the ventilating pressure. In newer ICU ventilators, the exhalation valve may "float," in which case pressures are less likely to rise with a patient cough.

TERMINATION OF THE INSPIRATORY PHASE: CYCLING MECHANISM

The phase variable measured and used to end inspiration is called the *cycle variable* (Figure 11-43). A breath can be pressure cycled, time cycled, volume cycled, or flow cycled (Box 11-11).

Pressure Cycling

A breath is considered pressure cycled when inspiratory flow ends and expiratory flow begins once a set pressure is

reached. Pressure cycling is not a common method used to cycle an ICU ventilator. The most frequent form of pressure cycling occurs when a ventilator reaches the upper pressure limit (high pressure limit) set above the peak inspiratory pressure used to ventilate the patient. This is typically accompanied by a visual and audible alarm, because it is considered an alarm event. Another kind of pressure cycle is used with intermittent positive-pressure breathing (IPPB) machines, which can also be used for

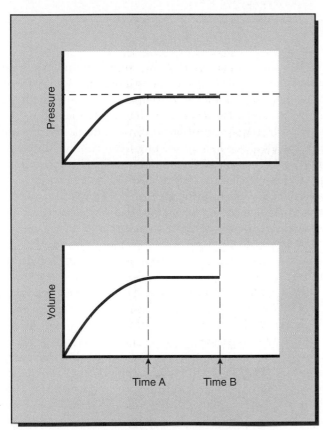

FIGURE 11-42 Pressure-time and volume-time waveforms illustrate a time-cycled, pressure-limited breath. The pressure peaks and the volume is delivered by time *A*. The pressure reaches the set limit and stays constant. No more volume enters the patient's lungs after time *A*. Between *A* and *B*, excess pressure is vented. Inspiration ends at time *B* (time cycled).

CLINICAL ROUNDS 11-7

A respiratory therapist observes the waveforms on the graphic display as an infant is being ventilated. The therapist notices that during inspiration, the pressure rises in a linear fashion and then plateaus before cycling into exhalation. The volume curve resembles the pressure curve. However, the flow curve rises rapidly to a constant value and then falls rapidly during inspiration and stays at the baseline flow until the ventilator finally cycles into exhalation. What are the limit and cycle variables for this breath?

See Evolve Resources for the answer.

BOX 11-10	Common Names for Maximum Safety Pressure Control

- Pressure limit
- Upper pressure limit
- Normal pressure limit
- High pressure limit
- Peak/maximum pressure

BOX 11-11	Cycling Variables

Volume cycling: The ventilator ends inspiration after a predetermined volume has been reached.
Pressure cycling: The ventilator ends inspiration after a predetermined pressure has been reached.
Time cycling: The ventilator ends inspiration after a predetermined time has elapsed.
Flow cycling: The ventilator ends inspiration after a predetermined flow has been achieved.

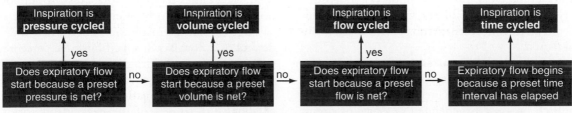

FIGURE 11-43 Criteria for determining the cycle variable during a breath on a mechanical ventilator. The determination is based on observation of the ventilator and ventilator graphics and on previous knowledge. (Modified from Chatburn RL, Volsko TA: Mechanical ventilators. In Wilkins RL, Stoller JK, Kacmarek RM: *Egan's fundamentals of respiratory care,* ed 9, St Louis, 2009, Mosby.)

delivery of aerosolized medications or for ventilating a patient. The operator sets a pressure and once the IPPB machine reaches that pressure, inspiratory flow ends and exhalation begins.

Time Cycling

When time is the phase variable used to end inspiration and allow expiratory gas flow to occur, the breath is said to be *time cycled.* Many current ICU ventilators are time cycled; the user sets a control called *inspiratory time,* which commonly determines the length of inspiration.

The set T_I can be changed in a few circumstances, depending on the other controls the user sets. First, setting an **inspiratory pause (inspiratory hold)** instructs the ventilator to deliver inspiration and close both the inspiratory and expiratory valves and "hold" the air in the patient for a fraction of a second (up to 2 seconds) before it opens the expiratory valve and allows expiratory flow to begin. Using inspiratory hold can extend the inspiratory time, depending on the ventilator used and how it is programmed.

Second, most ventilators have a maximum time limit for inspiration, for example, during a pressure-support (PS) breath (more on pressure support later in this chapter). If the breath is taking too long to delivery, the ventilator ends the breath based on a fixed time (e.g., 3 seconds). Therefore a PS breath in this instance could not have an inspiratory time longer than 3 seconds.

Volume Cycling

During volume ventilation, flow is delivered from the ventilator to the patient circuit and the patient until a specific volume has been delivered *from the ventilator.* As soon as the volume has been delivered, inspiratory flow ends and exhalation begins. Typically, contemporary ICU ventilators deliver a specific amount of flow over a certain period of time. Inspiration ends when the calculated tidal volume, based on the flow and time signals, has been delivered.

Even though the ventilator may measure a specific volume output during volume-cycled ventilation, the amount delivered to the patient may be less. This discrepancy can be due to leaks in the system or compression of some of the volume in the patient circuit (tubing compressibility). Leaks may occur in the patient circuit, especially where devices are added to the circuit, such as heat and moisture exchangers, filters, humidifiers, Y-sensors, capnometry devices, and nebulizers. Leaks can also occur around an uncuffed endotracheal tube or through a bronchopleural fistula.

Volume can also be lost as a result of a phenomenon called **tubing compressibility (tubing compliance factor).** The expansion of the patient circuit can easily be seen when high pressure is generated in a patient circuit during inspiration. The circuit expands during inspiration and returns to normal during exhalation. Part of the tidal volume delivered from the ventilator contributes to the expansion of the circuit. This amount of volume never

---

BOX 11-12	Tubing Compliance (Compressibility Calculation)

To calculate tubing compliance (C_T), perform the following procedure before connecting the ventilator to the patient:
1. Set the ventilator volume to 100 or 200 mL.
2. Select a low flow setting (e.g., 40 L/min).
3. Set the upper pressure limit to the maximum and the positive end-expiratory pressure (PEEP) to zero.
4. Occlude the patient's Y-connector.
5. Manually trigger the ventilator, record the measured peak inspiratory pressure (PIP), and measure the exhaled volume (V).

C_T equals the measured volume divided by the measured pressure ($C_T = V/PIP$).

---

reaches the patient. This "lost" volume is important in infants and small children. For this reason, infant patient circuits are much smaller in diameter and are made from a lower compliance plastic and thus expand less.

Most current ICU ventilators can automatically measure and calculate the loss of volume from tubing compressibility and compensate by increasing actual volume delivery. Others, such as the BEAR 1000, allow the operator to measure the tubing compliance (compressibility) and enter this number into the ventilator. The ventilator can then compensate for volume compressed in the tubing during inspiration. Box 11-12 gives an example of how to calculate tubing compliance for a ventilator that does not do so automatically.

Most adult ventilator patient circuits have a tubing compliance factor of 1 to 3 mL/cm H_2O. In other words, for every centimeter of water pressure generated during ventilation of a patient, 1 to 3 mL is lost (compressed) to tubing compliance. For example, if the **peak inspiratory pressure (PIP)** is 10 cm H_2O and the tubing compliance (C_T) is 2 mL/cm H_2O, the volume lost to the circuit is 10 × 2 mL/cm H_2O = 20 mL. If the tidal volume leaving the ventilator is 500 mL, only 480 mL reaches the patient. Clinical Rounds 11-8 provides exercises in determining loss of volume due to tubing compressibility.

Flow Cycling

Another criterion for terminating inspiration is flow cycling. With flow cycling, the ventilator ends inspiration when it measures a specific flow. Pressure-support ventilation (PSV) is the most common mode that uses flow cycling.[22,23] That is, inspiration ends when the ventilator detects that flow has dropped by some percentage of the peak flow measured during inspiration.

PSV is a patient-triggered, pressure-targeted, flow-cycled mode. Originally, PS breaths ended when gas flow dropped to about 25% to 30% of the peak inspiratory flow (e.g., BEAR 1000) or when a specific flow was measured. For example, in the Puritan Bennett 7200, when the inspiratory gas flow drops off at the end of inspiration to 5 L/min, inspiratory flow delivery ends.

CLINICAL ROUNDS 11-8

Calculating Tubing Compliance

Part I

Calculate the tubing compliance of a circuit. The volume was measured at 90 mL during the tubing compliance test, and the peak inspiratory pressure (PIP) was 45 cm H_2O. What is the tubing compliance?

If this circuit is used to ventilate a child with a set tidal volume of 300 mL and a PIP of 20 cm H_2O, how much volume is lost to the circuit? How much of the volume will go to the patient?

Part II

An adult patient circuit has a compliance of 3 mL/cm H_2O. During inspiration, the peak inspiratory pressure reaches 28 cm H_2O. The tidal volume is set at 640 mL on the ventilator. How much volume is lost to the circuit, and how much will reach the patient?

See Evolve Resources for the answers.

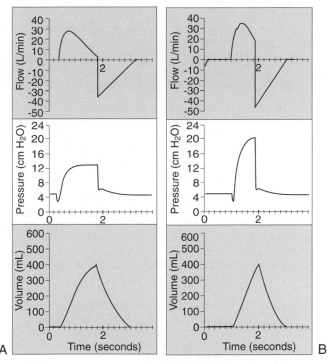

FIGURE 11-44 Effect of changes in termination flow (flow drop-off) during pressure-support ventilation. Termination flow is set as a small percentage of the peak inspiratory flow (**A,** *left panel*) and as a greater percentage of the peak inspiratory flow (**B,** *right panel*). (See text for further explanation.) (From Hess DR, MacIntyre NR, Mishoe SC, et al.: *Respiratory care: principles and practice,* Philadelphia, 2002, WB Saunders.)

(NOTE: Historically, PSV was the only mode that was flow cycled out of inspiration. Now some ICU ventilators allow pressure-limited, time-cycled breaths, also called pressure-controlled ventilation, to be flow cycled.)

Because not all patients have similar breathing patterns, fixed end points did not always synchronize with the patient's breathing pattern. Many of the current ICU ventilators, such as the Puritan Bennett 840 and the Maquet Servo[i], allow the operator to adjust the flow termination point. In some units this feature can be adjusted from 5% to 80% of the peak flow measured during inspiration, but the range varies, depending on the ventilator used. The clinician must carefully adjust the flow cycle value.[24,25]

Figure 11-44 illustrates two different PS breaths. In Figure 11-44A, the pressure is set at about 13 cm H_2O, the peak flow is about 30 L/min, and inspiration ends when the flow drops to about 5 L/min (about 17% of peak flow). The breath is long enough to reach its set value and produce a pressure plateau. In Figure 11-44B, the pressure is set at about 20 cm H_2O, peak flow is about 35 L/min, and inspiration ends when flow drops to about 20 L/min (about 57% of peak flow). Inspiration is short, and a visible pressure plateau does not occur.

Inspiratory Pause

The inspiratory time can be extended or delayed by keeping the expiratory valve momentarily closed, thus preventing gas flow from leaving the circuit. This maneuver is referred to by several different names, including *inspiratory pause,* *inflation hold,* and *inspiratory plateau.*

Inspiratory pause can occur in either pressure or volume ventilation. In volume ventilation, it is commonly used to obtain a reading of the **plateau pressure (P_{plat})** for estimation of the alveolar pressure and calculation of **static compliance** (C_s = Volume ÷ [P_{plat} − PEEP]) (Box 11-13) (Figure

BOX 11-13	Peak, Plateau, and Transairway Pressures

As volume is delivered, pressure rises to a peak (peak inspiratory pressure [PIP]) at the end of inspiration. PIP represents the pressure needed to overcome both airflow resistance and compliance.

When an inspiratory pause is selected, the volume is briefly held in the lungs at the end of inspiration, and the pressure reading drops to a plateau. The plateau, or static, reading indicates the pressure needed to overcome the static (lung) compliance alone.

The difference (PIP − P_{plat}) is the transairway pressure (P_{TA}), which is the pressure associated with airflow resistance. This value is used to calculate airway resistance:

$$R_{aw} = P_{TA} \div Flow$$

11-45). It can also be used to extend the T_I for the purpose of increasing the mean airway pressure and potentially improving a patient's oxygenation.

A control for this function is located on the operating panel. The inspiratory pause control enables the operator to select a time ranging from fractions of a second up to about 2 seconds.

During pressure ventilation, an *inspiratory hold pressure* can also be observed when T_I is sufficient to allow the

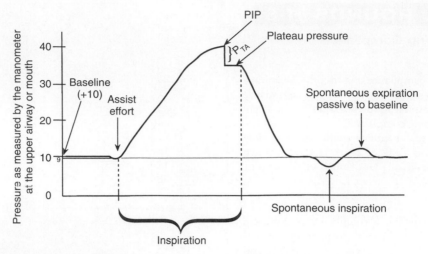

FIGURE 11-45 Volume breath with an inspiratory hold provides a pause before expiratory flow begins, allowing estimation of the plateau (alveolar) pressure. For this technique to be performed accurately, the patient cannot be making spontaneous breathing efforts. Also shown are the baseline pressure at a positive end-expiratory pressure (PEEP) of 10 cm H_2O, the transairway pressure (P_{TA}) (i.e., the peak inspiratory pressure [PIP] minus the plateau pressure [P_{plat}]; or $P_{TA} = PIP - P_{plat}$), and pressure changes during a spontaneous breath. (From Pilbeam SP, Cairo JM: *Mechanical ventilation: physiological and clinical applications,* ed 4, St Louis, 2006, Mosby-Elsevier.)

selected pressure to equilibrate with the patient's lungs. In this situation, inflation hold is not actually selected as a parameter on the control panel. Flow reads zero during this time, before expiratory flow is allowed to begin (see Figure 11-39B).

A similar phenomenon can be observed with infant ventilators when a pressure-relief valve is used to limit the pressure during inspiration. In this situation, the pressure-relief valve opens during the inspiratory phase and allows the pressure in the circuit to be maintained at a constant level. Excessive pressure is vented into the room. The pressure remains constant until the ventilator cycles into expiration (time-cycled ventilation, pressure limited) (see Figure 11-42).

EXPIRATORY PHASE: BASELINE VARIABLE

Normally, when inspiratory flow ceases during ventilation, the expiratory valve opens, allowing expiratory flow to begin. The expiratory phase is the time between inspiratory phases.

The baseline variable is the parameter controlled by the ventilator during exhalation. Typically pressure is the baseline variable.

Baseline Pressure

Baseline pressure is the pressure level from which inspiration begins. It generally is sustained throughout the expiratory phase. A zero baseline pressure is equal to atmospheric pressure.

Baseline pressures above zero are commonly called **positive end-expiratory pressure (PEEP)** or **continuous**

BOX 11-14	PEEP and CPAP

PEEP is the term most commonly used when mandatory ventilator breaths are delivered with a positive baseline pressure.

CPAP is the term most commonly used to describe the positive baseline pressure continuously applied to the airway of a spontaneously breathing patient. Patients doing well on CPAP alone do not require mandatory breaths from a ventilator.

---

positive airway pressure (CPAP) (Box 11-14) (see Figures 11-45 and 11-46).

Positive End-Expiratory Pressure

PEEP occurs because a resistance, applied during exhalation, limits lung emptying and increases functional residual capacity (FRC) to increase the mean airway pressure and to improve lung recruitment and oxygenation. The use of PEEP is described elsewhere and is beyond the scope of this text.[11] Increased pressure is accomplished by using a resistance device, which can be either a flow or threshold resistor, as described earlier in this chapter.

Continuous Positive Airway Pressure

CPAP is a technique in which a patient breathes spontaneously at an elevated baseline pressure (see Figure 11-46). As with PEEP, the expiratory pressure is accomplished with the use of some type of expiratory resistance device. CPAP can be achieved through a mechanical ventilator or a spontaneous breathing CPAP device, as described earlier in this chapter.

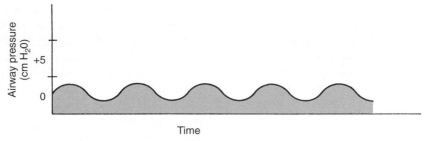

FIGURE 11-46 Curve of pressure and time for continuous positive airway pressure (CPAP). (From Pilbeam SP: *Mechanical ventilation: physiological and clinical applications*, ed 3, St Louis, 1998, Mosby.)

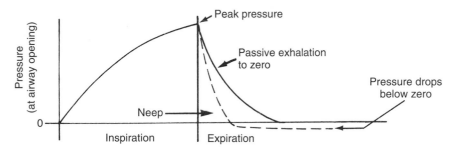

FIGURE 11-47 Pressure-time curve for a mandatory breath, showing normal passive exhalation to zero baseline *(solid line)* and exhalation using negative end-expiratory pressure (NEEP) *(dashed line)*. (From Pilbeam SP: *Mechanical ventilation: physiological and clinical applications*, ed 3, St Louis, 1998, Mosby.)

As with PEEP, CPAP can be used to increase the FRC, to increase the mean airway pressure (MAP), and to improve lung recruitment and oxygenation. It is also used for the treatment of sleep apnea (see Chapters 14 and 15).

Subambient Pressure (Negative End-Expiratory Pressure)

Historically, negative pressure during expiration was called **negative end-expiratory pressure (NEEP)** (Figure 11-47). One of the designs for NEEP used a Venturi at the upper airway to actively draw air from the airway. This older technique was intended to counterbalance the increase in mean intrathoracic pressures caused by positive-pressure ventilation, which can potentially reduce venous return to the heart. NEEP also allowed for more rapid respiratory rates in infants.

Negative pressure during expiration currently is used during high-frequency oscillation (see Figure 11-3). The ventilator actually creates a pressure drop, drawing air out of the circuit. It also is used to facilitate expiration in patients ventilated with the Venturi ventilator (Cardiopulmonary Corp.; see the Evolve Web site for this text). The Venturi provides a slight negative pressure at the very beginning of exhalation. This low negative pressure is believed to facilitate removal of air from the circuit and to reduce the patient's expiratory resistance.

Continuous Gas Flow During Exhalation

Ventilators that provide flow triggering to begin inspiration have a flow of gas passing through the circuit through-out expiration, called *base flow* or *bias flow*. In some ventilators this flow does not begin until about one third of the expiratory time has occurred, thus helping prevent resistance to exhalation. Because this bias flow is present in the patient circuit during the remainder of expiration, it provides immediate flow to a patient at the beginning of the next inspiratory effort.

In current ICU ventilators that use bias flow for flow triggering, the system is designed such that this flow does not increase the baseline pressure. The ventilator's software programming also eliminates this flow in the flow-time waveform so that the baseline flow during exhalation appears to be zero (see the expiratory flow waveform in Figure 11-40).

Expiratory Hold: End-Expiratory Pause

Expiratory hold or **end-expiratory pause** is a procedure performed to estimate the pressure in the patient's lung and ventilator circuit caused by trapped air. Air trapping, or **auto-PEEP**, can occur when a high minute ventilation is used (greater than 10 L/min). It also can occur in patients with obstructive airway disease in whom airway resistance is high and exhalation takes longer than normal, or when a patient is actively exhaling. In these cases, there is not enough time for the patient to exhale completely.

Normally, expiratory flow is finished about halfway through the expiratory phase. The second half of expiration is a period with no flow. In other words, the expiratory portion of a flow-time curve normally shows flow returning to zero during exhalation.

When a patient has air trapping (auto-PEEP), the expiratory flow does not return to zero. A new inspiration begins before the patient has had time to exhale completely. As a result, air remains trapped in the lungs. To be watchful of air trapping, the operator must be sure the flow curve returns to zero before the next breath. If it does not (as illustrated by arrow 3 in Figure 11-48), auto-PEEP is present. The operator then can perform an expiratory pause to determine how much pressure is being trapped.

The expiratory pause maneuver is performed at the end of exhalation after a mandatory breath. For this measurement to be accurate, the patient must not make any spontaneous breathing efforts, or a stable end-expiratory pressure reading cannot be obtained. Activating the expiratory pause control closes both the inspiratory and expiratory valves at the end of expiration and delays delivery of the next mandatory breath. This delay allows time for equilibration of pressures in the circuit and for the operator to obtain a reading of end-expiratory pressure. Current ICU ventilators typically display either the amount of auto-PEEP measured or the total PEEP measured, which can then be compared to the set PEEP value so that the difference can be determined.

To help eliminate auto-PEEP, the operator should try to use a lower minute ventilation if possible. Also, increasing inspiratory flow can shorten inspiratory time and allow more time for exhalation. The use of bronchodilators may help patients with bronchoconstriction by reducing airway resistance. The patient also should be checked (by auscultation) to determine whether the airway needs suctioning.

Time-Limited Exhalation

Time limiting of exhalation can be used as a safety feature during ventilation. Ventilators can be programmed with a minimum expiratory time so that the patient has an adequate amount of time to exhale. This is especially important for infants, who have very rapid respiratory rates that result in a very short total cycle time. Stacking of breaths can occur when exhalation is too short, and air trapping (auto-PEEP) can occur.

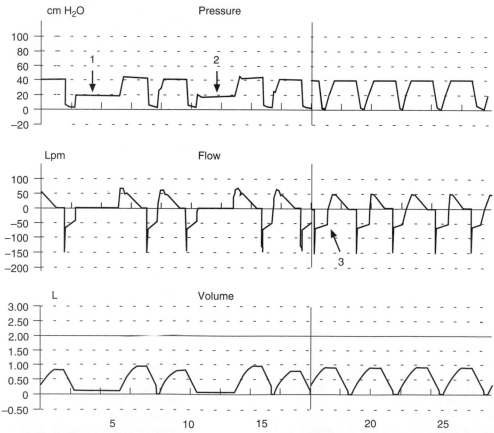

FIGURE 11-48 Pressure-time, flow-time, and volume-time curves showing the use of end-expiratory pause, allowing the estimation of auto-PEEP *(arrows 1 and 2)*. Without using a pause, the presence of auto-PEEP can be detected from the flow curve. Flow does not return to zero before the next mandatory breath *(arrow 3)*. (See text for a complete description.) (Redrawn from Nilsestuen JO, Hargett K: Managing the patient-ventilator system using graphic analysis: an overview and introduction to Graphics Corner, *Respir Care* 41:1105, 1996.)

PART III   BASIC MODES OF VENTILATION

KEY TERMS

adaptive support ventilation (ASV)	expiratory positive airway pressure (EPAP)	pressure-controlled ventilation (PCV)
airway pressure-release ventilation (APRV)	inspiratory positive airway pressure (IPAP)	pressure-limited ventilation
assist-control mode	intermittent mandatory ventilation (IMV)	pressure-regulated volume control (PRVC)
autoflow		pressure-support ventilation (PSV)
automatic tube compensation	mandatory minute ventilation (MMV)	proportional assist ventilation (PAV)
Automode	pendelluft	synchronized intermittent mandatory ventilation (SIMV)
bilevel positive airway pressure (BiPAP, bilevel pressure assist, bilevel pressure support)	pressure-controlled inverse ratio ventilation (PCIRV)	variable pressure control (VPC)
control mode		variable pressure support (VPS)

Modes of ventilation describe the pattern of breath delivery to a patient. The use of the terms associated with ventilator modes indicates the type of breath being delivered and how the breaths are triggered, controlled, and cycled. Most ventilator control panels (user interfaces) have a mode selection switch or screen. Unfortunately, the naming of modes varies among manufacturers, which causes confusion.

The *mode of ventilation* is the pattern of interaction between the ventilator and the patient. It should describe three essential components:
1. The breathing sequence and the control variables within a breath
2. The control type used between breaths
3. The control variables (detailed description)[7]

Part of the difficulty in teaching the modes of ventilation is that the terms used in the hospital setting and by ventilator manufacturers are substantially different from a more ideal way of explaining the actual description of a mode. Given these difficulties, the following section focuses first on a better method of classifying ventilator modes based on Chatburn's classification system. A later section reviews modes as they are commonly ordered by physicians in the hospital and explains how these orders translate to terminology specific to different brands of ventilators. For a discussion of the application of different ventilator modes and how they are set, the reader is referred elsewhere.[7,9,11]

CHATBURN'S CLASSIFICATION OF VENTILATOR MODES

For almost two decades, Robert L. Chatburn has struggled to bring consistency, accuracy, and acceptance to a ventilator classification system that clearly and concisely defines ventilator modes and breath delivery. This section reviews his approach to this concept.[2,3,5,7]

After studying the engineering, clinical aspects, and resources needed to train clinicians about ventilation modes, Chatburn reached four main conclusions:

1. The current names for modes of ventilation are outdated and confusing.
2. Confusion with names can lead to confusion about clinical application.
3. A ventilator mode classification system should be applicable to the modes available on any ventilator.
4. All terminology proposed for ventilator classification needs to be clearly defined.

A mode description includes a statement of how the ventilator controls pressure, volume, and flow during inspiration and also describes how breaths are sequenced.

Some of the concepts of Chatburn's system have already been presented, such as how the equation of motion describes the interaction between the patient and the ventilator. A key point of this equation is that for any mode of ventilation, only one variable (pressure, volume, or flow) can be controlled at a time.

Also presented earlier were the primary breath control variables of volume and pressure and the trigger, limit, and cycle variables of volume, flow, pressure, and time.

Box 11-15 presents the Chatburn classification scheme for ventilator modes. It can be seen that greater detail about a particular mode can be found by using the more detailed levels of the outline.

Breathing Pattern

The main breath-control variables are volume, pressure, and dual control (see Box 11-15, I, a). In volume control, volume remains constant but pressure can vary (see Figure 11-40). In pressure control, pressure remains constant but volume can vary (see Figure 11-39). A dual control, breath-variable mode allows the ventilator to switch from pressure control to volume control or vice versa *within a breath*.

BOX 11-15   Three-Level Classification Scheme for Ventilator Modes*

I. Breathing pattern
  a. Primary breath-control variable
    i. Volume
    ii. Pressure
    iii. Dual
  b. Breath sequence
    i. Continuous mandatory ventilation (CMV)
    ii. Intermittent mandatory ventilation (IMV)
    iii. Continuous spontaneous ventilation (CSV)
II. Control type
  a. Tactical control (within a breath)
    i. Set point
    ii. Auto set point
    iii. Servo
  b. Strategic control (between breaths)
    i. Adaptive
    ii. Optimal
  c. Intelligent control (between patients)
    i. Knowledge based
    ii. Artificial neural network
III. Operational algorithms
  a. Phase variables
    i. Trigger
    ii. Limit
    iii. Cycle
    iv. Baseline
  b. Conditional variables
  c. Computational logic

Modified from Chatburn R: Classification of ventilator modes: update and proposal for implementation, *Respir Care* 52:301, 2007.
*These elements can be used to characterize modes of ventilator operation. The specification of a mode should begin with and may be limited to a description of the mandatory breaths. However, a complete specification includes descriptions of both mandatory and spontaneous breaths.

For example, in pressure augmentation on the BEAR 1000 ventilator, a breath starts out as a pressure-controlled breath but switches to a volume-controlled breath if the desired tidal volume is not delivered during the first part of the breath.

Current ICU ventilators can automatically adjust the pressure limit over several breaths to achieve a target tidal volume. For example, in pressure-regulated volume control (PRVC) on the Servo[i] ventilator, the ventilator delivers a pressure-controlled breath but targets a set volume over several breaths. If the set volume is not achieved, the ventilator slowly adjusts the pressure level to accomplish delivery of the set volume. Autoflow on the Dräger EvitaXL is another example of pressure-controlled ventilation (PCV) with a volume target. A general and simpler term for this breath-to-breath automatic adjustment of set points is a *self-adjusting mode*.[7]

The three types of breath sequences (see Box 11-15, I, b) are continuous mandatory ventilation (CMV), intermittent mandatory ventilation (IMV), and continuous spontaneous ventilation (CSV). Figure 11-49 shows how to determine the breath sequence in use. With CMV, either

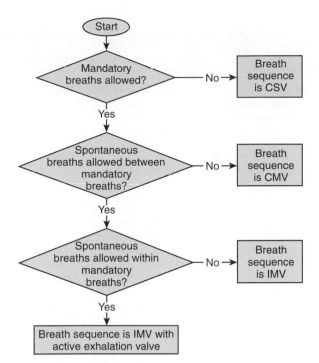

FIGURE 11-49 Algorithm for distinguishing among the three types of breath sequence: continuous mandatory ventilation (CMV), intermittent mandatory ventilation (IMV), and continuous spontaneous ventilation (CSV). (From Chatburn R: Classification of ventilator modes: update and proposal for implementation, *Respir Care* 52:301, 2007.)

time- or patient-triggered breaths are mandatory breaths. However, when spontaneous breathing is allowed between mandatory breaths, the breath sequence is IMV. This breath sequence is commonly called SIMV, meaning *synchronized* IMV, in which patient triggering can activate a mandatory breath. According to Chatburn, patient triggering can be specified in level III, a, i (see Box 11-15) and need not be specified by using the older term *SIMV;* IMV becomes a more appropriate terminology. With CSV all breaths are spontaneous. (NOTE: An assisted breath may be spontaneous or mandatory. See previous discussion of assisted breaths in this chapter.)

Control Type

Seven types of controls are used in mechanical ventilation (Table 11-1).[6,7] At the basic level, control emphasizes what happens within a breath. In *tactical control,* operator input to the ventilator is needed. At the next level, *strategic control,* the ventilator takes over some of the control normally adjusted by user input. The set points can be adjusted automatically by the ventilator over several breaths. The highest level is *intelligent control,* in which the input and control from the ventilator take over input from the user. This type of software programming uses the experience and input of experts.

Operational Algorithms

At the greatest level of detail, the description of the mode must include the exact instructions used by the ventilator's

control circuit to create a breathing pattern. This description includes the *phase variables* (see Box 11-15, III, a) described earlier in this chapter. For example, volume-controlled intermittent mandatory ventilation (VC-IMV) plus pressure support would be VC-IMV with a set point control of volume for mandatory breaths and a limit variable for spontaneous breaths of pressure above baseline pressure. This would indicate that spontaneous breaths are *assisted;* that is, during a spontaneous breath, the pressure rises above baseline during inspiration when the pressure-support level is set above zero.

Conditional variables (see Box 11-15, III, b) are used by software programs in the ventilator to evaluate a breathing pattern and then allow the ventilator to intervene or not intervene based on what is measured or evaluated. For example, if the ventilator determines that spontaneous minute ventilation has fallen below the minimum minute ventilation set by the operator, the ventilator can increase some parameter (volume, pressure, or respiratory rate) to increase the minute ventilation to the patient.

Very advanced control types use fairly complex instructions, which are referred to as *computational logic* (see Box 11-15, III, c). Computational logic is a description of the relationship between the settings selected by the operator, the monitored information fed back to the ventilator computer, and the final output or breathing pattern delivered. An example of a very advanced level of computational logic is **adaptive support ventilation (ASV),** which is used on the Hamilton GALILEO and G5 ventilators. The ventilator monitors lung mechanics, alveolar ventilation, dead space volume, expiratory time constant, ventilating pressures, and respiratory rate. It then strives to minimize the work of breathing for the patient and also protect the lung (see Chapter 12, section on the Hamilton GALILEO, for more information about this mode). In describing this mode based on Chatburn's classification system, the rules that govern breath delivery and the breath sequence would be part of the computational logic description.

Summary of Chatburn's Classification System for Ventilator Modes

Modes of ventilation named and used in the clinical setting and by ventilator manufacturers follow no standard set of rules. This can make communication about ventilator modes confusing. Table 11-2 provides a description of modes of ventilation available on a few of the ICU ventilators currently used in the United States based on Chatburn's system. Evaluation of this table and practice in using this system could improve clinicians' ability to communicate about modes of ventilation.*

*As respiratory therapist Tim Op't Holt has said, "I see this classification as the Rosetta Stone for the interpretation of mode hieroglyphics!"

TABLE 11-1

Basic Types of Controls Used in Current Mechanical Ventilators

Control Type	Characteristics	Description of Example Mode	Example Mode	Applicable Ventilators
Set point	The output of the ventilator automatically matches a constant operator-preset input value. Multiple set points are possible.	Mandatory breaths are pressure limited and time cycled, according to the operator-set values for peak inspiratory pressure and frequency.	Pressure-controlled intermittent mandatory ventilation (PC-IMV)	Bird VIP
Auto set point	The ventilator selects which operator-adjusted set points are enforced at the moment.	Inspiration starts in pressure control and switches to volume control. Inspiration starts in volume control and switches to pressure control.	Pressure augmentation Continuous mandatory ventilation (CMV) plus pressure-limited ventilation	BEAR 1000 Dräger Evita-4
Servo	The ventilator output automatically follows a varying input.	The instantaneous value of pressure is proportional to the instantaneous volume and/or flow generated by the patient.	Proportional assist Automatic tube compensation	Puritan Bennett 840 Dräger Evita-4
Adaptive	One ventilator set point is automatically adjusted to achieve another set point as the patient's condition changes.	Mandatory breaths are pressure limited, and the pressure limit is automatically adjusted between breaths to achieve the preset tidal volume. Inspiratory time is adjusted to maintain an inspiration to expiration ratio of 1:2 as the patient's breathing frequency changes.	Pressure-regulated volume control Adaptive I-time	Maquet Servo[i] VersaMed iVent
Optimal	One ventilator set point is automatically adjusted to optimize another set point according to some model of system behavior, and the output can be maximized or minimized dynamically.	Each breath is pressure limited, and the pressure limit is automatically adjusted between breaths (using ventilatory mechanics measurements) to minimize the work of breathing.	Adaptive support ventilation	Hamilton GALILEO
Knowledge based	Set points are automatically adjusted according to a rule-based expert system.	The pressure-support level for spontaneous breaths is automatically adjusted to maintain appropriate breathing frequency, tidal volume, and end-tidal carbon dioxide ($ETCO_2$), depending on the type of patient pathology.	SmartCare	Dräger EvitaXL
Artificial neural network	Set points are automatically adjusted by an artificial neural network. The actual rules are generally unknown. The relation between inputs and outputs is determined by weighting factors at neural nodes that change with learning.	The network inputs are the current ventilator settings and partial pressure of arterial blood gases and pH. Network outputs are the most appropriate ventilator settings projected to maintain blood gases within an acceptable range.	Experimental	Not available
Actual electrical activity of the diaphragm*	Set points are automatically adjusted based on electrical activity of the diaphragm and the level of response to the electrical activity as set by the operator.	The onset, intensity, and termination of diaphragm electrical activity determine the breath trigger, breath limit, and breath cycle of the ventilator. The operator sets the amount of response to the level of electrical activity.	Neurally adjusted ventilatory assist (NAVA)	Maquet Servo[i]

Modified from Chatburn R: Classification of ventilator modes: update and proposal for implementation, *Respir Care* 53(3):301-323, 2007.
*The eighth type of control has been added to Chatburn's original table.

TABLE 11-2

Some Common Modes Available on Five ICU Ventilators Used in the United States*

Ventilator	Mode Name (VC-CMV)	Breathing Pattern	MANDATORY BREATHS ONLY					SPONTANEOUS BREATHS
			Control Type	Trigger Variable	Limit Variable	Cycle Variable	Operational Logic	
XL	Continuous mandatory ventilation (and CMV + assist)	VC-CMV	Set point	F, T	F, V	T	N/A	
840	Volume control Assist control	VC-CMV	Set point	F, T	F	T	N/A	
Servo[i]	Volume control	VC-CMV	Set point	F, P, T	F, V	T	N/A	
Gold	Assist control Synchronized controlled Mandatory ventilation	VC-CMV	Set point	F, P, T	F, V	T	N/A	
AVEA	Volume Assist Control	VC-CMV	Set point	F, P, T	F, V	T	N/A	

Ventilator	Mode Name (PC-CMV)	Breathing Pattern	Control Type	Trigger Variable	Limit Variable	Cycle Variable	Operational Logic
XL	Continuous mandatory ventilation + pressure-limited ventilation	DC-CMV	Auto set point	F, V	F, V, P	T	Computational logic: Mandatory breaths start as volume controlled but switch to pressure controlled if airway pressure (P_{aw}) reaches the set maximum pressure (P_{max}).
840	Pressure control, assist control	PC-CMV	Set point	F, P, T	P	T	N/A
Servo[i]	Pressure control	PC-CMV	Set point	F, P, T	P	T	N/A
Gold	Pressure control, assist control (pressure controlled, controlled mandatory ventilation)	PC-CMV	Set point	F, P, T	P	T	N/A
AVEA	Pressure assist control	PC-CMV	Set point	F, P, T	P	T	N/A

Ventilator	Mode Name (VC-SIMV + PSV)	Breathing Pattern	MANDATORY BREATHS					SPONTANEOUS BREATHS	
			Control Type	Trigger Variable	Limit Variable	Cycle Variable	Operational Logic	Control Type	Trigger/Limit/Cycle
XL	SIMV + PSV	VC-IMV	Set point	F, T	F, V	T	Computational logic: Mandatory breaths are volume controlled. Spontaneous breaths occur between timed mandatory breath windows (time determined by rate).	Set point	P or flow trigger; P limit; P or flow cycle
840	SIMV + PSV	VC-IMV	Set point	F, P, T	F, V	T	(Same as above)	(Same as above)	(Same as above)
Servo[i]	SIMV (volume control) + PSV	VC-IMV	Set point	F, P, T	F, V	T	(Same as above)	(Same as above)	(Same as above)
Gold	SIMV + PSV	VC-IMV	Set point	F, P, T	F, V, P	P, T		(Same as above)	(Same as above)
AVEA	Volume SIMV	VC-IMV	Set point	F, P, T	F, V, P	P, T		(Same as above)	(Same as above)

Continued

TABLE 11-2
Some Common Modes Available on Five ICU Ventilators Used in the United States*—cont'd

Ventilator	Mode Name (PC-SIMV + PSV)	Breathing Pattern	MANDATORY BREATHS					SPONTANEOUS BREATHS
			Control Type	Trigger Variable	Limit Variable	Cycle Variable	Operational Logic	Control Type / Trigger/Limit/Cycle
XL	PC+	PC-IMV	Set point	F, T	P	T	Computational logic: Mandatory breaths are pressure controlled. Spontaneous breaths occur between timed mandatory breath windows (time determined by rate).	Set point / P or flow trigger / P limit / P or flow cycle
840	PC-SIMV	PC-IMV	Set point	F, P, T	P	T	(Same as above)	(Same as above)
Servo[i]	SIMV (pressure control) + PSV	PC-IMV	Set point	F, P, T	P	T	(Same as above)	(Same as above)
Gold	PC-SIMV + PSV	PC-IMV	Set point	F, P, T	P	T	(Same as above)	(Same as above)
AVEA	Pressure SIMV	PC-IMV	Set point	F, P, T	P	T	(Same as above)	(Same as above)

Ventilator	Mode Name (PC–Volume Target)	Breathing Pattern	MANDATORY BREATHS					SPONTANEOUS BREATHS
			Control Type	Trigger Variable	Limit Variable	Cycle Variable	Operational Logic	Control Type / Trigger/Limit/Cycle
XL	CMV + Autoflow	PC-CMV	Adaptive	F, T	P	T	Computational logic: Mandatory breaths are pressure controlled. If the target volume is not met, the pressure limit is automatically adjusted.	N/A
840	VC+	PC-CMV	Adaptive	F, P, T	P	T	(Same as above)	N/A
Servo[i]	PRVC	PC-IMV	Adaptive	F, P, T	P	T	(Same as above)	N/A
Gold	PC-assist control (PC, CMV) + adaptive pressure ventilation (or APV-CMV)	PC-CMV	Adaptive	F, P, T	P	T	(Same as above)	N/A
AVEA	PRVC	PC-CMV	Adaptive	F, P, T	P	T	(Same as above)	N/A

Ventilator	Mode Name (PC-SIMV–Volume Target)	Breathing Pattern	MANDATORY BREATHS					SPONTANEOUS BREATHS
			Control Type	Trigger Variable	Limit Variable	Cycle Variable	Operational Logic	Control Type / Trigger/Limit/Cycle (+PSV) then:
XL	SIMV + Autoflow	PC-IMV	Adaptive	F, T	P	T	Computational logic: Mandatory breaths are pressure controlled. If the target limit is not met, the pressure limit is adjusted. Spontaneous breaths occur between timed mandatory breath windows (time determined by rate).	Set point / P or flow trigger / P limit / P or flow cycle
840	VC + SIMV	PC-IMV	Adaptive	F, P, T	P	T	(Same as above)	(Same as above)
Servo[i]	SIMV-PRVC	PC-IMV	Adaptive	F, P, T	P	T	(Same as above)	(Same as above)
Gold	PC-SIMV + adaptive pressure ventilation (or APV-SIMV)	PC-IMV	Adaptive	F, P, T	P	T	(Same as above)	(Same as above)
AVEA	PRVC SIMV	PC-IMV	Adaptive	F, P, T	P	T	(Same as above)	(Same as above)

Ventilator	Mode Name (Spontaneous PS/CPAP)	Breathing Pattern	MANDATORY BREATHS Control Type	Trigger Variable	Limit Variable	Cycle Variable	Operational Logic	SPONTANEOUS BREATHS Control Type	Trigger/Limit/Cycle (+PSV) then:
XL	Pressure support and/or CPAP	PC-CSV	N/A	N/A	N/A	N/A	Computational logic: When PS pressure is set above zero baseline pressure, spontaneous breaths are "assisted." When PS is set at zero and spontaneous breaths are at a baseline pressure (CPAP), spontaneous breaths are unassisted.	Set point	Flow trigger Pressure limit P or flow cycle
840	Spontaneous (PS and/or CPAP)	PC-CSV	N/A	N/A	N/A	N/A	(Same as above)	(Same as above)	(Same as above)
Servo[†] Gold	Pressure support/CPAP Spontaneous (PSV, CPAP)	PC-CSV PC-CSV	N/A N/A	N/A N/A	N/A N/A	N/A N/A	(Same as above) (Same as above)	(Same as above) (Same as above)	(Same as above) (Same as above)
AVEA	CPAP-PSV	PC-CSV	N/A	N/A	N/A	N/A	(Same as above)	(Same as above)	(Same as above)

Ventilator	Mode Name (Airway Pressure-Release Ventilation [APRV] + PS)	Breathing Pattern	MANDATORY BREATHS Control Type	Trigger Variable	Limit Variable	Cycle Variable	Operational Logic	SPONTANEOUS BREATHS Control Type	Trigger/Limit/Cycle (+PSV) then:
XL	APRV	PC-IMV	Set point	F, T	P	T	Computational logic: Mandatory breaths are pressure controlled. Spontaneous breaths may occur during mandatory breath delivery or between mandatory breaths. Spontaneous breaths are unassisted.	Set point	Pressure Pressure Pressure
840	Bilevel	PC-IMV	Set point	F, T	P	T	Computational logic: Mandatory breaths are pressure controlled. Spontaneous breaths may occur during mandatory breath delivery or between mandatory breaths. When PS pressure is set above zero baseline pressure, spontaneous breaths are "assisted." When PS is set at zero and spontaneous breaths follow mandatory breaths and are at a baseline of zero, spontaneous breaths are unassisted.	Set point (above baseline pressure only)	F, P trigger P limited F, P cycle
Servo[†]	BiVent	PC-IMV	Set point	F, T	P	T	(Same as above)	Set point above mandatory breaths and/or between mandatory breaths	F, P trigger P limit F, P cycle
Gold	(N/A—see ASV, Chapter 12)								
AVEA	BiPhasic—APRV	PC-IMV	Set point	F, T	P	T	(Same as above)	(Same as above)	

*Presented so that comparable modes of different manufacturers are listed together.

†Specific details about each mode are available in Chapter 12 under the name of each ventilator.

Ventilator models: XL, Dräger EvitaXL; 840, Puritan Bennett 840; Servo, Maquet Servo[i]; Gold, Hamilton GALILEO Gold; AVEA, VIASYS AVEA. CMV, Continuous mandatory ventilation; CSV, continuous spontaneous ventilation; DC, dual control; F, flow; P, pressure; PC, pressure control; IMV, intermittent mandatory ventilation; V, volume; VC, volume control.

COMMON CLINICAL TERMINOLOGY FOR MODES OF VENTILATION

As mentioned previously, the names used for modes of ventilation in the clinical setting do not follow a sense of logic, as does Chatburn's classification system. However, for the student of mechanical ventilation, exposure to the clinical setting would become a confusing experience without some idea of the terms clinicians currently are using to discuss or follow ventilator orders. For that reason, the following section reviews terminology used in the acute care environment.

Controlled Mechanical Ventilation, or Control Mode

The **controlled mode** (volume-controlled continuous mandatory ventilation [VC-CMV] or pressure-controlled continuous mandatory ventilation [PC-CMV]) is the delivery of a preset volume (volume-targeted) or pressure (pressure-targeted) breath at set intervals (time-triggered breaths). Breaths are time or volume cycled and pressure or volume limited, and volume or time cycled. Each breath is mandatory. Controlled ventilation (VC-CMV or PC-CMV) generally is used when patients make no inspiratory effort, as with patients suffering from a drug overdose, neurologic or neuromuscular disorders, or seizure activities that require sedation and sometimes induced paralysis. Figure 11-50 shows the pressure, flow, and volume

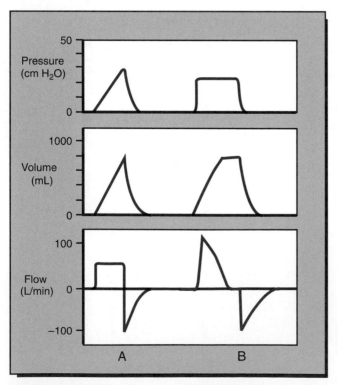

FIGURE 11-50 Pressure, volume, and flow scalars for volume-targeted ventilation with constant flow **(A)** and pressure-targeted ventilation **(B),** both in the control mode.

scalars for controlled ventilation. Figure 11-40A shows volume-targeted CMV, and Figure 11-50B shows pressure-targeted CMV.

Note that ventilation in which the patient cannot trigger a breath should not be deliberately selected on the operating panel. That is, the ventilator should not be insensitive to the patient's inspiratory effort. Generally, if a practitioner wants to eliminate spontaneous breathing, the patient must be sedated and paralyzed. Control of breathing can be provided by any CMV or IMV mode of ventilation. Most current ventilators do not have pure "control mode" options (i.e., a knob that says "control mode").

When practitioners in the clinical setting hear the term *control mode* or **assist-control mode** (described in the following section), they typically assume that volume ventilation is being used. This assumption has come about through the historical development of this breath type. The phrase **pressure-controlled ventilation (PCV)** is commonly assumed to mean time-triggered ventilation that is pressure targeted (pressure limited). Being specific about the meanings of terms is important so that misunderstandings do not occur.

Assist, Assist-Control Ventilation

Modes referred to in the clinical setting as assist and assist-control modes should more appropriately be called *continuous mandatory ventilation (CMV)* (either VC-CMV or PC-CMV), in which breaths are patient triggered. (NOTE: The use of the word "assist" here should not be confused with Chatburn's classification of an *assisted* breath.)

In a ventilator, sensing mechanisms are designed to detect a drop in pressure, flow, or volume in the circuit when a patient makes an inspiratory effort. Operators set a control called a *sensitivity* or *trigger (variable)*. The sensitivity setting determines how easy or how difficult it is for a patient's effort to trigger breath delivery. Operators also set a back-up mandatory breath rate when using patient triggering to ensure that a minimum number of breaths are delivered for patient safety if the patient becomes apneic.

When breaths are patient triggered, the pressure-time scalar shows a downward deflection at the beginning of breath delivery (Figure 11-51). Breath intervals may be irregular, but each breath delivers the set volume or pressure, regardless of how it was triggered. If the patient's rate drops below the set rate (i.e., if the time between patient-initiated breaths is longer than the ventilator cycle time [60 sec/set rate]), time-triggered breaths occur. Breaths continue at the mandatory rate (time triggered) until the patient's effort is detected before the next timed ventilator interval.

In summary, VC-CMV and PC-CMV (typically called assist or assist-control) are patient or time triggered, volume or pressure targeted, and usually volume or time cycled. In volume ventilation, breaths are volume or flow limited. In pressure ventilation, breaths are pressure limited.

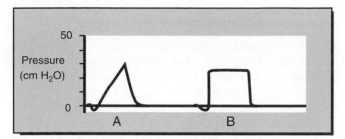

FIGURE 11-51 Pressure-time curves for volume and pressure ventilation in the assist-control mode. Note the deflection of the pressure below baseline before breath delivery.

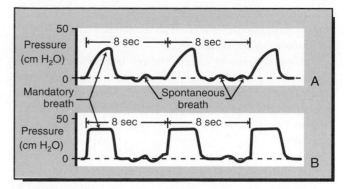

FIGURE 11-52 Pressure-time curves for volume ventilation **(A)** and pressure ventilation **(B)** with intermittent mandatory ventilation (IMV).

Pressure-Controlled Ventilation

Pressure-controlled (pressure-limited) continuous mandatory ventilation (PC-CMV) sometimes is referred to as pressure-controlled ventilation. It should be pointed out that PCV is not a "mode" of ventilation but a breath type. The operator sets a target pressure. Sensitivity is also set to allow for patient triggering. A rate and an inspiratory time are set to establish the total cycle time. The rate guarantees a minimum respiratory rate.

When the breath is triggered, the ventilator produces a rapid inspiratory flow to achieve the set pressure. When the pressure is reached and the lungs fill, the flow decreases (descending ramp). The breath ends when the inspiratory time has passed. Volume delivery varies with the set inspiratory time and the patient's lung characteristics and whether the patient is actively inspiring (see Figure 11-39). For example, when the patient's lungs are stiff, less volume is delivered for the same amount of pressure. As the lungs improve, less pressure is required to deliver the same volume. If the patient actively inspires, the ventilator increases flow delivery to maintain the set pressure, which can increase volume delivery. If the inspiratory time is too short, the ventilator does not have enough time to deliver all the set pressure to the lungs, and the volume may be lower than desired.

In its early development, PC-CMV was used with inverse inspiration to expiration (I:E) ratios and was termed **pressure-controlled inverse ratio ventilation (PCIRV).** Inverse ratios were used to increase the mean airway pressure, with the intent of improving oxygenation of the patient. (See the section on PCIRV later in the chapter.)

Another commonly used abbreviation is PC-SIMV, referring to pressure-controlled breaths (breath type) delivered intermittently. Some ventilator companies use labeling such as PC-SIMV or SIMV-PC to designate the breath type and mode selection (see Chapter 12).

Intermittent Mandatory Ventilation

Intermittent mandatory ventilation (IMV) is designed to deliver volume- or pressure-targeted breaths at a set minimum frequency (time triggered). Between mandatory breaths, the patient can breathe spontaneously from the ventilator circuit without getting the set volume or pressure from the ventilator itself. During this spontaneous breathing period, the patient breathes from the set baseline pressure, which may be ambient pressure or a positive baseline pressure (PEEP/CPAP). Spontaneous breaths can also be assisted by the use of pressure support (see the section on pressure support later in this chapter). Because patients have an opportunity to breathe spontaneously, they must assume part of the work of breathing. For this reason, IMV is commonly used for patients who can provide part of the ventilatory work.

Figure 11-52 shows the pressure-time graph for IMV with volume and pressure ventilation. During IMV with volume ventilation (IMV vol.), mandatory breaths are time triggered, volume targeted, and volume cycled. During IMV with pressure ventilation (IMV press.), mandatory breaths are time triggered, pressure targeted, and time cycled.

When IMV is used for weaning a patient from the ventilator, the mandatory breath rate can be progressively reduced, allowing for more spontaneous breaths from the patient. Historically, IMV circuits had to be added to the patient circuit to provide IMV ventilation. Only older generation home care ventilators provide IMV, and an IMV setup needs to be added. The Evolve Web site for this text includes a section on "Setting up a ventilator with IMV."

Synchronized Intermittent Mandatory Ventilation

Synchronized intermittent mandatory ventilation (SIMV) originally was added to ventilators about two decades ago. The distinguishing characteristic at the time was that with IMV, mandatory breaths were always time triggered. With SIMV, mandatory breaths could be either patient or time triggered. In addition, to use IMV, more circuitry had to be added to the ventilator by the operator. When SIMV was incorporated into the ventilator, this additional circuitry was built in.

SIMV describes synchronous breath delivery when a patient effort is detected (patient triggering). When the time for a mandatory breath occurs based on the set mandatory breath rate, the machine waits briefly for a patient effort. If the patient triggers the breath (patient effort detected), the ventilator *synchronously* delivers the mandatory breath. If no patient effort is detected, a time-triggered mandatory breath is delivered.

During the spontaneous period between mandatory breaths, the patient breathes from the baseline pressure, which may be ambient or positive (PEEP/CPAP). Spontaneous breaths can also be assisted by the use of pressure support (see the section later in this chapter on pressure support).

Most commonly used ICU ventilators have controls labeled SIMV. Sometimes these controls are labeled "SIMV(vol.)" and "SIMV(press.)" on the control panel to distinguish between volume- and pressure-targeted SIMV. Box 11-16 outlines how the controls are set for volume- and pressure-targeted breaths in either CMV or IMV/SIMV ventilation. Figure 11-53 illustrates volume and pressure SIMV.

BOX 11-16	**Operator-Selected Controls for Volume- and Pressure-Targeted Breaths in Assist-Control and Intermittent Mandatory Ventilation/ Synchronized Intermittent Mandatory Ventilation (IMV/SIMV)**

For volume-targeted breaths in assist-control and IMV/SIMV, the operator normally selects from two options:
1. With volume-cycled (or flow-time*) ventilators, the volume, flow, and rate are set.
2. With time-cycled ventilators, the volume, rate, and inspiratory time are set.

For pressure-targeted breaths in assist-control and IMV/ SIMV modes, the operator normally selects the following:
1. Pressure
2. Mandatory rate
3. Inspiratory time

---

*Flow and time are measured, and the ventilator cycles when it estimates that the set volume has been delivered.

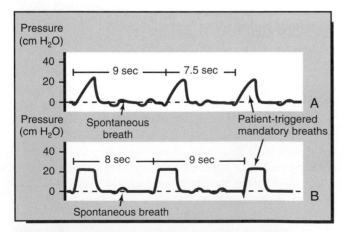

FIGURE 11-53 Pressure-time curves for volume ventilation (**A,** *top curve*) and pressure ventilation (**B,** *bottom curve*) with synchronized intermittent mandatory ventilation (SIMV). (See text for explanation.)

Pressure-Support Ventilation

Pressure-support ventilation (PSV), or PC-CSV, is a spontaneous breath type that allows the operator to select a pressure to support the patient's work of breathing. It is patient triggered, pressure limited, and flow cycled.[24,25] PSV can also be used to support the work of breathing for spontaneous breaths during IMV/SIMV ventilation. Figure 11-54 shows the waveforms for SIMV plus PSV for both volume- and pressure-targeted mandatory breaths.

In PSV, as in pressure-controlled continuous mandatory ventilation (PC-CMV or PC-IMV), the ventilator delivers a high flow of gas to the patient when a breath is triggered. As the lungs fill, the flow and the pressure gradient between the machine and the patient decrease. The flow curve appears as a descending waveform but never falls all the way to zero during inspiration because ventilators are programmed to measure the drop in flow during inspiration until it reaches a predetermined amount. Some ventilators end inspiration when flow drops to 25% of peak flow during inspiration. Others end inspiration at fixed rates (e.g., the Puritan Bennett 7200 (Covidien, Inc., Pleasanton, California) cycles when flow drops to 5 L/min). Still other ventilators provide flow cycling as an adjustable parameter. This allows the operator to change the cycle level (% flow) based on the type of patient being ventilated. Examples of these ventilators include the Hamilton GALILEO Gold, the Servo[i], and the Newport e500.

In the future, new software may automatically adjust the flow-cycling threshold by monitoring such factors as the pulmonary time constant at end-exhalation and the slope of the pressure waveform at end-inspiration. This monitoring may allow adjustment of the flow-cycling threshold by the ventilator.[26-29]

If a leak is present in the system, the ventilator increases the flow to maintain the set pressure. In this situation, the flow may not decrease to the flow-cycle value, and inspiration will be prolonged. As a safety feature, ventilators have a back-up time cycle that usually is a set time between 1 and 5 seconds, depending on the type of ventilator used.

The breath can also be pressure cycled if the pressure begins to rise higher than the set pressure, which might occur if the patient begins to actively exhale or cough. Typically, a PS breath pressure cycles at 2 to 3 cm H_2O above the set pressure. These safety back-up systems are available with any ventilator that provides PSV.

The volume delivery in PSV is determined by three factors: the set pressure, the patient's lung characteristics (resistance and compliance), and the patient's inspiratory effort.

PSV has two common uses. The first is to reduce the patient's work of breathing when resistance to breathing is increased because of an artificial airway and the ventilatory circuit. The work of breathing imposed by small endotracheal tubes can be a major contributor to fatigue. A review of Poiseuille's law illustrates the basic theory of pressure support when airway resistance (R_{aw}) is increased

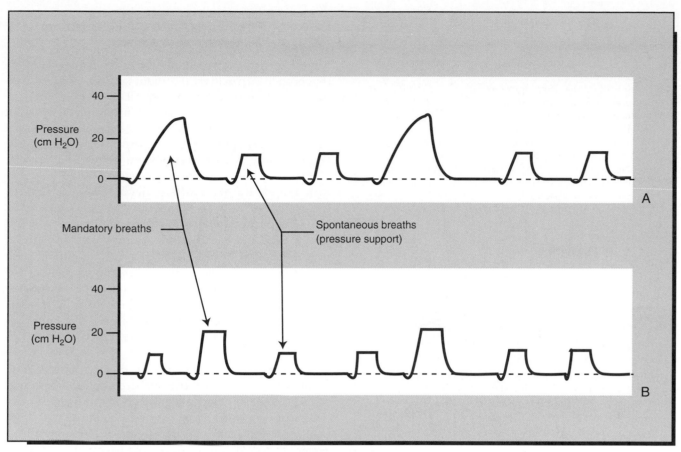

Mandatory breaths

Spontaneous breaths
(pressure support)

FIGURE 11-54 Pressure waveforms of SIMV(vol.) plus pressure-support (PSV) (**A**, top waveform) and SIMV(press.) + PSV (**B**). Note that the pressure-support ventilation (PSV) breaths both show a constant pressure delivery. Mandatory breaths in volume ventilation are different from mandatory breaths in pressure ventilation.

BOX 11-17	Use of Pressure-Support Ventilation with Increased Airway Resistance

Pressure support increases the pressure gradient for gas flow across a tube. Theoretically, if the pressure gradient across the tube is high enough, the effect of the increased resistance attributable to the tube is negated.

(see Chapter 1). Reducing the diameter of the airway significantly increases the resistance to gas flow, which can be a contributing factor to the difficulty of weaning some patients (Box 11-17).

When the increased work of breathing is associated with the artificial airway or the ventilator system, the initial PS level that is set does not have to be very high (a setting of 5 to 10 cm H_2O commonly is used). Another way to estimate the starting pressure level is to calculate the patient's transairway pressure, which is the difference between the peak pressure and the plateau pressure ($P_{TA} = P_{peak} - P_{plat}$). The P_{TA} reflects the pressure generated to overcome the resistance caused by the ventilator circuit, the endotracheal tube, and the patient's airways.[11] The P_{TA} value is a safe starting point for PS. The PS level can be adjusted after it is activated to fit the patient's needs.

Current ventilators, such as the Dräger EvitaXL and the Puritan Bennett 840, have an artificial airway compensation feature, called **automatic tube compensation.** When the type of artificial airway the patient has (endotracheal tube or tracheostomy) and the size of the tube are programmed into the ventilator, the ventilator calculates and delivers the amount of pressure support needed to compensate for the resistance through the artificial airway.

PSV also is used for spontaneously breathing patients who have intact respiratory centers. PSV can be adjusted so that much of the work of breathing is provided by the ventilator with a simple increase in the set pressure level. This result can be accomplished by measuring volume delivery while adjusting pressure. The desired tidal volume (V_T) is based on the patient's ideal body weight (IBW) and lung condition. For example, 5 to 6 mL/kg may be appropriate for a patient, but tidal volume needs vary with different lung conditions.[11,23] Box 11-18 lists the types of patients who might benefit from PSV; Clinical Rounds 11-9 and 11-10 provide exercises in PSV.

BOX 11-18	Patients Who Are Candidates for Pressure-Support Ventilation

- Patients with an artificial airway in place and any of the following conditions:
  - Airways smaller than optimum size
  - Spontaneous respiratory rates greater than 20 breaths/min (adults)
  - Minute ventilation greater than 10 L/min
- Patients supported with intermittent mandatory ventilation/synchronized intermittent mandatory ventilation (IMV/SIMV) or continuous positive airway pressure (CPAP) (with spontaneous breaths) and any of the following conditions:
  - A history of chronic obstructive pulmonary disorder (COPD)
  - Evidence of ventilatory muscle weakness requiring ventilatory support

CLINICAL ROUNDS 11-9

A patient has a peak pressure of 24 cm H_2O and a plateau pressure of 18 cm H_2O. What might be an appropriate initial setting for pressure support (PS) in this patient?

Assume that you have initiated pressure support on an 80-kg patient who is spontaneously breathing. What might be an appropriate volume to target with the PS mode?

See Evolve Resources for the answer.

CLINICAL ROUNDS 11-10

If the algorithm (computer program) that controls the ventilator's function determines the cycling criteria in pressure-support ventilation (PSV), how would you argue that this breath is classified as a spontaneous breath? Isn't the ventilator determining the cycling time and not the patient?

See Evolve Resources for the answer.

Bilevel Positive Airway Pressure (Bilevel Pressure-Assist)

Bilevel positive airway pressure is similar to CPAP in that both breath delivery techniques provide positive pressure during inspiration and expiration. With CPAP, the pressure tends to stay at a fairly constant baseline with a slightly negative pressure as the patient breathes in and a slightly positive pressure as the patient breathes out (see Figure 11-46). With bilevel positive airway pressure, the **inspiratory positive airway pressure (IPAP)** is higher than the **expiratory positive airway pressure (EPAP)** (Figure 11-55).

Bilevel positive airway pressure is referred to by several names, including bilevel positive airway pressure, **bilevel pressure-assist,** bilevel PEEP, bilevel CPAP, bilevel positive pressure, and **bilevel pressure-support.** One of the original companies to manufacture this mode was the Respironics Corporation, which named the mode *BiPAP.* The term **BiPAP,** although a brand name for this unit, has become the popular term used by clinicians to describe this method of ventilation.

BiPAP administered via a nasal or face mask is commonly used to treat obstructive sleep apnea. Units that provide BiPAP generate a high gas flow through a microprocessor-controlled valve. Operator controls for both IPAP and EPAP are available. Inspiration normally is patient triggered, but it can be time triggered when a rate control is provided. BiPAP units can be flow or time cycled. Hospitals also use these units for noninvasive positive-pressure ventilation (NIPPV) for patients who do not necessarily require intubation. Chapter 14 provides more detail about the Respironics BiPAP S/T and other devices that can provide bilevel pressure support and noninvasive ventilation.

Most BiPAP units also provide leak compensation. The normal interface between the unit and the patient is a mask. Because masks commonly have leaks around them during ventilation, these units can compensate for leaks. In many cases the unit can determine the amount of leakage and increase the flow output to compensate. It can

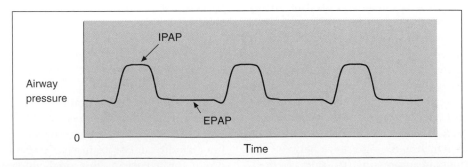

FIGURE 11-55 Bilevel positive airway pressure (BiPAP) showing inspiratory positive airway pressure (IPAP) and expiratory positive airway pressure (EPAP). Note that both pressures are higher than a zero baseline pressure. (From Pilbeam SP: *Mechanical ventilation: physiological and clinical applications,* ed 3, St Louis, 1998, Mosby.)

continue its normal triggering and cycling, even when a small leak is present.

ADDITIONAL MODES OF VENTILATION

The advent of faster computer systems, more sophisticated programming, and higher levels of technology in monitoring have provided for a variety of intelligent systems. These technologic advances have allowed for the development of additional modes of ventilation and breath delivery. As a result, in addition to the more commonly ordered modes of ventilation, such as CMV, IMV, BiPAP, and the spontaneous modes of PS and CPAP, several other, more sophisticated modes have become available. Some of these modes are adaptations of CMV, such as inverse ratio ventilation. Others are adaptations of IMV, such as airway pressure-release ventilation.

Still other modes and breath types have arisen to provide a solution to a problem. For example, during pressure-controlled continuous mandatory ventilation (PC-CMV) or pressure-controlled intermittent mandatory ventilation (PC-IMV), when the patient's lung characteristics change, the volume delivery also changes. This can affect the overall minute ventilation $\dot{V}_E$, acid-base status, and oxygenation (Historical Note 11-6). Two modes of ventilation were developed and became available in the 1990s to overcome this problem. One is a dual control mode, and the other is an adaptive mode.

Recall that a *dual control* mode allows the ventilator to switch from one control variable to another within a single breath. For example, the control variable can switch from pressure to volume within a breath. Examples of this are pressure augmentation on the BEAR 1000 and volume-assured pressure support (VAPS) on the Bird 8400. Another dual control mode switches from volume to pressure (e.g., the pressure-limited ventilation mode on the Dräger Evita-4).

With PC-CMV, volume is variable. Some clinicians want to have the benefits of a pressure breath and also a consistent volume delivery. One solution is the *adaptive* mode, in which the set point is adjusted automatically to achieve another set point; this occurs over several breaths rather than during a single breath. An example of this is pressure-regulated volume control (PRVC) on the Maquet Servo 300 and Servo^i and the VIASYS AVEA ventilators. In PRVC, the pressure is adjusted by the ventilator over several breaths to achieve the set tidal volume.

Both the dual control mode and the adaptive mode offer the benefits of pressure ventilation, including the ability to limit maximum pressure, allow a more patient-adaptive flow pattern, and provide better gas distribution with the descending flow delivery. At the same time, these modes still target a set volume.

Another adaptive, closed-loop mode that has been available since the 1970s is **mandatory minute ventilation (MMV),** which guarantees delivery of a set minimum minute ventilation ($\dot{V}_E$).[30] MMV has been used as a method of weaning as well as a method of backing up ventilation.

These and other modes are briefly described in the following section (Box 11-19). Chapter 12 provides more detail on each ventilator.

Inverse Ratio Ventilation

In the early 1970s, Reynolds reported success using mechanical ventilation in infants when the inspiratory phase exceeded the expiratory phase, using an inspiratory hold.[31,32] Since then, inverse ratio ventilation (IRV) has been used both in infants and adults. The primary purpose of this technique is to treat acute respiratory distress syndrome (ARDS). By extending the inspiratory time, the mean airway pressure is increased, and oxygenation can be improved. Sometimes air trapping (auto-PEEP) occurs, which increases or restores the functional residual capacity (FRC) of the lung. In this instance auto-PEEP can keep alveoli open that otherwise would collapse on exhalation. When IRV is used, auto-PEEP should be monitored and measured along with the PEEP levels selected by the operator so that alveolar pressures do not exceed 30 cm H_2O.

HISTORICAL NOTE 11-6

Volume Ventilation

Historically, respiratory therapists and physicians in the United States were trained to set a desired tidal volume and rate for a patient. Consequently, when pressure-controlled ventilation (PCV) was developed, clinicians at first were reluctant to use it as a common ventilator mode, because they could not guarantee a volume delivery. As a result, researchers and manufacturers struggled to develop ways to use pressure ventilation, which had certain advantages, but to guarantee volume delivery. Thus "volume-targeted" pressure-control modes became popular.

BOX 11-19	Servo-Controlled Modes of Ventilation

1. Mandatory minute ventilation, as in the BEAR 1000, the Hamilton Veolar, the Ohmeda Advent, and several others
2. Pressure-targeted ventilation with volume guaranteed every breath, as in pressure augmentation (P_{aug}) in the BEAR 1000 ventilator and volume-assured pressure support (VAPS) in the Bird T-Bird and the Bird 8400STi
3. Pressure-targeted ventilation with volume guaranteed over several breaths, as in pressure-regulated volume control (PRVC) in the Maquet Servo^i, VC+ on the Puritan Bennett 840, and Autoflow in the Dräger E-4 and EvitaXL, and volume support (VS) in the Maquet Servo^i, to name a few
4. Proportional assist ventilation (PAV) on the Puritan Bennett 840
5. Adaptive support ventilation (ASV) in the Hamilton GALILEO and Hamilton G5

Levels above this value are known to damage the lungs. The current recommendation is that pulmonary pressures be kept lower than 30 cm H_2O rather than risk potential lung injury.[33-36]

Inverse ratio ventilation is VC-CMV or PC-CMV with an I:E ratio greater than 1:1. When inspiration is time cycled, the inspiratory time is extended and the expiratory time shortened, assuming the ventilator can accommodate these settings. ICU ventilators normally are time cycled when PC-CMV is used. However, not all units have controls for the inspiratory time during volume ventilation. To extend the inspiratory time, the operator can reduce flow; use a descending ramp waveform, which extends the T_I in non-time–cycled volume ventilation; or use an inspiratory pause. Box 11-20 provides a list of equations describing the interrelationship of the inspiratory time, expiratory time, I:E ratio, flow, respiratory rate, and volume. For a more detailed explanation of the relationship among these parameters, the reader is referred elsewhere.[11]

Currently, rather than trying to improve oxygenation with IRV, the emphasis is on ventilating patients with low lung volumes (V_T less than or equal to 6 mL/kg of IBW), finding an optimum PEEP level, and preventing alveoli from collapsing and reexpanding.[33-36] These strategies are designed to reduce lung injury and improve oxygenation.

Airway Pressure-Release Ventilation

Airway pressure-release ventilation (APRV) provides two levels of CPAP and allows for spontaneous breathing at both levels. This mode was invented by Dr. Christine Stock and Dr. Jay Block in the late 1980s.[37] APRV was introduced as a means of controlling the mean airway pressure and improving oxygenation in patients with severe lung injuries, and it often uses inverse I:E ratios.[38]

APRV is available on ventilators such as the Dräger E-4 and EvitaXL, the Maquet Servo[i], the VIASYS AVEA, the Hamilton GALILEO Gold and G5, and the Puritan Bennett 840. APRV may be referred to by another name. For example, on the Puritan Bennett 840, it currently is called *Bilevel* ventilation, and on the Servo[i] it is called *BiVent*.

APRV is a time-triggered, pressure-limited, and time-cycled mode that allows for spontaneous breathing. Some ventilators even allow patient triggering and cycling. Currently, APRV is most frequently used for patients with ARDS and acute lung injury (ALI). APRV may benefit these patients by reducing the risk of lung injury and providing better ventilation-perfusion matching, cardiac filling, and patient comfort than other modes that do not provide for spontaneous ventilation.[38,39,40]

Patients are given an elevated baseline pressure that approximates their plateau pressure or their mean airway pressure (approximately 20 to 25 cm H_2O). The baseline pressure is periodically released to a lower level (usually zero) for a very brief period (about 0.2 to 1 sec).[38,39] The high CPAP level increases the mean airway pressure to improve oxygenation. The intervals during which pressure briefly drops to a lower CPAP level allow for ventilation (i.e., exhalation of carbon dioxide). As soon as this expiratory period is complete, pressures return to the higher CPAP level (Figure 11-56).

Pressure-Targeted Ventilation with Volume Guaranteed for Every Breath

Pressure augmentation (P_{aug}), found on the BEAR 1000 ventilator, and volume-assured pressure-support (VAPS), available on the T-Bird and Bird 8400st, are examples of dual control modes that provide **pressure-limited ventilation** with volume guaranteed for every breath. In P_{aug} and VAPS, the patient initiates a breath (patient triggering), and the pressure climbs to a set level. During inspiration, the ventilator monitors the V_T delivery. If volume is delivered before flow drops to its set value (value set on the flow

---

BOX 11-20	Interrelation of Tidal Volume, Flow Rate, Inspiratory Time, Expiratory Time, Total Cycle Time, and Respiratory Rate

I. The total cycle time (TCT) equals the inspiratory time (T_I) plus the expiratory time (T_E).
$$TCT = T_I + T_E$$
II. The respiratory rate (f) equals 1 min (60 sec) divided by the total cycle time.
f = 1 min/TCT = 60 seconds/TCT (seconds) = breaths/min
Calculate the TCT from f.
$$TCT = 60 \ sec/f$$
III. The inspiratory to expiratory ratio (I:E ratio) equals the inspiratory time divided by the expiratory time:
I:E = T_I/T_E.
Remember: $TCT = T_I + T_E$ and $TCT - T_I = T_E$
IV. Calculate the T_E from f and T_I.
$$f = 60 \ sec/TCT \ and \ TCT = T_I + T_E$$
$$T_E = TCT - T_I$$
V. Reduce the I:E ratio to its simplest form; divide the numerator and denominator by T_I.
$$I:E = (T_I/T_I)/(T_E/T_I)$$
VI. Determine the I:E ratio when inverse ratio ventilation is used.
In inverse ventilation, the I:E ratio equals the division of both the numerator and the denominator by the expiratory time:
$$I:E = (T_I/T_E)/(T_E/T_E)$$
VII. Calculate the T_I, T_E, and TCT from the I:E ratio and f.
$$TCT = T_I + T_E \ and \ f = 60 \ sec/TCT$$
$$f = 60 \ sec/(T_I + T_E)$$
$$T_I + T_E = 60 \ sec/f$$
VIII. Calculate the T_I from the tidal volume (V_T) and flow ($\dot{V}$).
$$T_I = V_T/\dot{V}$$
IX. Calculate the V_T from T_I and $\dot{V}$.
$$V_T = \dot{V} \times T_I$$
X. Calculate the $\dot{V}$ from V_T and T_I.
$$\dot{V} = V_T/T_I$$

Modified from Pilbeam SP, Cairo JM: *Mechanical ventilation: physiological and clinical applications*, ed 4, St Louis, 2006, Mosby/Elsevier.

control), then inspiration flow cycles. If volume is not delivered by the time flow drops to its set value, then flow continues at the amount set on the flow control until the set V_T is delivered. Inspiration then becomes volume cycled (based on measured flow and time elapsed). Figure 11-57 provides examples of these types of breaths.

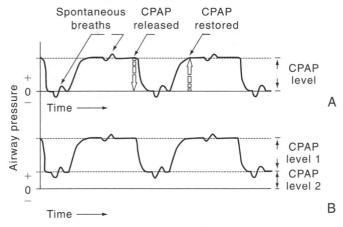

FIGURE 11-56 Pressure-time curve for airway pressure release ventilation (APRV). **A,** APRV when pressure is released to atmospheric pressure. **B,** APRV when pressure is released to above atmospheric pressure (CPAP level 2). (Redrawn from Dupuis Y: *Ventilators,* ed 2, St Louis, 1992, Mosby.)

Pressure-Targeted Ventilation with Volume Guaranteed over Several Breaths

An adaptive control mode of ventilation uses patient-triggered (or time-triggered), pressure-limited ventilation and adjusts the pressure level to achieve the set volume over several breaths. Examples of ventilators that provide this form of ventilation are the Maquet Servo 300 and Servo[i], the Hamilton GALILEO Gold, the Puritan Bennett 840, and the VIASYS AVEA. Other ventilators provide the same mode with slightly different names. For example, **Autoflow** mode is the name used on the Dräger E-4, VC+ is used on the Puritan Bennett 840, and **variable pressure control (VPC)** is the name used by Cardiopulmonary Corp.'s Venturi ventilator.

In **pressure-regulated volume control (PRVC),** breaths are patient or time triggered, pressure limited, and time cycled. The operator sets a maximum safety pressure and the desired V_T. The ventilator gives a test breath and calculates system compliance and resistance. The ventilator determines the pressure needed to deliver the set volume. As it ventilates the patient, the ventilator monitors pressure and volume. It adjusts pressure delivery to accomplish volume delivery in increments of 1 to 3 cm H_2O at a time, up to the maximum pressure, which equals the set

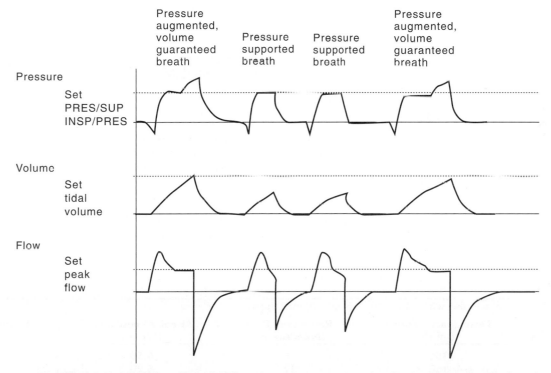

FIGURE 11-57 Examples of breath delivery in pressure augmentation (P_{aug}) with synchronized intermittent mandatory ventilation (SIMV) plus pressure-support ventilation (PSV). Note that the flow curve for a mandatory breath *(left)* rises rapidly, descends to the set flow value, and remains constant at the set flow until the volume is delivered. For PSV breaths *(two breaths in the center),* flow is a descending ramp–like curve and ends when it is about 30% of the peak inspiratory flow rate. The breath at the right is similar to the first breath delivered *(far left).* (Courtesy VIASYS Corp, Yorba Linda, Calif.)

upper pressure limit minus 5 cm H_2O (e.g., Servo[i]) or to a maximum pressure limit (e.g., VIASYS AVEA). Pressure delivery can go as low as the set baseline (PEEP level). If the volume cannot be delivered within these parameters, the ventilator sounds an alarm to alert the clinician.

Although this adaptive mode of ventilation targets the set breath delivery, it does not guarantee a constant V_T delivery. Whether this is a concern depends on the goals of the clinician and the patient's needs. When the patient has an increased effort, the ventilator may not be able to distinguish this from an improvement in compliance and thus reduce its support. Clinicians may find this mode beneficial but should be aware of its limitations.[41]

Mandatory Minute Ventilation

Mandatory (or minimum) minute ventilation is a closed-loop form of volume- or pressure-targeted ventilation used in patients who can perform part of the work of breathing and are progressing toward weaning from mechanical ventilation.[30] MMV guarantees a minimum $\dot{V}_E$ even though the patient's spontaneous ventilation may change. The minimum $\dot{V}_E$ set by the operator in MMV usually is less than the patient's projected spontaneous $\dot{V}_E$. When the measured $\dot{V}_E$ falls below a minimum level, the ventilator increases the pressure, rate, or volume to return the ventilator to the minimum $\dot{V}_E$. The Hamilton Veolar is an example of a unit that increases pressure using pressure-support breaths for MMV. The BEAR 1000 is an example of a unit that uses rate to adjust MMV during volume ventilation. The Servo 300 has volume-support ventilation that functions like MMV and increases the tidal volume to maintain the minute volume. The operator must set high rate and low tidal volume alarms on most units to indicate when the patient's rate rises too high and tidal volume falls too low (Clinical Rounds 11-11), which indicates an increased work of breathing, even if the patient could maintain the desired $\dot{V}_E$ (Table 11-3).

Volume-Support Ventilation

Volume-support ventilation (VSV) on the Maquet Servo 300 is similar to PRVC, except that there is no back-up rate with volume support. VSV is a purely assist mode. VSV is patient triggered, pressure limited, and flow cycled, which basically makes it a form of PSV except that volume delivery is targeted over several breaths.

As with PRVC, pressure increases and decreases within the same limits described to maintain V_T. If the patient's respiratory rate drops and the set $\dot{V}_E$ is not being maintained, the Servo 300 increases V_T delivery (up to 150%) in an attempt to achieve the set $\dot{V}_E$. Again, this aspect is similar to MMV.

If the patient becomes apneic, the ventilator automatically switches to PRVC, delivers whatever mandatory rate is set, and sounds an alarm to alert the practitioner. The patient may experience difficulty with breath synchrony with VSV.[42,43] The **variable pressure support (VPS)** mode available on the Cardiopulmonary Venturi ventilator is similar to VS on the Servo 300.

With a more recent version of the Servo, the Maquet Servo[i], volume support has changed. VSV in the Servo[i] is also PS with a volume target. However, unlike the Servo 300, the V_T delivery does not increase if the patient's respiratory rate drops. The Servo[i] is not minute ventilation based in VSV as is the Servo 300. If the patient becomes apneic, the ventilator switches to a back-up mode.

The operator needs to set appropriate alarms for high and low minute ventilation and high and low rates, as with any mode of ventilation, to be alerted to changes in these parameters. Modes similar to VSV are available on other ventilators, such as the VIASYS AVEA.

CLINICAL ROUND 11-11

A patient on mandatory minute volume (MMV) has a set minute ventilation of 4 L/min and a measured minute ventilation of 6 L/min (spontaneous V_T = 600 mL; spontaneous rate = 10 breaths/min). Over several hours, the patient's tidal volume drops to 300 mL, and the rate increases to 25 breaths/min. Will the ventilator increase ventilation delivery to reduce the patient's work of breathing?

See Evolve Resources for the answer.

TABLE 11-3

Constant Minute Ventilation with Changing Alveolar Ventilation

Tidal Volume (mL)	Dead Space Volume (mL)*	Respiratory Rate (breaths/min)	Alveolar Ventilation (L/min)	Minute Ventilation (L/min)
800	150	10	6.50	8.0
667	150	12	6.20	8.0
533	150	15	5.75	8.0
400	150	20	5.00	8.0
250	150	32	3.20	8.0

From Pilbeam SP, Cairo JM: *Mechanical ventilation: physiology and clinical applications,* ed 4, St Louis, 2006, Mosby/Elsevier.
*Assuming a constant anatomic dead space volume of 150 mL, minute ventilation can remain constant while alveolar ventilation decreases, the respiratory rate increases, and the tidal volume falls.

Switching Modes During Ventilation: Automode

Adaptive set point control ventilation has gone a step farther. Ventilators now can switch modes based on monitored information. For example, the Maquet Servo 300 and Servo^i have a control called **Automode.** When this feature is turned on, the ventilator can switch from volume control to volume support. In other words, it switches from VC-CMV to VC-CSV and back again based on how the patient is breathing.

Suppose the patient is in volume control (VC-CMV) with Automode activated. If no patient breaths are detected, the breaths are time triggered, volume limited, and time cycled. However, when the ventilator detects patient efforts, it switches to pressure support with the same set targeted volume (i.e., volume support). In VS, breaths are patient triggered, pressure limited, flow cycled, and volume targeted (adaptive control).

If the patient is in the pressure-control mode (PC-CMV) with Automode on and the ventilator does not detect a patient effort, breaths are time triggered, pressure limited, and time cycled. If patient efforts are detected, the ventilator switches to pressure support (i.e., patient-triggered, pressure-limited, flow-cycled breaths [PC-CSV]).

With Automode, the ventilator can switch from a more supportive breath to a more spontaneous breath, thus allowing the patient more control over his or her breathing. This feature now is available on other ventilators, although it has a different name. For example, on the Cardiopulmonary Venturi, the ventilator switches from VPC to VPS if the minute ventilation falls too low, or from SIMVpc to CPAP when spontaneous breathing improves. Each of these mode switches is described in more detail in the section on the ventilator in question (see Chapter 12).

Proportional Assist Ventilation

Proportional assist ventilation (PAV) is a method of assisting *spontaneous* ventilation in which the practitioner adjusts the amount of the work of breathing assumed by the ventilator. PAV provides partial ventilatory support in which the ventilator generates a rapid inspiratory pressure delivery in proportion to the inspiratory effort of the patient.[44] Currently PAV is available on the Puritan Bennett (PB) 840 ventilator. (See Chapter 12, section on the PB 840, PAV+.)

PAV is an approach to ventilatory support in which pressure, flow, and volume delivery at the airway increase in proportion to the patient's inspiratory effort. PAV augments the underlying breathing pattern of a patient who experiences increased work of breathing associated with worsening lung characteristics (increasing R_{aw} or decreasing compliance [C]). The more effort the patient exerts during inspiration, the more pressure and flow the machine provides.

PAV allows patients to reach comfortably whatever ventilatory pattern suits their needs. In studies comparing PSV with PAV, the two modes show comparable safe short-term effects on gas exchange and hemodynamics without adverse effects.[45-49]

The operation of PAV is based on the equation of motion previously described (see Box 11-7). The amount of pressure generated by the patient's own respiratory muscles is used as an index of inspiration effort:

$$P_{mus} = (V \times e) + (Flow \times R) - P_{aw}$$

where P_{mus} is pressure generated by the respiratory muscles, V is volume, e is elastance (L/compliance), R is resistance, and P_{aw} is airway pressure. P_{mus} can be calculated when e and R are known. The signal obtained from these variables can be used as a reference for the amount of pressure the ventilator needs to produce.[47]

Figure 11-58 shows an example of a device for delivering PAV. A cylinder, within which a rolling seal piston moves, is filled with air intended for a patient. The cylinder is connected to the patient through a patient circuit and an artificial airway. The piston operates on a very low resistance arm connected to an electrically powered motor. When the patient inhales, air moves from the cylinder toward the patient. The piston moves forward to assist the patient's inspiration. The air movement is sensed by a flow-measuring device, which generates flow and volume signals that are sent to a microprocessor. The microprocessor then signals the piston in a positive feedback manner. The greater the patient effort, the greater the piston force. The electric motor supplies current to the piston in proportion to the flow and volume signals. The sum of these two signals determines the amount of electric current going to the motor.

Gain controls determine how much pressure will be exerted based on where the gain is set. The gain set for the flow determines how much pressure is generated for each unit of flow (cm H_2O/L/sec [i.e., resistance units]). The gain set on the volume signal establishes how much pressure will result for each unit of the volume signal (cm H_2O/L [i.e., elastance units]).[45]

For a better understanding of the concept behind this technique, consider the following example. Suppose a patient is connected by endotracheal tube to a sealed rigid box. When the patient spontaneously inhales, the pressure inside the box decreases in proportion to the volume of air the patient inspires. The pressure drop inside the box represents an increased workload. If the box is replaced with a ventilator that provides instantaneous pressure delivery as soon as the patient breathes in, and does so in proportion to the amount of air inspired, then the ventilator basically "unloads" the amount of work. This response represents "volume" proportional assist. Figure 11-59 compares a patient on CPAP with a patient on volume proportional assist ventilation.[49]

Here is another example: A patient is connected by endotracheal tube to a narrow tube. When the patient inspires, pressure in the tube drops. In flow-proportional assist ventilation (flow-PAV), the ventilator increases

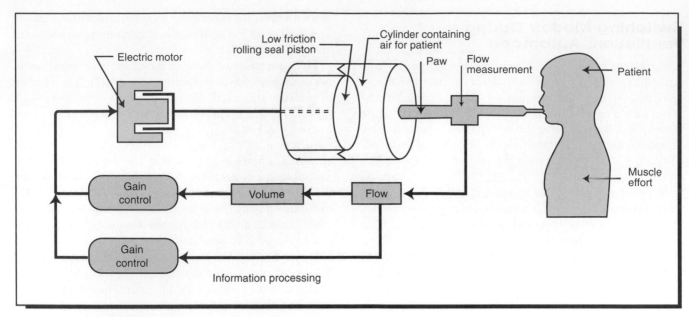

FIGURE 11-58 Simplified diagram of a proportional assist ventilation (PAV) delivery system. A piston is coupled to an electric motor that generates force in proportion to the supplied current. The current is determined by the measured rate of volume delivery and gas flow to the patient. The gain controls are set by the operator and determine what proportion of patient effort is assisted.

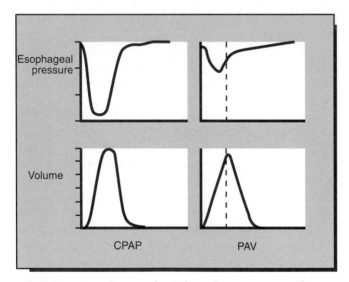

FIGURE 11-59 Volume and esophageal pressure curves for a continuous positive airway pressure (CPAP) breath and a proportional assist breath (volume gain). (Redrawn from Schulze A, Schaller P: *Am J Respir Crit Care Med* 153:671, 1996.)

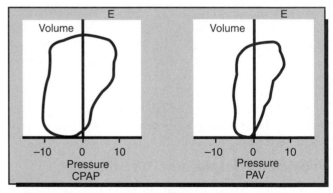

FIGURE 11-60 Pressure-volume loop changes comparing continuous positive airway pressure (CPAP) with proportional assist ventilation (PAV) and showing inspiration (I) and expiration (E). PAV reduces the work of breathing (WOB). Inspiratory WOB is the area within the loop to the left of the vertical axis. Expiratory WOB is the area within the loop to the right of the vertical axis. (Redrawn from Schulze A, Schaller P: *Am J Respir Crit Care Med* 153:671, 1996.)

pressure during inspiration in proportion to the rate of inspiratory flow generated by the patient. The increased pressure delivered by the ventilator has the effect of unloading the work (Figure 11-60).[49]

When volume- and flow-proportional assist ventilations are used together, they respond to both the elastance (1/C) and resistance (R) components of breathing and help unload the work of breathing in proportion to patient effort. The greater the volume and flow demand of the

patient, the higher the force (pressure) provided by the ventilator.[49-53]

For PAV, some of the settings established by the operator include (1) the baseline pressure, (2) the gain for volume (elastance component), and (3) the gain for flow (resistance component).*

*See the section on PAV+ in the Puritan Bennett 840 ventilator in Chapter 12.

BOX 11-21 | **Determining Proportional Assist**

Airway pressure using proportional assist can be determined using the following equation:

$$P_{aw} = (f1 \times Volume) + (f2 \times Flow)$$

Where:

P_{aw} is the airway pressure.

f1 is the ventilator supported load of elastance or the amount of volume assist.

Volume is the ventilating volume.

f2 is the ventilator support for resistance load or the amount of flow assist.

Flow is the flow during ventilation.

For example, if gain is set at 50% of the patient's elastance and 50% of the resistance, the ventilator will provide half the work performed by the patient required to overcome the forces of elastance and resistance (Box 11-21). If the patient makes no effort, the ventilator does no work. Thus PAV is better suited for patients with abnormalities in resistance and compliance and less so for those with neuromuscular weakness and chest wall deformities with an inability to generate a strong inspiratory effort.[49,51]

PAV, however, shares a common problem with the conventional partial ventilatory support modes. In mechanically ventilated patients, the respiratory system impedance may change over time. With pressure-limited modes, these changes may result in variation in the amount of assist and volume delivered to the patient by the ventilator. These changes may prevent the synchrony between the ventilator's output and the patient's inspiratory demand.[44,53]

Another difficulty with PAV occurs with excessive unloading. This may result in resonant oscillations and runaway pressures. It is important to determine the appropriate level of unloading that could be applied to clinical practice. The level of resistive unloading should not exceed the resistance of the patient and the artificial airway. The level of elastic unloading most likely should be limited to a level that targets the patient's elastance needs to that of a normal lung.[53]

In summary, PAV is an alternative mode of ventilation for spontaneously breathing patients. It has been shown to be a safe and effective method of ventilation in a variety of patients compared to PSV. When PAV is used, assessment of the compliance and resistance of the patient and endotracheal tube is important so that levels of unloading that fully compensate for the resistance and compliance levels can be avoided.

Adaptive Support Ventilation in the Hamilton GALILEO

Adaptive support ventilation (ASV) is an optimal control mode of ventilation. This mode is considered an optimal control type because the ventilator set point is adjusted automatically by the ventilator to optimize another set point based on some model of system behavior.[50] It is a mode in which the ventilator determines dynamic compliance ($C_D = V_T/[PIP - PEEP]$) and expiratory time constant (exhaled V_T/peak expiratory flow rate) for the patient and establishes a respiratory rate and V_T delivery based on monitored and set parameters. Its purpose is to target the respiratory rate and V_T to establish the least amount of work possible for the patient based on lung characteristics.[50]

Both mandatory and spontaneous assisted breaths are pressure limited. The pressure level is adjusted by the ventilator, based on measured parameters (e.g., expiratory time constant, compliance, pressure, and measured volume), to both minimize the work of breathing and protect the lung.[50]

The clinician sets the following parameters:

1. Patient's IBW and the percentage of $\dot{V}_E$ the operator wants the ventilator to supply
2. Maximum pressure limit and baseline pressure (PEEP)
3. Pressure or flow trigger
4. Rise time (pressure ramp)

When the patient is apneic, breaths are time triggered, pressure targeted, and time cycled (PC-CMV). Both the respiratory rate and V_T are calculated to establish the optimum $\dot{V}_E$ based on the patient's IBW and lung mechanics. The maximum pressure limit determines the upper limit of pressure delivery.

When the patient can perform some spontaneous breaths, patient-triggered breaths are supported at a calculated pressure using PSV (minimum $P = PEEP + 5$ cm H_2O) (in other words, PC-CSV with a volume target). The difference between the actual number of spontaneous breaths and the calculated number established by the ventilator equals the number of mandatory breaths delivered.

In spontaneously breathing patients with an adequate spontaneous rate, the ventilator adjusts pressure delivery to keep patients in the optimum calculated range for rate and V_T. The ranges for respiratory variables in ASV are presented in Table 11-4. Chapter 12 provides a more in-depth discussion of ASV and the Hamilton GALILEO ventilator.

Similar modes are being rapidly designed with the development of each new ventilator. Readers are advised to read about the specific ventilator they plan to use in Chapter 12 to learn more details about the newer closed-loop modes in use with each unit and also any literature available from the manufacturer (see Chapter 12, section on ASV on the Hamilton GALILEO).

TABLE 11-4

Adaptive Support Ventilation in the Hamilton GALILEO

Parameter	Range
Respiratory rate range	5 to 60 breaths/min
Tidal volume range	4.4 to 22 mL/kg
Inspiratory time	0.5 sec (or expiratory time constant [RCe]) to 2 × RCe or 3 sec

Neurally Adjusted Ventilatory Assist

Neurally adjusted ventilatory assist (NAVA) is a mode of ventilation based on neural respiratory input. NAVA is available as an option on the Maquet Servo[i] ventilator (see Chapter 12, section on NAVA with the Maquet Servo[i] ventilator). NAVA relies on detection of the electrical activity of the diaphragm (EAdi*) to control ventilator function.[54]

NAVA requires the use of a special nasogastric (NG) tube that is fitted with an electrode array. The catheter is positioned in the esophagus so that the electrical activity of the diaphragm can be detected by the electrode array. The clinician can use a monitoring screen on the Servo[i] during catheter insertion to determine where the electrode array is positioned in the esophagus in relation to the diaphragm. This helps in situating the NG tube correctly so that the sensors can most accurately detect diaphragmatic activity. (NOTE: The NG tube can also be used as a feeding tube.)

A cable connects the electrical array imbedded in the NG tube to the EAdi module of the ventilator, which in turn commands the ventilator's functions.

As the diaphragm depolarizes, the electrical signal is captured by the electrode array and transmitted to the EAdi module and the ventilator. The ventilator begins inspiration as soon as the diaphragm begins depolarization. The depth and length of the breath are also established by the diaphragm's electrical activity (i.e., the greater the electrical activity, the deeper the breath). When activity diminishes, inspiratory flow is stopped.

Besides establishing the intensity of diaphragm firing, the ventilator can be programmed to control the level of assistance. The operator sets a level of support proportional to the electrical activity of the diaphragm (range, 0 to 30 cm $H_2O/\mu V$). For example, if the operator selects 3 cm $H_2O/\mu V$ of muscle activity and the electrode array measures 5 μV (diaphragm depolarization), the potential pressure delivery is 15 cm H_2O. (NOTE: Simple numbers are used here just as an example and do not represent actual readings.) Theoretically, if the activity of the diaphragm increased to 10 μV, the pressure would increase to 30 cm H_2O. However, studies have demonstrated that the stretch receptors in the lungs sense the rise in volume with the rise in pressure and signal the brain to reduce the firing of the diaphragm. As a result, a lower pressure and lower volume are delivered than one would expect. Thus the lung is protected from excessive distention.[55]

Just as ventilator triggering and breath limitation are neurally controlled, breath cycling is controlled by the activity of the diaphragm. The breath ends when electrical activity decreases (neural cycling). In addition, if the patient becomes apneic, the ventilator automatically switches to a back-up mode of ventilation.

*Medical literature uses the abbreviation *EAdi* for electrical activity of the diaphragm; Maquet, manufacturer of the Servo[i] ventilator, uses *Edi* in its literature.

Potential benefits of NAVA include the following:
- Reduced work of breathing: Fewer patient trigger efforts are missed. Also, intrinsic PEEP does not affect triggering.
- Improved synchrony: The patient's neural and diaphragmatic electrical activity control the onset and breath delivery. Synchrony with the ventilator is an important part of unloading the work of the diaphragm during both inspiration and expiration.[56,57]
- Reduced need for sedation and/or paralysis: Allowing the patient basically to control the breathing pattern may reduce the need for sedation.
- Improvement in ventilation: Compared to standard methods, ventilation is improved by allowing neural triggering and neurally adjusted ventilator assistance, particularly in patients with severe airflow impairment.[58]
- Potential improvement in synchrony and oxygenation and a reduced incidence of barotrauma in the infant population.[58]
- Better ventilator regulation in noninvasive ventilation because of the ability of NAVA to ventilate despite variable leaks.[58]

Many patients with a variety of pulmonary disorders might benefit from NAVA as long as the respiratory center, phrenic nerve, and neuromuscular junction are functionally intact and there are no contraindications to or limitations on the use of the NG tube.[58]

NAVA probably represents the first applicable form of assisted ventilation in which the patient's respiratory center controls ventilation. Additional research is needed to verify some of the uses and possible side effects of this mode of ventilation.[59]

High-Frequency Ventilation

High-frequency ventilation (HFV) uses mandatory rates higher than normal and tidal volumes lower than normal. HFV generally is defined as any mode of ventilation that provides a mandatory rate of more than 100 breaths (pulses) per minute.[60] For particularly high rates, frequencies are usually given in Hertz (Hz) or cycles per second, with 1 Hz equaling 60 cycles (breaths)/min.

Five basic types of HFV are available:
1. High-frequency positive-pressure ventilation (HFPPV)
2. High-frequency jet ventilation (HFJV)
3. High-frequency oscillatory ventilation (HFOV)
4. High-frequency flow interruption (HFFI)
5. High-frequency percussive ventilation (HFPV)

The two most frequently used forms of HFV are HFJV and HFOV.[60]

High-Frequency Positive-Pressure Ventilation

HFPPV uses a conventional volume- or pressure-limited ventilator with a low-compliance patient circuit. With HFPPV, the airway is intermittently pressurized with gas with no air entrainment. Mandatory rates are about 60 to 110 breaths/min. As mentioned, breath rates are sometimes given in Hertz (1 Hz = 1 cycle/sec). In this case 60 to 100 breaths/min would be 1 to 1.8 Hz, respectively.

HFPPV was developed by Sjöstrand[61] in the late 1960s to minimize the cardiovascular side effects of positive-pressure ventilation. Animal studies also showed its effectiveness in eliminating intracranial pressure variations normally associated with breathing, thus providing a better surgical field for microneurosurgical procedures.

Early prototypes used an H-valve assembly in which the circuit was connected to an insufflation catheter attached to the endotracheal tube. The catheter was fitted with either a pneumatic (fluidic) valve (Figure 11-61) or a rapidly responding exhalation valve (Figure 11-62).

A problem can occur with HFPPV. The short inspiratory times and high rates may prevent adequate V_T delivery. Breath stacking may develop at these rates, because only passive exhalation occurs.[62,63] That is, when respiratory rates are this rapid, sometimes the air has enough time to enter the lungs but not enough time to leave. Breaths begin to "stack up" in the lungs, resulting in trapped air, which creates auto-PEEP. With other modes of HFV now more popular and the use of other techniques for the management of acute lung injury (e.g., permissive hypercapnia and open lung ventilation), HFPPV is not often used clinically.

High-Frequency Jet Ventilation

In 1977 Klain and Smith[64] developed a method of high-frequency jet ventilation (HFJV) that used a percutaneous transtracheal catheter. The catheter was connected to an air source that provided a jet injection of air controlled by a fluidic logic ventilator. Rates up to 600 breaths/min

(10 Hz) were used. Later this technique used a catheter that allowed for air entrainment.

HFJV offers rates of about 100 to 600 breaths/min (1.7 to 10 Hz, respectively) with a V_T smaller than anatomic dead space volume. (Historical Note 11-7 lists some of the earlier uses of HFJV.) In general, HFJV operates by passing gas from a high pressure source through a variable regulator that reduces the pressure to the desired working level. The gas then passes through a device, usually a solenoid or a fluidic valve, that governs the amount and duration of flow. The gas jet is then delivered through a specially made triple-lumen endotracheal tube (Figure 11-63A), which is similar to conventional endotracheal tubes except that two additional small lines are added. One is for delivering jet ventilation, and the other is for monitoring distal airway pressures. The jet stream exits the tube at about one third of the tube's length from the distal end. The pressure tube is located at the distal tip of the tube.

If a jet tube is not used, a special jet adapter can be attached to the endotracheal tube (Figure 11-63B). Another technique when a special jet tube is not in place is to use

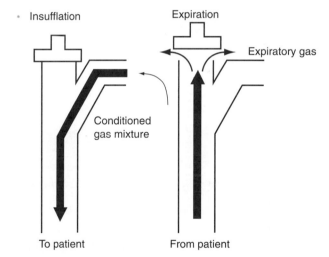

FIGURE 11-62 Modification of the H-valve for high-frequency positive-pressure ventilation (HFPPV) uses an expiratory valve that closes during inspiration to prevent gas leakage. (From Pilbeam SP: *Mechanical ventilation: physiological and clinical applications,* St Louis, 1986, Mosby.)

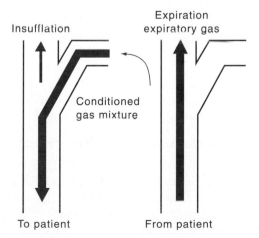

FIGURE 11-61 Pneumatic valve assembly used with high-frequency positive-pressure ventilation (HFPPV) introduces a gas mixture during inspiration. Because of the Coanda effect, the gas stream hugs the channel. No air entrainment occurs, and only a small amount of gas leaks from the expiratory limb. (From Pilbeam SP: *Mechanical ventilation: physiological and clinical applications,* St Louis, 1986, Mosby.)

HISTORICAL NOTE 11-7

Early Uses of High-Frequency Jet Ventilation
- To provide surgical fields undisturbed by ventilatory movement
- For use with bronchoscopy and laryngoscopy to provide better surgical field access while maintaining ventilation
- To reduce cardiovascular side effects associated with intermittent positive-pressure ventilation (IPPV)
- To reduce the risk of barotrauma
- To maintain ventilation when large air leaks are present (e.g., bronchopleural fistula)

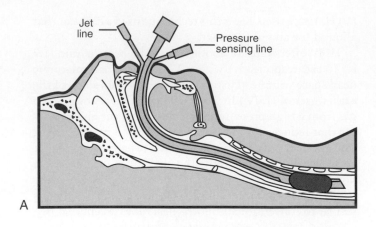

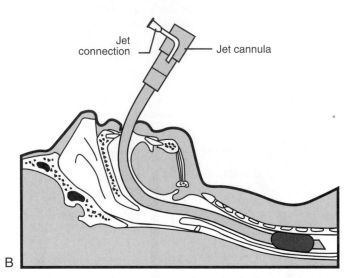

FIGURE 11-63 Diagram of an endotracheal tube used in high-frequency jet ventilation **(A)** and a jet connection with a jet cannula attached to a standard endotracheal tube **(B).**

a small catheter inserted either through a conventional endotracheal or a tracheostomy tube. Early studies showed that the best position for the jet is close to the proximal end of the trachea near the vocal cords.[64]

The operational principle of HFJV involves the delivery of short breaths or pulsations (20 to 34 msec) under pressure through a small lumen at high rates (4 to 11 Hz).[64] The tidal volume of the breath depends on four basic factors:

· Length of the pulsation
· Amplitude or driving pressure of the jet
· Jet orifice size
· Patient's lung characteristics

Under certain conditions, gas can be entrained around the jet through the physical process of jet mixing. It results from the viscous shearing of the jet gas layer with stagnant gas in the airway. This gas is dragged downstream in an entrainment-like effect. The volume of entrained gas can alter V_T delivery, depending on the patient's lung characteristics.[65] Examples of jet ventilators include the Bunnell

Life Pulse currently in use (Bunnell, Salt Lake City, Utah) and the Adult Star 1010, which is no longer being supported by the manufacturer. (See Chapter 13 for additional information on the Bunnell jet ventilator.)

High-Frequency Oscillatory Ventilation

High-frequency oscillatory ventilation (HFOV) currently is the most widely used form of HFV in adult patients. It also is frequently used in neonatal and pediatric patients. As a ventilatory technique, it has been shown to improve oxygenation and support gas exchange and provide more effective lung recruitment than conventional ventilation in patients with ARDS.[66-68]

HFOV uses a reciprocating pump to generate an approximation of a sine wave (see Figures 11-3 and 13-37). Examples of devices that provide this function are reciprocating pumps (usually pistons), diaphragms, and loudspeakers. Although not true oscillators, high-frequency flow interrupters (discussed in the following section) can be used in ventilators to provide a similar effect. These ventilators are called "pseudo-oscillators."

With HFOV, pressure is positive in the airway during the inspiratory phase (forward stroke) and negative during the expiratory phase (return stroke). Therefore both inspiration and expiration are active, and bulk flow rather than jet pulsations is produced. HFOV uses frequencies in the range of 1 to 50 Hz (60 to 3000 cycles/min), and V_T is less than the anatomic dead space volume. Some oscillators have a fixed I:E ratio, and others allow the I:E ratio to be adjusted.

HFOV is one of the most widely used forms of HFV in infants and pediatric patients. An example of an oscillator is the Sensormedics 3100A from VIASYS Critical Care (Yorba Linda, California) (Chapter 13). The 3100A uses a diaphragm-shaped piston that is powered magnetically, much like a stereo speaker (see Figure 13-38). The mean airway pressure control sets the tension on the diaphragm. Gas is oscillated back and forth by the action of the diaphragm. The amplitude of the wave set by the power control determines the forward and backward excursion of the piston, which helps determine the V_T. In the 3100A, rigid plastic circuits provide the bias flow of warmed and humidified air that is delivered to the patient.

High-Frequency Flow Interruption

High-frequency flow interruption (HFFI) is similar to HFJV but differs in its technical design. In HFFI a control mechanism interrupts a high-pressure gas source. A common mechanism is a rotating ball with a flow port in the center. Another example is a rotating bar with a slit through the center (Figure 11-64). Frequencies with HFFI are as high as 15 Hz. As in HFJV, the high-pressure bursts of gas can entrain static gas supplied by the addition of a bias flow circuit, which enhances volume delivery. An example of this device was invented by Emerson; their HFFI uses a spinning ball and consists of a conduit that conducts a gas flow. Inside the conduit is a ball with a flow port in the center. The ball is moved back and forth in the conduit by an electric motor at rates up to 200 cycles/min. As it moves, the ball interrupts the outflow of gas (Figure 11-65).[65] An example of a HFFI (a pseudo-oscillator) is the Infant Star ventilator.

High-Frequency Percussive Ventilation

Dr. Forrest M. Bird, a pioneer in ventilatory devices, designed a high-frequency percussive ventilation (HFPV) device in which he incorporated the beneficial characteristics of both a conventional positive-pressure ventilator and a jet ventilator. It operates in such a way that high-frequency breaths can be provided at ambient pressures. Figure 11-66A shows the rapid pressure waves representing high-frequency pulses with pauses following where these pulses are interrupted. High-frequency pulses (100 to 900 cycles/min) can also be superimposed on conventional positive-pressure breaths (5 to 30 cycles/min). In this case the pulses still occur, but the baseline rises as a positive-pressure breath is delivered (Figure 11-66B). These devices can be compared with time-cycled, pressure-limited ventilation when high-frequency pulsations are injected throughout the inspiratory phase. The resulting unit is called a high-frequency percussive ventilator.[69]

A ventilator that incorporates this principle is the Bird VDR-4 volumetric diffusive respirator (Percussionaire, Sandpoint, Idaho), which uses a sliding Venturi (Figures 11-67 and 11-68). At the mouth of the Venturi is a jet orifice. Around the jet is a continuous bias flow of warm, humidified air. During inspiration, a diaphragm connected to the Venturi fills with gas. This action slides the Venturi forward, toward the patient's airway, simultaneously blocking the expiratory port. During this time, the jet is activated and begins delivering short pulses of gas. At the same time, a large amount of air is entrained through the now open inspiratory ports, so that flow to the patient is high. The large gas flow is due to the pressure gradient between the jet and the patient connector. As inspiration progresses and pressure builds in the patient's airway, this gradient is reduced; therefore flow is reduced. However, the jet pulsations continue throughout inspiration. When the set inspiratory time is reached, inspiration ends. The diaphragm is no longer pressurized, and the Venturi slides

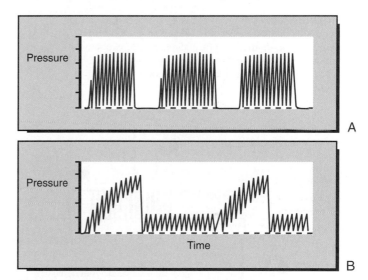

FIGURE 11-66 **A,** Example of a pressure-time waveform created during high-frequency percussive ventilation (HFPV). **B,** Example of a pressure-time curve during HFPV superimposed over standard positive-pressure breath delivery.

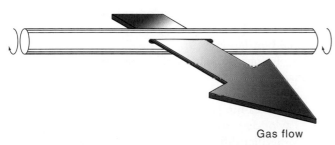

Gas flow

FIGURE 11-64 High-frequency flow interrupter. Flow is interrupted at high frequencies as a rotating metal bar allows flow to pass through during some portions of the breath and blocks it at others. (From Pilbeam SP: *Mechanical ventilation: physiological and clinical applications,* St Louis, 1986, Mosby.)

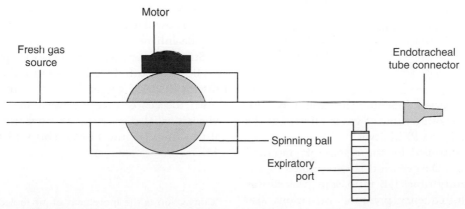

FIGURE 11-65 Example of a high-frequency oscillatory device, the spinning ball.

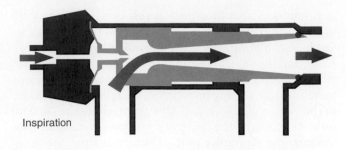

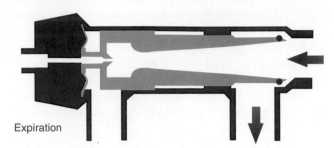

FIGURE 11-67 Design of the sliding Venturi for a high-frequency percussive generator used to provide high-frequency percussive ventilation (HFPV). (See text for explanation.) (From Pilbeam SP: *Mechanical ventilation: physiological and clinical applications,* ed 3, St Louis, 1998, Mosby.)

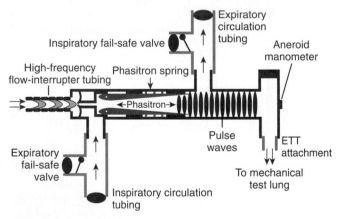

FIGURE 11-68 Schematic of the pulse generator (Phasitron), circulation tubing, and fail-safe valves. The open arrows denote airflow through the circuit. The bidirectional arrow denotes the sliding movement of the Phasitron component that creates the gas pulses. (From Allen PF, Thurlby JR, Naworol GA, et al: Measurement of pulsatile tidal volume, pressure, amplitude, and gas flow during high frequency percussive ventilation, with and without partial cuff deflation, *Respir Care* 52:45, 2007.)

back away from the patient, opening the expiratory port. During exhalation, a counterflow of gas is directed at the airway to maintain the set PEEP level.[66,69]

Ventilation is controlled by the respiratory rate and peak airway pressure. Oxygenation is determined by the PEEP level, inspiratory time, I:E ratio, and peak airway pressure. The high-frequency pressure oscillations also affect gas exchange, which makes clinical monitoring

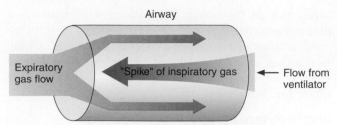

FIGURE 11-69 Effects of streaming in high-frequency jet ventilation (HFJV). Forward movement of the gas in the center, produced by pulsations from the jet, causes gas along the airway walls to be pushed backward. (From Pilbeam SP: *Mechanical ventilation: physiological and clinical applications,* ed 3, St Louis, 1998, Mosby.)

of these variables an important part of frequency adjustments.

The clinical benefits of HFPV may include facilitation of secretion removal.[70] HFPV has been used prophylactically in patients with thermal airway injury to help prevent pneumonia and atelectasis.[71-73]

Mechanisms of Action of High-Frequency Ventilation

The mechanisms of action of the various forms of HFV are not clearly understood; however, ventilation successfully occurs even when the V_T is less than the patient's anatomic dead space volume (V_D). Alveoli located close to the airways are thought to be ventilated by convection, just as in conventional ventilation.*

The following additional mechanisms may be responsible:

· Pendelluft
· Gas streaming or helical diffusion
· Taylor dispersion
· Molecular diffusion
· Spike formation

Pendelluft is the movement of gases from one area of the lungs to another as a result of differences in the compliance and resistance of various lung regions; this is also called out-of-phase ventilation. This movement occurs through normal anatomic channels (e.g., alveolar ducts, the pores of Kohn, and the canals of Lambert). When lung tissue is oscillated, as occurs with HFV, this phenomenon may be enhanced.

Streaming or asymmetric velocity profiles occur when gas flows in both directions at once through a conductive airway. Inspired gas is believed to move into the lungs down the center of the airways in a parabolic fashion, whereas exhaled gas tends to move near the walls and out of the lungs (Figure 11-69). This wall air movement may

---

*Convection is the movement of air molecules associated with the pressures of ventilation.

occur in a helical fashion and has been called *helical diffusion.*

Taylor dispersion is thought to occur in HFOV. It is the enhanced mixing of gases associated with the turbulent flow of high-velocity gases moving through small airways and their bifurcations. Taylor dispersion can occur where two gas streams meet. The erratic pattern of eddies and streams created is thought to enhance gas mixing and diffusion.

Simple molecular diffusion also occurs, at least at the terminal air spaces, and is another mechanism that adds to gas mixing. It is the result of the random thermal oscillation of molecules.

With regard to spike formation, one theory proposes that a spike (a parabolic-shaped front), a high-energy wave impulse of gas, travels rapidly through the center of the airway, much like a bullet. This gas movement may provide a larger area of gas mixing in the distal portions of the lungs.[74]

KEY POINTS

Many important aspects of mechanical ventilation must be understood before a practitioner begins managing a patient-ventilator system. Most common aspects of mechanical ventilation related to the physical characteristics and technical operation of ventilators have been reviewed in this chapter. The main focus has been on physical function and terms and explanations of fundamental concepts related to mechanical ventilation. Chapters 12, 13, and 14 review the use and operation of a variety of mechanical ventilators.

Additional information is available elsewhere on the management of patients receiving mechanical ventilation, the complications of ventilation, understanding ventilator graphics, and troubleshooting patient-ventilator dysfunction.[11]

▶ Ventilators are electrically powered, pneumatically powered, or pneumatically powered and microprocessor (electrically) controlled.

▶ Current ICU ventilators are primarily single-circuit ventilators. The source gas is the same as the gas that enters the patient's lungs.

▶ Three flow-controlling valves currently used in ventilators are proportional solenoids, stepper motors with valves, and digital valves with on/off configurations.

▶ Two key elements of fluidic devices are the Coanda effect and the flip-flop valve.

▶ The main parameter controlled by the ventilator is referred to as the *control variable.*

▶ The three variables the ventilator can control are volume, flow, and pressure. However, the ventilator can control only one of these variables at a time.

▶ Triggering begins a breath, and cycling ends a breath.

▶ A limiting variable limits the amount (value) a parameter (pressure, volume, flow) can reach during inspiration. However, the limit variable does not end the breath.

▶ The terminology used in the clinical setting to describe modes of ventilation can be confusing, because there is no logic or consistency to its application.

▶ During MMV, when the measured $\dot{V}_E$ falls below a minimum level, the ventilator increases the pressure, rate, or volume to return the ventilator to the minimum $\dot{V}_E$.

▶ The primary purpose of PCIRV is to treat acute respiratory distress syndrome so as to increase the mean airway pressure, restore the FRC, and improve oxygenation.

▶ PRVC is pressure-limited ventilation with a volume target.

▶ Volume support is pressure-support ventilation with a volume target.

▶ Automode is an adaptive set point control form of ventilation in which the ventilator can switch modes based on monitored information.

▶ Proportional assist ventilation is a method of assisting spontaneous ventilation in which the practitioner adjusts the amount of work of breathing assumed by the ventilator based on the patient's elastance and resistance characteristics.

▶ Adaptive support ventilation is considered an optimal control type, because the set point is automatically adjusted by the ventilator to optimize the patient's work of breathing and prevent lung injury associated with ventilation.

▶ With NAVA, the ventilator begins inspiration as soon as diaphragmatic depolarization is detected. The depth and length of the breath are also established by the diaphragm's electrical activity. When diaphragmatic activity ends, inspiration ends.

▶ The two most frequently used forms of high-frequency ventilation are HFJV and HFOV.

▶ High-frequency percussive ventilation may improve oxygenation, support ventilation, and assist with secretion clearance.

▶ Five different mechanisms may be responsible for gas movement during HFV. They include pendelluft movement, gas streaming, Taylor dispersion, molecular diffusion, and spike formation.

ASSESSMENT QUESTIONS

See Evolve Resources for the answers.

1. All of the following are potential sources of power for a mechanical ventilator *except*:
   a. Pneumatically powered
   b. Electrically powered
   c. Combined pneumatically and electrically powered
   d. Fluidically powered

2. A ventilator measures a drop in tidal volume during pressure ventilation and automatically increases the pressure to return the volume to its original value. This is best described as:
   a. Pressure control ventilation
   b. A closed-loop control system
   c. An open-loop control system
   d. A pneumatically controlled ventilator

3. During operation of a ventilator, the respiratory therapist sets the tidal volume at 500 mL, the respiratory rate at 10 breaths/min, and an inspiratory time of 1.2 sec. These settings are associated with what type of ventilation?
   a. Pressure-targeted, flow-cycled ventilation
   b. Volume-targeted, flow-cycled ventilation
   c. Volume-targeted, time-cycled ventilation
   d. Volume-targeted, pressure-cycled ventilation

4. Which of the following are used as names for pressure-targeted ventilation?
   a. Pressure-limited ventilation
   b. Pressure-controlled ventilation
   c. Pressure-targeted ventilation
   d. All of the above

5. Which of the following is/are volume control device(s) for mechanical ventilators?
   I. Rotary drive piston
   II. Proportional solenoid
   III. Bag-in-a-chamber
   IV. Stepper motor with valve
   a. I only
   b. II only
   c. I and III only
   d. I, III, and IV only

6. A jet stream passes through an opening with a wall adjacent to its left side; the jet deflects toward the wall. What fluidic principle does this describe?
   a. Slip streaming
   b. Coanda effect
   c. Flip-flop device
   d. Separation bubble

7. Classification and description of VC-CMV with a constant flow scalar in which a flow setting is required would include which of the following?
   I. Time triggered
   II. Volume limited
   III. Pressure cycled
   IV. Constant flow
   a. I and III
   b. II and IV
   c. I, II and IV
   d. I, II, III, and IV

8. The following waveforms are noted during ventilation of a patient: a descending flow pattern that returns to baseline before cycling into exhalation, and a constant pressure curve, in which the pressure decreases slightly below the baseline before the beginning of inspiration; volume delivery varies. This best describes what form of ventilation?
   a. Time-triggered, volume-variable ventilation
   b. Patient-triggered, pressure-limited, time-cycled ventilation
   c. Patient-triggered, volume-limited, flow-cycled ventilation
   d. Volume-triggered, pressure-limited, volume-cycled ventilation

9. A commonly used abbreviation for the mode described in question 8 is:
   a. PCV
   b. PSV
   c. VCV
   d. PRVC

10. What are all the possible trigger mechanisms in patient-triggered ventilation?
    I. Pressure
    II. Volume
    III. Time
    IV. Flow
    a. I and III
    b. I and IV
    c. II and IV
    d. I, II, and IV

11. During patient ventilation, the ventilator adjusts pressure to target the set tidal volume. This would be classified as:
    a. Adaptive
    b. Simple
    c. Set point
    d. Complex

12. A pressure scalar on a patient indicates that the difference between the peak inspiratory pressure and the plateau pressure is 5 cm H_2O. This value best describes:
    a. Static compliance
    b. Dynamic compliance
    c. Transairway pressure
    d. Airway resistance

13. An apneic patient is severely hypoxemic. The physician wants to use an elevated baseline pressure. What would be an appropriate recommendation for the respiratory therapist to make?
    a. CSV with CPAP
    b. IPPB
    c. VC-CMV plus PEEP
    d. Oxygen mask

ASSESSMENT QUESTIONS—cont'd

14. The flow-time curve for a paralyzed and sedated patient receiving PCIRV reveals that a mandatory breath occurs before flow returns to zero at the end of exhalation. Which of the following is present?
    a. Inflation hold
    b. PEEP
    c. Air trapping
    d. Patient triggering

15. A physician wants to use pressure ventilation that uses a long time at a high pressure with periodic releases of pressure. She wants to be sure that the lungs do not deflate during the release periods. Which of the following modes of ventilation would the respiratory therapist recommend?
    a. Pressure-regulated volume control
    b. Pressure augmentation
    c. Proportional-assist ventilation
    d. Airway pressure-release ventilation

16. What HFV technique provides an active inspiratory and expiratory phase?
    a. High-frequency positive-pressure ventilation
    b. High-frequency flow interruption
    c. High-frequency jet ventilation
    d. High-frequency oscillatory ventilation

17. A patient is being ventilated by means of a continuous-flow CPAP system set at 10 cm H_2O. The respiratory therapist notices that during spontaneous inspiration, the monitored inspiratory pressure is 5 cm H_2O and the expiratory pressure is 10 cm H_2O. To solve this problem, what should the therapist consider doing?
    a. Check the function of the one-way valve between the patient and the CPAP generator.
    b. Increase the flow to the system.
    c. Increase the pressure setting on the PEEP/CPAP valve.
    d. Check the system for leaks.

18. Which of the following are the four phases of a breath?
    I. End of exhalation/beginning of inhalation
    II. End of inhalation/beginning of exhalation
    III. Delivery of inspiration
    IV. The expiratory phase
        a. I and II
        b. II and IV
        c. III and IV
        d. I, II, III, and IV

19. The phase variables include which of the following?
    I. Trigger variable: begins inspiration
    II. Control variable: remains constant during inspiration (e.g., volume or pressure)
    III. Limit variable: places a minimum value on a variable (pressure, volume, flow, or time) during delivery of a breath
    IV. Cycle variable: ends inspiration.
        a. I
        b. II and III
        c. III and IV
        d. I, II, and IV

20. A patient on flow triggering has a base flow of 10 L/min and a flow trigger of 3 L/min. At what measured flow will the ventilator begin inspiration?
    a. When the expiratory flow drops from 10 L/min to 7 L/min
    b. When inspiratory sensitivity senses a rise in flow of 3 L/min
    c. When the expiratory flow increases from 10 to 13 L/min
    d. The answer cannot be determined from the information given.

21. While checking the ventilator graphics, the respiratory therapist notices no downward deflection of the pressure curve before inspiratory flow begins. The inspiratory flow curve is constant and has a fixed inspiratory flow time of 1 second. What are the trigger and cycle mechanisms and is this breath-volume or pressure targeted ventilation?
    a. Pressure-triggered, constant-flow, time-cycled ventilation
    b. Time-triggered, flow-limited, time-cycled ventilation
    c. Time-triggered, constant-pressure, flow-cycled ventilation
    d. Patient-triggered, volume-limited, time-cycled ventilation

22. During ventilation the flow rises sharply to a peak of 100 L/min and progressively decreases. The pressure-time curve shows a sharp rise to plateau. The respiratory therapist notices that volume varies over time. What type of ventilation is this?
    a. Volume-targeted ventilation
    b. Flow cycling
    c. PC-CMV
    d. APRV ventilation

23. During PSV ventilation (PC-CSV), what is the cycle variable?
    a. Time
    b. Flow
    c. Pressure
    d. Patient effort

24. Which of the following is the clinical name commonly applied to patient- or time-triggered, volume-targeted, and time-cycled ventilation?
    a. Assist-control
    b. Controlled ventilation
    c. PCV
    d. Pressure augmentation

25. PRVC is different from P_{aug} in terms of what primary characteristic?
    a. PRVC is pressure targeted.
    b. PRVC guarantees volume over several breaths.
    c. PRVC guarantees volume for every breath.
    d. PRVC is not a servo controlled mode.

ASSESSMENT QUESTIONS—cont'd

26. Which of the following modes responds by giving more flow and pressure when a patient demands more? In this mode the operator sets the amount needed to unload the work imposed by elastance and resistance.
    a. APRV
    b. PAV
    c. ASV
    d. PRVC

27. What type of ventilation relies on detection of diaphragm depolarization?
    a. NAVA
    b. PAV
    c. CSV
    d. HFV

28. During ventilation of a spontaneously breathing patient, the ventilator increases the respiratory rate so that the set minute volume is achieved. This best describes:
    a. IMV
    b. CPAP
    c. NAVA
    d. MMV

29. The Hamilton GALILEO ventilator has a closed-loop mode of ventilation that uses an advanced level of computational logic. This mode is called:
    a. Adaptive support ventilation
    b. Proportional assist ventilation
    c. Intermittent percussive ventilation
    d. Neurally adjusted ventilatory assist

30. Which of the following breath sequences are described by Chatburn's classification system?
    a. Continuous mandatory ventilation (CMV)
    b. Synchronized intermittent mandatory ventilation (SIMV)
    c. Intermittent mandatory ventilation (IMV)
    d. Continuous spontaneous ventilation (CSV)
    (1) I and IV
    (2) II and III
    (3) I, III, and IV
    (4) I, II, III, and IV

References

1. Mushin WW, Rendell-Baker L, Thompson PW, et al: *Automatic ventilation of the lungs,* Philadelphia, 1980, FA Davis.
2. Chatburn RL: *Classification of mechanical ventilation,* Dallas, 1988, American Association for Respiratory Care.
3. Chatburn RL: A new system for understanding mechanical ventilators, *Respir Care* 36:1123, 1991.
4. Branson RD, Hess DR, Chatburn RL: *Respiratory care equipment,* Philadelphia, 1995, JB Lippincott.
5. Chatburn RL, Primiano FP: A new system of understanding modes of mechanical ventilation, *Respir Care* 46:604, 2001.
6. Blanch PB, Desautels DA: Chatburn's ventilator classification scheme: a poor substitute for the classic approach, *Respir Care* 39:762, 1994.
7. Chatburn RL: Classification of ventilator modes: update and proposal for implementation, *Respir Care* 52:301, 2007.
8. Chatburn RL: Computer control of mechanical ventilation, *Respir Care* 49:507, 2004.
9. Chatburn RL: *Fundamentals of mechanical ventilation,* Cleveland Heights, Ohio, 2003, Mandu Press.
10. Chatburn RL, Volsko TA: Mechanical ventilators. In Wilkins RL, Stoller JK, Scanlan CL: *Egan's fundamentals of respiratory care,* ed 8, St Louis, 2003, Mosby/Elsevier.
11. Pilbeam SP, Cairo JM: *Mechanical ventilation: physiological and clinical applications,* ed 4, St Louis, 2006, Mosby/Elsevier.
12. Raniere VM: Optimization of patient-ventilator interactions: closed loop technology to turn the century (editorial), *Intensive Care Med* 23:936, 1997.
13. Branson RD: Dual control modes, closed loop ventilation, handguns and tequila (editorial), *Respir Care* 46:232, 2001.
14. Sanborn WG: Microprocessor-based mechanical ventilation, *Respir Care* 38:72, 1993.
15. Scanlan CL, Wilkins RL, Stoller JK: *Egan's fundamentals of respiratory therapy,* ed 7, St Louis, 1999, Mosby.
16. Dupuis Y: *Ventilators: theory and clinical application,* ed 2, St Louis, 1992, Mosby.
17. Branson RD, Hess DR, Chatburn RL: *Respiratory care equipment,* ed 2, Philadelphia, 1999, Lippincott Williams & Wilkins.
18. Morgan SE, Kestner JJ: Modification of a critical care ventilator for use during magnetic resonance imaging, *Respir Care* 47:61, 2002.
19. Banner MJ: Expiratory positive pressure valves and work of breathing, *Respir Care* 32:431, 1987.
20. Spearman CB: Positive end-expiratory pressure: terminology and technical aspects of PEEP devices and systems, *Respir Care* 33:434, 1988.
21. Nilsestuen JO, Hargett K: Managing the patient-ventilator system using graphic analysis: an overview and introduction to Graphics Corner, *Respir Care* 41:1105, 1996
22. MacIntyre N, Nishimura M: The Nagoyo conference on system design and patient-ventilator interactions during pressure support ventilation, *Chest* 97:1463, 1990.
23. Hess DR, MacIntyre NR: *Respiratory care: principles and practice,* Philadelphia, 2002, WB Saunders.
24. Chatmongkolchart S, Williams P: Evaluation of inspiratory rise time and inspiratory termination criteria in new-generation mechanical ventilators: a lung model study, *Respir Care* 46:666, 2001.
25. Williams P, Mueluer M: Pressure support and pressure assist/control: are there differences?: an evaluation of the newest intensive care unit ventilators, *Respir Care* 45:1169, 2000.
26. Hess DR: Mechanical ventilation strategies: what's new and what's worth keeping? *Respir Care* 47:1007, 2002.
27. Branson R: Understanding and implementing advances in ventilator capabilities, *Curr Opin Crit Care* 10:23, 2004.
28. Yamada Y, Du HL: Effects of different pressure support termination on patient-ventilator synchrony, *Respir Care* 43:1048, 1998.
29. Du HL, Ohtsuji M, Shigeta M et al: Expiratory asynchrony in proportional assist, *Am J Respir Crit Care Med* 165:972, 2002.

30. Hewlett AM, Platt AS: Mandatory minute volume: a new concept in weaning from mechanical ventilation, *Anaesthesia* 32:163, 1977.

31. Reynolds EOR: Effect of alterations in mechanical ventilator settings on pulmonary gas exchange in hyaline membrane disease, *Arch Dis Child* 46:152, 1971.

32. Reynolds EOR, Taghipadeh A: Improved prognosis of infants mechanically ventilated for hyaline membrane disease, *Arch Dis Child* 49:405, 1974.

33. Meade MO, Herridge MS: An evidence-based approach to acute respiratory distress syndrome, *Respir Care* 46:1368, 2001.

34. Hass CF: Lung protective mechanical ventilation in acute respiratory distress syndrome, *Respir Care Clin N Am* 9:363, 2003.

35. Acute Respiratory Distress Syndrome Network (ARDSnet): Ventilation with lower tidal volumes as compared with traditional tidal volumes for acute lung injury and the acute respiratory distress syndrome, *N Engl J Med* 342:1301, 2000.

36. Kallet RH, Corral W: Implementation of a low tidal volume ventilation protocol for patients with acute lung injury or acute respiratory distress syndrome, *Respir Care* 46:1024, 2001.

37. Stock MC, Downs JB: Airway pressure release ventilation: a new approach to ventilatory support during acute lung injury, *Respir Care* 32:517, 1987.

38. Foland JA, Martin J: Airway pressure release ventilation with a short release time in a child with acute respiratory distress syndrome, *Respir Care* 46:1019, 2001.

39. Frawley PM, Habashi NM: Airway pressure release ventilation: theory and practice, *AACN Clinical Issues* 12:234, 2001.

40. Myers TR, MacIntyre NR: Does airway pressure release ventilation offer important new advantages in mechanical ventilator support? *Respir Care* 52:452, 2007.

41. Branson RD, Chatburn RL: Should adaptive pressure control modes be utilized for virtually all patients receiving mechanical ventilation? *Respir Care* 52:478, 2007.

42. Sottiaux TM: Patient-ventilator interactions during volume-support ventilation: asynchrony and tidal volume instability—a report of three cases, *Respir Care* 46:255, 2001.

43. Keenan HT, Martin LD: Volume support ventilation in infants and children: analysis of a case series, *Respir Care* 42:281, 1997.

44. Grasso S, Ranieri VM: Proportional assist ventilation, *Respir Care Clin N Am* 7:465, 2001.

45. Kondili E, Xirouchaki N, Vaporidi K et al: Short-term cardiorespiratory effects of proportional assist and pressure-support ventilation in patients with acute lung injury/acute respiratory distress syndrome, *Anesthesiology* 105:703, 2006.

46. Schulze A, Rieger-Fackeldey E, Gerhardt T et al: Randomized crossover comparison of proportional assist ventilation and patient-triggered ventilation in extremely low birth weight infants with evolving chronic lung disease, *Neonatology* 92:1, 2007.

47. Younes M: Proportional assist ventilation: a new approach to ventilatory support. I. Theory, *Am Rev Respir Dis* 145:114, 1992.

48. Younes M et al: Proportional assist ventilation: results of an initial clinical trial, *Am Rev Respir Dis* 145:121, 1992.

49. Schulze A, Schaller P: Proportional assist ventilation: a new strategy for infant ventilation? *Neonatal Respir Dis* 6:1, 1996.

50. Otis AB, Fenn WO, Rahn H: Mechanics of breathing in man, *J Appl Physiol* 2:592, 1950.

51. Hart N, Hunt A, Polkey MI et al: Comparison of proportional assist ventilation and pressure support ventilation in chronic respiratory failure due to neuromuscular and chest wall deformity, *Thorax* 57:979, 2002.

52. Kondili E, Prinianakis G, Alexopoulou C et al: Respiratory load compensation during mechanical ventilation-proportional assist ventilation with load-adjustable gain factors versus pressure support. *Intensive Care Med* 32:692, 2006.

53. Leipälä JA, Iwasaki S, Lee S et al: Compliance and resistance levels and unloading in proportional assist ventilation, *Physiol Meas* 26:281, 2005.

54. Beck J, Sinderby C, Lindstrom L et al: Effects of lung volume on diaphragm EMG signal strength during voluntary contractions, *J Appl Physiol* 85:1123, 1998.

55. Sinderby C, Beck J, Spahija J et al: Inspiratory muscle unloading by neurally adjusted ventilatory assist during maximal inspiratory efforts in healthy subjects, *Chest* 131:646, 2007.

56. Beck J, Campoccia F, Allo JC et al: Improved synchrony and respiratory unloading by neurally adjusted ventilatory assist (NAVA) in lung-injured rabbits, *Pediatr Respir* 61:289, 2007.

57. Beck J, Tucci M, Emeriaud G et al: Prolonged neural expiratory time induced by mechanical ventilation in infants, *Pediatr Respir* 55:747, 2004.

58. Sinderby C, Navalesi P, Beck J et al: Neural control of mechanical ventilation in respiratory failure, *Nature Med* 5:1433, 1999.

59. Sinderby C: Ventilatory assist driven by patient demand (editorial), *Am J Respir Crit Care Med* 168:729, 2003.

60. Fessler HE, Hess DR: Does high-frequency ventilation offer benefits over conventional ventilation in adult patients with respiratory distress syndrome? *Respir Care* 52:595, 2007.

61. Sjöstrand U: High-frequency positive pressure ventilation (HFPPV): a review, *Crit Care Med* 8:345, 1980.

62. Calkins JM: High-frequency jet ventilation: experimental evaluation. In Carlon CG, Howlan WS, editors: *High-frequency ventilation in intensive care and during surgery,* New York, 1985, Marcel Dekker.

63. English P, Mason SC: Neonatal mechanical ventilation. In Hess DR, MacIntyre NR: *Respiratory care: principles and practice,* Philadelphia, 2002, WB Saunders.

64. Klain M, Smith RB: High-frequency percutaneous transtracheal jet ventilation, *Crit Care Med* 5:280, 1977.

65. Watson K: Ventilatory support in newborn and pediatric patients. In Pilbeam SP: *Mechanical ventilation: physiological and clinical applications,* ed 3, St Louis, 1998, Mosby.

66. Fessler DM, Weiler N, Heinrighs et al: High-frequency oscillatory ventilation for adult acute respiratory distress syndrome, *Intensive Care Med* 29:1656, 2003.

67. Bollen CW, van Well GT, Sherry T et al: High frequency oscillatory ventilation compared with conventional mechanical ventilation in adult respiratory distress syndrome: a randomized controlled trial. *Crit Care* 9:R430, 2005.

68. Bollen CW, Ulterwaal CS, vanVught AJ: Cumulative meta-analysis of high-frequency versus conventional ventilation in premature neonates, *Am J Respir Crit Care Med* 168:1150, 2003.

69. Allan PF, Thurlby JR, Naworol GA: Measurement of pulsatile tidal volume, pressure amplitude, and gas flow during high-frequency percussive ventilation, with and without partial cuff deflation, *Respir Care* 52:45, 2007.

70. Toussaint M, De Win H, Steens M et al: Effect of intrapulmonary percussive ventilation on mucus clearance in Duchenne muscular dystrophy patients: a preliminary report, *Respir Care* 48:940, 2003.

71. Velmahos GC, Chan LS, Tatevossian R et al: High-frequency percussive ventilation improves oxygenation in patients with ARDS, *Chest* 116:440, 1999.

72. Reper P, Wibaux O, Van Laeke P et al: High frequency percussive ventilation and conventional ventilation after smoke inhalation: a randomized study, *Burns* 28:503, 2002.

73. Salim A, Martin M: High-frequency percussive ventilation, *Crit Care Med* 33:S241, 2005.
74. English P, Mason SC: Neonatal mechanical ventilation. In Hess DR, MacIntyre NR: *Respiratory care: principles and practice,* Philadelphia, 2002, WB Saunders.

Internet Resources

American Association for Respiratory Care: www.aarc.org. Check "Resources," Clinical Practice Guidelines, and look for the following:
   a. Patient-Ventilator System Check
   b. Ventilator Circuit Changes
American Journal of Respiratory and Critical Care Medicine: http://ajrccm.atsjournals.org
Bird and BEAR ventilators: www.viasyshealthcare.com (NOTE: Recently purchased by Cardinal Health) (www.cardinalhealth.com)
Cardiopulmonary Corp.: www.cardiopulmonarycorp.com
Dräger ventilators: www.draegermedical.com
Hamilton Medical: www.hamilton-medical.com
Maquet (Servo ventilators): www.maquet.com
Medscape: www.medscape.com
National Board for Respiratory Care: www.nbrc.org
National Library of Medicine: http://text.nlm.nih.gov
Percussionaire: www.percussionaire.com
Philips Medical (owners of Respironics): www.philipsmedical.com
Puritan Bennett: www.PuritanBennett.com (now part of Covidien [www.covidien.com])
Respironics: www.respironics.com (now owned by Philips)
Society of Critical Care Medicine: www.sccm.org
Ventilator information: www.ventworld.com
VIASYS Health Care: VIASYS AVEA and Vela ventilators: www.viasyshealthcare.com. (NOTE: Recently purchased by Cardinal Health) (www.cardinalhealth.com)
Virtual Hospital: www.vh.org
   a. Look into Respiratory Problems
   b. Look into Radiology

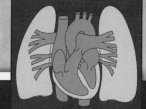

Chapter 12

Mechanical Ventilators: General-Use Devices

SUSAN P. PILBEAM

OUTLINE

Common Features of Ventilators
Distinguishing Different Models
Common Internal Mechanisms
Patient Monitoring
Parameters and Displays
Modes of Ventilation
Alarms
Understanding Individual Ventilators
Presentation of Specific Ventilators
Cardinal Health Ventilators
Cardinal Avea
Cardinal Bear 1000
Cardinal Bird 8400* Ventilator
Cardinal Bird T-Bird* Ventilator
Cardinal Vela
Dräger Ventilators
Dräger Evita*
Dräger Evita 2 Dura*
Dräger E-4 (Evita 4)
Dräger EvitaXL SW 6.0
Dräger Savina*

Hamilton Ventilators
Hamilton Veolar^{FT}*
Hamilton Galileo Gold
Hamilton Raphael
Maquet Ventilators
Maquet Servo 900C*
Maquet Servo 300
Maquet Servo^i Ventilator System
Maquet Servo^s Ventilator
Newport Ventilators
Newport Breeze E150*
Newport Wave E200
Newport e500
Puritan Bennett Ventilators
Puritan Bennett 840
Puritan Bennett 740
Puritan Bennett 760
Puritan Bennett 7200
Respironics Ventilators
Respironics Esprit Ventilator

This chapter has been designed in a slightly different manner from the other chapters in the text. In this chapter, each ventilator is treated as a separate section, with an outline, objectives, key terms, assessment questions, and references. The intention of this design is to allow the reader to examine all the relevant material for one ventilator without moving from one part of the text to another. The chapter provides detailed information about a number of multipurpose mechanical ventilators that can be used for both pediatric and adult patients. Emphasis is placed on ventilators used primarily in the intensive care unit. Each ventilator presented includes a concise description so that the reader could literally work through how to operate the device using the information provided. It is not the author's intention that this chapter be read from begin-

ning to end; rather, the reader should use it to gain knowledge about a specific ventilator or ventilators.

Every effort has been made to ensure that the information provided in this chapter is accurate. However, readers should always consult the operating manuals and instructions from the manufacturer whenever using medical devices for patient care. Readers also need to be aware of software changes and any options that may have been added to equipment they are using. They need to familiarize themselves with the changes.

Since the last edition of this text, an Evolve Resources has been made available as a text feature. The reader is referred to that site for information on some of the less frequently used or discontinued ventilator models. Some examples include the Dräger Evita, the Hamilton Amadeus, the Newport E150, the Bird 8400, and the Bird T-Bird. These ventilators, which were presented in the sixth and seventh editions of the text, have been moved from the text to the Web site. These changes have been introduced

*See Evolve Resources for a detailed description of this ventilator.

because of space constraints and also because although some facilities still have these ventilators, their use has declined significantly or they are no longer produced or supported by the manufacturer.

The incorporation of microprocessors into mechanical ventilators in the 1980s forever changed their design. Ventilators with microprocessing features can rapidly monitor, manage, and store information and even change machine function. Manufacturers can change or add new modes or features by simply adding new software, a circuit board, or maybe even a new interface to the device.

Buyouts are another phenomenon that has affected the character of ventilator purchases and use. For example, Bear Medical Corporation merged with Allied Health Corporation, which was then purchased by Thermo Electron Corporation, which also owns Bird Ventilator Products. The original Bird Company was owned by Dr. Forrest Bird, who sold it to the 3M Corporation. In 2001, the company changed the name of the Bear and Bird Ventilator division to Viasys Healthcare, Critical Care Division. In 2008, Cardinal Health purchased Viasys Healthcare and now owns their products. Likewise, Nellcor purchased the Puritan Bennett Corporation, as well as Infrasonics. In turn, Nellcor Puritan Bennett was bought out by Mallinckrodt, which was then purchased by Tyco. Some of the Tyco medical products were spun off to another division, Covidien. And so goes the buyout phenomenon, which ultimately affects the availability of ventilators.

Both the economic situation and technologic advances have resulted in a rapidly changing environment for mechanical ventilators. It is important for consumers to keep these factors in mind and to be aware that units used or purchased may not have the features they would desire or the expected manufacturer support.

COMMON FEATURES OF VENTILATORS

Fierce competition among manufacturers has created an advantageous situation for consumers. Because ventilators can be reprogrammed, whenever a manufacturer advertises a new feature, it is usually not long until other manufacturers offer a similar option. For example, the Puritan Bennett 7200 ventilator was one of the first to offer a backup mode of ventilation. This backup ventilation has preprogrammed parameters, such as tidal volume (V_T), rate, fractional inspired oxygen (F_IO_2), and flow, which are activated if the ventilator detects the presence of apnea. Most ventilators now used in acute care have a backup ventilation feature.

Distinguishing Different Models

Because programmable features can be added to a ventilator, clinical facilities can purchase a unit and then add new features as they are developed. This add-on concept has resulted in much confusion about the names and numbers given to various machines. For example, a hos-

pital initially purchases a unit called the Magnolia 500; however, after developing several new alarm or monitoring capabilities, the manufacturer now calls it the Magnolia 500a or maybe the Magnolia 500 version 2.0. Keeping track of all of the new features added after the initial purchase is truly an art for both the purchaser and the sales representative, not to mention authors of ventilator texts. This places an important responsibility on clinicians to learn about updates and to understand how they affect the functions of a particular ventilator. Ultimately it is the user's responsibility to follow the manufacturer's instructions and recommendations.

Common Internal Mechanisms

The internal mechanisms of many microprocessor-controlled machines have several similarities. For example, they usually require high-pressure air and oxygen gas sources for pneumatic power, as well as electricity to power the internal microprocessors and various electronically operated components. Gas entering the ventilator's internal circuit is filtered before its temperature and pressure are measured. The gas pressure then is regulated, and both gases are mixed. The mixture is sometimes fed into a holding tank or pressurized cylinder that acts as a reservoir for gas under pressure. The gas may then be routed to a microprocessor-controlled flow valve. Although these valves vary by manufacturer, they all provide rapid response for a variety of gas delivery methods. For example, they can give a constant flow and preset volume, or they can give a constant pressure while volume delivery varies. They can change the shape of the inspiratory flow waveform during volume ventilation and respond rapidly to a patient's spontaneous demand for gas flow. Chapter 11 provides additional information on the internal drive mechanisms of ventilators.

Historically, respiratory therapists (RTs) were required to learn the specific details of the internal parts of ventilators such as the Bird Mark 7 and the Emerson Post-Op ventilator. It was important for RTs to know this information so that they could disassemble and repair these devices. This is no longer the case. Trained technical specialists now repair the internal mechanism. For this reason, much of the discussion of the internal function of ventilators in this chapter is presented in an abbreviated fashion.

Patient Monitoring

Sophisticated new technology enables flow and pressure delivery to be monitored rapidly and accurately and allows a variety of monitors and alarms to be used. Pressure and flow are often measured internally, near the main ventilator outlet and return line (i.e., expiratory valve area); however, some ventilators monitor flow, pressure, or both at the patient's upper airway. Although types of monitors vary, their function usually is the same. For example, ventilators incorporate flow-measuring devices, which may be variable-orifice pneumotachographs or ultrasonic technology, depending on the manufacturer's preference. Chapter 8 reviews the function of several of these devices.

Ventilators usually have digital displays of the following parameters: V_T, rate (spontaneous and total), peak inspiratory pressure (PIP), plateau pressure (P_{plat}), positive end-expiratory pressure (PEEP), continuous positive airway pressure (CPAP), peak flow, oxygen percentage, and inspiratory to expiratory (I:E) ratio. Most ventilators also offer a graphic display screen for pressure-, flow-, and volume-time waveforms, as well as flow-volume and pressure-volume loops.

Parameters and Displays

Most ventilators now have light-emitting diode (LED) control panels, which show the operator the mode and parameters currently set and monitored, along with graphic information. Some display screens or control panels are touch sensitive. Most control panels include a display window that can provide the operator with a written message, such as an alarm message.

The range of available volume, pressure, and flow also tends to be very similar in current ventilators. For example, the V_T range for units used for pediatric and adult patients tends to be about 50 to 2000 mL (it may be lower than 50 mL in units that can volume ventilate infants). The typical range of inspiratory pressure limits is 0 to 120 cm H_2O, PEEP/CPAP values usually are 0 to 50 cm H_2O, and pressure-support pressure levels generally range from 0 to 100 cm H_2O.

Nearly every ventilator intended for use in acute care provides the following ventilatory modes: continuous mandatory ventilation (CMV) and intermittent mandatory ventilation (IMV) (either volume targeted or pressure targeted); and spontaneous, which includes PEEP/CPAP and pressure-support ventilation (PSV). Dual control modes and closed-loop intelligent modes also are available. (See Chapter 11 for further descriptions.)

Modes of Ventilation

Chapter 11 describes a method of defining ventilator breaths and modes of ventilation. Unfortunately, manufacturers do not follow a consistent method for naming breath types and modes, and this has resulted in a great deal of confusion. Each manufacturer may have a different name for the same mode and breathing pattern. This makes learning breath types and modes for each of the ventilators very difficult for the beginner. Appendix 12-1, at the end of this chapter, attempts to clear up some of this difficulty by providing the manufacturer's name for the mode, breathing pattern, control type, and operational logic. It also provides a list of the ventilators presented in this chapter and the modes of ventilation for each.

Alarms

Common alarms include high and low pressure, high and low oxygen percentage, high and low minute volume, high rate, and high and low PEEP/CPAP. Ventilators also have alarm-silencing buttons that usually silence audible alarms for 1 to 2 minutes. Sometimes the type of alarm that is active is shown in a display window. Some ventilators illuminate the LEDs next to the violated alarms to indicate which alarms are being or have been activated. Some units scroll through the chronologic order of the alarm events as the operator reads the display screen.

Critical alarms, such as low gas supply, loss of power, and ventilator inoperative alarms (i.e., critical internal error detected by the microprocessor), are available and cannot be silenced.

In the unit's memory, microprocessors can save information about which alarms have occurred or what changes have been made and can report these to the operator in some form. This information may be accessed under some type of trending screen.

New ventilators also have internal memory areas that cannot be accessed by the user, but only by company technical specialists. It is important to know this, because the user cannot erase essential memories that can be used to diagnose errors or serious events.

Understanding Individual Ventilators

Once clinicians have mastered the use of a newer, more sophisticated ventilator, they usually do not find it difficult to understand another brand. Manufacturers have tried to make their equipment user friendly and provide a wide variety of materials and services to explain their operation, such as training videotapes, Web-based information, instruction and operation manuals, trained technicians and clinical application specialists, CD-ROM interactive programs, and product specialists via telephone or Internet. And, as always, users are encouraged to read the directions.

Presentation of Specific Ventilators

It is assumed that readers have a basic understanding of the physical properties of ventilators as outlined in Chapter 11. The machines are presented in such a way as to help prepare readers to use them in a clinical setting; therefore the discussions do not focus in too much detail on internal function or classification.

Identifying the need for ventilation, setting initial ventilator parameters, adjusting settings based on the patient's response and arterial blood gas analysis, complications of ventilation, and discontinuing ventilation are subjects beyond the scope of this text. However, this information is available in other sources.*

---

*One such source is Pilbeam SP, Cairo JM: *Mechanical ventilation: physiological and clinical application,* ed 4, St Louis, 2006, Mosby.

CARDINAL HEALTH VENTILATORS

CARDINAL AVEA[1-3]

OUTLINE

Power Source
Internal Drive Mechanism
Controls
   Ventilator Set-Up
   Membrane Buttons and LEDs
   Primary Breath Controls
Modes of Ventilation
   Continuous Mandatory Ventilation (CMV)
   Synchronized Intermittent Mandatory Ventilation (SIMV)
   Pressure-Regulated Volume Control (PRVC) Breath
      Delivery
   Airway Pressure-Release Ventilation (APRV)/BiPhasic
   Time Cycled, Pressure Limited (TCPL)
   CPAP/PSV Mode
   Noninvasive Positive-Pressure Ventilation (NPPV)
   Apnea Back-Up Ventilation (ABV)
Advanced Settings
   Volume Limit
   Machine Volume

Inspiratory Rise
Flow Cycle
PSV Tmax
Waveform Feature
Sigh
Bias Flow
Pressure Trigger
Vsync
Vsync Rise
Monitors and Displays
Alarms and Indicators
Special Features
   Trends
   Heliox
   Respiratory Mechanics
   Independent Lung Ventilation (ILV)
   Neonatal Application
Troubleshooting

OBJECTIVES

Upon completion of this section, you will be able to:
- Explain the power sources of the AVEA.
- Describe the function of each of the membrane buttons.
- Identify indicators located on the ventilator front.
- Determine the current power source and battery status.
- Outline the parameter setup when NEW PATIENT is selected.
- Name the limit for the I:E ratio variable.
- Compare the trigger, target (limit), and cycle variables for the available modes of ventilation.
- Identify the icons and waveforms on the main screen.
- Recognize visual and audible alarm signals and the level of priority.
- Explain how to access the ventilator set-up, screen menu, main screen, advanced settings, alarm limits, and mode menu.
- Describe the purpose of each of the advanced settings.
- Explain how to access respiratory mechanics and the function of each of the respiratory mechanics.

KEY TERMS

Accumulator
Artificial airway compensation
   (AAC)

Internal scroll pump
Pressure-targeted ventilation
Pressure triggering

User interface module (UIM)
Variable-orifice pneumotachometer

The AVEA ventilator originally was developed by VIASYS Healthcare, Critical Care Division, Palm Springs, California (Figure 12-1). In 2008, VIASYS was purchased by Cardinal Healthcare's ventilator division, and the AVEA became part of Cardinal Health's Critical Care ventilator division. This purchase also included the acquisition of Bird, Bear, and Sensormedics ventilation products.

The AVEA is a servo-controlled, software-driven ventilator designed for neonatal to adult patients. The user interface is a full color, active matrix, LCD touch screen. Membrane buttons surrounding the touch screen give access to various screens and enable special functions. The AVEA can be used for conventional invasive or noninvasive positive-pressure ventilation.

Software upgrades can be uploaded to the ventilator when new product developments become available. The new software is electronically delivered to a laptop and then transferred to the ventilator; this process is performed by the company's technical support personnel.

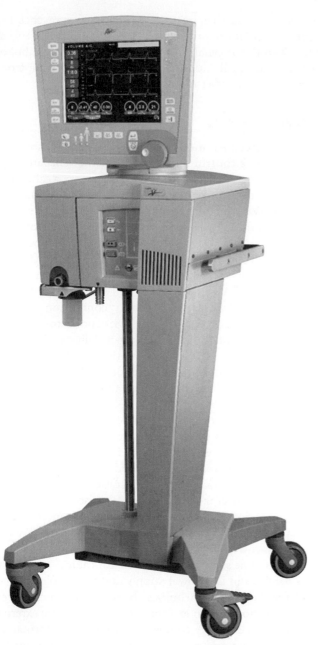

FIGURE 12-1 AVEA ventilator. (Courtesy Cardinal Health, Yorba Linda, Calif.)

POWER SOURCE

The AVEA is electrically and pneumatically powered. Gas power can be provided by external high-pressure wall or cylinder gas or by an internal compressor. Box 12-1 presents the gas source types and pressure ranges.

The ventilator's electric power is provided by a standard 110/120-volt AC power source (230/240-volt AC outside the United States). In emergencies, it uses a back-up 24-volt DC battery power supply.

When maximally charged, the internal battery can power the ventilator alone for 1 hour under normal operating conditions. When powering the ventilator and compressor together, the internal battery provides about 30 minutes of power. It takes about 4 hours to fully charge the internal battery.

An optional external battery is also available. When fully charged, the internal and external batteries combined can provide about 2 hours of operating time for both the ventilator and the compressor under normal operating conditions. Together they can power the ventilator alone for up to 7 hours. It takes about 12 hours to fully charge the batteries.

Box 12-2 and Figure 12-2 describe and illustrate the indicators used to provide information about the main power and battery charge status.

INTERNAL DRIVE MECHANISM

High-pressure gas input to the ventilator occurs by way of two gas sources: air and oxygen. A rigid **accumulator** serves as an internal reservoir to supply flow on demand to the patient.

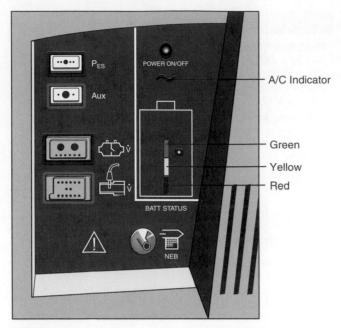

FIGURE 12-2 The Front Panel Display of the AVEA, located below the display screen, contains connectors for pressure and for flow and volume monitoring, as well as battery indicators. (See text for further description.) (Courtesy Robert Whitesides, MAQUET Inc., Bridgewater, N.J.)

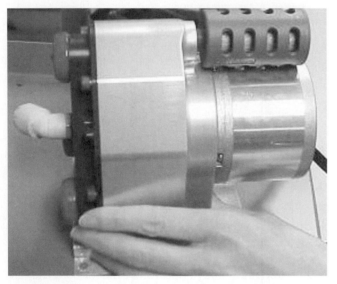

FIGURE 12-3 Compressor of the AVEA containing the scroll pump. (Courtesy Cardinal Health, Yorba Linda, Calif.)

When no high-pressure air source is available, the internal compressor operates to supply airflow. The **internal scroll pump** compressor was designed using technology similar to refrigerator compressors (Figure 12-3). In a cross-sectional view, the scroll pump looks like a nautilus shell on the inside. The scroll pump can be described as an orbital compressor in which one half is stationary and the other half moves in a circular fashion.

When the internal compressor is operating, the gas is drawn into the compressor. As the compressor rotates, the gas is moved farther into the scrolls until it reaches the center, where it exits the compressor to power the ventilator. When the internal compressor is active, the symbol of the nautilus shell illuminates; this appears on the front panel, below the user interface module.

CONTROLS

The **user interface module (UIM)** contains all software and electronic control mechanisms for the ventilator and communicates with the gas delivery engine via a cable connection on the rear panel. Other connections on the rear panel of AVEA include two diameter index safety system (DISS) gas inlet fittings, one for air and one for oxygen; analog input and output for synchronized independent lung ventilation (Figure 12-4); and input of up to two external signals to be displayed on the main screen of the user interface. A remote nurse call connection, the O_2 sensor cell, and an external battery connection also are found on the rear panel. The DISS connectors can be changed to adapt for helium-oxygen delivery. When the helium connector is added, the ventilator software adapts for the change in density and viscosity of the lighter gas so that parameter displays such as flow and volume are corrected.

Patient monitoring from the AVEA includes esophageal, tracheal, and proximal airway pressure monitoring. Proximal airway flow sensing with either a **variable-orifice pneumotachometer** or hot wire flow-sensing technology is available for measuring tidal volume delivery at the patient Y-connector (see Figure 12-2; also see Chapter 8 for information on pneumotachometers). Connections for each of these devices are color coded, labeled, and keyed to prevent incorrect attachments.

In this same section of the ventilator cabinet are indicators for AC and DC power supply and the nipple connection for the internal nebulizer. Beneath the touch screen are connections for an external printer, a separate external display device (SVGA connector), a medical information bus (MIB) port, and two RS-232 interface connections for data input and output.

Except for the on/off power switch, which is on the rear panel of the unit, all operator controls are on the front panel of the user interface. Before using the ventilator on a new patient or when the patient circuit is changed, the operator must perform a number of checks to ensure that the ventilator is functioning properly. Two different series of tests are run. The first series verifies general operations, and the second series verifies the alarm functions.

Ventilator Set-Up

After the start-up testing, the clinician can choose either RESUME CURRENT and continue ventilation at the current control settings, or NEW PATIENT can be selected, which clears the previous data (trends and saved loops). Ventilation begins at default values for the currently selected patient size (neonatal, pediatric, or adult) when the NEW

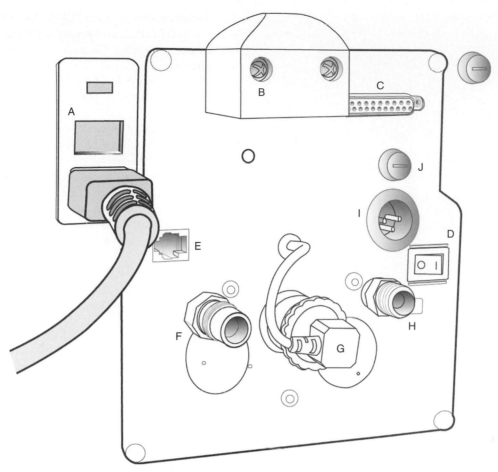

FIGURE 12-4 Rear panel of the AVEA ventilator. **A,** AC power connector. **B,** UIM connector. **C,** Analog input and output independent lung ventilation port. **D,** Power on/off switch. **E,** Nurse call system connector. **F,** Air DISS fitting. **G,** Oxygen sensor. **H,** Oxygen DISS fitting. **I,** External battery connector. **J,** External battery fuse. (See text for further explanation.)

PATIENT selection is accepted. The operator selects the appropriate patient size and, once accepted, the ventilator SET UP screen is selected (Figure 12-5).

The SET UP screen allows the clinician to enable certain features, including artificial airway compensation, leak compensation, and circuit compliance compensation (see Chapter 11 for an explanation of tubing compliance and its calculation).

When **artificial airway compensation (AAC)** is turned on, the ventilator adjusts the pressure delivered to compensate for the pressure drop across the artificial airway. The pressure delivered is based on a calculation that takes into account the flow, gas composition (air-oxygen or heliox), fractional inspired oxygen (F_IO_2), tube diameter, length, and pharyngeal curvature based on patient size (adult, pediatric, neonate). (NOTE: If AAC is activated during patient ventilation, a sudden increase in Ppeak and V_T occurs. Caution must be used to minimize the risk of excessive V_T delivery.)

Leak compensation is active during exhalation to help maintain baseline pressure in the circuit in the event of leaks. A flow control valve supplies flow when the pressure drops below its target, up to a maximum flow based on

patient size. In addition, the expiratory valve relieves pressure when the circuit pressure exceeds a target value. Both these functions help stabilize the baseline pressure during exhalation.

Body temperature pressure saturated (BTPS) correction for active (heated humidifier) or passive (heat and moisture exchanger) humidification systems, and an electronic self-test (EST) are also available. The patient's weight and a 24-character patient ID also can be entered. (NOTE: The patient's weight information is used to correct displayed monitored values for patient weight.) After all selections have been made, the operator presses SET UP and ACCEPT, and ventilation begins.

Membrane Buttons and LEDs

Figure 12-6 shows the membrane buttons and LEDs labeled 1 through 23 on the AVEA, moving counterclockwise around the screen.

The membrane buttons on the AVEA are as follows:

1. This LED flashes for high and medium priority alarms and stays on continuously for low priority alarms.

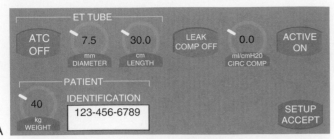

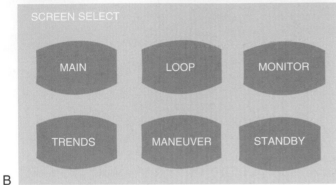

FIGURE 12-5 A, The ventilation SET UP screen of the AVEA allows selection of artificial airway compensation (previously called *automatic tube compensation [ATC]*), leak compensation, circuit compliance, humidifier type, and patient weight and identification number. **B,** The SCREENS SELECTION window allows display of the screens MAIN, LOOP, MONITOR, TRENDS, MANEUVER, and STANDBY. (See text for explanation.) (Courtesy Cardinal Health, Yorba Linda, Calif.)

2. The ALARM SILENCE button silences an alarm for 2 minutes.

3. The ALARM RESET button cancels visual indicators of resolved alarms.

4. The ALARM LIMITS button opens and closes the ALARM LIMITS window, where operator-adjustable alarm settings are located.

5. The MANUAL BREATH button delivers a single mandatory breath using current settings when pressed during the exhalation phase of a breath.

6. The SUCTION button with LED indicator initiates a DISCONNECT FOR SUCTION maneuver (Box 12-3).

7. The INCREASE O_2 button increases the O_2% for 2 minutes. The default increases O_2 to 100% in adult and pediatric patients. The O_2 increases to 20% above the set O_2% or to 100%, whichever is less, for neonates. If pressed again during the 2-minute interval, the maneuver is cancelled and the ventilator resumes its previous O_2% settings.

8. A DATA DIAL is used to change a highlighted field or control on the touch screen.

9. The ACCEPT button activates proposed changes to highlighted field or controls.

10. When the CANCEL button is pressed, the ventilator disregards proposed changes and reverts to the previous settings, which are still in effect.

11. The expiratory hold (EXP HOLD) button allows measurement of end-expiratory pressure for the

determination of auto-PEEP. The hold lasts up to 20 seconds in adult and pediatric patients and 3 seconds in neonates. (See Chapter 11 for an explanation of auto-PEEP.)

12. The inspiratory hold (INSP HOLD) button can be used to determine the plateau pressure (maximum, 3 seconds).

13. The NEBULIZER button provides nebulization for 30 minutes, synchronized with the inspiratory phase. Powering the nebulizer requires attachment of a high pressure air source and a total flow to the internal nebulizer of greater than 15 L/min (see Box 12-4 for further information).

14. PATIENT SIZE LED indicators show the currently selected patient size; there is no associated membrane button.

15. The panel lock (LOCK) button disables all front panel controls except MANUAL BREATH, INCREASE % O_2, ALARM RESET, ALARM SILENCE, and the panel lock (LOCK) button.

16. Pressing the PRINT button sends the current screen displays to an external printer.

17. The SET UP key opens and closes the VENTILATOR SETUP screen.

18. The ADV SETTINGS button opens and closes an ADVANCED SETTINGS window for feature activation or parameter adjustment.

19. The MODE button opens and closes the MODE menu. The MODE INDICATOR can also be used to access the MODE menu.

20. The EVENT button opens and closes a menu of event markers (e.g., ARTERIAL BLOOD GAS), which can be placed on the trend display.

21. The FREEZE button suspends real-time updating of data on the current graphics screen display until it is pressed again. With the screen frozen, the DATA DIAL can be used to scroll a cursor through waveform or loop graphics for examination of specific data points.

22. The SCREEN button opens and closes the screen MENU. The SCREEN INDICATOR can also be used to access this menu.

23. The MAIN button returns to the main screen display from any screen.

BOX 12-3	Disconnect for Suctioning Maneuver (AVEA)

When the SUCTION button is pressed, the ventilator:
1. Enables the INCREASE O_2% maneuver for 2 minutes (see INCREASE O_2 button)
2. Disables the demand system on loss of PEEP
3. Silences all alarms for 2 minutes
If the SUCTION button is pressed again during the 2 minutes, the maneuver is cancelled.

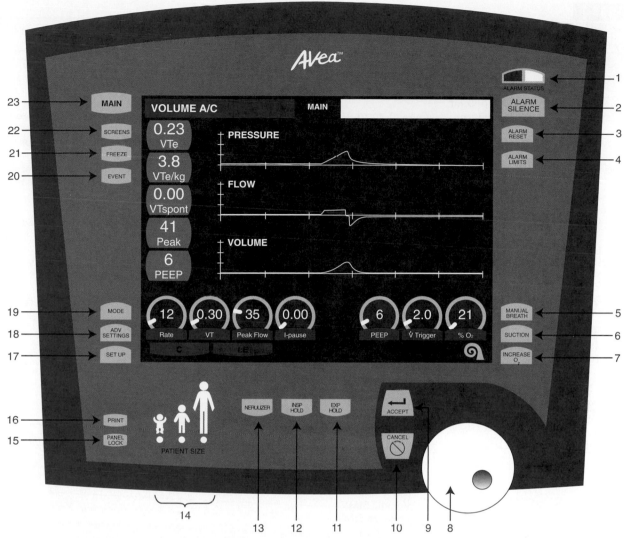

FIGURE 12-6 Front panel (user interface module) of the AVEA ventilator, showing the membrane buttons, the LEDs and indicators, the data dial, and the touch screen displaying the normal operating screen. (See text for explanation.) (Courtesy Cardinal Health, Yorba Linda, Calif.)

| BOX 12-4 | Nebulizer Function (AVEA) |

When the internal nebulizer is used, the ventilator decreases the flow to the patient by 6 L/min to compensate for the nebulizer output. However, because the internal nebulizer flow can be as high as 8 L/min, use of the nebulizer may still affect the tidal volume delivery. (NOTE: The nebulizer is inactive in neonatal modes.)

Use of an external flowmeter to power the nebulizer is not recommended; because it would have no compensation for volume, it is constant during both inspiration and exhalation, and it could affect the percent oxygen delivery.

Primary Breath Controls

Primary breath controls are rate, tidal volume, inspiratory pressure, peak flow, inspiratory pause, PEEP, pressure support, flow trigger, and F_IO_2. These controls are displayed along the bottom of the touch screen (see Figure 12-6). Only controls active for the current mode of ventilation are visible. For example, if volume assist control (VOLUME A/C) is selected, tidal volume is available as a primary control, but inspiratory pressure is not. Table 12-1 lists primary breath controls and their description.

To change a primary breath control, the operator touches the screen knob directly over the control. The control highlights (changes color), showing that it can now be changed. To change the setting, the operator turns the DATA DIAL clockwise or counterclockwise to increase or decrease the value. When the desired setting appears, the operator touches the screen knob again or presses the

TABLE 12-1

Primary Breath Controls—AVEA

Display Control (units)	Description
RATE (bpm)	Breath rate shown in breaths per minute: 1-120 bpm (adult), 1-150 bpm (pediatric/neonate)
V_T (mL)	Tidal volume in milliliters: 100-2500 mL (adult), 25-500 mL (pediatric), 2-300 mL (neonate) When the machine is operating only on the internal compressor, the maximum available V_T is 2000 mL.
INSP PRESS (cm H_2O)	Inspiratory pressure: 0-90 cm H_2O (adult/pediatric), 0-80 cm H_2O (neonate). Used during pressure ventilation as the target pressure (limited to total peak inspiratory pressure [PIP] of 90 cm H_2O).
PEAK FLOW (L/min)	Sets the peak inspiratory flow during volume ventilation: 3-150 L/min (adult), 1-75 L/min (pediatric), 0.4-30 L/min (neonate).
INSP TIME (sec)	Inspiratory time: 0.2-5 sec (adult/pediatric), 0.15-3 sec (neonate). Sets the maximum inspiratory time for all mandatory breaths and ends inspiration if the normal cycling criteria have not been met and when the time limit is reached.
INSP PAUSE (sec)	Sets inspiratory pause after volume delivery: 0.0-3 sec. Adds to the set inspiratory time.
PSV (cm H_2O)	Pressure-support ventilation: 0-90 cm H_2O (adult/pediatric), 0-80 cm H_2O (neonate) (limited to total PIP of 90 cm H_2O).
PEEP (cm H_2O)	Positive end-expiratory pressure: 0-50 cm H_2O.
FLOW TRIG (L/min)	Flow trigger sensitivity; sets the inspiratory flow trigger in liters per minute: 0.1-20 L/min. When enabled, sets a bias flow through the patient circuit during part of the expiratory phase.
% O_2	Controls the percentage of oxygen delivery: 21% to 100%.
PRES HIGH (cm H_2O)	In airway pressure-release ventilation (APRV), sets the maximum pressure target: 0-90 cm H_2O (limited to total PIP of 90 cm H_2O).
TIME HIGH (sec)	In APRV, sets the time during which maximum pressure is maintained: 0.2-30 sec.
TIME LOW (sec)	In APRV, sets the time during which minimum pressure is maintained: 0.2-30 sec.
PRES LOW (cm H_2O)	In APRV, sets the minimum pressure target: 0-45 cm H_2O.

TABLE 12-2

Modes of Ventilation—AVEA

Adult/Pediatric Modes	Neonatal Modes
Volume A/C	Volume A/C
Pressure A/C	Pressure A/C
PRVC A/C	TCPL A/C
Volume SIMV	Volume SIMV
Pressure SIMV	Pressure SIMV
PRVC SIMV	TCPL SIMV
APRV/BiPhasic	—
CPAP PSV	CPAP PSV

APRV, Airway pressure release ventilation; *PRVC,* pressure-regulated volume control; *TCPL,* time cycled, pressure limited.

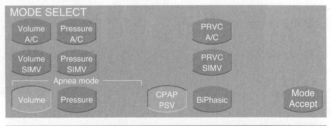

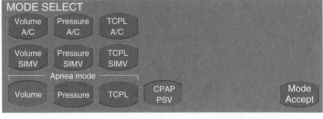

FIGURE 12-7 MODE SELECT screens for adult and pediatric patients **(A)** and neonatal patients **(B).** In the adult/pediatric screen, BIPHASIC recently was replaced by APRV. (See text for more detail.) (Courtesy Cardinal Health, Yorba Linda, Calif.)

ACCEPT button to accept the change. The control returns to its normal color, and ventilation continues with the new setting in effect. If the operator presses the CANCEL button rather than the ACCEPT button or does not accept the change within 15 seconds, the control returns to its normal color, and ventilation continues at the previous settings. The technique of touch—turn—accept applies to almost all user interactions with the touch screen display.

MODES OF VENTILATION

As do many currently available ventilators, the AVEA offers a selection of modes and breath types. Table 12-2 lists the ventilation modes for adult, pediatric, and neonatal patients. Noninvasive ventilation for pediatric and adult patients and nasal CPAP for infants have been added since the original release. (NOTE: See Chapter 11 for a description of the basic function of each of these modes.)

Selections are made from the MODE menu, which is accessed by pressing the MODE button or the MODE INDICATOR (Figure 12-7). The menu displays only the modes and breath types available for the currently selected patient size.

Continuous Mandatory Ventilation (CMV)

On the AVEA, CMV is provided when VOLUME A/C, PRESSURE A/C, or PRVC A/C is selected. During CMV, the set breath rate establishes the minimum mandatory breath rate. The patient can receive additional breaths above this set amount, but all breaths are mandatory (i.e., at the set pressure or volume). Breaths may be time or patient triggered. Flow triggering is the usual patient trigger. A/C breaths are pressure or volume targeted. When pressure-targeted A/C is selected, the breath commonly is time cycled based on the set inspiratory time (T_I). When volume-targeted A/C is selected, the common cycling mechanism is volume.

During a mandatory breath (pressure or volume targeted), the demand system is active and can provide additional flow or volume if demanded by the patient. VOLUME A/C is the default mode for adult and pediatric patients. It is automatically set when a new patient is selected if no other mode is activated.

Synchronized Intermittent Mandatory Ventilation (SIMV)

The SIMV mode provides mandatory breath delivery at the set mandatory rate and allows for spontaneous breathing from the baseline pressure between mandatory breaths. Mandatory breaths can be time or patient triggered, as with A/C ventilation. Mandatory breaths can be either pressure or volume targeted.

Spontaneous breaths in SIMV can be from a zero baseline or from a baseline with PEEP/CPAP added. Spontaneous breaths can also be supported with PSV.

Pressure-Regulated Volume Control (PRVC) Breath Delivery

PRVC is a pressure-targeted form of breath delivery that adjusts pressure to target a set tidal volume. Mandatory breaths are time or patient triggered, pressure targeted, and time cycled.

When PRVC is selected, the first breath is a volume-targeted breath with an inspiratory pause. This breath is evaluated by the ventilator to measure system compliance and resistance and provide a pressure target for the next breath. From that point on, breaths are pressure targeted. Adjustments are made in the pressure if the ventilator is not achieving the set volume. Pressure changes are made up or down in steps of 3 cm H_2O (see Chapter 11 for a further description of PRVC). The maximum tidal volume that can be delivered is determined by the setting on the VOLUME LIMIT control.

PRVC breath delivery is available in the adult and pediatric patient categories. It can be used in PRVC A/C and in PRVC SIMV.

Airway Pressure-Release Ventilation (APRV)/BiPhasic

APRV allows the patient to breathe spontaneously at two preset pressure levels. These two levels are set using the PRES HIGH and PRES LOW settings. The values for these are selected based on the patient's optimum PEEP/CPAP level to prevent both lung injury (PRES HIGH) and alveolar collapse (PRES LOW). The duration of the high pressure is established by the TIME HIGH setting. The duration of the

low pressure is based on the set TIME LOW value. Breaths, therefore, are both time triggered and time cycled. This mode also can allow for synchronization of the phase changes, if the advanced settings for TIME HIGH and TIME LOW synchronization periods are available on the unit.

With APRV/BiPhasic, a pressure support level can be set. The set PSV amount is the same for both the high and low pressure settings.

APRV/BiPhasic has very specific clinical uses, and patients must be monitored carefully when it is used. APRV is not available for the neonatal patient settings. Apnea backup ventilation is available during APRV ventilation. (See Chapter 11 for additional information on airway pressure-release ventilation.)

Time Cycled, Pressure Limited (TCPL)

TCPL ventilation is used only for neonatal patients. It can be used in A/C or SIMV modes. With TCPL-A/C, mandatory breaths are time or patient triggered, pressure or volume limited, and time cycled. With TCPL-SIMV, mandatory breaths are time or patient triggered, pressure or volume limited, and time cycled. Spontaneous breaths are similar to those with standard SIMV (i.e., patient triggered, pressure targeted, and flow cycled).

CPAP/PSV Mode

The CPAP/PSV mode is used for patients who are breathing spontaneously.

CPAP and PSV breaths are patient triggered, pressure limited, and flow cycled. If CPAP or PSV pressures are set at zero, 2 cm H_2O of PS is given during spontaneous breathing for adult and pediatric patients, and 0 cm H_2O is added for neonatal patients. This helps reduce the work of breathing by the patient through the system. PSV is active when the CPAP/PSV, SIMV, or APRV/BiPhasic modes are selected.

The default flow-cycle settings, called PSV CYCLE, are 25% (adult and pediatric patients) and 10% (neonatal patients). The PSV flow cycle can be adjusted from 5% to 45% using the ADVANCED SETTINGS menu. As a safety backup, PSV breaths time cycle out of inspiration if the T_I becomes too long. Time cycling is based on the PSV TMAX setting. The default values for PSV TMAX are 5 seconds for adults, 0.75 seconds for pediatric patients, and 0.35 seconds for neonates. Adjustments to PSV TMAX are also made in the ADVANCED SETTINGS window, described later in this section.

When CPAP/PSV is selected, apnea backup ventilation must also be set (see apnea backup ventilation later in this section).

Noninvasive Positive-Pressure Ventilation (NPPV)

NPPV can be performed using any mode and with the dual limb patient circuit (adult and pediatric sizes). Leak compensation must be turned on using the ventilator set-up screen when NPPV is selected. A nasal mask or face mask is connected to the patient as the noninvasive interface. NPPV nasal CPAP is available in the neonatal mode.

Apnea Backup Ventilation (ABV)

ABV is active in all SIMV, APRV/BiPhasic, and CPAP/PSV modes. When CPAP/PSV is selected, the operator must select the breath type and mode for ABV and set the primary controls.

If the set apnea time elapses before a breath is detected, apnea ventilation begins. After ABV begins, the ventilator delivers a mandatory breath. If no spontaneous effort is detected, the ventilator continues to deliver breaths. The audible alarm can be silenced temporarily, but it cannot reset until apnea ventilation stops.

Apnea ventilation ends when one of the following occurs:

· A spontaneous effort by the patient is detected.
· A manual breath is delivered.
· The mandatory breath rate is increased above the apnea interval setting.

If a patient remains apneic, apnea ventilation continues at the preset parameters. The operator may need to change the rate or the mode of ventilation to manage the patient more appropriately. (NOTE: The operator should also check the apnea time to be sure it is set correctly.)

The controls for the apnea breath type are no longer visible once the MODE ACCEPT button has been pressed during set up of apnea backup ventilation. To review ABV settings, the operator must open the mode window and select APNEA SETTINGS.

ADVANCED SETTINGS

Advanced settings are controls that allow the clinician to refine breath delivery beyond the scope of the primary breath controls. The ADV SETTINGS membrane button opens and closes the ADVANCED SETTINGS window. (NOTE: Advanced settings are associated with specific primary controls; however, not all primary controls have an associated advanced setting.) For example, suppose you are in TCPL with the neonatal patient size, and you want to set a volume limit. You press the ADV SETTINGS key to bring up the ADVANCED SETTINGS window. Then you touch the inspiratory pressure key (INSP PRESS), and the touch key for volume limit appears in the ADVANCED SETTINGS window. You can then adjust your volume limit and touch ACCEPT to activate the control.

Volume Limit

Volume limit (VOL LIMIT) is a feature active in pressure-targeted modes of ventilation, including pressure A/C, PRVC A/C and Vsync A/C, pressure SIMV, PRVC SIMV, Vsync SIMV, TCPL, and PSV breaths. Note: Vsync will be discussed later.

In neonatal ventilation, volume limit requires the use of a proximal flow sensor that connects at the patient Y-connector. When volume limit is activated, pressure-targeted breaths also become volume limited. That is, if the set volume limit (a maximum volume) is reached before the normal time-cycle or flow-cycle criteria for a breath, the breath is terminated (volume cycled.) If the set V_T is not delivered before the normal cycling mechanism (T_I set in A/C and pressure SIMV or the flow-cycle limit in PSV), ventilation continues at the set pressure and ends inspiration using the normal cycling criteria. The potential advantage of this feature is protection of the lungs from excessive volume delivery despite changing lung characteristics during pressure ventilation.

Machine Volume

Machine volume (MACH VOL) is another volume criterion that establishes a minimum volume delivery. It is active in pressure-targeted mandatory breaths, such as pressure A/C and pressure SIMV. When the MACH VOL feature is set, the machine delivers the set pressure and monitors volume delivery through the internal flow sensor. If the set MACH VOL is achieved during inspiration, the ventilator mode cycles via its normal cycling mechanism. If MACH VOL is *not* achieved before the set cycling criteria, the ventilator delivers the minimum tidal volume by transitioning to a continuous inspiratory flow to achieve the set volume within the set T_I. As a result of the increased flow requirements, airway pressure increases as well. The ventilator adjusts flow (and therefore pressure) to achieve the MACH VOL (minimum volume) for every breath delivered.

There are two conditions in which the ventilator will terminate the breath before the minimum volume is delivered. In the first case, if the high-pressure limit is met or exceeded before the minimum tidal volume is delivered, the high-pressure limit alarm activates and the breath is terminated. In the second case, if the volume limit is reached, inspiration ends and the ventilator displays VOLUME LIMIT on the status bar (Clinical Rounds 12-1).

Inspiratory Rise

The inspiratory rise (INSP RISE) control adjusts the rate at which pressure is delivered during inspiration during a mandatory pressure breath in the following modes: pressure A/C, pressure SIMV, PRVC A/C, PRCV SIMV, TCPL

CLINICAL ROUNDS 12-1

The AVEA ventilator is set in the adult category with the pressure A/C mode. The inspiratory pressure is 15 cm H_2O, and PEEP is set at 5 cm H_2O. The current Ppeak is 20 cm H_2O. The upper pressure limit is set at 35 cm H_2O. The delivered V_T for the patient is 0.39 L (390 mL). The therapist wants to guarantee a minimum V_T of 0.5 L (500 mL), so he selects MACH VOL under advanced settings, dials the MACH VOL to 0.5 L, and accepts the setting. What will happen to the peak inspiratory pressure and volume delivery?

See Evolve Resources for the answer.

A/C, TCPL SIMV, and Vsync. It is similar to the rise time or sloping feature in other ventilators. A setting of 1 is the most rapid rise in pressure, and a setting of 9 is the slowest. A separate control (PSV RISE) is available for adjusting the rise in PSV ventilation. It is adjusted in the same fashion as INSP RISE. (NOTE: Also see Vsync Rise in the following section.)

Flow Cycle

FLOW CYCLE allows adjustment of the percentage at which the ventilator flow cycles a breath during **pressure-targeted ventilation** (A/C and SIMV) and TCPL (A/C and SIMV). Therefore mandatory pressure breaths can be time or flow cycled (range, 0 to 45%). (NOTE: Flow cycling for PSV is adjusted using the PSV CYCLE feature.)

PSV Tmax

PSV TMAX sets the maximum length of inspiratory time allowed during a PSV breath (range, 0.2 to 5 seconds [adult/pediatric patients] and 0.15 to 3 seconds [neonates]).

Waveform Feature

The WAVEFORM feature allows the operator to select either a square wave (constant flow) or a decelerating (descending) ramp flow pattern during volume ventilation. The default is a descending ramp. With this waveform selected, the ventilator begins flow delivery at the set peak flow and decreases flow until 50% of the set peak flow is reached.

Sigh

The SIGH control allows the ventilator to deliver a sigh breath at 1.5 times the set tidal volume every 100 breaths for adult and pediatric patients.

Bias Flow

Bias flow is flow present in the patient circuit during the expiratory portion of a breath. This feature establishes the flow from which flow triggering is accomplished (range, 0.4 to 5 L/min, default, 2 L/min). (See Chapter 11 for an additional explanation of flow triggering.)

Pressure Trigger

Pressure triggering is available in addition to flow triggering on the AVEA. Both trigger mechanisms are always active (relative to their sensitivity setting). The ventilator responds to whichever trigger threshold is reached first. The range for pressure triggering is −0.1 to −20 cm H_2O, and the range for flow triggering is 0.1 to 20 L/min.

Vsync

Vsync changes volume breaths to pressure-limited, volume-targeted breaths. Vsync can be activated in volume modes (volume A/C and volume SIMV). When Vsync is selected, a single test breath with a pause is delivered to measure the end-inspiratory pressure (plateau pressure). System compliance and resistance are evaluated to determine the initial

---

CLINICAL ROUNDS 12-2

A patient is receiving pressure SIMV ventilation on the AVEA ventilator at a rate of 6 breaths/min. The inspiratory pressure is set at 25 cm H_2O, PSV is 10 cm H_2O, and CPAP/PEEP is 5 cm H_2O. PSV CYCLE is set at 20%, and FLOW CYCLE is set at 40%. T_I is set at 1.5 seconds. The peak inspiratory flow for a pressure-supported breath is noted from the flow-time waveform to be about 50 L/min. The inspiratory flow curve for a mandatory breath does not reach zero before inspiration ends.
1. What is the peak inspiratory pressure for a mandatory breath and for a pressure-supported breath?
2. Is a mandatory breath time or flow cycled?
3. At what flow will pressure-supported breaths cycle out of inspiration?

See Evolve Resources for the answer.

---

pressure needed to deliver the set volume. Each subsequent breath is delivered at a pressure sufficient to provide the volume. Should the volume be less than or more than the set volume, the inspiratory pressure is moved up or down in increments of no more than 3 cm H_2O on the next breath to ensure delivery of a set volume. (NOTE: Vsync is available only for adult and pediatric patients.)

Vsync Rise

Vsync rise, which is active only when Vsync is enabled, functions similarly to the inspiratory rise feature in adjusting the slope of the inspiratory pressure rise during breath delivery (range, 1 to 9, with 9 the slowest). Clinical Rounds 12-2 presents a problem using advanced settings.

MONITORS AND DISPLAYS

The AVEA has both digital and graphic monitoring displays. The main screen continuously displays up to five monitored parameters (see Figure 12-6, left column). The operator can customize these five main screen displays or an extended display of 15 on the monitor screen from a list of 55 items. The monitor screen is accessed by touching the SCREEN INDICATOR or by pressing the SCREEN button. Table 12-3 lists some of the monitored parameters.

A maximum of three waveform tracings can be displayed simultaneously on the main screen (see Figure 12-6). The operator can touch the WAVEFORM title bar, and a menu will appear with choices for airway pressure, esophageal pressure, tracheal pressure, flow, volume, and two analog input signals. All waveforms are graphed against a horizontal time axis. The vertical axis also can be touched. When the numbers on the axis change color, the dial knob can be used to change the scale of the graph. For example, if the y-axis is pressure and the range is −40 to 80 cm H_2O, you can change this to −20 to 40 cm H_2O.

The LOOP screen displays two real-time loops (e.g., flow-volume and pressure-volume loops). When loops are

TABLE 12-3

Commonly Selected Monitor Screen Displayed Data—AVEA

Displayed Data	Description
Vte	Exhaled tidal volume (mL)
Vte/Kg	Milliliters of Vte per kilogram adjusted for patient weight
Vti	Inspired tidal volume (mL)
Spon V_T	Spontaneous V_T (mL)
Spon V_T/Kg	Milliliters of Spon V_T per kilogram adjusted for patient weight
Mand V_T	Mandatory V_T (mL)
Mand V_T/Kg	Mandatory V_T per kilogram adjusted for patient weight
% Leak	Percent leakage; the difference between the inspiratory and expiratory volume in % difference
Ve	Calculated minute volume (L/min) based on set V_T and rate for volume breaths only
Spon Ve/kg	Spontaneous minute volume adjusted for patient weight
Rate	Respiratory rate (breaths/min)
Spon Rate	Spontaneous rate (breaths/min)
Ti	Inspiratory time (sec)
Te	Expiratory time (sec)
I:E	Calculated value for inspiratory to expiratory ratio, based on set rate, V_T, and peak flow for volume breaths, and rate, and inspiratory time for pressure, TCPL and PRVC breaths (range, 1:99.9 to 99.9:1)
f/V_T	Rapid, shallow breathing index (B/min/L); respiratory rate divided by tidal volume
Ppeak	Peak inspiratory pressure (cm H_2O)
Pmean	Mean airway pressure (cm H_2O)
Pplat	Plateau pressure (cm H_2O), if available
PEEP	Positive end-expiratory pressure (cm H_2O)
Air inlet	Air inlet pressure (psig)
O_2 Inlet	Oxygen inlet pressure (psig)
F_IO_2	Percent of oxygen displayed as a whole number
Cdyn	Dynamic compliance (characteristic) (mL/cm H_2O)
Cs (Cstat)	Static compliance (mL/cm H_2O); requires an inspiratory hold maneuver
Rrs	Respiratory system resistance (cm H_2O/L/sec); calculation is performed during an inspiratory hold maneuver
PIFR	Peak inspiratory flow rate (L/min)
PEFR	Peak expiratory flow rate (L/min)

Additional monitored values are listed in the operator's manual.

displayed, the waveforms (scalars) are no longer visible. Up to four loops can be saved at a time using the FREEZE function. Any saved loop can be selected as a reference loop for comparison with live loops (Figure 12-8).

The STANDBY mode is available for use when a patient is temporarily away from the ventilator. While in STANDBY, the ventilator supplies 2 L/min of gas continuously through the patient circuit to prevent damage to the circuit or overheating of the chamber water should a heated humidifier be left on. To go to STANDBY, press the SCREENS

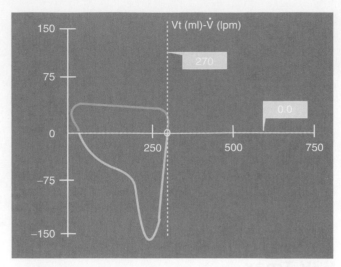

FIGURE 12-8 Graphic display showing a flow-volume loop in the FREEZE mode with the tidal volume (270 mL) and the flow (0 L/min) at the dotted line. The horizontal axis is volume, and the vertical axis is flow. (Courtesy Cardinal Health, Yorba Linda, Calif.)

key, and then press the STANDBY key. The screen will display the message, "Are you sure you want to stop ventilating this patient?" Pressing YES places the ventilator in standby. Ventilation can be resumed by pressing the RESUME button. Ventilation begins at the most recent control settings.

ALARMS AND INDICATORS

Alarms and indicators are used to notify clinicians when automatic and adjustable alarm limits are violated or when conditions affecting ventilator function are detected. All types of alarms have visual displays. Alarm messages appear in the ALARM INDICATOR at the upper right of the touch screen. When multiple alarms are activated, a white triangle appears to the right of the alarm message. This touch icon is used to open and close a drop-down display of up to nine alarm messages. The highest priority alarm is always displayed in the top position.

Alarm conditions result in visual and audible alarms at three different levels:

- High priority—Five tones are repeated with a flashing red alarm indicator.
- Medium priority—Three tones are repeated with a flashing yellow alarm indicator.
- Low priority—A single tone sounds with a solid yellow alarm indicator.
- Normal status—A solid green alarm indicator remains lighted.

Table 12-4 provides information on ventilator alarms. To set the limits for an alarm, the operator selects the ALARM LIMITS button, and the ALARM LIMITS screen appears (Figure 12-9). The operator presses the touch screen knob immediately over the alarm control. The knob highlights. The alarm value is adjusted by using the DATA DIAL until the control reaches the value required. Pressing the touch

TABLE 12-4	
Alarms—AVEA	
Alarm	**Description**
Vent Inop	Ventilator failure. The safety valve opens (SAFETY VALVE message appears). Spontaneously breathing patients can breathe room air.
Loss of Air	Wall or cylinder air below 18 psig. No compressor installed.
Loss of O_2	O_2 supply below 18 psig.
Loss of Gas Supply	All gas sources failed. Safety valve opens.
Low P_{PEAK}	Peak inspiratory pressure less than the set Low P_{PEAK} value.
High P_{PEAK}	Peak inspiratory pressure greater than the High P_{PEAK} value. Inspiration ends.
Ext High P_{PEAK}	High P_{PEAK} alarm has been active for longer than 5 seconds. Safety valve opens. No breaths are delivered.
Low PEEP	Baseline pressure drops below set Low PEEP level.
Low Minute Volume	Monitored exhaled Ve is less than set value for Low Ve alarm.
High Minute Volume	Monitored exhaled Ve is greater than set value for High Ve alarm.
High V_T	Monitored exhaled V_T is greater than set value for High V_T alarm.
Apnea	Ventilator does not detect a breath during set apnea interval.
High rate	Monitored total breath rate exceeds high rate value.
I-Time Limit	Inspiratory time exceeds set MAX I-time plus any set pause time (5 sec [adult/pediatric patient], 3 sec [neonate]).
I:E Limit	I:E ratio exceeds 4:1 for a mandatory breath. Inspiration ends.
Low F_IO_2	Delivered O_2 falls below set F_IO_2 minus 6% or falls below 18%.
High F_IO_2	Delivered O_2 rises above set F_IO_2 plus 6%.

screen knob or pressing the ACCEPT button sets the new alarm limit. To close the alarm screen, the operator can either press the MAIN (screen) button or press ALARM LIMITS again.

SPECIAL FEATURES

Some of the special features or special functions available for use with the AVEA include trends screens, heliox gas delivery, esophageal pressure monitoring, tracheal pressure monitoring, respiratory mechanics, and independent lung ventilation (ILV).

Trends

Pressing the TRENDS membrane button displays four trends' histograms and the trends' data spreadsheet. Trends can also be accessed by pressing the SCREENS key and then the TRENDS screen button.

For example, a histogram might be a graph of the mean airway pressure on the y-axis graphed against time on the x-axis. Parameters are trended as 1-minute averages over a 24-hour period.

Each of the histograms and columns on the spreadsheet can be configured as desired by touching the title of the histogram or the header of the spreadsheet to bring up a menu to scroll through possible parameter changes. To look at the histogram or spreadsheet over time, press the FREEZE button and use the DATA DIAL to move the cursor through the time line.

Pressing the EVENT membrane button opens a scrollable menu of event markers. These include arterial blood gas (BG), chest x-ray (CXR), suction (SXN), intubation (ETT), feeding (FEED), diagnostic procedure (DX), and therapeutic procedure (RX). Pressing the ACCEPT button places the event in the trend buffer. Marked events appear on the data spreadsheet in green text with an asterisk next to the time code.

Heliox

Heliox delivery is available on the comprehensive AVEA package and as an option on the standard AVEA ventilator. By changing a connector on the back of the ventilator (see

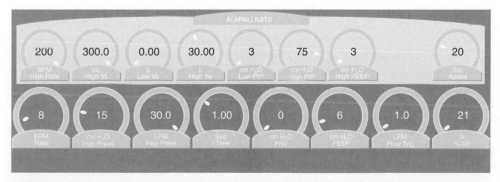

FIGURE 12-9 ALARM LIMITS screen, which appears above the screen display of ventilator parameters. This screen appears at the bottom of the touch screen. (Courtesy Cardinal Health, Yorba Linda, Calif.)

Figure 12-4), an 80/20 mixture of helium and oxygen can be attached to the ventilator and used in place of the air source. (NOTE: The heliox connector at the back of the AVEA is designed for use with an 80/20 mixture of helium [80%] and oxygen [20%] only. The ventilator identifies the gas input from this connection and adjusts to accommodate the change.) Volumes (numeric and graphic) are automatically compensated for accurate volume display.

Once the gas hoses are attached, the operator must allow 90 seconds for the accumulator to purge before beginning patient ventilation with heliox gas. (NOTE: A 100% helium cylinder should *never* be used because of the risk of hypoxia and death.)

Patients with severe airway resistance may benefit from the lower gas density of heliox compared with an air-oxygen mixture. The lower density allows volumes to be delivered at a lower airway pressure. In addition, lower density heliox allows gas to move past airway obstructions or restrictions more easily than air-oxygen mixtures.

Respiratory Mechanics

The AVEA can perform several respiratory mechanics maneuvers. These are accessed by pressing the SCREENS touch pad to view the SCREENS menu and selecting the MANEUVERS screen. Some of the mechanics maneuvers available include the following:

- Esophageal pressure measurement
- MIP/P_{100}
- Inflection point (Pflex)
- AutoPEEP

Information about the purpose of such measurements is available elsewhere.[4]

The esophageal maneuver screen is used when an esophageal balloon is inserted to measure esophageal pressure. This pressure measurement helps determine a patient's work of breathing. A balloon test is performed before insertion to verify the integrity and size of the balloon catheter. With this option activated, the ventilator empties and refills the balloon every 30 minutes to measure esophageal pressures.

The maximum inspiratory pressure (MIP) and P_{100} maneuver measure the negative deflection of the pressure scalar (pressure-time waveform) during an active patient inspiration when the inspiratory and expiratory valves are closed. The MIP is the maximum (negative) pressure the patient can generate during inspiration. Generally, the patient is coached for this procedure. The P_{100} requires no patient instruction. It measures the pressure drop that occurs 100 msec after the beginning of active inspiration.

The purpose of the Pflex maneuver is to determine two points on the pressure-volume (P/V) curve during a slow inspiration, the lower pressure (lower Pflex) and the upper pressure (upper Pflex). The lower Pflex indicates a change in the slope of the P/V curve at the beginning of a breath, where it is believed the lungs begin to be recruited (opening of the alveoli). The upper Pflex is believed to indicate a point at which the lungs become overdistended.[4] To execute the inflection point (Pflex) maneuver, the operator sets V_T, flow, PEEP, sensitivity, and PEEP equilibration time. Pflex values are used to help the operator establish appropriate PEEP levels to set during ventilation, which helps prevent alveolar collapse, and the upper Pflex, which should be avoided during inspiration to help prevent overinflation.

The AutoPEEP maneuver allows the measurement of intrinsic PEEP and total PEEP (intrinsic PEEP plus set PEEP). This can be done only on a patient who is not actively breathing. During this measurement, the ventilator closes the inspiratory and expiratory valves. Pressure in the patient's lungs and the ventilator circuit equilibrate. At the end of the measurement, the ventilator displays AUTO PEEP, or the total PEEP, and dAUTOPEEP, which is the actual intrinsic PEEP value (total PEEP minus the set PEEP.).

Pressures measured in the trachea can be used for some of the mechanics measurements. These pressures can be measured by the ventilator when a tracheal catheter is connected to the port on the front of the ventilator designed for this purpose (see Figure 12-2). Tracheal catheters can be placed through the endotracheal tube and into the airway. The catheter should be placed so that it does not extend beyond the tip of the endotracheal tube.

Independent Lung Ventilation (ILV)

For clinicians who want to provide ILV to a patient through a double-lumen endotracheal tube, the AVEA can be synchronized with another AVEA for this purpose. The ventilator provides an output (master) and an input (slave) for synchronization of the ventilators. The output connector supplies a 5-VDC logic signal synchronized to the breath phase of the master through a 25-pin connector on the rear of the ventilator. The operator's manual provides a table of pin functions.

Neonatal Application

A neonatal application option is available with the AVEA. This option is described in Chapter 13.

TROUBLESHOOTING

Before using the ventilator on a new patient or when the patient circuit is changed, the operator must perform a pretest using Operational Verification Testing. The first test reviewed is for general operations, and the second is for alarm function. These tests are performed to ensure that the ventilator is performing safely and accurately. The operator's manual provides more information on how to perform testing for individuals using the AVEA in the clinical setting.

Operators of the Cardinal AVEA should always defer to the operator's manual when using the equipment in their clinical facilities. Manufacturers frequently add options and software upgrades to their equipment, and the operator needs to be aware of the features and options available on the AVEA ventilators he uses.

KEY POINTS

▶ The AVEA can be used for conventional invasive or noninvasive positive-pressure ventilation and in neonatal, pediatric, and adult patients.

▶ The internal battery provides about 30 minutes of power when both the ventilator and the compressor are running.

▶ A DISS connector on the back panel can be changed to adapt for helium-oxygen delivery.

▶ Patient monitoring from the AVEA includes esophageal, tracheal, and proximal airway pressure monitoring.

▶ The artificial airway compensation feature adjusts the pressure delivery from the AVEA to compensate for the pressure drop across an artificial airway.

▶ NPPV can be performed using any mode for pediatric and adult patients.

▶ Apnea backup ventilation is available in all modes in which spontaneous ventilation is available (SIMV, APRV/BiPhasic, and CPAP/PSV modes).

▶ When the VOLUME LIMIT feature is activated, pressure-targeted breaths also become volume limited at the set volume (i.e., the maximum allowable volume).

▶ Machine volume (MACH VOL) establishes a minimum volume delivery when mandatory breaths are pressure targeted.

▶ Vsync changes volume breaths to pressure-limited, volume-targeted breaths.

▶ Respiratory mechanics that can be measured with the AVEA include esophageal pressure measurement, MIP/P_{100}, inflection point (Pflex), and AutoPEEP.

ASSESSMENT QUESTIONS

See Evolve Resources for answers.

1. A 2-year-old child is ventilated with the AVEA at 35% oxygen. The respiratory therapist presses the INCREASE O2 button before suctioning. The resulting oxygen delivery will be:
   a. 100% for 2 minutes
   b. 35% for 2 minutes
   c. 55% for 2 minutes
   d. 100% for 1 minute

2. The easiest way to determine whether the ventilator is connected to an AC power source is to:
   a. Check the on/off switch on the back panel
   b. Check the POWER ON indicator for a green light
   c. See whether the touch screen is on
   d. See whether the AC POWER indicator is illuminated green

3. When NEW PATIENT status is accepted after the AVEA is turned on:
   a. The ventilator resets all settings to the default values
   b. The ventilator begins working at the most recently stored values
   c. The operator is required to enter all new parameters
   d. Parameters are present based on the patient's body surface area

4. When volume-targeted breaths are activated, triggering is based on which of the following?
   I. Time
   II. Flow
   III. Pressure
   IV. Volume
      a. I
      b. II and III
      c. I and IV
      d. I, II, and III

5. To set a descending flow waveform in volume A/C and volume SIMV, the operator must:
   a. Go to the ADVANCED SETTINGS window and press the peak flow control
   b. Go to the MODE selection screen and pick WAVEFORM
   c. Touch the WAVEFORM icon on the lower portion of the touch screen whenever volume-targeted ventilation is active
   d. Do nothing, because the AVEA only has a descending flow waveform

6. When the tidal volume is set at 500 mL and the SIGH control is enabled, which of the following statements is/are true?
   I. A sigh volume of 750 mL will be delivered.
   II. The operator must also select the sigh frequency.
   III. A sigh breath occurs every 100 breaths.
   IV. The sigh tidal volume is set at twice the tidal volume setting.
      a. I only
      b. IV only
      c. I and III only
      d. II and IV only

7. Pressing the MAIN icon in the SCREENS selection window:
   a. Checks the main circuit breaker
   b. Displays the main screen
   c. Lists the main ventilator parameters
   d. Displays the main alarm limits

8. An alarm occurs accompanied by three audible tones and a yellow flashing bar in the upper right area of the touch screen. This indicates:
   a. A high priority alarm
   b. A medium priority alarm
   c. A low priority alarm
   d. A change in a ventilator parameter

ASSESSMENT QUESTIONS—cont'd

9. The maximum available I : E ratio for a mandatory breath is:
a. 1 : 1
b. 2 : 1
c. 3 : 1
d. 4 : 1

10. Which of the following features are available for use with the AVEA ventilator?
I. Esophageal pressure monitoring
II. Tracheal pressure monitoring
III. Heliox gas delivery capability
IV. Nitric oxide gas delivery capability
a. I and II
b. III and IV
c. I, II, and III
d. I, II, III, and IV

11. Which of the following statements is true regarding the measurement of respiratory mechanics with the AVEA?
I. Respiratory mechanics are accessed by pressing the SCREENS touch pad.
II. On the SCREENS menu, RESPIRATORY MECHANICS is chosen.
III. AutoPEEP is one of the available respiratory mechanics measurements.
IV. The maximum inspiratory pressure (MIP) can be measured.
a. I and III
b. II and III
c. I, II, and IV
d. I, III, and IV

References

1. Avea Ventilator Systems: Operator's manual, (revision A), L1523, Palm Springs, Calif, March, 2005, Cardinal Health (previously VIASYS Healthcare, Critical Care Division).
2. Clinical Education Materials, Monographs and Presentations, L1490 revision A, software disc, Palm Springs, Calif, Cardinal Health (previously VIASYS Healthcare, Critical Care Division).
3. Ross K, marketing products manager, VIASYS Healthcare, Critical Care Division: Personal communication, Yorba Linda, Calif, June, 2006.
4. Pilbeam SP, Cairo JM: *Mechanical ventilation: clinical and physiological application,* ed 4, St Louis, 2006, Mosby/Elsevier.

Internet Resource
www.cardinal.com

CARDINAL BEAR 1000

OUTLINE

Power Source
Internal Mechanisms
Controls and Alarms
  Control Panel
  Monitors and Alarms
  Alarms
Modes of Ventilation
  Changing Ventilator Modes
  Assist CMV

SIMV/CPAP (PSV)
Pressure Control
PC-SIMV with CPAP and PSV
Pressure Augment
Special Features
Graphics
Troubleshooting

OBJECTIVES

Upon completion of this section, you will be able to:
· Describe the major components of the internal mechanisms of the Bear 1000.
· Identify the controls and discuss the function of each.
· Explain how the controls are set.
· Discuss how the alarms are set.
· Assess what alarm-activated LEDs and alarm messages indicate, and state possible causes.
· Compare each of the modes of ventilation on the Bear 1000, including the trigger and cycle mechanisms and the target variable (pressure or volume).
· Evaluate a graph or a description of a graphic display that shows pressure sloping or pressure augmentation (Paug) to determine whether the ventilator is set appropriately.
· Explain the function of the COMPLIANCE COMP control.
· Identify a resource that can help determine the causes of a functional problem in the Bear 1000.

The Bear 1000 and 1000 T/ES ventilators[1,2] are manufactured by Cardinal Health (Palm Springs, California), formerly VIASYS, Critical Care Division. The Bear 1000 model is the primary focus of this section (Figure 12-10). Special features added for the Bear 1000 T/ES model are presented in the appropriate sections. The Bear 1000 can be programmed to provide ventilation for children and adults.

POWER SOURCE

The Bear 1000 is pneumatically powered and microprocessor controlled. It is normally connected to external high-pressure sources of air and oxygen (30 to 80 psig). An air compressor can be added to the unit so that the ventilator can operate from a high-pressure air source without external gas connections; however, this eliminates the ability to increase F_IO_2. The power switch for the unit is on the back of the ventilator.

The patient circuit has a proximal pressure line for monitoring of airway pressure at the Y-connector. The exhalation valve is mounted internally. Gas from the patient exits through the exhalation diaphragm and the external flow sensor, which is a hot wire anemometer (Box 12-5).

BOX 12-5	Exhalation Flow Sensor on the BEAR 1000

Remember from Chapter 8 that a hot wire anemometer measures gas flow as the rate of heat loss from the hot wire. Therefore the greater the flow, the greater the current needed to maintain a high constant temperature.

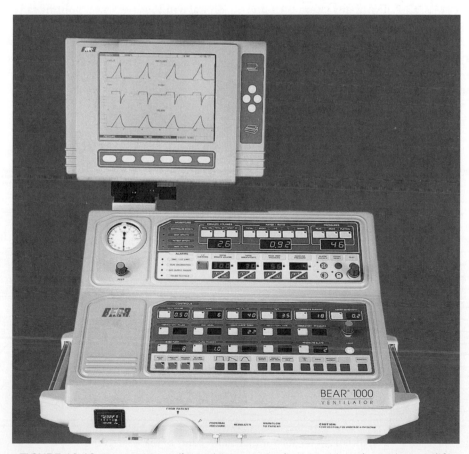

FIGURE 12-10 Bear 1000 ventilator. (Courtesy Cardinal Health, Palm Springs, Calif.)

INTERNAL MECHANISMS

Compressed oxygen and air enter the Bear 1000 through filters and check valves and is passed to regulators that reduce the pressures to an internal driving pressure of 18 psig. Gas passes to a blender and is then directed to an **accumulator.** The accumulator holds 3.5 L of gas under driving pressure (18 psig) and acts both as a mixing chamber to blend gases and as a source of high flow (greater than or equal to 200 L/min). Gas exits the accumulator and passes to a flow-control valve that is positioned by a stepper motor, so that rapid changes in flow are possible (see Chapter 11). The flow delivery logic of the microprocessor uses information from the monitors and the control panel to determine outflow from the valve.

Both control panel settings and patient flow demand determine the output from the flow-control valve. The flow-control valve allows for delivery of flows from 10 to 150 L/min for volume breaths and in excess of 200 L/min for pressure breaths or on patient demand. From the flow-control valve, gas travels through the **subambient overpressure-relief valve (SOPR)** and out of the ventilator through the outlet check valve.

CONTROLS AND ALARMS

The operating panel of the Bear 1000 is separated into two sections (Figures 12-11 and 12-12). The lower section contains the control functions, and the upper section contains the alarms and monitors. Both panels have a key and must be unlocked before any settings can be changed. Once unlocked, both panels have a CONTROL knob that adjusts the numeric value of any parameter selected. To select a parameter, the operator simply presses the touch pad for the parameter, and an LED illuminates and flashes to show that it has been selected.

Control Panel

The control panel is organized into four rows of controls (see Figure 12-12). With the exception of the CONTROL knob, each control variable (e.g., volume and rate) has a touch pad, a small LED to show when it is active, and a digital window to give the operator the selected value. A control can be selected and changed only if the LED for the variable is illuminated, and only those controls available in the current mode of ventilation illuminate. For example, to change V_T during volume ventilation, the touch pad next to the parameter is pushed, and the CONTROL knob at the far right on the second row of controls then is turned until the desired value for V_T appears. The change in the parameter's actual value occurs immediately.

The top row of controls on the control panel includes (from left to right) TIDAL VOLUME (100 to 2000 mL), RATE (0, or 0.5 to 120 breaths/min), FLOW (10 to 150 L/min), O_2% (21% to 100%), PRESSURE SUPPORT (0 to 80 cm H_2O), and ASSIST SENSITIVITY (0.2 to 5 cm H_2O).

Units programmed for lower volumes can provide lower tidal volumes (30 to 99 mL) and flows (5 to 150 L/min). To obtain these lower variables, the operator must press and hold the touch pad for V_T or flow while turning the CONTROL knob. When a P is displayed in the adjacent digital window, the lower volume range has been obtained. When a pediatric circuit is used, it is recommended that the PRESSURE SLOPE control (in the third row) be turned to 0 or P0. This control can be readjusted using the ventilator's graphic display after it is attached to the patient (see the discussion of pressure sloping).

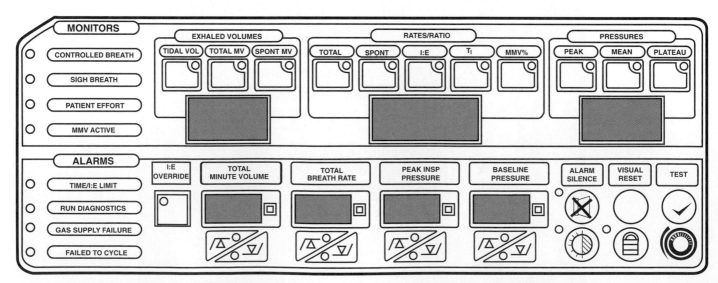

FIGURE 12-11 Monitor and alarm panel of the Bear 1000.

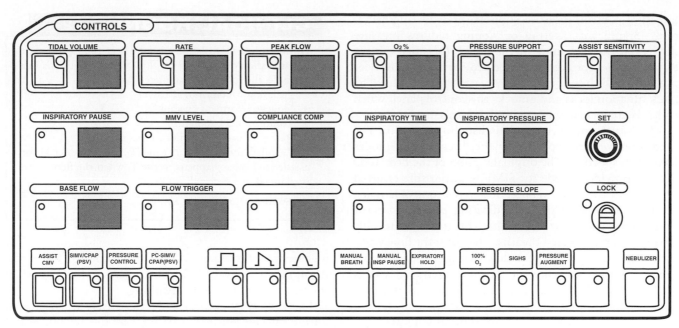

FIGURE 12-12 Control panel of the Bear 1000.

The second row of controls includes the INSPIRATORY PAUSE (0 to 2 seconds), MANDATORY MINUTE VOLUME (MMV) (0 to 50 L/min), COMPLIANCE COMP (compliance compensation) (0 to 7.5 mL/cm H_2O), INSPIRATORY TIME (0.1 to 5 seconds), INSPIRATORY PRESSURE (0 to 80 cm H_2O), and the CONTROL knob. With an inspiratory pause, both the inspiratory and expiratory valves close and hold the delivered breath in the patient and the patient circuit after inspiration. The inspiratory pause is commonly used to measure the plateau pressure for calculation of static compliance. The MMV control sets the minimum minute ventilation ($\dot{V}_E$) the operator wants the ventilator to provide for the patient (see the discussion of modes later in this chapter). The COMPLIANCE COMP control compensates for the volume lost as a result of tubing compressibility (tubing compliance). The operator enters the numeric value of tubing compliance for the patient circuit used. This value is obtained by performing a tubing test and calculation (see Chapter 11 for explanation). The ventilator adds volume to the set V_T (Equation 1) to establish volume output (Equation 2), so that the desired V_T is delivered to the patient. The monitor display of V_T (monitor and alarm panel) shows the measured exhaled V_T minus the additional volume (Equation 3).

Equation 1

Volume added = (COMPLIANCE COMP setting) × (PIP − PEEP)

where *PIP* is the peak pressure from the previous breath.

Equation 2

Volume output from ventilator = Volume added (for tubing compliance) + Set V_T

Equation 3

Volume displayed = Measured exhaled V_T − Volume added

When the INSPIRATORY TIME control is used with pressure-control ventilation (pressure control and PC-SIMV/CPAP[PS]), the breath is time cycled out of inspiration. The INSPIRATORY PRESSURE control sets the level of pressure that the ventilator will maintain during inspiration for **pressure-control ventilation (PCV)**. (These modes are reviewed in the discussion of modes later in this section.) On the original panel of the Bear 1000, the INSPIRATORY PRESSURE control was called PRES SUP/INSP PRES and controlled the pressure for pressure-support breaths, pressure-targeted breaths in PCV, and pressure augmentation. It was changed in the updated version so that SIMV could provide mandatory PCV and spontaneous PSV with different pressure levels for each. The CONTROL knob allows the operator to adjust the value of the selected parameter.

The third row of controls includes the BASE FLOW control (0, or 2 to 20 L/min), FLOW TRIGGER control (from 1 to 10 L/min), two blank controls for future updates, PRESSURE SLOPE control (from −9 to 9 for adult settings and P-9 to P9 for pediatric settings), and the LOCK control. Base flow is the flow added to the circuit during exhalation to provide flow triggering. Flow trigger is the amount the flow must drop from the base flow value to trigger a flow-triggered breath (see Chapter 11). The FLOW TRIGGER control can be set only if base flow is active. (NOTE: The unit can be set so that pressure and flow transducers for triggering a breath are active. The ventilator selects the signal that is most sensitive to patient effort and has the fastest response. The manufacturer calls this the SMART TRIGGER option.)

PRESSURE SLOPE provides control over the speed at which the inspiratory pressure level is achieved. The amount of slope can be monitored by observing how the pressure curve tapers at the beginning of a pressure breath (pressure control, pressure support, pressure augmentation). Significant tapering or sloping reduces pressure delivery at the beginning of the breath (negative values). Positive values for pressure slope provide rapid delivery of pressure at the beginning of the breath (Figure 12-13). The LOCK function locks and unlocks the control panel. When controls are locked, they cannot be changed.

The fourth row of controls is listed in Box 12-6. The mode controls are explained in the discussion of modes later in this section. The original version of the Bear 1000 did not provide a mode for SIMV with pressure-targeted breaths, but the newer version does. This control is called PC-SIMV/CPAP(PSV), with PSV indicating pressure-support ventilation. The FLOW WAVEFORM controls operate only during volume-targeted breaths. The constant flow waveform delivers flow at the peak flow setting. The descending ramp rapidly rises to the peak flow setting, then descends linearly until flow decreases to about 50% of peak. The sine flow progressively rises to peak flow and gradually falls to zero in a sinusoidal pattern (Clinical Rounds 12-3).

When activated during expiration, the MANUAL BREATH control delivers one mandatory breath in any mode based on the set values. (NOTE: The unit will not allow a manual breath to be delivered during inspiratory flow of another breath.) MANUAL INSPIRATORY PAUSE triggers a pause at the end of inspiration of the next volume breath and operates

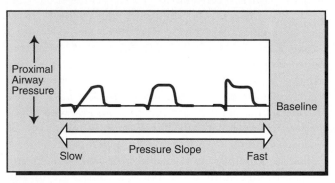

FIGURE 12-13 PRESSURE SLOPE function shown during pressure-support breaths on the Bear 1000; slow (−9) to fast (9). (See text for further explanation.) (Courtesy Cardinal Health, Palm Springs, Calif.)

BOX 12-6	Fourth Row of Controls on the Operating Panel of the BEAR 1000

MODE CONTROLS
ASSIST CMV, SIMV/CPAP (PSV), PRESSURE CONTROL, PC-SIMV/CPAP (PSV)

FLOW WAVEFORM CONTROLS
CONSTANT (rectangular), DESCENDING RAMP, SINELIKE WAVE

MISCELLANEOUS CONTROLS
MANUAL BREATH, MANUAL INSPIRATORY PAUSE, EXPIRATORY HOLD, 100% O$_2$, SIGHS, PRESSURE AUGMENT, blank control (for future option), NEBULIZER

---

for as long as it is depressed, up to a maximum of 2 seconds. It can be used to obtain a plateau pressure reading when the patient is not actively breathing.

EXPIRATORY HOLD delays breath delivery when pressed during the end of exhalation. It closes the expiratory and inspiratory valves at the moment the next mandatory breath would have been delivered and stops breath delivery for as long as it is pressed (up to a maximum of 9 seconds). It is used for measuring auto-PEEP.

The 100% O$_2$ knob delivers 100% oxygen through the patient circuit until it is pressed a second time or 3 minutes have passed, whichever comes first.

When the SIGH control is selected, a sigh breath is provided every 100th breath. The conditions of delivery vary with the mode. Sigh is not available with pressure control in either A/C or SIMV modes. With CPAP, only mandatory breaths are counted until the 100th mandatory breath; therefore sigh delivery is unlikely. The volume delivery is 150% of the set V$_T$. The pressure limit for sigh is 150% of the set pressure limit. When it is time for delivery, the sigh breath replaces the next volume breath. With assist/control (A/C), the **total cycle time (TCT)** is doubled. With SIMV, TCT does not change.

PRESSURE AUGMENTATION is another control in this row; it is reviewed in the discussion of modes of ventilation later in this section.

When the **NEBULIZER control** is selected, a 10-psig gas source is made available to the nebulizer port, which can be connected to a small-volume nebulizer for delivery of medication. Approximately 6 L/min of flow comes from this port. The ventilator automatically subtracts 6 L/min from the flow that would be delivered during inspiration so that V$_T$ delivery does not change significantly. In addition, the nebulizer operates only when the flow from the main inspiratory line exceeds 20 L/min, regardless of the mode, pressure slope, or waveform selected. The nebulizer port operates for 30 minutes unless the control is turned off first.

The PEEP control knob is located below the analog manometer. The PEEP control has no numeric values next to it; therefore adjustment is determined by the PEEP value indicated on the analog manometer. PEEP ranges from 0 to 50 cm H_2O and is available with all modes. If a leak occurs in the patient circuit when baseline is above zero, the ventilator increases flow through the circuit to try to maintain the selected PEEP level.

The **analog pressure manometer** reads from −10 to 120 cm H_2O and provides monitoring in all modes. It is a backup method of verifying digitally displayed pressure values (peak, mean, and plateau pressure).

Monitors and Alarms

The top panel of the Bear 1000 contains the alarms and monitors (see Figure 12-11). The first row of this section contains monitored information, and the second row contains alarm information. On the left of the panel is a list of four possible breath functions: CONTROLLED BREATH, SIGH BREATH, PATIENT EFFORT, and MMV ACTIVE. An LED adjacent to each of these illuminates to indicate the type of breath that has just been initiated. For example, the CONTROLLED BREATH LED lights up if a set volume or pressure breath is either patient or time triggered. It also lights up for a sigh breath or a manually triggered breath. The SIGH BREATH LED lights during the inspiratory phase of a sigh breath. The PATIENT EFFORT LED indicates that patient effort was equal to or greater than the set assist sensitivity or flow trigger. The MMV ACTIVE LED indicates that the ventilator is giving backup breaths to maintain a minimum level of ventilation (see MMV in the section under modes) and remains lit as long as the MMV backup is active.

The next section of the monitor panel is the exhaled volume section. There is one digital readout window and three potential volume readings: V_T, TOTAL $\dot{V}_E$, and SPONTANEOUS $\dot{V}_E$. The operator selects the desired displayed volume by pressing the touch pad below the volume. Volumes are measured by the flow sensor located near the main expiratory line. The expiratory flow sensor reads flow and converts it to volume readings at STPD (standard temperature [77° F, or 25° C], ambient pressure, dry gas). The microprocessor subtracts the volume attributed to humidity from the exhaled volumes to help correct readings.

V_T represents the most recent breath of any type. $\dot{V}_E$, total or spontaneous, is the average of the most recent breaths. Any changes represent the actual exhaled volumes accumulated over 1 minute. The V_T ranges from 0 to 9.99 L, and the $\dot{V}_E$ (both total and spontaneous) ranges from 0 to 99.9 L/min.

The next panel displays respiratory rate (total or spontaneous), I:E ratio, inspiratory time, or MMV %. Likewise, there is one digital display window; therefore the operator selects which parameter is to be displayed. Rate is an average of the most recent breaths and reflects a 60-second accumulated value. Available readings are 0 to 155 breaths/min. The total represents all breaths, and the spontaneous rate represents only the patient's spontaneous breaths for CPAP or pressure-support breaths.

The I:E ratio ranges from 1:0.1 to 1:99.9 and can be calculated with the following ratio: 1:(T_E/T_I). The reading

---

BOX 12-7	Calculating I:E Ratios on the BEAR 1000

A patient on A/C volume ventilation on the Bear 1000 has the following settings: V_T − 1.0 L; rate = 10/min; flow = constant; peak flow = 60 L/min. Calculate the I:E ratio.

$$TCT = 60/10 \text{ breaths/min} = 6 \text{ sec}$$
$$T_I = V_T/Flow$$

Change flow to L/sec.

$$60 \text{ L/min} = 1 \text{ L/sec}$$
$$T_I = V_T/Flow = 1 \text{ L}/(1 \text{ L/sec}) = 1 \text{ sec}$$
$$T_E = TCT - T_I = 6 - 1 \text{ sec} = 5 \text{ sec}$$
$$I:E = 1:5$$

(If you had trouble with this calculation, refer to Chapter 11.)

BOX 12-8	Measuring the Plateau Pressure

Plateau pressure measurement is an attempt to estimate the pressure in the patient's lungs at the end of inspiration; however, it really measures the pressure in both the lungs and the patient circuit.

When the plateau pressure is measured, a patient cannot be actively breathing. If the patient tries to breathe in or out against the closed valves, which is only natural, the plateau reading will be inaccurate.

---

is based on the last breath and updates at the beginning of the next inspiration. It does not measure spontaneous or pressure-support breaths (Box 12-7).

T_I displays the inspiratory time for the previous breath. Similar to the I:E ratio, it does not work for spontaneous or pressure-supported breaths. Its values range from 0 to 9.99 seconds.

The MMV % monitor (0 to 100%) displays the average percentage of time in the last 30 minutes that the MMV backup rate has been used instead of the normal breath rate control.

The pressure monitors include PEAK, MEAN, and PLATEAU. As with the other monitors, the operator must select which of the three is to be displayed. PEAK (0 to 140 cm H_2O) shows the PIP for the most recent breath but does not read spontaneous peak pressure. MEAN (0 to 140 cm H_2O) shows the average mean pressure at the Y-connector for the last breath. PLATEAU (0 to 140 cm H_2O) requires an inspiratory pause of at least 0.1 second. This can be done using the inspiratory pause control on the second row of controls or the manual inspiratory pause on the fourth row of controls. The window displays the plateau pressure of the previous breath. If no measurable plateau was present on the previous breath, it reads zero (Box 12-8).

Alarms

The alarms being monitored appear in the second row on the monitor and alarm panel. The left column of alarms represents built-in alarms. The TIME/I:E LIMIT alarm is activated under two circumstances:

· When T_I is greater than or equal to 5 seconds plus inspiratory pause time and T_I exceeds T_E

· When the I:E ratio exceeds 1:1 for mandatory breaths

For example, if an attempt is made to alter the ratio to 2:1, the alarm will sound. If these limits are exceeded, the ventilator ends inspiration. The first alarm condition cannot be disabled. To disable the second alarm condition, the operator must select the I:E override key, which is to the right of the TIME/I:E LIMIT alarm. When the LED for the I:E override key is on, the ventilator allows inverse ratios up to 4:1.

The RUN DIAGNOSTICS indicator tells the operator that the microprocessor has detected a system or electronic problem during the self-test or normal operation. A troubleshooting code can be viewed in the total minute volume digital display by pressing the test key.

The gas supply failure alarm activates if either source gas pressure falls below 27.5 psig. The ventilator will continue to operate from the remaining gas source, but this can alter F_IO_2 delivery.

The FAILED TO CYCLE alarm activates if the ventilator does not cycle because of an external or internal condition. The error code appears in the total minute volume digital display window. An internal safety valve opens, allowing the patient to breathe room air.

These four built-in alarms are both visual (flashing light) and audible. If any of these LEDs are lit but not flashing, the alarm condition occurred but was corrected. Pressing the VISUAL RESET pad near the right side of this row of alarms turns off the light.

Four sets of adjustable alarms are in the second row. The alarm sequence, from left to right, is TOTAL MINUTE VOLUME, TOTAL BREATH RATE, PEAK INSPIRATORY PRESSURE, and BASELINE PRESSURE. These alarms can all be adjusted in the same way. For each alarm panel, one digital display window is used for both the high and low settings of a particular alarm. To the right of the digital window is an LED that lights up when the alarm is violated. There are two touch pads below the digital window; the left one has an upward-pointing triangle and sets the upper limit; the right one has a downward-pointing triangle and sets the lower limit. To adjust either, the alarm panel must be unlocked with the LOCK control. Either the upper or lower limit touch pad is touched for the desired alarm parameter. For example, if the upper alarm key for total minute volume is touched, its current numeric value appears in the digital display window. At the same time, the touch pad light that was touched begins to flash and will do so for 15 seconds or as long as the CONTROL knob continues to be turned. While it is flashing, the touch pad light can be adjusted by turning the ALARM CONTROL knob on the far right side of the alarm panel. It is important to note that the alarm level changes as soon as the knob is turned, even while the alarm indicator is flashing. While the first selected alarm parameter is still flashing, the operator can select another alarm to adjust by repeating the same process.

Even though the indicators may be flashing, only one parameter can be adjusted at a time.

When the alarm parameters set by the operator have been exceeded, the small light to the right of the digital display (the alarm trigger indicator for that control) flashes and an audible alarm sounds. After the alarm condition is corrected, the alarm trigger indicator stays lit until the VISUAL RESET pad is pressed.

The high and low $\dot{V}_E$ alarms range from 0 to 80 and 0 to 50 L, respectively. High and low V_T rate alarms range from 0 to 155 and 1 to 99 breaths/min, respectively. The high and low PIP alarms are slightly more involved. The high PIP range is 0 to 120 cm H_2O, and reaching this alarm limit ends inspiration. For a sigh breath, the PIP is 150% of the set high PIP limit, or 120 cm H_2O, whichever occurs first. When a high PIP alarm occurs, the pressure in the proximal line must drop to within 5 cm H_2O of the PEEP level (baseline). If a kink is present in the main expiratory line, the line pressure may not be able to drop, and delivery of the next breath is delayed until pressure in the proximal line decreases. The range for the low PIP alarm is 3 to 99 cm H_2O; this value cannot be set below 3 cm H_2O. The alarm is not active for spontaneous breaths and is also inactive in PSV and PCV under the following condition:

$$[\text{PEEP} + (\text{Pressure support or Inspiratory pressure})]$$
$$\leq \text{to 3 cm } H_2O$$

If the abbreviation PRO appears in the PIP alarm display window, the machine pressure is greater than the sum of the high PIP alarm setting + 10 cm H_2O. The PRO alarm is most commonly caused by disconnection of the proximal pressure line from the machine or the patient circuit, but large leaks can also be responsible.

HIGH and LOW BASELINE PRESSURE alarms (0 to 55 cm H_2O and 0 to 50 cm H_2O, respectively) occur when monitored pressure limits are exceeded. Box 12-9 gives some examples of situations in which these events can occur.

Five touch pads and the CONTROL knob are to the right of the alarms in this row. The top three touch pads are as follows:

1. ALARM SILENCE—Silences audible alarms for 60 seconds or until pressed again; cannot silence the FAILED TO CYCLE alarm.

2. VISUAL RESET—Resets visual alarms after alarm conditions have been corrected.

BOX 12-9	Situations Affecting the Baseline Pressure

PEEP is set at 8 cm H_2O, and the high and low PEEP alarms are set at 13 and 3 cm H_2O, respectively. If a leak occurs and pressure during expiration falls to zero, the low baseline pressure alarm activates. If the patient actively exhales or coughs during expiration and prevents the pressure from falling to at least 8 cm H_2O, the high baseline pressure alarm sounds.

3. TEST—Has three functions: (1) activates the visual and audible indicators for 4 seconds during normal operation to check function; (2) displays any troubleshooting codes that might have occurred in the total minute ventilation digital window; and (3) if pressed before the ventilator is turned on and held while the power is turned on, it causes the ventilator to enter OPERATOR DIAGNOSTICS, and the operating manual should be consulted.

The bottom two touch keys are the DIMMER key and the LOCK key. The DIMMER key adjusts the brightness of the LEDs on the control panel, and the LOCK key locks the alarm control panel so that values cannot be changed accidentally. The LED near this key is lit when the panel is locked. Changes to alarm controls cannot be made until this key is pressed to unlock it.

MODES OF VENTILATION

The mode controls on the Bear 1000 include ASSIST CONTINUOUS MANDATORY VENTILATION (ASSIST CMV), SIMV/CPAP(PSV), PRESSURE CONTROL, PC-IMV/CPAP(PSV), PRESSURE AUGMENT, and MMV. Each of these will be reviewed.

Changing Ventilator Modes

The first four mode keys are on the lower left row of the control panel. The last, PRESSURE AUGMENTATION, is the farthest right control in this row. Mode keys have three conditions: OFF, SETUP, and ON. When an operating mode is changed on the Bear 1000, the following procedure is used: The operator first presses the mode key for the new mode desired: OFF to SETUP. This causes the LED by that mode's touch pad to flash while the original mode key's LED stays lit. The control panel illuminates the controls available for the new mode. The operator then adjusts each control variable for the new mode to the desired setting, along with all desired alarm settings. After everything is set, the operator presses the new mode touch pad a second time: SETUP to ON. It stays illuminated, and the old mode switches off.

Assist CMV

ASSIST CMV is **volume-targeted ventilation** that can be time or patient triggered, volume limited, and volume cycled. All of the control parameters are available for ASSIST CMV except MMV, inspiratory time, pressure support, or inspiratory pressure.

SIMV/CPAP (PSV)

SIMV/CPAP (PSV) is volume-targeted SIMV. The operator can provide a positive baseline (PEEP/CPAP) in this mode by using the PEEP control. Pressure support is also available for spontaneous breaths. Volume breaths can be patient or time triggered. Mandatory breaths are based on the V_T, rate, peak flow, and flow waveform selected.

Spontaneous breaths begin from the set baseline pressure. In addition, PSV can be provided for spontaneous

breaths based on the set pressure support level. The set PSV pressure is added to the PEEP level. For example, if the PEEP is 5 cm H_2O, and the PSV is set at 15 cm H_2O, PIP during a PSV breath will be 20 cm H_2O. The PSV breaths are patient triggered, pressure limited, and flow cycled at 30% of the peak inspiratory flow.

During SIMV, if the rate is turned to zero, the ventilator provides CPAP and/or PSV.

Pressure Control

Pressure control provides time- or patient-triggered, pressure-limited, time-cycled breaths. In addition to inspiratory pressure, the operator sets the rate, T_I, assist sensitivity and/or base flow and flow trigger, and pressure sloping. Most other controls, including the waveforms, sigh, and pressure augment, are not available. As in all modes, it is very important to set the upper pressure limit. Even though pressure is set, pressure can go above the set inspiratory pressure level. For example, if the patient coughs, the pressure may exceed the set value. A reasonable setting would be 10 to 15 cm H_2O above the set inspiratory pressure.

PC-SIMV with CPAP and PSV

PC-SIMV/CPAP(PSV) is ventilation in which mandatory breaths are pressure targeted and time cycled (Box 12-10; also see Chapter 11). Spontaneous breaths can occur with pressure support or simply from the set baseline (PEEP). As in pressure control, the operator sets the rate, inspiratory pressure, triggering mechanisms, and T_I. PEEP and pressure support can also be set. Both the inspiratory pressure setting and the pressure support setting are added to the PEEP level.

If rate is turned to zero, the ventilator allows the patient to breathe spontaneously at the set baseline (zero or PEEP/CPAP). If the sensitivity is set appropriately, the ventilator can monitor spontaneous breaths, which occurs when the patient's inspiratory effort meets or exceeds the set trigger value. These spontaneous breaths can also be pressure supported.

Pressure slope can also be used in this mode and can affect the rate of flow at the beginning of the breath during pressure-targeted mandatory pressure-support breaths, or spontaneous breaths.

BOX 12-10	Reviewing Definitions of Breath Types

Mandatory breath delivery is completely determined by the ventilator (i.e., triggering, delivery of inspiration, and cycling are ventilator controlled). Breaths are commonly volume or pressure targeted.

An *assisted breath* is patient triggered. The delivery of inspiration and the ending of inspiration (cycling) are determined by the ventilator.

With *spontaneous breaths*, the patient controls all phases of the breath.

Pressure Augment

Pressure augment, or pressure augmentation (Paug), is a dual control, closed-loop mode of ventilation that guarantees volume delivery for each breath.

Paug provides the benefits of pressure-targeted ventilation, such as high initial gas flows, a descending-ramp flow pattern, and a limited pressure, with the added feature that it can guarantee volume delivery. Key criteria for the use of pressure augmentation are (1) the patient must be able to initiate breaths and (2) the patient must have a consistent respiratory rate and a reasonable inspiratory effort.

Paug is designed to work in any patient-triggered volume breath. For this reason, it works only in ASSIST CMV and SIMV/CPAP (PSV). It is selected by pressing the pressure augmentation control so that it is illuminated. The operator also selects the V_T, rate, inspiratory pressure level above baseline, peak flow, and sensitivity setting. It also is important to set an appropriate pressure limit of about 10 cm H_2O above the inspiratory pressure plus PEEP. Regarding flow pattern, it is currently recommended that a constant flow pattern be selected to help keep T_I shorter.

Pressure augmentation operates in the following manner: When the patient triggers a breath, the ventilator provides a high inspiratory gas flow to achieve the set pressure level. As it delivers this flow, it monitors flow and volume delivery. From this point, one of two possible scenarios unfolds. If patient inspiratory flow demand and the set pressure are high, the ventilator recognizes that the

minimum volume is delivered quickly, and it does not need to take any action. Inspiration ends when the flow drops to 30% of measured peak flow. If the patient demand is modest, however, the ventilator may find that the volume has not been delivered by the time the measured flow has dropped to a value equal to the flow set on the peak flow control. In this case, it does not allow the flow to drop farther, but maintains flow at the set peak flow and continues to provide this flow until it determines that the minimum volume has been delivered, at which point the breath ends.

Figure 12-14 illustrates some of the potential outcomes of Paug. Waveform A is an example of a typical pressure-support breath instead of a pressure-augmented breath, so that readers can make some comparisons with pressure augmentation. In waveform A, the breath is patient triggered, pressure limited (25 cm H_2O), and flow cycled at 30% of the peak inspiratory flow, and the patient achieved a V_T of about 1 L.

In waveform B, the patient has a moderate inspiratory demand, and flow rises to reach and maintain the pressure (25 cm H_2O). Flow drops to the set value of 40 L/min, and the ventilator determines that the set volume of 0.8 L has not been reached. It maintains the flow at 40 L/min. Because more flow is going into the patient's lungs, the pressure rises above the set value. When the ventilator determines that the volume was delivered, the breath ends. This is a classic pattern of a pressure-augmented breath.

In waveform C, it appears that the set pressure of 25 cm H_2O is not adequate to quickly meet the volume setting for this particular patient. When the flow drops to the set

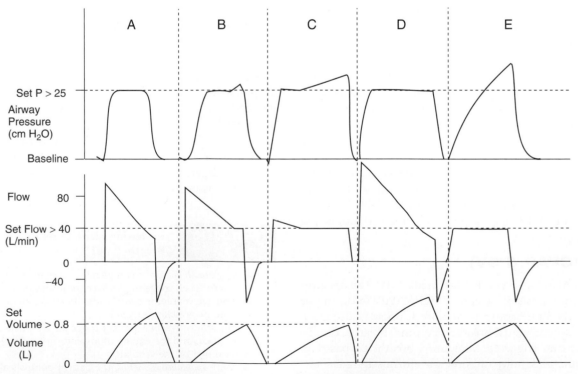

FIGURE 12-14 Various waveforms achievable with pressure augmentation. (From Pilbeam SP, Cairo JM: *Mechanical ventilation: physiological and clinical applications,* ed 4, St Louis, 2006, Mosby.)

value (40 L/min), it is maintained until the volume of 0.8 L is delivered. Notice how long inspiration is compared with waveforms A and B. To more appropriately provide pressure augmentation, the inspiratory pressure needs to be increased. The flow may need to be increased as well.

In waveform D, the patient has a high inspiratory demand, flow rises rapidly to reach and maintain the set pressure, the inspiratory pressure is set high, and minimum volume is surpassed. Volume delivery is high. In this situation, inspiration ends when the flow drops to about 30% of peak flow. Paug can provide whatever volume and flow the patient desires and still remain within a safe pressure limit.

In waveform E, no patient effort is detected. The ventilator delivers a typical volume breath at a constant flow setting. Pressure rises to a peak, which depends on the volume delivered and the patient's lung characteristics.

When Paug is used in ASSIST CMV, every breath is potentially augmented. With SIMV, only the patient-triggered mandatory breaths are augmented. It is strongly recommended that practitioners use the graphic waveforms for pressure, volume, and flow against time when adjusting Paug for a patient.

Because of its ability to perform pressure augmentation, the ventilator can also augment flow and volume. If patient inspiratory demand drops the measured airway pressure below the baseline pressure, the ventilator automatically increases flow to maintain the baseline. This augments flow to the patient and also increases volume delivery above the set value if the patient demands it. For example, in the CPAP mode or with SIMV + CPAP, if the baseline pressure during spontaneous breathing drops below the set value because of patient demand, the ventilator increases flow to the patient to maintain the baseline and augment the patient's needs.

MMV Feature

MMV operates in the SIMV and CPAP modes to ensure that a spontaneously breathing patient's minute volume does not drop below a set level. As long as the monitored total exhaled minute volume meets or exceeds the value set in the MMV setting, backup ventilator support is inactive. However, if the exhaled $\dot{V}_E$ falls below the set MMV, the breath rate automatically increases to ensure that the minimum $\dot{V}_E$ is delivered. The backup breath rate (breaths/min) is determined as follows:

$$\text{Backup rate} = (\text{MMV level})/V_T$$

The MMV ACTIVE indicator illuminates during inspiration and exhalation whenever the MMV mode is active. The MMV % indicator displays the percent of time during the last half-hour that the MMV backup rate has been in use instead of the rate set by the clinician.

The ventilator returns to operation at the clinician-set rate when the monitored $\dot{V}_E$ exceeds the set MMV by 1 L/min or 10%, whichever is greater. (NOTE: The MMV must be set to a value greater than the set $\dot{V}_E$ [Rate × V_T]. The TOTAL BREATH RATE alarm must be set appropriately to avoid high respiratory rates.)

SPECIAL FEATURES

The Bear 1000T/ES version of the Bear 1000 features some upgrades. Two more pressure transducer connectors have been added. One is intended for monitoring esophageal pressures (P_{ES}) and the second tracheal pressures (P_{TRACH}). The BALLOON button on the control panel is used to initiate the filling of the esophageal balloon. When pressed once, the button results first in a NEGATIVE LEAK TEST being performed, and the balloon then inflates to the proper fill volume (0.8 mL). When the button is pressed and held, the ventilator performs a DISTENSION MANEUVER, causing the balloon to fill beyond its normal measuring volume (5 to 5.5 mL for adults, 2 to 2.5 mL for pediatric patients). It then returns to the proper fill volume.

The 1000T/ES also determines the inflection points on a pressure/volume loop using algorithms to identify the upper and lower inflection points. The 1000T/ES provides calculations of the work of breathing and weaning data, which include the following:

· Ventilator, patient, and imposed work of breathing (Joules/L)
· AutoPEEPes (esophageal)
· AutoPEEPaw (airway)
· Maximum inspiratory pressure (MIP) (range, −60 to 0 cm H_2O)
· P_{100}, the pressure generated during the first 100 msec of inspiration (range, −20 to 0 cm H_2O)
· f/V_T ratio (rapid shallow breathing index; range, 0 to 300)
· Change in esophageal pressure during inspiration (range, −100 to 0 cm H_2O)

GRAPHICS

The Bear 1000 has a graphics monitor and program that can easily be added to the ventilator unit. The graphics panel has a viewing screen (see Figure 12-10), below which are six operating keys. To the right of the screen are two icons and four operating keys that look like arrow heads. The power switch for the screen is on the back panel of the unit, and the screen is activated by touching the icon that looks like pages of paper on the upper right corner of the panel to the right of the screen. The icon at the bottom of the panel looks like a printer and allows the information on the screen to be printed when the machine is connected to a printer. The four directional arrows have two main functions: they can change the lighting on the screen, and when used for functions, they can change the amplitude scale of the graphs. For example, if the range of a pressure graph is 0 to 10 cm H_2O, the arrows can be used to change the range to 0 to 100 cm H_2O.

The operator's manual provides information about setting the time and date and other start-up information.

Menus are provided at the top and bottom of the basic waveform pages of the screen. The top menu provides access to waves, loops, set-up, and time and has several blank positions for future updates. The bottom menu provides information about what parameter is on the screen (e.g., flow or volume) and allows it to be selected and changed. The bottom menu also can freeze a screen, mark a particular graph for reference, and scale the x-axis of the graph.

One to three graphs can be displayed on the screen. For example, the operator may want to view pressure, volume, and flow scalars. Loops or graphs can be provided by highlighting the options appearing on the top menu on the screen. The graphic display also has a mechanics page, which offers flow-volume and pressure-volume loops, as well as compliance, resistance, and work of breathing calculations.

TROUBLESHOOTING

The variety of alarms and monitors and the availability of graphic monitoring make everyday troubleshooting fairly simple. In addition, the operator's manual contains a troubleshooting section with a table of symptoms, possible causes, and corrective actions. For example, suppose the low baseline pressure alarm activates. Possible causes might be that the patient is disconnected from the ventilator, a leak is present in the patient circuit, or a leak is present in the exhalation valve diaphragm. Solutions would include reconnecting the patient, checking the circuit for leaks, and, finally, checking the diaphragm for holes or tears. After any problems are corrected, a leak test should be performed.

More than 20 possible problems are identified in the troubleshooting section of the operator's manual. It is beyond the scope of this text to cover all of them. Readers who intend to use this ventilator should consult that section for more information.

Radio frequency interference (RFI)/**electromagnetic frequency interference (EFI)** can affect the operation of the Bear 1000, just as it can any medical device that uses a microprocessor. Walkie-talkies and cellular phones should not be used near these types of medical devices.

It is important to be sure to check which system is in operation when troubleshooting a ventilator problem.

KEY POINTS

▌ The Bear 1000 is pneumatically powered and microprocessor controlled and can be used for pediatric to adult patients.

▌ The lower section of the operating panel of the Bear 1000 contains the control functions, and the upper section contains the alarms and monitors.

▌ A control can be selected and changed only if the LED for the variable is illuminated.

▌ A sigh breath is delivered every 100th mandatory breath in volume ventilation when the SIGH control is active.

▌ When the LED for the I:E override key is on, the ventilator allows inverse ratios up to 4:1.

▌ An alarm level changes as soon as the ALARM CONTROL knob is turned, even while the alarm indicator is flashing.

▌ To change a mode of ventilation, the operator presses the mode key and the control panel illuminates the controls available for the new mode. The operator presses the new mode touch pad a second time to activate the new mode.

▌ The Bear 1000 provides a dual control mode of ventilation called PRESSURE AUGMENT and a weaning mode called MINIMUM MINUTE VENTILATION (MMV).

ASSESSMENT QUESTIONS

See Evolve Resources for the answers.

1. The flow-control valve of the Bear 1000 is powered by which type of device so that rapid changes in flow are possible?
   a. An electronic flow transducer
   b. A linear-drive, microprocessor-controlled piston
   c. A proportional rotary microswitch
   d. A stepper motor

2. To adjust the V_T setting on the Bear 1000, which of the following should be performed?
   a. Turn the tidal volume knob to the desired value.
   b. Press tidal volume, key in the value on the numeric key pad, and press enter.
   c. Press the tidal volume touch pad and rotate the control knob (at the far right on the second row of controls) until the desired value for V_T appears.
   d. Reduce the $\dot{V}_E$ setting, then change the rate until the desired V_T appears in the message window.

ASSESSMENT QUESTIONS—cont'd

3. To set the high total $\dot{V}_E$ alarm on the Bear 1000, which of the following must be performed?
   I. Unlock the alarm panel.
   II. Touch the left upward-pointing triangle below the total $\dot{V}_E$ digital window
   III. Turn the alarm control knob until the desired value is displayed.
   IV. Press the activated touch pad to the right of the alarm.
      a. III only
      b. I and II only
      c. II and IV only
      d. I, II, and III only

4. An alarm sounds, and the respiratory therapist notes that the GAS SUPPLY FAILURE LED is illuminated. This indicates which of the following?
   a. One or more of the gas sources is less than 35 psig.
   b. One gas supply has lost pressure, but if another gas supply is still available, the ventilator will continue to operate.
   c. The measured F_IO_2 has dropped below the set value.
   d. Inspiratory pressure in the patient circuit is below the set value.

5. Which of the following statements about the Bear 1000 is/are true?
   I. The Bear 1000 requires at least one high-pressure gas source and an electrical power source.
   II. If an air compressor has been added to the unit, it can become a high-pressure gas source.
   III. If a compressor is the only high-pressure gas source available, the Bear 1000 will ventilate, but it cannot deliver a high oxygen percentage.
   IV. An internal rotary turbine provides the air source for the Bear 1000.
      a. IV only
      b. I and III
      c. I, II, and III
      d. I and IV

6. A nurse is trying to adjust the V_T on the Bear 1000 ventilator. Although the V_T reading is 0.5 L and the LED next to the V_T control is illuminated, turning the control has no effect. What could be the problem?
   a. The LOCK control may be active.
   b. The ventilator is in the pressure control mode.
   c. The tidal volume cannot exceed 0.5 L.
   d. The ventilator is in CPAP mode.

7. During MMV the patient's minute volume falls below the set value. This will result in:
   a. An increase in ventilating pressure
   b. An increase in the rate of ventilation
   c. An audible and visual alarm
   d. No change in ventilator function

8. The COMPLIANCE COMP control indicates a value of 3 cm H_2O. The set V_T is 0.7 L (700 mL) and the PIP is 25 cm H_2O. What volume will the ventilator add to the selected volume of 700 mL (0.7 L) if the compliance compensation feature is active?
   a. 25 mL
   b. 75 mL
   c. 700 mL
   d. It will not add any volume.

9. A patient is on pressure augmentation. The pressure-time graph shows a rapid rise to the set value, which is maintained constantly during inspiration. Flow rapidly rises to a peak, then progressively descends to 30% of peak flow and ends. The set volume is 0.5 L (500 mL), but the delivered volume is 0.75 L (750 mL). This best describes:
   a. Active inspiration by the patient
   b. Compliance compensation is active
   c. A pressure-augmented breath
   d. A volume-targeted breath

10. During SIMV/CPAP (PSV), the rate is turned to zero. PEEP is set at 5 cm H_2O, and PSV is set at 10 cm H_2O. Which of the following is/are true?
   I. The peak inspiratory pressure for a PSV breath will be 15 cm H_2O.
   II. All breaths will be patient triggered.
   III. The set volume will be delivered when the patient triggers a breath.
   IV. CPAP of 5 cm H_2O will be provided.
      a. I only
      b. I and II
      c. III and IV
      d. I and IV

References

1. Bear 1000 ventilator instruction manual, Pub No 50-10613-00, Palm Springs, Calif, 1995, and L-1575 and 6/2001 version A, Viasys Healthcare, Critical Care Division.

2. Pilbeam SP, Cairo JM: *Mechanical ventilation: physiological and clinical applications*, ed 4, St Louis, 2006, Mosby.

Internet Resource
www.cardinal.com

CARDINAL BIRD 8400 VENTILATOR

The Bird 8400STi ventilator is a second-generation unit derived from the Bird 6400. It previously was manufactured by Bird Medical Technologies and subsequently was purchased by VIASYS Healthcare, Critical Care Division. Viasys was purchased by Cardinal Health in 2008. Cardinal Health now owns the Bird 8400STi ventilator. Additional information about the Bird 8400 is available on the Evolve Resources Web site for this text.

CARDINAL BIRD T-BIRD VENTILATOR

The Bird T-Bird was once part of the Bird Medical Technologies ventilator fleet. As mentioned previously, Bird was purchased by VIASYS Healthcare, Critical Care Division, which was purchased in 2008 by Cardinal Health. Additional information on the Bird T-Bird is available on the Evolve Resources Web site for this text.

CARDINAL VELA

OUTLINE

Power Source
Internal Mechanism
Controls
    Preuse Testing
    User Interface Controls
    Monitors
Alarms
Modes of Ventilation
    Airway Pressure-Release Ventilation/BiPhasic
      (APRV/BiPhasic)
    Apnea Backup Ventilation (ABV)
    Noninvasive Ventilation (NIV)

Special Functions: Advanced Settings
    Assured Volume (on the Vela Comprehensive)
    Volume Limit
    Vsync
    Flow Cycle—Pressure-Control Breaths
    Selecting the Flow Pattern in Volume Ventilation
    Additional Options
Troubleshooting

OBJECTIVES

Upon completion of this section, you will be able to:
· Explain the function of the available oxygen sources of the Vela.
· Discuss the function of the internal turbine.
· Describe the leak compensation function.
· Compare the process for setting ventilator controls on the Vela to the process for the Avea.
· Perform a preuse test on the Vela.
· Describe how and when to set up apnea backup ventilation.
· Define Assured Volume, Volume Limit, Vsync, and Flow-Cycle.
· Explain the use of PSV during APRV/BiPhasic ventilation.

KEY TERMS

Antisuffocation valve	Assured volume	Subambient relief valve

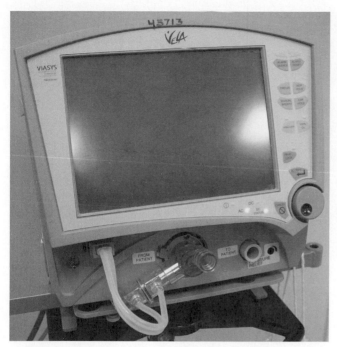

FIGURE 12-15 Vela ventilator. (Photograph courtesy Susan P. Pilbeam.)

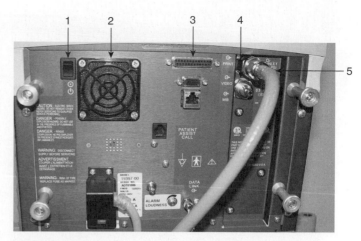

FIGURE 12-16 Back panel of the Vela ventilator. *(1)* On/off switch. *(2)* Air intake filter. *(3)* Standard connectors for printer, video, and medical information bus (MIB). *(4)* Low pressure oxygen connector. *(5)* DISS oxygen connector. (Photograph courtesy Susan P. Pilbeam.)

In 2001 Viasys Healthcare, Critical Care Division, released a ventilator called the Vela (Figure 12-15). In 2007 Cardinal Health purchased Viasys Healthcare. The Cardinal Vela is alike in function to the T-Bird ventilator and has similar modes, parameters, and alarms.* A major difference between the two is the touch screen flat panel user interface on the Vela. The Vela can be used for pediatric and adult patients for invasive and noninvasive ventilation.

Currently three versions are available: the basic model (the Vela), the Vela+, and the Vela Comprehensive. The basic model includes all the basic modes, functions, and basic waveform graphics. The Vela+ includes PRVC mode and Vsync, noninvasive ventilation, and leak compensation. The Vela Comprehensive additionally provides loops, trends, maximum inspiratory pressure (MIP), square waveform, APRV/BiPhasic mode, and Assured Volume ventilation.

This section reviews general information about the Vela, Vela+, and Vela Comprehensive package.[1]

POWER SOURCE

The Vela is a microprocessor-controlled unit. It requires an electrical source but does not require a gas source to operate (electrically powered ventilator). An internal turbine provides the gas source that flows to the patient (single circuit).

*Information on the Bird T-Bird is available on the Evolve Web site for this text.

The on/off switch is located on the back panel of the ventilator. When the switch is turned to the ON position, the ventilator emits an audible alarm that lasts until the unit is pressurized enough to be connected to the patient. Ventilation begins immediately. There is no standby position.

Oxygen can also be provided to the patient using either a high-pressure oxygen DISS connector (40 to 65 psig) or a low-pressure O_2 source. The connectors are located on the back panel of the unit (Figure 12-16). Low-pressure gas must be provided by an O_2 flowmeter and low-pressure oxygen tubing connected to the tapered connector at the back of the ventilator.

An internal battery can serve as a backup power source and has an operating capacity of approximately 6 hours.

INTERNAL MECHANISM

Ambient air enters the unit through the air filter, and oxygen enters through either the high-pressure or low-pressure oxygen connector. When high-pressure oxygen is attached, an internal blender mixes the gas based on the oxygen setting on the control panel. With low-pressure oxygen, the F_IO_2 depends on the flow setting of the oxygen flowmeter and the patient's minute ventilation. (NOTE: A formula for estimating the F_IO_2 when low-pressure oxygen is used is available with the operator's manual.) When low-pressure oxygen is supplied, the oxygen control must be set to 21% to prevent alarms associated with the oxygen supply pressure and the delivered oxygen concentration.

Blended gases from the oxygen source and the internal turbine are sent to an accumulator, which helps mix the gases and also helps reduce the noise generated by the built-in turbine. The microprocessor uses information about the pressure measured and the turbine speed to control the precise flow delivered to the patient.

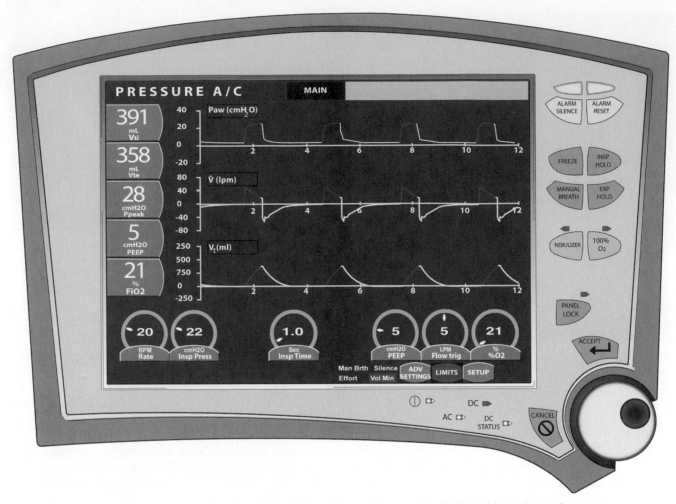

FIGURE 12-17 User interface of the Vela ventilator. (Courtesy Cardinal Health, Yorba Linda, Calif.)

An internal **subambient relief valve** or **antisuffocation valve** opens if the ventilator cannot provide adequate air during inspiratory demand. The patient can then inhale to open the valve and receive room air. For example, this might occur during a ventilator inoperative condition.

The ventilator also has internal transducers for measuring pressure. The expiratory flow transducer is a differential pressure transducer (see Chapter 8).

CONTROLS

The front portion of the Vela contains the connectors for the patient circuit, expiratory pneumotachometer, and user interface (Figure 12-17 and 12-18). The user interface consists of a touch screen color LCD and membrane controls or touch pads located to the right of the screen (Figure 12-17).

Preuse Testing

Before using the ventilator on a new patient or if the ventilator does not seem to be operating properly, the operator should perform an operational verification test. (NOTE: This test *cannot* be performed while the ventilator is connected to a patient.)

Flow Transducer

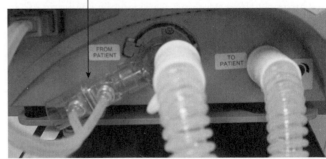

FIGURE 12-18 Vela ventilator, showing the connectors for the patient circuit (inspiratory and expiratory limbs) and the flow sensor connector between the expiratory valve body and the ventilator (*left*).

After disconnecting the patient or before connecting the patient, turn the ventilator OFF. Press and hold the ACCEPT button, and turn the ventilator ON. Continue holding the button until the ventilator completes the Power On Self-Test (POST). The button is released when the UVT START UP message appears on the screen. A menu appears on the

BOX 12-11	Unit Verification Test (UVT) Menu of Available Tests (Vela)

Lamp Test
Switch Test
Alarm Test
Filter Test
Leak Test
Extended Functions

screen that allows for selection of additional tests. Box 12-11 lists the available tests, and the operator's manual provides a description of each of the tests.

A patient circuit is connected to the ventilator before use, and the desired type of humidifier is selected and placed in the circuit. The ventilator set-up screen (activated by pressing the SETUP screen button) allows selection of the type of humidifier being used. Either active humidification (assumes 37° C) or passive humidification (assumes 25° C) can be chosen. The selection is used to calculate correctly the delivered and displayed volumes in body temperature pressure saturated (BTPS).

The variable-orifice flow sensor (pneumotachometer) is attached at the expiratory valve body on the lower front of the ventilator. The monitor line for the flow sensor is connected to the left (see Figure 12-18). The volume that flows through the exhaled flow sensor is displayed as the exhaled volume.

User Interface Controls

The user interface consists of the screen controls available on the membrane buttons and the touch screen controls.

Membrane Buttons

The membrane buttons are on the right panel of the operating unit (see Figure 12-17).

The ALARM SILENCE key disables the audible portion of an alarm for 60 seconds when pressed. Pressing it again restores the audible alarms. This button also functions as a VENT INOP alarm. (NOTE: The VENT INOP alarm activates if the ventilator fails because of a nonrecoverable condition, such as loss of power. The safety valve opens, allowing a spontaneously breathing patient to inhale room air.)

The ALARM RESET cancels the visual indicator for alarms that are no longer active.

The FREEZE button freezes the current screen, including the waveforms, and suspends the updating of data until it is pressed again. As with the AVEA ventilator, when the screen is frozen, the operator can scroll through the displayed waveforms and loops using the DATA DIAL to move the cursor. The DATA DIAL is located at the lower right corner of the unit. A vertical dotted line appears in the scalars screen (see Figure 12-8). Wherever the dotted line crosses a scalar, the value for that scalar appears in a balloon. The dotted line can be moved by scrolling with the DATA DIAL.

A loop can be saved by pressing FREEZE when a loop is displayed. A total of four loops can be saved at a time. The oldest is discarded when a fifth is added. When the operator is in the SAVED LOOP function, a window appears giving the dates of the saved loops.

When the inspiratory hold (INSP HOLD) button is pressed and held, the ventilator holds inspiration immediately after the preset volume has been delivered. It can be held up to 6 seconds.

The expiratory hold (EXP HOLD) button holds the expiratory phase for up to 6 seconds at the start of the next breath interval. When it is held the patient cannot breathe in or out. EXP HOLD can be used to measure intrinsic PEEP (see Chapter 11).

Pressing the MANUAL BREATH button during exhalation delivers a single mandatory breath based on current ventilator settings. No breath is delivered if the button is pressed during inspiration.

The NEBULIZER button provides flow to the nebulizer connector when it is activated. The connector is located at the lower left panel of the ventilator front. Nebulizer flow is synchronized with inspiration. To be operational, the ventilator must be connected to a high-pressure O_2 source. An inline nebulizer is attached, and the button is pressed. The ventilator delivers 6 L/min flow of 100% oxygen during inspiration through the nebulizer connector. Using the nebulizer affects the F_IO_2, volume delivery (in volume ventilation), and peak pressure. (NOTE: About 50 mL is added to the tidal volume every 0.5 second of inspiratory time.) A safe upper pressure limit should be set. Pressing the NEBULIZER button again (the membrane key on the right) stops nebulization (Clinical Rounds 12-4).

When the 100% O_2 button is pressed, the ventilator delivers 100% oxygen for 3 minutes. Pressing the button again cancels the maneuver and returns the ventilator to its previous settings.

The PANEL LOCK control disables all front panel controls except MANUAL BREATH, 100% O_2, ALARM REST, ALARM SILENCE, and the PANEL LOCK button.

The ACCEPT button allows the ventilator to accept data entered into a field on the touch screen.

Pressing CANCEL results in cancellation of data entered into a field on the touch screen. The ventilator continues to operate at current settings.

CLINICAL ROUNDS 12-4

A respiratory therapist decides to use the nebulizer port on the Vela to deliver a bronchodilator treatment. The patient settings are $V_T = 450$ mL, rate = 12, $F_IO_2 = 0.25$. However, the therapist notes that the measured F_IO_2 is 0.29, and the tidal volume is about 500 mL. How can the therapist maintain the same settings during the treatment?

See Evolve Resources for the answer.

Screen Controls

When the ventilator is on, the screen displays a variety of information. The mode of ventilation is shown at the top left corner of the screen. The top center indicates the operating window currently open on the screen, and the message window is located at the top right (see Figure 12-17).

The screen controls are used for patient set-up, mode and parameter selection, and alarm settings. The first screen to appear when the ventilator is turned on is the PATIENT SELECT screen. Ventilation of a current patient can be resumed (RESUME CURRENT), or a new patient can be selected (NEW PATIENT). Resuming ventilation continues ventilation at the most recent patient settings. Selecting NEW PATIENT clears all saved loops and trends and resets all parameters to the factory default values. (NOTE: The operator must touch PATIENT ACCEPT to accept either selection.) If NEW PATIENT is selected, ventilation begins at the default settings, and the set-up screen is displayed. MAIN is pressed to return to the main screen.

The SETUP screen can be accessed at any time by pressing the SETUP button on the bottom right corner of the touch screen (see Figure 12-17). The SETUP menu provides an optional LEAK COMPENSATION ON selection of humidifier types (discussed earlier), and the option to enter a patient identifier number. Once these steps have been completed, pressing SETUP ACCEPT activates the items selected.

Leak compensation is designed to compensate for leaks around an endotracheal tube. It compensates for small leaks up to 5 L/min. When noninvasive ventilation is used, leak compensation is activated automatically. During NIV, the compensation ensures that gas leakage around the mask can be compensated for up to 40 L/min. Leak compensation adjusts a bias flow through the ventilator circuit to maintain the set PEEP level and establish a baseline for patient breath triggering.

Mode selection is accessed by pressing the indicator at the top left of the touch screen, which names the current mode of ventilation. The menu displayed includes both invasive and noninvasive ventilation modes that are available. (See the section later on Modes of Ventilation.)

At the top center of the screen is the MAIN touch key. Pressing this key brings up the menu for SCREEN SELECT, which includes the following screens:

- MAIN—main menu
- LOOP—brings up loops (optional)
- MONITOR—monitor screen
- TRENDS—trends screen
- MANEUVER—to perform weaning functions such as negative inspiratory force (NIF) and vital capacity (VC)
- EXTENDED FUNCTIONS—extended functions menu

The EXTENDED FUNCTIONS menu allows access to stored data, performance calibrations, and customization of the front panel. To access this menu, touch the EXTENDED FUNCTIONS screen indicator. Box 12-12 provides additional information about these functions. More information is also available in the operator's manual.

BOX 12-12	Extended Functions and Alarm Ranges (Vela)

EXTENDED FUNCTIONS

Events—Stores data events for service evaluation and troubleshooting*

Transducer Data—Allows setting of the transducer analog outputs for service*

Transducer Test—Allows service testing of transducer function*

Version Info—Provides software version information and turbine serial number

Date/Time—Displays hours of operation and the date/time configuration

F_IO_2 Monitor Calibration—Permits calibration of the internal oxygen sensor[†]

Vent Setup—Allows setting and selection of the following: Low Min Vol OFF, Panel Lock, F_IO_2 monitor (ON/OFF), Units of Measure setting for altitude (feet/meters), Altitude setting for accurate volume measurement, Language buttons, Video Normal/Inverse (reverses graphic color configuration)

ALARM RANGES

High rate alarm range: 3 to 150 breaths/min or off
Low minute volume alarm: 0 to 99.9 L/min
Low peak pressure alarm: 0 to 60 cm H_2O
High peak pressure alarm range: 5 to 120 cm H_2O
Apnea interval: 10 to 60 sec

---

*Functions used by company technical support personnel.

[†]F_IO_2 calibration can be done using either ambient air or a 100% oxygen calibration. Either can be done on or off a patient, but it affects F_IO_2 delivery while it is being performed. Oxygen calibration takes about 4 minutes.

Screen Controls: Setting Ventilator Parameters

For each mode of ventilation, screen controls appear at the bottom of the screen for setting up the mode that has been selected. As seen in Figure 12-17, the parameters appear as circular screen controls. In this figure, the mode is PRESSURE A/C. The available parameters shown are rate (breaths/min), inspiratory pressure (cm H_2O), inspiratory time (seconds), PEEP (cm H_2O), flow trigger (L/min), and %O_2. (NOTE: The controls vary, depending on the mode of ventilation selected.) Table 12-5 lists the primary breath controls.

To change a parameter, the operator touches the screen directly over the control. This changes the screen control color. To change the value, the operator uses the DATA DIAL. Turning the dial in a clockwise direction increases the selected value, and turning it counterclockwise decreases it. To accept the displayed value, the operator either touches the screen directly over the highlighted control or presses the ACCEPT membrane button located near the DATA DIAL. The control color changes back to normal, and the ventilator begins operating with the new setting.

If the CANCEL button is pressed or the parameter is not actively accepted within 15 seconds, the ventilator continues at the previous settings.

Monitors

With a ventilation mode active, a column of five parameters is listed on the left side of screen (see Figure 12-17). These are the five currently selected monitored parameters. Each of these five positions has five available options. For example, the top position allows the selection of any of the following to be displayed in that position: exhaled tidal volume (Vte), inhaled tidal volume (Vti), spontaneous tidal volume (Spont Vt), mandatory tidal volume (Mand Vt), and minute volume (Ve). The operator can select the monitored parameter to be displayed in each of these five positions.

Table 12-6 lists all the available parameters that are monitored and the ranges for each. A monitor screen can also be activated to view 15 monitored parameters at one time.

TABLE 12-5
Primary Breath Controls—Vela

Control (Label)	Range (Default)
Breath rate (rate)	2-80 breaths/min (12 breaths/min)
Tidal volume (volume)	5-2000 mL (500 mL)
Inspiratory pressure (Insp Pres)	1-100 cm H_2O (15 cm H_2O)
Inspiratory time (I-Time)	0.3-10 sec (0.3 sec)
Peak flow (Peak Flow)*	10-140 L/min (35 L/min)†
Inspiratory pause (Insp Pause)	Off, 0.1-2 sec
PSV (Pressure Support)	Off, 1-60 cm H_2O (0 cm H_2O)
Positive end-expiratory pressure (PEEP)	0-35 cm H_2O (0 cm H_2O)
Inspiratory flow trigger (Flow Trig)	1-20 L/min, Off (2 L/min)

*Volume ventilation.
†Maximum available peak flow is 180 L/min.

TABLE 12-6
Monitored Parameters—Vela

Monitored Parameter	Range
Total breath rate (f)	0-250 breaths/min
Inspired tidal volume (Vti)	0-4000 mL
Spontaneous breath rate (f)	0-250 breaths/min
Mandatory exhaled tidal volume (Mand Vt)	0-4000 mL
Spontaneous exhaled tidal volume (spont Vt)	0-4000 mL
Exhaled minute volume (Ve)	0-99.9 L/min
Spontaneous exhaled minute volume (Spon Ve)	0-99.9 L/min
Mandatory exhaled minute volume (Mand Ve)	0-99.9 L/min
Peak inspiratory pressure (Ppeak)	0-140 cm H_2O
Mean airway pressure (Pmean)	0-99 cm H_2O
Positive end-expiratory pressure (PEEP)	0-99 cm H_2O
Inspiratory time (Ti)	0.01-99.99 sec
Expiratory time (Te)	0.01-99.99 sec
I:E ratio (I:E)	1:99-99:1
Oxygen-regulated pressure	0-100 psig
Percent oxygen	18% to 100%

ALARMS

Alarms available on the Vela include high- and low-pressure alarm limits, low–minute volume alarm, high-breath rate alarm, and apnea interval. Preset alarms for high and low regulated oxygen pressure are also available. Alarms are audible and visual. Alarm messages appear in the upper righthand corner of the screen.

To access the ALARM LIMITS set-up screen, the operator presses the LIMITS control in the lower right area of the screen (see Box 12-12 for information on alarm ranges).

MODES OF VENTILATION

Box 12-13 lists the modes of ventilation available for invasive and noninvasive ventilation. Available modes are continuous mandatory ventilation (CMV), referred to on the Vela as ASSIST/CONTROL (A/C), intermittent mandatory ventilation (IMV), referred to on the Vela as SIMV, and continuous spontaneous ventilation (CSV), labeled on the Vela as CPAP/PSV.

Breath control types include volume and pressure. Pressure-regulated volume control (PRVC) is a self-adjusting breath type. Breaths are pressure limited and volume targeted to the set volume. (See Chapter 11 for more information on PRVC.) PRVC can be selected in either the A/C or the SIMV mode.

Breath delivery in A/C can be patient or time triggered, volume or pressure limited, and time cycled. During SIMV, mandatory breaths are either patient or time triggered, volume or pressure limited, and time cycled. Spontaneous breaths during SIMV are patient triggered, pressure limited, and flow cycled.

In spontaneous ventilation (CPAP/PSV), selecting PEEP sets the CPAP level, and setting the pressure determines the pressure target for a PSV breath. The flow-cycling criteria for pressure support in the Vela is adjustable from

BOX 12-13   Modes of Ventilation (Vela)

INVASIVE MODES
Volume Assist/Control (Volume A/C)
Pressure Assist/Control (Pressure A/C)
PRVC A/C
Volume SIMV
Pressure SIMV
PRVC SIMV
CPAP/PSV
APRV/Biphasic

NONINVASIVE MODES
NPPV A/C
NPPV/SIMV
NPPV/CPAP PSV

APRV, Airway pressure release ventilation; *CPAP,* continuous positive airway pressure; *NPPV,* noninvasive positive pressure ventilation; *PRVC,* pressure regulated, volume controlled; *PSV,* pressure-support ventilation; *SIMV,* synchronized intermittent mandatory ventilation.

TABLE 12-7	
APRV/BiPhasic Parameter Ranges—Vela	
Parameter	**Range (Default)**
Pressure high (Pressure High)	0-60 cm H_2O (15 cm H_2O)
Pressure low (Pressure Low)	0-45 cm H_2O (6 cm H_2O)
Time High	0.3-30 sec (4 sec)
Time Low	0.3-30 sec (2 sec)

APRV, Airway pressure release ventilation.

5% to 30%. A unique feature of the Vela is that pressure control can be flow cycled (Off to 30%) as well as time cycled.

The baseline pressure in any mode is determined by the PEEP setting. Bias flow is adjustable from 10 to 20 L/min.

Airway Pressure-Release Ventilation/BiPhasic (APRV/BiPhasic)

In addition to traditional modes, the Vela also has APRV, as described in Chapter 11. The controls available for this mode are shown in Table 12-7. The TIME HIGH and TIME LOW settings are maximum time settings. Information about the use of APRV is available elsewhere.[2]

Pressure support can be added to either the high or low time periods. During TIME LOW, PSV is adjusted with the normal pressure-support controls. During TIME HIGH, PSV is adjusted with an advanced setting (T HIGH PSV). If T HIGH PSV is activated, the ventilator delivers the same level of pressure support during both TIME HIGH and TIME LOW.

The Vela can synchronize the change from PRESSURE LOW to PRESSURE HIGH. Advanced settings of TIME HIGH and TIME LOW allow the adjustment of a SYNC window to provide patient synchronization. SYNC is adjustable from 0 to 50%. The ventilator synchronizes the change from PRESSURE LOW to PRESSURE HIGH when it detects an inspiratory effort within the T LOW SYNC window. Transition from PRESSURE HIGH to PRESSURE LOW occurs with the end of inspiration detected after the T HIGH SYNC window opens. If the SYNC is set to zero (0%), transition between pressures is based on the time settings.

Apnea Backup Ventilation (ABV)

Certain modes rely on spontaneous ventilation from the patient when they are selected. These include the following:

- SIMV
- APRV/BiPhasic
- CPAP/PSV
- NPPV/CPAP PSV

When any of these spontaneous modes are selected, APNEA MODE choices appear on the screen. The apnea settings screen allows the operator to select the rate, volume (or pressure), flow (or Ti), pause, NPPV PSV, PEEP, flow trigger, and F_1O_2 for apnea backup ventilation. Apnea backup ventilation defaults to a breath rate of 12 breaths/

min, unless a higher rate is set. The operator must set the primary controls visible at the bottom of the touch screen for the selected apnea breath type before pressing the MODE ACCEPT button.

In SIMV, the apnea backup breaths are delivered at the current ventilator breath settings (volume or pressure). (NOTE: The controls for the apnea breath type are not visible once the MODE ACCEPT button has been pressed. Only during CPAP/PSV do the controls remain visible.)

Apnea ventilation activates if no patient effort is detected during the APNEA INTERVAL set in the ALARMS screen. A high priority alarm (audible and visual) occurs when ABV is initiated. During apnea backup ventilation, normal ventilation resumes at its current settings once the patient initiates two consecutive breaths or the ALARM RESET button is pushed.

Noninvasive Ventilation (NIV)

Noninvasive ventilation uses the same circuit as invasive ventilation on the Vela, but the patient interface changes to some type of mask (see Chapter 14). Masks used with the Vela should not have valves or leak vents (i.e., they should be nonvented masks). Adjusting the BIAS FLOW, along with using the LEAK COMPENSATION feature, can help overcome leaks and optimize the ventilator's sensitivity to a patient's efforts. If nuisance alarms occur, the low minute ventilation alarm can be deactivated in NIV (under the EXTENDED FUNCTIONS screen).

SPECIAL FUNCTIONS: ADVANCED SETTINGS

A variety of advanced settings may be used on the Vela, depending on the version of the ventilator available and the mode and primary breath controls that have been set. The advanced settings allow additional adjustments to be made to the primary breath control. Advanced settings are accessed by pressing the ADV SETTINGS button at the bottom right of the touch screen. When this button is pressed, the advanced settings available for the current mode and breath type appear.

Assured Volume (on the Vela Comprehensive)

Assured volume sets the minimum tidal volume for a pressure-targeted breath (e.g., PRESSURE A/C and PRESSURE SIMV). When a pressure-targeted (pressure-control) breath is delivered, if the set ASSURED VOLUME has not been met during the breath, the ventilator transitions to continuous flow to ensure that the set volume is delivered. If the tidal volume delivered equals or exceeds the set ASSURED VOLUME during delivery of a pressure breath, the ventilator time cycles out of inspiration (Clinical Rounds 12-5).

Volume Limit

Volume limit (VOL LIMIT) sets the maximum volume for a pressure breath. It is active for PRVC/Vsync breaths only.

CLINICAL ROUNDS 12-5

During PRESSURE A/C ventilation with the Vela ventilator, the therapist sets the pressure at 22 cm H_2O, the PEEP at 5 cm H_2O, and the inspiratory time at 1.1 seconds. The ASSURED VOLUME is set at 500 mL for the patient. Initial tidal volumes at the time were measured at 550 mL. Over a period of several hours, the patient's lung compliance progressively decreases. During patient assessment, the therapist notes that the inspiratory time is 1.5 seconds and the tidal volume is 500 mL. Explain what the ventilator is doing at this time.

See Evolve Resources for the answer.

If the measured volume meets or exceeds the set VOL LIMIT, inspiration ends (volume cycled). This is indicated by the ventilator alarm status indicator, which turns yellow, and the words VOLUME LIMIT are displayed. (NOTE: The alarm status indicator cannot be reset until a breath that does not meet the volume limit threshold is delivered.)

The operator's manual states that high inspiratory flow rates or the use of very compliant ventilator circuits may allow delivery of a tidal volume that exceeds the set VOL LIMIT. This can be caused by circuit recoil, with additional volume going to the patient. Because of this, delivered tidal volume should be monitored closely.

Vsync

VSYNC is available when VOLUME A/C and VOLUME SIMV modes are selected. When VSYNC is activated, volume breaths are delivered as pressure-limited breaths with the volume delivery targeted at the set volume. As with any pressure breath, the inspiratory flow pattern becomes a descending flow pattern.

The first breath that occurs when VSYNC is activated is a volume breath with an inspiratory pause (40 msec) that allows the ventilator to determine system compliance and resistance. With the available information, the ventilator targets the pressure for the next breath (a pressure-limited breath) so that the set volume is delivered. If the volume is not delivered, the ventilator increases pressure (3 cm H_2O) to achieve the set volume. If the volume is too high, the ventilator steps down the pressure. Maximum volume delivery is determined by the VOL LIMIT setting.

Flow Cycle—Pressure-Control Breaths

The FLOW CYCLE control allows the operator to set the percent of measured peak inspiratory flow at which the ventilator ends a pressure-control breath. The available range is 0 (off) to 30%, with 0 (off) being the default.

Selecting the Flow Pattern in Volume Ventilation

In the Vela Comprehensive, the operator has the option of selecting either a descending (DECEL) or constant (SQUARE) waveform. This option is available in volume breath delivery. The descending waveform is the default.

Additional Options

In addition to the features described, a few other features are available. These are explained in Box 12-14.

TROUBLESHOOTING

Alarms and messages help in troubleshooting most of the common problems that occur during ventilation with the Vela. In addition, the operator's manual provides information about alarm conditions.

BOX 12-14	Advanced Settings (Vela)

Sigh—When this function is on, the ventilator delivers a sigh breath 1.5 times the set tidal volume every 100 breaths or every 7 minutes, whichever occurs first.

Bias Flow—Adjustable from 10 to 20 L/min.

PC Flow Cycle—Sets the percent of peak inspiratory flow at which inspiration ends in a pressure-controlled breath (range, 5% to 30%; default, Off).

PSV Cycle—Sets the percent of peak inspiratory flow at which inspiration ends for a pressure support breath (range, 5% to 30%; default, 25%).

PSV Tmax—Determines the maximum inspiratory time of a pressure-support breath (range, 0.3 to 3 sec; default, 3 sec).

Time High—Available in APRV/BiPhasic mode only; sets the maximum time at the high pressure setting (range, 0.2 to 30 sec; default, 4 sec).

Time Low—Available in APRV/BiPhasic mode only; sets the maximum time at the low pressure setting (range, 0.2 to 30 sec; default, 2 sec).

KEY POINTS

▶ The Vela uses an internal turbine to provide a source of pressurized air for ventilation.

▶ Either a high-pressure (40 to 65 psig) oxygen source or a low-pressure O_2 source, from an O_2 flowmeter, can be used to provide oxygen.

▶ Using the nebulizer line provided by the Vela requires high-pressure O_2. It also results in an increase in V_T and peak pressure and a change in F_IO_2.

▶ LEAK COMPENSATION is automatically activated when noninvasive ventilation is used.

▶ The selection of the type of humidifier determines the calculation of volume displays (BTPS).

▶ The function of VSYNC used with volume ventilation is similar to pressure-regulated volume control (PRVC) ventilation.

ASSESSMENT QUESTIONS

See Evolve Resources for the answers.

1. When the Vela is using a low-pressure oxygen source, which of the following statements is/are true?
   I. The oxygen control must be set at the estimated oxygen delivery percentage.
   II. The Vela operator's manual provides a way to estimate the F_IO_2 delivery based on the flowmeter setting and the patient's minute ventilation.
   III. The flowmeter must be set to at least 10 L/min.
   IV. The ventilator is connected to an O_2 flowmeter by oxygen tubing.
   a. I
   b. II and III
   c. I and IV
   d. II and IV

2. When LEAK COMPENSATION is active, the ventilator displays what monitored exhaled volume?
   a. The volume that flows through the expiratory sensor
   b. The volume that flows out of the ventilator to the main inspiratory limb of the patient circuit
   c. The value for the inspired volume minus the leaked volume measured
   d. The volume that flows through the expiratory sensor plus the volume that leaks out of the circuit

3. For a preuse test on the Vela, which of the following are required?
   I. The patient must not be connected to the ventilator.
   II. The ventilator must be in the OFF position.
   III. The operator must press and hold the ACCEPT button and turn the ventilator ON.
   IV. The ACCEPT button is released only when the UVT START UP message appears on the screen.
   a. I and II
   b. II and III
   c. I and IV
   d. I, II, III, and IV

4. Which of the following statements is/are true regarding apnea backup ventilation?
   I. It is available whenever a spontaneous mode is selected.
   II. Apnea backup ventilation defaults to a breath rate of 12 breaths/min unless a higher rate is set.
   III. The operator must set the primary controls for apnea backup before pressing the MODE ACCEPT button.
   IV. In *all* modes, the controls for the apnea breath type are not visible once the MODE ACCEPT button has been pressed.
   a. I
   b. III and IV
   c. I, II, and III
   d. I, II, III, and IV

5. The function of VOL LIMIT is to:
   a. Ensure a minimum volume delivery during pressure ventilation
   b. Limit the volume for a pressure breath
   c. Limit the volume for any breath during spontaneous ventilation
   d. Guarantee a volume limit during APRV

References

1. Vela Ventilator Systems, Operator's Manual (Cardinal Health Care [previously VIASYS Respiratory Care]), part no. L1533 Revision F, June 2005, Dublin, Ohio.

2. Pilbeam SP, Cairo JM: *Mechanical ventilation: physiological and clinical application*, ed 4, St Louis, 2006, Mosby-Elsevier.

Internet Resource
www.cardinal.com

DRÄGER VENTILATORS

DRÄGER EVITA

The Dräger Evita was the first in a series of ventilators manufactured by Drägerwerk in Lübeck, Germany (represented in the United States by Dräger Corp., Telford, Pennsylvania). Information about the original Evita ventilator is available on the Evolve Resources Web site for this text.

DRÄGER EVITA 2 DURA

The Dräger Evita 2 Dura is a modification of the Evita 2, which was never marketed in the United States. The Evita 2 Dura is manufactured by Drägerwerk and represented in the United States by the Dräger Corp. There are many similarities between the Evita 2 Dura and the Dräger E-4 (Evita 4) ventilator. Because the E-4 is used more in the United States than the Evita 2 Dura, the E-4 is presented in detail here. Information about the Evita 2 Dura is presented on the Evolve Resources Web site for this text.

DRÄGER E-4 (EVITA 4)

OUTLINE

Power Source
Internal Mechanism
Patient Circuit
Controls and Alarms
   Peripheral Controls
   Overview of Standby Controls
   Monitors and Alarms
Modes of Ventilation
   Standard Settings of Ventilator Modes
   Continuous Mandatory Ventilation (CMV)
   SIMV and SIMV with Pressure-Support Ventilation
    (SIMV + PSV)
   Pressure-Control Ventilation Plus (PCV+)
   Pressure-Support Ventilation (PSV)
   Continuous Positive Airway Pressure (CPAP)
   Airway Pressure-Release Ventilation (APRV)

Mandatory Minute Volume Ventilation (MMV) and
   MMV with Pressure-Support Ventilation
   (MMV/PSV)
Apnea Ventilation
AutoFlow
Proportional Pressure Support (PPS)
NeoFlow
Special Functions
   Sigh (Intermittent PEEP)
   Intrinsic PEEP
   Occlusion Pressure
   Special Function Touch Pads
   Special Upgrades with Software Update 2.n
Ventilator Graphic Waveforms
Troubleshooting

OBJECTIVES

Upon completion of this section, you will be able to:
- Describe the front panel on the Dräger E-4.
- Discuss the function of each control on the E-4 front panel.
- Compare the set-up of a ventilator mode on the E-4 with that on another microprocessor-controlled intensive care unit (ICU) ventilator.
- Assess an alarm situation, describe its priority level, and suggest a possible cause and solution.
- Identify a pressure-time graph for a patient breathing spontaneously during PCV.
- Compare the upper Paw alarm limit to the Pmax pressure limit.
- Describe the method for setting PCV and APRV and compare it with the two modes of ventilation.
- Discuss the similarities and differences for AutoFlow and PRVC on the Servo 300 (see Chapter 11).
- List the features available when NeoFlow is added as an upgrade to the Dräger E-4.
- Explain the set-up and function of proportional pressure support.

KEY TERMS

Airway pressure-release ventilation
   (APRV)
Apnea ventilation
AutoFlow
Continuous mandatory ventilation
   (CMV)
Continuous positive airway pressure
   (CPAP)
Cyber knobs
Cyber pads
Electromagnetic servo valves

Flow trigger
Inspiratory hold
Inspiratory pause
Inspiratory time (T_I)
Mandatory breaths
Mandatory minute volume ventilation
   (MMV)
Maximum pressure limit (Pmax)
Microprocessor
Monitors
NeoFlow

Occlusion pressure (P0.1)
Pmax pressure limit
Pressure support (PS)
Pressure-support ventilation (PSV)
Proportional pressure support
   (PPS)
Sensitivity
Synchronized intermittent
   mandatory ventilation (SIMV)

Dräger Medical has been manufacturing a line of critical care ventilators for many years, including the Dräger Evita, Dräger Evita 2 (E-2) Dura, Dräger Evita 4 (E-4 and E-4 *edition*), and the Dräger EvitaXL. (NOTE: The company did not manufacture an Evita 3.) The Savina is an addition to the fleet that is intended for the low- to medium-level ICU.

The Dräger Evita (Evita 1) ventilator was the first in the series and was manufactured by Drägerwerk in Lubeck, Germany. The Evita is no longer available for purchase. Information on the features and operation of the Dräger Evita is available on the Evolve Resources Web site for this text.

The Evita 2 was a modified version of the Evita (Evita 1), but it was never marketed in the United States. A second version, the Evita 2 Dura, replaced the Evita 2 and was marketed internationally. The Evita 2 Dura can be purchased in a basic configuration, and options and software can be added to upgrade it to an E-4, if desired. For additional information on the Evita 2 Dura, see the Evolve Resources Web site for this text.

The Evita 4, or E-4, was the next version of the Evita series (Figure 12-19).[1,2] The manufacturer refers to the E-4 as the Dräger E-4 Pulmonary Work Station because it can monitor a variety of patient information. It also is available as the E-4 *edition,* the upgraded version of the original E-4. The Dräger EvitaXL followed the E-4. Both the E-4 and the E-4 *edition* can be upgraded to an EvitaXL. All these units are designed for use with neonatal to adult patients, primarily in the acute care setting.

The internal operative system of the Savina is similar to that of the Evita ventilators, but fewer of the optional features are available with the basic unit. The Savina can be used with pediatric and adult patients for both invasive and noninvasive ventilation. It is a much more compact unit than the Evitas and seems to be more popular for subacute and long-term care units or hospitals.

The following section reviews the function and features of the E-4. Because software and options can be upgraded or changed, readers are advised to check the software version of the E-4 they are using and check for any options that may have been added compared with those presented in this text. The user should always follow the warnings and safety precautions in the manufacturer's operating manual. The manual should be the primary source for operation of the ventilator.

DRÄGER E-4

The front panel of the Dräger E-4 has touch pads, a rotary (dial) knob, and a computer screen. The infrared touch screen uses light beam interruption technology. Images or icons are present on the screen. Some are shaped like knobs (soft knobs, or **cyber knobs**), and some are shaped like touch pads (soft pads, or **cyber pads**). All these dials and knobs (discussed later in this section) are used to control the unit.

Below the front operating panel are the connections for the main inspiratory and expiratory lines, the expiratory valve, and the nipple connector for the nebulizer line. The expiratory flow sensor is to the left of the expiratory valve. On the far right side, below the unit's main control knob (rotary knob), is a protective cover that hides the oxygen sensor and the ambient air filter.

POWER SOURCE

The E-4 normally uses two 50-psig gas sources (air and oxygen, ranging from about 40 to 87 psig). The unit can operate on a single gas source if the second is unavailable, but it will issue an alert when one gas source is used, because this alters oxygen-delivery capabilities. A standard AC 120-volt outlet is used to power the **microprocessor** and the electrical components. The on/off switch is located on the back panel of the unit.

INTERNAL MECHANISM

The internal mechanism is similar to those of many of the recently released ICU ventilators. The gas sources enter the

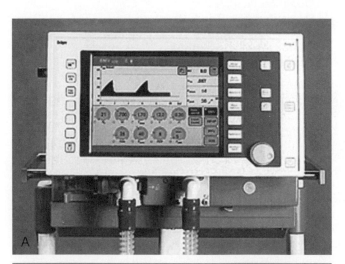

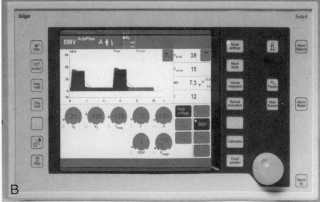

FIGURE 12-19 A, Dräger E-4 (Evita 4) ventilator. **B,** Full screen with controls. (Courtesy Dräger, Telford, Pa.)

unit through connections on the back panel and pass through filters. Their pressure is measured and reduced to a working pressure. The incoming flow is then directed to two flow-control valves. (NOTE: In the Dräger Dura and the E-4, these flow-control valves are high-pressure **electromagnetic servo valves.**) The function of these valves is controlled by the microprocessor, which uses information from the settings on the front panel, internal flow, pressure transducers, and the action of the valves themselves to control the flow to the patient. These valves regulate the amount of pressure and flow and the flow waveform of the gas delivered according to the selected modes and settings. The valves also control the F_IO_2 based on the set value, and the changes are instantaneous. (NOTE: Information on the flow-control valves and transducers can be found in Chapter 11.) From the flow-control valves, gas is directed to the patient.

A variety of pressure and flow transducers monitor internal gas flow, the output from the unit, and the gas return from the patient through the expiratory valve.

PATIENT CIRCUIT

Connections for the patient circuit are located just below the front panel (see Figure 12-19A). The inspiratory line is located on the right. Either a heated humidifier or a heat and moisture exchanger (HME) can be used with the Evita 4. (NOTE: The two should *never* be used together.) The expiratory line connection is below the front panel on the left. The expiratory valve assembly is connected to the ventilator near the main expiratory line connection.

CONTROLS AND ALARMS

A number of controls, **monitors,** and alarm settings are available on the Dräger E-4. Basically, the E-4 uses a single rotary knob, several hard touch pads on the side of the computer screen, and the touch-sensitive soft knobs (cyber knobs) and soft pads (cyber pads) on the computer screen (Figure 12-20).

Peripheral Controls

Several controls used during normal operation of the ventilator are located on both sides of the screen. Those on the left side of the screen include the nebulizer, suction 100% O_2, **inspiratory hold,** print, and several blank keys for future upgrades. These controls are reviewed in the discussion of special functions later in this section.

On the immediate right side of the computer screen are touch pads, which are used to select several operations. These include the following:

1. MODE SETTINGS
2. ALARM LIMITS
3. VALUES MEASURED
4. SPECIAL PROCEDURE
5. A blank key (for upgrades)

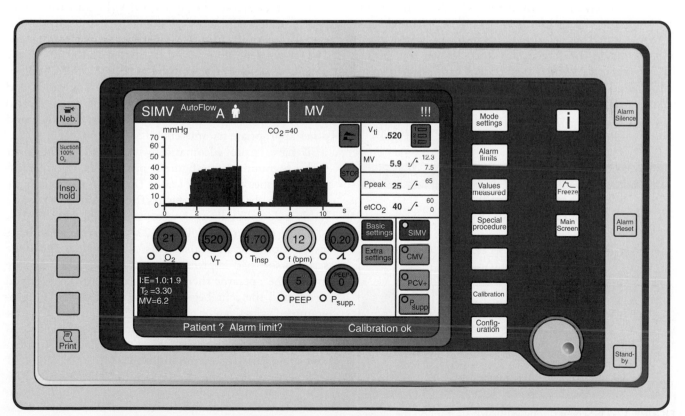

FIGURE 12-20 Front panel of the Dräger E-4 ventilator, showing the touch pad controls, the rotary knob, and the screen in a standard ventilating mode.

6. CALIBRATION
7. CONFIGURATION

The function of each touch pad is covered as the various controls and alarms are described.

Three more touch pads and the rotary knob are to the right of the screen. The touch pads include an information key (i), a freeze control to freeze graphic waveforms, and a main screen pad for selecting standard menus to appear on the computer screen.

The knob can be rotated to select numeric values for parameters and pressed to activate the new parameters. It also can be used to move the cursor (vertical line) on the screen when it appears under certain functions.

On the far right side of the front panel are the following additional touch pads:

1. ALARM SILENCE (2 minutes)
2. ALARM RESET
3. STANDBY (for switching between the standby and the operating modes)

Overview of Standby Controls

After the power switch is turned on, the unit runs a series of self-tests and a signal can be heard. After the tests are complete, the screen asks the operator to select adult, pediatric, or neonate (E-4 upgraded version 2.n software) by touching the desired soft pad (cyber pad) and entering the ideal body weight (IBW) of the patient (Figure 12-21). The available volumes and flows are different for each type of patient (Table 12-8). To set the IBW, the operator touches the screen soft knob for IBW, which highlights the knob and changes its color to yellow. The dial knob is then rotated to set the actual numeric value, which appears inside the screen soft knob. When the desired IBW appears, the knob is pushed to set the selected value; this changes the soft knob from yellow to green to show that the value has been set. These same actions (touching [the soft knob or cyber pad], turning [the rotary knob],

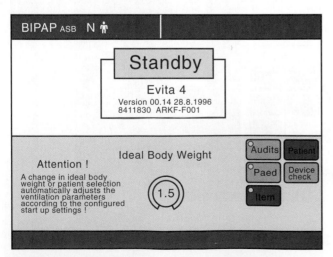

FIGURE 12-21 Screen during ventilator start-up on the Dräger E-4 version 2.n with NeoFlow. (Redrawn from Dräger, Telford, Pa.)

TABLE 12-8	
Parameter Ranges—Dräger E-4	
Tidal Volume	
Adult	0.1-2 L
Pediatric	20-300 mL
Neonate	3-100 mL
Flow	
Adult	6-120 L/min (to 180 L/min with Autoflow)
Pediatric	6-30 L/min (to 60 L/min with Autoflow)
Neonate	0.25-30 L/min
Neonate continuous flow	6 L/min
Variable Ranges for All Patients	
Respiratory rate	0-100 breaths/min
	0-150 breaths/min with NeoFlow
Inspiratory time	0.1-10 sec
Inspiratory pressure (set)	0-80 cm H$_2$O
Maximum pressure limit	0-100 cm H$_2$O
Percent oxygen	21% to 100%
PEEP	0-35 cm H$_2$O
Trigger sensitivity	0.3-15 L/min
Pressure support	0-80 cm H$_2$O
Rise time for PS	0-2 sec

and pushing [the rotary knob]) are how most controls are set. The manufacturer refers to this sequence as "touch, adjust, confirm."

The unit requests the patient's IBW because the microprocessor is programmed at the factory to begin ventilation automatically using CMV with factory-set parameters. The factory default V$_T$ is 7 mL/kg, based on the IBW of the patient. The respiratory rate is based on Radford's nomogram for the V$_E$ of a person that size.[3] The mode and parameters may be reconfigured, but the operator can also do a standard ventilator set-up and select the mode and other appropriate parameters.

To have the unit automatically start ventilating a patient with programmed (configured) parameters, the operator simply pushes the rotary knob. To set up the unit more specifically, the operator touches the STANDBY soft key and holds it down for about 3 seconds until the unit displays STANDBY ACTIVATED (Figure 12-22). The ventilation are shut off, but all adjustments can be made. The mode settings soft pad is pressed, and the desired settings are made. The operator then touches the STANDBY soft pad again, and the unit begins ventilation. (NOTE: The programmed values can be changed by "configuring" the unit so that some other mode and parameters are available as soon as ventilation is started. See the discussion of configuration in this section and in Box 12-15.)

Because of the design of the E-4 unit, the control knobs that appear on the screen vary for each mode of ventilation selected. For example, if the operator wants to use the **synchronized intermittent mandatory ventilation (SIMV)** mode in volume ventilation, only the controls

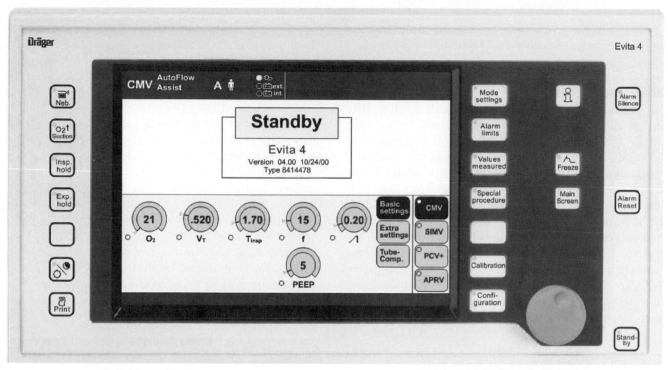

FIGURE 12-22 Standby screen showing controls for setting up CMV ventilation on the Dräger E-4. (Courtesy Dräger, Telford, Pa.)

BOX 12-15   Configuring the Ventilator, or Setting Parameters and Functions into Memory (Dräger E-4)

As with many computer programs, the Dräger E-4 microprocessor permits the operator to set a certain mode and its parameters. The operating manual provides a detailed description of each adjustment that can be made during configuration of the unit. A few examples are provided here.

To access the configuration function, press the configuration touch pad. The computer screen lists a menu of parameters or variables the operator can select, including values, curves, trends, sound, screen, ventilation, and system defaults. To adjust any available screen, touch the desired soft pad. For example, if you wish to change the values measured screen, touch the values soft pad to bring up a menu of current available values (e.g., MV, Pplat, C, R, and f).

To replace one value with another, touch the appropriate soft pad to highlight the value to be deleted. A column of all the available measured and calculated variables appears to the left. Using the dial knob, select

(highlight) the variable you want to be displayed. When it is highlighted, push the dial knob to replace the variable being deleted.

A similar procedure is available to change graphic waveforms, data trends, ventilation parameters, and system defaults. System defaults allow the unit to access specific external computer ports, such as the port that connects to a printer. System defaults also let you select computer variables, such as baud rate and parity check bits. System defaults provide a way to change the date, time, and language on the screen or the desired units of measurement (e.g., mbar [millibars] or cm H_2O).

If you want to change the ventilation mode and the parameters that automatically appear when the unit is turned on, you must enter an access code. The access code usually is given to the individuals in the department who have the authority to change this set function (e.g., the clinical specialist or the department head).

---

that are active in that mode appear on the screen. For this reason, it is easier to discuss the various controls as their uses or the specific modes are discussed. The available ranges for control parameters are listed in Table 12-8. If the operator goes beyond the range of normal ventilation for a parameter, the knob stops adjusting as it is turned. A message appears at the bottom of the screen telling the operator what needs to be done to continue. For example, if the operator selects a respiratory rate of 4 breaths/min in SIMV and the **inspiratory time (T_I)** is set at 1 second,

the knob will freeze and the message at the bottom will read I:E < 1:3 CONFIRM, followed by an icon for the rotary knob. When the operator presses the knob, the SIMV rate will drop below 4 breaths/min with a T_I of 1 second.

Monitors and Alarms

In every mode of ventilation, the E-4 provides monitored parameters at the top of the screen. A graphic may be present on the left side. On the top right are current values, such as O_2%, Ppeak, Pplat, and minute ventilation (MV).

Although these are the variables most commonly selected, they can be changed by the institution according to the standards of the clinical site. Box 12-16 describes the selection of ventilator parameters for display.

Measured Values

The VALUES MEASURED touch pad brings up a screen that displays values being measured or calculated by the unit, such as F_IO_2 (Table 12-9 and Figure 12-23). The ventilator has a built-in oxygen analyzer and does an automatic oxygen calibration every 24 hours. The unit optimally can include a mainstream carbon dioxide analyzer that provides information on end-tidal carbon dioxide (etCO_2), CO_2/time, and single-breath CO_2 (CO_2/volume). Calculated values include carbon dioxide production ($\dot{V}CO_2$) dead space (V_D), and V_D/V_T measurements. The analyzer normally is taken out of the circuit and calibrated before use. A special block built into the ventilator allows zero and reference calibration of the carbon dioxide analyzer (see the operator's manual for instructions).[1]

Alarms

Alarms can be set by pressing the ALARM LIMITS soft pad, which provides a screen display allowing adjustment of the available alarm values (Figure 12-24). For example, to set the HIGH RATE alarm, touch the soft pad (cyber pad) adjacent to the respiratory rate (f_{spn}). The soft pad changes from green to yellow. Using the rotary knob, set the desired high rate; the number appears inside the soft pad. Press the dial knob to activate the new setting; the soft pad changes back to green. Table 12-10 lists the ranges for the adjustable alarms. The limits for $O_2\%$ are set automatically by the ventilator (Table 12-10). The automatic alarm limit for low airway pressure is the set PEEP value plus 5 cm H_2O. For example, if PEEP is 5 cm H_2O, the low pressure limit is 10 cm H_2O and is not adjustable. When the upper Paw alarm limit is reached, an audible and visual alarm is activated, inspiratory flow delivery stops, and the expiratory valve opens, dropping pressure to baseline. This alarm is functional in all modes of ventilation

---

BOX 12-16	Selecting Displayed Parameters (Dräger E-4)

The E-4 allows graphed and digitally displayed information to be viewed. Available graphs include pressure, flow, volume, and end-tidal CO_2, graphed per unit of time. Any two graphs may be selected by touching the green soft (cyber) pad at the top right of the curve and then touching the particular curve.

  On the top right, digital measurements are displayed in three groups of four. Scroll through these measurements by touching the green soft pad at the top right of the measurements. O_2, V_T exhaled, MV, and f (frequency) are the most common. Pressures (Ppeak, Pplat, PEEP, and mean airway pressure) are the most common for Screen 2. End-tidal data often are placed on Screen 3.

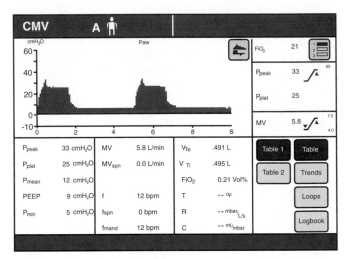

FIGURE 12-23 Example of a VALUES MEASURED screen on the Dräger E-4 ventilator. (Redrawn from Dräger, Telford, Pa.)

TABLE 12-9

Commonly Measured and Displayed Parameters—Dräger E-4

Parameter	Definition	Range
Ppeak	Peak pressure	0-99 cm H_2O
Pplat	Plateau pressure	0-99 cm H_2O
Pmean	Mean pressure	0-99 cm H_2O
PEEP	Positive end expir. press	0-99 cm H_2O
Pmin	Minimum pressure	0-99 cm H_2O
MV	Minute ventilation	0-99 L/min
MV$_{spn}$	Spontaneous MV	0-99 L/min
f	Total frequency	0-150 breaths/min
f$_{spn}$	Spontaneous frequency	0-150 breaths/min
fmand	Mandatory frequency	0-150 breaths/min
VTe	Exhaled tidal volume	0-3999 mL
VTi	Inhaled tidal volume	0-3999 mL
F$_IO_2$	Fractional inspired O_2	15% to 100%
T	Breathing gas temperature	18°-51°C
R	Resistance	0-600 cm H_2O/L/sec
C	Compliance	0-300 mL/cm H_2O

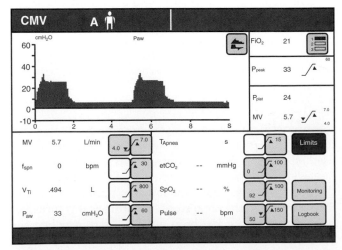

FIGURE 12-24 ALARM PARAMETER screen on the Dräger E-4. (Redrawn from Dräger, Telford, Pa.)

and is similar to the upper pressure limit on most ventilators. However, the Ppeak alarm is not to be confused with the Pmax pressure limit. The Pmax pressure limit is not an alarm; rather, it actually changes the way a breath is delivered during CMV, SIMV, and MMV ventilation. For this reason, Pmax is reviewed under the discussion of modes of ventilation.

Basically, the E-4 has three levels of alarm indicators:
· WARNING (top priority)
· CAUTION (medium priority)
· ADVISORY (low priority)

The function of each of these is listed in Table 12-11. After an alarm has been activated, the audible tone can be silenced with the ALARM SILENCE touch pad. The LED appears on the ALARM SILENCE pad when the audible alarms are inactive and is functional for 2 minutes. Once the problem has been corrected, the alarm is reset by touching the ALARM SILENCE soft pad (LED off). Medium and low priority messages do not need to be acknowledged after the problem is solved. However, high priority messages must be acknowledged by the operator to verify that the problem has been resolved; this is done by pressing the ALARM RESET touch pad. The message leaves the screen and is stored in memory. (NOTE: Access to the LOGBOOK func-

tion is available on the ALARM LIMITS and the MEASURED VALUES screens to recall any stored, top priority alarm messages.)

Examples of low priority alarms include AIR SUPPLY LOW, FLOW MONITORING OFF, and INSPIRATORY HOLD INTERRUPTED. Examples of medium priority alarms are AIR SUPPLY PRESSURE TOO HIGH, CHECK SETTINGS, and PRESSURE LIMITED. Examples of top priority alarms are numerous, such as APNEA, DEVICE FAILURE, and LOW O_2 SUPPLY. The operator's manual provides a list of all alarms.[1] After any top priority alarm, the operator must be absolutely certain that the patient is being ventilated. (NOTE: When a MIXER INOP alarm activates, the blender is defective, and the manufacturer advises that the patient be ventilated manually until the unit can be replaced. The problem unit should be removed from service until it is repaired by a service representative.)

MODES OF VENTILATION

Modes of operation available on the E-4 are listed in Box 12-17.

TABLE 12-10
Alarm Ranges—Dräger E-4

Parameter	Range
Minute ventilation	High MV: 0.5-41 L/min
	Low MV: 0-40 L/min
High f_{spn}*	0-120 breaths/min
High VTi*	30-4000 mL
High Paw	10-100 cm H_2O
Apnea time	5-60 sec
High end-tidal CO_2 (etCO_2)†	0-100 mm Hg
Low etCO_2†	0-99 mm Hg
Nonadjustable O2% Alarm	
O_2% less than 60%	Upper O_2% alarm: +4%
	Lower O_2% alarm: −4%
O_2% greater than 60%	Upper O_2% alarm: +6%
	Lower O_2% alarm: −6%

*No lower alarm limit available.
†Available only when CO_2 analyzer (capnograph) is added.

BOX 12-17   Modes of Ventilation (Dräger E-4)

CMV (continuous mandatory ventilation, an A/C mode)
SIMV (volume or pressure targeted)
SIMV + PSV
PCV+
PCV + PS
CPAP/PSV
APRV
BiPAP
MMV
MMV/PSV
Apnea ventilation
Autoflow*
PPS† (proportional pressure support)
NeoFlow*
Noninvasive ventilation (NIV)‡

*Available as an option.
†Available in parts of Europe.
‡Another available option on the E-4 (Evita 4) that is described in the section on the EvitaXL ventilator later in this chapter.

TABLE 12-11
Displayed Information with Priority Alarms—Dräger E-4

Alarm Light	Message* (on Screen)	Message (Background Color)	Audio	Alarm Level
Red flashing	Name of alarm followed by "!!!" (e.g., "APNEA!!!")	Red	Five tones; repeated twice every 15 sec	Warning; top priority
Yellow flashing	Name of alarm followed by "!!" (e.g., "O_2 PRESSURE HIGH!!")	Yellow	Three tones; repeated every 30 sec	Caution; medium priority
Yellow constant	Name of alarm followed by "!" (e.g., "FAN MALFUNCTION!")	Yellow	Two tones; occurs only once	Advisory; low priority

*Appears in the upper right corner of the screen.

Standard Settings of Ventilator Modes

When the ventilator is first turned on, the standard mode that is programmed (configured) is CMV (i.e., an assist-control [A/C] mode using volume ventilation). The institution purchasing the unit can change this by reconfiguring the unit. To change (reconfigure) the start-up mode, press CONFIGURE, then press the VENTILATION soft pad; enter the access code; touch MODES, select the desired start-up mode with the dial knob; and activate it by pressing the dial knob. The operator's manual provides a full description of how to configure the start-up modes and alarm settings.

If the operator wants to change the mode of ventilation, pressing the VENTILATION soft pad provides a screen that lists the available modes. When the new mode soft pad is pressed, the parameters that can be set in that mode appear on the screen, and the mode soft pad turns yellow. Parameters are set in a manner similar to the way in which alarm parameters are set. Touch the parameter soft knob that is to be changed (e.g., V_T). The soft knob changes from green to yellow. Turn the rotary knob to obtain the desired numeric value, which appears in the center of the soft knob. Then press the rotary knob to activate this setting. The old mode continues to operate until the new setting has been selected. When it is selected, the new mode soft pad changes to black. Inactive modes appear green.

The Dräger E-4 can provide flow triggering in all modes of ventilation. The flow-trigger level is set as follows:

- Touch the EXTRA SETTINGS soft pad
- Touch the FLOW-TRIGGER soft pad
- Touch the FLOW soft knob
- Dial in the desired flow-triggering value using the rotary knob
- Press the rotary knob to activate the newly set **flow trigger** value

Trigger **sensitivity** can be turned off only in CMV. However, situations in which sensitivity should be turned off are rare. PEEP/CPAP and $O_2\%$ can be selected in any mode. (NOTE: If the power fails or STANDBY is selected, the settings that were in effect before the interruption are again in effect when the unit is reactivated.)

Continuous Mandatory Ventilation (CMV)

The **continuous mandatory ventilation (CMV)** mode is an A/C volume ventilation mode. The operator sets V_T, flow, f (CMV), T_I, sensitivity, PEEP, F_IO_2, and the desired alarm settings. Breaths are patient or time triggered, volume targeted, and time cycled. All breaths deliver the set V_T.

Flow to the patient is constant at the flow setting value. If the flow is high and the V_T is delivered before T_I is achieved, the inspiratory valve closes (the expiratory valve is already closed), and the breath is held until the set T_I has elapsed. This can be identified by an **inspiratory pause** in

the pressure-time graph and flow returning to zero before the end of inspiration on the flow-time graph (Clinical Rounds 12-6; also see Figure 12-23). An inspiratory pause may also be identified by touching the I TIME or FLOW soft pad. When the pad is yellow, a blue **smart window** appears at the bottom left of the screen and displays the I:E ratio, T_E, and pause time. As the variable selected is changed, the new calculated values are displayed. For example, if the flow is decreased and T_I shortened, the pause time decreases.

The high peak pressures that may occur during volume ventilation can be avoided by using the Pmax pressure limit function. When Pmax is used, the pressure and flow delivery characteristics of the unit change (see the following discussion and Figure 12-25).

CLINICAL ROUNDS 12-6

You are setting up a patient on CMV with the Dräger E-4. The settings are as follows: V_T = 0.5 L (500 mL); f = 10 breaths/min; flow = 60 L/min; T_I = 2 seconds; and the waveform is constant.

Answer the following questions:
1. What is the I:E ratio?
2. How long does it take the ventilator to deliver the volume?
3. If the delivery time is shorter than the selected T_I, when does inspiration end?

See Evolve Resources for the answer.

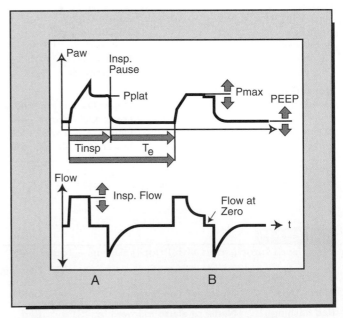

FIGURE 12-25 Pressure limit function on the Dräger E-4 operating during volume-targeted mandatory breaths. The top curve is a pressure-time curve, and the bottom curve is a flow-time curve. **A,** This breath shows a typical volume-delivered breath with a constant flow delivery. **B,** A second breath delivery illustrates when the pressure limit is selected. (See text for further explanation.) (Redrawn from Dräger, Telford, Pa.)

BOX 12-18	Pmax: Pressure Limit Function (Dräger E-4)

Pmax was the concept behind the first Evita ventilator. The manufacturer now believes that the AutoFlow function is superior to Pmax and should be the option of choice for pressure reduction. In Pmax, the operator may manually adjust it to within 3 cm H_2O of the plateau pressure (Pplat). In AutoFlow, the E-4 automatically brings the peak pressure (Ppeak) equal or close to the Pplat, as timing allows. In AutoFlow, the exhalation valve floats, but in Pmax it is closed. The manufacturer recommends that the Pmax be kept in the off position in machine configuration.[1]

Pmax Pressure Limit Function

Pmax pressure limit is a safety feature. It operates to control pressure during delivery of a volume breath in CMV, SIMV, and MMV modes (Box 12-18). To configure Pmax, the operator accesses CONFIGURE, then VENTILATION, enters the access code; touches MODES, and then PMAX.

When Pmax is operational, the ventilator limits the pressure delivered during a mandatory breath. During inspiration the pressure in the circuit rises quickly to the maximum pressure setting (PMAX). Inspiration continues for the set inspiratory time (time cycled), but the amount of pressure in the circuit does not go above this setting.

With Pmax, flow rises rapidly at the start of inspiration, along with pressure. Flow then plateaus at the set flow value. It remains constant at the set value until the set Pmax is reached, at which point flow descends to baseline. Pmax pressure is maintained throughout the remainder of T_I (see Figure 12-25).

Generally, the delivered V_T achieves the set value as long as flow drops to zero before the end of inspiration (i.e., an inspiratory hold). If flow does not drop to zero, the volume cannot be delivered, and a VOLUME NOT CONSTANT alarm activates.

It is recommended that the **AutoFlow** be used with this and any other volume mode so that patient flow is not restricted. When AutoFlow is used, it takes over the task of setting both INSP FLOW and PMAX, and these screen soft knob controls are no longer displayed (see the discussion of AutoFlow later in this section).

SIMV and SIMV with Pressure-Support Ventilation (SIMV + PSV)

As described in Chapter 11, SIMV provides a maximum number of **mandatory breaths** and allows the patient to breathe spontaneously between them. Mandatory breaths can be patient or time triggered, volume or pressure targeted, and time cycled. Spontaneous breaths can be assisted with **pressure support (PS),** in which case PS breaths are patient triggered, pressure targeted, and flow cycled.*

With SIMV, the operator selects the mandatory breath rate, which determines the time between mandatory breaths. For example, if the SIMV rate is 5 breaths/min, the time between mandatory breaths is 12 seconds (60 seconds/5 breaths/min). The patient can breathe spontaneously during the 12-second interval. All other adjustable parameters in SIMV are the same as those described in the previous section on CMV.

In the SIMV volume-targeted mode, the operator selects the target volume for the mandatory breaths. With SIMV *volume*-target, either Pmax or AutoFlow can also be used. With SIMV *pressure*-target, the operator sets the target pressure for mandatory breaths, but Pmax and AutoFlow are not active because breath delivery is already pressure targeted, and the ventilator controls these functions.

When SIMV is first activated, the patient has approximately a 5-second window during which to make an inspiratory effort and trigger a mandatory breath. If a patient effort is not detected, the first mandatory breath occurs at its set cycle. Using the previous example, if the SIMV rate is 5 breaths/min, the time between mandatory breaths is 12 seconds. Without a detected effort, the first mandatory breath would occur in about 12 seconds. The timing of mandatory breaths is similar in function to the Evita, which is described in the Evolve Resources for this text.*

Apnea ventilation can be activated during this mode and is reviewed later in this section.

Pressure-Control Ventilation Plus (PCV+)

PCV+ is a pressure-targeted mode. In PCV+ the patient can breathe spontaneously between mandatory breaths, meaning that the unit basically operates as SIMV. The patient can also breathe spontaneously during inspiration (Figure 12-26). Mandatory breaths are patient or time triggered, pressure targeted, and time cycled. Spontaneous breaths are patient triggered, pressure targeted, and pressure or flow cycled.

The operator sets the desired pressure (PINSP), a minimum respiratory rate, and a flow trigger. Time triggering is determined by the set rate and patient triggering by the flow-trigger setting. Peak pressure during a mandatory breath is equal to the PINSP pressure setting plus the set PEEP.

During PCV+, the unit functions as follows: When it is time for a mandatory breath (based on the rate setting) and the patient makes an inspiratory effort, a mandatory breath is delivered. During this time, the set pressure is achieved and held relatively constant, but the patient can still breathe spontaneously by receiving flow on demand (see Figure 12-26).

---

*Pressure-support breaths are described in the discussion on pressure support later in this section.

*For a detailed description of SIMV breath timing, see Modes of Ventilation for the Evita ventilator on the Evolve Resources Web site for this text.

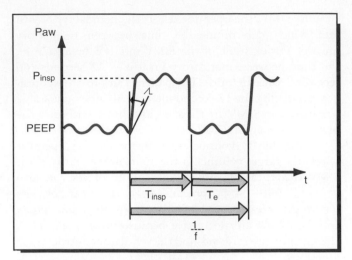

FIGURE 12-26 Pressure-time curve for a spontaneously breathing patient on PCV+. (Pinsp = inspiratory pressure setting; Tinsp = inspiratory time setting, and Te = expiratory time based on the total cycle time [TCT = 1 min/f, or 60 sec/f].) The angle drawn at the beginning of the first mandatory breath shows the potential for adjusting the slope using the RISE TIME control. (See text for further explanation.) (Redrawn from Dräger, Telford, Pa.)

Spontaneous breaths that occur between mandatory breaths can be assisted with pressure support by setting the desired PS level (PCV + PS). An elevated baseline (PEEP/CPAP) can also be set.

The RISE TIME control is used in this mode to slow flow and pressure delivery at the beginning of the breath.* RISE TIME is set by using the soft knob with the symbol for an ascending ramp below it on the computer screen. Pressure rise is adjustable from 0 to 2 seconds and represents the amount of time it takes the ventilator to achieve the set pressure from the beginning of inspiration. A rapid rise is appropriate for a patient with a high peak inspiratory flow. A slow rise is more appropriate for a small pediatric patient with less of a high flow demand. In Figure 12-26, the arrow at the beginning of the first mandatory breath shows the potential changes in pressure delivery that can occur with a change in rise time. The rise can be rapid (arrow pointing to left line from baseline pressure) or slow (arrow pointing to right line from baseline pressure). In most clinical settings, the default rise time of 0.2 seconds is adequate; it is seldom necessary to go above 0.4 seconds. If RISE TIME is being used, it affects both mandatory and PS breath delivery.

Because V_T and $\dot{V}_E$ may vary in this mode, the operator needs to set $\dot{V}_E$ alarm limits carefully. As with SIMV volume ventilation, apnea ventilation can be activated during this mode. Pmax and AutoFlow are not active during this mode because breath delivery is already pressure targeted, and the ventilator controls these functions.

Pressure-Support Ventilation (PSV)

The E-4 can provide PSV during SIMV, PCV+, MMV, and spontaneous (CPAP) ventilation. The target pressure is set using the PSUPP soft knob, which indicates the pressure above PEEP that will be delivered during a PS breath. PS breaths are patient triggered, pressure targeted, and flow cycled (25% of peak for adults; 6% of peak for pediatric and neonatal patients).* Patient triggering can be based on the flow trigger or on the volume trigger when the inspired volume exceeds 25 mL (12 mL in pediatric mode and 1 mL/32 msec for the neonatal setting), whichever occurs first. Whenever PSV is active, the pressure rise time control is also functional.

If the patient actively exhales or coughs during the start of a PS breath and the circuit pressure rises, inspiratory flow ends. This prevents excessive pressure from building in the circuit and can be identified by the flow going to zero or less than zero on the flow-time curve. Inspiratory flow during a PS breath time cycles out of the inspiratory phase if the inspiratory time exceeds 4 seconds (1.5 seconds for pediatric patients, but adjustable with the T_I control in neonatal patients). A prolonged T_I most often occurs if a leak is present. If the time-cycling criteria occur for three consecutive breaths, an alarm is activated to warn of a possible leak in the system. Apnea ventilation is available in the pressure-support mode.

Continuous Positive Airway Pressure (CPAP)

Spontaneously breathing patients often benefit from breathing at elevated baseline pressures **(continuous positive airway pressure [CPAP]),** which increases functional residual capacity. CPAP is available on the E-4 when the PS mode is selected. CPAP can be provided with or without PSV. CPAP can be selected alone by turning the PSV level to 0 cm H_2O, using its soft knob, and setting the PEEP soft knob to the desired CPAP level (cm H_2O). Apnea ventilation is available when CPAP is being used.

Airway Pressure-Release Ventilation (APRV)

Airway pressure-release ventilation (APRV) is a mode of ventilation in which two levels of CPAP are set. It operates very much like PCV+, except that the "expiratory" interval is very brief (Figure 12-27). After the APRV soft pad is selected, the upper pressure level is set using P_{HIGH}, and the lower level is set using P_{LOW}. The unit also times the length of both pressure levels. T_{HIGH} is the length of time that high pressure is provided, and T_{LOW} is the length of time that low pressure is provided. Both are intended for use with spontaneously breathing patients (see Chapter 11). The RISE TIME control can be used to taper the pressure

---

*RISE TIME can be set to control pressure delivery in any mode when pressure-targeted breaths are available.

*If a leak is present that prevents flow cycling, the unit will time cycle out of inspiration in 4 seconds.

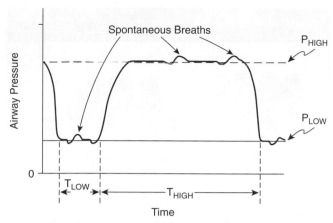

FIGURE 12-27 Pressure-time curve for airway pressure-release ventilation. (See text for further explanation.)

change from P_{LOW} to P_{HIGH}, but the length of rise time cannot be longer than the set T_{HIGH} time. Apnea backup ventilation is recommended when this mode is used.

Mandatory Minute Volume Ventilation (MMV) and MMV with Pressure-Support Ventilation (MMV/PSV)

Mandatory minute volume ventilation (MMV) is a closed-loop form of ventilation used in patients who can perform part of the work of breathing and who are progressing toward discontinuation of the ventilator. MMV guarantees a minimum $\dot{V}_E$, even with changes in the patient's spontaneous pattern. (See Chapter 11 for additional information on the uses of MMV.)

MMV is set by selecting that soft pad and then setting the MMV the patient is to accomplish using the V_T, flow, f, and T_I settings. A pressure-support level should be set to ensure that the patient has adequate support for spontaneous breaths.

As described in Chapter 11, with MMV the patient can breathe spontaneously and contribute all of the $\dot{V}_E$ with only PSV or CPAP with no mandatory breaths; or the patient might contribute only a portion of the $\dot{V}_E$. The difference between the spontaneous and the set $\dot{V}_E$ is provided by mandatory breaths at the set volume.

Pmax or AutoFlow can be used in MMV. (NOTE: It is important to set the high rate alarm to protect the patient from rapid, shallow breathing that would result in an equivalent $\dot{V}_E$ but would also increase the work of breathing and provide inadequate alveolar ventilation.)

Apnea Ventilation

Apnea ventilation supplies volume ventilation with a set respiratory rate and V_T in case the patient becomes apneic in SIMV, PCV, PS/CPAP, or APRV. If the patient stops breathing for the length of time set on the APNEA ALARM control, the alarm is activated and apnea ventilation begins. To set apnea ventilation, touch the EXTRA settings soft pad, then the APNEA VENT soft pad, and then the ON soft pad.

Set the desired volume and rate using the V_{TAPNEA} and F_{APNEA} soft knobs on the APNEA VENTILATION screen. When these parameters have been set, press the dial knob for activation. The baseline pressure, O_2%, trigger sensitivity, and other alarm parameters remain as they are in the current mode. (Additional information on apnea ventilation is available in the section on the EvitaXL.)

AutoFlow

AutoFlow is a dual mode of ventilation similar to pressure-regulated volume control and volume support in the Servo[i] ventilator. Use of AutoFlow provides pressure-targeted breaths with volume guarantee whenever volume ventilation (CMV, SIMV, MMV) is simultaneously selected (see Chapter 11). AutoFlow also alters the function of the inspiratory and expiratory valves, allowing patients to receive whatever inspiratory flow they demand (up to 180 L/min) in any volume mode, regardless of the volume settings. In addition, it makes the expiratory valve more interactive with the patient. For example, if the patient coughs or breathes during the set inspiratory time of a mandatory breath, the expiratory valve system allows the patient to inhale and exhale freely while maintaining the inspiratory pressure. Very little resistance or pressure builds up in the circuit when active patient breathing occurs. In AutoFlow, the circuit pressure rarely builds to the upper Paw alarm limit.

When AutoFlow is in use, the unit calculates the system compliance (C) and resistance (R) and establishes the minimum pressure needed to deliver the set volume. To access AutoFlow:

- Select extra settings on the screen
- Touch the AUTOFLOW ON soft pad
- Press the rotary knob to confirm that AutoFlow is activated

In AutoFlow the unit takes over the function of PMAX PRESSURE LIMIT and INSP FLOW, and the soft knobs for those functions are deleted from the screen. When AutoFlow is started, the ventilator delivers a volume-targeted mandatory breath and measures the plateau pressure during that breath. The plateau pressure is used as the starting ventilating pressure for AutoFlow (Figure 12-28). The unit delivers plateau pressure, measures delivered volume, and calculates the system C and R. If the delivered volume is lower than the set volume, the unit increases pressure delivery by a few centimeters of water pressure (cm H_2O) for the next breath. If the delivered volume is too high compared with the set volume, it reduces pressure delivery for the next breath. The pressure change between breaths is never greater than 3 cm H_2O.

Volume delivery may be higher than the set value if the patient is actively inspiring. If the patient continues to actively breathe in, the pressure level is slowly lowered accordingly. If the operator wants to avoid exceeding a specific V_T, the V_{Ti} UPPER LIMIT alarm can be used for this purpose. If the alarm is exceeded once, an advisory alert ("!") occurs, and V_T delivery is limited. If the alarm is exceeded three times, the following occur:

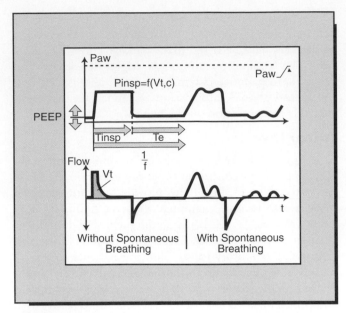

FIGURE 12-28 AutoFlow with a pressure-controlled, volume-guaranteed breath without spontaneous breathing *(left).* Flow drops to zero, and pressure delivery equilibrates with the pressure in the lungs. V_T has been delivered. During the second breath *(right),* the patient is spontaneously breathing during the plateau portion of the mandatory breath and afterward during the expiratory phase. (Redrawn from Dräger, Telford, Pa.)

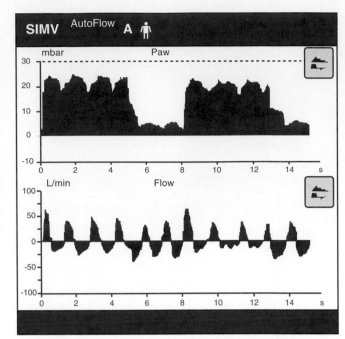

FIGURE 12-29 Volume-targeted SIMV with AutoFlow set. The patient can breathe spontaneously in all phases. (Redrawn from Dräger, Telford, Pa.)

1. A warning alarm is activated ("!!!," in red) with the message EXCEEDING $V_{TI} \times 3$.
2. V_T delivery is limited to the value of the V_{TI} UPPER LIMIT setting for all breaths.
3. The ventilator cycles into exhalation and drops airway pressure to the set baseline (set PEEP) if necessary for all breaths.

Whenever a spontaneous patient inspiratory effort is detected between mandatory breaths, the unit delivers whatever flow the patient demands. The patient can also breathe during the plateau phase of a mandatory breath (Figure 12-29). The inspiratory pressure is limited by the upper Paw limit setting minus 5 cm H_2O.

When AutoFlow is used, several types of breathing patterns can occur:

1. If the V_T is delivered and flow drops to zero before the unit time cycles out of a mandatory inspiration, the ventilator ensures that the patient can breathe spontaneously during the remaining inspiratory time. During this time, however, the pressure being delivered by the unit is maintained.
2. If the patient breathes in and out during a mandatory breath, the plateau delivery stays constant and does not fluctuate significantly. Flow is provided as needed to meet patient demand. The expiratory valve opens during spontaneous exhalation to avoid pressure build-up and resistance to exhalation while still maintaining plateau pressure (Figure 12-30).
3. If inspiration ends before flow drops to zero, the volume is delivered, but the pressure may be higher than the

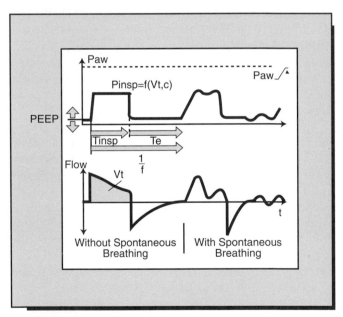

FIGURE 12-30 AutoFlow with a pressure-control breath in which the flow does not drop to zero before inspiration ends. The set pressure does not equilibrate with the lungs. V_T delivery is lower, because the T_I was not long enough to deliver the pressure. Remember that this pressure is calculated to be what is required, based on system compliance and resistance, to deliver the set V_T. (Redrawn from Dräger, Telford, Pa.)

true plateau. The unit may have to increase pressure and flow to deliver the V_T when T_I is short. The clinician may want to increase T_I, but it may be more appropriate to evaluate the patient before any change is made (Clinical Rounds 12-7).[4]

CLINICAL ROUNDS 12-7

A patient on AutoFlow has the following ventilator settings and monitored parameters: mode = SIMV; V_T (set) = 0.65 L (650 mL); f = 12 breaths/min; inspiratory pressure = 20 cm H_2O; T_I = 2 seconds; upper pressure limit = 30 cm H_2O.

The patient has done well on these settings for the past 4 hours. During the next hour, however, the respiratory therapist notices that inspiratory pause time (i.e., time when flow is zero) has become progressively shorter, and eventually there is no pause. Flow never goes to zero before the end of inspiration; the inspiratory pressure is now 25 cm H_2O. What do you think the therapist should do in this situation?

See Evolve Resources for the answer.

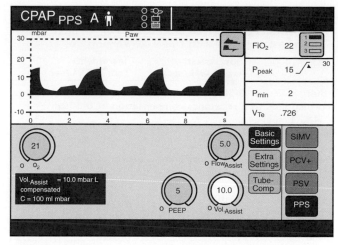

FIGURE 12-31 Screen during PPS on the Dräger E-4 (version 2.n). (Redrawn from Dräger, Telford, Pa.)

It is recommended that AutoFlow be activated whenever a spontaneously breathing patient is being volume ventilated, regardless of the volume mode chosen (CMV, SIMV, or MMV).

Proportional Pressure Support (PPS)[5]

Proportional pressure support (PPS) is a proportional assist ventilation mode that was described in Chapter 11.* PPS provides a positive feedback system of respiration; that is, the more the patient inspires, the more pressure the person receives. The amount of pressure provided is based on the volume assist and flow assist (explained later in this section) set by the operator.

Key points to remember about PPS include:

1. There is no support if there is no inspiratory effort from the patient. Therefore the patient must have an adequate inspiratory effort and ventilatory drive.
2. It is important to set minimum $\dot{V}_E$ and apnea alarms, as well as apnea backup ventilation, in case the patient stops breathing. Upper Paw and upper V_T alarm limits are also set to protect against high pressures and volumes.
3. This is a positive feedback system. The more actively the patient inspires, the more assistance the individual receives from the unit, and vice versa.
4. There must be no leaks in the system (cuff leaks, circuit connection leaks, or bronchopleural leaks).

When inspiration is strong during PPS, the unit supports the patient with a high pressure. With shallow, less forceful breaths, the unit provides a lower pressure. The amount of assistance provided during PPS is separated into the elastic (compliance) and the resistive components. Using VOL ASSIST, the operator decides how much work the unit will support for the elastic portion of the work of breathing. Using FLOW ASSIST, the operator determines how much work is provided by the unit to overcome resistive work.

The procedure for setting PPS is as follows:
· Touch the PPS soft pad on the ventilator screen (the standard screen for setting up ventilator modes)
· Touch the VOL ASSIST soft knob
· Set the desired value using the dial knob
· Press the dial knob for activation
· Touch the FLOW ASSIST soft knob and set the desired value using the dial knob (Figure 12-31)
· Press the dial knob for activation

The range of values for volume assist and flow assist are listed in Table 12-12. For example, if 10 cm H_2O/L is set, the unit compensates for the elastic work of breathing with a compliance of 100 mL/cm H_2O (Box 12-19). If 5 cm $H_2O/L/sec$ is set for the flow assist, the unit compensates for a resistance of 5 cm $H_2O/L/sec$ (see Box 12-19). The ventilator calculates the amount of airway pressure it needs to provide for both the volume and flow assist portions of the breath.

PPS has some limits. The maximum Paw is equal to the upper Paw alarm limit minus 5 cm H_2O; the maximum inspiratory V_T is equal to the upper alarm limit for V_{Ti}; the maximum T_I is limited to 4 seconds (1.5 seconds in pediatric patients; the neonatal setting is adjusted by the clinician with the T_I control [E-4 with NeoFlow]). PPS is a new mode of ventilation in the United States; therefore its effectiveness will be evaluated as the results of its use in clinical studies are made available.

NeoFlow[6,7]

NeoFlow is a mode of ventilation that can be added to the E-4 ventilator to enable it to be adapted for neonatal use (patient weight from 0.5 to 6 kg). NeoFlow requires the installation of a flow sensor between the end of the endotracheal tube and the Y-connector of the patient circuit. The other end is attached to the back of the ventilator unit.

*PPS currently is not available in the United States. It has been available in parts of Europe since 1997.

TABLE 12-12

Proportional Pressure-Support Ranges of Available
Settings—Dräger E-4 with Upgrade (Version 2.n)

	Flow Assist (cm H$_2$O/L/sec)	Increment (cm H$_2$O/L/sec)
Adult	0-30	0.5
(corresponds to a resistance compensation of 0-30 cm H$_2$O/L/sec)		
Pediatric	0-30	0.5
	30-100	5.0
(corresponds to a resistance compensation of 0-100 cm H$_2$O/L/sec)		
Neonatal	0-30	0.5
	30-300	5.0
(corresponds to a resistance compensation of 0-300 cm H$_2$O/L/sec)		

	Volume Assist (cm H$_2$O/L)	Increment (cm H$_2$O/L)
Adult	0-24.9	0.1
	25-99.5	0.5
(corresponds to a compliance compensation of infinity to 10 mL/cm H$_2$O)		
Pediatric	0-99	1.0
	100-1000	10.0
(corresponds to a compliance compensation of infinity to 1 mL/cm H$_2$O)		
Neonatal	0-30	0.5
	30-300	5.0
(corresponds to a compliance compensation of infinity to 0.5 mL/cm H$_2$O)		

BOX 12-19   Proportional Pressure Support

The setting for volume assist is a pressure/volume
measurement of elastance (cm H$_2$O/L). It is the inverse of
compliance. In this example, if elastance is 10 cm H$_2$O/L,
compliance is 1 L/10 cm H$_2$O, or 0.1 L/cm H$_2$O, or
100 mL/cm H$_2$O.

Flow assist is a measurement of resistance, where $R = \Delta P/Flow$. The setting for flow assist is cm H$_2$O/(L/sec).

The flow sensor must be calibrated when it is used for the
first time and then at least once every 24 hours (see the
operator's manual).

When the unit is turned on and the screen displays the
STANDBY mode, the operator selects the NEO soft pad for
neonatal ventilation. In the neonatal mode, the unit can
provide volume ventilation; AutoFlow; apnea backup
ventilation; pressure support with assisted spontaneous
breathing (ASB); continuous base flow; and measurements
of circuit leaks, airway pressure, and breath triggering. (See
Chapter 13 for additional information on NeoFlow on the
Dräger E-4.)

SPECIAL FUNCTIONS

A variety of features are available on the Dräger E-4, some
of which are similar to those on other ICU ventilators and
others that are unique to this unit. Some of these functions are reviewed here.

Sigh (Intermittent PEEP)

As with a normal sigh breath, the intended purpose of
intermittent PEEP is to open up or keep open areas of the
lung likely to become atelectatic. Sigh breaths are accomplished with the E-4 ventilator by intermittently increasing
the PEEP level in the CMV mode.

Intermittent PEEP, or "sigh" breaths, can be activated
by touching the EXTRA SETTING soft pad on the screen and
setting the value as for other parameters. The intermittent
PEEP knob is turned to the desired pressure level. The
baseline pressure (baseline PEEP) is increased by the value
set on the INT PEEP knob (0 to 35 cm H$_2$O) for two consecutive breaths every 3 minutes during CMV only (Figure
12-32). The function becomes active as soon as it is set,
and the top of the main monitoring screen reads INT PEEP
ACTIVE when it is selected.

During the sigh interval, the VOLUME NOT CONSTANT
alarm is deactivated. Because intermittent PEEP increases
the baseline, it is advisable to set the Pmax pressure limit
appropriately to prevent overdistention of the lungs during
regular breath delivery (see Figure 12-32).

Intrinsic PEEP

An estimate of the amount of auto-PEEP (intrinsic PEEP),
as well as an estimate of the trapped volume in a patient's
lungs, can be determined by using the intrinsic PEEP
(PEEPi) function. These measurements can be performed
only when the patient is not actively breathing during the
measurement.

To perform an auto-PEEP measurement, select the
SPECIAL PROCEDURE touch pad. From the computer screen,
touch the PEEPi soft pad. The maneuver is performed
automatically, and the waveform display is frozen. On the
screen, values for PEEP(set), PEEPi, and trapped volume
(Vtrap) are shown. Using the dial knob and the screen
cursor, the operator can select to view the auto-PEEP level
at any time on the pressure-time curve. The PEEPi values
appear above the waveform.

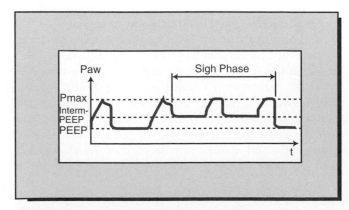

FIGURE 12-32 Intermittent PEEP for the delivery of sigh
breaths. (Redrawn from Dräger, Telford, Pa.)

Occlusion Pressure

Measurements of the **occlusion pressure (P0.1)** are used to evaluate a patient's neuromuscular drive.[4] This procedure can be performed automatically by selecting the SPECIAL PROCEDURES touch pad, the P0.1 soft pad, and the START soft pad.

At the beginning of inspiration, the ventilator occludes the inspiratory and expiratory valves 0.1 second after the beginning of inspiratory flow. The pressure measured at that time is displayed. The value for the occlusion pressure is shown on the screen. The normal value is about −3 to −4 cm H_2O. Values more negative than −6 cm H_2O may indicate impending exhaustion and respiratory muscle fatigue that may lead to respiratory failure, as in patients with chronic obstructive pulmonary disease. They also indicate forceful active inspiration.

As with PEEPi, the waveform is frozen on the screen. The rotary knob and screen cursor can be used to view the specific value for the occlusion pressure from the pressure-time curve at precise moments during the maneuver.

Special Function Touch Pads

As mentioned previously, a set of touch pads is located to the left of the screen on the front panel of the E-4. Their function is explained here.

Nebulizer Touch Pad

The nebulizer touch pad (NEB) switches on the nebulizer gas source and functions during adult ventilation only. Gas only flows through the nebulizer outlet during inspiration, and the unit automatically maintains the set $\dot{V}_E$ and approximates the set O_2%.

When the nebulizer is activated, the LED on the touch pad appears with a screen message, NEBULIZER ON. The nebulizer continues to operate for 30 minutes or until the pad is touched again. After its use, a FLOW CALIBRATION message appears, showing that the nebulizer is off and the flow transducer is automatically being cleaned and recalibrated to preserve accuracy (Box 12-20).

The expiratory flow sensor is a heated wire (see Chapter 8). To protect the sensor during the use of nebulized medications, a filter placed inline before the sensor may be helpful.

Suction 100% O_2

The SUCTION 100% O_2 touch pad is used to provide 100% O_2 for 3 minutes. The LED on the pad is illuminated, and the message O_2 ENRICHMENT 180 S appears at the bottom of the screen; the time remaining also is displayed.

A pressure of 4 cm H_2O is applied if a PEEP of less than 4 cm H_2O is set to help the ventilator identify when the circuit is disconnected and reconnected when an open suction procedure is used. All other parameters are unchanged. After disconnection has been identified, the unit provides 100% oxygen for 2 minutes during suctioning. During these 2 minutes, the audible alarm is silenced so that it is not a nuisance, and a flow of 4 L/min is provided through the circuit. This low flow is intended to reduce humidifier splash.

After the patient is reconnected, ventilation is resumed, and an additional 2 minutes of 100% oxygen are provided to the patient. The alarms are reactivated, and the E-4 returns to its normal operating mode. The main display screen reads FINAL O_2 ENRICH 120 S. Pressing the RESET/CONFIRM key at any time stops the oxygenation procedure, which cannot be restarted for 15 seconds. (NOTE: The oxygenation procedure is interrupted if the ventilator does not detect a disconnection within the first 3-minute period.)

During the 3-minute suction interval, the low $\dot{V}_E$ alarm is turned off (Clinical Rounds 12-8). For 2 minutes thereafter, 100% O_2 is provided, and the alarms are reactivated. (NOTE: If the patient is not disconnected after the 100% O_2 control is activated, the operator must touch the pad again to reactivate the alarm, or an undetected disconnect may occur.)

Inspiratory Hold

The inspiratory hold (INSPIR HOLD) touch pad provides an inflation hold maneuver when pressed and held down for as long as the inspiratory pause is desired (maximum of 15

BOX 12-20	Clinical Note: Caution During Nebulization

1. Do not use a heat and moisture exchanger (HME) during nebulization because it reduces medication delivery and may increase airway resistance by depositing medication on the HME.
2. Do not use filters on the nebulizer outlet, because they may increase resistance and impair ventilation.

CLINICAL ROUNDS 12-8

Clinical note on suctioning:
1. If the patient is not disconnected after the suction 100% O_2 pad is pressed, the unit continues to ventilate the patient in the set mode but uses 100% O_2. After 3 minutes, the O_2 program is terminated and the alarms are reactivated.
2. To stop SUCTION 100% O_2, press the pad again. The LED will flash for 15 seconds, and normal operation will resume. The oxygen enrichment cannot be restarted until the flashing stops.

Some institutions use closed-suction catheter systems and do not disconnect the patient before suctioning. Do you think the clinician should still disconnect the patient to activate the oxygen enrichment function?

See Evolve Resources for the answer.

seconds). When activated, either the current inspiration is held or a new mandatory breath is delivered and the inspiration is held. Inspiratory hold functions in all modes except CPAP when pressure support is set at zero.

Print

The PRINT function allows the microprocessor to print if a compatible printer is attached.

Special Upgrades with Software Update 2.n

The Dräger E-4 has a software version 2.n that includes the features discussed in the following sections. Additional updates include the option of noninvasive ventilation (NIV) for mask ventilation.

Compliance Compensation

The E-4 (version 2.n and higher) provides compensation for volume lost as a result of tubing compressibility. The unit adds the volume needed to compensate for the volume lost and subtracts this added volume from the measured expiratory volume to give a close measurement of the volume actually exhaled by the patient. The resistance and compliance of the patient circuit are determined when the patient circuit is changed (STANDBY mode) with the AIRTIGHT CHECK soft pad.

Support During Hose Change

When a patient circuit is changed, the ventilator can check the hose for leaks by using the STANDBY mode (select the AIRTIGHT CHECK soft pad). In addition, the resistance and compliance of the circuit are measured to provide compliance compensation for the volume lost as a result of tubing compliance (see the previous discussion of compliance compensation).

Automatic Tubing Compensation (ATC)

As a part of the breathing support package (software version 2.n and higher), an automatic tubing compensation (ATC) feature has been added to the E-4 to compensate for the airway resistance associated with small artificial airways. ATC can be used with all modes of ventilation. In CMV, SIMV, and MMV, tube compensation is active during expiration after a mandatory breath and during spontaneous breathing phases.

This ventilator function regulates airway pressure at the tracheal level (Box 12-21). When it is selected, the ventilating pressure during all breaths compensates for the resistance associated with varying size endotracheal tubes. This compensation depends on the direction of gas flow. The airway pressure is increased during inspiration and decreased during expiration. (NOTE: The expiratory portion can be switched off if the operator wants to compensate only for the inspiratory portion.) The pressure can be increased to a value equal to the upper Paw alarm limit minus 5 cm H_2O or reduced to a minimum of 0 cm H_2O.

The tube compensation function is set as follows:
1. During STANDBY mode, select the TUBE COMP soft pad.
2. Touch either the ET TUBE or the TRACH TUBE soft pad, depending on the type of artificial airway in use.
3. Use the ID 0 soft knob to set the size of the tube's inner diameter (with the dial knob) and confirm it by pressing the dial knob.
4. Use the COMP soft knob and the dial knob to set the percentage of compensation provided. For example, a reading of 70 inside the COMP soft knob provides 70% compensation for the artificial airway.

VENTILATOR GRAPHIC WAVEFORMS

The graphics monitor with the E-4 is part of the main computer screen during standard operation. Additional waveforms can be viewed simultaneously, and different waveforms may be displayed during its normal function (see Box 12-16; Box 12-22). Timed graphics can be frozen

BOX 12-21	Calculating the Tracheal Pressure (Dräger E-4 Upgrade Version 2.n)

The Dräger Evita 4 (2.n software version) calculates and displays tracheal pressure based on a mathematical equation:
$$P_{trachea} = P_{aw} - K_{tube} \times Flow^2$$
where $P_{trachea}$ is the pressure in the trachea, P_{aw} is the pressure at the Y-connector of the patient circuit, K_{tube} is the tube coefficient (listed in the operating manual), and $Flow$ is the patient flow (inspiratory flow is greater than zero, and expiratory flow is less than zero.)

An example of a tube coefficient is 6.57 cm $H_2O/L^2/sec^2$ for an endotracheal tube with an inner diameter (ID) of 8 mm.

For pressure support the equation is as follows:
$$\Delta P_{aw} = Comp \times K_{tube} \times Flow^2$$
where ΔP_{aw} is pressure support at the tube, $Comp$ is the degree of compensation (0 to 100%), K_{tube} is the tube coefficient, and $Flow$ is the patient flow.

BOX 12-22	Waveform Display (Dräger E-4)

1. Select the STANDARD PAGE computer screen by pressing the main screen touch pad. In the right field, four measured values are displayed. In the left field, two waveforms are displayed.
2. To select waveforms, touch the icon on the computer screen at the top right of the waveform area that looks like two tiny waveforms (see Figure 12-20). Touch the screen key that indicates the waveform desired.
3. To select loops, touch the VALUES MEASURED touch pad. The computer screen displays several selections on the lower right corner. Touch the LOOPS soft pad on the screen. Two different loops appear on the lower left part of the screen. To change the loop parameters, touch the waveform icon between them.

by pressing the FREEZE touch pad on the right side of the unit's front panel. The operator can view a measured numeric value for a given time on any graph by positioning the cursor on the computer screen and rotating the dial knob to the desired time on the curve. The value is shown on the screen above the waveform. The graph can be unfrozen by pressing FREEZE a second time.

The E-4 can also display trends of data. Select MEASURED VALUES and then TRENDS. In this setting, the operator can use the ZOOM IN or ZOOM OUT soft pads to narrow or widen the time frame for the data trend. Again, the operator can change the parameters viewed or trended by touching the waveform icon. This function can also be analyzed by using the cursor with a link to the LOGBOOK.

TROUBLESHOOTING

The alarms and monitored information sections offer assistance for solving most problems that might occur with the E-4. In addition, the operator's manual has a troubleshooting section that alphabetically lists all the alarm messages, gives their priority level, provides common causes, and recommends remedies. Covering this extensive material is beyond the scope of this text. Users are advised to consult the operator's manual. For additional information about Dräger products, check the company's Web site at http://www.draeger.com.

KEY POINTS

▶ The Dräger E-4 requires at least one high-pressure gas source and an electrical power source to operate.

▶ The E-4 can be configured to ventilate adult, pediatric, or neonatal patients.

▶ The ventilator has a built-in oxygen analyzer and does an automatic oxygen calibration every 24 hours.

▶ The unit optimally can include a mainstream carbon dioxide analyzer that provides information on end-tidal carbon dioxide, CO_2/time, and single-breath CO_2 (CO_2/volume).

▶ The Ppeak alarm functions separately from the Pmax pressure limit control. The Pmax limit is not an alarm, but rather actually changes the way a breath is delivered during CMV, SIMV, and MMV ventilation.

▶ When Pmax is operational, the unit guarantees the set V_T but limits the pressure delivered during the breath.

▶ In PCV+ the patient can breathe spontaneously both during inspiration and between mandatory breath delivery.

▶ AutoFlow provides pressure-targeted breaths with volume guarantee whenever volume ventilation (CMV, SIMV, MMV) is simultaneously selected.

▶ The E-4 (version 2.n and higher) provides compensation for volume lost as a result of patient circuit compressibility.

▶ Automatic tube compensation compensates for the airway resistance associated with small artificial airways.

ASSESSMENT QUESTIONS

See Evolve Resources for the answers.

1. A mode that is patient triggered, pressure targeted (pressure limited), and flow cycled is called:
   a. Airway pressure-release ventilation
   b. Pressure-regulated volume control ventilation
   c. Pressure-support ventilation
   d. Proportional assist ventilation

2. AutoFlow on the Dräger E-4 is similar to which mode on the AVEA?
   a. PRVC
   b. Pressure augment
   c. APRV
   d. VAPS

3. When the patient actively inspires during APRV, the E-4:
   a. Increases its support
   b. Maintains a constant pressure
   c. Slows flow delivery
   d. Limits maximum volume delivery

4. Which of the following accurately describe(s) the function of AutoFlow?
   I. AutoFlow allows spontaneous inspiratory flows up to 180 L/min.
   II. AutoFlow regulates inspiratory pressure delivery to achieve the set V_T.
   III. AutoFlow fixes flow delivery at the set flow value.
   IV. AutoFlow allows the patient to cough without significant buildup of pressure in the circuit.
      a. I only
      b. II only
      c. II and III only
      d. I, II, and IV only

5. During PCV ventilation with the E-4, the patient can breathe spontaneously at any time during a mandatory breath, even during the expiratory portion of the breath. True or False?

6. The Pmax pressure limit function of the E-4 is an upper airway pressure alarm. True or False?

ASSESSMENT QUESTIONS—cont'd

7. The function of NeoFlow on the E-4 is to provide flow triggering. True or False?
8. Describe the controls on the front panel of the Dräger E-4 ventilator.
9. Explain how to change the numeric value for a parameter, such as V_T, with the E-4.

10. An audible five-tone alarm is heard, and a red area is present at the top right corner of the E-4 computer screen. Inside the red area is a message that reads HIGH FREQUENCY!!! What priority level is this alarm, and what does it indicate?

References

1. Evita 4: Intensive care ventilation operating instructions 90 28 676-GA 5664.510, ed 1; and version 4.n, Telford, Pa, 2001, Dräger, Drägerwerk AG.
2. Technical data—Evita 4 edition, 90 50 818, Germany, 2006, Dräger Medical AG & Co, KG.
3. Pilbeam SP, Cairo JM: *Mechanical ventilation: physiological and clinical applications,* ed 4, St Louis, 2006, Mosby/Elsevier.
4. Lear GF: Personal communication, Telford, Pa, 2002, Dräger, Drägerwerk AG.
5. Breathing support package, proportional pressure support PPS, tube compensation, ATC, supplement to the instruc-tions for use of the Evita 4 as from software version 2.n 90 28 825-GA 5664.520 e, ed 1, Telford, Pa, 1996, and version 4.n, 2001, Dräger, Drägerwerk AG.
6. E-4 plus option NeoFlow NI 5664.515e/117D, Telford, Pa, 1997, Dräger.
7. NeoFlow: neonatal mode, supplement to the instructions for use of the Evita 4 as from software version 2.n ED 2077947.97, ed 2, Telford, Pa, 1997, and version 4.n, 2001, Dräger, Drägerwerk AG.

Internet Resource
www.draeger.com

DRÄGER EvitaXL SW 6.0

OUTLINE

OBJECTIVES

Upon completion of this section, you will be able to:
- Identify the specific areas of the EvitaXL front control panel.
- Explain the procedure for selecting and setting parameters and modes.
- Recognize the way to identify which electrical source is operating with the EvitaXL.
- List the modes of ventilation available for the Evita XL.
- Describe the following modes or functions as they operate with the EvitaXL: APRV, Pmax (PLV), AutoFlow, sigh.
- Compare the difference between the operating screens of the E-4 and the EvitaXL.
- Describe the measurements obtained with the expiratory hold, inspiratory hold, and occlusion pressure controls.
- Give one use for the reference loops available with the EvitaXL.
- Explain the purpose of the low-flow pressure-volume loop feature.
- Compare weaning using SmartCare and traditional methods of weaning.

KEY TERMS

Airway pressure-release ventilation (APRV)
Apnea ventilation
AutoFlow
Control panel
Electromagnetic servo valves
Expiratory hold
Expiratory hold maneuvers

Flow trigger
Inspiratory hold maneuvers
Inspiratory pause
Inspiratory time (T_I or Tinsp)
Mandatory minute volume ventilation (MMV)
NeoFlow
Occlusion pressure ($P_{0.1}$)

Pmax pressure limit
Pressure limit ventilation (PLV)
Screen keys
Screen knobs
Sensitivity
SmartCare/PS
Smart window

The Dräger EvitaXL (software version 6.0) is the most recent release of the Dräger Evita series of ventilators as of this writing. The two earlier versions, the Dräger E-4 and the Evita 2 Dura, were developed after the original Evita ventilator.* The Dräger E-4 (Evita 4) ventilator is described in the previous section.

The E-4 and the Evita 2 Dura can be upgraded with the XL option to provide them with the options and features available with the EvitaXL. This section explains the features of the Dräger EvitaXL (version SW 6.0). The EvitaXL is designed to be used for ventilation of adults, children, and infants (minimum, 3 kg). To use the EvitaXL for infants, the NeoFlow option must be added. NeoFlow is described in more detail in Chapter 13 (Box 12-23).[1]

The EvitaXL has a front **control panel** with touch pads, a dial (rotary) knob, and a computer screen (Figure 12-33). The operating screen (control panel) contains the information and controls needed for ventilation. On the right side of the screen are fixed keys that allow access to various functions. On the lower right of the control unit is a rotary dial knob for selecting and confirming settings on the operating screen or control panel. All of these dials and knobs are used to control the unit and are discussed later in this section. Below the front operating panel are the connections for the main inspiratory and expiratory lines, the expiratory valve, and the nipple connector for the nebulizer line. The expiratory flow sensor is to the left of the expiratory valve.

BOX 12-23	Operator Instructions for the Dräger EvitaXL

Operators of the EvitaXL should refer to the instruction manual for the particular version of the ventilator they are operating. Options and software upgrades may or may not be available on the unit they have. The operator should make sure to follow the warning and safety precautions provided in the manufacturer's operating manual, and this manual should be the primary source for operation of the ventilator.

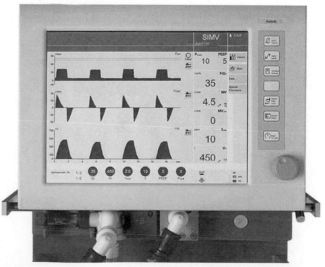

FIGURE 12-33 Front view of the Dräger EvitaXL ventilator. (See text for explanation.) (Courtesy Dräger Medical, Telford, Pa.)

*See the Web site for this text for information on the Evita and Evita 2 Dura.

POWER SOURCE

The EvitaXL normally uses two 50-psig gas sources (air and oxygen, at a range of 40 to 87 psig). The unit will operate on a single gas source if the second is unavailable, but it will issue an alert when only one gas source is used, because oxygen delivery is altered. A standard AC 120-volt outlet is used to power the microprocessor and the electrical components. An on/off switch is located on the back panel of the unit, beneath a protective cover.

The EvitaXL has alternative DC power sources:
· Two internal 12-volt, lead-acid gel batteries in the DC power pack
· Optional external rechargeable 12-volt or 24-volt lead-acid gel batteries

The external DC power source (or sources) can be used for in-hospital transport. The length of time power is available depends on the type and number of batteries used and their charge level.

The lower right corner of the operating screen displays the type of power in use:
· AC line power (electrical plug icon)
· External battery (battery icon with EXT)
· Internal battery (battery icon with INT)

If the AC power supply fails or is lost, the ventilator automatically switches to the available DC power source (external or internal). The internal battery provides up to 10 minutes of operation after a power failure. It is intended for use only as an emergency power source (Box 12-24).

INTERNAL MECHANISM

The internal operating mechanism that delivers gas to the patient is similar to the one used for the E-2 Dura and the E-4. The gas sources enter the unit through connections on the back panel. The gases are filtered, and their pressure is measured and reduced to an appropriate working pressure. The incoming flow is then directed to two high-pressure, flow-control **electromagnetic servo valves.** The function of the valves is controlled by the microprocessor, which uses information from the settings on the front panel, internal flow, pressure transducers, and the action of the valves themselves to control the flow to the patient. The valves regulate the amount of pressure and flow and the flow waveform of the gas delivered according to the selected modes and settings. The valves also control the F_IO_2 based on the set value. From the flow-control valves, gas is directed to the patient. A variety of pressure and flow transducers monitor internal gas flow, the output from the unit, and the gas return from the patient through the expiratory valve.

PATIENT CIRCUIT

Connections for the patient circuit are located just below the front panel (see Figure 12-33). The inspiratory line should be installed with an inline bacterial filter in place (not shown in the figure). Either a heated humidifier or a heat and moisture exchanger (HME) can be used with the EvitaXL. (NOTE: The two should *never* be used together.) The expiratory line connection is below the front panel on the left. The expiratory valve is to the left of the expiratory line connection. During normal maintenance, the expiratory valve assembly is removed for cleaning, but it should not be disassembled beyond removing the expiratory diaphragm. An expiratory flow sensor is located to the left of the expiration line connection.

OVERVIEW OF CONTROLS AND VENTILATOR START-UP

A number of controls, monitors, and alarm settings are available on the Dräger EvitaXL. As does the E-4, the EvitaXL uses a single rotary knob, several hard touch keys on the side the computer screen, and the touch-sensitive **screen keys** and **screen knobs** on the computer screen (Figure 12-34). The computer screen can display a variety of different pages, all of which display a similar layout (Figure 12-35).

Screen Page Selection

To select a specific screen (page), the operator touches the respective screen key (see Figure 12-35, item 8). For example, touching the main screen symbol selects the main screen. The VALUES icon allows the operator to choose a screen that permits the selection of different groups of measured values to be displayed. The DATA screen displays all measured values. SPECIAL PROCEDURES is used to select additional functions, such as nebulization and oxygenation before suctioning.

Peripheral Controls

Several controls used during normal operation of the ventilator are located on the right side of the screen. These touch pads or touch keys are used to select several operations as described in Figure 12-34.

BOX 12-24	Warning for Switch to DC Power (EvitaXL)

A caution message appears when the unit is switched to the internal battery: INT. BATTERY ACTIVATED !! The message must be acknowledged by the operator by touching the ALARM RESET key and pressing the dial knob to confirm.

When the ventilator has operated on the internal battery for about 8 minutes, a caution message is displayed: INT. BATTERY ONLY 2 MINUTES LEFT !! The unit must be reconnected to an AC power source or a fully charged external battery power source.

The final warning—INT BATTERY DISCHARGED !!!—indicates that the internal battery power has been operating for 10 minutes. To prevent loss of power, the operator must connect the unit to an alternative power source.

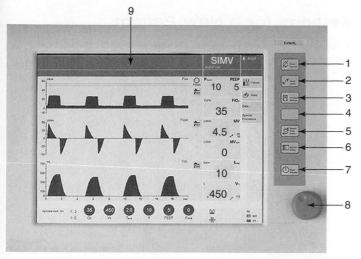

FIGURE 12-34 Details of the control panel on the EvitaXL. *(1)* Alarm silence key; *(2)* alarm limits setting key; *(3)* ventilator settings for ventilator modes and parameters; *(4)* unassigned key for future use; *(5)* sensor parameter key for calibrating sensors and activating and deactivating monitoring; *(6)* system setup key for configuring various ventilator functions; *(7)* start/standby control; *(8)* rotary dial knob for selecting and confirming settings; and *(9)* touch-sensitive screen for displaying various screen views. (Courtesy Dräger Medical, Telford, Pa.)

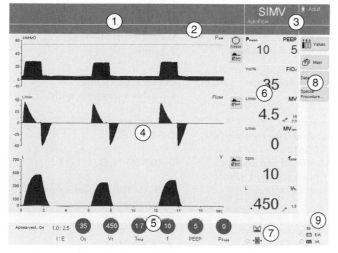

FIGURE 12-35 View of the typical screen display on the EvitaXL: *(1)* Space for display of alarm messages. *(2)* Space for display of operator prompts. *(3)* Mode of ventilation display, patient size selected (adult or child), and AutoFlow when selected. (AutoFlow is reviewed later.) *(4)* Graphic display of real-time waveforms, loops and trends, depending on the page selected. *(5)* Digital display of set ventilation parameters. *(6)* Display of measured values. *(7)* Humidification type and status selected. *(8)* Touch-sensitive screen keys available for the currently selected page. *(9)* Power supply indicator. (Courtesy Dräger Medical, Telford, Pa.)

On-Screen Controls

On-screen controls are touch sensitive. The round icons on the screen are screen knobs. The rectangular icons on the screen are screen keys. Parameter settings using screen knobs or keys are made and confirmed in three steps:

TABLE 12-13

Status of Screen Controls Based on Color—EvitaXL

Color	Status
Grey	Not available
Yellow	Ready for use
Pale green	May be adjusted but is not active
Dark green	May be adjusted and is active

1. Touch the desired screen knob to make it active (screen key turns yellow).
2. Turn the rotary control knob (lower right of the main screen).
3. Press the control knob to confirm the setting (screen key turns dark green).

The status of the screen controls is based on their color (Table 12-13). These same actions (touch [soft knob], turn [rotary knob], and push [rotary knob]) are how most controls are set. The manufacturer refers to this sequence as "touch, adjust, confirm."

The rotary knob on the lower right of the main screen can be rotated to select numeric values for parameters and pressed to activate them. It also can be used to move the cursor (vertical line) on the screen when it appears under certain functions.

Overview of Standby and Start-Up Controls

After the power switch is turned on, the unit runs a series of self-tests. A horizontal bar graph appears in the display window, providing the amount to time elapsed for the SELF TEST. The operator must wait for these tests to be completed before trying to operate the ventilator.

After the tests are complete, the EvitaXL displays an opening or start-up screen. The ventilator will automatically start ventilation using the configured settings unless values are changed or the STANDBY mode is activated within 30 seconds. In the opening screen, the operator presses the STANDBY screen key and then presses the dial knob within 30 seconds to confirm. STANDBY ACTIVATED!!! appears at the top of the screen where alarm messages are displayed. To reset this message, the operator presses the ALARM RESET screen key to the right of the message and presses the dial knob to confirm.

The ventilator's readiness for patient use must be checked before a new patient is connected to the ventilator. Once the ventilator is powered on and in the STANDBY setting, the screen displays the last date the device check was performed. When the operator touches the DEVICE CHECK screen key (vertical tab), a list of all the individual checks appears (Figure 12-36 and Box 12-25). (NOTE: A device check is not possible during calibration of the flow or O_2 sensor.) To start the test procedure, the operator touches the CHECK screen key. The ventilator guides the user through each test and requires "yes" or "no" responses by touching the respective screen keys. Additional information on the tests is provided in the operator's manual.

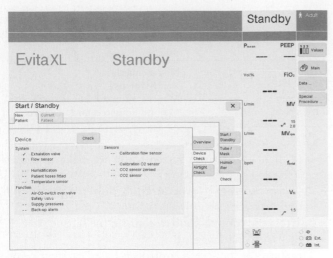

FIGURE 12-36 EvitaXL STANDBY screen with DEVICE CHECK tab open. (See text for additional information.) (Courtesy Dräger Medical, Telford, Pa.)

BOX 12-25	Tasks Performed During Readiness for Operation (Device Check) on the EvitaXL

System check
Expiratory valve test
Flow sensor (or neonatal flow sensor) fit
Type of humidifier
Completeness of patient circuit
Temperature sensor fit
Function
Gas supply pressure check
Safety relief valve test
Audible alarm test
Air/O_2 switchover valve test
Sensors
Calibration of flow sensor (adult or neonate)
Calibration of O_2 sensor
Zero and calibration of carbon dioxide (CO_2) sensor
Patient circuit leak test
Patient circuit compliance and resistance test

The results of the last patient circuit leak test display values for leakage, circuit compliance, and inspiratory and expiratory resistance of the circuit. The patient circuit leak test must be repeated under three circumstances:

· After the device check (readiness for operation) is performed
· When the patient circuit is changed or modified
· If the humidifier is changed

The leak test is done in the STANDBY mode using the AIRTIGHT CHECK screen key. In addition to checking circuit leaks, the patient circuit compliance (tubing compressibility factor) is also determined. The EvitaXL uses the calculated circuit compliance to correct automatically for patient circuit compressibility.

Settings for a New Patient

While in the START/STANDBY screen, the operator can select PREVIOUS PATIENT or NEW PATIENT. Touching PREVIOUS PATIENT restores the previous ventilator settings. Selecting NEW PATIENT allows the operator to select the new patient's size (adult or pediatric) (NOTE: The available volumes and flows are different for each patient size.) (Table 12-14). Next, the operator enters the ideal body weight (IBW) of the patient (Box 12-26).

The unit requests the patient's IBW because the microprocessor is programmed at the factory to automatically begin ventilation using the continuous mechanical ventilation (CMV) mode with factory default settings. (More on

TABLE 12-14	
Parameter Ranges—Dräger EvitaXL	

Tidal Volume (Body Temperature Pressure Saturated [BTPS] ± 10%)	
Adult	0.1-2 L
Pediatric	0.02-0.30 L
Neonate	0.03-0.10 L
Flow	
Adult	6-120 L/min (to 180 L/min with AutoFlow)
Pediatric	6-30 L/min (to 60 L/min with AutoFlow)
Neonate	0.25-30 L/min
Neonate continuous flow	6 L/min
Variable Ranges for All Patients	
Respiratory rate	0-100 breaths/min
	0-150 breaths/min with NeoFlow
Inspiratory time	0.1-10 sec
Inspiratory pressure (set) (Pinsp)	0-95 cm H_2O
Maximum inspiratory pressure limit (Pmax)	0-100 cm H_2O
Percent oxygen	21% to 100% (plus or minus 5% of set)
PEEP	0-50 cm H_2O
Trigger sensitivity	0.3-15 L/min
Pressure support	0-95 cm H_2O
Rise time for PS	0-2 sec

BOX 12-26	Setting the Ideal Body Weight (EvitaXL)

To set the ideal body weight (IBW), touch the screen soft knob for IBW, which highlights the screen knob and changes its color to yellow. Rotate the dial knob to set the actual numeric value, which appears inside the screen soft knob. When the desired IBW appears, push the dial knob to set the selected value, which changes the screen knob from yellow to green to show that it has been set. The EvitaXL determines the tidal volume (V_T) and respiratory rate (f) based on the entered IBW and displays these values. These settings go into effect when ventilation is switched on.

CLINICAL ROUNDS 12-9

A patient with an ideal body weight of 80 kg will be ventilated with the EvitaXL. The respiratory therapist sets the IBW during start-up of the ventilator. What will the patient's tidal volume be?

See Evolve Resources for the answer.

CMV later in this section.) The factory default for V_T is 7 mL/kg, based on the patient's IBW. The respiratory rate is based on Radford's nomogram for the $\dot{V}_E$ of a person that size.[2] To have the unit automatically start ventilating a patient with programmed (configured) parameters while in the STANDBY screen, the operator simply pushes the rotary knob (Clinical Rounds 12-9).

The operator can also do a standard ventilator set-up and select the mode and appropriate ventilation parameters, or the mode and parameters may be reconfigured so that some other mode and parameters are available as soon as the power switch is turned on.

The STANDBY screen (see Figure 12-36) also allows for selection of the type of patient interface (mask or endotracheal tube) and the type of humidifier in use:

- ACTIV HUMID indicates a heated breathing-gas humidifier
- HME/FILTER is a heat and moisture exchanger or similar filter

Control Knobs for Parameters of Ventilation

To set ventilation parameters while in the START/STANDBY computer screen, the operator presses the START screen key and then presses the dial knob. Once the new computer screen opens, the operator can adjust various parameters by selecting the VENTILATOR SETTINGS key. The VENTILATOR SETTINGS window appears in the lower left corner of the screen (Figure 12-37), allowing the operator to select and set the desired ventilator parameters, such as oxygen percentage ($O_2\%$), V_T, **inspiratory time (T_I or Tinsp),** respiratory rate (f), and so on. The control knobs that appear vary, depending on the mode selected. For example, if the SIMV mode is selected in volume ventilation, only the controls that are active in SIMV volume ventilation appear on the screen. (NOTE: If the power fails or STANDBY is selected, the settings that were in effect before the interruption are again in effect when the unit is reactivated.)

The available ranges for control parameters are listed in Table 12-14. If the operator tries to set a value beyond the normal available range for a parameter, the knob stops adjusting the numeric value as it is turned. A message appears at the bottom of the screen telling the operator what needs to be done to continue. For example, if the operator selects a respiratory rate of 4 breaths/min in SIMV and the T_I is set at 1 second, the knob will freeze and

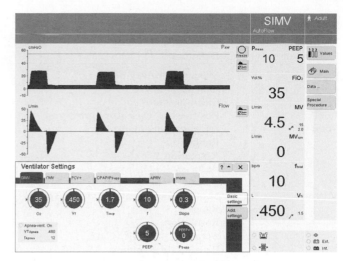

FIGURE 12-37 Lower left corner of this figure shows the ventilator settings available in the SIMV mode of ventilation on the EvitaXL. (Courtesy Dräger Medical, Telford, Pa.)

the message at the bottom will read, I:E < 1:3 CONFIRM, followed by an icon for the dial knob. When you press the knob, the SIMV rate will drop below 4 breaths/min with a T_I of 1 second.

MONITORS AND ALARMS

In every mode of ventilation, the EvitaXL provides monitored parameters on the right side of the screen. The active mode appears in the top right corner. Graphics are centrally located (see Figure 12-33). On the bottom is a row that displays the set parameters. Although these are the variables most commonly selected, the displayed variables can be changed.

Measured Values

The VALUES touch pad brings up a screen that displays values being measured or calculated by the unit, such as F_IO_2 (Table 12-15; also see Figure 12-37). Expiratory flow for the ventilator is measured with a hot wire pneumotachometer (see Chapter 8). The ventilator has a built-in galvanic oxygen analyzer and does an automatic oxygen calibration every 24 hours. The unit optimally can include a mainstream infrared carbon dioxide analyzer that provides information on end-tidal carbon dioxide ($etCO_2$), CO_2/time, and single-breath CO_2 (CO_2/volume). Calculated values include carbon dioxide production ($\dot{V}CO_2$), dead space (V_D), and V_D/V_T measurements. The analyzer normally is taken out of the circuit and calibrated before use (see the operator's manual for instructions).[1]

Alarms

Alarms can be set by pressing the ALARM LIMITS touch pad to the right of the display screen (see Figure 12-33). Alarm parameters should always be set appropriately for the patient. When ALARM LIMITS is pressed, a screen display appears that allows adjustment of the available alarm

TABLE 12-15

Commonly Measured and Displayed Parameters—Dräger EvitaXL

Parameter	Definition	Range
Ppeak	Maximum airway pressure	0-120 cm H_2O
Pplat	Plateau pressure	0-99 cm H_2O
Pmean	Mean pressure	0-99 cm H_2O
PEEP	Positive end-expiratory pressure	0 to 50 cm H_2O
Pmin	Minimum airway pressure	−20 to 99 cm H_2O
	Range	−45-100 cm H_2O
	Resolution	1 cm H_2O
	Accuracy	4% (cm H_2O)
MV	Minute ventilation	0-100 L/min
MVspn	Spontaneous breathed minute volume	
	Range	0-120 L/min (BTPS)
	Resolution	0.1 L/min or values < 1 L/min: 0.01 L/min
	Accuracy	±8% of measured value
VTe	Exhaled tidal volume	
	Range	0-6 L (BTPS)
	Resolution	1 mL
	Accuracy	±8% of measured value
f_{tot}	Breathing frequency	0 to 240 breaths/min
f_{spn}	Spontaneous frequency	
	Range	0-300 breaths/min
	Resolution	1 breath/min
	Accuracy	±1 breath/min
F_IO_2	Fractional inspired O_2 measured on inspiratory side	
	Range	15-100 vol.%
	Resolution	1 vol.%
	Accuracy	±3 vol.%
T	Breathing gas temperature	18° to 51°C
R	Resistance	0-600 cm H_2O/L/sec
C	Compliance	0-300 mL/cm H_2O

BTPS, Body temperature pressure saturated.

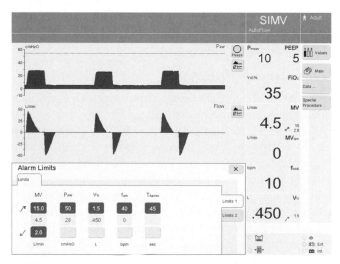

FIGURE 12-38 ALARM LIMITS window (lower left corner of the screen). (See text for further explanation.) (Courtesy Dräger Medical, Telford, Pa.)

values (Figure 12-38). For example, to set the HIGH RATE alarm, touch the screen key adjacent to the spontaneous respiratory rate (f_{spn}). The screen key changes from green to yellow. Using the rotary knob, set the desired high rate; the number appears inside the screen key. Press the dial knob to activate the new setting; the soft pad changes

back to green. Table 12-16 lists the ranges for the adjustable alarms.

The alarm limits for O_2% are set automatically by the ventilator (see Table 12-16). The automatic alarm limit for low airway pressure is the set PEEP value plus 5 cm H_2O. For example, if PEEP is 5 cm H_2O, the low pressure limit is 10 cm H_2O and is not adjustable. When the upper Paw alarm limit is reached, an audible and visual alarm is activated, inspiratory flow delivery stops, and the expiratory valve opens, dropping pressure to baseline. This alarm is functional in all modes of ventilation and is similar to the upper pressure limit on most ventilators. However, the Ppeak alarm is not to be confused with the **Pmax pressure limit.** The Pmax limit is not an alarm; rather, it actually changes the way a breath is delivered during CMV, SIMV, and MMV. For this reason, Pmax is reviewed under the discussion of modes of ventilation.

Basically the EvitaXL has three levels of alarm indicators:

- WARNING (top priority)
- CAUTION (medium priority)
- ADVISORY (low priority)

The function of each of these is listed in Table 12-17. After an alarm has been activated, the audible tone can be silenced with the ALARM SILENCE touch pad. The LED appears on the ALARM SILENCE pad when the audible alarms

TABLE 12-16

Alarm Ranges—Dräger EvitaXL

Parameter	Range and/or Description
Expiratory Minute Ventilation	
Alarm at upper alarm limit	If MV has exceeded the upper limit MV 41 to 0.1 L/min
Alarm at lower alarm limit	If MV falls below the lower limit 0.01 to 40 L/min
Setting range for NIV	1-60 L/min
Volume	
Alarm at lower alarm limit	If the set V_T could not be applied (alarm limit is linked to set V_T)
Alarm at upper alarm limit	If applied V_T exceeds the alarm threshold, inspiration is interrupted and the exhalation valve opens
Setting range	21-4000 mL
High f_{spn}*	5-120 breaths/min; the rate is exceeded during spontaneous breathing
Airway Pressure (P_{aw})	
Alarm at upper alarm limit	If P_{aw} high value is exceeded
Setting range	10-100 cm H_2O
Paw alarm at lower limit	If value of PEEP + 5 cm H_2O (linked to set PEEP value) is not exceeded for at least 96 msec in two consecutive ventilator breaths
Apnea Alarm Delay Time	If no breath is detected; range, 5-60 sec
End-Tidal CO_2 Alarm†	
High end-tidal CO_2 ($etCO_2$)	If the upper limit has been exceeded
Range	0-98 mm Hg (1-15 vol.%)
Low $etCO_2$	If the value drops below the lower alarm limit
Range	0-97 mm Hg (0-14.9 vol.%)
Inspired O2% Alarm	
Alarm at upper alarm limit	If O_2% exceeds the upper alarm limit for at least 20 sec
Alarm at lower alarm limit	If O_2% falls below the lower alarm limit for at least 20 sec
Range	Both alarm limits are linked to the set value: Threshold for settings below 60 vol.%: ±4 vol.% Threshold for settings above 60 vol.%: ±6 vol.%

f_{spn}, Spontaneous frequency; *NIV*, noninvasive ventilation.
*No lower alarm limit available.
†Available only when CO_2 analyzer (capnograph) is added.

TABLE 12-17

Displayed Information with Priority Alarms—Dräger EvitaXL

Alarm Light	Message* (on Screen)	Message (Background Color)	Audio	Alarm Level
Red flashing	Name of alarm followed by "!!!" (e.g., "APNEA!!!")	Red	Five tones; repeated twice every 7 sec	Warning; top priority
Yellow flashing	Name of alarm followed by "!!" (e.g., "O₂ PRESSURE HIGH!!")	Yellow	Three tones; repeated every 20 sec	Caution; medium priority
Yellow constant	Name of alarm followed by "!" (e.g., "FAN MALFUNCTION!")	Yellow	Two tones; occurs only once	Advisory; low priority

*Appears at the top of the screen.

are inactive and is functional for 2 minutes. Once the alarm situation has been corrected, the alarm can be reset by touching the ALARM SILENCE soft pad (LED off). Medium and low priority messages do not need to be acknowledged after the problem is solved, but high priority messages must be acknowledged by the operator to verify that the problem has been resolved. This is done by pressing the ALARM RESET touch pad. The high priority alarm message leaves the screen and is stored in memory. (NOTE: Access to the LOGBOOK function is available on the ALARM LIMITS and the MEASURED VALUES screens to recall any stored, top priority alarm messages.)

During an alarm, the operator can touch the ALARM INFO screen key to view all currently active messages. The dial knob can be used to select a message. By touching the "?" screen key, a screen is displayed that provides information about the possible cause and solution to the alarm that was selected (Figure 12-39).

Examples of low priority alarms include AIR SUPPLY LOW, FLOW MONITORING OFF, and INSPIRATORY HOLD INTER-

RUPTED. Examples of medium priority alarms are AIR SUPPLY PRESSURE TOO HIGH, CHECK SETTINGS, and PRESSURE LIMITED. Examples of top priority alarms are numerous. A few examples are APNEA, DEVICE FAILURE, and LOW O$_2$ SUPPLY. The operator's manual provides a list of all alarms.[1] After any top priority alarm, the operator must be absolutely certain that the patient is being ventilated. (NOTE: When a MIXER INOP alarm activates, the blender is defective; the manufacturer advises that the patient be manually ventilated until the unit can be replaced and that the problem unit be removed from service until repaired by a service representative.)

MODES OF VENTILATION

Modes of operation available on the EvitaXL are listed in Box 12-27.

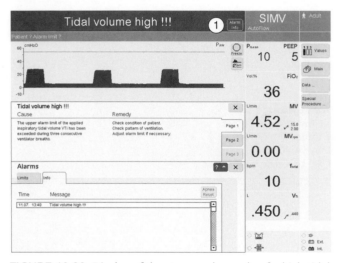

FIGURE 12-39 Display of the cause and remedy of a high tidal volume high priority alarm on the EvitaXL screen. The (1) indicates the alarm information screen key. (Courtesy Dräger Medical, Telford, Pa.)

BOX 12-27	Modes of Ventilation Currently Available on the EvitaXL

Continuous mandatory ventilation (CMV)
AutoFlow
Pressure limit ventilation (PLV or Pmax)
SIMV and SIMV with pressure-support ventilation
Pressure-control ventilation plus (PCV+)(BIPAP)
Pressure-support ventilation (PSV)
Continuous positive airway pressure (CPAP)
Airway pressure-release ventilation (APRV)
Mandatory minute volume ventilation (MMV) and MMV with PSV
Apnea ventilation
AutoFlow*
Noninvasive ventilation (NIV)*
NeoFlow*

*Available as an option.

BOX 12-28	Reconfiguring the Ventilator's Start-Up Mode (EvitaXL)

To change (reconfigure) the start-up mode, perform the following steps:
1. Press the SYSTEM SETUP key.
2. Press the VENTILATION screen key.
3. Touch MODES & SETTINGS and enter the access code 3032.
4. Touch the MODES screen key.
5. Select the desired start-up mode by touching STARTUP (screen key).
6. Select and confirm by using the dial knob.

NOTE: The operator's manual provides a full description of the process for configuring the start-up modes and alarm settings.

Standard Settings of Ventilator Modes

When the ventilator is turned on initially, the standard mode that is programmed (configured) appears. For example, CMV is an assist-control (A/C) mode that may be the default mode for the unit. The institution purchasing the ventilator can change the default mode by reconfiguring the unit. Box 12-28 describes how to reconfigure a ventilator mode.

To select a different mode of ventilation from the default mode, the operator presses the VENTILATION SETTINGS control to the right of the screen (see Figure 12-34). At the bottom of the screen, a small window will appear that includes various selections in the form of horizontal and vertical tabs, as on a catalog card (see Figure 12-37). The mode tabs are arranged horizontally across the top. BASIC SETTINGS and ADDITIONAL settings are the two tabs arranged vertically on the right.

When the new mode screen key is pressed, the parameters that can be set in that mode appear on the screen, and the MODE soft key turns yellow. Parameters are set in a manner similar to that in which alarm parameters are set. The operator touches the parameter screen knob (e.g., V$_T$). The screen knob changes from green to yellow. The rotary knob is turned to obtain the desired numeric value, which appears in the center of the screen knob. The rotary knob is then pressed to activate the setting. The old mode continues to operate until the new mode has been selected and confirmed.

Continuous Mandatory Ventilation (CMV)

The CMV mode is an A/C volume ventilation mode. The operator sets the V$_T$, flow, f(CMV), TINSP, **sensitivity,** PEEP, O$_2$%, and desired alarm settings. PEEP/CPAP and O$_2$% can be selected in any mode. Breaths are patient or time triggered, volume targeted, and time cycled. All breaths deliver the set V$_T$.

Flow to the patient is restricted to the flow setting selected. If the flow is high and the V$_T$ is delivered before

TINSP is achieved, the inspiratory valve closes (the expiratory valve is already closed), and the breath is maintained in inspiration. This event can be recognized from the pressure-time waveform. An **inspiratory pause** will be present. On the flow-time curve, the flow will return to zero before the end of inspiration (Figure 12-40). An inspiratory pause may also be adjusted by changing, for example, the TINSP. When the knob is touched and changes to yellow, a blue **smart window** appears at the bottom left of the screen and displays the I:E ratio, T_E, and pause time. As the variable selected (TINSP) is changed, the new calculated values are displayed. For example, if the TINSP is shortened for a fixed flow, the duration of the inspiratory pause will decrease (Clinical Rounds 12-10).

Two potential drawbacks exist with this type of mandatory breath. First, if the lungs are nonhomogenous, the resulting peak pressures may lead to overdistention in some areas of the lung. Second, both the inspiratory and expiratory valves are closed during the inspiratory pause, which may lead to patient-ventilator asynchrony if the patient makes a breathing effort during the pause time.

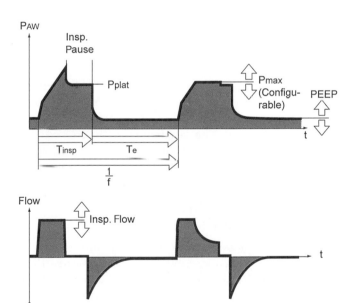

FIGURE 12-40 The pressure (Paw) curve *(top)* and the flow curve *(bottom)* on the left illustrate an inspiratory pause in which the flow decreases to zero before the end of the inspiratory phase. The Paw and flow curves on the right illustrate the function of Pmax (PLV). (See text for additional information.) (Courtesy Dräger Medical, Telford, Pa.)

CLINICAL ROUNDS 12-10

You are setting up a patient on CMV with the Dräger EvitaXL. The settings are as follows: V_T = 0.5 L (500 mL); f = 10 breaths/min; flow = 60 L/min (1 L/sec); and Tinsp = 1 second. Will there be an inspiratory pause with these settings? If yes, how can you shorten or eliminate the pause?

See Evolve Resources for the answer.

The rate of gas delivery at the beginning of the breath can be adjusted with the EvitaXL. The SLOPE key allows the rate of rise to the peak flow to be tapered. A setting of zero slope provides an immediate rise to the set flow, whereas any value greater than zero provides a more gradual rise to the set flow.

The Dräger EvitaXL can provide flow triggering in all modes of ventilation. The flow-trigger level is set by choosing the ADD SETTINGS screen key, which allows selection of the desired flow-trigger value using first the FLOW-TRIGGER screen key and then the FLOW screen key. As with other adjustments, the setting is confirmed by pressing the dial knob.

Two other functions that can be available when volume-targeted ventilation is used (CMV and SIMV) are AutoFlow and pressure limit ventilation. Both can be accessed through the selection of the ADD SETTINGS control, and both alter breath delivery during a volume-targeted breath.

AutoFlow

AutoFlow is a dual control mode of ventilation (see Chapter 11). It can be activated when a volume-targeted mode of ventilation is selected, such as CMV, SIMV, or MMV. AutoFlow provides pressure-limited breaths (pressure-controlled ventilation [PCV]) that are volume targeted. The ventilator monitors the exhaled (delivered) volume, compares it with the set volume, and adjusts the pressure level from one breath to the next to achieve the set volume (adjustments are made in increments of 1 to 3 cm H_2O).

As with any pressure-limited breath, AutoFlow uses a descending (decelerating) inspiratory flow pattern while it targets the set volume. When AutoFlow is used, it provides for automatic control of INSP FLOW and PINSP.

When AutoFlow is started, the ventilator delivers a volume-targeted mandatory breath with an inspiratory pause. It then measures the plateau pressure and delivered volume and calculates system compliance (C) and resistance (R). The next breath is a constant pressure breath with the lowest peak pressure determined to achieve the selected V_T (Figure 12-41).

As ventilation progresses in AutoFlow, if the delivered (exhaled) volume is lower than the set volume, the unit increases pressure during inspiration by a few centimeters of water pressure (cm H_2O) for the next breath to try to achieve the selected volume. If the delivered volume is too high compared with the set volume, the unit decreases pressure delivery for the next breath. The pressure change between breaths is never greater than 3 cm H_2O. During AutoFlow, the inspiratory pressure does not exceed the Paw limit minus 5 cm H_2O. For example, suppose the target volume is 500 mL, and this volume initially required 20 cm H_2O to deliver. Let us assume the Paw limit is set at 40 cm H_2O. Suppose there is a reduction in the patient's lung compliance. The ventilator would need to progressively increase pressure to deliver the set volume. Once the

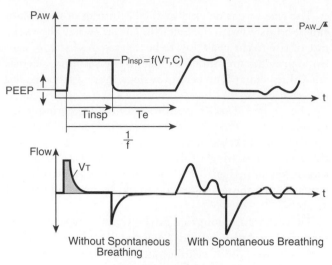

FIGURE 12-41 AutoFlow on the EvitaXL ventilator. The top curve represents pressure-time and the bottom curve flow-time. The breath on the left illustrates a pressure-targeted breath with the Paw calculated to achieve the set tidal volume. The breath on the right illustrates how a patient can breathe spontaneously at any time during AutoFlow. (Courtesy Dräger Medical, Telford, Pa.)

delivering pressure is 35 cm H_2O, the pressure limit is reached. The ventilator will display the message VOLUME NOT CONSTANT, and an audible alarm will be activated. The clinician should evaluate the patient and determine what intervention is appropriate. For example, the patient may need to be suctioned, or the TINSP may be set too short.

AutoFlow makes the expiratory valve more interactive with the patient. For example, if the patient coughs or breathes during the set inspiratory time of a mandatory breath, the valve system allows the patient to inhale and exhale freely while maintaining the inspiratory pressure. Very little resistance or pressure builds up in the circuit when active patient breathing occurs. Because AutoFlow alters the function of the inspiratory and expiratory valves, a patient is able to receive the inspiratory flow demanded up to 180 L/min in any volume mode, regardless of the volume settings. Therefore the "set" volume is not only a "target" volume but also a minimum volume.

To access AutoFlow, the operator performs the following steps:

1. Selects the ADD SETTINGS screen key in the respective ventilation
2. Touches the AUTOFLOW ON screen key
3. Presses the dial knob to confirm that AutoFlow is activated

Once AutoFlow is activated, the functions of PMAX PRESSURE LIMIT and INSP FLOW are no longer available.

When AutoFlow is used, several types of breathing patterns can occur:

1. The V_T is delivered and flow drops to zero before the unit time cycles out of a mandatory inspiration. During this time the pressure delivered by the unit is maintained until exhalation begins (see Figure

12-41). However, the patient can breathe spontaneously during any part of the inspiratory time.
2. If the patient breathes in and out during a mandatory breath, the plateau delivery stays constant and does not fluctuate significantly. Flow is provided as needed to meet patient demand. The expiratory valve opens during spontaneous exhalation to prevent pressure buildup and resistance to exhalation while maintaining plateau pressure (see Figure 12-41).
3. A TINSP that has been set too short can be identified from the flow-time curve. If inspiration ends before flow drops to zero, the volume is delivered, but the pressure may be higher than desired. The unit may have to increase pressure and flow to deliver the V_T when TINSP is short. The patient should be evaluated before any change is made.[3] The clinician may want to increase TINSP to reduce the peak inspiratory pressure.

In AutoFlow, the operator should always set a maximum tidal volume alarm limit, VTi, so that overdistention of the lungs does not occur if compliance decreases suddenly. If the V_T exceeds the high VTi limit, an alarm message is displayed and the ventilator goes into expiration. In addition, an inspiratory pressure alarm limit (Paw) that is appropriate for the patient should be set to prevent excessive pressure (Clinical Rounds 12-11).

When a patient is breathing very actively, volume delivery may be higher than the selected V_T value. If the patient continues to breathe actively, the pressure level is slowly lowered accordingly. The ventilator has interpreted the large volumes for the current pressure as an improvement in the patient's lung characteristics (C and/or R). In this case, AutoFlow may not be the best mode for the patient.

Pressure Limit Ventilation (PLV or Pmax)

The high peak pressures that may occur during volume ventilation can be avoided by using the **pressure limit ventilation (PLV)** function. PLV is a supplementary function or safety feature that can be used in CMV, SIMV, and MMV. Its purpose is to limit peak pressures during volume

---

CLINICAL ROUNDS 12-11

A patient on AutoFlow has the following ventilator settings and monitored parameters: mode = CMV; V_T (set) = 0.6 L (600 mL); f = 10 breaths/min; inspiratory pressure = 18 cm H_2O; T_I = 1.5 seconds; upper pressure limit = 40 cm H_2O.

The patient has done well on these settings for the past 4 hours. During the next hour, however, the respiratory therapist notices that the upper Paw limit alarm is activated. The inspiratory pressure is now 35 cm H_2O, and the V_T is 550 mL. What do you think the therapist should do in this situation?

See Evolve Resources for the answer.

BOX 12-29   **Setting Start-Up Defaults to Allow PLV (Pmax) on the EvitaXL**

To set start-up defaults to allow for pressure limit ventilation (Pmax), perform the following steps:
1. Press the SYSTEM SETUP key (VENTILATION and ADDITIONAL SETTINGS screen page).
2. Touch the VENTILATION screen key.
3. Touch MODES & SETTINGS screen key.
4. Enter access code 3032.
5. Touch ADD SETTINGS screen key.
6. Set PLV pressure using PMAX.
7. Press dial knob to confirm.

HISTORICAL NOTE 12-1

Pmax (Pressure Limit Ventilation)

Pmax was the concept behind the first Evita ventilator. In the EvitaXL, it is referred to as *pressure limit ventilation (PLV)*. The manufacturer now believes that the AutoFlow function is superior to the use of Pmax/PLV and that AutoFlow should be the option of choice for reducing ventilating pressures. In AutoFlow, the EvitaXL automatically brings Ppeak equal or close to the Pplat, as timing allows. In AutoFlow, the exhalation valve floats, but in Pmax/PLV it is closed. The manufacturer recommends that the Pmax/PLV be kept in the OFF position in machine configuration.[1]

---

ventilation. Box 12-29 describes the procedure for setting PLV as a start-up default. Historical Note 12-1 discusses PLV and Pmax.

When PLV is operational, the unit targets the set V_T but limits the pressure delivered during the breath. When it is active, the set Pmax value is drawn as a horizontal blue line in the pressure-time waveform. The PMAX screen knob also appears in the menu for VENTILATOR SETTINGS.

During volume ventilation with PLV, if the pressure in the circuit rapidly reaches the maximum pressure setting (PMAX), inspiration continues for the set inspiratory time (time cycled), but the amount of pressure in the circuit does not go above this setting (see Figure 12-40). Flow also rises rapidly at the start of inspiration to the set flow value. (NOTE: The set flow is based on the set inspiratory time and the volume selected.) The flow remains at the set value until the set Pmax is reached, at which point flow descends to baseline while the Pmax pressure is maintained throughout inspiration (see Figure 12-40). The V_T remains constant at the set value as long as flow drops to zero before the end of inspiration (i.e., an inspiratory hold). If flow does not drop to zero for the pressure provided by the unit, the volume cannot be delivered and a VOL NOT CONSTANT, PRESSURE LIMITED !! alarm is activated.

It is recommended that AutoFlow be used with any other volume mode so that patient flow is not restricted. When AutoFlow is used, it takes over the task of setting both INSP FLOW and PMAX, and these screen controls are no longer displayed (see the discussion of AutoFlow in the previous section).

SIMV and SIMV with Pressure-Support Ventilation (SIMV + PSV)

As described in Chapter 11, SIMV provides a maximum number of mandatory breaths and allows the patient to breathe spontaneously between them. Mandatory breaths can be patient or time triggered, volume or pressure targeted, and time cycled. Spontaneous breaths can be assisted with pressure support, in which case the pressure-support breaths are patient triggered, pressure targeted, and flow cycled. (Pressure-support breaths are described in the discussion on pressure support later in this section.)

With SIMV the operator selects the mandatory breath rate, which determines the time between mandatory breaths. For example, if the SIMV rate is 5 breaths/min, the time between mandatory breaths is 12 seconds (60 seconds/5 breaths/min). The patient can breathe spontaneously during part of the 12-second interval. All other adjustable parameters in SIMV are the same as those described in the earlier section on CMV.

In the SIMV volume-targeted mode, the operator selects the target volume for the mandatory breaths. Inspiratory flow can be set, along with inspiratory time (T_I). In the SIMV volume-targeted mode, either Pmax or AutoFlow also can be used.

In the SIMV pressure-targeted mode, the operator sets the target pressure for mandatory breaths, but Pmax and AutoFlow are *not* active because breath delivery already is pressure targeted, and the ventilator controls these functions.

When SIMV is activated, the patient has approximately a 5-second window (1.5 seconds in pediatric mode) in which to make an inspiratory effort and trigger a mandatory breath. If a patient effort is not detected, the first mandatory breath occurs at its set cycle. Using the previous example, if the SIMV rate is 5 breaths/min, the time between mandatory breaths is 12 seconds. Without a detected effort, the first mandatory breath occurs in about 12 seconds.

Apnea ventilation can be activated during this mode and is reviewed later in this section.

Pressure-Control Ventilation Plus (PCV+)(BiPAP)

PCV+, also known as BiPAP, is a pressure-targeted mode of ventilation in which the patient can breathe spontaneously at any time during the breath cycle (inspiration and expiration). It sometimes is described as two levels of CPAP (continuous positive airway pressure) with time cycling from one level of CPAP to the other (Figure 12-42). Mandatory breaths are patient or time triggered, pressure targeted, and time cycled. Spontaneous breaths are patient triggered, pressure targeted, and pressure or flow cycled.

The operator sets the pressure, a minimum respiratory rate, and a flow trigger. Time triggering is determined by

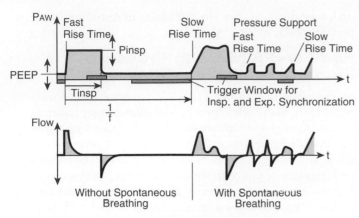

FIGURE 12-42 Pressure-time curve *(top)* and flow-time curve *(bottom)* for PCV+. Without spontaneous breathing, a mandatory PC breath is delivered. During spontaneous breathing *(breath on the right),* the patient is able to receive flow at any time during the breath delivery. (See text for additional information.) (Courtesy Dräger Medical, Telford, Pa.)

the set rate and patient triggering by the flow-trigger setting. Pressure during a mandatory breath is equal to the PINSP setting.

During PCV+, the unit functions as follows: When it is time for a mandatory breath (based on the rate setting) and the patient makes an inspiratory effort, a mandatory breath is delivered. During this time, the set pressure is achieved and held relatively constant, but the patient can still breathe spontaneously by receiving flow on demand (see Figure 12-42). The change from exhalation to inhalation and from inhalation to exhalation is patient synchronized when the patient is breathing spontaneously.

Spontaneous breaths that occur between mandatory breaths can be assisted with pressure support by setting the desired pressure-support level (PCV + PS). An elevated baseline (PEEP/CPAP) can also be set.

The RISE TIME control is used in this mode to slow flow and pressure delivery at the beginning of the breath.* RISE TIME is set by using the screen knob with the symbol for an ascending ramp. The rise time is adjustable from 0 to 2 seconds and represents the amount of time it takes the ventilator to achieve the set pressure from the beginning of inspiration. A rapid rise is appropriate for a patient with a high peak inspiratory flow. A slow rise is more appropriate for a small pediatric patient with less of a high flow demand. Figure 12-42 shows the slow rise time that tapers flow and pressure delivery on the second breath compared with the first. In most clinical settings, the default rise time of 0.2 seconds is adequate; it is seldom necessary to go above 0.4 seconds. If rise time is being used, it affects both mandatory and pressure-support breath delivery.

In the PCV+ mode, the V_T delivered is based on ΔP (Pinsp minus PEEP), patient effort, and the patient's lung characteristics. Because V_T and $\dot{V}_E$ may vary in this mode,

*RISE TIME can be set to control pressure delivery in any mode when pressure-targeted breaths are available.

the operator needs to set the $\dot{V}_E$ alarm limits carefully. As with SIMV volume ventilation, apnea ventilation can be activated during this mode. Pmax and AutoFlow are not active during this mode because breath delivery is already pressure targeted.

Pressure-Support Ventilation (PSV)

The EvitaXL can provide PSV during SIMV, PCV+, MMV, and spontaneous (CPAP) ventilation. The target pressure is set using the PSUPP screen knob. The setting selected determines the pressure above PEEP that will be delivered during a PS breath. PS breaths are patient triggered, pressure targeted, and flow cycled. Patient triggering generally is set at flow triggering. Whenever PSV is active, the RISE TIME control is also functional.

Inspiration normally ends when inspiratory flow decreases to a certain value, called the *flow-cycle criterion.* The flow-cycle criterion is 25% of peak inspiratory flow for adults and pediatric patients and 6% in neonatal patients. (See Chapter 11 for additional information on flow-cycle criteria.) Apnea ventilation is available in the pressure-support mode.

If the patient actively exhales or coughs during the start of a PS breath and the circuit pressure rises, inspiratory flow ends. This prevents excessive pressure from building up in the circuit and can be identified by the flow going to zero or less than zero on the flow-time curve. Inspiratory flow during a PS breath time cycles out of the inspiratory phase if the inspiratory time exceeds 4 seconds (1.5 for pediatric patients, but adjustable with the T_I control in neonatal patients). A prolonged T_I most commonly occurs if a leak is present. If the time-cycling criteria occur for three consecutive breaths, an alarm is activated to warn of a possible leak in the system.

Continuous Positive Airway Pressure (CPAP)

Spontaneously breathing patients may benefit from breathing at elevated baseline pressures (CPAP), which helps maintain or restore functional residual capacity (FRC). CPAP is available on the EvitaXL when the CPAP/P SUPP mode is selected. CPAP can be provided with or without PSV. CPAP alone can be selected by turning the PSV level to 0 cm H_2O and setting the PEEP to the desired CPAP level (cm H_2O). Apnea ventilation is available when CPAP is being used.

Airway Pressure-Release Ventilation (APRV)

In **airway pressure-release ventilation (APRV),** two levels of CPAP are set. This mode of ventilation operates very much like PCV+, except that the "expiratory" interval is very brief (Figure 12-43). APRV allows spontaneous breathing at a high level of CPAP with brief periods of pressure release to a lower pressure level.

After APRV is selected, the upper pressure level is set using P_{HIGH}, and the lower level is set using P_{LOW}. The unit

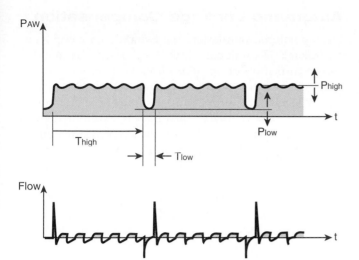

FIGURE 12-43 Pressure-time curve *(top)* and flow-time curve *(bottom)* for the APRV mode. The patient can breathe spontaneously at any time. (See text for additional information.) (Courtesy Dräger Medical, Telford, Pa.)

also times the length of both pressure levels. T_{HIGH} is the length of time high pressure is provided, and T_{LOW} is the length of time low pressure is provided. Both are intended for use with spontaneously breathing patients (see Chapter 11). The RISE TIME control can be used to taper the pressure change from P_{LOW} to P_{HIGH}, but the length of rise time cannot be longer than the set T_{HIGH} time. Apnea backup ventilation is recommended when this mode is used.

Mandatory Minute Volume Ventilation (MMV) and MMV with Pressure Support (MMV/PSV)

With **mandatory minute volume ventilation (MMV),** the ventilator provides mandatory breathing only if the patient's spontaneous breathing is not adequate and drops below the preselected MMV setting. MMV is set by selecting that screen tab and then setting the MMV appropriate for the patient using the V_T, flow, f, and T_I settings. A pressure-support level should be set to ensure that the patient has adequate support for spontaneous breaths. As described in Chapter 11, with MMV the patient can breathe spontaneously and contribute all of the $\dot{V}_E$ with only PSV or CPAP added and no mandatory breaths; or the patient might contribute only a portion of the $\dot{V}_E$. The difference between the spontaneous and the set $\dot{V}_E$ is provided by mandatory breaths at the set volume. If no spontaneous breathing is present, the mandatory breath rate and set respiratory rate provide the total $\dot{V}_E$. Pmax or AutoFlow can be used in MMV. (NOTE: It is important to set the high rate alarm to protect the patient from rapid, shallow breathing that would result in an equivalent $\dot{V}_E$ but would also increase the work of breathing and provide inadequate alveolar ventilation.)

The system is designed to prevent premature delivery of mandatory breaths in patients who have irregular spontaneous breathing patterns while at the same time providing an alarm in the event of an extended period of low $\dot{V}_E$.

Apnea Ventilation

Apnea ventilation supplies ventilation with a set respiratory rate and V_T in case the patient becomes apneic in SIMV, PCV+, PS/CPAP, or APRV. If the patient stops breathing for the length of time set on the APNEA TIME ALARM control (T_{Apnea}), the alarm is activated and apnea ventilation begins. The EvitaXL activates the apnea alarm if either no expiratory flow is detected or if insufficient inspiratory gas is delivered for the duration of the set apnea time delay.

Apnea ventilation is set by touching the ADD SETTINGS screen key, then the APNEA VENTILATION screen key, and then the VT and F screen knobs. When these parameters are set, the operator presses the dial knob to confirm. The operator then touches the ON or OFF screen key to activate or deactivate apnea ventilation. The baseline pressure (PEEP), O_2%, trigger sensitivity, and other alarm parameters remain as they are in the current mode. (NOTE: The caution message APNEA VENTILATION !! may be obscured by high priority alarm messages.) Once an apnea ventilation event has resolved, the operator can touch the ALARM RESET screen key and press the dial knob to confirm a return to the original mode of ventilation.

NeoFlow[1,4,5]

NeoFlow is a mode of ventilation that can be added to the EvitaXL ventilator to allow it to be adapted for neonatal use (patient weight from 0.5 to 6 kg). NeoFlow requires the installation of a flow sensor between the end of the endotracheal tube and the Y-connector of the patient circuit. The other end is attached to the back of the ventilator unit. The flow sensor must be calibrated when it is used for the first time and then at least once every 24 hours (see the operator's manual).

When the unit is turned on and the screen displays the STANDBY mode, the operator selects the neonatal option. In the neonatal mode, the unit can provide volume ventilation; AutoFlow; apnea back-up ventilation; pressure support with assisted spontaneous breathing (ASB); continuous base flow; and measurements of circuit leaks, airway pressure, and breath triggering. (See Chapter 13 for additional information on NeoFlow on the Dräger ventilator.)

Noninvasive Mask Ventilation (Option)

With the EvitaXL, the operator has the choice between selecting invasive or noninvasive ventilation. Noninvasive ventilation (NIV) uses a nasal or face mask as the patient interface. The patient must be breathing spontaneously to use this mode. All modes of ventilation except independent lung ventilation (ILV)* can be selected in the MASK

*See the EvitaXL operating manual for additional information on ILV.

mode. (NOTE: NIV, or MASK[NIV], is *never* used for intubated patients or patients with tracheostomies.)

To set MASK ventilation, the operator presses the START/STANDBY key. TUBE/MASK is then selected, which allows selection of the MASK(NIV) screen key. Pressing the dial knob confirms that the MASK ventilation mode has been selected. The message MASK VENTILATION appears in the top right message display area.

The EvitaXL compensates for leaks up to 30 L/min in the adult and 15 L/min in pediatric patients. When large leaks are present, it is recommended that PCV be selected as the NIV mode. To prevent alarms from artifact, the following alarms can be deactivated:

· Low minute volume alarm
· High inspiratory tidal volume alarm
· Apnea time (upper limit) alarm

However, alarms should not be switched off if the patient's safety is compromised.[1] A time delay due to a disconnection (TDISCONNECT) can be set for the low Paw alarm and adjusted between 0 and 60 seconds.

In NIV on the EvitaXL, apnea cannot be reliably detected. For this reason, use of external pulse oximetry oxygen saturation (SpO$_2$) monitoring is recommended.[1]

SPECIAL FUNCTIONS

A variety of special functions or features are on the Dräger EvitaXL, some of which are similar to other ICU ventilators and others that are unique to this unit. Some of these functions are reviewed here.

Compensation for Patient Circuit Compliance

The EvitaXL provides compensation for volume lost as a result of tubing compressibility. During the ventilator check before beginning patient ventilation, the EvitaXL determines the resistance and compliance of the patient circuit (STANDBY mode) with the AIRTIGHT CHECK soft pad.

The circuit compliance value (mL/cm H$_2$O) is used to adjust flow and volume delivery from the unit during ventilation. The unit adds the volume needed to compensate for the volume lost to the circuit during inspiration. It then subtracts this added volume from the measured (displayed) expiratory volume to give a close estimate of the volume actually exhaled by the patient. Thus the set and measured inspired and expired volumes more correctly reflect what is delivered to the patient.

Flow Trigger

The set **flow trigger** determines how sensitive the ventilator is to the patient's inspiratory effort. Based on this setting, the ventilator synchronizes breath delivery with the patient's inspiratory effort. This parameter is available in the ADD SETTINGS menu. The flow trigger screen allows the operator to turn this parameter on or off and to adjust the level of sensitivity. (See Chapter 11, section on patient triggering for more information.)

Automatic Leakage Compensation

During volume ventilation, the EvitaXL can compensate for leakage. The unit has a leak compensation feature that can be turned off or on. When leak compensation is activated, the ventilator compares delivered flow with exhaled flow. The difference provides a measurement of the amount of leakage. The ventilator then increases volume delivery from the unit to compensate for the leak measured on the previous breath. This correction also takes into account the patient circuit compliance and pressure delivery during inspiration.

During NIV, a maximum of 30 L/min of leakage in the adult and 15 L/min of leak in the pediatric mode can be compensated. (NOTE: The Evita XL compensates leaks up to 200% of set V$_T$ [maximum of 2 L] regardless of the mode of ventilation.)[1]

Sigh (Intermittent PEEP)

As with a normal sigh breath, the intended purpose of the sigh function on the EvitaXL is to open up or keep open areas of the lung that are prone to collapsing (atelectatic). Sigh breaths are accomplished in the EvitaXL ventilator by intermittently increasing the PEEP level to the set sigh pressure value for two consecutive breaths in the CMV mode. The range of baseline sigh pressure (PEEP) is 0 to 35 cm H$_2$O (Figure 12-44).

Intermittent PEEP, or "sigh" breaths, can be activated by touching the ADD SETTINGS screen key on the screen and is set like other parameters. The intermittent PEEP screen knob is turned to the desired pressure level using the dial knob. The function becomes active as soon as the ON screen key is selected and the dial knob is pressed. Once it is set, the main monitoring screen reads INT PEEP ACTIVE when it is selected.

During the sigh interval, the VOLUME NOT CONSTANT alarm is deactivated. Because intermittent PEEP increases the baseline, it is advisable to set the Pmax pressure limit appropriately to prevent overdistention of the lungs during regular breath delivery.

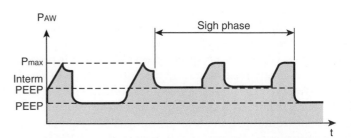

FIGURE 12-44 Example of the pressure-time waveform during the sigh mode with the EvitaXL. Pmax is maximum pressure, interm PEEP is the PEEP applied during the sigh phase, and PEEP is the regular setting for PEEP before and after the sigh. (See text for additional information.) (Courtesy Dräger Medical, Telford, Pa.)

Automatic Tubing Compensation (ATC)

An automatic tubing compensation (ATC) feature is available on the EvitaXL to compensate for the airway resistance associated with small artificial airways. ATC can be used with spontaneous breathing, PSV, PCV+, and CMV with AutoFlow activated. In CMV, SIMV, and MMV, tube compensation is active during expiration after a mandatory breath and during spontaneous breathing phases.

This ventilator function regulates airway pressure and flow at the tracheal level to reduce the work of breathing associated with endotracheal or tracheostomy tubes (Box 12-30).

When it is selected, the ventilating pressure during all breaths compensates for the resistance associated with varying size endotracheal tubes. This compensation depends on the direction of gas flow. The airway pressure is increased during inspiration and decreased during expiration. (NOTE: The expiratory portion can be switched off if the operator only wants to compensate for the inspiratory portion.) The pressure can be increased to a value equal to the upper Paw alarm limit minus 5 cm H_2O or reduced to a minimum of 0 cm H_2O.

To set the tube compensation function, the following should be performed:

1. During STANDBY mode, select the ADD SETTINGS screen key in the selected ventilation mode.
2. Touch the ATC screen key.
3. In the ATC set-up screen, touch either the ET tube or the TRACH tube screen key, depending on the type of artificial airway in use.
4. Use the ID 0 screen knob to set the size of the tube's inner diameter (with the dial knob) and confirm it by pressing the dial knob.
5. Use the COMP screen key and the dial knob to set the percentage of compensation provided. For example,

---

BOX 12-30   Calculating the Support Pressure During Automatic Tubing Compensation (EvitaXL)

The Dräger EvitaXL calculates and displays tracheal pressure based on a mathematical equation:

$$P_{trachea} = P_{aw} - K_{tube} \times Flow^2$$

where $P_{trachea}$ is the pressure in the trachea, P_{aw} is the pressure at the Y-connector of the patient circuit, K_{tube} is the tube coefficient (listed in the operating manual), and *Flow* is the patient flow (inspiratory flow is greater than zero, and expiratory flow is less than zero).

An example of a tube coefficient is 6.57 cm $H_2O/L^2/sec^2$ for an endotracheal tube with an inner diameter (ID) of 8 mm.

For pressure support, the equation is as follows:

$$\Delta P_{aw} = Comp \times K_{tube} \times Flow^2$$

where ΔP_{aw} is the pressure support at the tube, *Comp* is the degree of compensation (0 to 100%), K_{tube} is the tube coefficient, and *Flow* is the patient flow.

---

a reading of 70 inside the COMP screen key provides 70% compensation for the artificial airway.

Select either ON or OFF, and press the dial knob to confirm.

SPECIAL PROCEDURES

A variety of special procedures or special functions are available with the EvitaXL, including nebulization of medications, external flow compensation, preoxygenation and postoxygenation for suctioning, disconnecting for suctioning, **inspiratory hold maneuvers** and **expiratory hold maneuvers,** support during hose change, and sensor calibration.

Nebulization of Medications

The EvitaXL provides a nebulizer port connection that allows use of an internal pneumatic nebulizer. The nebulizer function is designed for nebulizers requiring a flow of 6 L/min at 29 psi. Using any other type of nebulizer may result in considerable variation in V_T and F_IO_2.[1]

In the adult mode, the nebulizer function can be used with every mode of ventilation. Flow through the nebulizer connector occurs during inspiration and requires a ventilator flow of at least 15 L/min. (NOTE: The nebulizer is switched off at flows less than 15 L/min.) The ventilator automatically maintains the set $\dot{V}_E$ and approximates the set O_2%.

In the pediatric mode, nebulization of medication requires a pressure control mode of ventilation or volume control with AutoFlow activated. In pediatrics the flow from the nebulizer port is continuous (inspiration and expiration). It is recommended that the nebulizer not be used at breath rates below 12 breaths/min.

To switch the nebulizer on, the operator selects the SPECIAL PROCEDURE screen function key and the ventilator displays the ADDITIONAL FUNCTIONS menu. The NEBULIZER screen key is then selected and activated by pressing the dial knob. The message NEBULIZER ON! appears on the screen. Nebulization automatically ends after 30 minutes. The expiratory flow sensor is automatically cleaned and calibrated after nebulization. The functioning of the flow sensor may be impaired by the accumulation of medications on sensors, filters, and heat and moisture exchangers.[1] Users are advised to check the function of these devices when ventilated patients are receiving nebulized medications. To protect the sensor during the use of nebulized medications, an expiratory filter can be placed inline before the sensor. Because filters also can accumulate moisture and residue from medications, they need to be checked and changed regularly.

External Flow Compensation

Sometimes practitioners power inline small-volume nebulizers by using an external gas source such as a separate flowmeter. To prevent alarms and ensure proper monitoring, the operator might adjust the minute volume alarms (high and low) and use an external SpO_2 monitor to monitor the patient's oxygen status for the duration of the treatment.

The EvitaXL can take the added external flow into account for the purpose of monitoring. Once the flow is added inline, the operator selects the FLOW menu and the MEASURE screen. The flow is measured by the flow sensor, and the value for this flow is displayed along with the date and time. The added flow cannot exceed 12 L/min, or the unit will interrupt calculation of the external flow. Once the flow has been calculated, the flow sensor and monitor take this additional flow into account. This helps prevent the FLOW MEASUREMENT INOP alarm, and the originally measured exhaled volume (before the added flow) is maintained. However, a higher value for VTe (exhaled volume) and minute volume is measured as a result of the higher flow. In volume-controlled ventilation, the delivered tidal volume is higher than the set value. The manufacturer recommends the use of pressure-controlled ventilation when an external flow source is used.[1]

Preoxygenation and Postoxygenation for Suction 100% O_2

To help reduce the risk of hypoxia during bronchial suctioning, a 100% O_2 support function is available. The 100 VOL% O_2 screen key is used to provide 100% O_2 for 2 minutes in adult patients. In pediatric patients, the oxygen concentration is 25% higher than the set F_IO_2 value. The message O_2 ENRICHMENT 180 S appears on the screen, and the time remaining is displayed. The preoxygenation lasts a maximum of 180 seconds.

To activate the suction function, the operator selects the SPECIAL PROCEDURE function key and the screen displays the menu ADDITIONAL FUNCTION. The operator then selects the O_2 ↑ SUCTION screen key and presses the dial knob to confirm, and the oxygenation program starts.

During the suction procedure, a pressure of 4 cm H_2O is applied if a PEEP of less than 4 cm H_2O is set to help the ventilator identify when the circuit is disconnected and reconnected when an open suction procedure is used. All other parameters are unchanged.

After disconnection has been recognized, the unit provides 100% oxygen for 2 minutes during suctioning. During these 2 minutes, the audible alarm is silenced so that it is not a nuisance, and a very small flow of gas is provided through the circuit to detect disconnection. The lower minute volume alarm is also deactivated during the suctioning procedure and for 2 minutes afterward. Other alarms are also switched off during suctioning, but for only 15 seconds afterward.

When the patient is reconnected within the time indicated, the disconnection phase is ended and ventilation resumes. If no reconnection occurs after 2 minutes, the preoxygenation program is interrupted. Alarms are reactivated (no longer silenced), and ventilation is again started. An additional 2 minutes of 100% oxygen are provided to the adult patient. In the pediatric patient, the F_IO_2 is 25% higher than the set value for 2 minutes. The main display screen reads FINAL O_2 ENRICHMENT 120 S, and the remaining time is counted down on the screen.

Pressing the O_2 ↑ SUCTION screen key at any time stops the oxygenation procedure, which cannot be restarted for 15 seconds.

Manual Inspiration (Inspiratory Hold)

The INSPIR HOLD touch pad displayed in the ADDITIONAL FUNCTION menu under SPECIAL PROCEDURE provides an inflation hold maneuver when pressed and held down for as long as the inspiratory pause is desired (maximum of 40 seconds). When activated, either the current inspiration is held, or a new mandatory breath is delivered and the inspiration is held. Inspiratory hold functions in all modes except CPAP when pressure support is set at zero.

Expiratory Hold

Expiratory hold (EXP HOLD) can be used to estimate the pressure in the circuit and the patient's lungs during exhalation. This can be used to determine intrinsic PEEP (auto-PEEP) or trapped air. The EXP HOLD screen key can also be used to measure negative inspiratory force (NIF), also known as *maximum inspiratory pressure (MIP)*. It is accessed under SPECIAL PROCEDURE, ADDITIONAL FUNCTION menu. By touching and holding the EXP HOLD screen key, the operator can keep the ventilator in the expiratory phase for up to 15 seconds. This procedure closes both the inspiratory and expiratory valves. (See the later section on negative inspiratory force.)

Support during Hose Changes—Leak Testing

When a patient circuit is changed, the ventilator can check the hose for leaks by using the STANDBY mode (i.e., selecting the AIRTIGHT CHECK soft pad). In addition, the resistance and compliance of the circuit are measured to provide compliance compensation for the volume lost as a result of tubing compliance (see the discussion of patient circuit compliance compensation).

DIAGNOSTIC FUNCTIONS

Intrinsic PEEP

An estimate of the amount of auto-PEEP (intrinsic PEEP) as well as an estimate of the trapped volume in a patient's lungs can be determined by using the intrinsic PEEP (PEEPi) function. These measurements can be performed only if the patient is not actively breathing during the measurement.

To perform an auto-PEEP measurement, select the SPECIAL PROCEDURE touch pad. From the computer screen, touch the PEEPi soft pad. The maneuver is performed automatically, and the waveform display is frozen. On the screen, values for PEEP(set), PEEPi, and trapped volume (Vtrap) are shown. Using the dial knob and the screen cursor, the operator can choose to view the auto-PEEP level at any time on the pressure-time curve. The PEEPi values appear above the waveform.

Occlusion Pressure

Measurements of the **occlusion pressure ($P_{0.1}$)** are used to evaluate a patient's neuromuscular drive.[6,7] This procedure can be performed automatically by selecting the SPECIAL PROCEDURES touch pad, the $P_{0.1}$ soft pad, and the START soft pad.

At the beginning of inspiration, the ventilator occludes the inspiratory and expiratory valves 0.1 second after the beginning of inspiratory flow. The pressure measured at that time is displayed. The value for the occlusion pressure is shown on the screen. The normal value is about −3 to −4 cm H_2O. Values more negative than −6 cm H_2O may indicate impending exhaustion and respiratory muscle fatigue that may lead to respiratory failure, as in patients with chronic obstructive pulmonary disease. They may also indicate forceful active inspiration.

As with PEEPi, the waveform is frozen on the screen. Using the rotary knob and screen cursor, the measured value for the occlusion pressure from the pressure-time curve can be viewed at precise moments during the maneuver.

Negative Inspiratory Force

Negative inspiratory force (NIF) is a measurement of the patient's maximum inspiratory effort against a closed system. As mentioned, it also is referred to as the *maximum inspiratory pressure*. Some clinicians use the maneuver to estimate the patient's ability to generate a strong inspiratory effort. The section on expiratory hold describes how to access this feature.

To measure NIF, the operator touches the EXP HOLD screen key and holds it (maximum, 15 seconds). The NIF is displayed on the ventilator NIP screen (SPECIAL PROCEDURE/DIAGNOSTICS).

Low-Flow PV Loop (Optional)

The low-flow pressure-volume (PV) loop is an optional feature available on the EvitaXL. Some clinicians use the low-flow PV loop to evaluate the upper and lower inflection points.[8-10] (For information on inflection points, see reference 2.) The low-flow PV loop technique can be performed only on a patient who is not breathing spontaneously (i.e., an apneic or a paralyzed patient). The patient must be monitored closely during the procedure, because it may compromise hemodynamic status. No leaks can be present in the system during the maneuver.

To begin the procedure, the operator selects SPECIAL PROCEDURE, then ADDITIONAL FUNCTION, and finally LOW FLOW PV-LOOP. The operator should read the screen information provided before proceeding with the test. The measurement is taken by touching PROCEDURE and selecting

the pressure from which the maneuver will start (PSTART), the maximum pressure to be reached (PLIMIT), the low flow setting (FLOW), and the maximum allowable volume (VLIMIT). Once the limits are established, the dial knob is pressed to confirm. The maximum duration of the procedure is displayed as TMAX. To record both inspiration and expiration, the operator touches the START INSP+EXP screen key and confirms by pressing the dial knob. If only the inspiratory portion of the loop is wanted, this option can be selected by using the START INSP ONLY screen key.

To end inspiration during the procedure, the STOP INSP control is selected. To stop the procedure immediately, the ABORT screen key is used and the dial knob is pressed to confirm.

Once the procedure has been completed, the EvitaXL displays the ANALYSIS screen (Figure 12-45). The operator can select a specific point on the curve by using the CURSOR 1 and CURSOR 2 controls. When the dial knob is used to position the cross-hair cursor over the designated point, the measured values for that point are displayed. Selecting two points on the curve displays a grey line between the two points that represents the compliance for that specific line (not shown in figure). An additional maneuver cannot be performed until a 60-second interval has passed since the end of the last procedure.

Additional Information Screens

The EvitaXL records and stores in memory setting changes, events, and alarms. These are listed in chronologic order by date and time in the logbook. The logbook can be seen by touching the DATA screen key and the LOGBOOK screen key. To view all setting changes in a single line entry, the operator turns the dial knob to select the desired time line.

Graphs of trended data are available by touching the DATA screen key and then TRENDS. The EvitaXL displays three trended parameters on the screen with a common time scale. Different trends can be selected for viewing, as well as a different time scale, including 1-, 3-, 6-, 12-, and 24-hour trend graphs.

VENTILATOR GRAPHIC WAVEFORMS

The graphics monitor with the EvitaXL is part of the main computer screen during standard operation. Additional waveforms can be viewed simultaneously, and different waveforms may be displayed during normal function. The operator can view a measured numeric value for a given time on any graph by positioning the cursor on the computer screen and rotating the dial knob to the desired time on the curve. The value is shown on the screen above the waveform. The FREEZE screen key can be used to freeze a current real-time waveform. The freeze mode ends automatically after 3 minutes.

Loops can be viewed as either two small loops, one on the left and one on the right, or as an enlarged loop on the

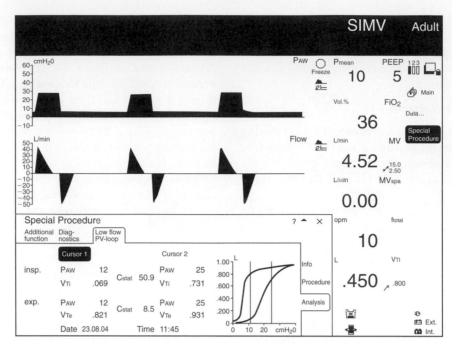

FIGURE 12-45 Lower portion of the screen display on the EvitaXL, showing the inspiratory (INSP) and expiratory (EXP) airway pressure (PAW), inspiratory V_T (VTi), expiratory V_T (VTe), and static compliance (Cstat) for the pressure-volume loop displayed. (See text for additional information.) (Courtesy Dräger Medical, Telford, Pa.)

left. Loops are accessed under the waveforms menu. Using the REF screen key allows a reference loop to be recorded (drawn in blue). The reference loop appears continuously in position as the current loop is recorded over it. This allows observation of the flow-volume loop, for example, before and after the administration of a bronchodilator. Loops, like waveforms, can be frozen for 3 minutes.

TROUBLESHOOTING

The alarms and monitored information offer assistance during operation for solving most problems that might occur with the EvitaXL. In addition, the operator's manual contains a troubleshooting section that alphabetically lists all the alarm messages, gives their priority level, provides common causes, and recommends remedies. Covering this extensive material is beyond the scope of this text. Users are advised to consult the operator's manual. Additional information about Dräger products is available on the company's Web site at http://www.draeger.com.

SMARTCARE/PRESSURE SUPPORT (PS) OPTION

SmartCare/PS is a ventilator option available with the Dräger EvitaXL. It is a closed-loop form of ventilation designed to shorten weaning time for intubated or tracheotomized patients who are ready for ventilator discontinuation. The focus of SmartCare is on control of assisted spontaneous breathing (ASB) with and without positive end-expiratory pressure (PEEP). The strategy of the software is to gradually reduce the level of assistance based on the patient's tolerance and comfort. The intent is to try to reduce the time on ventilation. The decision to use SmartCare for a particular patient is made by the patient's physician.[11]

The goal of SmartCare is to keep the patient within a "comfort zone." The comfort zone is defined as an acceptable respiratory rate, a V_T above a minimum threshold, and an end-tidal CO_2 below a maximum threshold (Table 12-18).[12]

SmartCare automatically adjusts pressure support as needed by 2 to 4 cm H_2O either upward or downward based on evaluation of the patient's spontaneous respiratory parameters (f_{spn}, V_T, PEEP, and etCO$_2$).[11] For example, with tachypnea the pressure is increased, whereas with bradypnea with a low etCO$_2$, the pressure is increased. The system is designed to accept transient instabilities in breathing. For example, it tolerates a short increase in the respiratory rate without changing the ventilator settings. (NOTE: The pressure assist support breath [P_{ASB}], or pressure support level, can be changed at any time by the user.)

Patient Criteria for Using SmartCare

SmartCare is appropriate for patients who have a stable spontaneous breathing drive and are ready for ventilator discontinuation. The patient should be hemodynamically stable and adequately oxygenated. An external SpO$_2$

TABLE 12-18

Ventilation Parameters—SmartCare (EvitaXL)

BODY WEIGHT > 35 KG		
Parameter	Abbreviation	Values
Lower limit, spontaneous breathing frequency	f_{spn} low	f_{spn} low: 15 breaths/min (all patients)
Upper limit, spontaneous breathing frequency	f_{spn} high	f_{spn} high: 30 breaths/min (patients without neurologic disorders) f_{spn} high: 34 breaths/min (patients with neurologic disorders)
Maximum limit spontaneous breathing frequency	f_{spn} max	f_{spn} max: 36 breaths/min (all patients)
Lower limit tidal volume	V_T low	V_T low: 250 mL (body weight ≤ 55 kg) V_T low: 300 mL (body weight > 55 kg)
Upper limit etCO$_2$	etCO$_2$ high	etCO$_2$ high: 55 mm Hg (patients without COPD) etCO$_2$ high: 65 mm Hg (patients with COPD)
Lower limit for P_{ASB}	P_{ASB}	When ATC is deactivated: $\quad P_{ASB}$ goal: 5 mbar (patient with tracheostomy with active humidifier) $\quad P_{ASB}$ goal: 7 mbar (patient with endotracheal with active humidifier) $\quad P_{ASB}$ goal: 9 mbar (patient with tracheostomy with HME/filter) $\quad P_{ASB}$ goal: 12 mbar (patient with endotracheal tube with HME/filter) When ATC is activated: $\quad P_{ASB}$ goal: 0 mbar (with active humidifier) $\quad P_{ASB}$ goal: 5 mbar (with HME/filter)
Upper limit for P_{ASB} above PEEP	P_{ASB} max	P_{ASB} max: 40 mbar
BODY WEIGHT 15 TO 35 KG; ENDOTRACHEAL TUBE AND ACTIVE HUMIDIFICATION		
Parameter	Abbreviation	Values
Lower limit, spontaneous breathing frequency	f_{spn} low	f_{spn} low: 18 breaths/min
Upper limit, spontaneous breathing frequency	f_{spn} high	f_{spn} high: 40 breaths/min
Maximum limit, spontaneous breathing frequency	f_{spn} max	f_{spn} max: 50 breaths/min (all patients)
Lower limit tidal volume	V_T low	V_T low: 6 mL (body weight setting)
Upper limit etCO$_2$	etCO$_2$ high	etCO$_2$ high: 55 mm Hg
Lower limit for P_{ASB}	P_{ASB}	P_{ASB} goal: 10 mbar
Upper limit for P_{ASB} above PEEP	P_{ASB} max	P_{ASB} max: 40 mbar

HME—heat moisture exchanger, ATC—automatic tube compensation, fspn—spontaneous respiratory rate, V_T—tidal volume, etCO$_2$—end-tidal carbon dioxide, P_{ASB}—pressure assist support breath.
From Dräger Medical (Telford, PA).

monitor with an alarm should be used when SmartCare is activated to monitor oxygenation status and to activate an alarm if a hypoxemic event occurs.

Activation and Set-Up of SmartCare

After the EvitaXL is turned on, it takes about 90 seconds for SmartCare to load. During this time it is not available for use. Once it is activated, the ventilator prompts the user to enter certain information and to set up the alarms.

To set SmartCare, the operator enters the patient's weight, the type of airway in use (endotracheal or tracheotomy tube), and the type of humidifier in use (active or heat and moisture exchanger [HME]), the patient's medical history (neurologic disorder [yes/no] or COPD [yes/no]), and NIGHT REST (yes/no and time), which enables the nighttime interval to be set for more support to allow for resting periods. Finally, PATIENT SESSION is selected. This allows the practitioner to turn on SmartCare. Box 12-31 provides a list of the conditions and guidelines that must be followed when SmartCare is used.

BOX 12-31   Patient and Ventilator Conditions to be Met with SmartCare (EvitaXL)

· Adult or pediatric patient with CPAP/PS profile
  · Weight range: 15 to 200 kg
· Requirements for patients weighing >36 kg
  · Endotracheal or tracheotomy tube
  · Active humidification or HME/filter
· Requirements for patient weighing 15 to 35 kg
  · Endotracheal or tracheotomy tube
  · Active humidification
  · Automatic tube compensation (ATC) deactivated*
Leakage compensation much be activated.
Apnea ventilation (backup) must be active and set appropriately.
CO$_2$ monitoring must be activated and blue CO$_2$ sensor (CapnoSmart) in use.
Flow monitoring (NeoFlow monitoring) activated.
PS (pressure-assisted spontaneous breathing [P_{ASB}]) above PEEP must be set at P_{ASB} of 5 mbar and 35 mbar.
PEEP must be set between 0 mbar and 20 mbar.

*With body weights >35 kg, ATC can be used with 100% compensation.

It is essential that the system have no leaks. Leaks may result in as much as a twofold increase in the patient's V_T.[11] The monitored exhaled tidal volumes are required to be above the lower limit V_T minimum setting. The lower limit for tidal volume (V_T low) is calculated based on the body weight entered for each patient. The higher tidal volume delivery caused by leaks may impede successful weaning. (NOTE: When SmartCare is used, the leak compensation feature must be activated.)

For patients weighing more that 35 kg, SmartCare requires that additional information be provided by the operator; for example, whether the patient has chronic CO_2 retention, as seen in COPD, because this will affect the adjustment of $etCO_2$ limits. Second, the type of airway (endotracheal or tracheostomy tube) and the type of humidifier (active humidification or HME) are needed. This information is used to establish the minimum pressure support at the end of the weaning process (5 to 12 mbar).

The setting NEUROLOGIC DISORDER provides a different value for the respiratory rate for the patient's comfortable zone for patients who weigh more that 35 kg. Remember that patients with damage to the brainstem may exhibit hyperventilation with an increased respiratory rate. SmartCare allows an elevated spontaneous respiratory rate up to 34 breaths/min in patients with neurologic disorders and still allows weaning to occur. Rates higher than this may indicate that the patient is not ready for weaning, and SmartCare may not be appropriate.

For patients weighing less than 35 kg, the SmartCare program assumes that the patient is intubated and has active humidification in use. The lower limit for tidal volume (V_T low) is calculated based on the body weight entered for each patient.

The clinician can adjust the F_IO_2, trigger sensitivity, and alarm limits for SmartCare. The pressure level (P_{ASB}) can also be adjusted, and the SmartCare program will continue therapy using the manually set value. PEEP can be adjusted, but the SmartCare program will not conduct spontaneous breathing trials for PEEP values of more than 5 mbar. However, the mode of ventilation cannot be changed, and PEEP cannot be adjusted above 19 mbar or the patient session is terminated. (NOTE: If the operator increases PS shortly before suctioning, SmartCare calls for a rapid reduction to avoid excessively high pressures.)

The top section of Table 12-18 provides the parameters and limits for patients weighing more than 35 kg, and the bottom of the table provides parameters for patients weighing 15 to 35 kg. (NOTE: These are set parameters and cannot be changed by the operator. They are thresholds defined within the software knowledge base.)

Monitoring Screen During SmartCare

Once the program is active, SMARTCARE appears in the upper portion of the screen and a separate color display is used. In SmartCare, measured values and settings are labeled with an SC, which appears in front of the parameter on the monitoring screen. For example SC-f_{spn} is the SmartCare spontaneous respiratory rate, and SC-V_T is the SmartCare tidal volume.

TABLE 12-19

Recommended Alarm Settings—SmartCare (EvitaXL)

Parameter	Alarm Limit
Low minute volume	−25% of current minute volume
High minute volume	+25% of current minute volume
High spontaneous rate	40 breaths/min (body weight > 35 kg)
	60 breaths/min (body weight ≤ 35 kg)
V_T /f ratio	12 mL/body weight (kg)
High Paw	42 mbar
Low $etCO_2$	18 mm Hg
High $etCO_2$	57 mm Hg (without chronic obstructive pulmonary disease [COPD])
High $etCO_2$	67 mm Hg (with COPD)
T_{Apnea}	60 sec

Alarm Settings

Once SmartCare is activated, the alarm settings can be selected appropriately for the patient. The SmartCare user's guide states that the alarm settings are the responsibility of the attending physician.[11] Table 12-19 provides a guideline based on current manufacturer-recommended alarm settings.

As SmartCare monitors the patient and adjusts pressure support above PEEP, the patient's weaning progresses. The size of the pressure change depends on the patient's monitored ventilation up to that time.

How SmartCare Changes Settings

As the patient breathes spontaneously and is monitored by the ventilator, SmartCare makes adjustments in pressure to accommodate changes in the patient's breathing. For example, if the rate is 31 to 34 breaths/min and the V_T and $etCO_2$ are acceptable, pressure is increased by 2 mbar. The ventilator is trying to increase pressure to improve V_T and reduce the patient's spontaneous respiratory rate. If the rate rises above 35 breaths/min, the ventilator increases the pressure by 4 mbar. This hopefully would increase V_T even more to help reduce the respiratory rate.

Suppose the patient is breathing deeply and has a spontaneous rate below 15 breaths/min with an acceptable $etCO_2$ (CO_2 is not elevated). The ventilator establishes that the patient is hyperventilating, and the pressure is reduced by 4 mbar.

When ventilation is inadequate and the V_T and $etCO_2$ are outside the defined range, the ventilator determines that the patient is hypoventilating, and pressure is increased by 2 mbar.

Ending SmartCare

Periodically the ventilator using SmartCare performs a weaning test, the spontaneous breathing trial (SBT). The SBT can be performed at any time and repeated as necessary. Once an SBT is evaluated as successful, the ventilator provides a message to the operator: SC:WEANING COMPLETED! Obviously, this is the point where the operator is prompted to disconnect the patient from the ventilator and evaluate the patient to see whether the person is ready to have the ventilator discontinued. (NOTE: The decision to extubate the patient must be assessed clinically by the physician or respiratory therapist.)

Troubleshooting SmartCare

The SmartCare operator's manual provides a table of messages, alarms, possible causes, and corrective actions to be taken during the use of SmartCare. The user is advised to refer to this manual for troubleshooting any problems encountered during a SmartCare session. For example, if no patient effort is detected, the message BREATHING CYCLE NOT DETECTED appears with a high priority alarm (!!!). The ventilator will continue to ventilate the patient (apnea ventilation), and the SmartCare session ends, but the operator must evaluate the patient to determine what corrective action needs to be taken.

Research Findings for Knowledge-Based Weaning

The use of knowledge-based weaning, such as the SmartCare system, is relatively new, but a few studies are available.

In one study, patients were ventilated successively with a computer-driven weaning process compared with standard manually adjusted pressure support.[12] In addition, the time spent in the "comfort zone" was significantly longer than with standard PS. The time spent with high airway occlusion pressure (high P0.1), which suggests an excessive work of breathing (WOB), was significantly lower with the automated PS system. Repeated periods of excessive WOB may actually slow weaning time. This is believed to be caused by diaphragm fatigue, which may aggravate diaphragmatic weakness.[12]

Compared with physician-controlled weaning guidelines, a computer-driven system has been shown in studies to reduce the duration of ventilation and the length of stay in the ICU.[13-15] However, not all studies have shown significant differences between standard weaning procedures and SmartCare in patients with chronic obstructive pulmonary disease (COPD).[16] Another benefit of a computer-driven weaning system is that it can continuously monitor and evaluate patient data. Clinicians cannot continuously be at the bedside to evaluate the patient, as a computer-driven system imbedded in a ventilator can do.[12,13]

To summarize, initial studies suggest that a knowledge-based, computer-driven ventilator system can shorten weaning time in certain patient populations compared with typical clinician-controlled weaning protocols.

KEY POINTS

- The EvitaXL (version 6.0) is designed to be used for ventilation of adults, children. and infants (minimum, 3 kg).
- With the EvitaXL, the operator can choose invasive or noninvasive ventilation.
- If the AC power supply fails or is lost, the ventilator switches to the available DC power source (external or internal); however, the internal battery provides a maximum of 10 minutes of operation and is intended for use only as a short-term emergency power source.
- Expiratory flow for the ventilator is measured with a hot wire pneumotachometer, and inspired oxygen concentrations are measured using a galvanic oxygen analyzer.
- As with the E-4, the EvitaXL can optimally include a mainstream carbon dioxide analyzer that provides information on end-tidal carbon dioxide, CO_2/time, and single-breath CO_2 (CO_2/volume).
- Available modes of ventilation include CMV, AutoFlow, PLV (Pmax), SIMV, PCV+, PSV, CPAP, APRV, MMV, and apnea ventilation.
- AutoFlow is a dual control mode that provides a pressure-limited, volume-targeted form of ventilation in which the ventilator adjusts the pressure to achieve the set volume.
- When pressure limit ventilation (PLV) is operational (with CMV, SIMV, and MMV), the ventilator targets the set VT but limits the pressure delivered during the breath.
- Special functions of the EvitaXL include compensation for patient circuit compliance, flow trigger, automatic leakage compensation, sigh (intermittent PEEP), and tubing compensation.
- Special procedures available are nebulization of medications, external flow compensation, preoxygenation and postoxygenation for suction 100% O_2, manual inspiration (inspiratory hold), expiratory hold, and support during hose change.
- Diagnostic functions available with the EvitaXL include measurement of intrinsic PEEP, occlusion pressure (P0.1), low-flow PV loop, and negative inspiratory force, which requires the use of the expiratory hold function.
- SmartCare/PS, an option available with the EvitaXL, is a closed-loop form of ventilation designed to shorten weaning time for intubated or tracheotomized patients who are ready for ventilator discontinuation.

ASSESSMENT QUESTIONS

See Evolve Resources for the answers.

1. Which of the following is/are specific area(s) of the EvitaXL front control panel?
   I. Fixed keys to allow access to various functions
   II. Rotary knob for selecting and confirming settings
   III. Operating screen (touch screen), which contains information and controls for ventilation
   IV. Four dial knobs below the screen to directly control the main parameters used in each mode
   a. III
   b. I and II
   c. II an IV
   d. I, II, and III

2. Which of the following statements about the power sources for the EvitaXL is true?
   a. When the AC power fails, the ventilator shuts down operation.
   b. An internal DC power source is available that provides 1.5 to 2 hours of power when AC power is lost.
   c. An internal DC power source provides about 10 minutes of power when AC power is lost.
   d. Two 50-psig gas sources are required for the EvitaXL to operate.

3. A mode in which the operator sets P_{HIGH}, P_{LOW}, T_{HIGH}, and T_{LOW} is called:
   a. Airway pressure-release ventilation
   b. Pressure-regulated volume control ventilation
   c. Pressure-support ventilation
   d. Proportional assist ventilation

4. When AutoFlow is activated on the EvitaXL which of the following occurs?
   a. Sensitivity to patient effort is reduced.
   b. Inspiration is flow cycled.
   c. A short release time (T_{LOW}) allows for exhalation.
   d. Breath delivery becomes pressure limited and volume targeted.

5. When comparing the EvitaXL with the E-4, the primary difference is/are the:
   a. Available modes provided
   b. Main screen or user interface
   c. Internal gas delivery system
   d. Monitoring system

6. To select and accept a ventilator parameter on the EvitaXL, the operator does all of the following *except*:
   a. Touch the screen knob
   b. Turn the dial knob
   c. Touch the screen knob to accept the setting
   d. Press the dial knob to confirm the setting

7. Using the expiratory hold function allows for measurement of which of the following parameters?
   I. Negative inspiratory force (NIF)
   II. Occlusion pressure
   III. Intrinsic pressure
   IV. Slow vital capacity
   a. I and III
   b. II and IV
   c. II and III
   d. I, III, and IV

8. The purpose for using the low-flow pressure-volume loop feature with the EvitaXL is to:
   a. Determine the length of an apnea period in a patient with apneic episodes
   b. Deliver nebulized medications at a slower breath rate
   c. Evaluate for the upper and lower inflection points
   d. Measure the slow vital capacity of the patient

9. A blue reference loop appears continuously on the screen while current loops (flow-volume) appear over the reference loop. The purpose of the reference loop is to allow:
   a. Observation of the flow-volume loop before and after a bronchodilator treatment
   b. Quantification of the pressure from air trapped in the lungs
   c. Verification that the patient is receiving a safe level of volume
   d. Recalibration of the loop while the patient is still receiving ventilatory support

10. SmartCare is best defined as:
    a. Training of the respiratory care staff from the Dräger Web site
    b. Respiratory care personnel who have passed the EvitaXL examination
    c. Making appropriate ventilator adjustments while using PSV for weaning
    d. A closed-loop form of ventilation designed to shorten weaning time

References

1. EvitaXL: Intensive care ventilator software 6.1n operating instructions, ed 1, November, 2005, 90 38 733 – GA 5664.660, Dräger Medical AG & Co. KG; Telford, Pa, Dräger, Drägerwerk AG.
2. Radford EP, Ferris BG, Kriete BC: Clinical use of a nomogram to estimate proper ventilation during artificial respirations, *N Engl J Med* 251:877, 1954.
3. Pilbeam SP, Cairo JM: *Mechanical ventilation: physiological and clinical applications,* ed 4, St Louis, 2006, Mosby/Elsevier.
4. E-4 plus option NeoFlow NI 5664.515e/117D, Telford, Pa, 1997, Dräger.
5. NeoFlow: neonatal mode, supplement to the instructions for use of the Evita 4 as from software version 2.n ED 2077947.97, ed 2, Telford, Pa, 1997, and version 4.n, 2001, Dräger, Drägerwerk AG.
6. Capdevila XJ, Perrigault PF, Perey PJ et al: Occlusion pressure and its ratio to maximum inspiratory pressure are useful predictors for successful extubation following T-piece weaning trail, *Chest* 108:482, 1995.
7. Scott GC, Burki NK: The relationship of resting ventilation to mouth occlusion pressure: an index of resting respiratory function, *Chest* 98:900, 1990.

8. Gama AM, Meyer EC, Gaudencio AM et al: Different low constant flows can equally determine the lower inflection point in acute respiratory distress syndrome patients, *Artif Organs* 25:882, 2001.

9. Albaiceta GM, Piacentini E, Villagra A et al: Application of continuous positive airway pressure to trace static pressure-volume curves of the respiratory system, *Crit Care Med* 31:2514, 2003.

10. Servillo G, DeRobertis E, Maggiore S et al: The upper inflection point of the pressure-volume curve: influence of methodology and of different modes of ventilation, *Intensive Care Med* 28:842, 2002.

11. SmartCare/PS—knowledge-based system for automating clinical guidelines, software 1.1, supplement to the instructions for use for EvitaXL from software version 6.n onwards, ed 1, 90 38 416 – GA 5664.630 en, Dräger Medical AG & Co. KGaA, Germany, July 2004.

12. Dojat M, Harf A, Touchard D et al: Clinical evaluation of a computer-controlled pressure support mode, *Am J Respir Crit Care Med* 161:1161, 2000.

13. Lellouche F, Mancebo J, Jolliet P et al: A multicenter randomized trail of computer-driven protocolized weaning from mechanical ventilation, *Am J Respir Crit Care Med* 174:894, 2006.

14. Shahsavar N, Ludwigs U, Blomqvist H et al: Evaluation of a knowledge-based decision-support system for ventilator therapy management, *Artif Intell Med* 5:37, 1995.

15. Bouadma L, Lellouche F, Cabello B et al: Computer-driven management of prolonged mechanical ventilation and weaning: a pilot study, *Intensive Care Med* 31:1446, 2005.

16. Jiang H, Yu SY, Wang LW: Comparison of SmartCare and spontaneous breathing trials for weaning old patients with chronic obstructive pulmonary diseases (in Chinese), *Zhonghua Jie He He Hu Xi Za Zhi* 29:545, 2006.

Internet Resource
www.draeger.com

DRÄGER SAVINA

The Dräger Savina, introduced in the United States in 2001, is an intensive care ventilator for use in adult and pediatric patients. The ventilator can be used in recovery rooms, ICUs, subacute care facilities, and transport inside and outside the hospital.

Its function is similar to the other Evita ventilators, but fewer options are available with this unit, making it more cost-effective for some critical care facilities. Additional information about the Savina is available on the Evolve Web site for this text.

HAMILTON VENTILATORS

HAMILTON VEOLAR^{FT}

The Hamilton VEOLAR[FT] is an early generation ventilator marketed by Hamilton Medical (Reno, Nevada). Because newer modes, such as the Galileo Gold, are available, the discussion on this model has been moved to the Evolve Web site for this text.

HAMILTON GALILEO GOLD[1]

OUTLINE

Power Source
Internal Function
Patient Circuit
Controls and Alarms
    Configuration of T_I, Peak Flow, or I:E
    Adjustable Control Parameters
    Alarms
    Upper Pressure Limit (Pmax)
    Monitoring
    Real-Time Monitoring
    Front Panel Touch Keys
Modes of Ventilation
    Assist/Control (A/C)
    Synchronized Intermittent Mandatory Ventilation (SIMV)
    Spontaneous Mode (CPAP and PSV)
    Pressure-Targeted Assist-Control Ventilation (P-A/C)

Pressure-Control Ventilation Plus Adaptive Pressure
    Ventilation (P-A/C + APV)
Pressure-Control/SIMV (P-SIMV)
Pressure-Control/SIMV Plus Adaptive Pressure
    Ventilation (P-SIMV + APV)
Adaptive Support Ventilation (ASV)
Adaptive Tidal Volume Support (AvtS)
Dual Positive Airway Pressure Mode (DuoPAP) and
    Airway Pressure-Release Ventilation (APRV)
Noninvasive Ventilation (NIV)
Special Features
Sigh
Backup Ventilation
Tube Resistance Compensation (TRC)
Pressure-Volume (P/V) Tool
Troubleshooting

OBJECTIVES

Upon completion of this section, you will be able to:
· Describe the function of the two knobs on the front of the GALILEO ventilator.
· Explain how to select a ventilator mode and the parameters for that mode.
· Explain how to select the alarm screen and set the alarms.
· Compare the addition of APV to standard PCV.
· Discuss how the microprocessor selects V_T, $\dot{V}_E$, and rate values for a patient receiving ASV.
· Describe the method the ventilator uses when starting ASV.
· Assess a patient case representing one of the three common scenarios that describes the function of ASV to determine how the ventilator will function.
· Troubleshoot a problem when an alarm indicator is activated.
· Describe backup ventilation in the GALILEO.

KEY TERMS

Adaptive tidal volume support	Internal reservoir tank	Variable-orifice differential pressure
Apnea backup ventilation (ABV)	Pneumotachograph	transducer
Electromagnetic flow-control valve	Tube resistance compensation (TRC)	Variable-orifice expiratory threshold
Expiratory trigger sensitivity (ETS)	Upper pressure limit (Pmax)	resistor

The GALILEO Gold is manufactured in Switzerland by Hamilton Medical and was first introduced in the United States in December, 1998, as the GALILEO (Figure 12-46). It is marketed by Hamilton Medical of Reno, Nevada. The unit is intended for use with adults, pediatric patients, and infants weighing 3 kg or more. The GALILEO Gold adds several new options to the original ventilator. These options are described later in this section.

The GALILEO is described in this section with enough detail to give the reader a good understanding of how the ventilator is operated. However, the reader is advised always to refer to the operator's manual when using the ventilator clinically, because software upgrades and available options may vary from time to time and from one device to another.

POWER SOURCE

The GALILEO is a microprocessor-controlled unit that requires high-pressure gas and electricity for power. It normally operates from air and oxygen wall outlets (pressure range, 29 to 87 psig). An additional external compressor can be purchased as an option and can provide the required gas power source if no other sources are available. A 110-volt standard electrical outlet can provide the electrical power needed to operate the unit (range, 100- to 240-volt alternating current [AC]). The main power on/off switch is on the back panel.

When the GALILEO is equipped with a specific performance package, the ventilator contains an internal battery. If AC power fails, the ventilator automatically switches to internal battery power. This battery can provide about 1 hour of operating time when fully charged. Battery indicators provide information and the amount of charge remaining. A green indicator means the internal battery is full. A yellow indicator shows that the battery is partly charged.

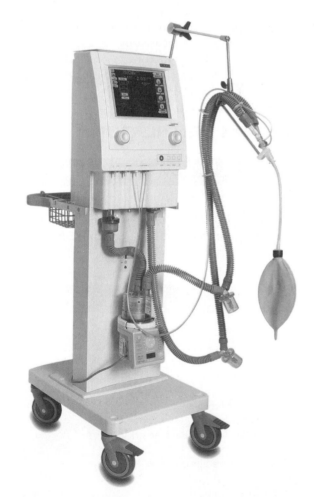

FIGURE 12-46 Hamilton GALILEO ventilator. (Courtesy Hamilton Medical, Reno, Nev.)

A red indicator means the internal battery charge is low. An audible alarm activates with a low battery charge, and this alarm cannot be silenced. The ventilator needs to be connected to an AC power source. A battery test can be run to determine the charge level. This test should be performed before the patient is connected to the ventilator.

INTERNAL FUNCTION

Two medical gas sources, air and oxygen, enter the internal circuit, where their pressures are reduced. If one source becomes unavailable, the unit switches to the remaining gas source but remains functional; however, this affects delivery of the fractional inspired oxygen (F_IO_2).

During normal operation, the gases are blended at the set F_IO_2 and stored under pressure in an **internal reservoir tank,** which holds up to 8 L under pressures of up to 350 cm H_2O. This pressurized gas allows for an uninterrupted flow, even at moments of high flow demand. After exiting the reservoir tank, gas is directed to an **electromagnetic flow-control valve.** The flow-control valve regulates the pattern of gas delivery to the patient and is in turn controlled by the microprocessor unit.

Modes and parameters selected by the operator are monitored, along with information received from the proximal airway monitor. This information governs the function of the flow-control valve, the expiratory valve, and other internal operating mechanisms. In addition, the GALILEO has a built-in galvanic fuel cell for analyzing and monitoring delivered oxygen concentrations.

PATIENT CIRCUIT

The main patient circuit consists of an inspiratory limb and an expiratory limb. A humidification system has been added to the inspiratory limb in Figure (Figure 12-46). The expiratory line is shown with an inline water trap. Exhaled gas is conducted to an expiratory valve. The expiratory valve uses a **variable-orifice expiratory threshold resistor** similar to the valve in the VEOLAR[FT]. (See the Evolve Web site for information on the VEOLAR[FT].)

The patient circuit has a proximal airway sensor that uses a **variable-orifice differential pressure transducer** to monitor and measure flow, volume, and pressure at the proximal airway (Figure 12-47). The pressure transducer is a variable-orifice **pneumotachograph,** the same type as that used in the VEOLAR[FT].*

Four small nipple connectors are located in an area above the attachment of the main patient circuit (see Figure 12-46; Figure 12-48). The two right connectors are attachments for the proximal airway pressure transducer lines. The next connector will power a small-volume nebu-

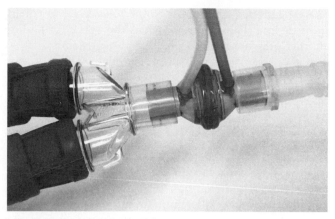

FIGURE 12-47 Flow sensor for the Hamilton GALILEO. (Courtesy Hamilton Medical, Reno, Nev.)

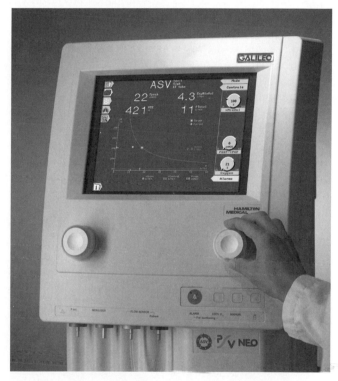

FIGURE 12-48 Front panel of the GALILEO. (Courtesy Hamilton Medical, Reno, Nev.)

lizer from a 15-psig independent compressor built into the ventilator. The far left connector is for auxiliary pressure monitoring.

When the nebulizer is available, it can provide 6 L/min of flow. (NOTE: The nebulizer should be placed in the inspiratory limb close to the Y-connector; placing the nebulizer between the flow sensor and the endotracheal tube increases dead space ventilation.) Use of the nebulizer results in a small increase in volume delivery but does not affect the F_IO_2. The set-up screen shows whether the nebulizer option has been added to a particular unit; in the CONFIGURE mode, the nebulizer settings will be visible (the set-up screen will be reviewed later in this section).

*See the Evolve Web site for this text for information on the VEOLAR[FT]; also see Chapter 8 for information on pneumotachometers.

As mentioned, the far left connector is for an auxiliary pressure line (Paux). This provides the option of adding another pressure monitor line for measurements such as carinal or esophageal pressures. The auxiliary pressure line in the GALILEO is comparable to the optional (OPT) pressure line in the VEOLAR^FT.

CONTROLS AND ALARMS

The control panel for the GALILEO is a simple design. It uses two knobs to control the color-active matrix computer screen. The right knob is called the *C* (control) knob, and the left knob is called the *M* (monitor) knob (see Figure 12-48). These knobs allow the operator to scan, select, and control all variables for operating and monitoring the ventilator.

The terms MODE, CONTROL, and ALARM are visible as menu items on the right side of the screen during normal operation (Figure 12-49). (NOTE: The active mode of ventilation appears at the top of the screen.) As the operator scrolls through the items listed on the screen using the C knob, each is highlighted in yellow. Once the desired option is highlighted, it is selected by pushing the C knob. For example, if MODE is the option chosen and the C knob is pushed, the unit opens a window displaying the ventilator mode screen, which lists all the modes available (Figure 12-50). The desired mode is selected by rotating the C knob through this menu until the desired mode is highlighted and then the C knob is pushed to select the mode. The operator must choose the CLOSE option on the same menu to verify the selection. This action automatically opens the controls window.

Each mode has its own control window (not shown), which contains only the parameters that can be adjusted in that mode. Initial default settings are displayed for the specific mode; thereafter the operator can select and adjust all the variables that need changing. The controls appear on the screen as icons (drawings) of ventilator knobs. For example, in pressure ventilation using assist-control (A/C), the operator has control over parameters such as Pcontrol, rate, PEEP, $O_2\%$, and % I time. Just as with mode selection, scrolling through each parameter icon allows selection of the various functions.

When the desired knob icon is highlighted (yellow), it is selected by pushing the C knob. The icon then changes to activated (red). Once activated, the numeric value of the parameter is changed by rotating the C knob either clockwise (to increase) or counterclockwise (to decrease). For example, if the pressure icon (knob) is highlighted, turning the C knob can change its value from 5 cm H_2O to 100 cm H_2O. After the desired value is selected, it is confirmed by pushing the C knob. A selected control knob automatically deactivates after 60 seconds if the operator does nothing to change it (Box 12-32).

After the operator has adjusted all the control parameters, the confirm icon must be selected to verify and activate the ventilator mode and parameters. The control window showing parameters for that mode disappears,

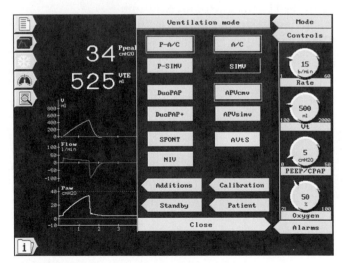

FIGURE 12-50 Hamilton GALILEO Gold ventilator window, showing the mode selections. (Courtesy Hamilton Medical, Reno, Nev.)

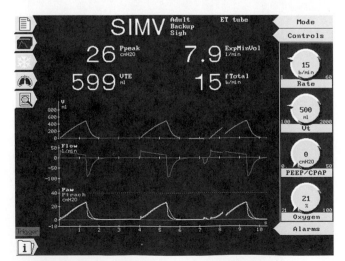

FIGURE 12-49 Normal operating window for ventilation with the Hamilton GALILEO (the SIMV mode screen is shown). (Courtesy Hamilton Medical, Reno, Nev.)

BOX 12-32	Activating a New Mode on the GALILEO

After any control menu has been chosen, the operator has a 60-second time limit. If the C knob is not used and no selections are made within that time, the normal operating menu returns. In this way, the operator is not required to close a menu if no action is taken. This also holds true for changing a parameter during ventilation. Suppose a respiratory therapist changed the set rate from 8 to 10 breaths/min. If the change is not confirmed, it would not take place even though the numeric value on the rate icon went from an 8 to a 10. If the change is not activated, the ventilator screen returns to 8 breaths/min after 30 seconds, and the rate actually never changes.

BOX 12-33	General Rules for Using Control Knob C on the GALILEO

The C knob is rotated either to highlight an item on a menu or to change the numeric value of a parameter. It is pushed to select (activate) the highlighted option.

Operating controls that are yellow can be selected. Controls change from yellow to red when they are selected (by a push of the C knob) and are then active (i.e., the operator can change their numeric values). After the desired value appears on the screen near the active icon, pushing the C knob again locks in the value.

The general rule is as follows: Rotate to locate, push to select, rotate to desired value, and push to confirm.

and the new mode becomes active. (NOTE: The control window must be closed [close icon] before the new mode becomes active.)

Depending on the mode selected, two to four parameter knob icons remain in a column on the right side of the normal operating screen. These icons display the parameters most often changed or manipulated in that mode of ventilation. For example, in the synchronized intermittent mandatory ventilation (SIMV) mode, respiratory rate, tidal volume (V_T), PEEP/CPAP, and O_2% appear (see Figure 12-49). Thus the control window does not have to be reopened to make common changes. Box 12-33 summarizes the general rules for using the C knob.

Configuration of T_I, Peak Flow, or I:E

The GALILEO allows the user to program (configure) a basic function into the unit. This function relates to the cycling of a breath in volume ventilation modes. The operator can choose any of the following three options:
- % T_I (adults), T_I (neonatal/pediatric patients)
- Peak flow
- I:E ratio

Notice that each of these options relates to the timing of breath delivery. For example, individuals who are used to ventilating patients with a set T_I would select the T_I option.

This programming option is available only during the start-up of the unit. The operator must press the M knob when the ON switch is turned on. The configuration screen appears and allows the operator to select one of the three options. After a choice is made and confirmed, the selected parameter becomes the control that appears on the normal operating screens.

For example, if T_I is selected, mandatory breaths are time cycled regardless of the mode. If peak flow is selected, the inspiratory flow for volume-targeted breaths in A/C and SIMV is determined by the peak flow setting, and in this case T_I would be based on peak flow and tidal volume. (NOTE: If peak flow is chosen, T_I still operates in pressure-control ventilation [P-A/C] and SIMV pressure-targeted [P-SIMV] modes. Mandatory breaths in these modes

CLINICAL ROUNDS 12-12

Answer each of the following questions in relation to breath cycling.
1. The GALILEO is configured to keep the % T_I constant. The respiratory therapist is using volume-targeted A/C ventilation. The V_T is 0.5 L, the rate is 10 breaths/min, and the % T_I is set at 25%. Calculate the T_I and the inspiratory flow (assume a constant flow pattern).
2. Assume that the rate is increased to 12 breaths/min but that V_T and T_I are the same as in the previous question. What is the new T_I and the new flow?
3. For this question, the GALILEO is configured to keep peak flow constant at the set peak flow during volume ventilation.
   · The respiratory therapist is using volume-targeted SIMV with a rate set at 15 breaths/min and a V_T of 0.8 L. The peak flow is set at 60 L/min. What is the T_I?
   · The therapist switches the mode to P-SIMV. What is the new T_I?
4. The GALILEO is configured for I:E constant. The respiratory therapist is using PCV or P-A/C. The I:E is 1:3, the rate is 15 breaths/min, and Pcontrol is set at 15 cm H_2O.
   · What is the T_I?
   · What is the peak flow?
   · Imagine that an inspiratory pause of 0.5 second is added. Does the pause increase the T_I when the unit is configured for a constant I:E ratio? How would using a pause affect breath delivery in this case?

See Evolve Resources for the answer.

remain time cycled.) If I:E is selected, the I:E ratio remains constant in all volume modes, regardless of changes in flow or pause time (Clinical Rounds 12-12).

Adjustable Control Parameters

The C knob provides access to several adjustable control parameters for each mode of ventilation (Box 12-34).[1] After all the necessary control parameters have been selected and confirmed, the control parameter menu is closed and the normal operating screen reappears.

Alarms

When ALARMS is selected on the operating screen (controlled by the C knob), the alarm menu appears on the screen (Figure 12-51). Alarms can be set automatically by the ventilator. The operator simply selects and activates AUTO from the alarms menu. The computer is programmed to provide high and low alarm defaults for all available options in each mode.* The operator can choose to adjust high and low alarms manually to whatever value is desired

*Values for the high and low alarm defaults are available from the manufacturer.

BOX 12-34	Adjustable Control Variables for the GALILEO

Rate Control: Sets the mandatory respiratory rate and determines the TCT for the mandatory breath.

Tidal Volume Control: Sets the desired volume delivery for a mandatory breath.

Pressure Control (Pcontrol): Determines inspiratory pressure above baseline during inspiration for a mandatory pressure breath (e.g., pressure-targeted breaths in A/C and SIMV modes (range, minimum of PEEP + 5 cm H_2O, maximum of 100 cm H_2O).

Maximum Pressure Limitation: Sets the maximum pressure above baseline during adaptive support ventilation (ASV) and adaptive pressure ventilation (APV) modes.

Pressure Support (Psupport): Establishes the pressure above baseline delivered during inspiration for Psupport.

PEEP/CPAP Control: Adjusts the amount of positive baseline pressure applied to the patient's airway in all modes of ventilation.

Oxygen Control: Adjusts the percentage of inspired oxygen delivery.

I:E Control: Fixes the I:E ratio for mandatory breaths. This ratio is based on the relationship of the set rate, $T_I/\%T_I$, and inspiratory pause (Pause/Tip control), which establish the time cycling of a mandatory breath. Patient triggering can shorten T_E and modify the I:E ratio for that breath, but it does not change the set value (see Clinical Rounds 12-12).

Ti/%Ti Control: Determines the time allotted to deliver V_T. $T_I/\%T_I$, + inspiratory pause determines I:E ratio.

Inspiratory Pause (Pause/Tip) Control: Keeps the exhalation valve closed for the set time following V_T delivery.

Peak Flow Control: Sets peak flow delivery for volume-targeted breaths. Peak flow plus inspiratory pause determines the I:E ratio when the unit is configured for peak flow.

Flow Pattern (Flow-P) Control: Allows the selection of the desired inspiratory gas flow pattern during volume ventilation (four patterns available: constant, full descending ramp, 50% descending ramp, and sine).

Flow Trigger/Pressure Trigger/Trigger Off (V'TR/ΔPTR/Trigger Off) Control: Allows the operator to adjust how sensitive the unit is to patient inspiratory effort. The measurement is performed at the proximal flow sensor (differential pressure transducer) located at the Y-connector. An automatic leak compensation is linked with flow trigger. The flow trigger is linked to the expiratory base flow to initially satisfy flow demand by the patient.

Percentage Minute Ventilation (%MinVol) Control: Used to set the minimum $\dot{V}_E$ delivered by the ventilator. Total target $\dot{V}_E$ is calculated as 0.1 L/min/kg IBW for adults and 0.2 L/min/kg for infant and pediatric patients.

Ideal Body Weight (Body Wt) Control: Allows the operator to enter the patient's IBW in kilograms.

Target Volume (Vtarget) Control: Sets the desired (targeted) V_T delivered during a mandatory pressure-controlled breath in the APV mode.

Pressure Ramp (Pramp) Control: Determines the rise time of pressure delivery during pressure-targeted breaths (either pressure control, pressure support, adaptive support ventilation or adaptive pressure ventilation).

Expiratory Trigger Sensitivity (ETS) Control: Allows the operator to adjust the percentage of peak flow at which a pressure-support breath will flow cycle (i.e., end inspiration). The range is 5% to 70% of measured peak inspiratory flow, in increments of 5%. For example, suppose peak flow during PSV is 100 L/min. If the operator sets the ETS at 10%, inspiration will end when flow drops to 10 L/min, and exhalation then begins.

---

within the available range. The alarms appear on the menu as bar graphs. Selecting a particular alarm, such as low V_T, illuminates that bar graph (orange) to indicate that it has been selected. Pushing the C knob activates the selected alarm, changing it to red. After the alarm is activated, turning the C knob allows the alarm value to be adjusted to the desired numeric value. Pushing the C knob when the desired number is present sets and verifies the alarm value.

A green horizontal line appears on the graph for each alarm bar graph (the line appears white in Figure 12-51). This line indicates the actual value measured for that parameter. Suppose that the high pressure limit alarm is selected; the green line shows the actual measured pressure value that is occurring for each breath. To the left of the green line, the numeric value for pressure also appears (green). This information is available whenever the alarm menu is active so that the operator can visually adjust the alarm range around the current value and also know the set value of each alarm parameter.

When an alarm event occurs, an audible alarm sounds and the red indicator on the left side of the alarm silence

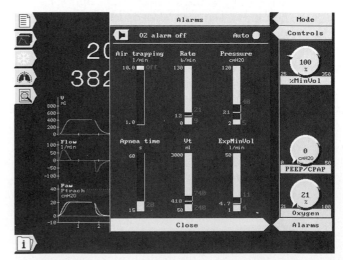

FIGURE 12-51 Alarm window on the Hamilton GALILEO. (See text for description.) (Courtesy Hamilton Medical, Reno, Nev.)

key blinks. A message is displayed on the bottom of the screen (message bar), and the active alarm symbol is displayed. If more than one alarm limit was violated, the active alarm symbol is visible on the screen. This indicates that messages are in the active alarm buffer. The operator can check the other active alarms by selecting the alarm buffer. In some software versions of the GALILEO, the alarm buffer is an icon that looks like an "i" inside a folder (see Figure 12-51). If there are no current active alarms, selecting the "i" gives the operator the last six alarms. Any time there is an active alarm, the "i" changes to a red bell inside a folder. Selecting this icon gives the operator a list of all currently active alarms. The alarm window scrolls alarm messages, and the alarm buffer provides a list of alarms. On the GALILEO Gold, the operator accesses the buffer by first closing any open window, selecting the active alarm symbol, and pressing the M knob.

The most recent alarm message is at the top of the list. The alarm buffer lists up to six alarm conditions in order of occurrence and gives the date and time of each alarm. The information about current alarms remains in the buffer as long as the condition that caused each alarm persists. If an alarm condition is corrected, it is stored in the unit's memory, and the GALILEO automatically resets the alarm. Information about active and reset alarms, along with other clinically significant events, is also stored in the event log.

Alarms of different priorities are given different sounds, which helps the practitioner distinguish those requiring immediate attention from those that are less critical. Using the ventilator and listening to the various alarms help the operator learn the different audible signals.

Adjustable and nonadjustable alarms for adults are listed in Table 12-20. Box 12-35 lists user attention messages for the GALILEO.

Upper Pressure Limit (Pmax)

Because of its importance in ventilator function, the high pressure alarm and its setting are worth reviewing. It is common for respiratory therapists to set an **upper pressure limit (Pmax)** 10 to 15 cm H_2O above the peak ventilating pressure. This should be set for all modes, whether pressure or volume targeted. For example, in pressure-controlled ventilation (PCV), the set pressure may be 20 cm H_2O, but what happens if the patient coughs? The pressure can rise above 20 cm H_2O (assuming that the high pressure alarm is set above the PCV level). For safety purposes, the high pressure limit should always be set about 10 to 15 cm H_2O above the ventilating pressure. When the high pressure limit is reached, inspiratory flow ends and the expiratory valve opens.

In the GALILEO, the high pressure limit (Pmax) also serves another function when adaptive support ventilation (ASV) or adaptive pressure ventilation (APV) is selected. When ASV or APV is used, the ventilator does not deliver pressures any higher than the upper pressure limit *minus* 10 cm H_2O (Pmax − 10 cm H_2O). Pressures can become

---

TABLE 12-20

Alarm Specifications for Adults—GALILEO

Alarm System	Adult Range
Adjustable Alarms	
Low/high minute ventilation	0-50 L/min
Low/high pressure	0-110 cm H_2O
Low/high V_T	0-3000 mL
Low/high rate	0-130 breaths/min
Apnea time	15-60 sec
Air trapping	1-10 L/min end-expiratory flow
Nonadjustable Alarms	
High pressure during sigh	
Exhalation obstruction	
Oxygen and air supply low	
Internal pressure low	
Check flow sensor tubing	
Disconnection on ventilator side	
Disconnection on patient side	
Oxygen concentration (high/low)	
No O_2 cell in use	
O_2 cell defective	
Turn the flow sensor (placed in the wrong direction)	
Oxygen supply, air supply (<28 psig)	
Loss of PEEP (3 cm H_2O below baseline for 10 sec)	
Check settings (inappropriately set)	
Loss of power supply	
Ventilator inoperative	

BOX 12-35   User Attention Messages (Galileo)

Flow sensor calibration needed
O_2 cell calibration needed
Check trigger
Check % MinVol/Pmax
Check rate
Check V_T
Check PEEP/Pcontrol
Check Psupport/Pcontrol
Check PEEP/Psupport
Check I : E
Check rate/T_I
Check V_T/T_I
Check T_I
Check %Ti
Check peak flow
Check Vtarget/Pmax
Check pause
Check flow pattern
Check Pramp
Check controls for sigh
Nebulizer inactive
Power alarm
If the message TECHNICAL FAULT appears and is followed by a number, the ventilator is experiencing technical difficulties and needs to be replaced. The manufacturer's service engineer should be called and given the number of the technical fault.

higher than Pmax – 10 cm H₂O in the circuit if, for example, the patient coughs. However, they can never go higher than the upper pressure limit setting (see the pressure bar graph in Figure 12-51 and "cough" Figure 12-52. (Pmax is displayed with a color not shown in the figure.)

Monitoring

During normal operation, four parameters are always displayed on the screen. A typical display might include peak pressure, mean airway pressure, expired minute volume, and total respiratory rate. These four can be customized to the user's preference by accessing the configuration window. In addition to these, several monitoring options appear on the upper left side of the screen (Figure 12-53) that are controlled by the M knob on the left side of the front panel (see Figure 12-48). The five main options appear as small icons in the monitoring menu. These options can be changed periodically by the manufacturer. One version of the available monitoring menus has a sheet of paper, a waveform, a snowflake, a pair of lungs, and a sheet of paper with a magnifying glass over it.

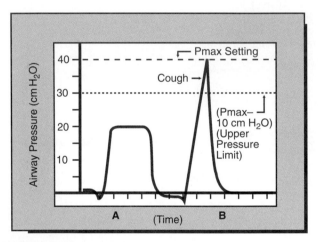

FIGURE 12-52 Pressure-time graph showing the Pmax pressure setting *(dashed line)*, the upper pressure limit (Pmax – 10 cm H₂O), a normal pressure breath **(A)** delivered during P-A/C + APV, and pressure noted during a cough **(B)**.

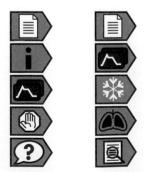

FIGURE 12-53 Monitor options on the Hamilton GALILEO and the GALILEO Gold. **A,** Original monitor options. **B,** Updated Gold version. (See text for description.)

When the sheet of paper icon is selected, its menu displays three icons: two sheets of paper, ASV, and a pressure icon (Paw/Paux). Selecting the sheets of paper provides information on the 26 parameters being measured and calculated, including peak pressure, V_T, PEEP/CPAP level, expired minute volume ($\dot{V}_E$), total respiratory rate, mean airway pressure, percentage of oxygen, static compliance, inspiratory airway resistance, pulmonary mechanics, pressure-time products, rapid shallow breathing index, I:E ratio, T_I, expiratory time (T_E), work of breathing (WOB), time constants, and so on. This screen lists the monitored parameters that are measured and calculated breath to breath but are not constantly displayed on the standard screen. The monitoring screen can be kept open continually to allow the display of all monitored parameters.

Paw and Paux provide monitored information on pressures measured either from the standard pressure measurements made with the flow sensor at the Y-connector (Paw) or from the auxiliary pressure sensor connector. Recall that a small nipple connector (Paux) allows use of a pressure monitor other than the one at the patient Y-connector. For example, the operator may want to monitor transpleural pressure using an esophageal balloon or carinal pressure using a special endotracheal tube or tube adapter. The user is advised to contact the manufacturer to find out the most appropriate auxiliary pressure monitoring equipment to use with the GALILEO.

The waveform icon in the monitoring menu pulls up a menu with four selections:
1. Real-time waveforms: Pressure-, flow-, and volume-time scalars.
2. Loops: Pressure-volume, flow-volume, and flow-pressure. (NOTE: In the loops menu, the operator can also choose Paux or Paw versus volume to observe total pressures compared with volume and pressures in the airway or in the esophagus versus volume.)
3. Trend curves: These can be configured for 1, 12, and 24 hours.
4. ASV target graphics screen: This screen provides information about adaptive support ventilation when the mode is operational. For example, in the ASV mode, the screen provides the target values for rate, V_T, $\dot{V}_E$, and inspiratory pressure above PEEP; it also displays the actual measured V_T, rate, and $\dot{V}_E$. The target values can be provided only if the operator has selected ASV and completed the necessary set-up (see ASV in the discussion of modes of ventilation).

The icon for freeze frame (snowflake) allows freezing of the current waveforms or trends and activates the cursor measurement.

The icon of the lungs has two items in its menu, a stop sign with a hand inside and a P/V (pressure-volume) curve icon. The stop sign allows selection of end-inspiratory and end-expiratory hold. Selecting the desired function results in the ventilator automatically performing the function. For example, in the inspiratory hold maneuver, the unit waits until the next inspiratory breath delivery to activate the hold. (NOTE: The ventilator provides up to a 10-second hold for adults and pediatric patients and a 3-second hold for infants.) Selection of the P/V icon provides a pressure-volume curve maneuver (see Special Features section).

The magnifying glass icon opens the events log, which shows up to 1000 events, including alarms and setting changes.

Real-Time Monitoring

The parameters measured by the proximal flow sensor and those calculated by the microprocessor are listed in Box 12-36.[2]

Front Panel Touch Keys

At the lower right corner of the control panel are four touch controls (see Figure 12-48). The alarm touch pad (left) silences the audible portion of the alarm system for 2 minutes. It can be reactivated by touching it again. The highest priority alarms cannot be silenced with this control; that is, the audible alarm for the following cannot be silenced:

1. Loss of source gas pressure.
2. An internal technical error that can be life-threatening or cause catastrophic problems.
3. Loss of battery power. When the ventilator is operated by battery power and the battery reaches the lowest charge level, the low battery alarm cannot be silenced. (NOTE: Loss of electrical power can be silenced with the separate alarm silence button on the battery panel.)
4. Apnea during an alarm silence.

The next touch pad is the 100% O_2, which provides 100% oxygen for 2 minutes. This is useful in procedures such as oxygenation before suctioning. If pressed a second time, the set oxygen percent is quickly resumed.

The manual touch pad delivers a manually triggered mandatory (pressure or volume) breath. To avoid auto-PEEP after a manual mandatory breath, the unit waits until it recognizes a period of 0.2 second of no expiratory gas flow. In earlier versions of the GALILEO, the fourth touch pad was a print pad, which when pressed could print the current computer screen when the ventilator was connected to a compatible printer. In the latest version, the fourth key activates the nebulizer function described previously.

MODES OF VENTILATION

The modes of ventilation currently available for the GALILEO are listed in Box 12-37. A backup rate is active whenever apnea is detected during any mode of ventilation with spontaneous breathing available. Whenever the mode screen is opened, in addition to a list of the modes, four items listed at the bottom of this menu can be used to open additional functions. They are: ADDITIONS, CALIBRATION, STANDBY, and PATIENT SELECTION. The ADDITIONS

BOX 12-36	Parameters Monitored and Calculated by the GALILEO

BREATH-TO-BREATH MEASUREMENT

Pressures
Peak pressure (Ppeak), minimum pressure (Pminimum), plateau pressure (Pplateau), PEEP/CPAP pressure, and mean airway pressure (Pmean, calculated value).

Flows
Inspiratory (Insp Flow) and expiratory (Exp Flow) flows.

Expiratory Tidal Volume (VTE)
Measured as exhaled air from the patient at the proximal airway pressure monitor.

T_I is the actual inspiratory time (in seconds) for a mandatory breath, measured from the beginning of inspiration to the end of the inspiratory pause. For a spontaneous breath, it is measured from the beginning of inspiration until the ETS (flow cycling) criteria are met.

T_E is the actual expiratory time in seconds; it is the time between the beginning of exhalation and the start of inspiration.

I : E Ratio
I : E ratio is expressed as 1 : X for normal I : E ratios and X : 1 for inverse ratios, where X is the relative expiratory time for a measured breath and is updated with each breath (minimum, 1 : 9; maximum, 4 : 1).

Oxygen
Measured inspiratory oxygen concentration.

EIGHT-BREATH AVERAGE

Expired Minute Volume (ExpMinVol)*
Measured at the airway; the sum of 8 consecutive measured breaths extrapolated to 1 full minute and updated after each breath.

fTotal* is the sum of spontaneous and mandatory breaths.

fSpont* is the sum of only spontaneous breath frequency.

Leakage Volume (VLeak)*
The difference between inspired and expired V_T measured at the patient's airway.

CALCULATED PARAMETERS OTHER THAN MEAN AIRWAY PRESSURE
Rinsp (inspiratory airflow resistance) and Rexp (expiratory airflow resistance) result from the patient's airway and the endotracheal tube and are measured in all modes and types of breaths.

Cstat† (static lung-thorax compliance) is measured using least squares fit from the exhaled V_T (in liters) and measured pressures (in cm H_2O).

RCInsp (inspiratory time constant) and RCExp (expiratory time constant) are calculated from the peak expiratory flow and volume.

WOBInsp (inspiratory work of breathing), auto-PEEP†, $P_{0.1}$ (occlusion pressure), PTP (inspiratory pressure-time product), and RSB (rapid shallow breathing index) are other calculated parameters.

---

*Measured at the airway; the sum of 8 consecutive measured breaths extrapolated to 1 full minute and updated after each breath.
†Calculated using least squares fit.[2]

BOX 12-37	Modes of Ventilation on the GALILEO Gold

ADULT/PEDIATRIC
Assist/Control, A/C [also called (S)CMV]
P-A/C (also called P-CMV)
SIMV
P-SIMV
SPONT
APVcmv (also called P-AC + APV)
APVsimv (also called P-SIMV + APV)
ASV
AVtS
DuoPAP
APRV
NIV

INFANT
P-A/C (P-CMV)
P-SIMV
SPONT
APVcmv
APVsimv
AVtS
DuoPAP
APRV

BOX 12-38	Parameters That Can Be Adjusted by the Operator in SIMV (Volume or Pressure Ventilation) on the GALILEO

Respiratory rate
V_T or pressure (Pcontrol above PEEP)
PEEP/CPAP
O_2%
I:E ratio or %T_I (T_I infants) or peak flow in volume ventilation
Flow or pressure trigger ($V'_{TR}/\Delta P_{IR}$)
Pressure support (for spontaneous breaths)
Flow pattern and pause (in volume ventilation)
Pressure ramp (P_{ramp}; in pressure control and pressure support only)
Expiratory trigger sensitivity (ETS; in PSV only)
Target volume (in APV)

menu allows the setting of sigh breaths, backup ventilation, and tubing resistance compensation (TRC) (these three functions are reviewed later).

The STANDBY feature places the ventilator in a waiting mode that allows the operator to maintain current patient settings while the ventilator is not performing any ventilatory functions. The STANDBY feature might be used if the patient is to be disconnected from the ventilator for any length of time.

The CALIBRATION function allows for calibration procedures that are performed before the patient is connected to the ventilator. Finally, the PATIENT SELECTION menu allows the operator to choose the correct patient size (i.e., adult, pediatric, or infant).

Assist/Control (A/C)

The assist-control mode on the Galileo is a standard A/C volume-targeted mode that offers time or patient triggering (flow or pressure). The breath can be time or volume cycled. The term *volume cycling* is used here to mean that inspiration ends when the measured flow and time are used to calculate that the set volume has been delivered. The parameters that can be adjusted in this mode are similar to other ventilators and include V_T; rate, peak flow, or % T_I or I:E; flow pattern; sensitivity (pressure or flow triggering); O_2%; and PEEP/CPAP.

Synchronized Intermittent Mandatory Ventilation (SIMV)

As with most ventilators, the SIMV mode can be time or patient triggered and volume targeted. Inspiration is time or volume cycled, as in A/C. Breaths can be delivered with an elevated baseline (PEEP/CPAP). The patient can breathe spontaneously between mandatory breaths. Pressure-support ventilation (PSV) can be added to spontaneous breaths (see the discussion of the spontaneous mode). Box 12-38 lists parameters that can be selected on the control menu and adjusted by the operator in SIMV when this mode is activated.

On the GALILEO during SIMV, the mandatory breaths have a maximum total cycle time (TCT) of 4 seconds, which is equal to a set rate of 15 breaths/min. If the rate is set higher, the TCT is shorter. For example, at 20 breaths, the TCT is 3 seconds. If the rate is lower than 15 breaths/min (e.g., 10 breaths/min [TCT = 6 seconds]), the TCT for a mandatory breath is still 4 seconds. A time of 4 seconds or less is used as a trigger window for the mandatory breath. If no triggering occurs inside this 4-second window, a mandatory breath is delivered (time triggered) at the end of the 4 seconds. If the ventilator is in a time-cycled mode, the T_I also is determined by the 4-second time frame. For example, in SIMV with a T_I set at 25%, the T_I is 1 second. At a T_I of 50%, it will be 2 seconds. (NOTE: The expiratory time may vary. If a patient triggers a breath, this can shorten the T_E, and the TCT is shortened as well.)

Spontaneous Mode (CPAP and PSV)

The spontaneous mode is used when the patient can breathe spontaneously but still requires some support or monitoring with alarms. The operator can adjust pressure support, CPAP, % O_2, triggering (flow or pressure trigger), pressure ramp (Pramp), PSV, and expiratory trigger sensitivity (the expiratory trigger sensitivity is for PSV breaths only; also see section on ETS and Pramp). The ventilator provides flow to meet patient demand while maintaining the desired baseline pressure and pressure support.

On the GALILEO, PSV is set above the PEEP/CPAP level. For example, if the clinician sets 10 cm H_2O of pressure support and the patient is receiving 5 cm H_2O of CPAP, the pressure during inspiration reaches 15 cm H_2O (PS + CPAP). The ventilator provides 2 cm H_2O of pressure support within the system, even when PSV is set at zero. This is done to reduce the work required by the patient to initiate flow from the demand system. (NOTE: This functionality is true of most microprocessor-controlled ventilators, not just the Hamilton GALILEO.)

Another important feature of PSV that the GALILEO offers is the ability to adjust the flow percentage at which the unit cycles out of inspiration. This feature is called the **expiratory trigger sensitivity (ETS).** The GALILEO is preprogrammed to flow cycle at 25% of peak for adults and 15% of peak for pediatric patients, but it allows this value to be adjusted from 5% to 70% of peak flow.[1] For example, if the peak flow during a pressure-support (PS) breath is 100 L/min and ETS is set at 30%, a PS breath ends inspiration when flow decreases to 30 L/min.

In case there is a leak in the system during PSV, a safety backup is available. The inspiratory time cannot exceed 3 seconds. With an infant, the maximum T_I is set by the operator. Therefore, if a leak exists around an uncuffed endotracheal tube, it does not interfere with cycling. The GALILEO also cycles out of a PS breath if the pressure reaches more than 2 cm H_2O above the set pressures. This pressure rise might occur if the patient coughs.

Whenever pressure-targeted breaths are selected with either PSV or PCV, the GALILEO allows the operator to adjust the slope or rise of the pressure curve using the PRAMP feature. Pramp determines the amount of time it takes from the very beginning of inspiratory flow until the set pressure is reached. The pressure curve can be tapered so that pressure does not abruptly enter the upper airway. Pramp is available in PSV, PCV, PCV+, APV, AVtS, and ASV. (See Chapter 11 for more details about ramping, sloping, or rise time.)

Pressure-Targeted Assist-Control Ventilation (P-A/C)

Pressure-targeted assist-control ventilation, as it is called on the GALILEO, is commonly called *pressure-controlled ventilation*. In P-A/C, the ventilator is time or patient triggered (flow or pressure trigger). The breath is pressure targeted at the set pressure-control level and time cycled out of inspiration. The V_T varies with the T_I, set pressure, patient effort, and changes in the patient's lung conditions. For this reason, setting the exhaled $\dot{V}_E$ alarm levels is especially important. As with PSV, the Pcontrol value is added to PEEP. For example, if Pcontrol is set at 15 cm H_2O, and PEEP is 10 cm H_2O, the maximum pressure generated by the ventilator during inspiration is 25 cm H_2O. In this example, it is advisable to set the upper pressure limit (Pmax) between 30 and 35 cm H_2O to limit the amount of pressure that could build up in the circuit if the patient coughs or forcibly exhales. The amount of pressure control cannot be set lower than 5 cm H_2O above the baseline pressure (PEEP).

Pressure-Control Ventilation Plus Adaptive Pressure Ventilation (P-A/C + APV)

The operator can also select APV when using pressure control (P-A/C + APV). On the upper portion of the screen, P-A/C APV is displayed. (NOTE: On some versions of the GALILEO, this mode is called *pressure-controlled mandatory ventilation with adaptive pressure ventilation [APVcmv].* The difference in terminology is determined by the selection of the English version used during configuration. Either United Kingdom or United States English is available.)

With this selection the operator sets a target volume (VTarget) instead of a target pressure. This is a dual control mode of ventilation that is a servo-controlled, or closed-loop, mode of ventilation. Through the automatic control of inspiratory pressure and flow, the specified target volume is generated with the lowest pressure possible under the current lung conditions. The ventilator reaches and maintains pressure at the target pressure, and the breath time cycles out of inspiration. If the exhaled V_T is less than the set value (VTarget), pressure adjusts upward to deliver the desired volume for the next breath. If V_T is more than VTarget, pressure is reduced. Pressure changes are made in increments of 1 to 2 cm H_2O.

Maximum pressure is determined by the upper pressure alarm limit setting (Pmax). The upward adjustment in pressure that is performed by the ventilator to correct V_T cannot exceed the Pmax value *minus* 10 cm H_2O. (NOTE: The manufacturer currently recommends a high pressure alarm limit setting of at least 10 cm H_2O above the peak pressure.) The amount of pressure control cannot be set lower than 5 cm H_2O above the baseline pressure (PEEP). When the ventilator has to go beyond these pressure limitations to achieve VTarget, audible and visible alarms occur and a message appears at the bottom of the screen indicating that the ventilator has now reached "pressure limitations." The target volume may not be delivered with the current setting for Pmax. The clinician must then decide either to reduce the target V_T or increase Pmax, depending on the patient's condition. (NOTE: P-A/C is similar to PRVC described in Chapter 11.) Clinical Rounds 12-13 provides a problem related to P-A/C + APV.

CLINICAL ROUNDS 12-13

A patient is being set up on P-A/C + APV on the GALILEO. The ventilator parameters are as follows: rate = 10 breaths/min, T_I = 1.5 seconds, PEEP = 5 cm H_2O, Pmax = 35 cm H_2O, F_IO_2 = 0.5, V_{target} = 0.6 L (600 mL).

A ventilating pressure of 25 cm H_2O is required to deliver the target volume for this patient. A few breaths after the mode is initiated, the respiratory therapist hears an audible alarm and sees a message indicating that ventilation is on PRESSURE LIMITATION. What changes should the therapist make?

See Evolve Resources for the answer.

Pressure Control/SIMV (P-SIMV)

The GALILEO can provide SIMV using pressure-targeted mandatory breaths (P-SIMV). This mode is very similar to conventional SIMV. Mandatory breaths are patient or time triggered, pressure targeted, and time cycled. Tidal volumes vary, depending on the set pressure, T_I, patient lung characteristics, and any patient effort that might be present. As with volume-targeted SIMV, a positive-pressure baseline (PEEP/CPAP) can be applied. Spontaneous breaths can be aided with the use of pressure support.

Pressure Control/SIMV Plus Adaptive Pressure Ventilation (P-SIMV + APV)

P-SIMV can also be altered using the APV function. At the top of the screen, P-SIMV + APV appears. (NOTE: Newer versions of the GALILEO also refer to this as APV_{SIMV}.) In P-SIMV + APV, mandatory breaths are still pressure breaths, but they become volume targeted to the set V_T. The ventilator adjusts pressure delivery during these mandatory breaths to achieve the volume target using the lowest possible inspiratory pressure; this is similar to P-A/C + APV. The primary difference is that a patient can breathe spontaneously between mandatory breaths at the set baseline and PS level in P-SIMV + APV.

Adaptive Support Ventilation (ASV)

ASV is a servo-controlled (closed-loop) technique that functions using pressure-targeted breaths to ensure a target minute ventilation while establishing protective lung strategies. The goal of ASV is to provide $\dot{V}_E$ and at the same time minimize the work of breathing and avoid potentially detrimental patterns of breathing (rapid, shallow breathing, excessive dead space ventilation, breath stacking, and excessively large breaths[2]).

ASV adapts to the changing capabilities and lung conditions of the patient. The GALILEO automatically alters its performance to match the patient's demands, from full support to spontaneous breathing. The more work the patient is able to perform, the less work the ventilator provides. ASV can ventilate the patient from an acute stage to a weaning stage.

Normally, when respiratory therapists or physicians first establish ventilation in a patient, they calculate the initial settings of $\dot{V}_E$, rate, and V_T. These settings are calculated from equations that have been established through clinical research that uses variables such as ideal body weight (IBW); patient height and gender; and any abnormal conditions that may be present.[3] For example, $\dot{V}_E$ may be based on body surface area (BSA), calculated from the patient's weight and height and adjusted for abnormal body temperature.[3,4]

ASV also follows specific algorithms or formulae on which it determines optimum ventilation and the best way to deliver volume and rate. Some of these rules are hard, and some are soft.[2] An example of a hard rule is the high pressure

limit set by the operator. In ASV the ventilator does not exceed the high pressure limit, even if it is unable to achieve its set goals. Soft rules are based on clinician input and on the patient's respiratory mechanics. Soft rules usually have a range of variability and may change with time or with operator input. An example of a soft rule is establishing the low V_T limits that are equal to 4.4 mL/kg of IBW. The lower V_T limit ensures that the minimum V_T is at least twice normal dead space and is based on the patient's weight.[2]

ASV is such a new approach to ventilation that an explanation of its operation is divided into several different sections:

1. Ventilator programming to establish respiratory parameters in ASV
2. Setting up the ventilator for ASV
3. Initial test breaths
4. Variations in breath delivery

Ventilator Programming to Establish Respiratory Parameters in ASV

ASV is programmed to calculate an overall minute ventilation for the patient. It uses pressure-targeted breaths to accomplish delivery of the minute ventilation. Breaths are a combination of PC breaths (time-triggered and time-cycled breaths) and PSV breaths (any patient-triggered breaths are pressure limited and flow cycled, as with a PS breath). Both types of pressure-limited breaths are also volume targeted. The volume target is established by the ventilator, as is the respiratory rate.

Some clinicians are concerned because the ventilator is performing many of the functions that normally are the clinician's purview. However, the GALILEO uses well-established equations and safe boundaries as guides for determining the minute ventilation, tidal volume, and rate (f).[2-9]

Minute Ventilation. The ventilator uses the following equations to calculate the minute ventilation[4-9]:

Equation 1 (Adults)

IBW > 15 kg: $\dot{V}_E$ target = 100 × (% Min vol/100) × IBW (kg)

Equation 2 (Pediatric patients)

IBW < 15 kg: $\dot{V}_E$ target = 200 × (% Min vol/100) × IBW (kg)

For example, an adult patient with an IBW of 70 kg set at 100% min vol will have a target $\dot{V}_E$ of 7000 mL/min or 7 L/min. This $\dot{V}_E$ can be achieved using a number of combinations of V_T and f. However, not all combinations are safe for the patient. Figure 12-54 shows how the GALILEO places limits on the potential V_T and rate combinations to make them safe for the patient. (NOTE: The operator always determines the absolute boundaries. For example, setting the high pressure alarm limit sets the boundary on high pressure.)

The $\dot{V}_E$ is divided into optimum targets for respiratory rate and V_T; these targets are determined using Otis's least work of breathing equation (Box 12-39).[6] The equation assumes that if the optimum breathing pattern results in

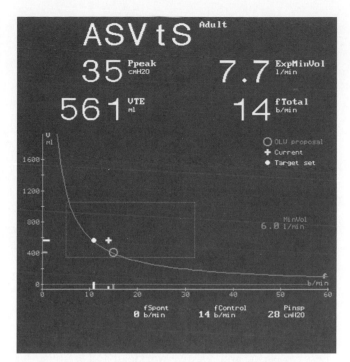

FIGURE 12-54 Operating screen of the GALILEO during adaptive support ventilation (ASV). The curved white line on the graph represents all the possible combinations of V_T and respiratory rate (f) that will result in a $\dot{V}_E$ of 6 L/min. The rectangle *(dotted line)* within the graph represents the safest boundaries for protecting the lungs. The top horizontal boundary protects against high V_T and high pressures. The lower horizontal boundary protects against hypoventilation. The right vertical boundary helps to prevent hyperinflation or breath stacking. The left vertical boundary helps prevent apnea. (Courtesy Hamilton Medical, Reno, Nev.)

BOX 12-39	Otis's Least Work of Breathing Formula

Total respiratory frequency (f):

$$f = \frac{\sqrt{1 + 4\pi^2 RCe\left(\dfrac{\dot{V}_E - f \times V_D}{V_D}\right)} - 1}{2\pi^2 RCe}$$

where *RCe* is the expiratory time constant, $\dot{V}_E$ is the minute ventilation, and V_D is the dead space volume (the GALILEO estimates dead space as 1 mL/pound IBW using Radford's nomogram).

the least work of breathing, it also results in the least amount of pressure during ventilation of a passive patient (Clinical Rounds 12-14).[2,6]

Tidal Volume. Tidal volume limits are determined by both hard and soft rule boundaries.[2]

The maximum V_T can be established by using the hard boundary for low breath rate and the calculated $\dot{V}_E$. For example, a $\dot{V}_E$ of 7 L/min with a minimum available rate of 5 breaths/min would establish a maximum boundary for V_T at 1.4 L (1400 mL).

The IBW is used to establish the soft boundaries for both high and low V_T.[2] High V_T is always less than 22 mL/kg. The lower V_T boundary assumes that V_T will be at least

CLINICAL ROUNDS 12-14

Problem 1

An adult patient has an IBW of 60 kg. The operator sets the $\dot{V}_E$ at 100%. What $\dot{V}_E$ will be established by the ventilator for the patient?

Problem 2

If an infant has an IBW of 5 kg and the operator sets the $\dot{V}_E$ at 50%, what $\dot{V}_E$ will the ventilator deliver for the infant?

See Evolve Resources for the answer.

twice normal dead space, which is about 2.2 mL/kg. Thus the lower V_T limit is set at 4.4 mL/kg. For example, in the 70-kg patient, a low V_T based on the IBW would be 2.2 mL/kg × 70 kg = 308 mL.

High tidal volume would also be affected by the upper pressure alarm limit setting. If delivery of a high tidal volume violates this limit, the alarm would activate, ending inspiration and reducing V_T delivery.

Rate. The % MIN VOL setting determines the soft rule for the maximum breath rate. Maximum breath rate is based on one of the following two equations[2,7-8]:

Equation 1

IBW > kg: Max f = 22 breaths/min × % Min vol/100

Equation 2

IBW < 15 kg: Max f = 45 breaths/min × % Min vol/100

For example, the 70-kg patient described previously (target $\dot{V}_E$ = 7 L/min, 100% Min Vol setting) would have a maximum rate of 22 breaths/min.

A hard boundary for the respiratory rate is set at 5 breaths/min for a low rate and 60 breaths/min for the maximum rate.[2] The low rate in turn affects the potential maximum V_T. For example, in a 70-kg patient, with % min vol set at 100%, the maximum V_T would be the $\dot{V}_E$/(5 breaths/min) or 7 L/(5 breaths/min) = 1.4 L or 1400 mL $V_T$max.

As a safety feature to allow sufficient time for exhalation if the respiratory rate is high, the ventilator measures the patient's expiratory time constant (RCexp) and makes sure that the expiratory time is at least equal to 2 × RCexp.

Patient Lung Characteristics. In addition to the internal equations for $\dot{V}_E$, V_T, and rate, ASV takes into consideration the patient's lung characteristics, which change with differences in pathology. For example, pulmonary edema results in reduced lung compliance. Low lung compliance is associated with a bodily response of a higher rate and lower V_T. The ventilator makes an effort to reduce the work of breathing by providing a rate and a V_T that reflect the patient's lung condition (lung compliance [C] and airway resistance [R]), but it stays within its limits (Table 12-21).

The ventilator is constantly analyzing the T_I, T_E, total rate, inspired $\dot{V}_E$, expiratory time constant (RCexp), R, C,

TABLE 12-21

Safety Limits in Adaptive Support Ventilation

Parameter	Value
Minimum pressure	PEEP + 5 cm H_2O
Maximum pressure	Pmax setting − 10 cm H_2O
V_T minimum	4.4 mL/kg IBW ($2 \times V_D$)
V_T maximum	22 mL/kg IBW ($10 \times V_D$)
Minimum mandatory rate	5 breaths/min
Maximum mandatory rate	60 breaths/min
Minimum T_I	RCexp,* or 0.5 seconds
Maximum T_I	$2 \times$ RCexp, or 3 seconds
Minimum T_E	$2 \times$ RCexp
Maximum T_E	12 sec

*RCexp, Expiratory time constant.

BOX 12-40 — Static Compliance and Airway Resistance (GALILEO)

Calculation of static compliance by the GALILEO does not require the operator to select an inspiratory pause (inflation hold) to get a static pressure reading. Static compliance is calculated mathematically using the least squares fit method. The unit performs 200 measurements per second of flow, pressure, and volume and then does a linear regression calculation to estimate static compliance and airway resistance. The analysis of pressure, flow, and volume is based on a mechanical model of the respiratory system.[2]

and ventilating pressures (Box 12-40).[9] It uses all this information, plus the input from the operator, to establish an appropriate breathing pattern that at all times tries to reduce the work of breathing and to balance the patient's spontaneous and mandatory breaths.

Setting Up the Ventilator for ASV

As in all cases, before connecting the patient to the ventilator, the operator performs preoperational procedures and tests to ensure optimum ventilator performance. The practitioner then provides some specific input information.

First, a high pressure alarm limit is set (ALARMS window). The manufacturer suggests a beginning high pressure limit of 45 cm H_2O. The maximum inspiratory pressure during ASV is always 10 cm H_2O below the set high pressure alarm limit. At a set value of 45 cm H_2O, this would be a maximum of 35 cm H_2O.

Second, the operator enters the patient's IBW (range, 10 to 200 kg). The IBW is used to determine the anatomic dead space of the patient at 2.2 mL/kg using Radford's nomogram.[4] The use of mechanical devices, such as a heat and moisture exchanger (HME), increases dead space and may also need to be considered in the decision on an IBW setting. As a rule of thumb, the operator should increase the body weight setting by 10% when an HME is used.[2]

Third, the percent of minute ventilation (% min vol) is set by the operator (range, 10% to 350%). A safe starting point is 100%. If the patient is hyperthermic, the percentage may be increased by 5% per degree F (10% per degree C). In high altitude conditions, the % $\dot{V}_E$ may be increased by 5% per 500 m above sea level.

Fourth, the operator can then select appropriate values for PEEP, trigger sensitivity, F_IO_2, Pramp, and ETS and confirm the initial settings. PEEP/CPAP and oxygen percentage aid patient oxygenation. Trigger sensitivity adjusts the ease of breath triggering. Pressure ramp and ETS tailor PS breaths.

Initial Test Breaths

The GALILEO assesses the patient by providing three test breaths (pressure breaths), starting at a minimum pressure just above baseline and gradually increasing the pressure. (NOTE: During ASV, pressure cannot go below PEEP/CPAP plus 5 cm H_2O or above the upper pressure limit alarm minus 10 cm H_2O.)

During the test breaths, the ventilator performs its measurements and calculations of V_T, f, C, R, and time constants. From these measurements the ventilator can assess the elastic and resistive workload and establish the optimum breath pattern (i.e., the ventilatory pattern that represents the least work of breathing for the patient). Table 12-21 lists the safety limits autoprogrammed by the unit to avoid complications associated with mechanical ventilation, including auto-PEEP, lung tissue injury associated with excessive volume (volutrauma), and excessive pressure (barotrauma), apnea, and tachypnea.

After a stable breathing pattern has been established, the operator needs to adjust alarm parameters appropriately.

Variations in Breath Delivery

The ventilator begins to deliver the optimum breathing pattern using pressure-targeted breaths.* It adjusts the inspiratory pressure and mandatory rate to achieve a given minimal $\dot{V}_E$ based on Figure 12-55. In this graph the horizontal and vertical axes (dashed lines) represent the measured respiratory rate and tidal volume, respectively. The white dot at the center is the optimum target for V_T and f. Each of the four quadrants represents the adjustments the GALILEO will make in inspiratory pressure (PI) and mandatory breath rate (fmand) to attain the optimum target.

- Upper left quadrant (I): The V_T is high, and the rate is low. ASV will reduce the PI to reduce V_T, and it will increase the rate.
- Lower left quadrant (IV): The V_T is low, and the rate is low. ASV will increase the PI and rate to correct the problem.
- Upper right quadrant (II): The V_T is high, and the rate is high. ASV will reduce the PI and rate.
- Lower right quadrant (III): The V_T is low, and the rate is high. ASV will increase the PI and reduce the rate.

*These breaths are like pressure-controlled breaths, but they are also volume targeted to achieve the optimum calculated V_T.

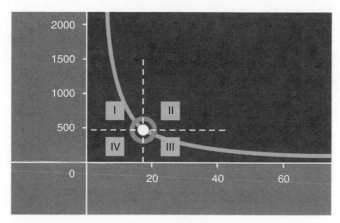

FIGURE 12-55 Graph representing the measured respiratory rate (*x*-axis), the measured V$_T$ (*y*-axis), and the target rate and volume *(center white dot)*. Each quadrant shows how ASV will adjust ventilator parameters to bring the ventilator toward the target. (See text for explanation.) (Courtesy Hamilton Medical, Reno, Nev.)

If compliance, resistance, or spontaneous breathing efforts change, ASV measures these changes and adjusts the inspiratory support and rate to maintain protective lung strategies. It allows the patient to resume spontaneous breathing when the person is able. Remember that although the mode provides a minimum selected V̇$_E$, patients can achieve a higher V̇$_E$ if they so choose.

Three common scenarios can occur that help describe the function of ASV.

1. If the patient is not breathing spontaneously, P-SIMV breaths are delivered. The ventilator provides the % V̇$_E$. Breaths are time triggered and pressure targeted to achieve the desired volume, as well as time cycled. As lung conditions change, the pressure level is adjusted between minimum and maximum to deliver the calculated V$_T$ with the least amount of pressure.

   If the patient assists a breath after having been apneic, the ventilator delivers a PS breath at the same pressure used for the pressure-controlled breath. This is logical, because the ventilator has calculated this to be the pressure required to deliver the optimum V$_T$.

2. If the patient is providing some but not all of the work of breathing, patient-triggered breaths are pressure-support breaths. Time-triggered breaths are pressure-control breaths. The ventilator calculates the difference between the spontaneous breathing rate and volume delivery, and the calculated rate (missing breaths) and volume delivery. The missing breaths are provided as added (time-triggered) pressure-controlled breaths designed to achieve the desired V̇$_E$.

3. If the patient is breathing spontaneously and triggering all breaths, these are pressure-support breaths with the pressure adjusted to maintain optimum ventilation.

In spite of the advanced intelligence of the GALILEO's closed-loop ventilation with ASV, the clinician is still required to monitor the patient carefully. This evaluation includes reviewing the patient's arterial blood gas values, breathing pattern, and breath sounds, to name but a few assessment parameters.

Sometimes adjustments to the % min vol will need to be made based on the findings for arterial blood gases (ABGs). For example, if ABGs are normal, the % min vol could remain the same, or weaning could be considered as long as the spontaneous breathing pattern was acceptable.

If the pH is below 7.3 and the partial pressure of arterial carbon dioxide (PaCO$_2$) is high, the clinician might consider an increase in the % min vol while monitoring the inspiratory pressure. If the PaCO$_2$ is low, the clinician might consider decreasing the % min vol as long as the spontaneous breathing pattern is acceptable.

With a low oxygen level (low PaO$_2$ and SpO$_2$), the clinician might consider increasing PEEP/CPAP and the F$_I$O$_2$. Many possibilities for abnormal ABGs and breathing patterns exist. The clinician needs to evaluate the patient and the ventilator parameters carefully when making decisions about ventilator management.

To summarize, ASV is a servo-controlled (closed-loop) mode of ventilation that delivers pressure breaths targeted to achieve the desired, ventilator-calculated volume. Time-triggered breaths are in PCV, and patient-triggered breaths are in PSV. The ventilator continually monitors patient lung characteristics and breathing patterns and calculates an optimum V$_T$ with the required pressure delivery and rate to optimize ventilation and minimize the patient's work of breathing. Patients may be completely controlled when first connected to the ventilator, but as they begin to recover and are able to breathe spontaneously, fewer mandatory breaths are required. Eventually patients breathe with only pressure-supported breaths. The ventilator continues to monitor all parameters and adjust its performance as needed.

Adaptive Tidal Volume Support (AVtS)

Adaptive tidal volume support is a modified form of ASV. AVtS was the mode of ventilation offered with the GALILEO Gold before ASV was approved by the U.S. Food and Drug Administration (FDA) in 2007.

When the AVtS mode is first set up for patient use, the operator enters the tidal volume, IBW, and % min vol. The clinician-set % min vol and IBW define the target minute volume, which is shown in the VENTILATOR ANALYZER window. The rectangular space that defines the VENTILATOR ANALYZER window in the main screen is similar to the one seen on the main screen for ASV (see Figure 12-54).

In AVtS the main screen display shows the set values for V$_T$ and rate (solid dot), along with the current measured values (cross), and the values proposed by the ventilator (open circle) based on the calculation for the least work of breathing (Figure 12-56). The least work of breathing calculation, as with ASV, is based on the Otis formula (see Box 12-39). The clinician can use the VENTILATOR ANALYZER window to determine the best rate and V$_T$ pattern for the patient. The inspiratory pressure and mandatory rate are then continuously adjusted by the ventilator to meet the clinician's preset ventilation settings.

As shown in Figure 12-56, the dotted rectangle drawn on the main screen shows all combinations of V_T and R that are compatible with lung protective strategies, just as in ASV. A curved line, which is green on the actual ventilator screen, shows all the possible combinations of V_T and f that result in the calculated minute volume.

The primary difference between AVtS and ASV is that ASV automatically targets the tidal volume based on Otis's least work of breathing calculation, whereas in AVtS the operator must select the V_T.

Dual Positive Airway Pressure Mode (DuoPAP) and Airway Pressure-Release Ventilation (APRV)

DuoPAP and APRV are similar forms of pressure ventilation designed to support spontaneous breathing on two levels of CPAP. These two modes were added to the Gold version of the GALILEO, which is the current operating model of the ventilator.

DuoPAP

In DuoPAP the operator sets a P-high (high pressure), the PEEP/CPAP (baseline pressure), T-high (time at high pressure), and rate. P-high is the target pressure provided during the time frame set by T-high. The rate establishes the TCT. For example, suppose the following parameters are set: P-high = 20 cm H_2O, PEEP = 0 cm H_2O, T-high = 1 sec, and rate = 10 breaths/min. The TCT will be 60 sec/rate, or 6 seconds. A P-high of 20 cm H_2O will be applied to the airway for 1 second and PEEP of 0 cm H_2O for 5 seconds (TCT − T-high = Remaining time). During either

of these time intervals, the patient can breathe spontaneously. A change from P-high to PEEP and PEEP to P-high can be either patient or time based.

With DuoPAP, pressure support can be added to the baseline (PEEP) setting. For example, if PS is set at 20 cm H_2O and PEEP is 5 cm H_2O, the peak pressure when the patient is breathing from baseline will be 20 + 5, or 25 cm H_2O (Figure 12-57).

Spontaneous breaths at the P-high level are supported with PS only when the PS plus PEEP setting is greater than P-high. In the previous example, with a P-high of 20 cm H_2O, if PS were set at 20 cm H_2O and PEEP equal to 5 cm H_2O, a spontaneous breath from the patient would result in pressure rising to 25 cm H_2O during peak spontaneous inspiration (5 cm H_2O above P-high; see Figure 12-57A). The use of DuoPAP by clinicians undoubtedly will evolve as clinical research demonstrates its many potential uses.

Airway Pressure-Release Ventilation (APRV)

APRV was described in Chapter 11. This mode, like DuoPAP, allows spontaneous ventilation at two levels of PEEP/CPAP. On the GALILEO, the operator sets APRV by setting P-high and P-low with corresponding time intervals of T-high and T-low. As with DuoPAP, pressure support can be added, and it follows the same pattern as that described for DuoPAP; that is, PS spontaneous breaths would appear above the P-high plateau only if PS + PEEP were greater than P-high.

Clinically, APRV has most commonly been used with long T-high times (time at high pressure) and short T-low times (time at low pressure or PEEP), establishing what is similar to an inverse I:E ratio. Spontaneous breathing is done mostly at the upper pressure level, usually with a short T-low interval. As with DuoPAP, the change from P-high to P-low to P-high can be based on the set time or it can be synchronized with the patient's spontaneous breathing rate (see Figure 12-57B).

Noninvasive Ventilation (NIV)

NIV is available with the GALILEO Gold version and is intended for use in the acute care environment for adult and pediatric patients; it is not intended for home care use. NIV is designed for spontaneously breathing patients who require only face masks or nasal masks as the patient interface. (NOTE: NIV should not be used for patients with irregular or absent breathing.)

The operator sets the noninvasive spontaneous mode, baseline pressure (PEEP/CPAP), pressure-support level, Timax, and ETS. Because leaks will be present, it is important to set breath cycling criteria and avoid long inspiratory times. It probably is more comfortable for the patient when the ventilator cycles are based on the ETS setting (flow cycle) rather than the Timax limit. A suggested starting point for ETS is 50%, and it probably should not be set below 30%. However, because of leaks, the ventilator may never reach the flow-cycle criteria, even when ETS is set as carefully as possible. Setting a Timax enables the ventilator

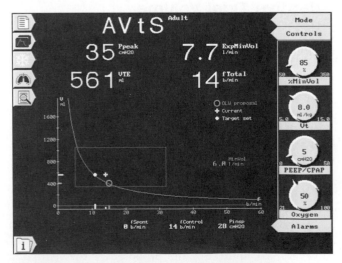

FIGURE 12-56 Graph representing AVtS with the measured respiratory rate (*x*-axis) and the measured V_T (*y*-axis). The target rate and volume are shown as a solid white dot. The current values are shown as a small cross or plus sign. The open circle represents the proposed V_T and rate. (See text for explanation.) (Courtesy Hamilton Medical, Reno, Nev.)

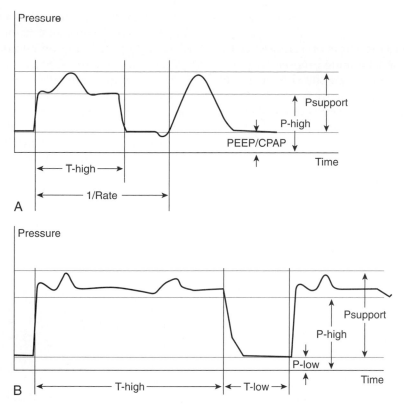

FIGURE 12-57 Pressure-time curves for DuoPAP **(A)** and airway pressure-release ventilation (APRV) **(B)**. (See text for explanation.) (Courtesy Hamilton Medical, Reno, Nev.)

to cycle into exhalation even when a leak is present, thus preventing a prolonged inspiratory phase. Timax should be long enough (about 1.5 seconds) to give ETS the chance to cycle the ventilator. This function is also available with the neonatal settings.

The LOW V_T and EXP MIN VOL alarms should be set low to avoid nuisance alarms. Because of leaks around the mask, the DISCONNECTION PAT SIDE alarm, which is based on volume criteria, is disabled, as is the EXHALATION OBSTRUCTED alarm. The DISCONNECTION VENT SIDE alarm remains enabled.

Because NIV is a pressure-targeted mode, it is important to pay particular attention to the pressure alarms. The low pressure alarm should be set above PEEP/CPAP and within about 5 cm H_2O of the Psupport setting. If the PEEP and inspiratory pressures can be maintained, the ventilator is sufficiently compensating for leaks. It is recommended that the peak inspiratory pressure not exceed 28 cm H_2O, because higher values may result in opening of the esophageal sphincter, forcing gas into the stomach.[3]

SPECIAL FEATURES

The Gold version of the GALILEO has an infant application for patients weighing less than 10 kg, with use of the infant flow sensor. Another special feature in the GALILEO Gold package is the P/V tool, which is described later.

Three additional items on the GALILEO Gold that are available under the ADDITIONS menu are sigh, backup ven-

tilation, and tubing resistance compensation. (NOTE: In the earlier version of the GALILEO, the additions menu listed sigh, standby, and nebulizer.)

Sigh

In all modes except ASV, a sigh breath can be applied every 100 breaths. In volume-targeted modes, the sigh function increases the V_T by 50% of the set value to a maximum of 2000 mL. In pressure-targeted modes, sigh increases the inspiratory pressure by up to 10 cm H_2O as allowed by the maximum pressure setting (Pmax). In ASV, a sigh is delivered every 50 breaths at a pressure 10 cm H_2O higher than nonsigh breaths.

Backup Ventilation

Backup ventilation is recommended in all modes in which spontaneous breathing is possible, but it actually is not necessary in ASV. The operator can select the desired backup ventilation (ADDITIONS menu) and apnea time (ALARMS window). If the set apnea time is exceeded, the **apnea backup ventilation (ABV)** becomes active. A medium priority alarm sounds, and the screen displays apnea ventilation. Breath delivery in ABV is either volume or pressure targeted.

If ABV becomes active, the message CHECK BACK-UP CONTROLS is displayed. The operator can check the active settings for ABV by opening the controls window. Settings for ABV will be displayed for reviewing and confirming. To change a setting, the operator follows the procedure for making any parameter change described earlier in this section.

To prevent backup ventilation from occurring when the patient is disconnected for suctioning or a similar procedure, the operator presses the ALARM SILENCE touch pad; this prevents ABV from becoming active for 2 minutes. In addition, whenever the ventilator mode is changed or ventilator calibration procedures are performed, backup ventilation is automatically suppressed for 30 seconds.

Tube Resistance Compensation (TRC)

TRC is intended for use in spontaneously breathing patients. It can be set to reduce the patient's work of breathing associated with the flow resistance imposed by an endotracheal tube or a tracheostomy tube. TRC is active during exhalation in volume modes and in both inspiration and exhalation in other modes.

From the ADDITIONS window, the operator opens the TRC window. The selections for tube type include ET-TUBE (endotracheal tube), TRACHE-TUBE (tracheostomy tube), or DISABLE TRC. After a tube type is selected, the tube size can be dialed in. A 100% compensation setting means that the maximum practical compensation is provided. The percent compensated can be adjusted below this value. Pressing confirm enables the TRC settings that were chosen. (NOTE: Setting TRC may result in autotriggering of the ventilator requiring resetting of values or disabling of TRC.)

Pressure-Volume (P/V) Tool

The P/V tool is an automatic method of performing the supersyringe technique of evaluating pulmonary mechanics by using nearly static conditions (very low flow). The technique is used in patients who have conditions such as acute respiratory distress syndrome (ARDS). It is contraindicated in patients with abnormalities such as open pneumothorax with chest tubes in place. Two P/V tools are available, the basic inspiratory P/V tool (PV Tool 1) and the advanced tool (PV Tool 2) that looks at a full, slow P/V loop, providing an optional end-inspiratory pause.

The basic, inspiratory P/V tool performs as follows[1]:

1. The expiratory phase of the current mandatory breath is prolonged and pressure is reduced to zero to ensure complete lung emptying before P/V testing.
2. The breathing circuit is slowly pressurized to a predefined peak pressure (range, 20 to 40 cm H_2O) at the selected ramp speed, such as 4 cm H_2O/sec (range, 2 to 5 cm H_2O/sec). Real-time pressure-volume values are plotted as the P/V technique is applied (Figure 12-58).
3. The fully automated maneuver is initiated by the operator.
4. At the end of the maneuver, pressure is released to baseline levels. The expiratory time is set to 3 × RCexp (the value obtained from the previous breath).
5. Normal ventilation is resumed.

Review of the P/V curve allows the clinician to examine the patient's pulmonary mechanics closely and to estimate lower and upper inflection points of the slow inspiratory P/V curve (see Figure 12-58).

The inspiratory-expiratory advanced P/V loop (P/V Tool 2) is different in several ways from the P/V Tool 1. The advanced P/V loop performs both an inspiratory and expiratory maneuver. In addition, it allows the operator to start the maneuver at a baseline PEEP rather than full exhalation (range, 0 to 20 cm H_2O).[1] As with P/V Tool 1, Ptop and ramp speed can be controlled, but the range for Ptop is different (the range is 25 to 60 cm H_2O). A control provides an end-inflation pause (T-pause; range, 0 to 30 seconds) and the ending PEEP value can also be chosen (EndPEEP; range, 0 to 20 cm H_2O) (Figure 12-59).

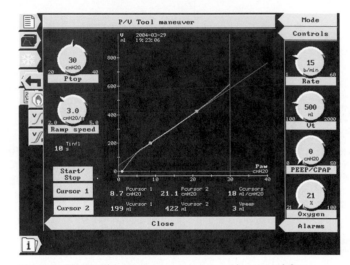

FIGURE 12-58 The inspiratory pressure-volume tool for automatically performing an inspiratory pressure-volume curve. Controls for setting Ptop and ramp speed are shown on the left side of the screen. (See text for additional information.) (Courtesy Hamilton Medical, Reno, Nev.)

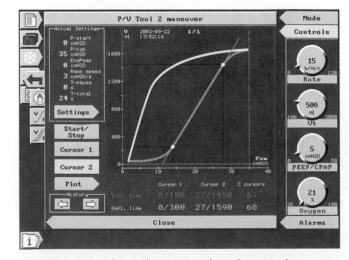

FIGURE 12-59 Advanced pressure-volume loop on the GALILEO Gold for automatically performing a slow inspiratory-expiratory pressure-volume loop. (See text for additional information.) (Courtesy Hamilton Medical, Reno, Nev.)

The additional controls available with the advanced P/V loop provide more flexibility in recruiting the lung and establishing points of lung overinflation and lung collapse (derecruitment).

TROUBLESHOOTING

The monitor, alarm, and message systems for the GALILEO provide important resources in solving common problems encountered during ventilation of a patient. The operator's manual also provides extensive and valuable information on troubleshooting common problems.

If a technical message appears, the operator should record the number indicated with the message and contact Hamilton Medical technical support about the problem. Any ventilator with a technical error problem should be removed from service immediately and replaced by another unit.

Additional information can be found in the operator's manual and by checking the company's Web site at www.hamilton-medical.com.

KEY POINTS

▶ An audible alarm will sound that cannot be silenced when the internal battery charge is low. The ventilator must be connected to an AC power source immediately.

▶ The GALILEO has a built-in galvanic fuel cell for analyzing and monitoring delivered oxygen concentrations.

▶ Using the optional nebulizer results in a small increase in volume delivery but does not affect F_IO_2.

▶ The general rule for using the C knob is: rotate to locate, push to select, rotate to desired value, and push to confirm.

▶ During the use of ASV or APV, the ventilator will not deliver pressures any higher than the upper pressure limit *minus* 10 cm H_2O (Pmax – 10 cm H_2O).

▶ The P-A/C + APV mode, also called APV_{CMV} or pressure-controlled mandatory ventilation, is a dual control mode of ventilation in which the operator sets a target volume (VTarget) instead of a target pressure, and the pressure is adjusted by the ventilator to achieve the set V_T.

▶ The functions set by the operator for ASV are (1) the high pressure alarm limit, (2) the patient's IBW (range, 10 to 200 kg), (3) the percent of minute ventilation (a safe starting point is 100%), and (4) appropriate parameter values for PEEP, trigger sensitivity, F_IO_2, Pramp, and ETS.

▶ AVtS mode is similar to ASV but requires that the operator set a V_T instead of this value being adjusted by the ventilator.

▶ During noninvasive ventilation with the GALILEO, a suggested starting point for ETS is 50%. A Timax should also be set and should be long enough (about 1.5 seconds) to give ETS the chance to cycle the ventilator. Setting a Timax enables the ventilator to cycle into exhalation even when a leak is present.

ASSESSMENT QUESTIONS

See Evolve Resources for the answers.

1. To select and set a specific ventilator control on the GALILEO, which of the following should be performed?
   I. Scroll through screen options or ventilator parameters using the C knob.
   II. Select a highlighted option (parameter) by pressing the C knob.
   III. After an icon turns red, rotate the C knob to change the numeric value.
   IV. Press the C knob to select the newly set value.
   a. III only
   b. I and IV only
   c. II and III only
   d. I, II, III, and IV

2. All of the following options can be configured as a cycling mechanism in volume ventilation in the GALILEO *except:*
   a. % TI (adult)
   b. Peak flow
   c. TCT
   d. I : E

3. An apneic patient is being ventilated with ASV on the GALILEO. Which of the following best describes the breath delivery in this situation?
   a. Flow- or pressure-triggered PS breaths that are volume guaranteed
   b. Pressure-triggered, volume-targeted breaths with a constant flow delivery
   c. Time-triggered, volume-targeted breaths with a constant flow delivery
   d. Time-triggered, pressure-targeted breaths that are volume guaranteed

ASSESSMENT QUESTIONS—cont'd

4. The control which determines the normal cycling of a pressure-support breath is called:
   a. Pressure termination
   b. Flow-cycle percent
   c. Expiratory trigger sensitivity
   d. Timax

5. An audible alarm activates and cannot be silenced, indicating that the internal battery charge is low. The respiratory therapist should immediately:
   a. Change ventilators
   b. Manually ventilate the patient
   c. Change the internal battery
   d. Connect the GALILEO to an AC power source

6. Which of the following is true when the operator uses the nebulizer provided as an option for the GALILEO Gold?
   a. F_IO_2 may vary slightly.
   b. V_T may increase a small amount.
   c. Inspiratory flow is limited to 15 L/min.
   d. The maximum nebulization time is 5 minutes.

7. During the use of ASV or APV, the GALILEO Gold ventilator will not deliver pressures any higher than:
   a. The upper pressure limit
   b. The Pmax value
   c. The upper pressure limit *minus* 10 cm H_2O (Pmax −10 cm H_2O)
   d. The lower pressure alarm limit plus the set PEEP

8. Which of the following statements is/are true about the P-A/C + APV mode?
   I. It is also called APVCMV.
   II. Another description for it is pressure-controlled mandatory ventilation.
   III. It is a dual control mode of ventilation.
   IV. The operator sets a target volume (VTarget), and the pressure is adjusted by the ventilator to achieve the set V_T.
   a. I and IV
   b. II and III
   c. I, II, and III
   d. I, II, III, and IV

9. When the viewing screen is in the ALARMS menu, how can the actual (current) value for airway pressure be determined?
   a. The actual alarm value for pressure is represented by a green horizontal line on the bar graph for pressure.
   b. The value is viewed on the main screen next to the pressure measurement.
   c. It can be seen by viewing the pressure alarm tab.
   d. The actual value appears as a blinking white horizontal line on the pressure bar graph.

10. Explain how a ventilator parameter, such as V_T, is adjusted on the Hamilton GALILEO.

References

1. Hamilton Medical: Operating manual: GALILEO, 610 175/00, 1997 and Galileo Intensive Care Ventilator, 610862/00 (version 3), Bronduz Switzerland, 2000, Hamilton Medical.
2. Branson RD, Johannigman JA, Campbell RS, et al: Closed-loop mechanical ventilation, *Respir Care* 47:427, 2002.
3. Pilbeam SP, Cairo JM: *Mechanical ventilation: physiological and clinical applications,* ed 4, St Louis, 2006, Mosby.
4. Radford EP, Ferris BG, Kriete BC: Clinical use of a nomogram to estimate proper ventilation during artificial respirations, *N Engl J Med* 251:877, 1954.
5. Iotti GA, Johannigman JA, Campbell RS, et al: Respiratory mechanics by least squares fitting in mechanically ventilated patients: applications during paralysis and during pressure support ventilation, *Intensive Care Med* 21:406, 1995.
6. Otis AB, Fenn WO, Rahn H: Mechanics of breathing in man, *J Appl Physiol* 2:592, 1950.
7. Brunner JX, Johannigman JA, Campbell RS, et al: Simple method to measure total expiratory time constant based on the passive expiratory flow-volume curve, *Crit Care Med* 23:1117, 1995.
8. Laubscher TP, Johannigman JA, Campbell RS, et al: The automatic selection of ventilation parameters during the initial phase of mechanical ventilation, *Intensive Care Med* 22:199, 1996.
9. Laubscher TP, Johannigman JA, Campbell RS, et al: Automatic selection of tidal volume, respiratory frequency and minute ventilation in intubated ICU patients as startup procedure for closed-loop controlled ventilation, *Int J Clin Monit Comput* 11:19, 1994.

Internet Resource
www.hamilton-medical.com

HAMILTON RAPHAEL[*1]

OUTLINE

Power Source
Internal Function
Controls
Alarms and Monitoring
   High (Upper) Pressure Limit (Pmax)
   Monitoring
   Real-Time Monitoring

Special Functions
Modes of Ventilation
   BiPhasic Concept of Ventilation
Troubleshooting

*This section was authored by Melissa Turner.

OBJECTIVES

Upon completion of this section, you will be able to:
- State the size of patient who can be ventilated with the RAPHAEL.
- Name the power sources required for use of the RAPHAEL.
- Explain the operation of the internal battery in the event of an AC power failure.
- Discuss the effect of using the nebulizer that comes installed with the RAPHAEL on tidal volume and the fractional inspired oxygen (F_IO_2).
- Review the function of the MODE control.
- Explain how a control parameter can be adjusted or changed.
- Describe how to identify an alarm when an alarm event occurs.
- Compare the Pmax alarm available during the use of (S)CMV+ or SIMV+ to the high pressure limit alarm used during other modes of ventilation.
- Name the function of the touch pad identified with the lung icon.
- Discuss what occurs if the STANDBY control is activated while a patient is still connected to the RAPHAEL ventilator.

KEY TERMS

Proximal airway pressure transducer

Tube resistance compensation (TRC)

The RAPHAEL ventilator is manufactured in Switzerland by Hamilton Medical and was first introduced in the United States in October 2003 (Figure 12-60). It is marketed by Hamilton Medical (Reno, Nevada). Currently two models are available, the RAPHAEL Color and the RAPHAEL XTC. The RAPHAEL XTC, the latest version, has a 10.4-inch color screen; the RAPHAEL Color has a 5.7-inch color screen. The Raphael ventilator is intended for use with adults and pediatric patients weighing 5 to 200 kg.

POWER SOURCE

Like the GALILEO, the RAPHAEL is a microprocessor-controlled unit that requires high-pressure gas and electricity for power. It normally operates from air and oxygen wall outlets (pressure range, 29 to 86 psig). If no gas power source is available, an optional external compressor is available. The main power on/off switch is on the back of the unit. The RAPHAEL uses a 110-volt standard electrical outlet (range, 100- to 240-volt alternating current [AC]).

In the event of an AC power failure, the RAPHAEL automatically switches to the internal backup battery source. The internal battery can provide power for about 1 hour. The battery charge status can be seen by opening the utilities window while the RAPHAEL is operating from an AC power source or by observing the battery symbol while running on battery power. A green battery symbol in the lower bottom right-hand corner of the screen indicates the charge level while the RAPHAEL is operating on battery power. The RAPHAEL provides a low battery alarm, which activates when approximately 10 minutes of battery power remain. In addition, a capacitor-driven backup buzzer sounds for at least 2 minutes when battery power is completely lost. Battery power should be checked before a patient is connected to the ventilator (Clinical Rounds 12-15).

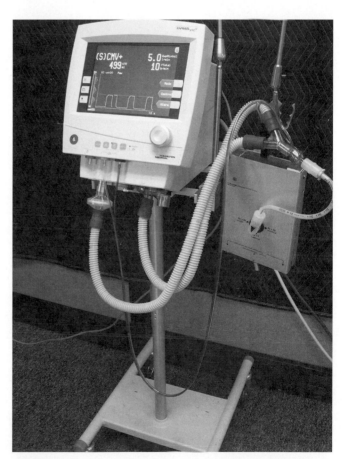

FIGURE 12-60 RAPHAEL ventilator with patient circuit, humidifier, and test lung attached. (Courtesy Hamilton Medical, Reno, Nev.)

The patient circuit for the RAPHAEL is identical to the circuit used with the GALILEO (see Figures 12-46 and 12-47). Delivered oxygen concentrations are analyzed and monitored by a built-in galvanic fuel cell. Three small nipple connectors are located on the bottom front panel

CLINICAL ROUNDS 12-15

During in-hospital transport of a patient ventilated with the Hamilton RAPHAEL, the respiratory therapist (RT) hears an alarm indicating that 10 minutes of internal battery power remain. Although every effort is made to access an AC power source quickly, the therapist subsequently hears a buzzer that cannot be silenced. What does this indicate, and what should the RT do to solve this problem?

See Evolve Resources for the answer.

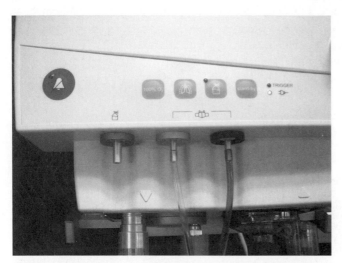

FIGURE 12-61 Nipple connectors below the front panel of the Hamilton RAPHAEL. (Courtesy Hamilton Medical, Reno, Nev.)

(Figure 12-61). The two nipple connectors on the right connect to the **proximal airway pressure transducer.** The nipple connector on the left will power a small-volume nebulizer. When the nebulizer is used, the adaptive volume controller takes the added volume of the nebulized gas into account in determining tidal volume delivery. Use of the nebulizer has no effect on the oxygen concentration.

INTERNAL FUNCTION

Two medical gas sources, air and oxygen, enter the RAPHAEL through water traps with integrated high-efficiency particle filters. Once inside the ventilator, the gas enters the pneumatic system, where an electronic mixer combines the oxygen and air according to the user-set F_IO_2. This gas concentration fills a reservoir tank, which is maintained at a constant pressure. If one of the gas sources becomes unavailable, the unit switches to the remaining gas source and remains operational, but the F_IO_2 is affected.

In the reservoir tank, the pressurized gas allows for an uninterrupted flow even during high flow demand. As the gas mixture is delivered to the patient, the pressure drops and the reservoir is continually refilled.

This is done as the high-pressure oxygen and air inputs are switched on and off as needed to maintain the pressure in the reservoir.

The nebulizer is also supplied by the reservoir. The gas from the reservoir tank supplies an inspiratory valve, which is controlled by the microprocessor. The microprocessor tells the inspiratory valve how much it should open and for how long to meet the user's settings. The opening of the inspiratory valve is constantly adjusted based on feedback from monitored data.

Modes and parameters that are operator selected are monitored, along with additional information received from the proximal airway monitor. This information controls the function of the inspiratory valve, the expiratory valve, and other internal operating mechanisms.

CONTROLS

The control panel (or user interface) for the RAPHAEL uses key pads and a dial knob. Use of the dial knob in conjunction with the key pads allows the operator to open and close operating windows, select and confirm parameters, and activate functions.

The controls labeled MODE, CONTROL, and ALARM are visible on the right side of the screen adjacent to a key pad. Pressing a key pad opens the menu for that key. If the key corresponding to MODE is pressed, a menu displays the available ventilator modes (Figure 12-62). (NOTE: The active mode of ventilation appears at the top of the screen.) The dial knob is then used to scroll through the modes. Each mode is highlighted as the knob is turned. When the desired mode is highlighted, the operator pushes the knob to select the mode. When a mode is selected, OK is automatically highlighted. The operator must confirm the choice by pressing the dial knob while OK is highlighted or by pressing the MODE key. This action automatically opens the control menu.

The CONTROL menu shows the parameter controls available in the selected mode, along with the default settings. The operator can select and adjust all parameters as needed. At the bottom of the menu are numbered tabs. Once the controls in the current tab are set, the operator may select the next tab for more control settings and options. To move to the next tab, the operator uses the dial knob to highlight the tab and then presses either the knob or the CONTROL key. When the settings and options on all tabs have been chosen, the operator confirms them by highlighting OK and pressing the dial knob or the CONTROL key. Once confirmed, the ventilator mode and parameters are activated.

A control parameter can be changed while in the same mode by pressing the CONTROL key to open the CONTROL menu. The operator selects the parameter to be changed and uses the dial knob to make the change. Setting changes that do not require a mode change take effect immediately after the operator presses the knob to confirm the change. (NOTE: Selecting OK merely closes the menu.)

TABLE 12-22

Tubing Resistance Compensation

Parameter	Definition	Range or Selection
Tubing resistance compensation (TRC)	Used to offset the resistance associated with an artificial airway.	
Tube type/TRC disabled	Allows selection in the TRC option of endotracheal (ET) tube or tracheostomy (Trach) tube, or TRC off.	ET tube Trach tube TRC Off
Tube size	Inner diameter of the tube (artificial airway).	4-10 mm
Compensation	Percent of compensation where 100% is the maximum practicable compensation based on given conditions.	0-100%

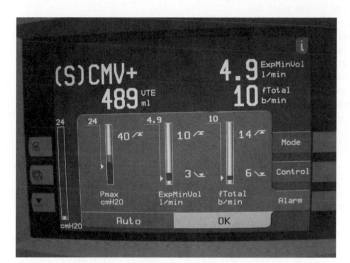

FIGURE 12-62 Hamilton RAPHAEL alarm window. (Courtesy Hamilton Medical, Reno, Nev.)

Tube resistance compensation (TRC) is also available in the CONTROL menu. Please refer to the description of *Tube Resistance Compensation (TRC)* in the section on the Hamilton GALILEO in this chapter (Table 12-22).

ALARMS AND MONITORING

When the ALARM key is pressed, the ALARM menu appears on the screen (Figure 12-62). The operator can have the unit set the alarms automatically. The operator simply highlights AUTO in the ALARM menu and selects it. The computer is programmed to provide high and low alarm defaults for all available alarms. The operator can also choose to set the alarm limits manually. The alarms appear on the menu as bar graphs with the numeric upper and lower settings to the right side of the bar. Each limit can be selected by highlighting it using the dial knob and then pressing the knob to select and turn to the desired setting. The knob is pressed once again to confirm the setting, and then OK is selected to close the window. The current measured value is shown to the left of the alarm bar, and the current alarm limits are shown to the right. When an alarm becomes active, the alarm bar is red.

When an alarm activates, an audible alarm sounds and the red indicator on top of the alarm silence key blinks. A message is displayed on the top (message) line of the screen. If more than one alarm limit was violated, only messages with the highest priority are displayed. If multiple messages of the same priority are necessary, they alternate. The event log icon may be selected at the top right of the screen; this shows the most recent alarms and setting changes. These data include the dates and times of occurrences. If the alarm condition is corrected, the RAPHAEL automatically resets the alarm. This information is also stored in the event log.

Alarms of different priorities produce different sounds, which helps the practitioner distinguish those that require immediate attention from those that are less critical. Becoming familiar with the ventilator and listening to the different alarms help the operator learn to distinguish the different audible signals.

Adjustable and nonadjustable alarms are listed in Table 12-23. Box 12-41 lists user attention messages for the RAPHAEL (Clinical Rounds 12-16).

BOX 12-41	User Attention Messages (RAPHAEL)

100% O$_2$ activated
Apnea backup ended
Connect patient
Disconnect patient
Flow sensor test failed
Flow sensor test in progress
Flow sensor test OK
IRV
Last setup activated
O$_2$ calibration failed
O$_2$ calibration in progress
O$_2$ calibration OK
Tighten system
Tightness test failed
Tightness test OK
Turn flow sensor
If the message TECHNICAL FAULT appears and is followed by a number, the ventilator is experiencing technical difficulties and needs to be replaced. The manufacturer's service engineer should be called and given the number of the technical fault.

TABLE 12-23

Adjustable and Nonadjustable Alarms—Hamilton RAPHAEL

ADJUSTABLE ALARMS

Alarm	Range	Automatic Setting	Default Setting	Resolution
Apnea	15-60 sec	Not applicable	Set during configuration	1
ExpMinVol Low	0.1-50 L/min	Measured ExpMinVol × 0.6 if measurement available; otherwise, (S)CMV + rate × V_T × 0.6	Based on rate and V_T	0.1
ExpMinVol High	0.1-50 L/min	Measured ExpMinVol × 2 if measurement available; otherwise, (S)CMV + rate × V_T × 2	Based on rate and V_T	0.1
Pmax	15-80 cm H_2O	Measured Pmax of last breath + 15 cm H_2O when auto-set active. When manually set, Pmax is the measured Pinsp of last breath +15 cm H_2O. Minimum of 40 cm H_2O if measurement available; otherwise, 40 cm H_2O or as set in configuration mode	Set during configuration	1
fTotal, low	0-99 breaths/min	Measured fTotal × 0.6 if measurement available; otherwise, (S)CMV + rate × 0.6 (minimum as set in configuration mode)	Set during configuration	1
fTotal, high	0-99 breaths/min	Measured fTotal × 1.4 if measurement available; otherwise, (S)CMV + rate × 1.4 (minimum as set in configuration mode)	Set during configuration	1

NONADJUSTABLE ALARMS

Alarm	Trigger Conditions
Air/oxygen supply	Input pressure for air or oxygen < 29 psi
Apnea backup	Ventilation in apnea backup mode due to no patient effort detected (no breath trigger) for the set apnea times in the following modes: Spont, SIMV+, PSIMV+, DuoPAP, DuoPAP+, and NIV modes
Battery low	Minimum of 10 minutes of battery power remaining.
Disconnection	For two consecutive breaths, any of the follow is true: VTexp < 1/8 delivered volume for V_T setting of more than 50 mL (all modes except NIV) Pmax < (PEEP + Pcontrol) − 5 cm H_2O Ptank < 750 cm H_2O for more than 2.5 sec The alarm is reset when both of the following are true for two consecutive breaths: Airway pressure > 3 cm H_2O or expiratory flow "50 mL/sec Ptank ≥ 750 cm H_2O for at least 500 msec
Exhalation obstructed	Monitored PEEP/CPAP > (set PEEP/CPAP + 5 cm H_2O) for 2 consecutive breaths
Check flow sensor	Sensing lines disconnected or occluded
High oxygen	Monitored oxygen ≥ (O_2 setting + 5% of setting)
High tidal volume	Delivered inspiratory tidal volume = 1/5 × set V_T
Inverse ratio	Monitored or set I : E ratio > 1 : 1
Low oxygen	Monitored oxygen < (O_2 setting − 5% of setting); minimum, 18%
Oxygen cell defective	Monitored oxygen < 18%
Oxygen and air supplies	Input pressures of both gas supplies < 29 psi
Pressure limitation	Pinsp + PEEP/CPAP ≥ (Pmax − 10 cm H_2O)
Volume measurement inaccurate	VTE > 2 × Delivered volume (for delivered volumes > 20 mL) or (VTE − Delivered volume) for delivered volumes > 20 mL
Others	Fan failure, flow sensor missing, main power loss (switching to battery), oxygen cell missing, replace clock battery

CLINICAL ROUNDS 12-16

During use of the RAPHAEL, a CHECK FLOW SENSOR alarm condition occurs. The respiratory therapist should take what action to determine the cause of the problem?

See Evolve Resources for the answer.

High (Upper) Pressure Limit (Pmax)

Because of its importance in ventilator function, the high pressure alarm setting is worth reviewing. For safety purposes, respiratory therapists commonly set the upper pressure alarm approximately 10 to 15 cm H_2O above the peak ventilating pressure in all modes. If the high pressure alarm limit is reached, inspiratory flow ends and the expiratory valve opens to allow exhalation.

In the RAPHAEL, the high pressure alarm setting also serves another function when used in two specific modes:

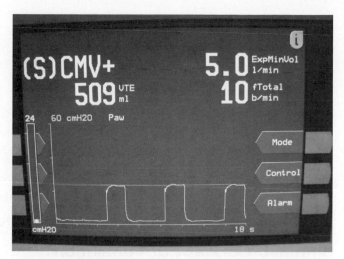

FIGURE 12-63 RAPHAEL screen during (S)CMV+ ventilation, showing the function of the high pressure alarm limit (Pmax). Although volume ventilation has been selected, the pressure-time waveform displayed shows the pressure "plateauing" (staying constant) during inspiration because the pressure has reached the pressure limitation value (high pressure alarm limit – 10 cm H_2O). Breath delivery is continued with the pressure remaining constant until inspiratory time ends the breath. The horizontal line across the tops of the P-T waveforms represents the pressure limitation, and the horizontal line 10 cm H_2O above it represents the high (upper) pressure limit (Pmax).

- Synchronized continuous mandatory ventilation ([S]CMV+)
- Synchronized intermittent mandatory ventilation (SIMV+)

During the use of (S)CMV+ or SIMV+, the ventilator will not deliver pressures any higher than the high pressure alarm setting minus 10 cm H_2O (Pmax – 10 cm H_2O). (Pmax is the same as "peak pressure alarm.") At 10 cm H_2O below the high pressure alarm setting, a *pressure limitation* alarm, which is nonadjustable, is activated. This pressure limitation allows breath delivery to continue at the set pressure limit (high pressure alarm – 10 cm H_2O [±2 cm H_2O]). The target tidal volume may not be achieved, but the patient is not subject to the immediate cycling off of all pressure and flow that would occur with a traditional high pressure alarm function.

Pressures can become higher than the pressure limitation in the circuit (e.g., if the patient coughs). However, the ventilating pressure can never go higher than the upper (high) pressure alarm setting (Figure 12-63).

Monitoring

During normal operation, four parameters are always displayed on the screen: expired minute volume, total respiratory rate, exhaled tidal volume and, on the left side, the bar graph with the peak airway pressure. The bar graph with the peak airway pressure is always displayed, but the other three monitored parameters can be changed in the configuration mode before a patient is connected to the ventilator. Only three parameters, besides the bar graph, may be

chosen for display at any time. In addition to these parameters, other monitoring options appear on the left side of the screen with the first two keys. The first is the numeric patient data key, identified by a sheet of paper, and the second is the graphic selection key, identified by a waveform icon (see Figure 12-62).

When the patient data key is selected, a window opens showing monitored parameters. Three tabs can be opened in the monitored parameters window. This window lists all monitored parameters that are measured breath to breath. A total of 19 parameters that are being calculated and measured can be viewed in this window.

Selecting the graphic selection key opens a window that allows the operator to choose different graphic displays, including data curves, dynamic loops, or trend curves. The data curves are displayed as real-time waveforms. The operator may choose pressure-time, flow-time, or volume-time scalars. When displaying dynamic loops, the operator may choose pressure-volume, pressure-flow, or volume-flow loops.

When choosing to display a trend, the operator may select monitored parameters as a 1-, 12-, or 24-hour trend. In the trend screen, numeric values can be examined at points along the trend curve. Only one parameter may be selected for trending at one time, although in certain cases a pair of parameters are automatically trended together, such as expiratory minute volume and spontaneous minute volume, total respiratory rate and control respiratory rate, and peak airway pressure and PEEP/CPAP.

The last key on the left side of the screen with a down arrow icon is the utilities key (see Figure 12-62). Selecting this key allows the user to perform a tightness test (leak test), a flow sensor test, and O_2 cell calibration; to adjust the loudness of audible alarms; to view the software version; to view options and operating hours; and to check battery status.

Real-Time Monitoring

The parameters measured by the proximal flow sensor, the oxygen cell, and those calculated by the microprocessor are listed in Table 12-24. The only parameter not measured on a breath-by-breath basis is the breath rate, which represents a running eight-breath average.

SPECIAL FUNCTIONS

At the lower left corner of the front panel are five touch controls (see Figure 12-61). The ALARM touch pad (left) silences the audible portion of the alarm system for 2 minutes. The indicator light is illuminated during alarm silence, and a symbol is displayed in the lower right corner of the screen. The alarm silence can be cancelled by pressing it again. (NOTE: A technical fault alarm cannot be silenced.)

The next touch pad is the 100% O_2, which provides 100% oxygen for 5 minutes. This is useful in procedures such as preoxygenation before a patient is suctioned. To

TABLE 12-24

Measured Parameters and Ranges—Hamilton RAPHAEL

Parameter	Range
MV Spont (spontaneous expiratory minute volume)	0-50 L/min
Oxygen (measured by O_2 cell, not flow sensor)	18% to 105%
PEEP/CPAP	−10-100 cm H_2O
Pinsp (inspiratory pressure)	−10-100 cm H_2O
Pmean (mean airway pressure)	−10-100 cm H_2O
Ppeak (peak pressure)	−10-100 cm H_2O
RCexp (expiratory time constant)	0-10 sec
Rinsp (inspiratory flow resistance)	0-999 cm H_2O/L/sec
TE (expiratory time)	0-60 sec
TI (inspiratory time)	0-30 sec
VTE (expiratory tidal volume)	−9000 to 9000 mL

terminate delivery of 100% oxygen before it stops automatically, the operator presses the 100% O_2 touch pad again.

The touch pad identified with the lung icon is used to perform an inspiratory hold, deliver a manual breath, and start breath delivery during a disconnection. To perform an inspiratory hold, the operator holds down the lung icon touch pad during any breath phase until the hold is performed. An inspiratory hold is performed for 15 seconds or until the touch pad is released. To deliver a manual breath, the operator presses and releases the touch pad during *exhalation*. To start a breath, the operator presses and releases the touch pad. The ventilator delivers a mandatory breath based on the current settings. Another use for manual breath delivery with this icon is after ventilator disconnection. For example, after the patient is reconnected to the ventilator, a manual breath can be delivered to start ventilation. Thus ventilation can be started immediately rather than waiting for a patient trigger or any slight delay for a time-triggered breath.

The nebulizer touch pad enables the pneumatic nebulization function for 30 minutes or until the touch pad is pressed again, whichever is first. The indicator key is lit while nebulization is active. As noted earlier, the nebulizer is powered directly from the reservoir tank.

The STANDBY touch pad places the RAPHAEL in STANDBY mode. During standby the operator can maintain ventilator settings while the RAPHAEL is not performing any ventilatory functions. This function is useful when preparing the ventilator before a patient is connected to it and during circuit changes. The operator must make sure that no patient is attached to the ventilator before putting it in the standby mode. Once the ventilator is placed in STANDBY mode, if it determines within 10 seconds that the patient is not disconnected, it will resume ventilation with the previous settings. Also, the RAPHAEL consumes oxygen in the STANDBY mode, therefore when an oxygen cylinder is used, care should be taken to make sure the oxygen source is not depleted.

MODES OF VENTILATION

The modes of ventilation currently available for the RAPHAEL are listed in Box 12-42. Back-up ventilation is available whenever apnea is detected during any mode of ventilation in which the patient is allowed to breathe spontaneously. (NOTE: The RAPHAEL uses flow triggering to sense a patient's inspiratory effort in all modes. Pressure triggering is not available.)

The sigh function can deliver a sigh breath once every 50 breaths. A sigh consists of a breath delivered at a pressure 10 cm H_2O higher than the current breaths when the sigh function is activated. (NOTE: Sigh is not available in DuoPAP or DuoPAP+ modes.)

BiPhasic Concept of Ventilation

The pneumatic design of the RAPHAEL uses a biphasic concept of ventilation, which relies on the use of an active

---

BOX 12-42   Modes of Ventilation Available on the RAPHAEL

SYNCHRONIZED CONTROLLED MANDATORY VENTILATION [(S)CMV+]
A mandatory mode of ventilation that provides volume-targeted, pressure-adapted mandatory breaths only. This mode functions in the same manner as APV_{CMV} in the GALILEO Gold ventilator. Refer to Pressure-Control Ventilation Plus Adaptive Pressure Ventilation (P-A/C + APV) in the section on the Hamilton GALILEO. (NOTE: Pressure trigger is not applicable in the RAPHAEL.)

PRESSURE-CONTROLLED VENTILATION (PCV+)
A mandatory mode. Please refer to Pressure-Targeted Assist/Control Ventilation (P-A/C) in the section on the Hamilton GALILEO.

SYNCHRONIZED INTERMITTENT MANDATORY VENTILATION (SIMV+)
Please refer to the APV_{SIMV} mode in the section on the Hamilton GALILEO.

PRESSURE CONTROL SYNCHRONIZED INTERMITTENT MANDATORY VENTILATION (PSIMV+)
Please refer to the P-SIMV mode in the section on the Hamilton GALILEO.

SPONTANEOUS MODE (SPONT)
Please refer to the spontaneous mode (SPONT) in the section on the Hamilton GALILEO.

DUAL POSITIVE AIRWAY PRESSURE MODE (DUOPAP) AND DUAL POSITIVE AIRWAY PRESSURE MODE WITH EXTENDED I:E TIMES (DUOPAP+)
Please refer to Dual Positive Airway Pressure Mode (DuoPAP) and Airway Pressure Release Ventilation in the section on the Hamilton GALILEO.

ADAPTIVE SUPPORT VENTILATION (ASV)
ASV is available on the RAPHAEL in the United States. Refer to ASV in the section on the Hamilton GALILEO.

NONINVASIVE VENTILATION (NIV)
Please refer to Noninvasive Ventilation in the section on the Hamilton GALILEO. (NOTE: Low tidal volume alarm is not applicable for the RAPHAEL.)

exhalation valve. The RAPHAEL has a special valve control system independent of any trigger mechanism. Gas can flow freely into and out of the patient at anytime, regardless of ventilator settings or the phase of the breath (inspiration or exhalation). In this way, the ventilator never forces air into a patient based on a preset rate or breath type. Instead, it responds to the patient's spontaneous breathing pattern.

TROUBLESHOOTING

The monitor, alarm, and message systems for the RAPHAEL provide important resources in solving common problems encountered during ventilation of a patient. The operator's manual also provides extensive and valuable information on troubleshooting common problems.

If a technical message appears, the operator should record the number indicated with the message and contact Hamilton Medical technical support about the problem. Any ventilator with a technical error problem should be removed immediately from service and replaced by another unit.

Additional information can be found in the operator's manual and by checking the company's Web site at www.hamilton-medical.com.

KEY POINTS

▶ The internal battery of the RAPHAEL can provide power for about 1 hour.

▶ The five touch controls include the ALARM touch pad, the 100% O$_2$, the lung icon, the nebulizer touch pad and the standby touch pad.

▶ The touch pad for the lung icon is used to perform an inspiratory hold, deliver a manual breath, and start breath delivery during a disconnection.

▶ After a patient is reconnected to the ventilator, a manual breath can be delivered to start ventilation immediately rather than waiting for a patient trigger or any slight delay for a time-triggered breath.

▶ The nebulizer receives gas directly from the internal reservoir.

▶ If it determines within 10 seconds of the ventilator being placed in standby that the patient is not disconnected, the RAPHAEL will resume ventilation using the previous settings.

▶ The RAPHAEL consumes oxygen in the standby mode, therefore when using an oxygen cylinder, care should be taken to make sure the oxygen source is not depleted.

▶ The modes of ventilation on the Raphael are the same as those available on the Hamilton GALILEO, although the names may differ slightly.

ASSESSMENT QUESTIONS

See Evolve Resources for the answers.

1. Which of the following statements about the Hamilton RAPHAEL ventilator are true?
   I. The RAPHAEL XTC has 10.4-inch color screen.
   II. It is intended for use with adults and pediatric patients weighing 5 to 200 kg.
   III. The RAPHAEL requires a high-pressure gas source to operate.
   IV. Electrical power is *not* required to use the RAPHAEL.
      a. I and III
      b. II and IV
      c. I, II and III
      d. II, III, and IV

2. Which of the following statements is true regarding the power sources in the RAPHAEL?
   a. In the event of an AC power failure, an alternative AC power source must be found.
   b. An internal battery can provide power for about 1 hour.
   c. To determine the status of the internal battery charge, the operator *must* open the utilities window.
   d. The RAPHAEL provides a low battery alarm, which signals that approximately 20 minutes of battery power remain.

3. Which of the following is true with regard to use of the nebulizer that comes installed with the RAPHAEL?
   a. The V$_T$ will increase slightly.
   b. The oxygen concentration will not change.
   c. The nebulizer receives its gas supply from an independent nebulizer compressor.
   d. Nebulization is adjustable from 15 to 30 minutes.

4. When the MODE control is pressed, the ventilator:
   a. Changes the mode of ventilation to the next mode on the list.
   b. Returns to the last mode of ventilation used.
   c. Opens a menu displaying the ventilator modes available.
   d. Displays the controls that can be adjusted in the current mode.

5. To change a control parameter while in a particular mode of ventilation, the operator:
   a. Presses the CONTROL key to open the CONTROL menu
   b. Selects the parameter to be changed
   c. Uses the knob to make the change
   d. All of the above

ASSESSMENT QUESTIONS—cont'd

6. Which of the following statements are true regarding alarm events that might occur with the RAPHAEL?
   I. When an alarm event occurs, an audible alarm sounds and the red indicator on top of the alarm silence key blinks.
   II. A message is displayed on the top (message) line of the screen.
   III. If more than one alarm limit was violated, the alarm message displays the first alarm that occurred.
   IV. If multiple messages of the same priority are necessary, they alternate.
   V. The event log icon may be selected to review the most recent alarms and setting changes, including dates and times of occurrences.
      a. I and V
      b. II, III and IV
      c. I, II, IV and V
      d. I, II, III, IV, and V

7. Which of the following statements is true regarding the high pressure alarm setting in the RAPHAEL?
   a. The Pmax function is available in any mode of ventilation.
   b. During the use of (S)CMV+ or SIMV+, the ventilator will not deliver pressures any higher than the high pressure alarm setting minus 10 cm H_2O (Pmax − 10 cm H_2O).
   c. Respiratory therapists usually set the high pressure alarm 5 cm H_2O above the current peak airway pressure.
   d. In the (S)CMV+ and SIMV+ modes, the ventilator holds the ventilating pressure at the set value for the high pressure alarm if that pressure is reached during inspiration.

8. Which of the following statements is true with regard to the operator's choices in displaying a trend?
   a. The operator may select monitored parameters as a 1-, 2-, 4-, 8-, or 12-hour trend.
   b. In the trend screen, numeric values can be examined at points that occur every 15 minutes on the trend curve.
   c. Only one parameter may be selected for trending at one time.
   d. Monitored parameters on the trend screen are always displayed individually.

9. The touch pad for the lung icon is used for which of the following functions?
   a. Perform an inspiratory hold
   b. Deliver a manual breath
   c. Start breath delivery during a disconnection
   d. All of the above

10. A respiratory therapist activates the STANDBY mode while a patient is still connected to the RAPHAEL. Which of the following will occur?
    a. The ventilator will go into standby, and the patient will not be ventilated.
    b. There is no standby function on the RAPHAEL.
    c. If the ventilator determines within 10 seconds that the patient is not disconnected, it will resume ventilation.
    d. A high priority "disconnect patient" alarm will activate.

Reference

1. Hamilton Medical: Raphael operator's manual (US), 624008/01, Software version 3, February, 2006, Hamilton Medical AG, Via Crusch 8, CH-7402 Bonduz, Switzerland.

Internet Resource
www.hamilton-medical.com

MAQUET VENTILATORS

MAQUET SERVO 900C

The Servo 900C ventilator was released in the United States in 1981 and continues in use today in some facilities. As of 2011, it will no longer be supported by the manufacturer. This represents a 30-year history of ventilation for this unit. The Servo 900C was designed for use in infant, pediatric, and adult ventilation. Additional information on the Servo 900C is available on the Evolve Web site for this text.

MAQUET SERVO 300

OUTLINE

Power Source
Internal Mechanism
Controls and Alarms
  Patient Range Selection
  Airway Pressures
Mode Selection
  Respiratory Pattern Settings
Volume Settings and Displays
  Oxygen Concentration
Alarms, Messages, and Alarm Silence/Reset
  Pause Hold

Modes of Ventilation
  Pressure Control
  Volume Control
  Pressure-Regulated Volume Control
  Volume Support
  Synchronized Intermittent Mandatory Ventilation
    (SIMV VOL CONTR) + Pressure Support
  SIMV (PRESS CONTR) + Pressure Support
  Pressure Support–CPAP
  Automode
Graphics Display Screens
Troubleshooting

OBJECTIVES

Upon completion of this section, you will be able to:
- Label a diagram of the control panel of the Servo 300.
- Explain the function of the controls on the operating panel of the Servo 300 and compare measured with set digital display values.
- Recommend a safe method for changing rate and V_T settings on the Servo 300.
- Assess an alarm situation and recommend an action to correct the problem.
- Compare each of the modes of ventilation on the Servo 300, including a review of triggering and cycling mechanisms and breath delivery (volume versus pressure).
- Explain the use of the select parameter guide (SPG) for setting up controls when switching to a new mode of ventilation.
- Describe the function of volume support, PRVC, and Automode.

KEY TERMS

Automode	Radio frequency interference (RFI)	Trigger sensitivity
Diodes	Total cycle time (TCT)	Upper pressure limit

The Servo 300 ventilator[1,2] is manufactured by Maquet (Bridgewater, New Jersey) primarily for use in the intensive care unit for neonatal, pediatric, and adult patients. It consists of two sections connected by a 2.9-m cable. One section is the control or operating panel. The other is the patient unit, which connects directly to the patient circuit. The patient circuit consists of a main inspiratory and a main expiratory line.

The control panel contains the electronic circuits that control ventilator function (Figure 12-64). It also contains the touch pads and dials the operator uses to select specific patient settings. The control panel provides illuminated information about selected parameters (green digital display) and measured parameters (red digital display). The patient unit controls the flow of gas to the patient. Flow and pressure are continually measured in the patient unit, compared with the control panel settings, and adjusted as needed. Practitioners often purchase the graphics monitor and an end-tidal carbon dioxide module as important additional items for monitoring patients.

POWER SOURCE

A standard 110- or 120-volt electrical outlet provides power to the display unit and the microprocessor-controlled unit. Two 50-psi gas sources (range, 29 to 94 psi) for air and oxygen are also normally used to power the Servo 300 and to provide flow to the patient (single-circuit ventilator). (NOTE: The unit can function with a single high-pressure gas source, but O_2% delivery may be altered.) This ventilator also has two internal 12-volt batteries that provide backup electrical power. The discussion of alarm features in this section reviews ventilator operation when either the electrical power or the gas supply fails.

The ON power switch is on the front panel at the top center of the ventilator control panel; this is the same control that allows the operator to switch modes of ventilation (see Figure 12-64). Switching to any of the ventilator modes activates the ventilator. Switching from any mode back to the VENTILATOR OFF BATTERY CHARGING setting turns off the ventilator but also activates an audible alert.

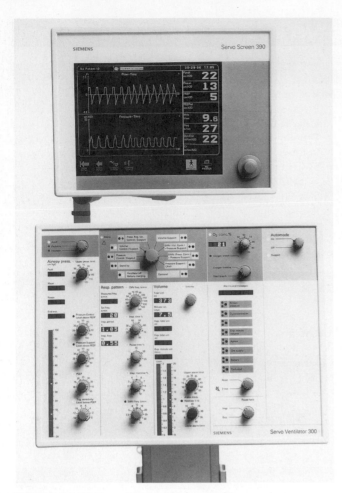

FIGURE 12-64 Servo 300A with the graphics monitor on top. (Courtesy MAQUET Inc., Bridgewater, N.J.)

In older models, the failure alarm box (FAB) alarm control was on the top left side of the ventilator, and the operator pressed it to deactivate it. In newer models the FAB alarm is internal and does not require deactivation.

INTERNAL MECHANISM

The flow delivery of gas to the patient is controlled by a high-performance, rapid response (4 to 6 msec) solenoid valve. Figure 12-65 shows the internal components of the Servo 300. The air and oxygen sources enter through separate gas inlets (*1* and *2*). They pass through bacterial filters and enter the gas modules, where pressures are monitored (*3*). The two gas sources leave their respective modules and enter a mixing chamber, and the pressure is again measured (*4*). Knowing the pressures in the modules and mixing chamber, the flow solenoid can determine the operation of the pin or needle valve that controls gas flow into the unit. The exiting gas is again measured for pressure (*5*) as it enters the inspiratory line (*6*). The inspiratory line houses a pressure-release or safety valve (maximum, 120 cm H_2O), the housing for the oxygen analyzer (*7*), and the main outlet for gas going from the ventilator to the patient (*8*).

The patient's expired gas passes into the ventilator through the connector for the main expiratory line (*9*), where expiratory gas flow (*10*) and pressure (*11*) are measured. (NOTE: Patient circuit pressures are monitored by both the inspiratory [*5*] and the expiratory [*11*] pressure transducers. Transducers also monitor flow for flow triggering.)

Gas then passes through the expiratory valve (*12*), which helps control the phasing of a breath (inspiration/expiration) and the level of PEEP present in the expiratory line. The expiratory valve, also called a *gate valve*, contains a soft, compressible tube that passes between two rollers. These rollers float and come together to adjust resistance to expiration when PEEP is used, and they also open and close to allow phasing of a breath. The gas then passes out of the ventilator through the expiratory one-way valve.

CONTROLS AND ALARMS

The control panel of the Servo 300 has nine sections (Figure 12-66):

1. PATIENT RANGE SELECTION
2. AIRWAY PRESSURES
3. MODE SELECTION
4. RESPIRATORY PATTERN
5. VOLUMES
6. OXYGEN CONCENTRATION
7. ALARMS, MESSAGES, and ALARM SILENCE/RESET
8. PAUSE HOLD
9. AUTOMODE

Patient Range Selection

The PATIENT RANGE SELECTION knob at the upper left corner lets the operator pick the appropriate setting based on the patient's size: ADULT, PEDIATRIC, or NEONATE. This selection affects several ventilator parameters (Table 12-25).

Airway Pressures

The left panel has four pressure controls, one control for **trigger sensitivity,** four digital monitors for airway pressure, and a bar graph display of monitored pressure.

The four pressure controls are:

1. UPPER PRESS LIMIT (16 to 120 cm H_2O)
2. PRESSURE-CONTROL LEVEL ABOVE PEEP (0 to 100 cm H_2O)
3. PRESSURE-SUPPORT LEVEL ABOVE PEEP (0 to 100 cm H_2O)
4. PEEP (0 to 50 cm H_2O)

The **upper pressure limit** is for patient safety; it limits the maximum airway pressure in all modes of ventilation. If the upper pressure limit is reached during breath delivery, inspiration ends and an audible alarm activates. The pressure control knob is active in two modes of ventilation: pressure control and SIMV (PRESS CONTR) + pressure support. The pressure-support knob is active in three modes: pressure support, SIMV (VOL CONTR) + pressure

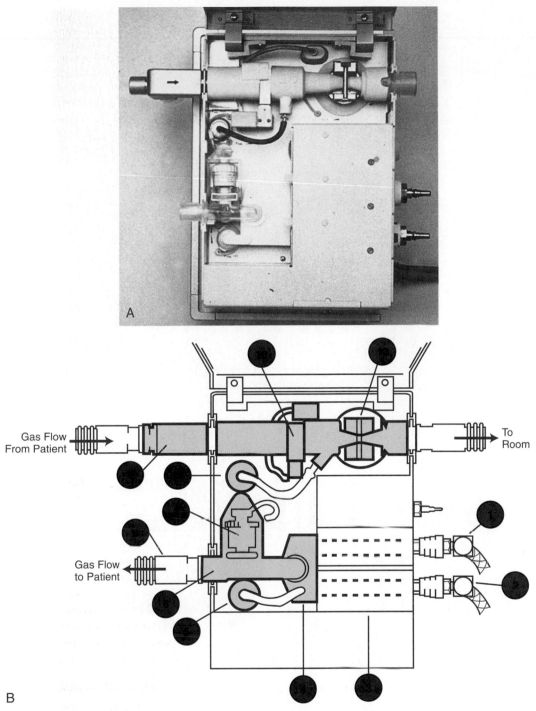

FIGURE 12-65 Internal components of the Servo 300. **A,** Photograph of the internal components. **B,** Diagram of the internal components. (See text for explanation.) (**A** courtesy MAQUET Inc., Bridgewater, N.J.)

support, and SIMV (PRESS CONTR) + pressure support. These are discussed in the following section on mode selection. PEEP sets pressure during exhalation in any mode currently available.

The TRIG SENSITIVITY LEVEL BELOW PEEP knob determines the patient effort required to trigger a breath and is active in all modes. It provides flow or pressure triggering. Pressure triggering is set by turning the knob counter-

clockwise to the indicated pressures (–17 to 0 cm H_2O). This reduces the sensitivity, making triggering more difficult. The flow-triggering setting is indicated by the green and red (most sensitive) markings on the dial. When flow triggering is selected, a low flow of gas passes through the patient circuit only during the expiratory phase and is monitored by both the inspiratory and expiratory flow transducers. Flow triggering of a breath occurs when the

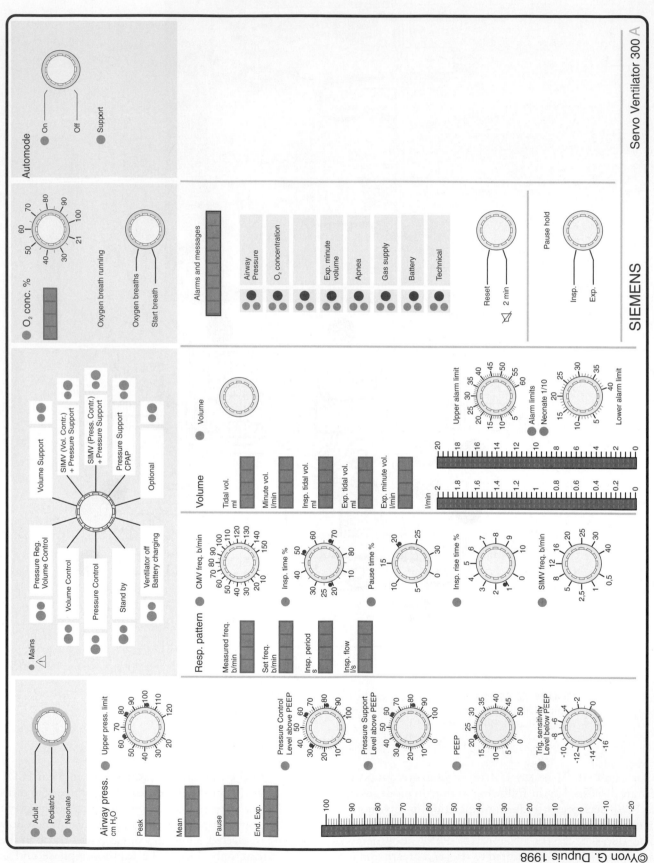

FIGURE 12-66 Front control panel of the Servo 300A. (See text for explanation.) (Courtesy Yvon Dupuis.)

©Yvon G. Dupuis 1998

Parameters and Functions Affected by Patient Range Selections—Servo 300

Continuous Flow Through the Circuit During Exhalation

Adult setting	2 L/min
Pediatric setting	1 L/min
Neonatal setting	0.5 L/min

Maximum Inspiratory Peak Flow

Adult setting	200 L/min
Pediatric setting	33 L/min
Neonatal setting	13 L/min

Maximum Measured Tidal Volume

Adult setting	3999 mL (range, 0-4000 mL)
Pediatric setting	399 mL (range, 0-400 mL)
Neonatal setting	39 mL (range, 0-40 mL)

Apnea Alarm Time

Adult setting	20 sec
Pediatric setting	15 sec
Neonatal setting	10 sec

Flow Trigger Range

Adult setting	0.7-2 L/min
Pediatric setting	0.3-1 L/min
Neonatal setting	0.17-0.5 L/min

Upper Alarm Limit—Minute Ventilation

Adult setting	0-60 L/min
Pediatric setting	0-60 L/min
Neonatal setting	0-6 L/min

Lower Alarm Limit—Minute Ventilation

Adult setting	0.3-40 L/min
Pediatric setting	0.3-40 L/min
Neonatal setting	0.06-4 L/min

From Siemens Medical (MAQUET Inc., Bridgewater, N.J.).

expiratory flow transducer measures a drop in flow (see flow triggering in Chapter 11). The set bias flow in the Servo 300 is based on the patient size selected (adult, pediatric, or neonatal; see Table 12-25). For example, when ADULT is selected on the patient selection switch, 2 L/min flows through the circuit during exhalation. The flow-trigger range for an adult is 0.7 to 2 L/min, depending on where the operator sets the triggering sensitivity dial. The closer the dial is set to the red area, the less the amount of flow that must be removed and the more sensitive the triggering.

The airway pressure monitors provide illuminated red digital readouts of measured values for peak, pause, and end-expiratory pressures and a calculated value for mean airway pressure. Peak inspiratory pressure is the highest pressure reached during inspiration and is measured by the inspiratory pressure transducer. Peak pressure is displayed on the pressure bar graph (described later in this section). However, the digital display value of pressure is actually the pressure measured by the expiratory pressure transducer.

Mean pressure is a calculated value based on the pressure measured during each complete breath cycle (inspiration plus expiration).

Pause pressure displays the pressure measured by the expiratory pressure transducer when a pause time is selected on the PAUSE TIME % control or when the manual inspiratory pause (INSP) is held during inspiration long enough for a pause to occur. It can be activated whenever a mandatory volume or pressure breath occurs in synchronized intermittent mandatory ventilation (SIMV) or assist-control (A/C) modes. The end-expiratory pressure display shows the pressure at the end of each breath and is also measured by the expiratory pressure transducer. When an expiratory pause is manually activated, both the inspiratory and expiratory valves close and this window displays the value for total PEEP ($PEEP_I + PEEP_E$) as measured by the ventilator.

The airway pressure bar graph has flashing **diodes** of various colors that monitor several pressure values. The diodes on the left side are red. The diodes on the right have different colors, depending on the pressure level. The right diodes are yellow for values less than 0 cm H_2O; green for values from 0 to 40 cm H_2O; yellow for values from 40 to 60 cm H_2O; and red for values from 60 to 100 cm H_2O. The upper pressure limit is indicated by four diodes that flash (two on the left, two on the right) when the pressure limit is reached or when it is set above 100 cm H_2O. The lower diodes on the bar graph indicate the pressure settings.

The actual airway pressure is shown by two side-by-side flashing diodes. The left one shows the pressure measured by the inspiratory transducer, and the right one shows the pressure measured by the expiratory pressure transducer. Because these pressures are measured at different places, the operator will see separations between the two when they reflect pressure variations, such as the rebound of pressure in the patient circuit or resistance to expiratory flow in the circuit. The value for the peak pressure digital display corresponds to the right illuminated diode (Figure 12-67). The pressure control (PC), pressure support (PS), and PEEP settings are shown by two diodes. If pressure support is set higher than pressure control, the diodes indicating both controls start flashing. PEEP is the lowest set of diodes, because PC and PS are additive to the set PEEP value.

A patient-triggered breath is indicated on the bar graph by two red and yellow flashing diodes that appear on the bottom right.

MODE SELECTION

At the top center of the control panel is a rotating knob with nine different positions (see Figure 12-66). These include VENTILATOR OFF BATTERY CHARGING, STAND BY, PRESSURE CONTROL, VOLUME CONTROL, PRESSURE REG VOLUME CONTROL, VOLUME SUPPORT, SIMV (VOL CONTR) + PRESSURE SUPPORT, SIMV (PRESS CONTR) + PRESSURE SUPPORT, PRESSURE SUPPORT—CPAP, and OPTIONAL.

VENTILATOR OFF BATTERY CHARGING is the off position for the ventilator. Keeping the ventilator plugged into an electrical outlet with the knob in this position recharges

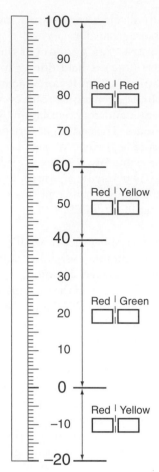

FIGURE 12-67 Airway pressure bar graph for the Servo 300 ventilator. This is an enlargement of the lower left section of the main panel. (See text for explanation.) (Courtesy MAQUET Inc., Bridgewater, N.J.)

CLINICAL ROUNDS 12-17

The respiratory therapist decides to use inverse ratio ventilation (IRV) on a patient who is difficult to oxygenate with the Servo 300 in volume control. The INSP TIME % control is turned to 80%, and the PAUSE TIME % to 10%. The yellow light next to the PAUSE TIME % control begins to flash. What does this indicate?

See Evolve Resources for the answer.

modes are set on the mode selection knob. The range of breath frequency is 5 to 150 breaths/min. The CMV FREQ B/MIN knob setting determines the **total cycle time (TCT)** for all modes. The ventilator does not allow the inspiratory time (T_I) to exceed 80% of the TCT. Because CMV FREQ B/MIN controls the TCT and the maximum T_I, it should be set appropriately for the patient being ventilated. In addition, CMV FREQ B/MIN is the backup rate for volume support if the patient becomes apneic.

INSP TIME % determines the percentage of time spent providing inspiratory gas flow (10% to 80%) based on the TCT. All mandatory breaths in either volume- or pressure-control ventilation are time cycled in either A/C or SIMV modes.

PAUSE TIME % (0 to 30% of TCT) provides an inspiratory pause (no inspiratory gas flow) and increases the length of inspiration for a volume-controlled breath. The sum of inspiratory time and pause time can never exceed 80% of the TCT, as determined by the rate set on the CMV FREQ B/MIN knob, regardless of the ventilator mode (Clinical Rounds 12-17). If the sum of these two settings exceeds 80%, the adjacent yellow indicator light flashes.

INSP RISE TIME % determines the time (% of TCT) in which the flow or pressure gradually rises to the set value in any mode of ventilation. INSP RISE TIME % is considered a patient comfort feature in adults and a lung protective strategy in newborns, because it prevents pressure overshoots. As long as the value is set above zero (range, 0 to 10% of TCT), the delivery of pressure and flow is tapered and does not instantly increase to the set value at the beginning of inspiration. Figure 12-68 shows how sloping affects pressure and flow delivery. At the zero setting there is no sloping, and pressure and flow rise rapidly. This can be uncomfortable for a patient and can cause oscillations or ringing in the patient circuit (see Figure 11-86). The maximum rise time setting of 10% gives the maximum time for tapering flow and pressure delivery, as well as a more gradual rise to the set parameters.

SIMV FREQ B/MIN determines the minimum number of breaths per minute when either SIMV mode is selected (range, 0.5 to 40 breaths/min). It must be set at a value lower than the CMV FREQ B/MIN control or the ventilator will default to the frequency set on the CMV FREQ B/MIN and the yellow light adjacent to the SIMV FREQ B/MIN control will flash.

the internal battery. The manufacturer recommends this as the best option for the ventilator when it is not in use. When the ventilator is in the STAND BY position, the electrical circuits are supplied with power and the expiratory flow transducer can warm up to its operating temperature (104° F [40° C]). Patient settings can be selected for use while the ventilator is in STAND BY. The seven ventilator modes are described in the discussion of modes of ventilation later in this section.

The OPTIONAL position of the mode knob has no function but can be used to add future upgrades.

Respiratory Pattern Settings

The respiratory pattern and inspiratory time controls and display are in the center area of the front panel. There are five control knobs: CMV FREQ B/MIN, INSP TIME %, PAUSE TIME %, INSP RISE TIME %, and SIMV FREQ B/MIN. There are also four digital display panels: MEASURED FREQ B/MIN, SET FREQ B/MIN, INSP PERIOD S, and INSP FLOW L/S.

The control marked CMV FREQ B/MIN sets the number of mandatory breaths per minute when volume control, pressure control, or pressure-regulated volume control

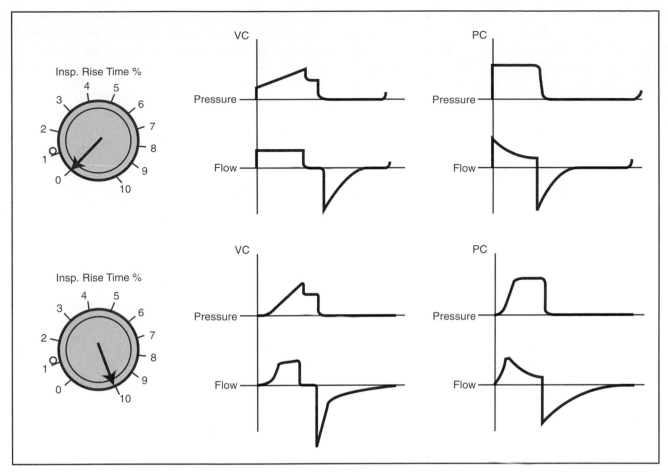

FIGURE 12-68 Inspiratory rise time percentage. During volume-control ventilation *(left curves)*, flow is normally constant when the inspiratory rise time percentage is set at zero *(top left)*. The use of inspiratory rise time tapers the beginning of the flow curve *(bottom left)*. During pressure ventilation *(right curves)*, flow is normally a descending ramp *(top right)*. Use of an inspiratory rise time percentage above zero tapers the beginning of the flow curve *(bottom right)*.

The display panels in this section provide information about the respiratory pattern. MEASURED FREQ B/MIN indicates in red the total of all breaths (spontaneous and mandatory) measured by the ventilator. SET FREQ B/MIN shows the set rate in green for A/C and SIMV modes. INSP PERIOD S provides the calculated T_I (in seconds) for mandatory breaths. INSP FLOW L/S shows the calculated flow (in liters per second) based on the TCT, set volume, and T_I for mandatory volume breaths.

The TCT, flow (in L/min), and the set I:E ratio can be obtained from the ventilator without manual calculations. The operator simply touches the pad with the two dots next to the STAND BY setting and immediately afterward touches the pad (two dots) next to the MODE setting selected for the patient. (NOTE: The operator does not need to press hard on these touch pads, because they are light sensitive, not touch or pressure sensitive.) This causes the digital display windows in this panel to read as follows:

1. SET FREQ B/MIN shows "(t)s" alternating with a numeric display of the calculated TCT (in seconds).
2. INSP PERIOD S shows "I:E" alternating with a numeric display of the set I:E ratio. (NOTE: This is the set ratio

and not a measurement of the I:E ratio. If the patient triggers a breath, this can shorten the expiratory time [T_E] and alter the set I:E ratio.)

3. INSP FLOW L/S shows "/min" alternating with a numeric display of the calculated flow (in L/minute). (NOTE: This is only shown when volume ventilation modes are in use.) In addition to these readings, the yellow light indicators adjacent to functional controls in the selected mode flash. To return to the normal display function, the operator touches the STAND BY touch pad again. The normal display also resumes if a minute passes without any operator intervention.

VOLUME SETTINGS AND DISPLAYS

The tidal volume (V_T) and expired minute volume ($\dot{V}_E$) are set using the volume control, which is active during the volume control, pressure-regulated volume control, volume support, and SIMV (VOL CONTR) + pressure support modes. The available V_T range can vary, depending on the patient size selected (see Table 12-25). All measured flows and set and indicated volumes are referenced to standard conditions (1013 mbar, 760 mm Hg). The operating manual provides the conversion calculations and necessary tables to obtain a reading of ambient conditions. This provision might be significant at high-altitude environments (e.g., 5000 to 10,000 feet); the reader is referred to the operator's manual.

Two volume reading displays are available for the set values. TIDAL VOL ML shows the set V_T (mL) as a green digital number. MINUTE VOL L/MIN shows the set $\dot{V}_E$ (in L/min) as a green number for volume ventilation in A/C (volume control) or SIMV (SIMV [VOL CONTR] + pressure support). Also provided are values for $\dot{V}_E$ (green) in pressure-regulated volume control (PRVC) and volume-support modes of ventilation.

Measured volumes are provided by the following three windows, which give digital values illuminated in red:

1. INSP TIDAL VOL ML provides the volume of each breath as measured by the inspiratory flow transducer during delivery from the ventilator outflow port. The monitored range is 50 to 3999 mL for adult settings, 10 to 399 mL for pediatric settings, and 2 to 39 mL for neonatal settings. If the measured value exceeds the range for the patient size selected (see Table 12-25), the number flashes and an over-range alarm occurs (see the discussion of alarms later in this section).

2. EXP TIDAL VOL ML displays the volume measured by the expiratory flow transducer for each breath coming back through the ventilator's expiratory port connection. Monitored ranges are the same as those for inspired V_T. As with inspired volumes, if the value exceeds the set range, the number flashes. When no leaks are present, inspiratory and expiratory values are approximately equal.

3. EXP MINUTE VOL L/MIN indicates the measured exhaled $\dot{V}_E$ in red numbers. The display range is 4 to 60 L/min for adults, 1 to 5 L/min for pediatric patients, and 0.2 to 1.5 L/min for neonatal patients (Box 12-43).

In this same section of the control panel are indicators and controls for the minute ventilation alarms. The Servo 300 has upper and lower minute volume alarm controls, the scale of which varies, depending on the patient range selected (according to size) (see Table 12-25). A volume bar graph provides indicators for various minute ventilation parameters. Colored diodes are red on the left side of the bar and green on the right. The set upper alarm limit is indicated by two red and two green diodes and is read at the lower two diodes. When the upper minute ventilation limit is set above 20 L/min, the lower two diodes start flashing. When the upper $\dot{V}_E$ alarm is exceeded, all four diodes flash. The monitored (measured) $\dot{V}_E$ is shown by one red and one green flashing diode. The set $\dot{V}_E$ is shown by one red and one green nonflashing diode. The measured $\dot{V}_E$ is superimposed on the set $\dot{V}_E$ when these values are equal. The lower $\dot{V}_E$ alarm limit is indicated by two red and two green diodes at the bottom of the volume bar graph. When the set lower alarm limit is violated, the diodes flash. (NOTE: The lower $\dot{V}_E$ alarm functions as the disconnect alarm. If the measured $\dot{V}_E$ falls below the lower alarm limit, the diodes flash.)

Oxygen Concentration

In the upper right section of the control panel is a control knob for adjusting the fractional inspired oxygen (F_IO_2) delivery (0.21 to 1). Upper and lower F_IO_2 alarms are automatically set internally by the microprocessor at 0.06 (6%) above and below the selected F_IO_2. The absolute minimum alarm limit is 0.18 (18%). The set oxygen concentration is digitally displayed. An internal oxygen analyzer continuously monitors oxygen delivery.

Near the oxygen control is a knob marked OXYGEN BREATHS/START BREATH. When the switch is turned to OXYGEN BREATHS, the ventilator provides 100% oxygen for 20 breaths or for 1 minute, whichever comes first, and then switches back to the current oxygen delivery setting. A yellow indicator light labeled OXYGEN BREATH RUNNING lights up when this control has been activated, and the display window reads O₂ CONC %. This 100% oxygen delivery can be canceled by turning the switch to OXYGEN BREATHS again before 20 breaths or 1 minute has passed (Box 12-44).

The other side of this knob is the START BREATH control, which is similar in some ways to the manual breath control on other ventilators. When activated, a breath based on the set control values is delivered. In the SIMV mode, this activates a mandatory breath. It is important to allow the patient time to exhale before activating this breath delivery.

BOX 12-43	Important Clinical Note on the Servo 300

The Servo is primarily a $\dot{V}_E$-based ventilator. This affects V_T delivery when the rate (CMV FREQ B/MIN) is adjusted. For example, suppose $\dot{V}_E$ = 5 L/min (V_T = 0.5 L and f = 10 breaths/min). If f is decreased to 5 breaths/min, the V_T will increase to 1 L to maintain the $\dot{V}_E$. When the mandatory rate needs to be reduced, it is recommended that the V_T be reduced first, by one half to one third.

BOX 12-44	Oxygen Breaths Control on the Servo 300

When the OXYGEN BREATHS function is activated, the following alarms are silenced for a maximum of 55 seconds:
· Oxygen alarm
· Expired $\dot{V}_E$ alarm
· Apnea alarm
· Technical alarm for over-range

ALARMS, MESSAGES, AND ALARM SILENCE/RESET

The ALARM section is on the right side of the patient control panel. Small lights in this section are yellow or red. A steady yellow light indicates two possible conditions: a high priority alarm condition that has been corrected and the alarm condition has been stored in memory, or certain alarm limits have been overridden and the alarm has been turned off manually. Another indicator is an audible caution (ticking) sound that occurs under a few special conditions and acts as a reminder to the user. For example, ticking occurs under the following conditions:

· The oxygen cell is disconnected.
· An error is detected in either a flow or a pressure transducer.
· The ventilator is placed in the STAND BY mode.
· The ventilator is operating on battery power.
· Only one high-pressure gas source is being used.

A red flashing light and a sound signal that a high priority alarm condition has occurred, requiring immediate attention. Table 12-26 lists the high priority alarms in order of importance.

The unit has seven alarm indicators (eight in some versions [i.e., CO_2 concentration]) in this section of the control panel: AIRWAY PRESSURE, OXYGEN CONCENTRATION, EXPIRATORY MINUTE VOLUME, APNEA ALARM, GAS SUPPLY, BATTERY, and TECHNICAL. The message display window at the top of this panel provides information about a current or recent alarm. This window normally displays the measured oxygen concentration.

If more than one alarm is active at a time, the highest priority alarm is displayed. The operator can display the alarm text for any of the seven alarm indicators by touching the light diode to the left of the desired alarm indicator. For example, if a yellow light next to an alarm indicator is constantly lit, a recent alarm condition for this parameter may have occurred. A message will appear in the display window showing the reason for the caution, but it will alternate with the oxygen concentration reading.

If more than one yellow light is present, the operator can sequentially select each illuminated light and check the alarm memory for that parameter. The lights can be turned off by using the RESET control or changing to another ventilatory mode.

Alarm conditions for the other seven parameters are listed in Table 12-27, which describes the more common causes for such conditions. Historical Note 12-2 provides a description of one of the original alarms. Box 12-45 provides information about the safety switches on some of the control knobs.

Besides resetting visual alarms, the RESET/2 MIN control can be used to silence some high priority alarms by turning it to the 2 MIN position for longer than 2 seconds, thus providing 2 minutes of silence. If the knob is turned to RESET before the end of 2 minutes, the alarm sounds again. For example, before disconnecting a patient for suctioning

TABLE 12-26

High Priority Alarm Functions on the Servo 300 (in Order of Priority)

TECHNICAL ERRORS—TRY RESTARTING UNIT

Power failure test
Internal RAM (random access memory) test
Internal ROM (read-only memory) test
Internal CPU (central processing unit) test
Ref and timing micromodule (MM) error
Mixer MM error
Panel MM error
Range switch error
Mode switch error

Operating Error	Check Function
Airway pressure	Airway pressure too high
Apnea	Apnea alarm
Expired $\dot{V}_E$	$\dot{V}_E$ too low/high
O_2 concentration	O_2 concentration too low/high
O_2 cell disconnect	O_2 sensor
No battery capacity left	No battery capacity
Limited battery capacity left	Limited battery capacity
High battery voltage	Internal battery voltage too high
Main failure	Battery
Pressure transducer error	Check tubing
Power failure	Technical error (see operating manual)
O_2 potentiometer error	Technical error (see operating manual)
Out of gas	Check pneumatic power source
Gas supply air	Check pneumatic power source
Gas supply O_2	Check pneumatic power source
High continuous pressure	High continuous pressure
CMV potentiometer error	Technical error (see operating manual)
Servo control module (SCM)	Technical error (see operating manual)
Microprocessor Error	
Over-range	Over-range: Select pediatric/adult
Barometer error	Technical error (see operating manual)
Regulation pressure limited	Limited pressure

BOX 12-45 — Safety Features on the Servo 300

· Measured values are shown as red digital displays. Set values are shown as green digital displays.
· Yellow lights that are constantly illuminated indicate active controls that must be set by the operator in the selected mode. A flashing yellow light indicates that a control has been set incorrectly.
· Safety catches are indicated by small black markings that appear on the number scale of certain control knobs or dials (e.g., UPPER PRESS. LIMIT, PRESSURE CONTROL LEVEL ABOVE PEEP, PRESSURE SUPPORT LEVEL ABOVE PEEP, PEEP, INSP. TIME %, and O_2 CONC). To turn a dial past a safety catch, the operator must push in the top of the knob while rotating it past the safety catch.

TABLE 12-27

Alarm Parameters, Messages, and Causes—Servo 300

Airway Pressure

Upper press limit	Set upper pressure limit has been reached, and inspiration ends.
Airway pressure too high	Airway pressure exceeds the upper pressure limit.
Limited pressure	Inadequate pressure to deliver volume support or pressure-regulated, volume-controlled breaths.
High continuous pressure	Continuous pressure > 15 cm H_2O plus PEEP level; continuous for more than 15 sec.

Oxygen Concentration

O_2 conc too low/high	F_IO_2 measured at above or below 0.6 of set F_IO_2, or F_IO_2 < 0.18; alarm inactive during and for 1 min after oxygen breaths are activated.
O_2 sensor	Oxygen cell is not connected.

Expired $\dot{V}_E$
(Must be set correctly for each patient size: adult, pediatric, or neonate.)

Exp minute volume too high	Expired $\dot{V}_E$ exceeds alarm setting.
Exp minute volume too low	Expired $\dot{V}_E$ is below alarm setting.

Apnea Alarm

Apnea alarm	No breaths, spontaneous or mandatory, detected: 20 sec (adult), 15 sec (pediatric), 10 sec (neonate).

Gas Supply Alarm

Air supply pressure too low/high Air: x.x bar O_2 x.x bar	Air supply is out of range (<29 to >100 psi). Ventilator defaults to use available gas source.
O_2 supply pressure too low/high Air: x.x bar O_2 x.x bar	Oxygen supply is out of range. Ventilator defaults to use available gas source.
Air O_2 supply pressure too low/high Air: x.x Bar O_2 x.x bar	Both gas sources have failed. Internal safety valve and expiratory valve open so patient can breathe room air if able.

Battery
(If the main power source fails, the ventilator switches to battery power and this alarm activates [yellow light]. The graphic screen turns off.)

Limited battery capacity left internal: xx v	High-priority alarm if remaining voltage ≤23 V.
No battery capacity left	Voltage ≤21 V (this alarm cannot be silenced).
See operating manual	At 18 V, safety valve opens.

Technical Alarms
(These generally are corrected by the technical staff. The Check Tubings alarm can be corrected by the clinician.)

Check tubings	Inspiratory/expiratory pressure difference ≥25%, or at least 5 cm H_2O for 20 sec. Causes: Disconnected pressure transducer tubings, transducer error, clogged bacterial filter, or any blockage in the breathing system.

or a similar procedure, turn the RESET/2 MIN control to 2 MIN. A short beep and the message ALARMS MUTED indicate that the alarms are silenced. The audible alarms for MINUTE VENTILATION, OVERRANGE, and APNEA can be silenced for 2 minutes in this manner. (The UPPER PRESS LIMIT alarm cannot be silenced with the 2 MIN knob.)

Pause Hold

At the lower portion of the right section is a manual control used to provide an inspiratory or expiratory pause. When an INSP PAUSE HOLD is activated, the inspiratory and expiratory valves close at the end of inspiration, preventing expiratory gas flow. The valves remain closed until the control is released or held for a maximum of 5 seconds. Using this control gives an opportunity to check the plateau pressure during this pause time.

When EXP PAUSE HOLD is activated, the inspiratory and expiratory valves close at the end of exhalation, just when another mandatory breath would have occurred. The valves remain closed as long as the control is held or up to a maximum of 30 seconds. This extended expiratory time allows expiratory pressure to be measured, which may facilitate estimation of the auto-PEEP level.

When a Servo 300 includes the available graphic monitor screen (see Figure 12-64), the inspiratory and expiratory pause controls can be used to have the microprocessor calculate a patient's static compliance (Cs). To perform this procedure, the operator turns the inspiratory pause control until the graphic screen displays the message MEASURING STATIC COMPLIANCE at the top center. Immediately the inspiratory pause is switched to the expiratory pause position for a few seconds and then is released. After a few seconds the calculated Cs value appears on the graphic screen. This calculation takes into account the PEEP level but not the tubing compliance factor.

HISTORICAL NOTE 12-2

In the original version of the Servo 300, a separate backup alarm was available that mounted on the left side of the ventilator; this was called the *failure alarm box (FAB)*.

If a 24-volt power failure occurred or if the ventilator mode control was turned to the ventilator OFF position, this audible and visible (red) alarm was activated and could not be silenced until the button on the FAB was pressed. This alarm also was activated briefly as a self-test when the ventilator was first turned on, and after a few seconds it became silent on its own.

This failure alarm prevented the electrical power from being disconnected or the ventilator from being turned off, either accidentally or deliberately, unless it was done by someone familiar with the FAB alarm who knew how to silence it.

In newer versions of the Servo 300, the FAB alarm is incorporated internally and is self-tested when the unit is turned on. When the ventilator is turned off, this alert chirps and then is silenced automatically.

MODES OF VENTILATION

The mode of ventilation is set with the MODE SELECTION switch. Appropriate settings for a mode can be achieved in two ways. First, if the patient is not yet connected to the ventilator, the patient settings can be selected (using the set parameter guide [SPG]) while the MODE SELECTION switch is in the STAND BY position (Box 12-46). The second method of mode selection is commonly used when the patient is already being ventilated and the operator wants to switch the mode. The operator touches the light diode to the left of the desired ventilator mode. The light next to the desired mode flashes, the parameters that are set for the desired mode illuminate, and those for the current active mode are turned off. When the pad next to the desired mode is touched a second time, the same sequence as the SPG can be followed, which essentially walks the operator through each control that needs to be set in the desired mode. To actively change to the desired mode, the operator turns the mode control switch to the new mode.

A word of caution needs to be added, because changing any parameter or control that is active in current mode takes effect immediately. To distinguish between the active and inactive controls, those that are currently active flash rapidly, and those that will be active in the new mode flash at a normal speed. For example, the INSP TIME % control adjusts T_I in both volume- and pressure-control mode. In either of these two modes, if the inspiratory time is increased while the SPG is followed, the T_I increases as soon as it is adjusted (i.e., changes do not wait for the new mode to be activated). Box 12-47 provides a word of caution.

The mode selection switch has a left half and a right half. Modes on the left (PCV, VCV, and PRVC) are A/C

BOX 12-46   Using the Set Parameter Guide (SPG) on the Servo 300

1. Before connecting the patient to the ventilator, use the mode selection switch to set the standby mode.
2. Touch the light diode next to the desired mode (e.g., next to the volume control). It will illuminate the controls or parameters to set for that mode.
3. Touch the light diode a second time; the first control parameter that needs to be set will flash, and the others will be off. For example, the light next to the patient range selection switch will flash, telling you to set that control.
4. Touch the light diode next to the mode (e.g., volume control) again, and the next control that needs to be set (e.g., upper pressure limit) will flash.
5. Continue setting controls when they flash and touching the light next to the desired mode until all appropriate parameters have been set.
6. Upon completion of the SPG, the ventilator will beep three times to indicate that the process has been completed. The mode is now ready to be operational or active.

(NOTE: If the patient is already connected to the ventilator and the clinician decides to use the SPG feature, any control that is active in the current mode of ventilation will be immediately changed. For example, a patient is in volume control mode at a rate of 12 breaths/min. The clinician uses SPG to switch the patient to SIMV at a rate of 12 breaths/min. If the CMV frequency knob is turned to 30 breaths/min so that it is higher than the SIMV frequency, the rate immediately goes to 30 breaths/min.)

BOX 12-47   Note of Caution on Use of the Servo 300

It is strongly recommended that whenever a patient is connected to a Servo 300 for the first time, all appropriate parameters be selected from the start-up. For example, even if volume ventilation will be used, the appropriate inspiratory pressure for pressure-control and pressure-support settings must still be set. This way, even if the mode switch is accidentally changed, the parameters appropriate for the patient are already within a reasonable setting range, and the inadvertent change will pose no danger to the patient.

---

modes and provide a clinician-selected volume or pressure for every patient breath. Modes on the right (VS, SIMV[VC] + PSV, SIMV[PV] + PSV, and PSV/CPAP) allow for spontaneous breaths. Not all patient-triggered breaths are mandatory.

Remember that regardless of the mode selected, certain things are always true. Pressure cannot exceed the UPPER PRESS LIMIT setting. If the limit is reached, volume delivery is reduced. T_I cannot exceed 80% of TCT (based on the CMV frequency setting). Flow and volume delivery can vary if a patient's active inspiration drops pressure below the baseline. For example, during pressure ventilation, such as during pressure control, the flow pattern is commonly a descending flow curve, and flow and volume delivery can vary. During volume ventilation, flow is usually constant, and there is no control knob with which to select a particular inspiratory flow curve (e.g., constant flow or a descending flow waveform) during volume ventilation. The only control the operator has over the flow waveform is the sloping or tapering feature provided by the INSPIR RISE TIME % control or by changing the inspiratory time. The patient, however, can obtain as much flow as desired (up to 180 L/min) during any mode of ventilation when airway pressure drops below the baseline (PEEP setting). This results in a flow-time curve that varies, depending on patient demand. Because a patient can obtain increased flow, volume can vary, even during volume ventilation. For example, when the volume-control mode is used, the selected volume normally is delivered, and this represents a minimum volume. If the patient so desires, additional volume can be obtained with an active inspiration.

Each of the modes is reviewed, with particular emphasis on some of the newer ventilatory methods available with the Servo 300.

Pressure Control

Pressure control allows patient or time triggering and provides pressure ventilation that is time cycled based on the T_I %. Inspiratory pause cannot be used in this mode. Flow delivery usually follows a descending curve, and minimum respiratory rate is set with the CMV frequency control.

Volume Control

Volume control is patient or time triggered and provides volume-targeted ventilation with time cycling. Flow delivery is normally constant. V_T is calculated based on CMV frequency and $\dot{V}_E$ settings as follows:

$$V_T = \dot{V}_E \div f$$

The minimum respiratory rate is set with the CMV frequency control. T_I is determined by the inspiratory time % and the pause time % controls.

Pressure-Regulated Volume Control

Pressure-regulated volume control is a servo-controlled (closed-loop) mode of ventilation that is very similar to the pressure-control ventilation (PCV). Breaths are patient or time triggered, pressure targeted, and time cycled. The main difference is that the ventilator can target volume delivery while still using pressure ventilation. It does this by constantly calculating system and patient compliance, volume delivery, and the pressure limits within which it has to operate.

When PRVC is activated, the ventilator begins by giving a breath with an inspiratory pressure of 10 cm H_2O (5 cm H_2O on older models). It then measures the volume delivered and calculates system compliance. The next three breaths are delivered to provide a pressure that delivers approximately 75% of the set V_T. (NOTE: The V_T is determined by the minute ventilation and rate settings and is displayed in the V_T window.) For each subsequent breath, the ventilator calculates the compliance of the previous breath and adjusts the inspiratory pressure level to achieve the set V_T on the next breath (Figure 12-69).

For example, suppose the set volume is 500 mL and the measured volume is 525 mL at a pressure of 23 cm H_2O (C = 22.8 mL/cm H_2O). In this case, the pressure might drop to 22 cm H_2O to deliver the 500 mL. The pressure is reduced until the set and monitored volumes are the same. On the other hand, if the measured volume is too low, the pressure level is increased. The ventilator will not change the pressure more than 3 cm H_2O from one breath to the next. This protects the patient from large changes in pressure. The maximum pressure that can be delivered is equal to the upper pressure limit setting minus 5 cm H_2O. The minimum pressure limit is the baseline setting. If the pressure reaches the UPPER PRESS LIMIT minus 5 cm H_2O, the message window will read LIMITED PRESSURE, and an alarm sounds. The operator must then decide whether to increase the UPPER PRESS LIMIT, and thus allow the ventilator to increase pressure to achieve the set V_T, or accept a lower V_T setting to prevent pressure from going too high.

One reason PRVC was designed was to provide the advantages of PCV, such as a descending flow ramp waveform to help improve gas distribution, an inspiratory flow rate that can vary with patient demand, and a limited pressure to prevent excessive pressures in the lungs. More important, however, PRVC provides another valuable feature: it guarantees a volume delivery.

Suppose a patient is being ventilated with volume control, and the operator wants to switch to PRVC. The operator should follow these steps:

1. Make sure the UPPER PRESS LIMIT is set appropriately. A starting value about 5 to 10 cm H_2O above the patient's current plateau pressure might be appropriate. This is a safe range and could be adjusted if necessary once PRVC is activated.
2. As long as no changes to other parameters are indicated (e.g., T_I, V_T, f, baseline pressure, or F_IO_2), they can remain the same.
3. The mode control switch is rotated to PRVC to activate the mode, and the ventilator self-regulates within the parameters set.

As long as safe limits for pressure and other parameters have been set, the patient is safe.

Volume Support

Volume support (VS) is also a servo-controlled mode that might be considered the weaning counterpart to PRVC and volume control. It is a mode of ventilation that provides breaths that can best be compared with pressure-support breaths. That is, they are normally patient triggered, pressure targeted, and flow cycled (5% of measured peak flow). The flow waveform normally is a descending ramp-like curve. The primary function is that a minimum V_T can be targeted. As in PRVC, the ventilator runs a series of test breaths beginning with one breath at

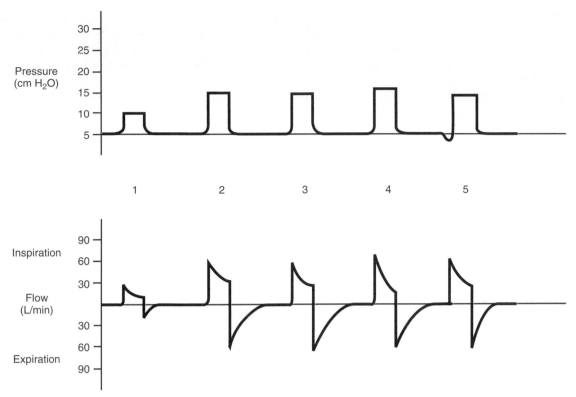

FIGURE 12-69 Test breaths in pressure-regulated volume control (PRVC). (See text for explanation.)

10 cm H_2O (5 cm H_2O in older models). It then gives three breaths at approximately 75% of the pressure calculated to deliver the V_T. Finally, the pressure is provided to give the appropriate volume.

As with PRVC, breaths are constantly monitored, and pressure increases when the volume reading is low or decreases if the volume reading is high, in increments of no more than 3 cm H_2O. Also as in PRVC, pressure can rise as high as the upper pressure limit setting minus 5 cm H_2O to deliver the set minimum volume. If the pressure reaches this limit, the message LIMITED PRESSURE appears in the message window, and an alarm sounds. Baseline pressure represents the minimum pressure level.

There are a few important differences between volume support (VS) and PRVC. First, there is no backup rate in VS. If the patient becomes apneic, the ventilator automatically switches to PRVC and the light diode next to that mode flashes. An alarm sounds, and the message window indicates that apnea has been detected. For this reason, only spontaneously breathing patients who have intact respiratory centers should be placed on this mode. Another important difference has to do with the minute ventilation setting. The Servo 300 tries to maintain the minute ventilation that the operator has set on the ventilator. Clinical Rounds 12-18 provides an exercise with an example of how the ventilator responds in volume support.

Because VS breaths are really pressure-support breaths, one might wonder why volume support is used. The reason, of course, is that the ventilator can target a minimum

CLINICAL ROUNDS 12-18

A patient is on volume support; the rate is set at 12 breaths/min, and the minute ventilation is at 6 L/min. V_T is targeted at 500 mL. The ventilator is able to maintain this volume within the pressure limitations, but the patient's spontaneous rate drops. How will the ventilator respond to the drop in the patient's respiratory rate (to 8 breaths/min)?

See Evolve Resources for the answer.

volume delivery. If a patient is ready for pressure support, volume support is also appropriate. An advantage of VS is the operator does not have to constantly adjust pressure levels, as sometimes occurs with PSV. The ventilator adjusts the pressure as the patient's condition changes. In addition, if the patient becomes apneic, the ventilator switches to a mode that provides continuous ventilation (e.g., PRVC).

Synchronized Intermittent Mandatory Ventilation (SIMV VOL CONTR) + Pressure Support

The SIMV (VOL CONTROL) + pressure support (SIMV VOL CONTR + PSV) mode provides mandatory breaths similar to those in volume control. During SIMV, the mandatory rate and SIMV cycle time are determined in the following way: The SIMV frequency control must be set lower than the CMV frequency to correctly establish the desired SIMV mandatory breath rate. If it is not, the ventilator defaults to the CMV FREQ B/MIN setting, and the yellow indicator next to the CMV frequency control flashes. Cycling times are determined as follows: The SIMV cycle time is calculated by dividing the SIMV frequency into 60 seconds. For example, with the SIMV FREQ B/MIN set at 4 breaths/min, the SIMV cycle time is 15 seconds. The SIMV cycle time has two phases. The first phase is the SIMV period, and the second is the spontaneous period. The SIMV period equals the CMV FREQ B/MIN setting divided into 60. For example, if the CMV frequency is set at 10 breaths/min, the SIMV period is 6 seconds. The spontaneous period is equal to the SIMV cycle time minus the SIMV period (e.g., 15 seconds − 6 seconds = 9 seconds).

The three equations are summarized here:
- SIMV cycle time = 60 seconds/(SIMV frequency)
- SIMV period = 60 seconds/(CMV FREQ B/MIN)
- Spontaneous period = SIMV CYCLE TIME − SIMV PERIOD

When a mandatory breath is triggered, the SIMV cycle begins. After delivery of the mandatory breath, the patient has 9 seconds to breathe spontaneously without receiving a mandatory breath (spontaneous period). At the end of 9 seconds, the 6-second SIMV period begins. The patient has 6 seconds in which to make an inspiratory effort and get a mandatory breath. If the patient fails to take a breath, then a time-triggered breath occurs at the end of the 6 seconds. This is very much like SIMV in the Servo 900C (Clinical Rounds 12-19).

SIMV (PRESS CONTR) + Pressure Support

SIMV (PRESS CONTR) + pressure support is SIMV in which mandatory breaths are pressure-controlled breaths. Pressure support can be added for spontaneous breaths. The only difference between SIMV (VOL CONTR) and SIMV (PRESS CONTR) is that mandatory breaths are volume controlled in the former and pressure controlled in the latter. The operator sets the pressure control level above PEEP.

Pressure Support–CPAP

The pressure support–CPAP setting is intended for spontaneously breathing patients. Breaths are patient triggered when spontaneous breaths can be detected at a set baseline

pressure (0 to 50 cm H_2O). Pressure support can also be set for all spontaneous breaths. The pressure is added to the baseline pressure (pressure-support level above PEEP). At PS greater than zero, inspiration is pressure limited and flow cycled at 5% of the measured peak flow. No minimum guaranteed rate or volume is provided in this mode.

Automode[2]

In 1997 a new feature for the Servo 300, Automode, was introduced in the United States. The on/off control for this mode is at the upper right corner of the updated operating panel (see Figures 12-64 and 12-66). This mode is designed to switch from a control mode to a support mode of ventilation if the patient triggers two consecutive breaths. The ventilator remains in the support mode as long as the patient keeps triggering breaths. Table 12-28 shows the control and support modes that are operational in Automode.

Automode works as follows: Suppose the patient is in the PRVC mode, and Automode is on. When the ventilator detects two consecutive patient efforts, it delivers one more mandatory PRVC breath on the second breath, and the next (third) patient-triggered breath is a VS breath. The ventilator continues to provide volume support as long as the patient continues to trigger the breath. If the patient stops triggering breaths, within a short period of time the ventilator switches back to delivering mandatory breaths. For adults, this period is 12 seconds; for pediatric patients, it is 8 seconds; and for neonates, it is 5 seconds.

If the patient is in volume control and the same conditions occur, the ventilator switches to volume support in a similar fashion. The first VS breath in this situation (volume control to volume support) is delivered at a pressure level equal to pause pressure. If no pause time is set, the ventilator uses the following formula to determine the inspiratory pressure for volume support:

$$\text{set P} = [(\text{PIP} - \text{PEEP}) \times 0.5 + \text{PEEP}]$$

The ventilator does not run through the series of test breaths it normally performs when the mode switch is turned to volume support.

If the patient is in pressure control with Automode and two patient efforts are detected, the switch to pressure support occurs on the third breath. The operator must have previously selected a pressure-support level above PEEP, because that is the pressure that will be delivered by the ventilator when it switches to pressure support.

CLINICAL ROUNDS 12-19

A patient on SIMV (VOL CONTR) + pressure support has a set CMV frequency of 15 breaths/min and an SIMV frequency control setting of 3 breaths/min. What are the SIMV cycle time, the SIMV period, and the spontaneous period for these settings?

See Evolve Resources for the answer.

TABLE 12-28		
Control and Support Modes in Automode—Servo 300		
Control Mode		**Support Mode**
Volume control	⟷	**Volume support**
Pressure control	⟷	**Pressure support**
Pressure-regulated volume control	⟷	**Volume support**

The purpose of Automode is to adapt the ventilator's status to a patient's spontaneous inspiratory efforts. The benefit of Automode obviously lies in its ability to monitor patient breathing effort. For this reason, it is essential that triggering sensitivity be set appropriately and that auto-triggering is not occurring. Autotriggering is detected as a patient-initiated breath without the patient actually making an effort. If autotriggering occurs, the trigger sensitivity needs to be adjusted.

GRAPHICS DISPLAY SCREENS

The graphics display screen provides the standard scalars for flow-time, volume-time, and pressure-time, in addition to several loops, including flow-volume and volume-pressure. From one to four different graphs can be viewed at any time. The right side of the graphics display has spaces for digital display of parameters, including peak pressure, mean pressure, dynamic compliance, and static compliance. Static compliance can be measured by using the PAUSE HOLD control, described in the earlier discussion about ventilator controls. Data screens on which the operator can custom design the monitored parameters to be displayed are also available. An example of an available option is the I:E ratio, which is the actual value on this screen as measured by the ventilator.

A carbon dioxide analyzer module can be attached to the Servo 390 graphics screen to display capnographic waveforms and calculations, including end-tidal carbon dioxide, carbon dioxide production, and dead space.

TROUBLESHOOTING

As noted previously, whenever the mandatory breath rate is reduced in a volume-controlled mode, the V_T delivery is increased because the ventilator is designed to deliver a specific $\dot{V}_E$. It is recommended that the volume be reduced by about one half before any large decrease in rate is performed.

Because many of the safety features base their function on clinician-selected settings, it is advisable to set all available parameters and alarms before beginning ventilation on a patient. For example, the ventilator will never allow the T_I to exceed 80% of the TCT. This is the TCT based on the CMV frequency. The ventilator has many safety features to limit this type of error that were reviewed in the discussion of controls and alarms in this section.

The operating manual contains a section that reviews common alarms and associated problems. **Radio frequency interference (RFI)** and electromagnetic frequency interference (EMI) can affect the function of medical devices using microprocessors. The Servo 300 is specially shielded to ensure protection against RFI and EMI interference. This shielding meets current safety standards.

KEY POINTS

▶ The Servo 300 is minute ventilation based.
▶ The ON power switch is the same control that allows the operator to switch modes of ventilation.
▶ The patient range selection knob affects several ventilator parameters and should be set based on the patient's size: ADULT, PEDIATRIC, or NEONATE.
▶ Because many of the safety features base their function on clinician-selected settings, it is advisable to set all available parameters and alarms before beginning ventilation on a patient.
▶ The patient effort required to trigger a breath is determined by the TRIG SENSITIVITY LEVEL BELOW PEEP.
▶ When the upper pressure limit is reached or when it is set above 100 cm H_2O, the four diodes flash (two on the left, two on the right).
▶ The available ventilator modes include VENTILATOR OFF BATTERY CHARGING, STAND BY, PC, VC, PRVC, VS, SIMV (VOL CONTR) + PS, SIMV (PRESS CONTR) + PS, and PS–CPAP.
▶ There are five control knobs: CMV FREQ B/MIN, INSP TIME %, PAUSE TIME %, INSP RISE TIME %, and SIMV FREQ B/MIN.
▶ The SIMV frequency control must be set lower than the CMV frequency to correctly establish the desired SIMV mandatory breath rate.

▶ The CMV FREQ B/MIN knob should be set appropriately because it determines the total cycle time for all modes.
▶ The ventilator does not permit the T_I to exceed 80% of the TCT.
▶ The sum of inspiratory time and pause time can never exceed 80% of the TCT, as determined by the rate set on the CMV FREQ B/MIN knob, regardless of the ventilator mode.
▶ The CMV FREQ B/MIN is the backup rate for volume support if the patient becomes apneic.
▶ The patient can obtain as much flow as desired (up to 180 L/min) during any mode of ventilation when airway pressure drops below the baseline (PEEP setting).
▶ When PRVC is activated, the ventilator begins by giving a breath with an inspiratory pressure of 10 cm H_2O (5 cm H_2O on older models) and then calculates system compliance. The next three breaths are delivered to provide a pressure that will deliver approximately 75% of the set V_T.
▶ In VS, if the patient becomes apneic, the ventilator switches to PRVC, an alarm sounds, and the message window indicates that apnea has been detected.
▶ Automode is designed to switch from a control mode to a support mode of ventilation if the ventilator detects two consecutive patient triggers.

ASSESSMENT QUESTIONS

See Evolve Resources for the answers.

1. As air and oxygen high-pressure gases enter the Servo 300, they pass to a:
   a. Large pressurized reservoir
   b. Pair of servo-controlled stepper motors
   c. Mixing chamber
   d. Spring-loaded bellows

2. The Servo 300 can be pressure or flow triggered in which of the following modes of ventilation?
   I. Pressure control
   II. SIMV (VOL CONTR)
   III. Pressure support
   IV. PRVC
      a. II only
      b. I and IV only
      c. II and III only
      d. I, II, III, and IV

3. A patient is switched from volume-control ventilation to SIMV (VOL CONTR). The SIMV frequency is set at 9 breaths/min, but only 8 mandatory breaths are being delivered. The yellow indicator next to the CMV frequency control flashes. The most likely cause of this condition is that:
   a. The CMV rate control is set at 8 breaths/min.
   b. The mode change was not activated correctly.
   c. The SIMV rate control is out of calibration.
   d. The patient has become apneic.

4. Which of the following modes guarantees volume delivery using pressure-targeted breaths and has a minimum set respiratory rate?
   a. Pressure-regulated volume control
   b. Volume support
   c. Automode
   d. SIMV (PRESS CONTR) + PS

5. An adult patient is being ventilated in volume support and becomes apneic. Which of the following will occur?
   I. The ventilator switches to VC.
   II. A light diode flashes next to the PRVC control.
   III. After 60 seconds the apnea alarm activates.
   IV. The ventilator will begin to ventilate the patient at the set rate.
      a. I only
      b. III only
      c. II and IV only
      d. I, II, III, and IV

6. A patient is in the pressure-support mode. The rate is set at 12 breaths/min. The patient's endotracheal tube cuff becomes deflated and a leak develops, preventing flow cycling. In this situation, what will end inspiratory flow?
   I. It will not end, but an apnea alarm will sound.
   II. It will end after 4 seconds (80% of TCT).
   III. It will switch to PRVC, and the apnea alarm will sound.
   IV. It will end when the circuit pressure reaches the upper pressure limit.
      a. II only
      b. I and III only
      c. II and III only
      d. I, II, and IV only

7. A digital display of volume is in red. This indicates which of the following?
   a. A measured value
   b. A set value
   c. An alarm condition
   d. An error in set-up

8. The Servo 300 uses what type of inspiratory flow valve?
   a. Stepper motor
   b. Spring loaded
   c. Scissor valve
   d. Solenoid valve

9. A patient on PRVC has a set V_T of 450 mL. The PIP is 18 cm H_2O. The upper pressure limit is 30 cm H_2O. The delivered tidal volume is 400 mL. How will the Servo 300 respond to this situation?
   a. It will not make any changes.
   b. It will increase pressure by 3 cm H_2O.
   c. An alarm will activate, producing the message PRESSURE LIMITED.
   d. The unit will switch to VS.

10. During volume-support ventilation, the following parameters are noted: upper pressure limit setting = 35 cm H_2O, set V_T = 0.6 L, PEEP = 10 cm H_2O, CMV frequency = 10 breaths/min. The pressure required to deliver the V_T rises to 31 cm H_2O. Which of the following answers is/are appropriate in this situation?
   I. The ventilator will sound an alarm.
   II. The message LIMITED PRESSURE will appear in the window.
   III. The respiratory therapist should assess the patient.
   IV. The ventilator will switch to PRVC.
      a. I and III
      b. I and IV
      c. I, II, and III
      d. IV only

References

1. Siemens Medical Solutions: Siemens Servo Ventilator 300 operating manual 6.0, s-171 95; part no 60 27 408 E313E, 1997, Solna, Sweden, Siemens, Elema AB, Siemens.

2. Siemens Medical Solutions: Siemens Servo Ventilator 300^A, Automode, order no 64 08 897 E315E, Solna, Sweden, 1997, Siemens.

Internet Resource

www.maquet.com

MAQUET SERVO[i] VENTILATOR SYSTEM[1,2]

OUTLINE

Power Source
Internal Drive Mechanism
Setting up a New Patient
Controls
 Fixed Keys
 Touch Screen Controls
 Nebulizer
 Text Message and Patient Trigger Indicator Field
 Waveforms
 Measured Value Boxes
 Parameter Controls
Modes of Ventilation
 Activating a Mode
 Volume Control
 Pressure Control
 Pressure-Regulated Volume Control

 Volume Support
 Pressure Support
 Spontaneous Breathing/CPAP
 Synchronized Intermittent Mandatory Ventilation
 Automode
 Backup Ventilation
Neonatal/Pediatric Application
Noninvasive Ventilation
Open Lung Tool
Special Features
 Trending of Data
 User Interface and Graphics
 Suction Support
 MRI Conditional Servo[i]
 Neurally Adjusted Ventilatory Assist
Troubleshooting

OBJECTIVES

Upon completion of this section, you will be able to:
· Identify the power source being used with the Servo[i].
· Recognize the amount of time available on the batteries.
· Describe the function of the modes available on the Servo[i], including VC, PC, PRVC, PS/CPAP, SIMV-VC, SIMV-PC, SIMV-PRVC, BiVent, and Automode.
· Explain the function of the ultrasonic nebulizer available with the Servo[i].
· Compare the two methods of setting ventilator parameters on the Servo[i], including use of the direct access knobs and use of the touch screen.
· Describe the alarm profile screen and the alarms available with the Servo[i].
· Identify the cause of an alarm situation.
· Explain the control settings for PSV.
· Recognize an increase in patient flow demand during VC.
· Discuss the accessing of trended data, alarm history, and the event log.
· List the modes of ventilation available with NIV for adults and for infants.
· Name the parameters graphed on the Open Lung Tool.

KEY TERMS

Automode
Inspiratory cycle off control (INSPIR CYCLE OFF)
Inspiratory rise time (T INSPIR RISE)

Neurally adjusted ventilatory assist (NAVA)
O$_2$ breaths
Occlusion pressure (P0.1)

Spontaneous breathing index (SBI)
Start breath

The Servo[i] ventilator system originally was released in the United States in 2002. The Servo[i] ventilator can be used in acute care facilities and for transport in the hospital and also outside the hospital. (It is approved for use in ambulances, fixed wing aircraft, and helicopters.) It is intended for patients ranging in size from neonates, infants (0.5 to 30 kg), and adults (10 to 250 kg) (Figure 12-70).[1]

Since its development, a number of options and features have been added (Box 12-48). For example, the Servo[i] can now be used not only for invasive ventilation, but also for noninvasive ventilation. In 2006 a feature called **neurally adjusted ventilatory assist (NAVA)** was approved

BOX 12-48	Available Options (Servo[i])
Nebulizer	
Automode	
Open Lung Tool	
CO$_2$ Analyzer	
Noninvasive ventilation (NIV)	
Y Sensor Measuring	
Nasal CPAP	
Status Window	
Neurally Adjusted Ventilatory Assist (NAVA)	
MRI Conditional Package	
Heloix Delivery System	

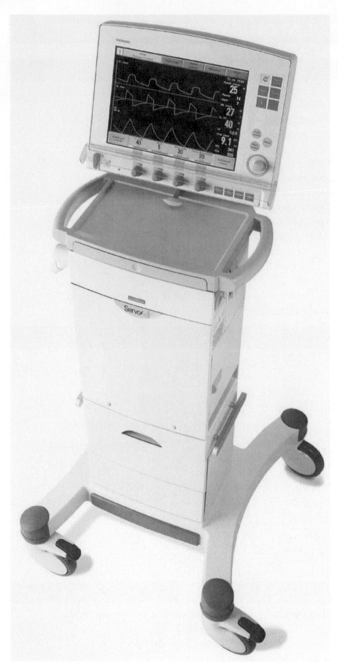

FIGURE 12-70 Patient unit and user interface *(top)* of the Servo[i]. (Courtesy MAQUET Inc., Bridgewater, N.J.)

The Servo[i] consists of two main parts: a patient unit, where gases are mixed and delivered to the patient, and a user interface (front panel), where the ventilator settings are selected and information is monitored (see Figure 12-70).

Three different configurations can be purchased, which differ primarily by the patient size selected. The Servo[i] Infant includes SIMV(PC) + PS, PS/CPAP, and PC (modes are reviewed later in this section). The Servo[i] Adult has SIMV(VC) + PS, PS/CPAP, and VC. The Servo[i] Universal includes all modes as well as pressure-regulated volume control (PRVC) and volume support.

The Servo[i] can be upgraded; therefore even if an adult version is purchased, infant features can be added. Upgrades are accomplished with personal computer (PC) cards, which are programmed by the company and inserted into a PC card slot on the side of the user interface (Figure 12-71). The cards can also be used to add additional modes, such as BiVent (airway pressure-release ventilation) (see Chapter 11 for an explanation of mode function).

Other options can also be added, including noninvasive ventilation (NIV), capnography, Y-sensor monitoring, **Automode,** a nebulizer option, NAVA, and an option called the *Open Lung Tool (OLT)*. The OLT option can be used to identify specific pressure points, such as the pressure at which the lung is overdistended or the pressure at

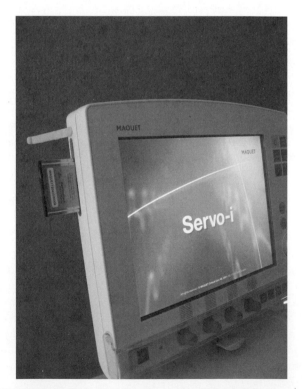

FIGURE 12-71 Side panel on the user interface of the Servo[i] allows a personal computer (PC) card to be inserted. Patient data can be saved to this card, and this same slot can be used by Maquet personnel to upload new software or check ventilator function and records. (Courtesy Amy Houck, sales representative, MAQUET Inc., Bridgewater, N.J.)

by the U.S. Food and Drug Administration (FDA) for use on the Servo[i] (see Chapter 11, section on NAVA.) In 2007, a magnetic resonance imaging (MRI) conditional model was also made available (see Special Features later in this section).

Now available is an option that will allow the use of helium and oxygen with the ventilator, although some hospitals currently are using helium and oxygen with the Servo[i] in an off-label manner. (NOTE: *Off-label* means the use of medical equipment in a way that was not originally intended. Off-label use of the Servo[i] for heliox therapy is not an unusual practice.)[2]

which significant lung compartments collapse in patients with acute respiratory distress syndrome (ARDS). The OLT also can be used to monitor a lung recruitment maneuver. The OLT tracks volumes, compliance, peak pressures, positive end-expiratory pressure (PEEP), and volumetric carbon dioxide (CO_2) changes (see the discussion of the Open Lung Tool later in this section).

An additional feature is the ability to save information from the ventilator for research or education purposes. To accomplish this, a *record card* can be inserted in the PC card slot and used to save data or screen shots. The information on the PC card can then be transferred to a personal laptop computer for study and evaluation.

The following discussion focuses on the functionality of version 3.1 of the Servo[i].

POWER SOURCE

The Servo[i] is electrically and pneumatically powered. It is recommended that the ventilator operate from a high-pressure air and oxygen source (approximately 50 psi). It will operate from one high pressure gas source, but this will affect delivery of the fractional inspired oxygen (F_IO_2).

The electrical power sources for the Servo[i] ventilator include AC power and 12-volt DC internal batteries. The status indicator for the power source is a STATUS pad in the upper right corner of the touch screen, which is part of the user interface (Figure 12-72). Besides indicating the current power source, the STATUS pad serves other functions (Box 12-49).

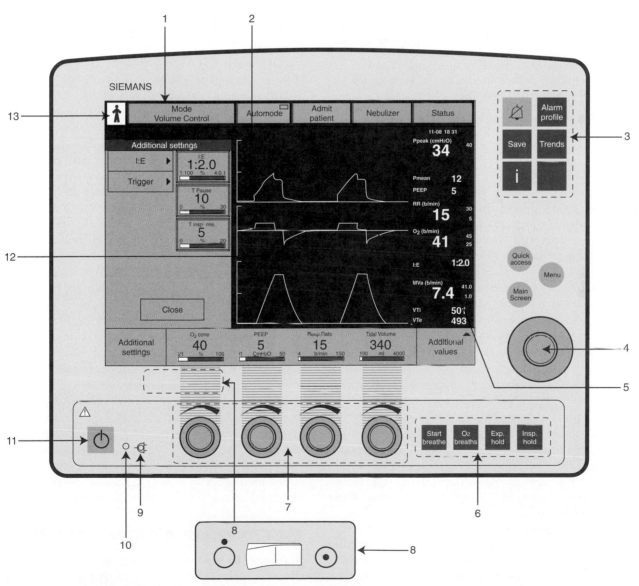

FIGURE 12-72 Control panel (user interface) of the Servo[i] ventilator. (See text for further description.)

BOX 12-49	Status Window (Servo^i)

When the STATUS pad in the upper right corner of the touch
screen is pressed, a list appears showing the following:
- General system information, including software
  version
- Status of O$_2$ cell/O$_2$ sensor
- Status of expiratory cassette
- Status of batteries
- Status of CO$_2$ module (if available)
- Status of Y sensor measuring (if available)
- Installed options
- Status of preuse check

BOX 12-50	Battery Module on the Servo^i

The Servo^i has an external battery module capable of
holding six 12-V rechargeable and interchangeable
batteries. A minimum of two batteries are locked into the
battery module. These batteries are automatically
charged when the ventilator is connected to an AC power
supply.

The battery module is used as a backup power source
should AC power fail and can also be used during
transport. Each battery provides approximately 30
minutes of power. When fully discharged, each battery
requires 3 hours to fully recharge.

The STATUS key on the touch screen of the front panel
of the Servo^i displays the minutes remaining in battery
backup time.

If the main power fails, the ventilator automatically
switches to battery operation. If no battery module has
been inserted or connected, a high priority alarm sounds,
and the inspiratory and expiratory valves open to allow
spontaneous breathing of room air. Box 12-50 describes
the battery module.

If the ventilator is to be used for transport and is currently ventilating a patient, the operator should ensure
that adequate battery power is available. (NOTE: To do this,
the operator touches the STATUS key and checks the amount
of time available on the batteries when the STATUS menu
is displayed on the screen.) If adequate battery power is
available, the operator can simply disconnect the AC power
cord from the wall. An alarm will sound, indicating the
switch to battery power. Touching the ALARM SILENCE
touch pad once brings up a screen message asking if the
operator wants to silence the audible alarm during transport. Pressing the "yes" selection silences the battery alarm.
The amount of time available on the batteries is displayed
under the word STATUS in the upper right corner of the
ventilator's LCD screen.

The Servo^i has two gas modules, one for a high-pressure
air source and one for high-pressure oxygen. (NOTE: During
operation, if the air and O$_2$ pressures are too low, the safety
valve and expiratory valve open and an alarm sounds.) The
ventilator can be operated from a single gas source, but
this alters F$_I$O$_2$ delivery.

All ventilator settings are made using the front panel,
also called the *user interface*. The ventilator can be operated
using the touch screen and the main rotary dial or the
direct access knobs when applicable.

INTERNAL DRIVE MECHANISM

The internal drive mechanism of the Servo^i consists of two
gas modules for air and O$_2$, which regulate the precise gas
flow in the ventilator. As air and O$_2$ enter the ventilator,
each gas is filtered and the temperature and pressure are
measured. In the gas module, flow is controlled by a proportional solenoid valve. The amount of current supplied
to the inspiratory solenoid is regulated so that the gas
module delivers a gas flow to the patient based on the
values set on the user interface (Figure 11-13).[3] A differential pressure transducer in the gas modules calculates flow
delivery.

The gases exit the gas modules and are mixed in the
main inspiratory channel. The oxygen concentration can
be measured using either a galvanic O$_2$ cell or an O$_2$ sensor
that uses ultrasonic technology. Both of these options are
available with the Servo^i. (NOTE: The galvanic O$_2$ cell
receives a two-point calibration during the preuse check.
The ultrasonic O$_2$ sensor is very stable, seldom requires
calibration, and has a much longer life than a galvanic cell.)
The pressure of the mixed gases delivered to the patient is
measured by an inspiratory pressure transducer. Gas then
flows through the main inspiratory limb of the patient
circuit to the patient (Figure 12-73, top).

Exhaled gases from the patient pass through the main
expiratory limb of the patient circuit and into what the
manufacturer refers to as an expiratory cassette. In the
expiratory cassette, expiratory flow is measured by ultrasonic transducers and expiratory pressure is measured by
a pressure transducer (Figure 12-73). (NOTE: The expiratory cassette can be removed and exchanged between Servo^i
ventilators. However, a preuse check must be performed
after the cassette is exchanged.)

Inspiratory and expiratory flow and pressure are continuously measured with transducers and ultrasonic
devices and controlled by the feedback system in the patient
unit. Information is compared with the front panel settings. Differences between set and measured values result
in adjustment of gas delivery based on the set target variable and the mode selected. For example, volume control
is an open-loop system that does not make any changes
based on monitored data. On the other hand, PRVC is a
closed-loop adaptive mode that adjusts settings based on
measured values. (See Chapter 11, modes of ventilation.)

SETTING UP A NEW PATIENT

Whenever the Servo^i will be used on a new patient, preuse
checks are performed. These are described in the operator's
manual and shown on the user interface during the operation. When the preuse check window appears on the screen,

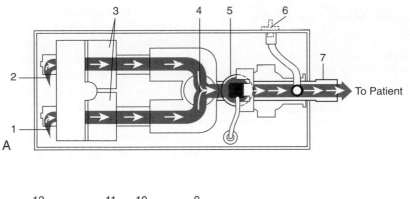

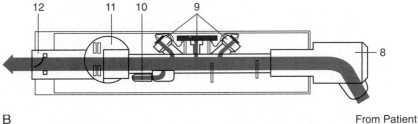

FIGURE 12-73 Top figure shows the inspiratory portion of ths Servo¹ air and O₂ inlets *(1) and (2)* gas modules; *(3)* mixing chamber; *(4)* O₂ analyzer; *(5)* pressure connecting line; *(6)* inspiratory connector to patient; *(7)* Expiratory cassette (bottom figure) showing the expiratory tube connection; *(8)* the ultrasonic transducers; *(9)* the connection for the pressure transducer; *(10)* the expiratory valve that controls the PEEP level; *(11)* the outlet where exhaled gas exits. (Courtesy MAQUET Inc., Bridgewater, N.J.)

it provides a "yes" or "no" option. The preuse check feature evaluates internal technical functions, such as pressure and flow transducers, the O₂ cell, safety valve, internal battery, internal leaks, and the patient circuit for leaks and for circuit compliance. The ventilator screen lists the 11 tests being performed and advises the operator when each test is passed. For part of the preuse check , the operator is instructed to disconnect and then reconnect the power source. As a final test, the operator is instructed to attach the patient circuit and occlude the patient Y-connector. This checks the circuit for leaks and for circuit compliance. As each consecutive test is passed, the screen indicates the "passed" status.

During the preuse check, the operator can elect to activate the tubing compliance function. This function adjusts the delivered V_T in all modes to correct for the loss of volume associated with the compressibility of the patient circuit (Box 12-51). (See Chapter 11 for an explanation of tubing compressibility [tubing compliance].)

After testing is completed, new patient data can be entered. Touching the PATIENT DATA or ADMIT PATIENT pad in the top bar of the screen allows the operator to enter patient information, including the patient's name, identification number, date of birth, date of admission, height, and weight. (NOTE: The operator must be sure to save the previous patient's data to a ventilator record card [a computer memory disk, shown in Figure 12-71] to avoid erasing data [Box 12-52].) As a privacy issue, the operator needs to be aware that if a patient's name is entered, that name will appear at the top of the operating screen. It may be more appropriate to use an identifying number.

BOX 12-51	Compensate for Circuit Compliance: Yes or No?

During the preuse check, the ventilator establishes the tubing compliance. If the compliance compensation is turned on (activated), the ventilator corrects volume delivery so that the volume the patient receives is the volume set. (See Chapter 11 for more information on compressible volume and tubing compliance factors.)

Some circumstances require that the compensation for circuit compliance feature be turned off.

First, the feature is not available in noninvasive ventilation because leaks are present during this form of ventilation. Leaks may trigger a low expiratory minute ventilation alarm if the compliance compensation is activated.

Second, when infants with uncuffed endotracheal tubes are being ventilated with small volumes, the low expired minute ventilation alarm may activate, even when set at its lowest value (0.01 L, or 10 mL). This occurs because in the presence of system leaks, low volumes, and active tubing compensation, the flow through the expiratory channel is very low and may be detected as a low $\dot{V}_E$ situation. The manufacturer suggests turning off the circuit compliance compensation feature.

The STAND BY window allows the operator to select a patient category (i.e., infant or adult) and either "invasive" or "noninvasive," depending on the features available on the ventilator being used. Selecting the appropriate patient size is important, because some parameter ranges and default categories are based on the patient's size. For example, in synchronized intermittent mandatory ventilation (SIMV), the default mandatory breath rate is 20

BOX 12-52 | **Ventilation Record Card for the Servo^i**

The ventilation record card allows the transfer of patient data from the ventilator system to a personal computer. Accessible data include the patient's name and identification code, logged events, trends, technical log, test results, and service log. Data can be copied to the card in the standby mode or during ventilation. The card is inserted into the front panel (user interface). Copying of the information must be confirmed by the operator. The card can then be inserted into a personal computer and accessed using the Windows Excel format.

---

breaths/min for infants and 5 breaths/min for adults. As another example, the range for the respiratory rate in continuous mandatory ventilation (CMV) is 4 to 100 breaths/min for an adult and 4 to 150 breaths/min for an infant. (The operator's manual provides a table containing the full range of available parameters.)

CONTROLS

The user interface, or front panel, consists of a touch screen and several knobs and touch keys for selecting and adjusting ventilator parameters. Figure 12-72 shows the major components of the front panel. The controls include the following:

(1) A menu touch pad area
(2) Text and alarm messages
(3) Fixed keys
(4) Main rotary dial
(5) Measured values boxes
(6) Special function keys
(7) Direct access knobs
(8) On/off switch (back panel of machine)
(9) Service connector
(10) Main indicator (green)
(11) Start ventilation/stop ventilation (standby)
(12) Waveform area
(13) Patient category

The Servo^i has four ways to access functions: touch screen panel functions, main rotary dial control, direct access knobs, and fixed keys. Using the touch screen, the operator can activate a particular menu by simply pressing the menu touch pad. Ventilator parameters can be selected and set by pressing the touch pad on the screen (enables parameter; turns white) and using the main rotary dial to "turn to" the desired value for the selected parameter. Pressing the parameter touch pad again confirms the setting (turns from white to blue). However, to finally accept the setting, the operator must press the ACCEPT pad. (NOTE: Pressing CANCEL cancels the setting and returns the parameter to the previous value.)

The items on the touch screen can also be set using the main rotary dial. Turning the dial causes the items on the screen to be highlighted sequentially, like scrolling through a computer menu. When the desired parameter is highlighted, pressing the dial confirms the selection. Turning the dial again changes the parameter value. To enter the selected value, the operator presses the main rotary dial. To activate the new setting, the operator turns the dial to highlight ACCEPT on the screen and again presses the dial.

Just below the screen is a bottom row of controls beginning with the START VENTILATION/STOP VENTILATION (STAND BY) key (left side), four direct access knobs located directly beneath the touch screen, and four special function keys on the right.

The START VENTILATION/STOP VENTILATION key can be used to place the ventilator in a standby condition to maintain the "warm-up" state of the ventilator electronics or after a preuse check has been completed. The unit will stop ventilating the patient if the operator presses the START VENTILATION/STOP VENTILATION touch pad and then the "yes" pad when a message appears asking if the operator wants to stop ventilation. Pushing the START VENTILATION/STOP VENTILATION key again begins ventilation.

The direct access knobs are for immediate adjustment of ventilator parameters. When a specific mode of ventilation is in use, four parameter boxes related to that mode appear in a row at the bottom of the screen just above the direct access knobs. They include the O_2 concentration, PEEP, rate, and volume or pressure. The knob just below each parameter allows the operator to change the setting. Color-coding of the set value provides information about the parameter limits. White is considered a safe setting range. Yellow is an advisory indicating that the setting is too low or too high for what are considered safe limits. Red indicates a setting outside of safe limits and the patient's response should be monitored closely. The color indicator for each setting advises the user that a level is being set that should be monitored closely, because it could lead to patient injury or inappropriate ventilation.

The special function keys to the right of the direct access knobs include **START BREATH, O_2 BREATHS,** EXPIRATORY HOLD, and INSPIRATORY HOLD. Pressing the START BREATH key results in a manually activated breath using the set parameters. The O_2 BREATHS key provides 100% O_2 for 1 minute and 2 minutes of alarm silence unless the key is pressed again, which returns the F_IO_2 to its set value. When the EXPIRATORY HOLD key is pressed, an expiratory hold results at the end of expiration for as long as the key is pressed (up to 30 seconds). Pressing the INSPIRATORY HOLD key provides an inflation hold that begins at the end of inspiration and lasts as long as the key is pressed (maximum, 30 seconds).

Fixed keys are located in the upper right corner of the front panel. There are two kinds of fixed keys: those used for shortcuts to a function or screen and those that start special ventilator functions. The latter require continuous direction by the operator when used.

Fixed Keys

The fixed keys include ALARM SILENCE, ALARM PROFILE, SAVE, TRENDS, INFORMATION (I), and a blank key. The blank key can be used for the NAVA option (see Chapter 11). Pressing ALARM SILENCE provides 2 minutes of silence for all alarms except for the NO BATTERY CAPACITY alarm if the ventilator is not connected to AC wall electricity and the batteries have no remaining power.

Pressing ALARM PROFILE results in the alarm screen appearing. This screen displays the settings for the upper and lower alarm limits for all applicable alarms. The alarm screen can also be used to change alarm settings. Additional information about alarms is provided later.

When pressed, the TRENDS key displays a screen showing trended values. Trends can be recorded for up to 24 hours with values being saved every 60 seconds. All saved events and system changes, such as running preuse ventilator checks, are shown as event "stamps" on the screen. The TRENDS screen provides controls for locating the time and type of an event, scrolling up and down the screen between event graphs, finding an explanation of an event, changing the resolution of the time axis, and closing the window.

Three round keys are located just below the square fixed keys. These include the MAIN SCREEN key, MENU key, and QUICK ACCESS key. Pressing the MAIN SCREEN key is a shortcut to return to the main view screen. The MENU key brings up a list of items when pressed (Table 12-29). Pressing the QUICK ACCESS key brings up a menu for loops and scales and the OLT option if it has been installed.

Touch Screen Controls

The touch screen area contains several areas for controlling functions and viewing information. Across the top is a row containing the following, from left to right (see Figure 12-72):

- Patient category—displays current selection (infant or adult)
- Current mode of ventilation
- Automode [on/off] (an option)—turns Automode on and off
- Admit patient/enter patient data—gives quick access to the patient data field
- Nebulizer [on/off] (an option)—turns the nebulizer function on and off (see the following section)
- System status—indicates the current source of power

Automode and the nebulizer are optional features.

Nebulizer

The Servo[i] ventilator has an optional ultrasonic nebulizer for the delivery of medications. For the nebulizer to function, the ventilator must be operating from an AC power source. Pressing the nebulizer pad brings up a TIME pad on the touch screen. The operator sets the time for the treatment by using the main rotary dial. Pressing the ACCEPT pad begins nebulization. After it is enabled, the nebulizer

operates continuously, regardless of the mode of ventilation or settings. No extra gas volume is added to the tidal volume; therefore F_iO_2 and minute ventilation remain unchanged.

The nebulizer assembly is fitted into the patient circuit with a T-piece (Figure 12-74). Medications are placed in a disposable 10-mL medication cup through an injectable cap. The medication cups are designed so that the airflow in the inspiratory limb of the patient circuit passes through the area where medications are nebulized. The bottom of

TABLE 12-29

Items on the Menu Screen—Servo[i]

Item*	Details
Alarm	Alarm profile, alarm history, and alarm mute
Review	Accesses trends, recorded waveforms, event log, and view configuration
Options	Lists installed optional features
Compliance circuit compensation	Indicates compensation for circuit compliance when performed during preuse check
Copy data	Copies data to ventilation record card
Biomed	Provides access to display of default configurations and other functions
Panel lock	Locks panel settings (e.g., during transport); can be unlocked using MAIN SCREEN control
X	Changes patient category

*An arrow next to a screen item indicates that submenus are present and will open when the screen item is touched. A sheet icon next to an item on the list indicates that there is no submenu for that item.

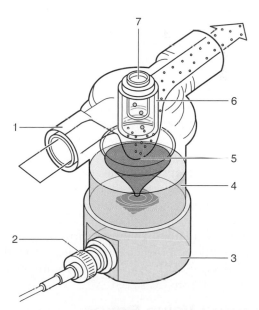

FIGURE 12-74 Ultra Nebulizer assembly of the Servo[i], showing (1) the main gas flow connector (from the ventilator to the patient); (2) the power cable from the ventilator; (3) the ultrasonic generator; (4) the water chamber (couplant cup); (5) the medication cup; (6) a T-piece adapter containing baffles; and (7) the injection membrane. (See text for further description.) (Courtesy MAQUET Inc., Bridgewater, N.J.)

the medication cup sits within another chamber that contains sterile water. The water is in direct contact with the ultrasonic generating crystal and the bottom of the medication cup. The T-piece has a mechanical baffle that ensures a mass median diameter (MMD) of 4 μm. (NOTE: The nebulizer cannot be used without sterile water in contact with the ultrasonic generator crystal, or the crystal may break.) Chapter 4 presents an explanation of ultrasonic nebulizer technology.

In addition to the Servo[i] Ultra Nebulizer, another nebulizer that produces small particles of nebulized medication that does not add to the volume delivery or change the F_IO_2 delivered is the Aeroneb Professional Nebulizer System (Aeroneb Pro) (see Chapter 4). This device can also be used to provide physician-ordered nebulized medication during ventilation with the Servo[i].

It is recommended that an expiratory filter be added to the expiratory inlet of the ventilator. These filters prevent nebulized medications from entering the environment, and they also reduce sediment on the expiratory diaphragm. Build-up of medication on the filter necessitates that the filter be changed on a regular basis to prevent an increase in expiratory resistance.

Text Message and Patient Trigger Indicator Field

Just below the top row of functions is a second row with two fields. On the left is a box that provides text messages. When a purple symbol (a T in a circle) appears near the area of this box, the most recent breath was patient triggered. (NOTE: Time-triggered breaths have no similar display.) The field on the right is the area for displaying alarm messages.

Below the two top rows is a large area of touch screen. The left is for displaying the real-time waveforms, and the right shows measured values and set alarm limits.

Waveforms

Three scalars are shown simultaneously in the operating screen: pressure-time (yellow), flow-time (green), and volume-time (light blue). The sweep and vertical axes can be individually or automatically adjusted. Pressure-volume and flow-volume loops are also available. (NOTE: To bring up loops, the operator presses the QUICK ACCESS pad and then the LOOPS pad.) In LOOPS, one or two reference loops can be recorded.

When the ventilator is equipped with the optional CO_2 monitor module, a fourth scalar can also show the CO_2 measured as a graphic. If so desired, the volume-time scalar can be removed from the screen.

Measured Value Boxes

Measured values boxes are normally displayed numerically on the right side in the touch screen. The values that appear can be customized by the operator (Table 12-30). They can be either a measured or a calculated value such as tidal volume (V_T), airway pressure (Paw), peak inspira-

TABLE 12-30

Measured Values Shown—Servo[i] and Servo[s]

Value	Definition
Default Values	
P_{peak}	Maximum inspiratory pressure
P_{mean}	Mean airway pressure
PEEP	Total positive end expiratory pressure
RR	Respiratory rate
$\dot{V}_{EE}$	End-expiratory flow
I:E	Inspiratory-to-expiratory ratio (only during controlled ventilation)
Ti/T_{tot}	Duty cycle or ratio of inspiration time to total breathing cycle time (only during spontaneous breathing)
O_2	Oxygen concentration in percentage
MV_e	Expiratory minute volume
VT_i	Inspiratory tidal volume
VT_e	Expiratory tidal volume
Additional Measured Values	
P_{plat}	Pressure during end-inspiratory pause
$PEEP_{tot}$	Intrinsic positive end-expiratory pressure
MV_i	Inspiratory minute volume
Cstatic	Static compliance, respiratory system
E	Elastance
C dyn	Dynamic characteristics
R_i	Inspiratory resistance
R_e	Expiratory resistance
WOBp	Work of breathing, patient
WOBv	Work of breathing, ventilator
Tc	Time constant
SBI	Shallow breathing index

From Siemens Medical (MAQUET Inc., Bridgewater, NJ.).

tory pressure (PIP), and so on. Also located in this area are the lower and upper alarm limits. If a value in the box is outside the acceptable range, three asterisks appear in the box.

In the lower right corner of the touch screen is an ADDITIONAL (MEASURED) VALUES control that can be used by the operator to selected preferred values for display.

On the lower left corner of the touch screen is a box for ADDITIONAL SETTINGS. This control provides a shortcut for adjusting parameter values. When the ADDITIONAL SETTINGS pad is pressed, the touch screen brings up a window showing all available settings for the current mode. As with other parameters, colors indicate a suggested level of safety of the parameter setting (white, yellow, and red) (Figure 12-72).

Parameter Controls

When a mode is selected, a touch screen window appears showing only the parameters available in that mode. Available parameters include respiratory rate, tidal volume, pressure control above PEEP (PC above PEEP), pressure support above PEEP (PS above PEEP), inspiratory rise time, I:E ratio, pause time, trigger sensitivity, PEEP, inspiratory cycle-off, breath cycle time, SIMV rate, trigger timeout, and O_2 concentration.

A few of the more unique parameters are described.

Inspiratory Rise Time

The inspiratory rise time control adjusts the rate of rise to full inspiratory flow or pressure at the beginning of a breath. This function is similar to sloping or ramping in other ventilators (see Chapter 11). **Inspiratory rise time (T INSPIR RISE)** can be adjusted either as a percentage of the total cycle time or in seconds.

Trigger Sensitivity

The Servo^i uses flow and pressure triggering to respond to a patient's inspiratory efforts. The trigger sensitivity box that appears on the touch screen displays a horizontal bar graph (Figure 12-75 and Box 12-53). This bar graph provides a visual indicator of the required patient effort.

When sensitivity is set above zero (rotating the control knob clockwise), breaths are flow triggered. The more the bar appears to the right side, the more sensitive the flow-trigger function. The sensitivity bar is green for normal settings and red for settings that are very sensitive (auto-triggering is possible). The default is 5, and the value is a reference number only, having no unit value.

When sensitivity is set below zero (to the left side of the bar; rotating the control knob counterclockwise), the ventilator becomes pressure triggered rather than flow triggered. A yellow bar indicates pressure triggering is set. The negative pressure required to begin inspiration appears as a digital value in the trigger sensitivity box. The most sensitive pressure setting is at zero (0) cm H_2O.

Inspiratory Cycle-Off Function

In supported modes of ventilation, such as pressure support and volume support, inspiration is flow cycled. In invasive ventilation, the flow-cycling variable, inspiratory cycle off, is adjustable from 1% to 40% of the peak flow measured during inspiration. In noninvasive ventilation, the range is 1% to 70%. When the calculated flow value is

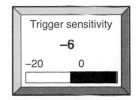

FIGURE 12-75 Trigger sensitivity box on the Servo^i. (See text for additional information.) (Courtesy MAQUET Inc., Bridgewater, N.J.)

BOX 12-53   Trigger Sensitivity Bar (Servo^i)

When the trigger sensitivity bar (see Figure 12-75) is displayed, colors are also displayed but are different from those of ventilator parameters. If the trigger sensitivity bar is green, this indicates a normal setting for flow triggering. If the bar is red, the risk of self-triggering is present (overly sensitive). If the bar is yellow, pressure triggering is being used.

---

measured by the ventilator, the inspiration for the support breath ends.

Breath Cycle Time

Breath cycle time is the total cycle time in a mandatory breath in SIMV (inspiratory time plus pause time plus expiratory time). It is set in seconds.

Trigger Timeout

Trigger timeout is the maximum allowed apnea time in Automode. In other words, it is the maximum amount of time that can elapse between two breaths. After this time period has elapsed, the ventilator switches back to a control ventilation mode. Trigger timeout is not a constant amount of time; rather it varies, depending upon how much spontaneous breathing the patient is doing. The more consecutive spontaneously triggered breaths that occur, the longer the timeout becomes up to a maximum of the set value. This means that for the spontaneously triggering patient, the timeout increases successively during the first 10 breaths. (See Automode later in this section.)

Alarms

All alarms on the Servo^i are audible and visual. The three alarm categories are high priority, medium priority, and low priority. High priority alarms result in a red background. The background turns yellow after the alarm condition ceases, but the alarm message remains on the screen until manually reset. Medium priority alarms are indicated with a yellow background, as are low priority alarms. The latter can be cleared from the screen even if the alarm condition remains.

Alarm limits are set by first pressing the ALARM PROFILE key, which brings up control pads on the touch screen for adjustable alarm limits. The operator presses the alarm limit desired, turns the main rotary dial to select the new value, and confirms the setting by pressing the parameter touch pad or by pressing the main rotary dial. Table 12-31 lists the available alarms and their defined values. The operator can use a recommended set of alarm limits in volume control, pressure control, and PRVC modes by pressing AUTOSET. Autoset uses measured values from patient data and provides safe, reasonable alarm settings based on the measured information. (NOTE: Autoset cannot be used during standby. The function needs to obtain patient values to propose values from calculated patient data.) Pressing the ACCEPT key activates the new alarm limits.

Pressing the DISPLAY CURRENT ALARMS key (bell icon) results in the appearance of a screen list of current alarm conditions in order of priority. Alarms that have occurred can be viewed by touching the MENU key and then selecting ALARM and ALARM HISTORY.

MODES OF VENTILATION

The modes of ventilation available on the Servo^i are the same as those available on the Servo 300 with the addition

TABLE 12-31

Alarms and Alarm Ranges—Servo[i]

Alarms	Range
Airway Pressure (Upper)	
Adult	16-120 cm H_2O
Infant	16-90 cm H_2O
Airway Pressure (Upper) During NIV	
Adult	16-60 cm H_2O
Infant	16-60 cm H_2O
High continuous pressure	Set PEEP + 15 cm H_2O exceeded for > 15 sec
O_2 concentration	Set value ± 6% or ≤18%
Expired Minute Volume (Upper Alarm Limit)	
Adult	0.5-60 L/min
Infant	0.01-30 L/min
Expired Minute Volume (Lower Alarm Limit)	
Adult	0.5-40 L/min
Infant	0.01-20 L/min
Apnea	
Adult	15-45 sec
Infant	5-15 sec
Gas supply	<2 kPa × 100 and > 6.5 kPa × 100
Respiratory rate	1-160 breaths/min
Battery	Limited battery capacity: 10 min
No battery capacity: Less than 3 min	
High end-expiratory pressure (or CPAP)	0-55 cm H_2O
Low end-expiratory pressure (or CPAP)	0-47 cm H_2O (setting alarm to zero is alarm off position)
Technical	See Operator's Manual chapter on Patient Safety.
Autoset (Alarm Limits) Specifications	
High airway pressure	Mean peak pressure + 10 cm H_2O or at least 35 cm H_2O
Upper minute volume	Expiratory minute volume plus 50%
Lower minute volume	Expiratory minute volume minus 50%
Upper respiratory rate	Breathing frequency plus 40%
Lower respiratory rate	Breathing frequency minus 40%
Low end exp. press.	Mean end expiratory pressure plus 3 cm H_2O

of SIMV PRVC + PS. Only changes made to the Servo[i] regarding the modes are included in this section.

The Servo[i] modes include four basic mode categories: controlled ventilation, supported ventilation, spontaneous ventilation, and combined ventilation. A special feature called *Automode* is also available and is the same feature as the Automode available on the Servo 300. The apnea criteria can be set and the Automode feature is activated after one breath, rather than two breaths with the Servo 300A. Trigger timeout also adds an additional safety to make sure the patient is ready for Automode. The timeout setting represents the maximum apnea time permitted during Automode. The control and assist/control (A/C) modes are volume control (VC), pressure control (PC), and PRVC. The support modes are volume support (VS) and pressure support (PS). SPONTANEOUS BREATHING/CPAP represents the spontaneous mode. The combined modes are any of the SIMV modes (SIMV-VC, SIMV-PC, and SIMV-PRVC). Each of these allows the addition of pressure support and/or CPAP. An optional available mode is BiVent, which is similar by definition to airway pressure-release ventilation (see Chapter 11).

Activating a Mode

To select a mode of ventilation, the operator first touches the mode pad (the pad that shows the current mode setting at the upper left corner of the screen) and then touches the mode pad with the down arrow to display the available modes. A menu of available modes appears on the touch screen (Figure 12-76). Pressing the touch pad for the desired mode results in all the related parameters for that mode appearing on the screen. Parameter variables can then be selected and adjusted (Figure 12-77). (NOTE: The direct access knobs at the bottom of the screen are inhibited when the parameter window is opened from the mode menu.)

Volume Control

Volume control is similar to A/C with a volume target. During volume ventilation on the Servo[i], the flow is normally constant based on the V_T, rate, and inspiratory time (based on the I : E ratio). If no patient effort occurs during inspiration, flow remains constant. However, if a patient effort is detected during inspiration, the ventilator switches to pressure support to satisfy the patient's flow demand. Thus the patient can actually receive a volume higher than the set value and additional flow. Clinical Rounds 12-20 provides an example of the application of volume control.

Pressure Control

Pressure control on the Servo[i] is similar to pressure control on the Servo 300. All breaths are delivered at a set pressure and can be time or patient triggered and time cycled. The rate of inspiratory flow and pressure delivery can be adjusted using the inspiratory rise time. PEEP can be used to elevate the baseline pressure.

CLINICAL ROUNDS 12-20

A patient on volume control ventilation with the Servo[i] is actively inspiring during mandatory breath delivery. The set V_T is 600 mL, the rate is 10 breaths/min, and the I : E is 1 : 2. The flow curve rises sharply after flow triggering of the breath, and then flow plateaus. After the plateau, the flow rises and falls like a sine wave and plateaus again. Inspiratory flow then ends.

1. Why is the flow not constant during breath delivery?
2. What will cycle the breath out of inspiration in this situation?
3. Will the set V_T be delivered?

See Evolve Resources for the answer.

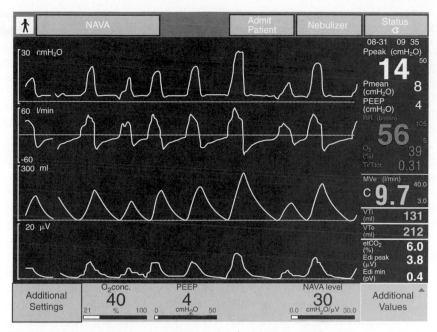

FIGURE 12-76 Mode selection screen of the Servo[i] ventilator, showing all current available modes (except NAVA). (Courtesy MAQUET Inc., Bridgewater, N.J.)

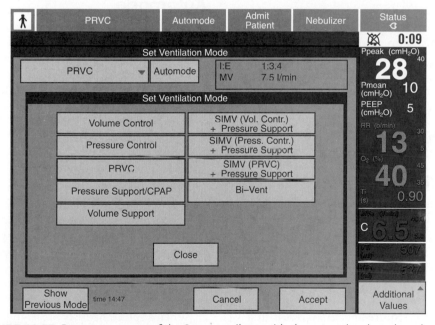

FIGURE 12-77 Parameter screen of the Servo[i] ventilator with the currently selected mode. (Courtesy MAQUET Inc., Bridgewater, N.J.)

Pressure-Regulated Volume Control

Pressure-regulated volume control is available on the Servo[i] and functions in the same manner as it does on the Servo 300 (see Chapter 11 and the section on the Servo 300 earlier in this chapter). The difference is that in the Servo[i], the first breath of a start sequence is a volume breath, using the set V_T, with a 10% pause time. The plateau pressure measured during the pause is used to determine the compliance and resistance. The ventilator then uses the plateau pressure level measured for the following breath. In PRVC each inspiration is delivered at a constant pressure (pressure targeted). However, the pressure can change from one breath to the next, because the Servo[i] endeavors to achieve the set tidal volume as its target. Changes occur in increments of 3 cm H_2O, up to a maximum pressure equal to the upper pressure limit minus 5 cm H_2O. Breaths can be patient or time triggered. Inspiratory flow and pressure delivery can be adjusted using the inspiratory rise time feature. Inspiration is time cycled based on the set inspiratory time.

Volume Support

Volume support is a patient-initiated breathing mode. Volume support on the Servo^i is basically pressure support with a volume target based on the set V_T. (NOTE: Pressure support is patient triggered, pressure limited, and flow cycled.) The operator does not set the minute volume when setting up VS on the Servo^i; therefore VS is not the same as on the Servo 300. The inspiratory pressure level is constant during a single breath. The pressure changes from one breath to the next, in increments of 3 cm H_2O, to achieve the set V_T. All breaths are patient triggered. The rate of inspiratory flow and pressure delivery can be adjusted using the inspiratory rise time. Inspiration is flow cycled based on the set percent of peak inspiratory flow. An alarm sounds if the pressure level required to achieve the set V_T reaches the upper pressure limit minus 5 cm H_2O.

In VS (and in PS) it is advisable to set an appropriate apnea time and to set the low and high rates and expired minute volume alarms for the patient in the event that spontaneous breathing changes significantly.

Pressure Support

PS on the Servo^i is similar to PS on the Servo 300. Pressure-support breaths are patient triggered, pressure targeted, and flow cycled. The inspiratory pressure and flow delivery can be adjusted with the inspiratory rise time function. One notable difference between the Servo^i and the Servo 300 is that the flow-cycling variable can be adjusted using the **inspiratory cycle off control (INSPIR CYCLE OFF).** The flow cycle is 5% of peak flow for the Servo 300; for the Servo^i, the flow cycle range is 1% to 40% in PS. For noninvasive ventilation PSV, the flow cycle range is 1% to 70%.

Spontaneous Breathing/CPAP

Spontaneous breathing, or breathing without added pressure delivery during inspiration, occurs under three conditions:

1. In VS when the target volume is maintained without requiring an added pressure from the ventilator. In other words, the patient's inspiratory effort triggers the ventilator to deliver flow to meet the person's demand. This flow requirement may result in a V_T delivery greater than the set value at a pressure near baseline.
2. In PS when the inspiratory pressure is set at zero.
3. When X is the function in Automode when either of the above conditions is met (see later discussion of Automode).

A spontaneous breath ends when flow decreases to the set percent of peak flow or if the upper pressure limit is exceeded (Clinical Rounds 12-21).

Synchronized Intermittent Mandatory Ventilation

As with other ventilators, SIMV on the Servo^i provides mandatory breaths at a set rate, and the patient can breathe

spontaneously between mandatory breaths. Mandatory breaths can be synchronized with the patient's spontaneous effort. In the Servo^i during SIMV, the mandatory breaths can be of three different types: PRVC, VC, or PC. Each of these breath types' function was described earlier. Spontaneous breaths are from the baseline pressure (PEEP/CPAP) and can be supported with PS.

Automode

The **Automode** feature is similar to the Servo 300 Automode. This mode facilitates weaning by allowing the patient to control his or her own pattern (pressure support) as long as the individual breathes spontaneously. The ventilator adapts to the patient's breathing pattern.

Initially, if the patient is apneic, the ventilator starts in a control mode (VC, PC, or PRVC). If the patient triggers a breath, the ventilator reacts by delivering a support breath. For example, in VC, the ventilator switches to VS; in PRVC, it switches to VS; and in PC, it switches to PS. (NOTE: In the Servo^i, Automode is activated as soon as the patient triggers one breath, whereas in the Servo 300, the ventilator waits for two consecutive patient-triggered breaths before switching to the support mode.)

If the patient is adequately maintaining ventilation, the support mode continues. However, if the patient fails to make an inspiratory effort, the ventilator switches back to the control mode.

When a spontaneously breathing patient regularly initiates breaths, the ventilator allows more time to elapse before it delivers a mandatory breath if no patient effort is detected. This is called the *trigger timeout,* described earlier. The operator can set a maximum trigger timeout. (NOTE: If the patient meets criteria for 10 cycles and is still spontaneously breathing, the ventilator uses the trigger timeout [apnea time] set by the operator to determine the switch back to a control mode if the patient becomes apneic.)

Backup Ventilation

In case the set apnea time (15 to 45 seconds for adults; 5 to 15 seconds for infants) is exceeded in volume- or pressure-support modes, a safety backup mode is enabled. Backup ventilation uses default settings. In VS the ventilator switches to VC. In PS/CPAP the ventilator switches to PC. The default settings used are an I:E ratio of 1:2, a rate of 15 breaths/min in adults and 30 breaths/min in infants, and an inspiratory rise time of 0.05 second. For pressure support switching to pressure control, the backup pressure level is either the set PS above PEEP or 20 cm H_2O, whichever is higher with the same backup rates.

NEONATAL/PEDIATRIC APPLICATION

The Servo^i can ventilate patients weighing 0.5 kg to 250 kg. Unlike the Servo 300, the Servo^i has two patient categories, infant and adult. The overlap in the parameter ranges, such as tidal volumes, flows, and respiratory rates, allows the clinician to more easily select between the two categories. For example, in the infant category, the V_T range is 2 mL to 350 mL, whereas the adult V_T range is 100 mL to 4000 mL. This allows a flexible overlap between the two.

Infant ventilation allows for both invasive and noninvasive ventilation. Additional information about using the Servo^i for neonatal/pediatric ventilation is presented in Chapter 13.

NONINVASIVE VENTILATION

One of the options available with the Servo^i is noninvasive ventilation for both adults and infants. As in any form of NIV, use of a well-fitting mask is important to successful application. A key component of NIV with the Servo^i is the requirement for a nonvented mask. The Servo^i uses a non-vented mask because, unlike other NIV ventilators, the Servo^i allows the patient's exhaled gas flow to return to the ventilator. This function allows for the monitoring of exhaled volumes and pressures. It also allows for alarm monitoring not typically available in NIV (Box 12-54).

If a vented mask is used by mistake, the patient's exhaled gas passes to the room and does not go back to the ventilator. The gas that is lost through this "leak" causes a discrepancy in the volume of exhaled gas returning to the ventilator. Unwanted alarms can occur, such as an excessive leak alarm. The practitioner therefore should always make sure that a nonvented mask is used with this ventilator.

To activate the NIV option, the ventilator must be in the STAND-BY mode. When NONINVASIVE is selected from the STAND-BY screen, portions of the ventilator screen change to orange to distinguish it from invasive ventilation.

The available NIV modes include PS and PC. Nasal mask CPAP (NCPAP) is available as an NIV optional mode in ventilators equipped for infant ventilation. Typically, the PS mode is selected for adults. The parameters to be adjusted are accessed and adjusted in the same manner as for invasive ventilation. In PS, the control labeled PS ABOVE PEEP represents an inspiratory positive airway pressure (IPAP) setting. The PEEP control represents an expiratory positive airway pressure (EPAP) setting. The PIP equals PS ABOVE PEEP plus PEEP. For example, if PS ABOVE PEEP is set at 12 cm H_2O and PEEP is set at 5 cm H_2O, the peak pressure will be 17 cm H_2O.

Additional settings in PS include F_IO_2, inspiratory rise time, inspiratory cycle-off, NIV backup rate, and backup inspiratory time (T_I). The backup rate is 4 to 20 breaths/min in adults and 4 to 40 breaths/min in infants. The T_I is adjustable from 0.5 to 2 seconds in adults, and 0.3 to 1 second in infants. Sensitivity is automatically set by the ventilator. If the patient lowers the pressure below PEEP or if the patient causes a decrease in expiratory volume, the ventilator delivers a breath.

Once the patient is ready to be connected to the device, the practitioner presses the START VENTILATION button (lower left corner below the main screen). The ventilator begins a 2-minute waiting position. This waiting period allows the clinician to adjust the mask for the patient and connect the ventilator circuit to the patient's interface. Ventilation begins, in this case, as soon as the ventilator detects a patient effort or when the user presses the soft key in the screen window that says START VENTILATION.

During NIV, the ventilator automatically compensates for leaks to maintain the set pressures. The amount of leak is displayed as a percent of delivered volume that is lost as a result of leakage. This value is shown in the lower right corner of the monitored data. If the leakage is excessive (more than 50 L/min for adults and more than 15 L/min for infants), as might occur with a patient disconnect, the ventilator does three things:
- Pauses ventilation
- Reduces flow to 7.5 L/min through the circuit
- Activates an alarm: LEAKAGE TOO HIGH. VENTILATION PAUSED. PLEASE CHECK PATIENT CIRCUIT.

The pause helps prevent patient discomfort that might result from excessive flows to the patient's face and eyes.

Once noninvasive ventilation has begun, the clinician can adjust ventilator parameters and alarms as needed to best suit the safety and comfort of the patient.

BOX 12-54	Alarm Function in Noninvasive Ventilation on the Servo^i

As with invasive ventilation, the following alarms are available during noninvasive ventilation:
- High Pressure
- High and Low Minute Volume
- High and Low Respiratory Rate
- High and Low End Expiratory Pressure

The unique feature is that all except the High Pressure alarm can be silenced. A small bell icon to the right of the alarm can be pressed to silence that alarm. A crossed bell indicates that the alarm has been silenced.

The apnea alarm can be turned off in Nasal CPAP by increasing the apnea alarm past the 45-second maximum. When the apnea alarm is turned off, a message to that effect appears on the screen.

OPEN LUNG TOOL

Ventilator-induced lung injury (VILI) is associated with both overdistention of the lungs and with allowing the lungs to collapse and re-expand during tidal breathing. This may occur in patients with acute lung injury (ALI) and ARDS, in which the lungs are in an unstable condition.[4-6] The pressures at which a patient's lungs become overdistended and at which they collapse can be determined in a variety of ways.[4,7] One method is the use of slow lung inflation while recording the pressure-volume curve (see the section on the Hamilton GALILEO Gold ventilator). However, this method requires heavy sedation or paralysis of the patient. Another method is to increase the pressure in the lung progressively while allowing the patient to continue breathing and to measure the compliance of the lungs at various changes in pressure.[7]

The Servo[i] ventilator has an optional feature, the Open Lung Tool (OLT), designed to help determine the pressure end-points of overdistention and lung collapse. The OLT can be accessed by pressing the QUICK ACCESS key. Once the key is activated, a screen appears showing scalars for pressure, volume, dynamic compliance, and volume of exhaled CO_2 (V_TCO_2) if it is available.[4] Every breath delivered to the patient is evaluated and plotted as a point on the scalars (Figure 12-78). At the same time, the normal monitoring area on the right side of the screen continually monitors normal parameters.

The OLT allows the operator to select any method of evaluating the pressure of overdistention and the pressure that occurs when the lung collapses. It also allows for con-tinuous monitoring of data during a recruitment maneuver. The flexibility of the OLT permits the patient to be ventilated during the procedure without requiring paralysis. Additional information on the use of the OLT is available from the manufacturer.[7]

SPECIAL FEATURES

A number of additional features are available with the Servo[i] ventilator. A few of these are reviewed here.

Trending of Data

The Servo[i] can trend up to 27 different ventilator parameters, including pressures, volumes, minute volumes, respiratory rate, leakage, measured oxygen concentration, CO_2 values, compliance, elastance, resistance, work of breathing, **occlusion pressure (P0.1),** and **spontaneous breathing index (SBI).**[4] These values can be accessed by pressing the TREND key or by going to MENU and selecting TRENDS. Each dot on the trend graph represents 1 minute. Whenever a parameter or alarm is changed or an event occurs, a green hash mark appears at the top of the trend screen. The screen cursor can be used to scroll to an event marker (green hatch mark) or any moment in time on the trend graph. When the cursor is placed at a specific point, all the monitored information that occurred at that minute of time can be read to the right of each trend line as a digital value.

In addition to the trended information, an event log is also available. The event log can be accessed by pressing the MENU key, selecting REVIEW, and then selecting EVENT

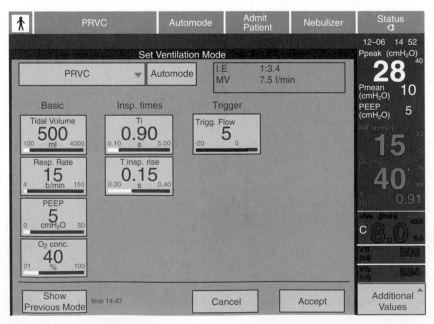

FIGURE 12-78 Open Lung Tool window on the Servo[i] ventilator. The top graph displays the end-inspiratory pressure (EIP) and PEEP. The middle graph shows the inspired tidal volume (V_Ti) and expired tidal volume (V_Te). The bottom graph shows the dynamic compliance (Cdyn) and can also display the volume of exhaled carbon dioxide (V_TCO_2) when it is available. (Courtesy MAQUET Inc., Bridgewater, N.J.)

LOG. Events are listed in chronologic order. The event log lists any changes that are made, along with any alarm that occurs.

User Interface and Graphics

The user interface of the Servo[i] is significantly different from the earlier generation Servo 300. The user interface connects to the patient unit by an 8-foot cord. It can be removed from the patient unit and attached directly to a patient's bed or a monitor pole. This adds to the Servo[i] portability. For example, the patient unit can be inserted into a bed mount and hung on a bed during transport, and the interface can be clamped to a bedrail.

The graphic display has been incorporated directly into the front panel. The graphic display remains the same; that is, the pressure curve is at the top, flow is in the middle, and volume is the lowest curve. Each graph is color-coded to correspond to the displayed monitored data (digital format) on the right side of the screen. For example, the pressure curve is yellow, and digital display of PIP, PEEP, and Pmean are all in yellow as well.

In addition to the standard scalars of pressure, flow, and volume, end-tidal CO_2 can also be graphed when the optional capnograph module is added. The CO_2 curve appears at the bottom of the screen.

Loops can be accessed and displayed on the left side of the screen by pressing the QUICK ACCESS key and selecting LOOPS. Reference loops are also available for evaluating the patient's condition before and after bronchodilator therapy.

Suction Support

A function called SUCTION SUPPORT allows the operator to disconnect the ventilator, resulting in the ventilator going into a pause mode without alarms and without causing continuous flow of gas from the unit. This is advantageous when the clinician must briefly disconnect the patient from the ventilator to change a filter, turn the patient, or perhaps use an open suction procedure to obtain a sputum sample.

Suction support can be activated by pressing the QUICK ACCESS key and then pressing SUCTION SUPPORT. A window appears that allows the user to adjust the F_IO_2 to be delivered for oxygenation before disconnection. Once accepted, a 120-second time frame begins during which the selected F_IO_2 is delivered. The ventilator waits for the patient to be disconnected. When the patient is disconnected, the ventilator recognizes the disconnect and pauses ventilation. It also silences the following alarms:

- Apnea
- Minute Volume
- Frequency
- $EtCO_2$
- PEEP

Ventilation of the patient resumes when either the patient is reconnected to the ventilator or the user presses the START VENTILATION soft key that appears on the screen.

(NOTE: If no disconnection occurs within 120 seconds, the ventilator resumes ventilation at the original F_IO_2 setting.)

After reconnection, the ventilator delivers the same F_IO_2 as in the preparation phase. After 60 seconds of postoxygenation, the oxygen concentration returns to the previous set value. Suction support is not intended for use with closed suction systems. In addition, suction support is not available during NIV or when the O_2 BREATHS button has been activated. Nebulization is temporarily paused when suction support is in use.

MRI Conditional Servo[i]

As mentioned previously, the Servo[i] can be adapted for use in an MRI environment using up to a 3-Tesla magnet; this makes an intensive care unit (ICU) ventilator available in the MRI suite. Servo[i] ventilators that have been more recently manufactured can be converted to an MRI conditional Servo[i]. This is done by the manufacturer and involves removing the metal drawers and insulating some of the components, such as the user interface, the power cord, and the cord that connects the user interface to the patient unit.

The Servo[i] that is MRI conditional can be identified by the decal on the front, which is a yellow triangle with the letters MRI in the center. Operators must make sure they are trained in the use of the ventilator in the MRI environment. For example, a line on the floor of the MRI suite marks a 200 Gauss line. The ventilator cannot be taken closer than this line or the force of the magnet may affect components of the ventilator. In addition, if the MRI Servo[i] is used outside the MRI suite, any equipment that has been added that includes metal parts must be removed. This includes removing the patient circuit support arm, any humidifier or humidifier bracket, heated wire circuits, Y-sensor modules, CO_2 sensor modules, and so on. Batteries are left in place, and it is recommended that battery power be used during image acquisition.

The MRI conditional availability of the Servo[i] adds a valuable tool for the clinician who must transport a critically ill patient requiring ventilatory support to the MRI suite. All the modes and features available with the standard Servo[i] become available even during MRI imaging conditions.

Neurally Adjusted Ventilatory Assist (NAVA)

Neurally adjusted ventilatory assist is a mode of ventilation based on neural respiratory output. NAVA is available as an option on the Servo[i]. NAVA relies on detection of the electrical activity of the diaphragm (Edi) to control the timing and level of assistance delivered.[8] NAVA requires the use of a special nasogastric (NG) tube that is fitted with an array of miniaturized sensors. (NOTE: The NG tube can also be used as a feeding tube.)

To activate NAVA, the clinician selects the NEURAL ASSESS pad, which is located directly under the TRENDS pad on the right side of the screen panel. It can also be selected under the mode selection screen. (NOTE: The NAVA option must be installed in the Servo[i] for this touch pad to be available.) Once NAVA is activated, a window appears on the left side of the main screen. The operator selects the ventilator Edi CATHETHER POSITIONING from the screen menu. At this point, it is time to prepare for catheter insertion.

Before insertion, the catheter is dipped in water to activate its coating so that it can more easily pass into the esophagus. The catheter is connected to the Edi cable. The cable connects the sensors' wires imbedded in the NG tube to the Edi module of the ventilator, which in turn commands the ventilator's functions. The catheter is then inserted into a nostril and advanced into the esophagus.

After insertion, the clinician uses the monitoring screen on the Servo[i] to determine where the array of sensors is located in the esophagus in relation to the diaphragm (Figure 12-79). Using the screen helps the operator correctly position the NG tube so that the sensors can most accurately detect activity from the diaphragm.

On the left side of the insertion screen, the image of the catheter's insertion position can be visualized. In the main part of the screen, electrocardiographic (ECG) waveforms are displayed as the catheter is advanced through the esophagus and toward the stomach (see Figure 12-79).

A total of eight electrodes are positioned along the lower portion of the catheter. The length of the electrode array is important. The electrodes have to include a large enough area along the length of the NG tube so that when the diaphragm moves during contraction, the electrodes still detect its electrical activity.

Once the electrode array is near the diaphragm, the screen displays the Edi signal (bottom waveform; see Figure 12-79). Ideally, the P-wave of the lowest visible ECG waveform should be flattened or inverted, indicating the catheter electrode array is in a good position to detect diaphragmatic activity.

The operator then goes to the main NAVA screen to check that pressure and flow detections are in synchrony with the Edi curve (Figure 12-80). As the diaphragm depolarizes, the electrical signals are captured by the sensors and transmitted to the Edi module and the ventilator.

The ventilator begins inspiration as soon as the diaphragm first begins depolarization. The operator can set the level of sensitivity by using the TRIGGER EDI SETTING (range, 0 to 2 µV). The depth of the breath is also established by the diaphragm's electrical activity (i.e., the greater the electrical activity, the deeper the breath). The cycle-off criterion that ends the breath depends on the decay of the diaphragm's electrical activity. Normally the breath ends when the peak Edi signal decays to 70% of the peak. If the signal is less than 2 µV, the cycle-off criterion is 40% of the peak signal. Thus, when diaphragmatic activity ends, inspiratory flow is stopped.

The operator can also provide instruction to the ventilator to control the level of assistance. The operator sets a level of support proportional to the electrical activity of the diaphragm (range, 0 to 30 cm H_2O/µV). For example, if the operator selects 2 cm H_2O/µV of muscle activity and the sensors are measuring 2 µV (diaphragm depolarization), the potential pressure delivery is 4 cm H_2O. Theoretically, if the diaphragmatic activity increased to 10 µV, the pressure would increase to 20 cm H_2O. However, studies have suggested that the stretch receptors in the lungs, the load receptors in the chest wall, and the muscles sense the rise in volume with the rise in pressure and signal the brain to reduce the firing of the diaphragm.[9] As a result, a lower pressure and a lower volume are delivered than would be

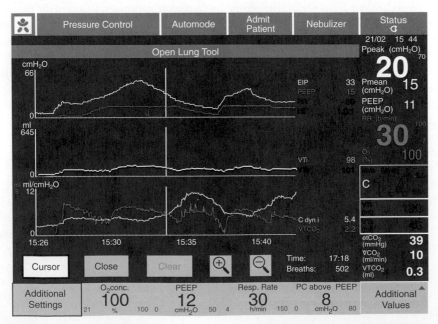

FIGURE 12-79 Edi catheter positioning window on the Servo[i] ventilator with the NAVA option installed. (See text for additional information.) (Courtesy MAQUET Inc., Bridgewater, N.J.)

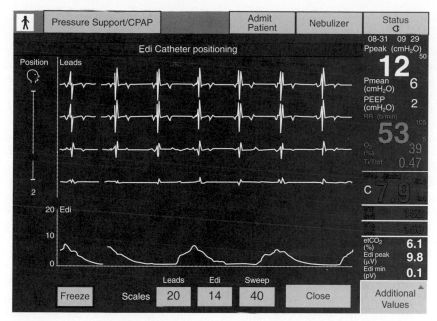

FIGURE 12-80 NAVA ventilation screen on the Servo[i] ventilator. The Edi signal is the bottom curve on the screen. The pressure curve is at the top, flow is the second curve, and volume is the bottom curve. The right column is monitored data. The NAVA level is one of the controls used by the operator. (See text for additional information.) (Courtesy MAQUET Inc., Bridgewater, N.J.)

expected with increasing NAVA levels. The lung may be protected from excessive distention.[9] Upper pressure limits are also set in case a large inspiratory effort (e.g., a sigh) is made by the patient. The upper pressure limit provides an additional method to protect the patient's lungs.

If the patient becomes apneic, the ventilator automatically switches to a backup mode of ventilation. NAVA switches to pressure support if the Edi signal is below the set Edi trigger level for 50% of the set apnea time. If no signal is detected and apnea is present, the backup NAVA mode is pressure control.

The alarm profile allows the clinician to adjust the upper pressure limit, high and low minute ventilation, high and low tidal volume, and high and low end-expiratory pressure alarms.

NAVA probably represents the first applicable form of assisted ventilation in which the patient's respiratory center controls ventilation. Currently, NAVA is specifically intended for use during invasive ventilation. Additional research is needed to verify some of the uses, determine possible side effects, and evaluate future applications of this mode of ventilation.[10]

TROUBLESHOOTING

Most alarm events are easily solved using the displayed messages that provide a description of the problem involved. For example, the RESPIRATORY RATE: LOW message suggests that the patient's respiratory rate has fallen below the alarm limit. The operator's manual contains a complete description of each alarm message, possible causes, and remedies, which are beyond the scope of this text. The reader is referred to that manual for additional information.[1]

KEY POINTS

▶ The Servo[i] can be upgraded through the use of personal computer cards. The PC card is inserted into a slot on the side of the user interface.

▶ The amount of time available on the batteries is displayed under the word STATUS on the upper right corner of the ventilator's LCD screen.

▶ In the gas module, flow is controlled by a proportional solenoid valve.

▶ The galvanic O_2 cell receives a two-point calibration during the preuse check. The ultrasonic O_2 sensor is very stable, seldom requires calibration, and has a much longer life than a galvanic cell.

▶ To accept selected ventilator settings when using the touch screen, the operator must press the ACCEPT pad. Pressing CANCEL cancels the setting and returns the parameter to the previous values.

KEY POINTS—cont'd

▶ The START VENTILATION/STOP VENTILATION key must be pressed to begin ventilation of a patient.

▶ The direct access knobs are for immediate adjustment of ventilator parameters.

▶ It is recommended that an expiratory filter be added to the expiratory inlet of the ventilator, especially when nebulized medications are administered through the ventilator circuit.

▶ The Servo^i uses flow or pressure triggering to respond to patient's inspiratory efforts.

▶ An optional available mode is BiVent, which is similar to airway pressure-release ventilation.

▶ To select a mode of ventilation, the operator touches the mode pad once and then touches the mode pad with the down arrow to display the available modes.

▶ PRVC is a pressure-limited mode with a volume target.

▶ Volume support is patient triggered, pressure limited, and volume targeted.

▶ Automode facilitates weaning by allowing the patient to control his or her own breathing pattern (pressure support) as long as the individual is spontaneously breathing.

▶ The Servo^i uses an unvented mask during NIV, because the Servo^i uses the patient's exhaled gas flow to the ventilator for monitoring and alarms.

▶ The Open Lung Tool allows the operator to select any method of evaluating the pressure of overdistention and the pressure that occurs when the lung units collapse.

▶ The Servo^i trends up to 27 different ventilator parameters.

▶ A function called SUCTION SUPPORT allows the operator to disconnect the ventilator and send it into a pause mode without alarms and without causing a continuous flow of gas from the unit.

▶ The Servo^i can be adapted for use in an MRI environment using up to a 3-Tesla magnet.

▶ Neurally adjusted ventilatory assist is a new option that uses the diaphragm's electrical activity to trigger and control spontaneous breaths. NAVA requires placement of a special monitoring NG tube.

ASSESSMENT QUESTIONS

See Evolve Resources for the answers.

1. The battery package in the Servo^i being used with a 68-year-old patient contains three fully charged batteries. The respiratory therapist must transport the patient still connected to the ventilator from the intensive care unit to the radiology department, which will take 20 to 30 minutes. How can the therapist determine how long the batteries will last?
    I. By estimating about 30 minutes of power for each battery
    II. By disconnecting the ventilator from the wall AC power and observing the number of minutes in the STATUS window
    III. By touching the STATUS key and viewing the battery status and time
    IV. By reading the amount of time displayed on each battery
        a. I only
        b. II only
        c. III and IV
        d. I, II, and III

2. When Automode is activated on the Servo^i, a spontaneously triggered breath becomes:
    a. Pressure support when the active mode is pressure control
    b. Volume support when the active mode is volume control
    c. Volume support when the active mode is PRVC
    d. All of the above

3. A patient in the radiology department is being ventilated with the Servo^i and requires a stat aerosol treatment with bronchodilators. The respiratory therapist connects Servo^i Ultra Nebulizer inline with the patient circuit but is unable to activate the nebulizer function. A possible cause of this is:
    a. There is no medicine in the nebulizer cup.
    b. The patient circuit has a leak.
    c. The ventilator is operating from battery power.
    d. The Servo^i does not have a built-in nebulizer function.

4. A quick method for increasing F_iO_2 delivery to a patient being ventilated with the Servo^i is to use the:
    I. Direct access knob adjacent to the F_iO_2 screen parameter
    II. Main rotary dial to proceed through the necessary steps
    III. Touch screen controls
    IV. O_2 BREATHS button on the lower right panel
        a. I only
        b. II and III
        c. I and IV
        d. IV only

5. A respiratory therapist is changing the pressure for a patient on pressure-control ventilation. As he reduces the PC ABOVE PEEP control, the screen area begins to illuminate with a red color and a low expiratory minute volume alarm occurs. The most likely cause of this is:
    a. A low pressure alarm
    b. An apnea alarm
    c. The patient has triggered inspiration
    d. The therapist has set the pressure too low to maintain $\dot{V}_E$ above the alarm level

ASSESSMENT QUESTIONS—cont'd

6. Which of the following controls sets the percent of peak inspiratory flow that cycles the ventilator out of inspiration during PS and VS?
   a. Inspiratory cycle-off
   b. Inspiratory rise time
   c. Peak flow control
   d. Trigger timeout

7. A patient being ventilated with the volume-control mode is actively breathing and frequently inspires deeply during the inspiratory phase of the breath. This will result in:
   a. A concave dip in the inspiratory pressure curve to below baseline pressure
   b. An increase in flow and volume delivery
   c. No change in the constant (square) inspiratory flow waveform
   d. Triggering of another breath

8. A nurse reports to the respiratory therapist that an alarm has been activating all evening on a patient being ventilated on the Servo[i]. However, the RT notes that there is no alarm message on the screen and no active alarm. The RT can determine what alarm occurred by doing which of the following?
   a. Pressing the ALARM PROFILE key
   b. Viewing the TRENDS screen
   c. Touching the MENU key and selecting ALARM HISTORY
   d. Pressing and holding the ALARM SILENCE key for 5 seconds

9. Which of the following modes of ventilation is/are available with NIV for infants on the Servo[i]?
   a. Pressure control
   b. Pressure support
   c. Nasal CPAP
   d. BiVent
      (1) II only
      (2) I, II, and III
      (3) I and IV
      (4) II and III

10. The Open Lung Tool on the Servo[i] can trend which of the following parameters?
    a. Peak pressure
    b. PEEP
    c. Dynamic compliance
    d. Tidal volumes
       (1) III only
       (2) I and II
       (3) III and IV
       (4) I, II, III, and IV

References

1. Maquet: User's manual (U.S. Version), ventilator system Servo-I V3.1, Maquet Critical Care, order no. 66-00-261, Solna, Sweden, 2007, Maquet.
2. Pilbeam SP, Barraza P, Wolff R et al: Special techniques in ventilatory support. In Pilbeam SP, Cairo JM: *Mechanical ventilation: physiological and clinical application*, ed 4, St Louis, 2006, Mosby/Elsevier.
3. Maquet: Servo education, study guide, Maquet Critical Care, order no. 66-72-817, Solna, Sweden, 2007, Maquet.
4. Pilbeam SP: Improving oxygenation and management of ARDS. In Pilbeam SP, Cairo JM: *Mechanical ventilation: physiological and clinical application*, ed 4, St Louis, 2006, Mosby/Elsevier.
5. Marini JJ, Gattinoni L: Ventilatory management of acute respiratory distress syndrome: a consensus of two, *Crit Care Med* 32:250, 2004.
6. Villar J, Kacmarek RM, Perez-Mendez L et al: A high positive end-expiratory pressure, low tidal volume ventilatory strategy improves outcome in persistent acute respiratory distress syndrome: a randomized, controlled trial, *Crit Care Med* 34:1311, 2006.
7. Maquet: *Lung recruitment: pocket guide,* Maquet Critical Care, order No. 66 61 271, Solna, Sweden, 2004, Maquet.
8. Beck J, Sinderby C, Lindstrom L et al: Effects of lung volume on diaphragm EMG signal strength during voluntary contractions, *J Appl Physiol* 85:1123, 1998.
9. Sinderby C, Beck J, Spahija J et al: Inspiratory muscle unloading by neurally adjusted ventilatory assist during maximal inspiratory efforts in healthy subjects, *Chest* 131:646, 2007.
10. Sinderby C: Ventilatory assist driven by patient demand (editorial), *Am J Respir Crit Care Med* 168:729, 2003.

Internet Resource

www.maquet.com

MAQUET SERVO^S VENTILATOR

OUTLINE

Power Source
Internal Drive Mechanism
Controls and Alarms

Modes of Ventilation
Monitors and Displays
Troubleshooting

OBJECTIVES

Upon completion of this section, you will be able to:
· State the size of the patient who can be ventilated with the Servo^S.
· List the primary differences between the Servo^S and the Servo^i.
· Discuss the battery operation and battery alarms.
· Explain how parameters are set and activated.
· Describe how to perform a preuse check.
· Name the power sources required for operation of the Servo^S.

KEY TERMS

Expiratory cassette   Safety valve

The Servo^S ventilator system from MAQUET Inc. (Bridgewater, New Jersey) is a critical care ventilator with the capacity to ventilate pediatric and adult patients.[1,2] The Servo^S can be used for either invasive or noninvasive ventilation. It is very similar to the Servo^i ventilator described in the preceding section. The primary differences are in the design of the carts, the location of the batteries, and the fact that the Servo^S cannot be used for neonatal ventilation. In addition, the Servo^S currently cannot be configured for use in a magnetic resonance imaging (MRI) suite.

As does the Servo^i, the Servo^S has two main parts: the user interface, where settings are selected and monitored data are visible, and a patient unit, where gases are mixed and delivered to the patient (Figure 12-81). The Servo^S has an optional cart for mounting the unit and an optional air compressor. This section provides a brief overview of the Servo^S.

POWER SOURCE

Like the Servo^i, the Servo^S requires at least one high-pressure gas source (air or oxygen), but it is intended to be used with both high-pressure air and oxygen (29 to 94 psi). It also requires an electrical power source, which can be a battery with an alternating current ([AC] 100- to 120-volt; 220- to 240-volt) or a direct current ([DC] 12- to 14-volt). Unlike in the Servo^i, the internally mounted batteries of the Servo^S are not accessible without removing the external cover from the patient unit. The internal batteries can provide up to 60 minutes of operating power.

INTERNAL DRIVE MECHANISM

The internal drive mechanism of the Servo^S is the same as for the Servo^i and is located inside the patient unit. Two gas modules (air and oxygen) regulate gas flow into the inspiratory mixing section. The gas mixture is then directed through the main gas inspiratory channel to the inspiratory line of the patient circuit.

As does the Servo^i, the Servo^S uses an **expiratory cassette,** in which gas flow is measured by ultrasonic transducers. In fact, the expiratory cassette design is identical for the two units (see Figure 12-73).

The manufacturer recommends that the preuse check be performed (this takes approximately 3 minutes) before the Servo^S is connected to a new patient. For this check, the Servo^S is connected to high-pressure air and oxygen and an electrical outlet (120-volt AC in the United States). During the preuse check, the ventilator evaluates internal functions such as the flow transducers, **safety valve,** oxygen cell, internal battery, internal leaks, and the integrity and compliance of the patient circuit. When the check is finished, the unit is ready for patient use.

The Servo^S has the same flexibility for adding software options as the Servo^i. A programmed computer card can be inserted into the slot at the side of the user interface (see Figure 12-71). This feature also allows new programs to be added by the manufacturer as they become available.

CONTROLS AND ALARMS

The user interface (front panel) of the Servo^S is identical to that of the Servo^i (see Figure 12-72). The on/off switch is on the back side of the user interface. The main touch key for starting ventilation or placing the ventilator in the standby position is on the lower left corner of the interface. The unit also has a touch screen for setting parameters and alarms. As on the Servo^i, fixed keys for accessing specific functions are located in the upper right section of the user interface, and four special function keys are in the lower right area. A main rotary dial and four direct access knobs are used to make ventilator changes. For a full description

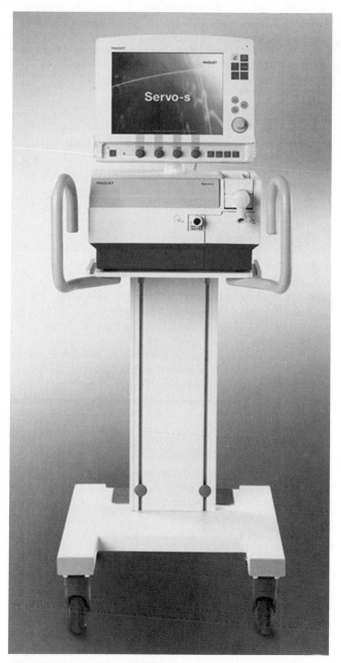

FIGURE 12-81 Servo^S ventilator, showing the user interface permanently mounted on the patient unit.

TABLE 12-32	
Alarms—Servo^S	
Alarm	**Alarm Range**
Adjustable Alarms	
Upper airway pressure (invasive)	16-120 cm H$_2$O
Upper airway pressure (noninvasive)	16-60 cm H$_2$O
End-Expiratory Pressure	
High alarm range	0-55 cm H$_2$O
Low alarm range	0-47 cm H$_2$O
Expiratory Minute Volume	
Upper alarm limit	0.5-60 L/min
Lower alarm limit	0.5-40 L/min
Respiratory Rate	
Upper alarm limit	1-160 breaths/min
Lower alarm limit	1-160 breaths/min
Apnea time	15-45 sec
Nonadjustable Alarms	
High continuous pressure	Set PEEP level + 15 cm H$_2$O (for longer than 15 sec)
Oxygen concentration	Set value ± 6% or < 18%
Gas supply	< 29 or > 94 psi
Battery	
Limited battery capacity	10 min
Low battery voltage	
No battery capacity	3 min

Technical alarms and additional alarms—see operator's manual.

of the operation of the controls and alarms, the reader is referred to the section on controls for the Servo^i.

The procedure for setting ventilator parameters is the same as for the Servo^i. The operator can use the direct access knobs to change the most commonly changed parameters in a mode, or the parameter screen can be used. Touching the mode of ventilation (upper left corner of the screen) displays the parameter window (see Figure 12-72). Touching the desired screen parameter highlights the item. Turning the control knob adjusts its value. The value can be accepted by pressing the control knob or touching the screen parameter pad again. As with the Servo^i, once all the desired parameters have been set, the operator must touch the ACCEPT key at the bottom of the parameter window to activate all the parameters.

The alarms for the Servo^S are listed in Table 12-32. Settings for the upper pressure limit, high and low minute volume, high and low rate, and high and low end-expiratory pressure alarms are easily accessed through the alarm profile control. For a description of an alarm, see the section on alarms in the discussion of the Servo^i ventilator.

MODES OF VENTILATION

The modes of ventilation for the Servo^S are listed in Box 12-55. These modes function in the same way as the Servo^i. The reader is referred to the section on modes of ventilation on the Servo^i for a full explanation of these modes.

MONITORS AND DISPLAYS

The monitored and displayed data are the same as for the Servo^i. Monitored data are displayed on the right side of the screen. As on the Servo^i, three pages of displayed data can be accessed by touching the ADDITIONAL VALUES screen pad at the bottom of the monitored data display. Table 12-30 lists the monitored values displayed. Monitored data can also be viewed on the trends screen. The trends screen allows viewing of data graphed over time. As on the Servo^i, an event log is available that displays the most recent ventilator changes and alarms.

BOX 12-55	Modes of Ventilation (Servo^S)

STANDARD INVASIVE VENTILATION MODES
Controlled ventilation
Volume control (VC)
Pressure control (PC)
Supported ventilation
Pressure support (PS) and
Continuous positive airway pressure (CPAP)
Combined ventilation (synchronized intermittent positive airway pressure [SIMV])
SIMV (VC) + PS
SIMV (PC) + PS

NONINVASIVE MODES
Pressure support
Pressure control

OPTIONAL MODES AVAILABLE
Pressure-regulated volume control (PRVC)
SIMV (PRVC) + PS
BiVent

As does the Servo^i, the Servo^S provides a graphic display of real-time waveforms of pressure, flow, and volume in the center of the screen adjacent to the monitored data (see Figure 12-71). In addition, data can be displayed as loops for volume-pressure and flow-volume.

TROUBLESHOOTING

Most alarm events are easily solved using the displayed messages that provide a description of the problem involved. The operator's or user's manual provides additional information on troubleshooting problems.

KEY POINTS

▶ The Servo^S and Servo^i are identical in functional design and user operation.
▶ The Servo^S can be used for pediatric and adult patients but not for neonatal patients.
▶ Currently the Servo^S cannot be configured for use in a MRI suite.
▶ The modes of ventilation available on the Servo^S are the same as those available on the Servo^i for both invasive and noninvasive ventilation.

ASSESSMENT QUESTIONS

See Evolve Resources for the answers.

1. The Servo^S can be used in which of the following patient populations?
    I. Neonatal
    II. Pediatric
    III. Adult
    IV. Geriatric
        a. I only
        b. II and III
        c. III and IV
        d. II, III, and IV
2. The Servo^S has the following features in common with the Servo^i *except:*
    a. User interface
    b. Patient unit
    c. MRI conditional cart
    d. Standard modes of ventilation
3. During battery operation, the Servo^S gives an initial low battery alarm when approximately how many minutes of battery power remain?
    a. 10 minutes
    b. 60 minutes
    c. 3 minutes
    d. 30 minutes

4. Which of the following is/are required to perform a preuse check on the Servo^S?
    I. High-pressure air source
    II. High-pressure oxygen source
    III. Electrical power supply
    IV. External oxygen analyzer
        a. III only
        b. I and II
        c. II and IV
        d. I, II, and III
5. To accept all changes in parameter settings on the Servo^S, the operator must:
    a. Press the control knob
    b. Touch the ACCEPT key at the bottom of the parameter window
    c. Touch the parameter pads a second time
    d. Touch the unlabeled control on the bottom left corner of the user interface

References

1. Maquet: User's manual, ventilator system Servo^S V3.1 (US Version), order no. 6664549, Solna, Sweden, 2006, Maquet.

2. Maquet: Data sheet, ventilation Servo^S (US Version), order no 6670112, Solna, Sweden, 2006, Maquet.

Internet Resource
www.maquet.com

NEWPORT VENTILATORS

NEWPORT BREEZE E150

The Newport Breeze E150 is an earlier generation Newport ventilator. The E150 can be used for neonatal, pediatric, and adult patients. Additional information is available on the Evolve Web site for this text.

NEWPORT WAVE E200

OUTLINE

Power Source
Internal Mechanisms
Controls and Alarms
Ventilator Settings
  Mode
  Bias Flow
  Sensitivity
  Pressure Support (Spontaneous)
  Pressure Control (Mandatory)
  PEEP/CPAP
  Inspired Minute Volume Alarm
  Fractional Inspired Oxygen (F_IO_2)
  Flow
  Inspiratory Time
  Respiratory Rate
Alarms and Monitors
Circuit Connections and Nebulizer Control

Back Panel Controls
Modes of Ventilation and Breath Types
  Volume-Targeted Ventilation
  Pressure-Targeted Ventilation
  Assist/Control
  Synchronized Intermittent Mandatory Ventilation (SIMV)
  Spontaneous Mode
  Pressure Support
  Sigh
Graphic Display Screens
Special Features
  Suctioning a Patient
  Pressure-Relief Valve
  Remote Alarm Silence
  Newport Compass Ventilator Monitor
Troubleshooting

OBJECTIVES

Upon completion of this section, you will be able to:
· Name the power sources required to operate the Wave E200.
· Describe the internal components.
· Explain the function of the controls on the front panel.
· Identify an alarm situation and suggest a possible cause and solution.
· Assess a problem associated with using bias flow and trigger sensitivity during spontaneous ventilation and recommend a solution.
· Solve a problem related to use of the low pressure alarm.
· Describe the available modes of ventilation.
· Explain the function of the nebulizer control.
· Compare the setting of pressure-targeted modes with that of volume-targeted modes.
· Identify a situation in which the pressure-relief valve is operating.

KEY TERMS

Accumulator tank   Bias flow   Electromagnetic poppet valve

The Newport Wave E200[1-3] is a general purpose ventilator designed for use with neonatal, pediatric, and adult patients (Figure 12-82). An accessory, the Compass Expiratory Monitor, can be added to enhance the ventilator's capabilities. The Navigator Graphics Monitor was available on earlier models. Air compressors are also available to power this unit. NOTE: The Newport E200 is no longer manufactured by Newport Medical.

POWER SOURCE

The Wave E200 is a microprocessor-controlled, pneumatically and electrically powered ventilator. It requires high-pressure air and oxygen gas sources (35 to 90 psig, optimum of 50 psig) and a standard AC electrical outlet (110 or 240 volts).

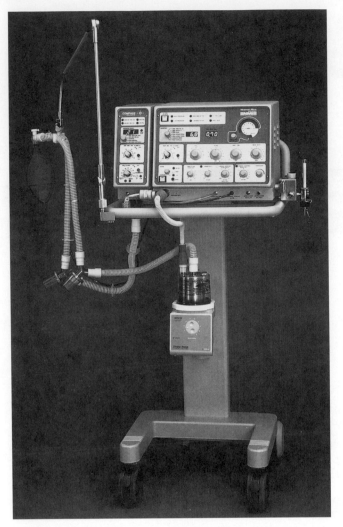

FIGURE 12-82 Newport Wave E200 ventilator. (Courtesy Newport Medical Instruments, Newport Beach, Calif.)

The air and oxygen high-pressure hoses are connected to the back of the unit. The E200 operates from a single gas source if one becomes disabled, but this may affect oxygen delivery. (NOTE: If both gas sources fail, a spontaneously breathing patient can obtain room air through the internal emergency intake valve. This requires an inspiratory effort of about −2 cm H_2O. In such a situation, the patient should be immediately ventilated by another method.)

The electrical on/off power switch is on the back panel of the machine. When the power switch is turned on, an alarm sounds temporarily and is followed by a brief self-test.

INTERNAL MECHANISMS

Source gases (air and oxygen) enter the internally mounted gas mixer. Blended gas leaving the mixer (28 psig) enters an accumulator tank and is pressurized to 2 atm. The accumulator helps provide a high gas flow to meet the patient's peak inspiratory flow needs during spontaneous breath-

ing, with or without pressure support. From the **accumulator tank,** flow is directed to the high-speed servo-controlled valve, which is also called a *metering valve.* This valve is an **electromagnetic poppet valve** (see Chapter 11). Its function is controlled by a microprocessor, which establishes the pattern of flow to the patient based on ventilator settings on the control panel. From the servo-controlled valve, gas is directed through a flow sensor, which is a differential pressure transducer, and then to the patient.

If the optional Compass monitor is not in use, the expiratory valve is mounted externally and is connected to the main unit's exhalation valve connector by a small-bore tube. The exhalation valve is a balloon diaphragm. The internal pressure on the balloon is determined by gas from the main flow manifold or by the flow from the PEEP control valve. Pressure within the exhalation valve is monitored by an electronic pressure transducer.

CONTROLS AND ALARMS

The front panel is divided into several sections (Figure 12-83). The top portion contains monitors, alarm indicators, and the high and low pressure alarm settings. The central portion houses the controls for ventilator settings and the $\dot{V}_E$ alarm control. The bottom section includes the connectors to the patient circuit and the nebulizer control button. Adjacent to many of the controls are LEDs that light up to alert the operator that the control is activated.

VENTILATOR SETTINGS

Mode

At the left of the bottom row is the control for selecting a ventilator mode (e.g., spontaneous, SIMV, A/C, and A/C + sigh).

A manual breath button is in this section as well. Pressing the manual button delivers gas flow at the set flow value for as long as the button is pressed (maximum, 3.8 seconds). Pressure is limited to the pressure-relief valve setting or, if pressure control is engaged, the set pressure target, whichever is lower. If the inflation causes the airway pressure to reach the upper pressure limit alarm setting, the unit cycles into exhalation.

Bias Flow

Bias flow (expiratory) provides flow in the circuit during the expiratory phase (0 to 30 L/min). Bias flow washes out any exhaled carbon dioxide, making fresh gas immediately available when the patient inhales. In addition, it reduces the ventilator's response time for pressure triggering a breath.

Immediately after delivery of a breath (either mandatory or spontaneous) there is a brief period of no bias flow. The absence of bias flow at this time allows the patient to exhale without added resistance. When pressure in the circuit is within 2 cm H_2O of baseline, the bias flow resumes at the flow rate set. (NOTE: Anytime airway pressure is elevated more than 2 cm H_2O above baseline, there is no bias flow.)

A recommended starting level for bias flow on adult patients is 2 to 5 L/min. The adult range is marked in green. For neonatal and pediatric patients, the starting level is about 2 to 3 L/min. In general, it is recommended that the least amount of bias flow possible be used. If it is set too high, it is more difficult for a patient effort to be detected by the trigger sensor.

Sensitivity

The sensitivity setting adjusts the airway pressure change required for a patient to trigger a mandatory or spontaneous breath (–5 to 0 cm H_2O). The sensitivity setting is also used to detect all breaths for monitoring. The total rate count is displayed in the monitor section. (NOTE: If a patient effort is not detected by the trigger sensitivity, it will not be counted in the monitored total rate, and the inspiratory V_T and the $\dot{V}_E$ will not be measured and displayed. If the Compass monitor is in use and the expiratory V_T and the $\dot{V}_E$ are not measured and displayed, the bias flow is set too high or the sensitivity trigger setting is set too low. Thus the ventilator may not be responding to patient effort because of inappropriate settings.)

Sometimes patients have leaks around the endotracheal tube, such as occurs with uncuffed infant tubes. In this situation, it is recommended that the bias flow be increased to help compensate for the leak and stabilize the baseline pressure. First, however, the operator should confirm the integrity of the patient circuit by performing a leak check. Sometimes, even when the patient circuit is not leaking but a small airway leak is present, the ventilator appears to autotrigger, and the baseline pressure may be unstable. In this situation, the operator should set the trigger sensitivity to –0.5 cm H_2O and increase the bias flow in 1 L/min increments until the autotrigger condition ceases. A severe leak may require that the ventilator be made less sensitive to autotriggering by reducing the trigger sensitivity to a more negative value.

Pressure Support (Spontaneous)

Use of the PRESS SUPPORT (spontaneous) setting provides pressure-support ventilation (PSV) for spontaneous breaths in the spontaneous and synchronized intermittent mandatory ventilation (SIMV) modes. Pressure support in the Wave E200 offers automatic inspiratory slope control, as well as a self-adjusting, variable breath termination (cycling-off criteria). The pressure range setting for PSV is "off" up to 60 cm H_2O. This pressure setting is additive to the baseline or PEEP/CPAP level (see the discussion of modes in this section).

Pressure Control (Mandatory)

The PRESS CONTROL (pressure control [PC]) knob adjusts the pressure provided during inspiration for pressure-targeted mandatory breaths (ranges, 0 to 75 cm H_2O or off). When activated, all mandatory breaths in assist-control (A/C) and SIMV are pressure targeted. If FLOW is set to the maximum level during PC, the unit automatically manages the inspiratory slope of all mandatory breaths (see the discussion of modes in this section).

PEEP/CPAP

The baseline pressure is adjusted using the PEEP/CPAP control. Because it is not numbered, the operator must watch the pressure displayed in the monitor window to view the selected baseline level. Baseline pressure ranges from 0 to 45 cm H_2O.

Inspired Minute Volume Alarm

The INSP MIN VOL ALARM control is the first one on the left in the next row of the ventilator setting section. It is used to adjust both high and low $\dot{V}_E$ alarms (in L/min). This knob is a dual control, with the higher (white) portion setting the high $\dot{V}_E$ alarm, and the lower (black) portion setting the low $\dot{V}_E$ alarm. The minute volume alarm has two possible ranges. With the 0-5 button unlit (i.e., not pressed) the range is 0 to 50 L/min. When the 0-5 button has been pushed and is green, the range is 0 to 5 L/min. Box 12-56 explains this alarm further. The expiratory $\dot{V}_E$ alarms are located on the Compass monitor.

The high $\dot{V}_E$ alarm can detect a leak or a disconnection in the patient circuit if the baseline pressure is set to a positive value. When proximal pressure drops because of a leak or disconnection and the drop in pressure repeatedly activates the trigger, the measured inspiratory $\dot{V}_E$ may increase in comparison with the patient's actual $\dot{V}_E$.

The low $\dot{V}_E$ alarm can be used to detect apnea when the spontaneous ventilation mode is in use or when obstructions occur in the airway during pressure-targeted ventilation.

Fractional Inspired Oxygen (F_IO_2)

Oxygen delivery can be adjusted from 0.21 to 1. The delivered oxygen concentration should be checked using an

---

BOX 12-56	Inspiratory Minute Volume Alarm on the Wave E200

The inspiratory minute volume alarm is based on the rate of volume delivered from the ventilator, not including bias flow. When the bias flow is on, the LOW MIN. VOL alarm may sound if the patient's efforts do not cause the ventilator to trigger, because it will not detect any volume.

For the alarm to work effectively, bias flow should be set as low as possible or at about 2 to 3 L/min. For example, suppose the bias flow is set at 15 L/min, and the patient is in the spontaneous mode with a CPAP level of 10 cm H_2O. With so much flow, the patient's efforts may not result in enough of a pressure and flow drop to meet the trigger sensitivity setting. The ventilator will not "see" the patient's V_T; therefore the low $\dot{V}_E$ may be violated.

oxygen analyzer. One is included in the optional Compass monitor.

Flow

The flow (1 to 100 L/min) provides a constant gas flow at the set value during volume ventilation and sets the maximum flow available during pressure-targeted mandatory breaths. It is recommended that the flow be set to the maximum (100 L/min) during pressure-targeted ventilation so that the Wave's microprocessor can automatically adjust the inspiratory rise (slope) during mandatory breath delivery.

Inspiratory Time

Mandatory breaths, either pressure or volume targeted, are time cycled. The inspiratory time (T_I) setting ranges from 0.1 to 3 seconds.

Respiratory Rate

This control sets the rate for mandatory breath delivery in either A/C or SIMV modes. The rate ranges from 1 to 100 breaths/min.

ALARMS AND MONITORS

In addition to the $\dot{V}_E$ alarm already reviewed, the top panel has a high and low pressure alarm control located adjacent to the pressure gauge (–10 to 120 cm H_2O). The high and low pressure alarm settings are indicated by illuminated green segments on the pressure gauge. (NOTE: The low pressure alarm segment turns dark when its set value is exceeded by the current airway pressure level.) Rotating the knob to its normal position sets the low and high pressure alarms in tandem. To set only the high alarm, the operator pulls out the knob before rotating it. If the pressure does not exceed the low pressure setting during a mandatory inspiration, an audiovisual alarm occurs. The low pressure alarm is also violated if the airway pressure drops below the sensitivity pressure setting for 3 seconds in any mode or for half of the expiratory time (T_E) for two consecutive breaths in the SIMV mode, whichever is shorter. Clinical Rounds 12-22 presents a problem concerning this situation.

The pressure displayed on the pressure gauge must reach the HIGH PRESSURE alarm setting for the HIGH PRESSURE alarm to sound.* When the patient circuit pressure reaches the set value, the ventilator cycles into exhalation. For the HIGH PRESSURE alarm, the pressure is measured near the main flow outlet port just inside the ventilator. If a HIGH PRESSURE alarm event occurs and the patient circuit pressure does not drop to at least 5 cm H_2O above baseline, no more mandatory breaths are delivered. An additional safety feature is the pressure-relief valve, which is reviewed in the discussion of special features later in this section.

*The unit has some built-in high pressure alarms as well.

CLINICAL ROUNDS 12-22

The following are the monitored pressures and pressure alarms set on the Wave for a patient receiving volume ventilation:

· Peak pressure = 30 cm H_2O
· PEEP = 10 cm H_2O
· High pressure alarm = 40 cm H_2O
· Low pressure alarm = 25 cm H_2O
· Trigger sensitivity = –0.5 cm H_2O (below baseline)

The low pressure alarm activates. You note the pressure gauge reads 7 cm H_2O during exhalation, and peak pressure is now 28 cm H_2O. The sensitivity trigger light flickers on, even though the patient does not appear to be inhaling. What do you think is causing the pressure drop? Why has the low pressure alarm activated?

See Evolve Resources for the answer.

TABLE 12-33

Alarm Indicators—Wave E200

Alarm	Triggering Condition
High pressure	Airway pressure exceeds high-pressure alarm setting.
Low pressure	Airway pressure does not achieve low-pressure alarm setting during a mandatory breath.
High $\dot{V}_E$	Measured inhaled $\dot{V}_E$ exceeds set high $\dot{V}_E$ alarm.
Low $\dot{V}_E$	Measured inhaled $\dot{V}_E$ is lower than low $\dot{V}_E$ alarm.
T_I too long	T_I has exceeded setting based on I:E ratio limit setting of switch on back panel (manufacturer uses "IT" to abbreviate inspiratory time).
Vent. Inop.	Microprocessor has detected a malfunction. The ventilator goes into exhalation. (Sometimes turning the unit off and then back on allows it to reset. If it does not, find another machine to ventilate the patient and call a service representative.)

From Newport Medical Instruments. (Newport Beach, Calif.)

At the top left corner of the front panel is a section containing an ALARM SILENCE button (60 seconds) and six LED indicators. Conditions resulting in illumination of these indicators are listed in Table 12-33.

Figure 12-83 shows a rotating knob with a list of measured and calculated parameters, as well as a digital display window in the upper portion of the front panel. Box 12-57 lists each parameter.

A window in the central portion of the E200 displays the set tidal volume (V_T) during volume-targeted breaths. This is based on the flow and T_I settings and is not a measured value. The measured inspiratory V_T is displayed in the monitor window, and the measured expiratory V_T is displayed in the monitor window of the optional Compass monitor.

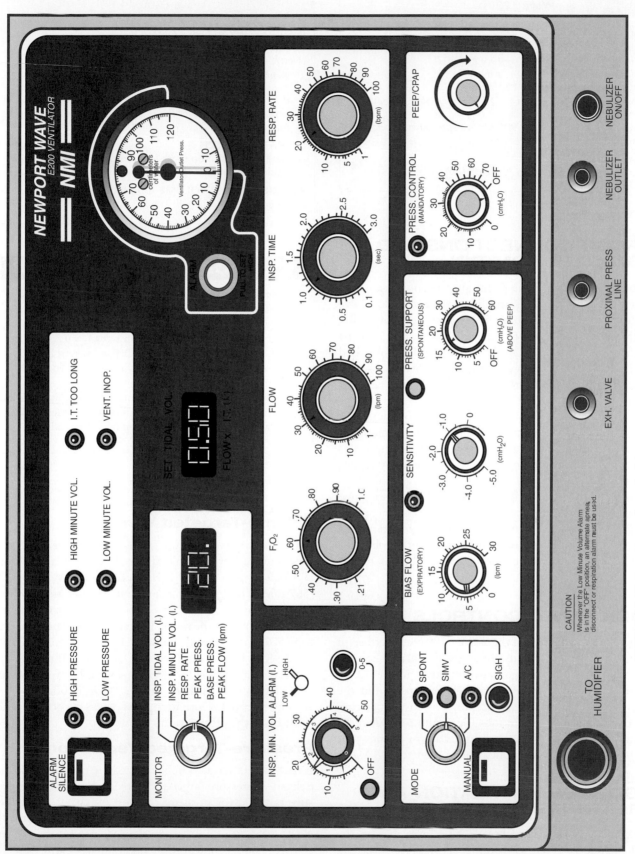

FIGURE 12-83 Front control panel of the Newport Wave E200. (See text for description.)

BOX 12-57	Monitored Parameters on the Wave E200

MEASURED VALUES
Inspired tidal volume (0 to 9.99 L)
Inspired minute volume (0 to 99.9 L/min)
Respiratory rate (0 to 999 breaths/min)
Peak airway pressure (0 to 120 cm H_2O)
Base pressure (0 to 120 cm H_2O; measured at the exhalation valve)
Peak inspiratory flow (0 to 999 L/min; spontaneous and mandatory)

CALCULATED VALUE
Mean airway pressure (0 to 120 cm H_2O)

BOX 12-58	Back Panel Controls on the Wave E200

INSPIRATORY PAUSE CONTROL
Can be set at 0% (off), 10%, 20%, of 30% of T_I.
(NOTE: During a pause, T_I for the Wave is constant at the value set on the front panel. Therefore, using inspiratory pause does not increase T_I but encroaches on the time during which inspiratory flow occurs. As a result, flow actually increases over the set value, and peak pressures may increase.)

I : E RATIO SWITCH
Allows I : E ratios of up to 3 : 1 or limits I : E ratios to 1 : 1 before alarming.

AUDIBLE ALARM VOLUME CONTROL
Adjusted

CIRCUIT CONNECTIONS AND NEBULIZER CONTROL

Just below the main front panel are the connections for ventilator output to the humidifier, the exhalation valve line connector, the proximal airway pressure monitoring line (receives purged gas to reduce obstruction), and the nebulizer line connector. Each connection is color-coded and sized differently to prevent accidental interconnection of lines. The NEBULIZER ON/OFF control is on the far right side.

Turning on the nebulizer control results in about 6 L/min (15 psig) of gas coming from the nebulizer outlet during each mandatory volume-targeted inspiration. The nebulizer does not function in PSV, PCV, or spontaneous breaths.

While the nebulizer is on, the flow from the ventilator is reduced by the amount delivered through the nebulizer line. This is to keep actual V_T and $\dot{V}_E$ delivery constant. The operator must remember to turn off this control when the treatment is finished; there is no automatic shut-off for the nebulizer.

BACK PANEL CONTROLS

The back panel controls of the Wave E200 are described in Box 12-58. Two additional, nonadjustable alarms are the mixer alarm, which sounds continuously if the air or oxygen inlet gas pressure drops below 31 psig, and the power supply alarm. If the AC power is lost or disconnected, this alarm is continuous for 5 minutes. When the ventilator is turned off, a continuous alarm sounds that may be silenced with the ALARM SILENCE button.

MODES OF VENTILATION AND BREATH TYPES

Modes of ventilation and breath types available on the E200 include A/C (either volume or pressure targeted), SIMV (either volume or pressure targeted), and spontaneous (including PSV).

CLINICAL ROUNDS 12-23

The respiratory therapist is attending a patient who is ventilated with the Wave E200. The current settings are: mode = A/C, flow = 60 L/min, T_I = 0.75 second, pressure control = off, rate = 10 breaths/min, F_IO_2 = 0.5, bias flow = 4 L/min, and PEEP = 5 cm H_2O. The current blood gas values are: pH = 7.38, $PaCO_2$ = 44 mm Hg, and PaO_2 = 56 mm Hg.

The physician wants to improve oxygenation and asks the therapist to increase the T_I to increase the mean airway pressure. How would the therapist respond to this request?

See Evolve Resources for the answer.

Volume-Targeted Ventilation

During volume ventilation, the V_T is determined by the set flow and T_I. For example, if the flow is set at 80 L/min (1.33 L/sec) and the T_I is 0.5 second, the V_T is 0.667 L (667 mL). The V_T value appears in the set tidal volume display. The I : E ratio is based on the respiratory rate and T_I. For example, if the rate is 20 breaths/min, the total cycle time (TCT) is 3 seconds (60 sec/[20 breaths/min]) if the T_I is 0.5 second, the T_E is 2 seconds, and the I : E ratio is 1 : 4. Clinical Rounds 12-23 gives an example of a problem related to V_T adjustment on the Wave E200. (NOTE: In volume-targeted ventilation, the PRESS CONTROL knob must be in the off position.)

Pressure-Targeted Ventilation

If the PRESS CONTROL knob is turned on, mandatory breath delivery is pressure targeted. There is no selection for pressure targeted (or pressure control) on the MODE switch. Changing to this mode is accomplished by setting the PRESS CONTROL knob to the desired inspiratory pressure setting. The set tidal volume digital display will read "−." As one would expect, flow is delivered in a descending, exponential manner as pressure at the airway increases toward the set value. Volume delivery varies with changes in patient lung compliance and airway resistance. Real-time V_T and $\dot{V}_E$ should be monitored.

If a slight leak exists in the circuit during pressure ventilation, the leak supplement function activates. With this function, the ventilator increases flow to maintain the set pressure. The operator should be sure to carefully monitor and assess the patient, as well as ventilator parameters, to ensure that volume and pressure delivery are adequate during pressure-control ventilation (PCV).

The maximum available flow during PCV is based on the flow setting. If a low flow value is set, it takes longer for the ventilator to achieve the set peak inspiratory pressure (PIP). A high flow setting achieves the set PIP more quickly. As mentioned, for best results the highest flow value is set (100 L/min). This allows the microprocessor to set the automatic slope control to adjust the rise time or slope.

If the flow is set manually, it must be set high enough to achieve the set pressure before the end of inspiration. In addition, as the T_I is increased, the amount of time that the pressure plateaus during inspiration increases (see Chapter 11). This will increase the mean airway pressure.

High Pressure Alarm in Pressure Ventilation

When pressure is set on the PRESS CONTROL dial, an automatic high pressure alarm limit is set at 10 cm H_2O above that value and terminates inspiration when exceeded. If the pressure fails to fall to less than or equal to 5 cm H_2O below baseline during exhalation, no additional mandatory breaths are delivered. (NOTE: In PCV, obstruction of the endotracheal tube cannot be detected by the high pressure alarm system during inspiration. An obstructed tube does not require much flow to achieve the pressure; therefore the high pressure alarm would not sound. An obstructed tube is detected as a drop in the minute ventilation and activates the LOW MINUTE VOL alarm. However, a HIGH PRESSURE alarm is activated if the patient tries to actively exhale during inspiration with PCV.)

Low Pressure Alarm in Pressure Ventilation

During pressure-targeted ventilation (PRESS CONTROL set), an automatic LOW PRESSURE alarm is set at half of the set pressure value. If the airway pressure does not exceed this value during inspiration, the alarm activates. The LOW PRESSURE alarm also activates if the airway pressure falls and remains below the trigger sensitivity pressure setting for 3 seconds in any mode or half of the expiratory time for two consecutive breaths in the SIMV mode, whichever is shorter. This usually indicates a leak in the circuit.

Assist/Control

In A/C, breaths are patient or time triggered, volume or pressure targeted, and time cycled. All breaths are mandatory.

Synchronized Intermittent Mandatory Ventilation (SIMV)[3]

In SIMV, mandatory breaths are patient or time triggered, volume or pressure targeted, and time cycled. Spontaneous breaths are patient triggered, pressure limited, and pressure cycled. PSV can be added to spontaneous breaths.

In SIMV, mandatory breaths are synchronized with a patient's spontaneous efforts based on the sensitivity setting. The mandatory breath interval (MBI) equals 60 seconds divided by the set breaths rate. For example, if the rate is 10 breaths/min, the MBI is 6 seconds. In the first MBI, if no patient effort is detected, then at the beginning of the next MBI, a time-triggered mandatory breath is delivered. In this example, a period of 12 seconds would elapse and then a mandatory breath would occur. The patient can breathe spontaneously throughout the remaining time of the MBI.

Spontaneous Mode

In the spontaneous ventilation mode, bias flow, F_IO_2, PEEP/CPAP, pressure support, and sensitivity are set. The patient breathes gas provided either by the bias flow control or by demand flow. The patient can also obtain gas at the set pressure when PSV is active. No mandatory breaths are delivered.

If the patient's effort causes airway pressure to decrease by the amount set on the sensitivity control, the ventilator provides additional flow or pressure support. Once the breath is detected, the internal servo-controlled flow valve delivers whatever flow the patient demands or whatever flow is needed for pressure support, up to 160 L/min. For this reason, it is important to set the sensitivity appropriately, so that the patient's work of breathing is not increased (Box 12-59). Spontaneous breaths that are detected are counted and displayed by the rate monitor.

If a high bias flow is set, this may provide a substantial part of the patient's flow requirements. In this case, the patient's inspiratory effort may not meet the trigger sensitivity setting, and the internal flow control valve will not open. No pressure support would be available. If this is a problem, the bias flow should be set lower. This is another reason it is important to set the sensitivity appropriately for the patient.

BOX 12-59	Setting Bias Flow and Sensitivity in the Spontaneous Mode on the Wave E200

It is very important to carefully adjust both bias flow and sensitivity in the spontaneous mode. The patient's inspiratory effort must exceed the sum of the pressure produced by the bias flow and the pressure required to trigger the sensitivity, or the internal flow valve will not open.

In the spontaneous mode, when CPAP is applied, the LOW PRESSURE alarm is automatically set based on the reading from the proximal pressure line. If the patient circuit pressure falls below the trigger sensitivity level for 3 seconds or longer, the low pressure alarm sounds.

Pressure Support

The PRESS SUPPORT control adjusts the PSV level for spontaneous breaths in the spontaneous and SIMV modes. The LED lights up when this mode is active. In either the volume- or pressure-targeted SIMV mode, PSV is available between mandatory breaths.

Pressure support (PS) breaths are patient (pressure) triggered, pressure targeted, and flow cycled. The flow that ends inspiration in PSV is calculated by the microprocessor. This calculation is based on a formula using target pressure, maximum flow delivered, and time. The longer any PS breath lasts, the higher the percentage of peak flow required to end (cycle) the breath. Inspiratory flow during PSV also ends if one of the following conditions occurs:

· V_T reaches 4 L
· PIP is 2 cm H_2O greater than the PSV pressure setting
· T_I is longer than 3 seconds

Sigh

The Wave E200 can provide sigh breaths in either volume- or pressure-targeted ventilation. The sigh function is selected by pressing the small green SIGH button next to the mode selector (active, lit; inactive, unlit). A sigh breath is given every 100 breaths when it is selected. For volume-targeted ventilation, the V_T delivered during a sigh breath is 1.5 times the set V_T. For pressure-targeted ventilation, the set peak pressure is achieved, just as with a normal breath, but it is sustained (1.5 times the set T_I). For either volume- or pressure-targeted ventilation, the T_I during a sigh breath is 1.5 times the set T_I. The HIGH PRESSURE alarm limit does not change for the sigh breath. The operator may want to take this into account when setting this alarm and the sigh function.

GRAPHIC DISPLAY SCREENS

The Navigator Graphics Monitor can no longer be purchased as a separate unit but was previously available with the Wave E200 or the Breeze E150 ventilators. Some ventilators still have the Navigator Monitor; therefore it will be described here.

In addition to providing real-time scalars of volume, flow, and pressure over time and loops for flow-volume and pressure-volume, the monitor can automatically perform measurements of compliance and resistance. It also monitors the respiratory rate, inspiratory and expiratory $\dot{V}_E$, inspiratory and expiratory V_T, peak inspiratory and expiratory flows, inspiratory and expiratory times, leak percent, and dynamic compliance and resistance. Alarm functions are also available for respiratory rate, $\dot{V}_E$ PIP, and apnea.

SPECIAL FEATURES

A few special features are available with the Newport Wave E200 ventilator, and these are reviewed here.

Suctioning a Patient

The E200 has a special feature that allows the ventilator to be placed into temporary standby for suctioning a patient. Box 12-60 lists the steps involved in this procedure.

Pressure-Relief Valve

On the side panel of the E200 is a pressure-relief valve that limits pressure delivery through the patient circuit during any mode but does not end inspiration. This safety pop-off is adjustable from 0 to 120 cm H_2O. Turning the knob clockwise increases the pressure limit; turning it counterclockwise lowers it.

During normal operation, the operator should set the pop-off pressure about 10 cm H_2O above the high pressure alarm setting. This control must be set before patient use. It is accomplished as follows:

1. Set the PRESS CONTROL knob to the OFF position.
2. Set the flow to a normal level for the patient.
3. Set the high pressure limit at 120 cm H_2O.
4. Occlude the patient Y-connector.
5. Press the manual button, and observe the pressure gauge.
6. Rotate the pressure-relief valve until the pressure plateaus at the desired value.
7. Return the ventilator controls to the proper settings.

BOX 12-60	Procedure for Suctioning with the Wave E200

1. Press and hold the ALARM SILENCE key for 3 seconds; a beep will sound.
2. During the next 10 seconds, the alarm silence light is on and the ventilator continues to function normally as it waits for a circuit pressure change.
3. When airway pressure drops below the trigger sensitivity pressure during exhalation or when a low pressure alarm condition occurs during a mandatory breath, the E200 switches into the suction standby mode.
4. In this mode, the following occur:
   · The LOW-PRESSURE alarm indicator flashes.
   · The alarm silence lamp remains lit for 60 seconds, after which the audible alarm sounds.
   · Bias flow is delivered through the circuit. When the HIGH-RANGE MINUTE VOLUME alarm is set, flow is 20 L/min. When the LOW-RANGE MINUTE VOLUME alarm is set, flow is 10 L/min.
   · Pressure-targeted breaths (PC and PS) are disabled.
5. Reconnecting the patient and eliminating major leaks from the circuit cancel the suction standby mode and return the ventilator to normal operation.
(NOTE: If suction standby is enabled by pushing the ALARM SILENCE button for 3 seconds but the circuit is not disconnected, nothing happens. After 10 seconds, the alarm silence is canceled.)

Remote Alarm Silence

The E200 has a REMOTE ALARM SILENCE control. This control is a long cable that connects to the back panel. The button on the end of the cable can be used to silence alarms for 60 seconds. This is helpful when a patient is suctioned from the side of the bed opposite the ventilator.

Newport Compass Ventilator Monitor

A separate monitor unit, called the Compass, can be attached to the Wave E200 to monitor expired gases. The unit can be mounted directly onto the left side of the ventilator. The analyzer for F_IO_2 can be hooked directly into the patient circuit or into the optional flush valve that mounts on the other side of the Wave E200. The Compass contains a heated, filtered exhalation system with its own exhalation valve. When it is in use, the externally mounted valve is not needed. Instead, the expiratory valve line on the Wave is attached to a small connector near the bottom of the Compass. The exhalation system provides alarms for high and low expired $\dot{V}_E$, and high and low F_IO_2. It also monitors the expired V_T, $\dot{V}_E$ I:E ratio, F_IO_2 (analyzed), and expired peak flow.

TROUBLESHOOTING

In addition to the alarms, monitors, and indicators available, the operating manual contains additional tips on troubleshooting. There is also a laminated card containing this information that can be hung on the side of the ventilator. The Wave E200 performs self-zeroing on all sensors and transducers at timed intervals and whenever it is turned on, although it still may be possible for a component to require calibration. Malfunctions of electrical components or transducers can occur when such devices are out of calibration or failing. Keeping a regular maintenance schedule is essential to preventing such problems. The user should refer to the service manual in such circumstances or contact a service representative.

Because the Wave is microprocessor controlled, radio frequency–emitting devices, such as cellular phones, pagers, and walkie-talkies, should not be used in the vicinity of the ventilator.

Because ventilators can be upgraded or changed by the manufacturer at any time, the user is advised always to defer to the operator's manual and operating instructions when using the Newport Wave E200.

KEY POINTS

- Pressing the manual breath button delivers gas flow at the set flow value for as long as the button is pressed (maximum, 3.8 seconds).
- A recommended starting level for bias flow is 2 to 5 L/min for adult patients and 2 to 3 L/min for neonatal/pediatric patients.
- The baseline pressure (PEEP/CPAP) control is not numbered. The operator must watch the pressure displayed to determine the baseline pressure.
- During volume ventilation, the V_T is determined by the set flow and T_I.
- If there is a slight leak in the circuit during pressure ventilation, the leak supplement function activates and increases the flow to maintain the set pressure.
- The initial available flow during PCV is based on the flow setting. A low flow takes longer to reach the set pressure.
- An obstructed endotracheal tube during PCV is detected as a drop in the minute ventilation and activates the LOW MINUTE VOL alarm. A high pressure limit alarm does not typically activate.

ASSESSMENT QUESTIONS

See Evolve Resources for the answers.

1. The Wave E200 uses which internal flow delivery device?
   a. Electromagnetic poppet valve
   b. Stepper motor with a scissors valve
   c. Linear-drive piston
   d. Internal bellows device

2. During volume ventilation of a patient with the E200, the airway pressure reaches the pressure limit set on the pressure-relief valve before it reaches the HIGH PRESSURE alarm. Which of the following statements about this situation are true?
   I. The operator should have set the pressure-relief valve higher than the high pressure alarm.
   II. An audible alarm will sound, and the high pressure alarm LED will illuminate.
   III. The pressure will plateau, but inspiration will not end.
   IV. Volume delivery will remain the same.
      a. I and III only
      b. II and IV only
      c. I, III, and IV only
      d. I, II, III, and IV

ASSESSMENT QUESTIONS—cont'd

3. During PCV using the E200, the respiratory therapist wants to give a nebulized medication treatment to a patient. What should she do?
   a. Select an external flowmeter to power the nebulizer and (while it is on) set the pressure-relief valve 1 cm H_2O above the set pressure.
   b. Until the treatment is finished, switch to a volume-targeted mode and use the pressure-relief valve to limit pressure.
   c. Connect the nebulizer line to the device and press the nebulizer button on the lower panel of the ventilator.
   d. Change the patient to another ventilator.

4. When the sigh function is selected, which of the following is/are true?
   I. A sigh breath is delivered every 100 breaths.
   II. This function can only be used in volume-targeted A/C.
   III. Sigh V_T is 1.5 times the set V_T.
   IV. Sigh T_I is 1.5 times the set T_I.
   a. I only
   b. II only
   c. III and IV only
   d. I, III, and IV only

5. The operator sets up the Wave E200 for volume-targeted A/C ventilation. However, it is noted that the pressure only rises to 10 cm H_2O, and the desired volume is not achieved. No alarms are active. What could be the problem?
   I. The pressure control knob is not in the off position.
   II. There is water in the circuit.
   III. The pressure is being released through the pressure-relief valve.
   IV. The bias flow is set too low.
   a. I only
   b. III only
   c. I and III only
   d. II and IV only

6. The respiratory therapist wants to use inverse ratio PCV on a patient being ventilated with the Wave. The rate is set at 12 breaths/min, and the T_I is 2 seconds. The T_I is increased to 3 seconds, and an audible alarm sounds. The IT TOO LONG LED illuminates. How can this problem be solved?
   a. Reduce the flow instead of increasing the T_I.
   b. Change the setting of the I:E ratio switch on the back panel.
   c. Increase the pressure setting for PCV.
   d. Increase the bias flow to 10 L/min.

7. During PCV, which of the following statements is/are true regarding the initial flow to the patient?
   I. The maximum available flow during PCV is based on the flow setting.
   II. If a low flow value is set, it takes longer for the ventilator to achieve the set PIP.
   III. A high flow setting achieves the set PIP more quickly.
   IV. For best results, the highest flow value should be set to allow the microprocessor to automatically adjust the rise time or slope.
   a. I only
   b. II and III
   c. I and IV
   d. I, II, III, and IV

8. During PCV, the respiratory therapist increases the T_I. How will this affect the pressure delivery during inspiration?
   a. The amount of time the pressure plateaus during inspiration increases.
   b. This will reduce mean airway pressure.
   c. Increasing the inspiratory time has no effect on pressure delivery.
   d. The rate of flow delivery will decrease, lengthening the time it takes to achieve the set pressure.

9. Which of the following is true regarding the high pressure alarm limit during PCV?
   a. Reaching the high pressure alarm limit does not end inspiration, but it limits the pressure delivered.
   b. The therapist needs to set an appropriate high pressure limit (10 to 15 cm H_2O above the set pressure).
   c. No high pressure alarm limit needs to be set because the set pressure cannot be exceeded in the patient circuit.
   d. An automatic high pressure alarm limit is set at 10 cm H_2O above the set inspiratory pressure.

10. During pressure-targeted ventilation (PCV) (set P = 20 cm H_2O), a large leak results in only 8 cm H_2O being reached during inspiration. This would result in which of the following?
    I. The ventilator will increase flow into the circuit.
    II. An automatically set LOW PRESSURE alarm will activate.
    III. A lower delivered V_T will result.
    IV. A high PEEP alarm will activate.
    a. I only
    b. II and IV
    c. I and III
    d. I, II, and III

ASSESSMENT QUESTIONS—cont'd

11. Which of the following is/are true regarding PSV?
 I. The longer a PS breath, the lower the percentage of peak flow required to end (cycle) the breath.
 II. Inspiratory flow during PSV will end when V_T reaches 4 L.
 III. A pressure support breath will cycle if the peak pressure increases to 2 cm H_2O higher than the set pressure.
 IV. A PSV breath will end if the T_I is longer than 4 seconds.
  a. I and II
  b. III
  c. II and III
  d. I, II, III, and IV

References

1. Newport Medical Instruments: Newport Wave ventilator operating manual, model E200, version 1.5, 1993, Newport Beach, Calif, 1993, Newport.
2. Pilbeam SP, Payne FR: Mechanical ventilators. In Burton GG, Hodgkin JE, Ward JJ, editors: *Respiratory care: a guide to clinical practice,* ed 4, Philadelphia, 1997, JB Lippincott.
3. Miller C: Personal communication, July 2006, Newport Beach, Calif.

Internet Resources
www.newportnmi.com
www.ventilators.com

NEWPORT e500[1-3]

OUTLINE

Power Source
 Power on Self-Test
 Battery Operation and Indicators
On/Standby Control and Patient Circuit
Internal Drive Mechanism
Ventilator Set-Up Procedure
 Leak Test
 Leak Compensation
 Additional Set-Up Features
Controls
 Using Ventilator Controls
 Ventilator Parameter Controls
 Sloping
 Monitored Data Section
Alarms
 Adjustable Alarms
 Nonadjustable Alarms
 Alarm Controls

Breath Types for Modes of Ventilation
 Breath Type in Volume Control
 Breath Type in Pressure Control
 Breath Type in Biphasic Pressure-Release Ventilation
 Breath Type in Volume-Targeted Pressure Control (VTPC)
 Breath Type in Volume-Targeted Pressure-Support Breaths
Modes of Ventilation
 Assist/Control (A/CMV) Ventilation
 Synchronized Intermittent Mandatory Ventilation (SIMV)
 Spontaneous (SPONT) Mode
 Noninvasive Ventilation (NIV)
 Back-Up Ventilation (BUV)
Special Feature: Newport e500 Graphic Display Monitor
 Setting Up the Graphic Display Monitor
 Waveforms and Loops
Troubleshooting

OBJECTIVES

Upon completion of this section, you will be able to:
· Describe the power sources and power indicators for the Newport e500.
· Explain the function of the controls on the Newport e500 front panel.
· Compare flow delivery during pressure control, volume control, and automatic flow adjustment by the ventilator during inspiration.

The Newport e500 ventilator (Newport Medical Instruments, Costa Mesa, California) is intended for use with infants, pediatric patients, and adults requiring a tidal volume of 20 to 3000 mL. It can be used for noninvasive and invasive positive-pressure ventilation (Figure 12-84).

POWER SOURCE

The Newport e500 requires an electrical power source and a high-pressure gas source for operation. The rear panel contains DISS connectors for high-pressure air and oxygen sources, as well as an AC power cord connector, a DC power source input connector, and two electronic cable connectors that attach to the control panel and the graphics display module. Figure 12-85 shows the rear panel of the e500. Table 12-34 describes each of the panel connectors and devices.

Power on Self-Test

When the ventilator is turned on, a power on self-test (POST) verifies the integrity of the software-controlled indicators, displays, audible alarm, and memory. Additional tests and calibrations are performed on an ongoing basis during operation. These include verification of software "watchdog" signals, flow and pressure transducer autozeroing, and oxygen analyzer calibration. The ventilator begins ventilation with the last set ventilator parameters used.

Battery Operation and Indicators

The internal battery can provide about 30 minutes of backup power when fully charged, and ventilation remains fully functional. The e500 can also use an external (DC) battery as a power source if the AC power source fails.

On the center left side of the front panel is an indicator section, which provides information about the batteries and power sources. The word CHARGING illuminates to show that the internal battery is recharging and the ventilator is connected to an AC power source. (NOTE: The internal battery will charge whenever the ventilator is plugged into an AC source, whether the unit is on or in the standby mode.) The INT BATTERY indicator illuminates, and the ventilator beeps every 5 minutes when the e500 is operating off the internal battery and not an AC source. The battery

TABLE 12-34

Rear Panel of the Gas Delivery Unit—Newport e500

Item	Description
1	Serial port for interface to central monitoring systems (RS-232C connector)
2	DISS high-pressure oxygen connector
3	DISS high-pressure air connector
4	Alarm beeper
5	Alternate site for electrical grounding equipment
6	Hour meter displays ventilator's operating hours (power on)
7	Connector for external battery
8	AC power module (replaceable fuses are located above the connector port)
9	Fan filter housing (with cover)
10	Remote alarm connector to interface with hospital nurse call system
11	Connector for e500 Control Panel to GDU
12	Alarm loudness control
13	Connector for e500 Graphic Display Monitor to GDU
14	Connection for external alarm silence cable
15	Bleed port (diffuser head) for gas exhaust from the ventilator pneumatic system

charge bar on the right of this section shows the relative charge remaining on the internal battery. The MAINS light illuminates when the ventilator is operating on AC power. (NOTE: The charge light will also be illuminated.)

The EXT BATTERY lights when an external battery is in use. The charge remaining is *not* indicated for the external battery.

ON/STANDBY CONTROL AND PATIENT CIRCUIT

The ON/STANDBY control switch is located on the left side of the front of the ventilator gas delivery unit (GDU), where the patient circuit connectors are located (Figure 12-86). The main inspiratory and expiratory lines of the patient circuit should have bacterial filters installed. A bacterial filter is placed between the inspiratory limb and the inspiratory port (TO PATIENT) to prevent contaminants in exhaled gases from entering the inspiratory line in the event of a **Device Alert** shutdown (Box 12-61).

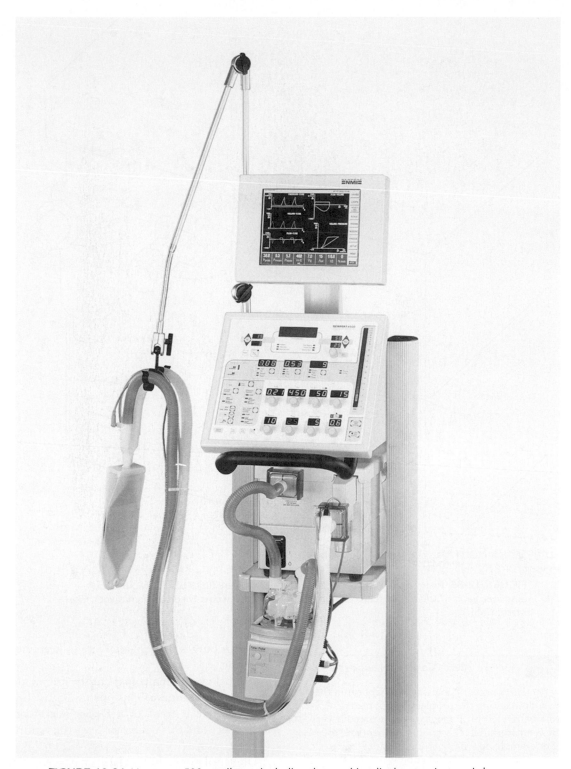

FIGURE 12-84 Newport e500 ventilator, including the graphics display monitor and the patient circuit. (Courtesy Newport Medical Instruments, Costa Mesa, Calif.)

A bacterial filter is used between the expiratory limb and the expiratory port (FROM PATIENT) to prevent exhaled gas contaminants from entering the exhalation system. The exhalation valve assembly is heated to prevent moisture in exhaled air from condensing on the expiratory flow sensor. The exhalation assembly has low resistance to allow for rapid return to baseline pressure after a positive pressure breath and reduce the potential for auto-PEEP resulting from expiratory resistance.

A proximal pressure connector is located between the inspiratory and expiratory connectors on the front of the GDU. This connector is used to attach a line from the ventilator to the patient Y-connector for monitoring proximal airway pressure. A small amount of flow from the

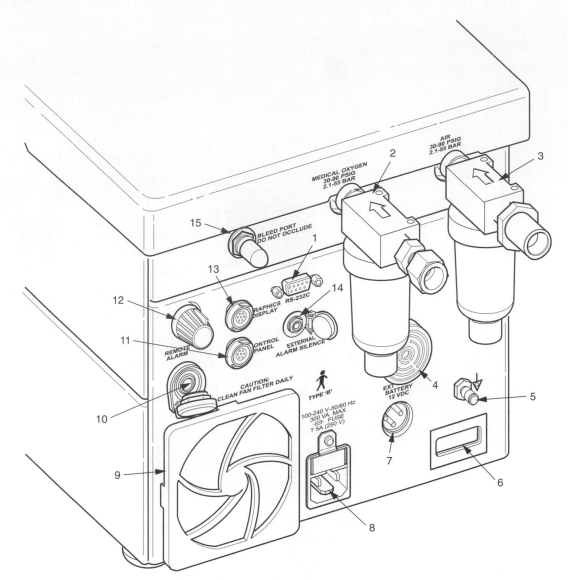

FIGURE 12-85 Rear panel of the e500 ventilator gas delivery unit (GDU). Table 12-34 describes each of the numbered components. (Courtesy Newport Medical Instruments, Costa Mesa, Calif.)

ventilator purges the proximal line to keep moisture from collecting.

Just below the main inspiratory line connector is an **emergency air intake.** This opening must be kept unobstructed. In the event of a Device Alert condition (see Alarms section), this opening allows the venting of patient circuit pressure.

The ventilator includes a built-in oxygen analyzer, which provides automatic high and low fractional inspired oxygen (F_IO_2) alarms and is automatically calibrated when the e500 is turned on, recalibrated every 30 minutes for the following hour, and every 8 hours of operation thereafter.

INTERNAL DRIVE MECHANISM

The e500 features an electronically controlled inlet gas mixing system, which blends and delivers gas with sufficient flow to accommodate a high inspiratory flow demand

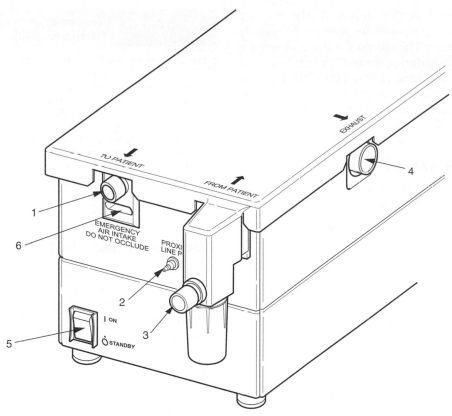

FIGURE 12-86 Front panel of the e500 ventilator patient unit, showing the connections for the patient circuit and the on/off switch. *(1)* Inspiratory port; *(2)* proximal pressure line port; *(3)* expiratory port; *(4)* exhaust outlet, which allows exhaled gases to vent to room air; *(5)* ON/STANDBY switch; and *(6)* emergency air intake opening. (See text for further explanation.) (Courtesy Newport Medical Instruments, Costa Mesa, Calif.)

from the patient (180 L/min for adults, 100 L/min for pediatric/infant patients).

The gas mixing system allows a quick change of F_IO_2. This occurs with the next breath when the F_IO_2 control is adjusted or within 3 minutes when the 100% button is pressed. When the F_IO_2 is set at 0.21, the e500 can operate with a single gas source (compressed air gas supply [greater than 10 psig]).

VENTILATOR SET-UP PROCEDURE

Before the e500 is used, a few tests or calculations should be performed. Before running these, the operator must make sure the patient circuit and humidification system are attached. A test lung is placed at the patient Y-connector. While pressing the PRESET VENT SETTINGS button, the operator turns the power switch (front of the GDU) to the ON position. This procedure allows entry to the USER SET UP routine. (NOTE: Pressing and holding the PRESET VENT SETTINGS button while in USER SET UP causes the e500 to enter normal ventilating conditions. To turn off the USER SET UP routine at this point, the operator must turn the power switch to the STANDBY position and press the ALARM SILENCE button.)

The set-up procedure allows selection of any of the following:

· Choosing a language
· Choosing the pressure measurement units (cm H_2O or mbar)
· Performing a leak test on the patient circuit
· Calculating and enabling circuit compliance compensation (volume and pressure ventilation)
· Selecting the circuit and humidifier type (high output, middle output, or heat and moisture exchanger [HME])
· Enabling a 90-second slow inflation (provides a pressure-volume curve for evaluating inflection points)
· Setting the time and date
· Adjusting for operation at ambient altitude
· Selecting the communication port protocol
· Viewing the violation message record

Leak Test

Before initiating mechanical ventilation with a new patient, the operator should be sure to use the LEAK TEST to ensure the integrity of the patient circuit and select the COMPLIANCE COMPENSATION feature.

To perform the leak test, the operator rotates the trigger knob until "c1" is displayed in the trigger window. The directions are followed as they appear in the message window. The operator is required, for example, to occlude the patient Y-connector. The criteria for this leak test are based on a pressure drop during the test. The final message will be either NO LEAK or LEAK TEST FAILED. If the leak test is failed because of an excessive drop in pressure during the test, the operator must be sure to check the circuit and any attached accessories for potential leak sites and correct these before repeating the test.

Leak Compensation

In addition to the leak test, the e500 features an automatic **leak compensation** to stabilize the baseline pressure when a small leak is present. The leak compensation during ventilation adjusts breath by breath, with a maximum of 15 L/min for adults and 8 L/min for pediatric/infant patients. The adjustment for leak compensation is based on flow measurement at end-exhalation. Leak compensation helps minimize the chance of autotriggering.

When the noninvasive ventilation feature is activated, automatic leak compensation increases to 25 L/min to accommodate leaks from nonvented masks.

As with the leak test, the compliance compensation calculation should be run whenever the patient circuit is changed. The patient cannot be connected during this procedure. (NOTE: Chapter 11 reviews volume loss associated with tubing compliance [compressibility factor] and its standard calculation.) To have the ventilator perform this calculation, the operator rotates the trigger knob to display "c2" in the trigger window. When the message window displays COMPLIANCE COMP TEST HIT EXP HOLD, the operator presses EXP HOLD. The operator then follows the directions in the message window as they are displayed.

The breathing compensation factor may be viewed by selecting V_TE in the monitor section of the control panel and reading the digital information displayed in the adjacent window. If the circuit compliance is outside the acceptable range, the message window will display CC TEST FAILED CC > 10 mL/cm H_2O. This typically indicates a significant leak in the patient circuit. The operator should check the integrity of the exhalation system, breathing circuit, and accessories before repeating the compliance test. After the test is passed, the new compliance compensation value is saved by pressing INSP HOLD. To enable or disable compliance compensation, the operator rotates the trigger knob to display "c3" and follows the on-screen instructions. When compliance compensation is enabled, the ventilator will automatically compensate for loss of volume associated with tubing compressibility based on the new saved value. The CCOMP indicator illuminates during the inspiratory phase of a volume- or pressure-controlled breath when this feature has been enabled.

The humidifier selected will affect monitored values for tidal volume (V_T) and minute volume. To check or change the humidifier selection, the operator rotates the control knob until "c4" appears in the trigger window. The window displays directions for making the change.

BOX 12-62	Slow Inflation Function (Newport e500)

The SLOW INFLATION function is enabled and disabled under the USER SET UP. When SLOW INFLATION is enabled and the ventilator is in adult volume ventilation, with the flow set at 1 to 2 L/min, pressing the MANUAL INFLATION key delivers a slow manual inflation that can last up to 90 seconds as long as the airway pressure does not reach the high Paw limit or 60 cm H_2O. A slow inflation allows clinicians to view the upper and lower inflection points on the monitor for evaluation of a PEEP setting and maximum safe distending pressure.

Additional Set-Up Features

The ADDITIONAL SET UP window features, such as ALTITUDE compensation, can also be reviewed or checked while the USER SET UP feature is in operation. The Newport e500 operating manual provides a detailed explanation of these items. As an example, Box 12-62 reviews the slow inflation technique, available in USER SET UP, which is used to obtain a pressure-volume curve and establish points on the curve where changes in lung compliance are occurring.

To start ventilation once USER SET UP has been completed, the operator presses and holds the PRESET VENT SETTINGS button. The next step is to select the appropriate patient category (adult or pediatric/infant) and then the breath type and mode, and adjust parameters as needed for the patient. Controls, breath type modes, and alarms are reviewed.

CONTROLS

The front control panel of the e500 has three main areas: a control section, a monitored data section, and an alarm and message section (Figure 12-87). The control section is subdivided into a left-hand box with the mode keys and a few other controls. The right-hand section contains the commonly set ventilator parameters, such as the respiratory rate control.

The mode control box includes a button for selecting the patient size, either adult or pediatric/infant (Ped/Infant). An indicator light shows the selected category. Changing the patient size selection affects the range of parameters. For example, the adult tidal volume range is 100 to 995 mL (5 mL resolution) or 1 to 3 L (0.01 mL resolution). The Ped/Infant range for tidal volume is 20 to 1000 mL (0.01 mL resolution).

The VOLUME CONTROL button is used to select volume-targeted breaths for assist/control (A/CMV), SIMV, or spontaneous (SPONT). An indicator illuminates to show the breath type and mode. To the right is the PRESSURE CONTROL button, which allows selection of pressure-targeted breaths in A/CMV, SIMV, or SPONT modes. Again, an indicator light illuminates to show the selected breath type and mode. The final mode and breath type panel is the

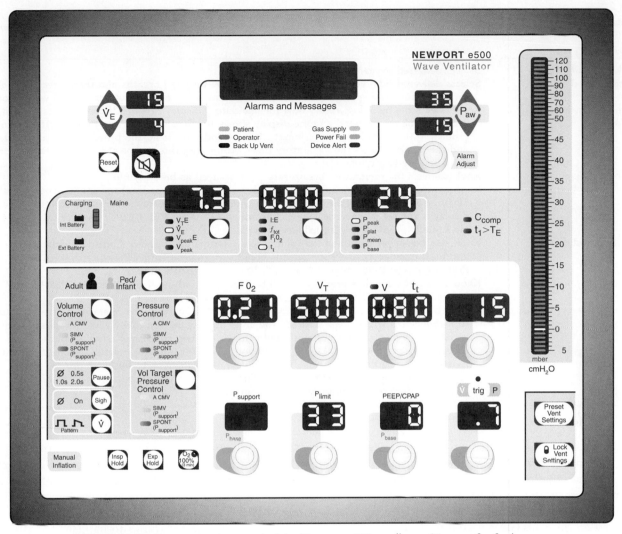

FIGURE 12-87 Front operating panel of the Newport e500 ventilator. (See text for further description.) (Redrawn from Newport Medical Instruments, Costa Mesa, Calif.)

VOLUME TARGETED PRESSURE CONTROL button. When this mode and breath type are selected, pressure ventilation is adjusted breath by breath to achieve the user-set volume. These controls are reviewed more extensively under the section on modes of ventilation and breath types.

The volume control section also includes a PAUSE control, a SIGH control, and a FLOW WAVEFORM control. The PAUSE button is for setting an inspiratory pause during volume-targeted breaths (off, 0.5, 1, and 2 seconds). The SIGH button activates sigh breath delivery with a sigh tidal volume equal to 1.5 times the set tidal volume. Sigh breaths occur every 100 breaths. The FLOW WAVEFORM control allows selection of either constant (square) or descending ramp flow waveforms during volume-targeted breath delivery.

Below the mode section are four additional controls: MANUAL INFLATION, INSPIRATORY HOLD, EXPIRATORY HOLD, and 100% OXYGEN DELIVERY (3 min). When pressed, the MANUAL INFLATION button delivers a manual inspiration that is up to 5 seconds long (or ends when a high Paw

alarm limit occurs). In pressure-controlled A/CMV and SIMV modes, MANUAL INFLATION is pressure targeted at the set pressure limit. In volume-targeted, pressure-controlled A/CMV and SIMV modes, MANUAL INFLATION is pressure targeted at the last pressure limit used by the software. In SPONT mode (all breath types), MANUAL INFLATION delivers a breath with a target pressure of PEEP/CPAP plus 15 cm H_2O. (NOTE: The maximum time for manual inflation is affected by the slow inflation control [see USER SET UP section].)

When the inspiratory hold button (INSP HOLD) is pressed, it starts an inspiratory hold at the end of inspiration for up to 5 seconds after a positive-pressure breath. This allows estimation of the plateau pressure (P_{plat}). If INSP HOLD is pressed during an exhalation, the hold takes place during the next positive-pressure breath until the button is released or until 5 seconds elapses. The measured plateau pressure is displayed in the P_{plat} display until the end of the next inspiration. A reading of "- -" means the ventilator was unable to obtain a stable reading (usually resulting from a

TABLE 12-35

Ventilator Control Parameters—e500

Control and Type	Description
F_1O_2 knob and display	Selects delivered oxygen concentration (0.21-1).
V_T knob and display	Selects delivered tidal volume for mandatory volume-targeted breaths and the target tidal volume for mandatory and spontaneous breaths in volume-targeted, pressure-controlled ventilation.
$\dot{V}/t_i$ indicator, knob, and display	Knob selects the peak inspiratory flow for mandatory display breaths. If the $\dot{V}$ indicator is lit, the breath is volume targeted and the display shows the flow setting. Flow range: 1-180 L/min (adult); 1-100 L/min (pediatric/infant). If the t_i indicator is lit, the breath is pressure targeted and the display shows the inspiratory time setting. Inspiratory time range: 0.1-5 sec (adult), 0.1-3 sec (pediatric/infant).
f knob and display	Knob controls the mandatory breath rate (f), displayed as breaths/min.
Psupport knob and display	Knob controls the pressure-support level (above PEEP/CPAP setting) for spontaneous breaths in SIMV or SPONT settings in either breath type (Volume Control or Pressure Control). The display is the set pressure level, which is added to the set PEEP/CPAP level. PS range: 0-60 cm H_2O (adult); 0-50 cm H_2O (pediatric/infant).
P_{limit} knob and display	Knob sets target pressure and the value display. This is for Pressure Control mandatory breaths and both mandatory and spontaneous breaths in Volume Target Pressure Control mode. Pressure range: 0-80 cm H_2O (adult); 0-70 cm H_2O (pediatric/infant).
PEEP/CPAP knob and display	Knob selects the baseline pressure for all breath types and modes and displays PEEP/CPAP. Range: 0-45 cm H_2O (adult), 0-30 cm H_2O (pediatric/infant).
Trigger indicator, knob, and display	Trigger button selects either flow ($\dot{V}$) or pressure (P) triggering. The operator presses the button to highlight the trigger type desired. The knob adjusts the sensitivity value for either trigger variable. The display shows the selected setting. The trig indicator flashes when the ventilator recognizes a patient effort. During exhalation, the e500 uses a ventilator-set bias flow, which is functional during flow triggering. The bias flow also functions to flush exhaled CO_2 and stabilize temperature, humidity, and baseline pressure in the patient circuit. The bias flow is turned off during an expiratory hold maneuver.

spontaneous breathing effort by the patient). P_{plat} is also displayed on the e500 GDM numeric screen with a time stamp indicating the time the measurement was made. The measurement of P_{plat} allows the e500 to calculate lung compliance and resistance when applicable. These are also displayed on the e500 GDM with time stamps.

Pressing the expiratory hold button (EXP HOLD) starts an expiratory hold maneuver at the end of the current exhalation for up to 20 seconds. This allows an estimated measurement of the auto-PEEP level. If pressed during inspiration, the hold takes effect during the next exhalation until the button is released or 20 seconds has elapsed. Selecting EXP HOLD can be used to detect auto-PEEP as long as the patient is not making any spontaneous breathing efforts. If a stable reading is obtained, the total PEEP (auto-PEEP plus set PEEP) is shown in the P_{base} display. Otherwise, the display remains unchanged. "PEEPtot-STAT" is displayed on the e500 GDM, along with a time stamp. This value is also used in the calculation of static compliance (Cstat), which is also time stamped.

The 100% OXYGEN DELIVERY (3 min) button delivers 100% O_2 for 3 minutes when activated. The indicator on the O_2 100% (3 min) button lights when 100% oxygen is delivered. Pressing the button again cancels 100% oxygen delivery.

Using Ventilator Controls

Adjusting any of the basic ventilator parameter controls is basically the same for all variables. The adjacent knob for any parameter is adjusted until the display window above the knob shows the desired setting. The ventilator retains the settings in memory within 10 seconds of selection. If the ventilator is turned off (placed in STANDBY), these values are retained in memory and used when the unit is powered up again. Setting a parameter outside of the available range causes three things to happen. The OPERATOR indicator blinks, an audible alarm sounds, and the message window describes which parameter is out of range.

Ventilator Parameter Controls

The right-hand area of the controls section contains F_1O_2, V_T, $\dot{V}_E$ or t_I, frequency (f), Psupport, P_{limit}, PEEP/CPAP, and trigger: $\dot{V}_E$ or P trigger. Table 12-35 describes each of these controls.

Below the pressure manometer on the right side of the control panel are two additional controls: LOCK VENT SETTINGS and PRESET VENT SETTINGS.

The LOCK VENT SETTINGS button does just that; it locks and unlocks all the buttons and knobs in the control section except for the MANUAL INFLATION control and the O_2 100% (3 min) control. The lock indicator illuminates when the lock is in effect.

Pressing the PRESET VENT SETTINGS button as the ventilator is turned on enters the USER SET UP procedure and suspends ventilation. The PRESET VENT SETTINGS function can also be used during ventilation. Pressing the PRESET VENT SETTINGS button during ventilation allows selection of ventilation parameters for a different mode/breath type without affecting current ventilator settings. The operator follows these steps:

1. Presses PRESET VENT SETTINGS.
2. Selects the desired breath type/mode. (NOTE: The preset breath type/mode indicator flashes, but the ventilator continues ventilation in the currently selected breath type and mode [current breath type/mode indicator remains steadily lit].)
3. Sets the desired ventilator parameters.
4. To exit the PRESET state, presses the PRESET VENT SETTINGS button again or waits 5 seconds after the last ventilator setting adjustment.
5. The ventilator saves the settings selected during PRESET as long as the ventilator is on.
6. After the new breath type/mode is selected, the settings that have been changed by the operator become effective.

Box 12-63 describes the safety benefit of setting parameters for ventilator modes not currently in use (NOTE: If a new breath type/mode is not selected in the PRESET state or if a ventilator parameter change is made before a new breath type/mode is selected, the changes to settings become immediate for the current breath type and mode.) (Clinical Rounds 12-24).

Sloping

Many ventilators have a separate sloping or rise time feature that adjusts the rate of pressure delivery during breath delivery. With the e500, the user can choose to adjust sloping manually or to allow the microprocessor to select the amount of slope. When AUTO is selected, the e500 adjusts sloping based on the real-time response of the system. During pressure-targeted breaths of any type, the ventilator delivers a flow at a software-optimized rate to quickly achieve and maintain the set pressure until the end of inspiration. Flow is adjusted to provide automatic sloping (rise) for every breath. The program is designed to avoid overshooting the set pressure for the breath (see Chapter 11 for a description of sloping or rise time).

Monitored Data Section

The center portion of the front panel contains the monitored data section. On the far left are the battery and power indicators described earlier. The first data monitoring display is for volume and flow information. By pressing the button adjacent to the available list, any of the following can be displayed:

- V_{TE}—expiratory tidal volume (mL)
- $\dot{V}_E$—expiratory minute volume (L)
- $\dot{V}_E$peakE—peak expiratory flow (L/min)
- $\dot{V}_E$peakI—peak inspiratory flow (L/min)

An indicator lights to show which variable is being displayed.

The second set of data displayed is timing and F_IO_2 data. Pressing the button displays any of the following:

- I:E ratio (inspiratory to expiratory ratio)—Displays 99:1 to 1:99. In SPONT mode, this display shows "- -". It displays the set I:E ratio while the inspiratory time, tidal volume, or rate is adjusted.
- f_{tot}—total breath rate in breaths/min.
- F_IO_2—measured fractional inspired oxygen concentration. The display will show "- -" if the oxygen supply pressure is below minimum or if the ventilator is connected to air only and the F_IO_2 is set at 21%. It will also display "- -" if the oxygen sensor is disconnected, defective, or not calibrated since power up or if oxygen sensor calibration is in progress.
- t_I—measured inspiratory time displayed in seconds and updated after each spontaneous or mandatory breath. It displays the set inspiratory time while tidal volume or flow is adjusted.

An indicator light shows which variable is currently being displayed in this section.

The third section of the display data is for patient pressure information. Using the adjacent button allows display of one of the following:

- P_{peak}—peak airway pressure (cm H_2O) updated after each positive-pressure inflation (range, 1 to 120 cm H_2O).
- P_{plat}—plateau pressure (cm H_2O) displayed at the end of an inspiratory hold or pause (range, 0 to 120 cm H_2O). The display shows "- -" if there is no PAUSE or INSP HOLD or the ventilator cannot measure a stable plateau pressure.

BOX 12-63	Patient Safety and Preset Vent Settings (Newport e500)

To ensure patient safety, it is advisable to use the PRESET VENT SETTINGS button to set safe values for all parameters for the patient. Should the ventilator inadvertently be changed to a different breath type or mode, the parameters for the new breath type or mode would still be appropriate for the patient. For example, if an adult patient is being pressure ventilated, a tidal volume is not set, although the volume can be viewed. Assume the ventilator holds in memory a V_T of 100 mL. If the mode were changed from pressure to volume, a V_T of 100 mL might not be appropriate for the patient currently being ventilated.

The ventilator has a built-in delay in delivering the new breath type that is intended to give the user more time to assess new settings before they are activated. It is advisable to adjust the breath and mode type and their variables to protect the patient.

CLINICAL ROUNDS 12-24

A respiratory therapist is ventilating a patient with pressure control SIMV with the e500 at a mandatory rate of 6 breaths/min. The therapist presses the PRESET VENT SETTINGS button, selects volume control with SIMV as the breath type and mode, and sets the respiratory rate to 2 breaths/min. How will the ventilator respond?

See Evolve Resources for the answer.

CLINICAL ROUNDS 12-25

A respiratory therapist presses the INSP HOLD button to obtain a plateau pressure reading for calculation of lung compliance. The P_{plat} display in the pressure section of the monitored data window shows "- -" and does not provide a value. What is the problem?

See Evolve Resources for the answer.

See Evolve Resources for the answer.

BOX 12-64	Range of High and Low Minute Volume and Pressure Alarms (Newport e500)

High minute volume alarm range: 2 to 80 L/min (adult), 0.2 to 60 L/min (pediatric/infant)
Low minute volume alarm range: 1 to 50 L/min (adult), 0.01 to 30 L/min (pediatric/infant)
High peak airway pressure alarm range: 5 to 120 cm H_2O (adult), 5 to 100 cm H_2O (pediatric/infant)
Low peak airway pressure alarm range: 3 to 95 cm H_2O (adult), 3 to 75 cm H_2O (pediatric/infant)
Tachypnea alarm: Off or 10 to 110 breaths/min

- P_{mean}—mean airway pressure (cm H_2O), the average pressure in the patient circuit for the past 30 seconds (range, 0 to 120 cm H_2O).
- P_{base}—baseline pressure (cm H_2O) (range, 0 to 99 cm H_2O)

As with the other monitored variables, a light indicator shows the current parameter on display. Clinical Rounds 12-25 presents an exercise related to pressure monitoring.

Toward the right of the monitor displays are two light indicators. The C_{COMP} indicator illuminates when the ventilator is correcting for patient circuit compliance. When C_{COMP} is used, the ventilator adjusts volume delivery for volume-controlled breaths to allow for the compliance of the patient circuit.

The $t_I > t_E$ indicator illuminates when inverse I : E ratios are present (inspiratory time is longer than expiratory time). To the far right of the monitor data section is a pressure bar graph. This provides a continuous display of real-time pressure measured in the patient circuit in cm H_2O or mbar (millibars). The display range is −5 to 120 cm H_2O or 5 to 117 mbar. The desired units of measure are set using the USER SET UP procedure.

ALARMS

For all alarms except the tachypnea alarm, the alarm controls and indicators of the e500 are located in the upper section of the front panel. The alarm system can be divided into three basic sections: adjustable alarms, nonadjustable alarms, and controls.

Adjustable Alarms

Adjustable alarms include the high and low minute volume and high and low peak airway pressure and tachypnea (high respiratory rate). The minute volume alarm control is located in the upper left section of the alarm area. Pressing the center $\dot{V}_E$ button selects between the high and low $\dot{V}_E$ alarm limit for adjustment of the high and low $\dot{V}_E$ values (Box 12-64 shows the alarm range). The low $\dot{V}_E$ alarm may be turned off when noninvasive ventilation is being used. Pressing the button once selects the high alarm limit, twice selects the low alarm limit, and three times exits alarm setting conditions. The adjacent display for the selected alarm limit flashes, and the message window describes the selected alarm. While the display is flashing, the operator rotates the ALARM ADJUST knob at the right side of the alarm section to set the desired value. The alarm limit is adjusted until the display shows the desired value. Once adjusted, the adjacent display windows show the high and low $\dot{V}_E$ alarm limits setting. When a violation of these settings occurs, an indicator above or below the button blinks red, and an alarm sounds.

The high and low airway pressure alarm indicators and control button are located on the right side of the alarm section. As with the minute volume alarm, the button is pressed to select between the high and low pressure alarm setting and to set the pressure alarm limits in the same manner as the minute ventilation alarm limits are set. The display windows to the left show the value for the high and low peak airway pressure alarms (see Box 12-64 for alarm range). The indicator above or below the selector button blinks red, and an alarm sounds to indicate a high or low airway pressure condition.

Nonadjustable Alarms

Table 12-36 lists the nonadjustable, patient-related alarms and the related message that appears in the ALARMS AND MESSAGE window at the top center portion of the front operating panel.

Alarm Controls

In addition to the high and low pressure and minute ventilation alarm controls described previously, there are five additional alarm controls.

- Tachypnea alarm—This control, located on the graphic display monitor, allows the operator to set a high respiratory rate alarm value. It may be turned off in any mode or breath type.
- Alarm silence—This button mutes audible alarms for 1 minute, including alarms that occur after the silent period begins. Pressing the ALARM SILENCE button again turns off the silence function. A Device Alert alarm cannot be silenced by this button unless the e500 is powered down first (see Box 12-61).
- Alarm silence suction/disconnect function—Holding down the ALARM SILENCE button for 1 second or longer enables a disconnection function. A short audible beep will occur when the button is held down. If the ventilator

TABLE 12-36

Nonadjustable Alarms and Related Messages*—e500

Message	Condition
Apnea	No patient effort detected or breath delivered for 20 sec.
F_IO_2 High	Measured $F_IO_2 > 0.07$ (7%) above set F_IO_2.
F_IO_2 Low	Measured $F_IO_2 < 0.07$ (7%) below set F_IO_2.
High Baseline Pressure	Monitored $P_{base} >$ (set $P_{base} + 5$ cm H_2O) for 2 consecutive breaths.
Low Baseline Pressure	Monitored $P_{base} <$ set P_{base} by a software-determined amount for longer than 0.5 sec for 2 consecutive breaths.
Prox Line Disconnect	Outlet pressure from the ventilator is greater than the proximal pressure when proximal pressure is near zero.
Sustained High Baseline	Monitored P_{base} has been ≥ 8 cm H_2O above set PEEP/CPAP for longer than 10 sec (adult) or 6 sec (pediatric/infant).

OPERATOR-RELATED ALARMS

(THE OPERATOR INDICATOR BLINKS, INDICATING AN ATTEMPT TO SELECT AN INVALID SETTING, WHEN THE MESSAGE WINDOW DISPLAYS THE FOLLOWING MESSAGES.)

Alarm	Description
Insp Time Too Long	Inspiratory time > 5 sec
Insp Time Too Short	Inspiratory time < 0.1 sec
I:E Ratio Inverse Violation	Inverse ratio > 4:1
P_{limit} Below P_{base}	Current P_{limit} setting is lower than the P_{base} (PEEP/CPAP) setting.
Low Paw Below P_{base}	Current low Paw alarm setting is lower than the P_{base} (PEEP/CPAP) setting.
Vol Target Not Met	Set volume target is not met before the breath ends.
Out of Range	An alarm or setting is out of range for the selected patient category.
Back Up Ventilation	Back Up Vent indicator blinks and a message appears, "Back Up Ventilation" indicating that backup ventilation is occurring in response to a Low $\dot{V}_E$ alarm.
Gas Supply Alarms	Gas Supply indicator blinks and the message window displays an alarm message if one or both gas supplies are below the operational pressure level of 10 psig. (NOTE: If the F_IO_2 is set at 0.21, this alarm is active only if air is lost.)
Power Fail Alarm	The Power Fail indicator blinks and the message window displays an alarm message with loss of AC power or a low internal battery power level.
Device Alert	Device Alert blinks when the ventilator is inoperative or less than 10% of the internal battery charge remains during battery operation. The emergency intake/relief and exhalation valves open, and a spontaneously breathing patient can receive room air. If available, 8 L/min of air is delivered through the proximal pressure tubing of the breathing circuit.

*The Patient indicator blinks when the Message window displays any of these alarm messages and an audible alarm occurs.

detects a circuit disconnection within 20 seconds, a suction disconnect function results. VENTILATION SUSPENDED appears in the message window. The automatic leak compensation is suspended, and a bias flow of gas is delivered through the circuit (10 L/min for adults, 5 L/min for pediatric/infant patients). Ventilation resumes only when the breathing circuit is reconnected or when 3 minutes elapse, whichever occurs first.

· Alarm reset button—Pressing this button clears visual indicators and messages for alarms that are no longer active.

· Alarm loudness knob—This knob adjusts the audible alarm volume (located on the rear panel of the GDU).

BREATH TYPES FOR MODES OF VENTILATION

The Newport e500 provides three breath types: volume-, pressure-, and volume-targeted pressure-control breaths (VTPC). These three breath types are available in A/CMV, SIMV, and SPONT modes of ventilation.

Breath Type in Volume Control

During volume ventilation, the ventilator delivers mandatory breaths based on the set V_T, flow, $\dot{V}_E$, frequency (f), PEEP/CPAP, F_IO_2, Pause, Sigh, and flow pattern setting. A constant (square) flow pattern and a descending ramp flow pattern are available for volume breaths. For a descending ramp, inspiration begins at the flow setting, decreases at a constant rate to 50% of the flow setting, and ends inspiration when the tidal volume has been delivered (volume cycled) unless a pause is set. Patient demand does not result in additional flow from the ventilator; therefore the operator must set a flow appropriate to the patient's needs.

Breath Type in Pressure Control

During pressure control ventilation, mandatory breaths are provided that are based on the set pressure (P_{limit}), inspiratory time (T_I), frequency (f), PEEP/CPAP, and F_IO_2 settings. The ventilator adjusts the flow during inspiration using either the operator-selected slope value or the AUTO selected feature. When AUTO is used, the ventilator adjusts the flow during inspiration to best achieve an immediate rise in the pressure delivery to the P_{limit} without overshooting the pressure. During pressure control the ventilator adjusts flow in response to patient demand to maintain the set pressure. Inspiratory flow ends when the set inspiratory time has elapsed (time cycled) or sooner if alveolar pressure reaches the target pressure.

Breath Type in Biphasic Pressure-Release Ventilation

Biphasic pressure-release ventilation (BPRV) is a breath type that affects pressure-control breaths in the A/CMV and SIMV modes of ventilation. BPRV is accessed using the open exhalation valve control under the extended features menu. When the pressure-control mode is not in use, this selection has no impact on ventilation.

BPRV mandatory breaths may be patient or time triggered. The airway pressure rises from the baseline pressure (PEEP/CPAP) setting to the pressure limit setting for the duration of the T_I setting. A small amount of flow is continually vented through the open (floating) expiratory valve. Flow and pressures are rapidly adjusted to accommodate the patient's spontaneous efforts. The T_I setting determines when the pressure drops to the baseline setting. Dropping to the baseline setting marks the beginning of the expiratory phase.

In A/CMV all patient- or time-triggered breaths are pressure targeted. A minimum mandatory breath rate is set on the respiratory rate control. In SIMV, the set rate determines the maximum mandatory breath rate. Spontaneous breaths between mandatory breaths can be supported with pressure support. The slope controls the rate of pressure rise for pressure support breaths. The automatic or manual adjustment of expiratory flow-cycle setting controls the inspiratory cycle for a PS breath.

Breath Type in Volume-Targeted Pressure Control (VTPC)

During VTPC ventilation, the e500 ventilator delivers mandatory breaths based on set values for P_{limit}, T_I, V_T, f, PEEP/CPAP, and F_IO_2. This breath type is similar to pressure control, but unlike pressure-control ventilation, the set pressure limit is the maximum allowable target pressure. The pressure varies to achieve a set V_T. Unlike volume ventilation, the V_T is a target and is not guaranteed for each breath. The ventilator determines the pressure needed to achieve the set V_T and increases or decreases the pressure by a maximum of 6 cm H_2O (up or down) per breath as needed. This is similar to pressure-regulated volume control (PRVC), described in Chapter 11. Clinical Rounds 12-26 provides an example problem using VTPC.

The target pressure of the first breath is 40% of the set P_{limit} or P_{base} plus 5 cm H_2O, whichever is higher. The maximum pressure permitted during this mode is the P_{limit} value. The minimum pressure is P_{base} plus 5 cm H_2O.

CLINICAL ROUNDS 12-26

A patient is ventilated with volume-targeted pressure control. The set tidal volume is 500 mL, the PEEP/CPAP is 10 cm H_2O, and the P_{limit} is 35 cm H_2O with a rate of 10 mandatory breaths/min. After the first few breaths, the peak pressure is 25 cm H_2O, and the exhaled V_T is 460 cm H_2O.

1. How will the ventilator respond to these measured values?
2. What is the maximum pressure to which the ventilator will rise?

See Evolve Resources for the answer.

If the set V_T is not achieved by the end of inspiration for three consecutive breaths when the target pressure equals P_{limit}, an operator alarm occurs and the message window will display VOL TARGET NOT MET. The operator should investigate the cause of higher pressures being required and try to correct any problem that may have changed the patient's lung compliance or airway resistance. It is also possible that the V_T, P_{limit}, T_I, or sloping is set inappropriately.

Volume-targeted pressure control is available in A/CMV and SIMV modes. In the A/CMV mode, all breaths are patient or time triggered, time cycled, and volume targeted. In the SIMV mode, the same target V_T and P_{limit} apply to both mandatory and spontaneous breaths. However, mandatory breaths are time cycled, and spontaneous breaths are flow cycled, based on the same flow-cycling threshold adjusting feature as standard pressure support described in the following section.

Breath Type in Volume-Targeted Pressure-Support Breaths

As with VTPC breaths, the e500 can also target a tidal volume during pressure-support breaths. Because pressure-support breaths are always spontaneous breaths, volume-targeted pressure support (VTPS) is available whenever the patient can maintain spontaneous nonmandatory breaths at an acceptable level or rate. This includes volume-targeted pressure control SIMV and SPONT (spontaneous) modes.

As with VTPC, the target pressure in VTPS for the first breath is 40% of the set P_{limit} or P_{base} plus 5 cm H_2O, whichever is highest. The ventilator delivers a flow to achieve and maintain the pressure. The lowest available pressure is the P_{base} setting plus 5 cm H_2O. The highest pressure is the set P_{limit}.

The e500 establishes a target pressure after each breath with the goal of meeting the set V_T. Pressure is adjusted up or down by a maximum of 6 cm H_2O breath by breath to achieve the set V_T. The set V_T may not be achieved with every breath but is still targeted.

Three criteria end a VTPS breath:

BOX 12-65	Flexcycle

A flow-cycling feature called *Flexcycle* is being used for flow-cycling pressure-support (PS) and VTPS breaths. Flexcycle uses pulmonary time constants calculated at end-exhalation and the slope of the pressure waveform at end-inspiration to automatically adjust the flow-cycling off threshold to specifically suit the patient's needs. It is adjusted on a breath-by-breath basis by the microprocessor.

- The patient stops demanding flow (flow decays to the flow cycling-off threshold).
- The pressure rises above the ventilator's current target level plus a small time-varied margin.
- The inspiratory time reaches a maximum value (2 seconds for adults, 1.2 seconds for pediatric/infant patients).

The standard cycling mechanism for VTPS and Psupport is flow cycling. It is adjustable from 5% to 55% of measured peak flow (Box 12-65), or the user may choose to have it automatically adjusted by the ventilator.

If the target pressure is equal to the P_{limit} (the maximum permitted pressure) and the target V_T is not reached by the end of a breath for three consecutive breaths, an operator alarm will activate and the message window will display VOL TARGET NOT MET. The operator should assess the patient to determine the cause of higher pressures being required to deliver the volume. Changes in the patient's lung compliance or airway resistance may have occurred. It is also possible that the V_T, PLIMIT, sloping, or expiratory flow cycle criteria are set inappropriately. The advantage of this breath type is the use of pressure-targeted ventilation and the automatic adjustment of pressure target for the lowest level that accommodates volume delivery.

MODES OF VENTILATION

Assist/Control (A/CMV) Ventilation

In A/CMV ventilation, all breaths are mandatory. Inspiration is patient or time triggered. Patient triggering can be either by flow or by pressure. The set rate establishes the minimum breath rate. The breath can be volume control, pressure control, or VTPC. Inspiration normally ends as follows:

- Volume breaths are time cycled.
- Pressure breaths are time cycled.
- VTPC breaths are time cycled.

Synchronized Intermittent Mandatory Ventilation (SIMV)

In SIMV the set breath rate establishes the maximum mandatory breath rate. The patient can breathe spontaneously between mandatory breaths. Mandatory breaths can be volume control or pressure control or VTPC. The mandatory breath is time or patient triggered and volume cycled (volume-targeted breaths) or time cycled (pressure-targeted breaths).

The baseline is the set PEEP/CPAP level. Spontaneous breaths in volume- or pressure-targeted SIMV can be supported with pressure support (Psupport) or set at zero Psupport. If zero is set, the ventilator actually delivers 1.5 cm H_2O of pressure above the set P_{base} during spontaneous inspiration to provide a low flow of gas to the patient for breath triggering.

If Psupport is set, the ventilator delivers the software-optimized flow (see Sloping, described earlier) to achieve the set pressure change. Inspiratory flow ends when one of three criteria occurs:

- The patient stops demanding flow (flow decays to the flow cycling-off threshold).
- The pressure rises above the PS target pressure level plus a small time-varied margin.
- The inspiratory time reaches a maximum value (2 seconds for adults, 1.2 seconds for pediatric/infant patients).

If VTPC is selected, spontaneous breaths are volume targeted and pressure supported (VTPS), as described previously. In this case, the maximum target pressure is less than or equal to P_{limit} for both the VTPC mandatory breaths and the VTPS breaths. The distinguishing feature between these breaths is that VTPC breaths are time cycled, and VTPS breaths are flow cycled. (NOTE: The nonsupported spontaneous breath type is not available when VTPC is selected. Only A/CMV, SIMV, and SPONT VTPS are available.)

Spontaneous (SPONT) Mode

When SPONT is selected, the operator sets the F_IO_2, PEEP/CPAP, Psupport or V_T, and P_{limit} (VTPS), sloping, expiratory cycle criteria, and trigger sensitivity for patient-triggered breaths. The patient's spontaneous efforts determine the rate, flow, volume, and cycling of each breath except for VTPS breaths. VTPS can be used in the SPONT mode (see previous discussion of VTPS).

Noninvasive Ventilation (NIV)

Noninvasive ventilation is available with the e500 and allows for patient ventilation using a mask or device as an interface. NIV is accessed through the extended features menu.

When activated, NIV provides leak compensation with a bias flow (range, 3 to 15 L/min for adults, 3 to 8 L/min for pediatric/infant patients). The bias flow is activated by turning on the LEAK COMP feature. If there is no leak, bias flow remains at 3 L/min. The bias flow is able to manage leaks up to 25 L/min.[4]

When the automatic slope rise feature is used with NIV, it tailors the inspiratory flow to meet the needs of a patient breathing through a mask rather than an endotracheal or tracheostomy tube.

(NOTE: During NIV, the low minute volume alarm can be turned off.)

Backup Ventilation (BUV)

When the ventilator detects that the low minute ventilation alarm setting has been violated, BUV begins. The BACK-UP VENT indicator blinks, and the message window displays BACK UP VENTILATION. If the current mode is volume- or pressure-targeted A/CMV or SIMV or volume-targeted pressure control A/CMV or SIMV, the ventilator uses the current control panel settings except for the respiratory rate. The rate increases to 1.5 times the current setting, or 15 breaths/min minimum and 100 breaths/min maximum.

For the SPONT breath type, the ventilator delivers pressure-targeted breaths with the following settings: P_{limit} (target pressure), 15 cm H_2O above the current PEEP/CPAP setting; T_I, 1 second for adults, 0.6 second for pediatric/infant patients; and respiratory rate, 12 breaths/min for adults, 20 breaths/min for pediatric/infant patients.

The normal ventilation settings resume when the patient's minute ventilation rises to the low minute volume alarm setting plus 10%.

SPECIAL FEATURE: NEWPORT e500 GRAPHIC DISPLAY MONITOR

The graphic display monitor (GDM) is designed for use with the Newport e500 ventilator (see Figure 12-84; Figure 12-88). The GDM connects to the ventilator via a serial communication interface. The GDM receives power from the ventilator when the e500 is connected to an AC power source. (NOTE: The GDM switches off during battery operation to conserve power.)

The GDM uses pressure and flow signals from the e500 to produce real-time graphics of pressure, volume, and flow measured by the ventilator. The screen is touch sensitive and allows the operator to select a waveform or loop to display in addition to offering freeze screen with cursor, scaling and autoscaling, reference loops, overtracing of loops, trends, and printing features (right column controls). In addition to the control features, a row of measured and calculated numeric data is displayed at the bottom of the screen (see Figure 12-88). Three predetermined sets of numeric data plus the extended functions settings are available. The "basic set" is normally displayed on power-up. A separate screen allows viewing of all the numeric values on one screen. It is accessed through selection of the NUMERIC button.

Setting Up the Graphic Display Monitor

To set up the GDM, select the SETUP button. The following can be set: date, time, patient information, units of measure, units of weight, breath averaging, slope/rise, manual or automated, and expiratory threshold manual or automatic, tachypnea alarm, and noninvasive ventilation. Some of these features are located in the extended functions menu. To set these variables, the operator performs the following:

1. Touches the desired item to be set up
2. Selects the value (keypad or alpha keys)
3. Presses ENTER to update

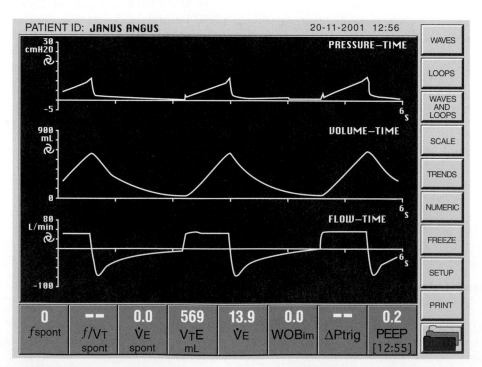

FIGURE 12-88 Newport e500 graphic display monitor screen. (See text for further description.) (Courtesy Newport Medical Instruments, Costa Mesa, Calif.)

To view the set-up parameters, the operator touches the SETUP button, and the current settings are displayed. To exit without changing any date, the operator can press ENTER or touch any command button at the right edge of the screen.

Waveforms and Loops

Pressure, volume, and flow scalars and volume-pressure and flow-volume loops can be selected for display. The screen can feature three scalars and two loops simultaneously. The FREEZE function suspends current plotting of graphs and holds the current display for extended viewing (FREEZE/START button). When FREEZE is on, a green vertical dashed cursor appears in the center of the screen. Left and right touch-sensitive arrow buttons allow the cursor to be moved. Numeric values are displayed for each point on a waveform or loop intersected by the cursor.

In addition to freezing a screen for reviewing, the GDM allows a reference loop to be saved. Touching LOOP and then REFERENCE LOOPS MENU accesses this function. A loop can be stored in memory and later used for comparison with other loops to evaluate changes in patient lung characteristics, for example, after bronchodilator therapy. Active loops can also be displayed overlying previous loops. The One Touch feature automatically plots and freezes a quasi-static volume-pressure curve when the operator performs a manual slow inflation maneuver. The movable cursor allows for estimation of lower and upper inflection points on the curve.

Trends functions can save up to 24 hours of selected trending parameters. The two trends screens can display the following:

TREND (SCREEN) 1
V_TE/flow, $\dot{V}_E$/time, f_{tot}/time, % leak/time
TREND (SCREEN) 2
P_{peak}/time, P_{mean}/time, P_{base}/time, f/V_T spont/time

TROUBLESHOOTING

The alarms and indicators on the front panel can help the operator solve most problems that might occur during operation. In addition, the operator's manual provides regular users with a symptom-driven table that identifies common problems, along with possible causes and solutions. For example, if a POWER FAILURE alarm sounds, any of the following might be the problem: disconnected power cord, open fuse, loss of AC power, battery completely discharged, or hardware failure. If checking the fuses and power sources does not correct the problem, the user should contact a qualified service technician.

A few troubleshooting situations are reviewed here:

1. If a Device Alert alarm occurs, the emergency intake/relief valve opens. If a bacterial filter is not in use, the inspiratory gas line of the patient circuit may be exposed to expiratory gas and its potential contaminants. Clean and sterilize the inspiratory gas delivery system after this event.

2. If monitored values for exhaled flows or volumes differ from set values, the flow sensor screen may be dirty or not calibrated correctly or a leak may be present in the circuit.

3. When monitored F_IO_2 values do not match set values, the oxygen or air pressure source(s) may be too low or a leak may be present in the pneumatic system for F_IO_2 monitoring.

4. If a HIGH BASELINE PRESSURE alarm message is present and the PATIENT indicator flashes, this means the measured baseline pressure has been greater than or equal to 5 cm H_2O above the set PEEP/CPAP for two consecutive breaths. Check the breathing circuit for kinks or obstructions. Evaluate the ventilator settings, and make any necessary adjustments.

5. An I:E RATIO INVERSE VIOLATION alarm occurs (OPERATOR indicator flashes) when ventilator settings (t_I, f, flow, V_T) would result in an inverse I:E ratio greater than 4:1. The ventilator will not permit an I:E ratio greater than 4:1. The operator should be sure to check flow, t_I, frequency, and so on.

6. When an INSP TIME TOO LONG alarm sounds and the OPERATOR indicator flashes, the ventilator settings have resulted in an inspiratory time longer than 5 seconds. Check and correct the V_T, flow, f, t_I, and pause settings.

7. An inspiratory time less than 0.1 second, excluding any pause or inspiratory hold, is not permitted. An INSP TIME TOO SHORT alarm indicates this condition. Evaluate and readjust V_T and flow settings as needed.

8. A PROX LINE DISCONNECT alarm (PATIENT indicator flashing) occurs when the ventilator outlet pressure is higher than the measured proximal pressure and the proximal pressure is near zero. Check the proximal pressure line connection and the patient to be sure the patient circuit is not disconnected or leaking. The ventilator will continue to ventilate the patient and monitors the ventilator via the ventilator outlet pressure rather than the proximal pressure line.

9. A SUSTAINED HIGH BASELINE PRESSURE alarm (PATIENT indicator flashing) means an obstructed or kinked breathing circuit, a restricted or defective exhalation valve, or a malfunctioning exhalation system. The monitored baseline pressure has been greater than or equal to 8 cm H_2O above the set PEEP/CPAP for longer than 6 seconds (pediatric/infant patient) or 10 seconds (adults).

The ventilator opens the emergency intake/relief and exhalation valves. The practitioner should provide alternative ventilation for the patient. Check the patient circuit for kinks or obstructions. Make sure the exhalation valve is functioning properly, and replace the exhalation filter if necessary. Evaluate ventilator settings, and make appropriate adjustments. If the alarm recurs, remove the ventilator from service and provide another means of ventilation to the patient. Contact a qualified service representative.

10. When the VENTILATION SUSPENDED message appears and no alarm is heard, the ventilator detects a circuit disconnect, and the SUCTION DISCONNECT FUNCTION is enabled. The ventilator will resume normal operation when it detects that the circuit is reconnected or when 3 minutes elapse, whichever happens first. The alarm will resume after 1 minute.

The e500 GDM monitor and the e500 ventilator are protected from common electromagnetic environments.

However, the e500 may be adversely affected by some high-frequency surgical devices or radiofrequency-transmitting devices, such as cell phones, cordless phones, and citizen band radios. The ventilator and monitor should not be used near magnetic resonance imaging (MRI) equipment.

Because ventilators can be updated and new features can be added, users of the Newport e500 should defer to the manufacturer's operating manual for the unit they are using for final determination of ventilator function.*

KEY POINTS

▶ The Newport e500 requires an electrical power source and a high-pressure gas source for operation.

▶ A proximal pressure connecter is used to monitor proximal airway pressure.

▶ When a patient has a high inspiratory flow demand, the e500 will provide up to 180 L/min flow for adults and up to 100 L/min of flow for pediatric/infant patients.

▶ The results of the leak test and compliance compensation values are not saved if the ventilator is turned off.

▶ Leak compensation helps minimize the chance of autotriggering.

▶ A reading of "- -" during an attempt to measure the plateau pressure means the ventilator was unable to obtain a stable reading.

▶ During auto-PEEP measurement, when a stable reading is obtained, the total PEEP (auto-PEEP plus set PEEP) is shown in the P_{base} display.

▶ Setting a parameter outside of the available range causes the OPERATOR indicator to blink, an audible alarm to sound, and the message window to describe which parameter is out of range.

▶ The ventilator will not permit an I:E ratio greater than 4:1.

▶ When the ventilator outlet pressure is higher than the measured proximal pressure, a PROX LINE DISCONNECT alarm occurs.

ASSESSMENT QUESTIONS

See Evolve Resources for the answers.

1. Which of the following statements is/are true when an external battery is used to power the Newport e500 ventilator?
   a. The amount of charge time remaining on the external battery is displayed on the charge indicator bar.
   b. The external battery icon illuminates.
   c. The CHARGING indicator illuminates.
   d. The e500 cannot use an external battery source.

2. When the MANUAL INFLATION button is pressed, it will:
   a. Deliver a breath as long as it is pressed (up to 5 seconds)
   b. *Not* deliver a manual breath in the spontaneous mode
   c. *Not* provide a slow inflation breath
   d. Deliver a breath at the set ventilator parameters

3. Which of the following statements is/are true regarding flow delivery in the e500 ventilator?
   I. During a pressure breath, flow delivery depends on patient demand.
   II. Two flow waveform patterns are available with volume breaths, square and descending.
   III. The available flow depends on the patient size selected.
   IV. During pressure breaths, flow is determined by the value set on the flow control.
   a. I only
   b. II and IV only
   c. I, II, and III only
   d. II, III, and IV only

4. When the e500 ventilator is turned on:
   a. The default values for ventilator parameters become active
   b. The last ventilator parameters used are available in memory for use
   c. The ventilator automatically goes into a new patient set-up mode
   d. All display windows read "- -" and require setting

---

* Newport Medical released the e360 ventilator in the United States in 2006. Information on this product is available on the company's Web site at www.newportnmi.com.

ASSESSMENT QUESTIONS—cont'd

5. To provide sloping (ramping) of a pressure breath on the e500:
   I. The operator uses the % rise time feature
   II. A slope control is adjusted from 1 to 19 (minimum slope/maximum slope)
   III. Flow is adjusted by the ventilator to provide automatic sloping (rise) for every breath
   IV. The operator enters the setup screen and selects inspiratory ramp
   a. II and III
   b. IV
   c. I and II
   d. II and IV

6. The F_IO_2 display in the monitored data section of the e500 displays "- -" under which of the following circumstances?
   a. The oxygen supply pressure is below acceptable limits.
   b. The ventilator is connected to oxygen only and the F_IO_2 is set at 100%.
   c. The oxygen sensor needs to be calibrated.
   d. The oxygen sensor is disconnected, defective, or has not calibrated since power-up.

7. The PRESET VENT SETTINGS control on the e500:
   a. Can only be accessed when the ventilator is powered on
   b. Is normally used to adjust current breath and mode parameters
   c. Should be used to set breath type and mode parameters for patient safety
   d. Is the first window to appear when the ventilator is turned on

8. During VTPC assist/control ventilation, the message window displays the message VOL TARGET NOT MET, and an audible alarm sounds. What is one control the respiratory therapist could adjust to correct the problem?
   a. Set V_T
   b. P_{limit}
   c. Set pressure
   d. Baseline pressure

9. An INSP TIME TOO SHORT alarm occurs during ventilation of a patient. The respiratory therapist should:
   a. Review and readjust V_T and flow settings as needed
   b. Increase the upper pressure limit
   c. Check for an obstruction in the circuit
   d. Evaluate the patient for hiccups

10. A SUSTAINED HIGH BASELINE PRESSURE message appears, an audible alarm sounds, and the PATIENT indicator is flashing. A possible cause of this problem might be:
    a. The set PEEP/CPAP is higher than the PEEP/CPAP upper pressure limit
    b. The operator has tried to set the baseline pressure higher than the available range for the patient size
    c. There is a kink in the patient circuit or a possible obstruction in the exhalation valve
    d. The patient is having a severe coughing episode

References

1. Newport Medical Instruments: Operating manual, Newport e500 Wave ventilator, OPR500 revision A, version 1.5, Costa Mesa, Calif, 2001, Newport.
2. Newport Medical Instruments: Operating/service manual, Newport e500 GDM graphic display monitor, OPRGDM 1900 revision B, Costa Mesa, Calif, 2001, Newport.
3. Miller C, director of clinical education, Newport Medical Instruments: Personal communication, June 2006, Newport Beach, Calif.
4. Miller C: Automatic leak compensation in the e500 ventilator, *Respir Ther* 1:53, 2006.

Internet Resources
www.newportnmi.com
www.ventilators.com

PURITAN BENNETT VENTILATORS

PURITAN BENNETT 840

OUTLINE

OBJECTIVES

Upon completion of this section, you will be able to:

· Explain the three primary functions of the expiratory filter.
· Identify a situation in which the battery has become operational in the backup power source.
· Describe how a short self-test (SST) is run by the operator.
· List the tests performed during SST.
· Analyze a problem in ventilator cycling during pressure-support ventilation (PSV).
· Provide a definition of the parameter settings in the lower screen.
· List the information contained in the upper screen.
· Describe the indicator lights on the Status Indicator Panel and the Breath Delivery Unit.
· Compare the vertical and horizontal adjustments on the available waveforms and loops.
· Identify the potential causes of problems during measurement of respiratory mechanics.
· Explain the function of rise time percent and expiratory sensitivity.
· Define the modes of ventilation available, including trigger, limit, and cycle parameters.
· Contrast the function of the expiratory valve during pressure-control (PC) and volume-control (VC) ventilation.
· Define PAV+.
· Explain the setup and operation of PAV+.
· Describe volume runaway during PAV+.
· Compare apnea ventilation with safety ventilation.

KEY TERMS

BiLevel ventilation
Extended self-test (EST)
Power on self-test (POST)

Proportional assist ventilation plus (PAV+)
Short self-test (SST)

Volume control plus (VC+)

The Puritan Bennett 840 ventilator (Figure 12-89) is owned and manufactured by Covidien (Mansfield, Massachusetts).[1-4] In 2007, Covidien separated from Tyco Healthcare, the company that previously owned Puritan Bennett. The Puritan Bennett ventilator line moved with Covidien and has relocated from Pleasanton, California, to Boulder, Colorado.

The 840 is designed to ventilate neonatal, pediatric, and adult patients and is most commonly used in the acute care setting. The ventilator includes a breath delivery unit (BDU) that controls ventilation and connects to the patient circuit. Above the BDU is a liquid crystal display (LCD) touch-sensitive interface screen. The screen, called the *graphic user interface* (GUI), displays monitored patient data and ventilator settings and information.

POWER SOURCE

The 840 is both electrically and pneumatically powered. It is electrically powered by a 120-volt AC current. The on/off switch is located on the center front of the BDU. A green indicator adjacent to the switch lights up when the unit is

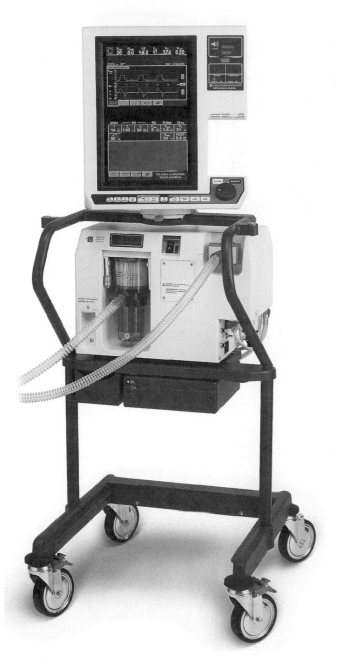

FIGURE 12-89 Puritan Bennett 840 ventilator, showing the graphic user interface and the breath delivery unit. (See text for description.) (Courtesy Puritan Bennett, a division of Covidien, Mansfield, Mass.)

The indicator for the battery or backup power source (BPS) is located in the upper right-hand portion of the front panel in the status indicator section. A yellow light indicates that the BPS is operating and the AC power is off or inadequate. A green light indicates that the ventilator is operating and the BPS has at least 2 minutes of charge available.

Battery charging indicators are located on the BPS panel itself, below the breath delivery unit. When the ventilator is operating on main power, the top BPS charging indicator (the green indicator next to the gray battery icon) shows that the BPS is fully charged. When the bottom yellow indicator (next to the gray battery icon) is illuminated, the BPS is still charging.

fier. It is intended for emergency power if AC power is lost or falls below an acceptable minimum. Keeping the ventilator plugged into an AC outlet when not in use charges the backup battery (Box 12-66).

Patient Circuit

The patient circuit includes a main inspiratory line, patient connector, and main expiratory line connected to an internally mounted exhalation valve. There are inspiratory and expiratory filters as well. The expiratory filter is heated and comes with a collector vial for liquid condensate from exhaled gas. The filter can be autoclaved for cleaning. The ventilator periodically checks the resistance through this filter during the short self-test.

Compressor

A separate compressor can be purchased for the unit. It can provide up to 200 L/min of flow and a minute ventilation of 50 L/min on room air. The compressor is attached to the ventilator by a high-pressure air hose, data communication cable, and electrical power cord. However, even if the compressor is attached, when the ventilator high-pressure air connector is attached to wall or cylinder air, the ventilator switches to the wall air source.

Indicators for the compressor are located in the Status Indicator Panel (SIP) in the upper right section of the GUI (Figure 12-90). There are two indicators for the compressor: READY and ON. When the green light is illuminated next to the READY indicator, the compressor is available. When the green light is on next to the ON indicator, the compressor is supplying air to the ventilator.

Self-Tests

Self-tests on the 840 include the **power on self-test (POST), extended self-test (EST),** and **short self-test (SST).** For any self-test, *the ventilator must be disconnected from the patient,* and the Y-connector must be uncapped. The POST runs automatically to check the microprocessor when the ventilator is powered on. The EST is a more

turned on. (NOTE: To turn the unit off, simply flip the switch to off; no additional action is required.) The unit also has a backup battery power source. It is pneumatically powered by two gas sources, compressed air and oxygen (35- to 100-psig sources). The unit is intended for use with these two gases only.

Battery

The 840 has an internal backup battery (802 backup power source), which provides power to the BDU and screen but does not power the compressor (optional) or the humidi-

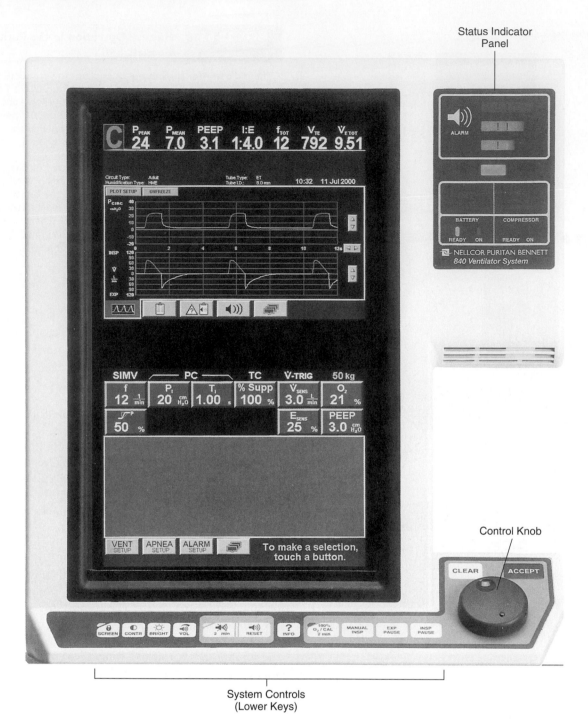

FIGURE 12-90 Puritan Bennett 840 graphic interface unit (GIU) with the DualView screens, status indicator panel, lower row of system control keys, and the control knob. (Courtesy Puritan Bennett, a division of Covidien, Mansfield, Mass.)

extensive test and generally is run by a qualified service technician.

The SST takes 3 minutes and verifies proper ventilator operation, checks the patient circuit for leaks, measures circuit compliance and resistance, and checks the exhalation filter resistance. The SST should be run when a new circuit or humidifier is added, between patient uses, and at least every 15 days during use. The SST can only be run immediately after the ventilator is turned on. Box 12-67

provides further instructions. After the SST is complete, the operator can begin normal ventilation by touching EXIT SST and then ACCEPT. The ventilator reruns the POST and then displays the start-up screen.

CONTROLS AND ALARMS

The controls and alarms are managed by the graphic user interface.

BOX 12-67	Performing the Short Self-Test (SST) on the Puritan Bennett 840

When the START UP screen is displayed, the SST selection is pressed. (NOTE: The operator must be sure the patient connector is not capped, or the ventilator will go into SAFETY BACK-UP VENTILATION.) The operator must then press the TEST button on the side of the ventilator within 5 seconds. Waiting longer cancels SST.

When the CURRENT SST SETUP screen appears, the patient circuit is selected (i.e., adult, pediatric, or infant). Then the humidifier type is selected (i.e., HME [heat and moisture exchanger], nonheated expiratory tube, or heated expiratory tube). The operator sets the humidifier volume when applicable. Pressing ACCEPT begins the SST, and the screen provides instructions to the operator as it is being preformed. (NOTE: The operator must pay special attention to the messages in the lower right corner of the bottom screen. For example, part of the test requires connecting and disconnecting parts of the circuit and capping the patient's Y-connector.)

After the test, the screen provides an alert about the ventilator's status. Should an error occur, a review of the operator's manual can help determine the procedure that needs to be followed. The operator's manual provides a table listing SST outcomes and how to proceed in each case.

BOX 12-68	A Spray of Particles (Puritan Bennett 840)

During a patient disconnect on earlier ventilators (e.g., the Puritan Bennett 7200), the loss of pressure in the circuit when PEEP was used resulted in the ventilator trying to compensate for the pressure drop. These ventilators produced a continuous surge of flow through the circuit to try to maintain pressure. The rapid flow would hit the water typically condensed in the circuit and create an aerosol, which was then released into the patient's room. This posed a risk of everyone in the vicinity inhaling these potentially contaminated particles.

Graphic User Interface (GUI)

The graphic user interface has three basic sections: a Dual-View touch-sensitive screen, the status indicator section (upper right portion), and the control function keys and control knob along the bottom of the unit below the touch screen.

DualView Screen

The DualView touch-sensitive screen (see Figure 12-90) is divided into two sections. The upper screen displays patient data in both digital and waveform formats. The lower screen shows the actual settings, provides an information and instruction area, and also has the SandBox. The SandBox allows the therapist to select several changes at one time and view these before they are actually activated.

Upper Screen

The upper screen holds patient information only and displays four areas: patient data, alarms and ventilator status, miscellaneous data, and graphics (see Figure 12-90). No ventilator settings can be changed in this area.

The patient data at the very top of the GUI are provided in abbreviations. (NOTE: $P_{E\ END}$ is displayed as PEEP on updated units.) The patient data area gives information about monitored parameters such as total breath rate, inspiratory to expiratory (I:E) ratio, tidal volumes, positive end-expiratory pressure (PEEP), and minute volume. The manufacturer occasionally uses abbreviations that may be unfamiliar to the practitioner. Fortunately, these can be defined immediately by touching and holding the abbreviation for the information needed. The full definition appears in a field at the bottom left corner of the lower screen. This disappears when the abbreviation is no longer being touched by the operator.

Below the monitored patient data on the top of the upper screen is a section that displays alarm messages when they occur. Alarms are grouped together by conditions that cause them and are accompanied by the help message, along with some suggestions for remedying the problem. For example, the CIRCUIT DISCONNECT alarm suggestions are NO VENTILATION, CHECK PATIENT, and RECONNECT CIRCUIT. These appear in red, and an audible, high priority alarm sounds simultaneously. A digital timer indicates the accumulated time of the nonventilation period. During this alarm message, the gas flow in the circuit is reduced to 5 L/min. This is an IDLE mode. The reduction in flow helps prevent a spray of aerosolized particles (Box 12-68).

The alarm display section can list the two highest priority alarms at any time. Any others that might be present are displayed in another section called MORE ALARMS in the MISCELLANEOUS window (more on that later).

Below the ALARMS window is the graphics display area, which typically monitors waveforms such as pressure-time and flow-time scalars. Additional graphs and loops are available below the display screen in a row of five icons (see Figure 12-90). These include:

- Waveforms
- More information (a clipboard)
- Alarm log (a triangle and clipboard with a picture of a speaker)
- More alarms (picture of a speaker)
- Other screens (picture of screens)

The WAVEFORM icon is the control that allows access to other scalars and loops. Under the more information CLIPBOARD are data not commonly displayed at the top of the screen, such as the spontaneous minute volume and measured oxygen percentage. The ALARM LOG icon displays the last 80 alarm events. The data displayed in this section are deleted when a new patient is set up for ventilation. The MORE ALARMS icon displays active alarms not included in the upper alarm message section, near the top of the screen,

TABLE 12-37

Other Screens for Upper Data Window—Puritan Bennett 840

Diagnostic Code Log	Extensive History of Last 80 Alarms and the Results of the EST Test
Ventilator Configuration	Serial number and software version for the ventilator
Installed options	List of installed options available
Operational Time Log	Compressor time and total ventilator operation time
Test Summary	Displays last short self-test (SST) and extended self-test (EST)
SST Results	Results of each test performed in SST

TABLE 12-38

Four Function Keys on the Lower Screen—Puritan Bennett 840

Function Key	Description
Vent Setup	Used to activate the SandBox and make several changes at one time. Changes will not activate until the Accept key is touched.
Apnea Setup	Allows changes to be made for the apnea ventilation mode, such as pressure or volume ventilation, tidal volume or set pressure, flow or inspiratory time (or I:E), flow waveform, oxygen percentage, and apnea interval.
Alarm Setup	Shows actual values of a parameter and adjustable values on a bar graph scale. Alarms are automatically set up based on the patient's entered ideal body weight information but can be adjusted.
Other Screens	Communication set-up for communicating with external devices and print set-up
	Time/Date changes
	More settings: Humidifier type, O_2 sensor enable/disable, and Dsens (disconnect sensitivity)

that displays the two highest priority alarms. Finally, the OTHER SCREENS icon allows access to the items in Table 12-37.

Lower Screen

The lower screen has five areas: the primary settings, the SandBox, the set-up keys, the symbol definition area, and the prompt area.

The primary settings appear at the top of this screen and are the current set parameters. They may include the trigger sensitivity, mode, mandatory rate, and volume, depending on the mode being used.

Below this is the subscreen area, which is accessed when the operator wants to change the mode or several settings all at one time. This is the SandBox, which allows changes to be made without the changes becoming active until the ACCEPT key is pressed. The available ventilator modes for the 840 are reviewed in a later section. (NOTE: Newer versions of 840 software allow batch changes to be made in the primary settings area as well.)

In the lower right corner is the Prompt area. It displays information to guide the operator in the use of ventilator functions. In Figure 12-90 the prompt area reads, "To make a selection touch a button," meaning a *screen button*. To the left of the prompt area is a row of four screen buttons: VENT SETUP, APNEA SETUP, ALARM SETUP, and MORE SCREENS. Table 12-38 provides information about these four functions.

Status Indicator Panel

The Status Indicator Panel, a separate panel to the right of the upper touch screen, provides information about the status of alarm indicators, ventilator inoperative condition, safety valve open, battery status, and compressor status.

Alarm indicators show the level of alarm priority. High level alarms are indicated by the symbol "!!!", which is displayed in red, blinks rapidly, and emits a tone during a high priority alarm situation. A medium alarm ("!!") is displayed in yellow, beeps three times, and blinks slowly if active. A low priority alarm "!" is a steady yellow light, and the alert gives a two-tone alert.

The VENT INOP indicator indicates that the unit cannot ventilate the patient and must be taken out of service. The safety valve open (SVO) means that only a spontaneously breathing patient can breathe room air through this valve. During a VENT INOP condition, the operator must find an alternative method of ventilating the patient until the unit can be replaced.

System Controls Lower Keys

The touch keys across the bottom of the GUI, just below the lower touch screen, serve several important functions. From left to right they are:

1. The SCREEN LOCK key—Appears yellow when the screen is in the locked position. When it is locked, touching the screen has no effect on the ventilator's function; this prevents accidental changes in settings and displays and allows for cleaning of the screen. The screen can be unlocked by touching the control again. The screen automatically unlocks during alarm conditions.

2. The DISPLAY CONTRAST key and the DISPLAY BRIGHTNESS key—Alter contrast and brightness in the original black and white screen, but have no function with the color GUI and are nonfunctional in newer versions of the GUI display.

3. The ALARM VOLUME key—Changes the alarm volume when the operator holds down this key and turns the control knob.

4. The 2 MIN ALARM SILENCE key—Turns green and produces a 2-minute alarm silence period when touched. It is reactivated in three conditions:

- When the 2 minutes elapse
- If the ALARM RESET key is pressed
- If a new high urgency alarm condition occurs

5. The RESET alarm key—(1) Clears active alarms, (2) clears autoreset high urgency alarms so that they are no longer illuminated, (3) cancels an active alarm silence, and (4) records any active alarms in the unit's memory. However, a DEVICE ALERT alarm cannot be reset because of the danger to the patient (more about these alerts later).

6. The QUESTION MARK (?) key—Displays basic operating information about the ventilator in the upper display window.

7. The 100% O$_2$/CAL 2 MIN key—Delivers 100% oxygen for 2 minutes when the ventilator is connected to an oxygen source; it lights up green during this period. Pressing it again restarts the 2-minute interval.

8. The MANUAL INSPIRATION key—Delivers a manually triggered breath based on the current mandatory settings. To prevent breath stacking, it can be activated only during the latter part of a mandatory exhalation.

9. The EXPIRATORY PAUSE key—Used to estimate the end-expiratory pressure and auto-PEEP (Box 12-69).

10. The INSPIRATORY PAUSE key—Used to estimate the end-inspiratory pressure. Pressing and holding this key pause inspiration for up to 8 seconds. This freezes the pressure-time waveform and shows the value for the plateau pressure (PPL), compliance (C), and resistance (R).

At the far right of the row of keys is the control knob. This is used to adjust the values for a setting, such as tidal volume. Once a parameter has been selected for change, touching the screen button for that item on the lower screen highlights the button. When the button is highlighted, turning the control knob clockwise increases the value, and turning it counterclockwise decreases the value. Instructions appear in the lower right corner. Adjacent to the knob are two touch pads. The CLEAR pad clears the change. The ACCEPT pad accepts the new setting, and thereafter the ventilator operates using the new setting.

Breath Delivery Unit (BDU) Indicators

Besides the normal status indicator screen, indicators are located on the front of the breath delivery unit (see Figure 12-89). These illuminate red under serious conditions. The left indicator is a VENTILATOR INOPERATIVE indicator; when active, it cannot be reset. The ventilator must be taken out of service and another method of ventilating the patient provided. The middle alert is SAFETY VALVE OPEN (SVO), which indicates that the patient is able to breathe room air spontaneously. This happens if the ventilator is inoperative, in which case the valve opens automatically. The right indicator alerts to a loss of the GUI. When it illuminates red, a malfunction is present in the GUI and the information displayed is unreliable. The ventilator must be taken out of service.

Alarms

The manufacturer refers to the alarm system as the Smart-Alert system. The ventilator is equipped with the normal alarms, such as high pressure, high and low tidal volume, high rate, prolonged inspiratory time, high and low oxygen percentage, apnea, power loss, and circuit disconnect. When these occur, a description of the alarm condition and possible remedies for the problem appear in the monitored data screen. The operator's manual provides a complete description of the available alarms.

An APNEA ALARM occurs when a patient's inspiratory efforts are not detected after a timed apnea period. The ventilator goes into apnea ventilation (AV), and the AV screen is displayed. To resume normal ventilation, the operator presses the RESET button. Normal ventilation will also resume after the patient takes two spontaneous breaths.

The DEVICE ALERT indicates that a background check detects a problem; this is a serious situation. The ventilator will reset only when an EST is run and passed.

When a PROCEDURE ERROR is detected, the ventilator begins SAFETY VENTILATION. For example, a procedure error occurs if a patient is attached to the ventilator before the set-up process is complete. In this case, the PROCEDURE ERROR alarm activates the SAFETY VENTILATION function. A procedure error also occurs if power is removed from the ventilator for 5 minutes or longer.

Safety ventilation consists of pressure-control mandatory breaths with a set pressure of 10 cm H$_2$O, a rate of 16 breaths/min, an inspiratory time of 1 second, a fractional

---

BOX 12-69	Expiratory Pause Key Function (Puritan Bennett 840)

The EXPIRATORY PAUSE key is pressed to activate expiratory pause. When the key is pressed, the ventilator waits until the end of the next mandatory inspiration and then closes the patient circuit. Closing the circuit involves closing the inspiratory and expiratory valves. An expiratory pause maneuver is started.

For an automatic pause (the key is pressed and released), the ventilator performs the pause, waits until the pressure in the circuit stabilizes, and then takes a reading. An automatic pause lasts 0.5 to 3 seconds.

For a manual pause (the key is pressed and held), the ventilator takes its measurement as soon as the pressure stabilizes or the pause ends. The pause cannot last longer than 20 seconds, at which time the patient circuit automatically opens. The manual pause is recommended for patients with suspected air trapping (auto-PEEP).

The graphics are displayed on the screen to allow visualization of pressure stabilization. Of course, the expiratory pause cannot be performed if the patient is making any ventilatory efforts, or the pressure will not be able to stabilize. At the end of the maneuver, the values for intrinsic or auto-PEEP (PEEP$_I$) and for total PEEP (PEEP$_{TOT}$ = set PEEP + [PEEP$_I$]) are displayed.

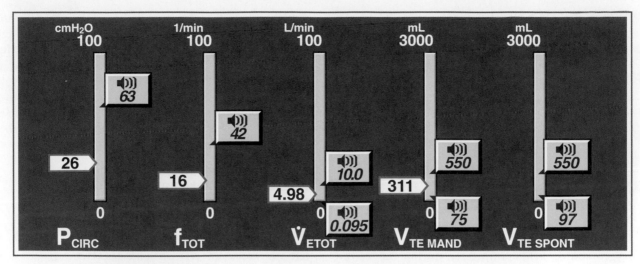

FIGURE 12-91 Puritan Bennett 840 alarm setup screen, which appears in the lower panel. Touching the ALARM icon and turning the control knob adjust the alarm level. The arrows to the left of the bars indicate the current value for that parameter. (See text for description.) (Courtesy Puritan Bennett, a division of Covidien, Mansfield, Mass.)

inspired oxygen concentration (F$_I$O$_2$) of 1, and a PEEP of 3 cm H$_2$O.

To set the alarm limits, the operator selects the alarm screen (ALARM SETUP button, lower screen). A window opens showing bar graphs, which indicate the current settings of the alarms and the measured value for the parameters (Figure 12-91). To change an alarm setting, the operator presses the desired alarm screen icon. (NOTE: This icon is shaped like a box containing a speaker.) When the alarm is highlighted, the value is changed with the control knob. Pressing the ACCEPT button activates the changes.

To view the alarm history, the operator selects the ALARM LOG in the monitored patient data screen. To reset the alarms, the operator touches the RESET key in the bottom row of controls, below the viewing screen.

Basic Parameter Changes—Touch, Turn, and Accept

To make ventilator changes, the operator selects a setting or mode on the lower screen. When the desired parameter is on the lower screen, the operator touches it to highlight the item, adjusts the value using the control knob, and presses ACCEPT. The new setting immediately becomes operational.

Starting a New Patient

When the ventilator is turned on, a POST runs, and the start-up screen appears with the following items listed:
- Same patient (use previous settings)
- New patient
- SST

To begin ventilation of a new patient, the operator presses that selection and then is prompted to enter the patient's ideal body weight (IBW). Values for the IBW are available in the operator's manual or can be calculated

BOX 12-70	Calculating Ideal Body Weight[5]

Ideal body weight (IBW) can be estimated in pounds as follows:

For males IBW = 106 + 6[Ht − 60] where *Ht* is the height in inches

For example, for a 5′ 8″ (68″) male: IBW = 106 + 6(68-60) = 106 + 6(8) = 154

To convert to kilograms, divide the weight in pounds (154) by 2.2, 154/2.2 = 70 kg

For females IBW = 105 + 5[Ht − 60] where *Ht* is the height in inches

For example, for a 5′ 6″ (66″) female: IBW = 105 + 5(66-60) = 105 + 5(6) = 135

To convert to kilograms, divide the weight in pounds (135) by 2.2, 135/2.2 = 61.5 kg

(Box 12-70).[5] After entering this information, the operator presses the CONTINUE button to bring up the next screen.

After the IBW has been entered, the operator selects the mode by touching the mode button and using the control knob to scroll through the options. The available modes are assist/control, synchronized intermittent mandatory ventilation (SIMV), spontaneous (SPONT), BiLevel (optional), and PAV+ (optional).

After selecting the mode, the operator chooses the mandatory breath type (volume controlled, volume controlled plus, or pressure controlled), or the spontaneous breath type (pressure support, volume support, or none), where appropriate, and the trigger sensitivity (pressure or flow). When the CONTINUE button is touched, the proposed settings appear in the SandBox (lower screen). The SandBox allows access to the settings available for the mode and breath type selected. Values calculated by the computer based on the entered IBW appear. These values can be accepted or changed by touching the parameter and adjusting the value with the control knob. To begin ventilation once all the settings have been selected, the operator presses the ACCEPT key. The settings can be canceled by pressing the RESTART key.

Apnea Ventilation Screen Adjustment

When the ventilator has been set up and the new patient connected, the unit begins ventilating using the assigned values. The next screen to appear is the APNEA VENTILATION screen. The initial IBW-based parameters are also automatically set in the AV mode. The operator may want to adjust the apnea time interval (TA; range, 10 to 60 seconds).

AV, a backup mode, is activated when the apnea time interval has been exceeded without the ventilator delivering a breath. An AV display appears in the upper panel where the waveforms screen normally appears. The AV display is not an active touch screen. In addition to displaying AV parameters, this screen also displays two messages: how to adjust AV, and how to deactivate the current apnea ventilation state. (NOTE: If the operator touches one of the icons, such as the graphics icon, the APNEA screen disappears.) To deactivate AV, the operator presses the ALARM RESET control. If the patient is still apneic, another alarm alert (!!) occurs. To silence the alarm, the operator presses ALARM SILENCE.

Alarm Limits

The initial alarm limits for the patient are adjusted automatically based on the IBW. However, the operator should check them to make sure they fit the desired values.

Making a Single Parameter Change

To quickly change a single parameter, the operator touches the screen button for the parameter in question. It becomes highlighted, and the breath timing bar appears on the screen (more information is provided in a later section). As the operator turns the control knob, the digitally displayed value of the setting changes. The numbers appear red to indicate that the value is different from the one that is currently active. After the new value has been selected, it is activated by pressing the ACCEPT key.

Breath Timing Bar

The breath timing bar (Figure 12-92) shows the results of parameter setting changes on the I:E ratio. This allows a visual representation of the effects of the changes. For example, in volume ventilation, if the flow is increased, the inspiratory time (T_I) shortens for the same volume and rate (Figure 12-92A). The green indicates the T_I, and the yellow indicates the expiratory time (T_E). (The colors are not shown in the figure.) The actual value in seconds appears inside the bar for both the T_I and T_E. The total cycle time (TCT) is shown at the right end of the bar. The minute

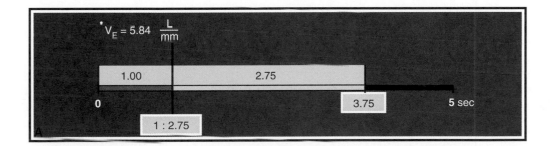

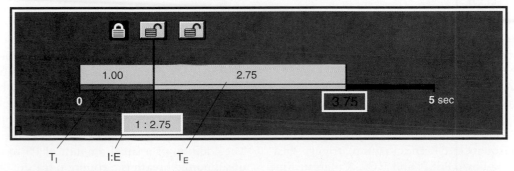

FIGURE 12-92 A, Breath timing bar for volume ventilation with a T_I of 1 second, a T_E of 2.75 seconds, and a TCT of 3.75 seconds on a time line of 5 seconds on a Puritan Bennett 840. The I:E ratio is 1:2.75, and the $\dot{V}_E$ is 5.84 L/min. **B,** Bar for pressure ventilation. Although the values are the same as in **A,** the first lock above the bar is locked; therefore the T_I is constant. (See text for description.) (Courtesy Puritan Bennett, a division of Covidien, Mansfield, Mass.)

CLINICAL ROUNDS 12-27

Breath Timing Bar

Part I

Assume that the current breath timing bar shows T_I = 1.00, T_E = 2.75 with a tidal volume (V_T) of 365 mL, a constant flow of 22 L/min, and a rate (f) of 16 breaths/min. Notice the total cycle time (TCT) is 3.75 seconds ($T_I + T_E$ = TCT). What will be the new values for the T_I and T_E if the flow is increased to 30 L/min?

Part II

During PC ventilation, the T_I is locked; it is 1 second. The rate is 16 breaths/min with a TCT of 3.75 seconds, and the T_E currently is 2.75 seconds. The respiratory rate is changed to 10 breaths/min. What will happen to the T_I, T_E, and TCT? Then the T_I is changed to 2 seconds. Will this change occur with T_I locked?

See Evolve Resources for the answer.

ventilation, based on the set rate and tidal volume, appears above the bar (Clinical Rounds 12-27, Part I).

During pressure ventilation (Figure 12-92B), three icons that look like locks appear above the breath timing bar. The left lock, if activated, keeps the T_I constant. (NOTE: Touching the lock activates it.) Any changes in rate may affect the I:E ratio and T_E, but the T_I remains constant. If the second lock is activated, the I:E ratio becomes constant, and the T_I and T_E can change. The right lock, when activated, keeps the T_E constant, and T_I and I:E ratio vary. A possible reason for fixing the T_E is if some concern exists that the patient might have air trapping and the respiratory therapist wants to make sure that the T_E is long enough for complete exhalation. Clinical Rounds 12-27, Part II, provides an exercise in pressure ventilation with the T_I constant.

MODES OF VENTILATION

Assist/Control

Assist/control (A/C) ventilation is available as volume or pressure targeted. In this mode, all breaths delivered have a preset volume (VC), **volume control plus (VC+),** or preset pressure (PC).

In volume A/C (ACVC), breaths can be either time or patient triggered (pressure or flow), volume limited, and volume cycled (see Chapter 11). The parameters that can be set are the tidal volume (V_T), mandatory rate, peak flow, flow waveform (square or descending ramp), trigger sensitivity (pressure or flow), PEEP, and F_IO_2. A plateau time (T_{PL}) for an inspiratory hold or pause may be selected, as can an upper pressure limit (Pcirc). The expiratory valve is closed during inspiration. This is different from the PC mode in which the expiratory valve floats. A cough results

in a pressure rise in the circuit, and the pressure may go as high as the set maximum pressure limit, at which point inspiratory flow ends.

In VC+, the breath is time or patient triggered (pressure or flow), pressure limited, volume targeted, and time cycled. The parameters set are the V_T, minimum mandatory rate, T_I, F_IO_2, trigger sensitivity (pressure or flow), PEEP, rise time % (sloping), and upper pressure limit; T_I, T_E, or the I:E ratio can be set as a constant (see earlier discussion of the breath timing bar). In VC+, the ventilator delivers a single standard volume test breath with a brief inspiratory pause to determine the relative lung compliance. In subsequent breaths, if the V_T is either higher or lower than the set V_T, the ventilator automatically adjusts the pressure to achieve the set volume. (NOTE: VC+ is similar to pressure-regulated volume control [PRVC], described in Chapter 11.) In VC+, the delivered pressure cannot exceed the upper pressure limit minus 5 cm H_2O. For example, if the upper pressure limit is 45 cm H_2O, the ventilator gives an alert if the pressure reaches 40 cm H_2O. V_T limits also can be set to end a breath if the V_T rises above the set volume end-points. Flow is delivered in a descending wave form, as in any pressure-limited mode.

In pressure A/C ventilation, or PC, the breath is time or patient triggered (pressure or flow), pressure limited, and time cycled. The parameters set are the V_T, minimum mandatory rate, T_I, F_IO_2, trigger sensitivity (pressure or flow), PEEP, rise time % (sloping), and upper pressure limit; T_I, T_E, or the I:E ratio can be set as a constant.

Synchronized Intermittent Mandatory Ventilation (SIMV)

In SIMV, mandatory breaths can be either volume or pressure targeted. These breaths have the same set parameters as in A/C. For the spontaneous breaths, the patient can breathe at a zero baseline or with PEEP/CPAP added. Spontaneous breaths can also be aided with PS or VS. For PS, the additional parameters set are the support pressure (P_{SUPP}), rise time percent (RT %), and expiratory sensitivity (E_{SENS}). (RT % and E_{SENS} are described in the section on special features.)

Spontaneous Mode

A spontaneous mode (SPONT) setting allows the operator to provide the desired F_IO_2, sensitivity, baseline pressure (PEEP/CPAP), rise time %, expiratory sensitivity, and high pressure limit. As in SIMV, spontaneous breaths can be aided with pressure support. When PS is not applied, each spontaneous breath receives pressure support of 1.5 cm H_2O above PEEP to reduce the work of breathing. (NOTE: The addition of a small amount of PS to a spontaneous unsupported breath is a common feature in most current intensive care unit [ICU] ventilators.) Volume support is actually pressure-support ventilation with a volume target. In VS, breaths are patient triggered (flow or pressure), pressure limited, and flow cycled. The ventilator automatically adjusts the pressure limit to achieve the set V_T. As in VC+, the pressure cannot exceed the set upper pressure limit minus 5 cm H_2O. For apnea ventilation, VC or PC with associated parameters must be chosen.

BiLevel Ventilation

BiLevel ventilation is a form of augmented pressure ventilation similar to airway pressure-release ventilation (APRV), described in Chapter 11. The pressure scalar for BiLevel resembles SIMV-PC.

BiLevel allows unrestricted spontaneous ventilation and synchronization of breathing with the patient's inspiratory and expiratory pattern. The operator uses the control knob to select BiLevel as the mode of ventilation. As does APRV, BiLevel provides two levels of PEEP or CPAP, designated $PEEP_H$ for the high level of PEEP (range, 5 to 90 cm H_2O) and $PEEP_L$ for the low level (range, 0 to 45 cm H_2O). $PEEP_L$ must be set at least 5 cm H_2O lower than $PEEP_H$. These two pressures are independent. For example, if $PEEP_L$ is 5 cm H_2O and $PEEP_H$ is 10 cm H_2O, the highest pressure reached is 10 cm H_2O.

The operator also sets the breath rate and the length of time $PEEP_H$ and $PEEP_L$ are applied (T_H and T_L, respectively). For example, if BiLevel is set up to function as APRV, the T_H might be set at 5 seconds and the T_L at 0.8 second.[5-8] T_L levels are targeted to keep the alveoli open. $PEEP_H$ is set to prevent overinflation. Figure 12-93A shows how spontaneous breathing can occur at both levels of PEEP. When no pressure support is set, a spontaneous effort receives 1.5 cm H_2O of pressure to reduce the work of breathing.

In addition, spontaneous breaths can be augmented with pressure support. If the PS level is set higher than $PEEP_H$, the upper portion of the PS breath actually appears above the $PEEP_H$ level (Figure 12-93B). The PS breath can also be seen during T_L, because the T_L is at a longer value in this part of the figure. Box 12-71 lists some of the potential benefits of BiLevel ventilation.

Proportional Assist Ventilation Plus (PAV+)

In **proportional assist ventilation plus (PAV+),** a method of breath delivery,[9] the PAV+ software option provides a specific spontaneous breathing pattern that is intended for use with invasive ventilation of spontaneously breathing

BOX 12-71	Potential Advantages of BiLevel Ventilation[1] (Puritan Bennett 840)

- Increased patient comfort
- Reduced requirement for sedation
- Improved monitoring of all volumes, spontaneous and mandatory
- Prevention of alveolar collapse and overdistention

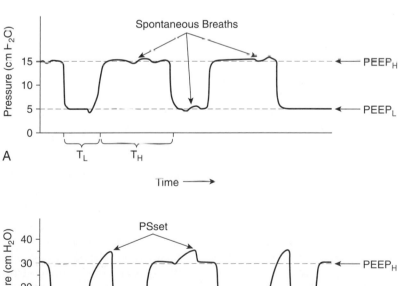

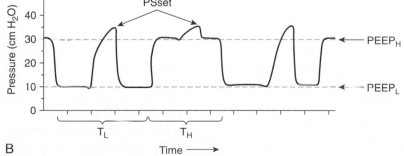

FIGURE 12-93 A, Puritan Bennett 840 pressure-time curve during BiLevel ventilation, showing spontaneous breaths superimposed over $PEEP_H$ and $PEEP_L$ levels. **B,** Set pressure support (PSset) at 35 cm H_2O with PEEPH$_H$ of 30 cm H_2O and $PEEP_L$ of 10 cm H_2O. Notice how PSset is clearly visible in T_L time frames but is superimposed on $PEEP_H$ during the T_H time frames.

BOX 12-72   **Intended Use of PAV+ (Puritan Bennett 840)**

- Adult patient (minimum 25 kg)
- Patient intubated with an endotracheal or tracheostomy tube (6 to 10 mm)
- Circuit and airway free of leaks
- Nonsilicone patient circuits (silicone circuits may cause pressure-flow oscillations, resulting in underestimation of patient resistance)

---

adult patients.* Because this is a relatively new mode of ventilation in the United States, the set-up and use of this mode are reviewed here.

In PAV+, patient efforts and the ventilator combine to perform 100% of the work of breathing. The proportion assist (PA) breath targets a pressure based on the selected percentage of support (% SUPPORT) set by the operator and the flow and volume readings from the patient.

During PAV+, the ventilator pressure increases in proportion to the instantaneously measured inspiratory volume and flow generated by the patient. As long as the patient is able to maintain a stable and adequate ventilatory pattern, PAV+ rhythmically unloads the respiratory muscles, allowing the patient to have a relatively normal breathing pattern. Box 12-72 lists the intended uses of PAV+.

Flow and volume are measured every 5 msec during the inspiratory phase. These measurements, along with ongoing estimates of the patient's resistance and compliance, allow the ventilator to calculate the pressure needed to assist the patient's spontaneous effort. The level of assistance is based on the % SUPPORT setting. If the patient stops breathing, PAV+ also stops.

The PAV+ algorithm uses the estimates of R and C to derive a value for elastance (E; 1/compliance), which must be known for the function of PAV+. However, because the actual resistance and elastance are estimated rather than truly known, overestimations of R and E could result in the ventilator generating more pressure than is needed to ventilate the patient at the desired settings (see the section on troubleshooting).

How PAV+ Works

During PAV+, the ventilator acts as an inspiratory amplifier; that is, it *proportionally* assists the inspiratory muscles. The software for PAV+ is based on the equation of motion (see Chapter 11).

Assuming that the patient is supplying all the work of breathing, the inspiratory muscle pressure (Pmus) is described by the following equation:

$$Pmus = (\dot{V}_L \times R) + (V_L \times E_{LUNG-THORAX})$$

---

*Proportional Assist and PAV are registered trademarks of the University of Manitoba and are used under license by Puritan Bennett. All other trademarks belong to Covidien, previously Tyco Healthcare Group, or an affiliate.

BOX 12-73   **Determination of Muscle Pressure and Ventilator Pressure**

The instantaneous value of muscle pressure (P^i_{mus}) is estimated with instantaneous measures of flow ($\dot{V}^i_L$), resistance (R^i), and volume (V^i_L):

$$P^i_{mus} = (\dot{V}_L) \times R^i \times K_1) + (V^i_L \times E^i_{PAV} \times K_2)$$

where *I* is the instantaneous value of pressure, flow, or airway resistance and K_1 and K_2 are the constants for R_{PAV} and E_{PAV}, respectively.

The % SUPPORT setting (S), along with measures of flow and volume, determines the amount of pressure applied by the ventilator at the Y-connector (P^iY).

The equation for P^i_{mus} shown above can be rewritten as follows:

$$P^iY = S (\dot{V}^i_L) + S (\dot{V}^i_L \times K_1) + S (\dot{V}^i_L)$$

where P^iY is the pressure generated by the ventilator at the Y-connector in response to the instantaneous measured values of lung flow and lung volume and *S* is the % support setting/100 (range, 0.05 to 0.95).

This value is the sum of three individual pressure elements (in parentheses) in the above equation.

The pressure gradient resulting in gas flow into the patient's lungs is the sum of P^iY and the patient's inspiratory effort, thus:

$$\Delta P^i_{GRADIENT} = P^iY + P^i_{mus}$$

---

where $\dot{V}_L$ is the flow through the resistance elements and into the lungs; *R* is the resistance elements (artificial plus patient airways); V_L is the inspiratory volume of the lungs; and $E_{LUNG-THORAX}$ is the elastance of the lung and thorax (i.e., $1/C_{LUNG-THORAX}$).

This equation assumes that the PAV+ estimates of patient resistance and elastance remain fairly stable over a short interval. The instantaneous value of muscle pressure (P^imus) can be estimated when the instantaneous values for inspiratory flow, airway resistance (estimated from flow and resistance of the artificial airway), and volume are also known (Box 12-73). The ventilator can then calculate an appropriate amount of pressure to apply at the Y-connector (see Box 12-73).

Set-Up Procedure for PAV+

PAV+ requires the attachment of an adult circuit to the ventilator. Before activation of PAV+, an SST is performed. Once the SST is passed, PAV+ can be set up from the NEW PATIENT SETUP screen or the current ventilation screen. For a new patient, the operator enters the value for the patient's IBW using the IBW button. Under the MODE button, the operator selects the SPONT mode and then the PA spontaneous breath type.

When PAV+ is selected, the default settings for PAV+ appear in the Sandbox in the lower screen. The operator then selects the type and internal diameter of the artificial airway the patient has in place (Clinical Rounds 12-28).*

---

*Additional information on IBW and ET/Trach size selection is available in the PAV+ addendum to the Puritan Bennett 840 operator's manual.

The appropriate % SUPPORT is also selected (see the following section). Inspiration is either flow (default) or pressure triggered. Inspiration is flow cycled (inspiration ends) based on the expiratory sensitivity setting. The default E_{SENS} is 3 L/min, although this can be adjusted from 1 to 10 L/min. During PAV+, E_{SENS} represents the actual flow value (L/min) measured at end-inspiration and not the percentage of peak flow, as is used in pressure-support ventilation (PSV). A slight delay in the ending of inspiration may occur as a result of the normal control system delay time that is present in all ventilators.[10]

Determining the % Support Setting

The setting range for the % SUPPORT control is 5% to 95%. For example, at the minimum setting of 5%, the patient provides 95% of the work of breathing (WOB) and the ventilator provides 5% of the WOB.

The 840 has a WOB bar that provides a guide for the user. The green area of the bar represents the optimum WOB. The % SUPPORT setting can be adjusted to maintain the patient's WOB (WOBpt) in the green area. If the WOBpt is to the left of the green area, the patient is being oversupported by the ventilator; if it is to the right of the green area, the patient may be undersupported.

A high level of support (i.e., a setting higher than 80%) is not recommended for initial settings, because it can be uncomfortable and inappropriate for the patient. A setting that is too high may also result in a "runaway" (described later). It probably is appropriate to start at 80% and gradually reduce the amount of support, evaluating the patient's response. In one study, when PAV+ was reduced from 80% to 50%, the patient's inspiratory effort and WOB increased to maintain comparable ventilation. This is different from PSV, in which an increased inspiratory effort is always assisted with a constant pressure.[11]

Once PAV+ has been accepted and ventilation begins, it is appropriate to wait 10 to 15 breaths for the patient to adapt to the new breath type. This also allows the ventilator to determine a stabilized response to the new settings. Waiting 10 to 15 breaths also holds true for any subsequent changes in the % SUPPORT level.

It is not uncommon to find that patients are actually oversupported in their current mode of ventilation (e.g.,

SIMV with PS). It may take a minute or two after switching to PAV+ for the patient's partial pressure of arterial carbon dioxide ($PaCO_2$) to return to a more normal level and for the patient to begin spontaneous efforts. For example, a patient who is on PS before switching to PAV+ may have too high a level of support provided; or, the ventilator may be autotriggering, resulting in a high respiratory rate and a lower than normal $PaCO_2$ for that patient. When the patient is switched to an appropriate level of PAV+, it may take a few moments before the $PaCO_2$ level increases enough to stimulate the respiratory center.

After beginning PAV+, the ventilator displays the APNEA SETUP screen, where the operator can select the appropriate apnea ventilation settings. (NOTE: The APNEA SETUP screen appears only when ventilation is started on a new patient.)

Finally, additional alarms can be adjusted according to the specific patient's needs. Appropriate alarm settings might include the high inspired spontaneous V_T alarm, the high total frequency alarm, the high inspiratory pressure limit alarm, and the low exhaled minute volume alarm. (NOTE: During PAV+, the low spontaneous V_T alarm is turned off to reduce nuisance alarms.)

Initiating PAV+ Ventilation

When PAV+ is first activated, the message PAV STARTUP flashes in the upper right corner of the waveform screen. During the start-up time, the ventilator makes an initial determination of the patient's compliance and resistance based on four consecutive PAV+ breaths. The initial four breaths are deliberately conservative, and each has an inspiratory pause. (NOTE: It is assumed that the patient's respiratory control center does not detect the pause.)[9]

The first breath is delivered based on the predicted R of the artificial airway selected and also on estimates of the patient's C and R using the patient's entered IBW. Measurements during and immediately after the pause for the next three breaths are used to estimate the patient's compliance and resistance. The C value is converted to elastance, where $E = 1/C$.

The fifth PA breath uses final estimations of C and R, along with the clinician-set % SUPPORT value. Thereafter, the ventilator randomly performs an inspiratory pause every 4 to 10 breaths to recalculate the C and R. It constantly updates values by averaging new values with previous values.

During the start-up period, if a 45-second interval occurs without a valid estimate of resistance and compliance, a low urgency alarm activates. The alarm increases in urgency if this condition continues for 90 seconds (medium urgency) or 120 seconds or longer (high urgency). Low minute volume and high rate alarms also occur under these conditions.

In a similar way, if resistance and compliance cannot be updated with valid values for a 15-minute interval after a successful start-up of PAV+, a low urgency alarm occurs. This progresses to a medium urgency alarm if it persists.

Findings in PAV+

With PAV+, V_T typically is highly variable, which indicates an increased ability on the part of the patient to control the V_T in response to changes in respiratory demand.[11] Because the amount of pressure applied to the airway with PAV+ is proportional to the pressure from muscle exertion (Pmus), the total pressure (Paw + Pmus) and V_T remain under the patient's control. In contrast, with PSV there is no automatic link between the end of the patient's effort and the end of the cycle. An increased inspiratory effort during PSV does not produce a difference in pressure from the ventilator. Pressure delivery in PSV is constant and is controlled by the operator and not the patient.[12]

When PAV+ is reduced (e.g., from 80% mechanical unload to 50%), this adjustment results in an increase in the patient's inspiratory effort and WOB to maintain a comparable level of ventilation, as would be expected.[11]

Monitored Information During PAV+

During PAV+, the 840 displays a variety of monitored parameters in the MORE PATIENT DATA and waveform screens. These monitored values are shown in Box 12-74.[9]

Alarms Associated with PAV+

The alarms available with PAV+ are shown in Box 12-75. During PAV+, if the pressure at the Y-connector reaches

---

BOX 12-74	Monitored Values Displayed During PAV+ (Puritan Bennett 840)

Patient compliance (C_{PAV})*: Change in volume per change of airway pressure when measured during zero flow. Estimated during a PAV+ pause maneuver.

Elastance (E_{PAV})*: Calculated value from the inverse of C_{PAV}.

Intrinsic PEEP (PEEPi): Estimate of pressure remaining in the lungs at end exhalation (range, 0 to 130 cm H_2O).

Patient resistance (R_{PAV})*: The calculated difference between the estimated total resistance and the resistance of the artificial airway.

Total resistance (R_{TOT})*: Estimated fraction of pressure/flow for both the ventilator system and the patient's airways at the peak of expiratory flow.

Spontaneous inspired tidal volume ($V_{TI SPONT}$): Display of inspired V_T (body temperature and pressure saturated [BTPS] value). Updated at the beginning of the following expiratory phase.

Normalized rapid shallow breathing index (RSBI) (f/V_T/kg): Available for PA breaths only. (NOTE: Normalizing of the f/V_T based on weight minimizes the variation in RSBI due to differences in V_T due to ideal body weight [IBW].)

Total work of breathing (WOB_{TOT}): The estimated WOB (Joules/L) of the patient and the ventilator during inspiration. (NOTE: Graphic displays of patient WOB are not measurements but filtered, model-based, calculated estimates.)

---

*If values for compliance, elastance, or resistance exceed the expected IBW-based limits, the value appears in parentheses, indicating a questionable value. The estimated value flashes if it exceeds its absolute limit.

BOX 12-75	Alarms Associated with PAV+ (Puritan Bennett 840)

High Peak Pressure: Violation of high set inspiratory pressure limit.

High Ventilation Pressure: Inspiratory pressure ≥100 cm H_2O.

PAV Startup Too Long: Software for PAV+ is unable to estimate initial valid values for C and R; possibly due to a short, spontaneous T_I or the type of humidifier selected.

PAV R & C NOT ASSESSED: PAV+ startup was successful, but later assessments were not; possibly due to short spontaneous T_I or the type of humidifier selected.

High Spontaneous Inspired Tidal Volume: Delivered inspiratory V_T ≥ the set inspiratory limit. Check for patient agitation or circuit air leaks and consider reducing the % SUPPORT.

---

the high peak pressure limit minus 5 cm H_2O or 35 cm H_2O (whichever is less), inspiration ends.

Graphics Display

Two pressure scalars are displayed on the ventilator's graphics screen. The first graph shows the measured circuit pressure. The second shows a shadow tracing of the estimated lung pressure during ventilation. The shadow display is not an actual measurement; rather, it is derived from filtered, model-based estimates (Figure 12-94).

Troubleshooting PAV+

Two unique problems can occur with PAV+: "runaway" and large leaks.

"Runaway" is a delay in ending the flow of gas from the ventilator. This can occur if the % SUPPORT is set at a high value and the ventilator overestimates the true values for R and E. The ventilator consequently provides more support than the patient needs.

For example, the ventilator detects a high resistance, although the actual R value is lower. If an estimated resistance were to exceed the actual value of the airway resistance at a high % SUPPORT setting, the pressure provided at the upper airway would exceed the actual amount needed to overcome the resistance of the artificial airway and the patient's airway. This could also result in hyperinflation or overinflation of the lungs. Fortunately, flow runaway is less of an issue than volume runaway. Flow peaks at the beginning of inspiration and decreases progressively during inspiration. Therefore, because flow declines, this condition may be self-limiting, although it could become uncontrolled.

Volume runaway is another matter. The stability of PAV+ is based mainly on the relationship between the true lung elastance and the true lung volume. As long as the estimated elastance and the true elastance are equal and the estimated volume and actual volume are equal, the pressure recoil of the lungs will be higher than the pressure provided at the upper airway, even at high values of %

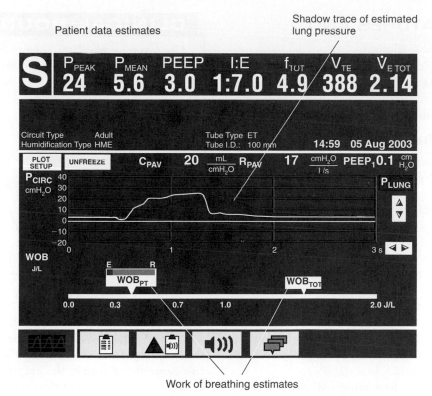

FIGURE 12-94 Graphics displays in PAV+. The shaded area of the pressure-time scalar represents a shadow tracing of estimated lung pressure. (See text for further explanation.) (Courtesy Puritan Bennett, a division of Covidien, Mansfield, Mass.)

SUPPORT (85% to 95%). Volume runaway occurs when the estimated value of lung elastance exceeds the actual value of lung elastance. The ventilator thinks it must deliver a higher pressure than is actually needed.

Recall that V_T delivery begins at functional residual capacity (FRC) and continues to increase during inspiration until it reaches a maximum V_T at end-inspiration. In volume runaway, if no restrictions were present, the inspiratory pressure would always exceed the recoil pressure (elastance) generated by the lung. Only the increase in lung stiffness near full inspiration might stop overinflation. For this reason, measured values for volume are compared with valid estimates for the patient's IBW. If valid estimates are not obtained, the PAV+ will not start or, after start-up, will not have reliable values. This reduces the possibility of underestimating a patient's compliance (overestimating elastance), which can lead to possible overinflation, although this finding was not supported in a study by Kondili et al.[13]

For safety purposes, the specification of a pressure threshold limit blocks an overpressure condition, just as the high pressure limit prevents overpressure breaths during conventional ventilation.

Another safeguard that can reduce the risk of this problem is setting an inspiratory V_T limit. If the high V_T limit is reached, the ventilator ends its part of flow delivery. Only an active inspiration by the patient would allow any additional flow and volume delivery from the ventilator.

In addition to the potential for runaway, large leaks can affect the function of PAV+ by interfering with the accuracy of the C and R measurements. For this reason, leaks in the patient circuit or endotracheal (ET) tube cuff may interfere with the performance of PAV+. For example, a leak around the ET tube during inspiration signals a higher flow and volume to the ventilator flow sensor than is truly entering the lung. This may cause an increase in ventilator pressure that is out of proportion to the actual inspiratory flow and volume entering the lung. Ventilator software algorithms for PAV+ can help reduce the response to this "leak effect." However, a major leak may still alter the pressure delivery during PAV+. For this reason, an excessive ET tube leak is one contraindication to the use of PAV. It may be appropriate to change the ET tube to facilitate use of PAV+.[14]

Summary of PAV+

The theoretical advantages of PAV+ are improved unloading of inspiratory muscles and better patient-ventilator synchrony. PAV+ relies on the rapid measurement of respiratory mechanics to make immediate adjustments in elastance and resistance unloading. Potential drawbacks might include increased WOB for the patient when insufficient unloading is provided, runaway, and the unfamiliarity of personnel with its use.[15]

SPECIAL FEATURES AND OPTIONS

Several features and options are available with the Puritan Bennett 840, including noninvasive ventilation, graphics, neonatal application, respiratory mechanics, rise time %, an active exhalation valve, and expiratory sensitivity.

Noninvasive Ventilation

The 840 can provide noninvasive ventilation (NIV) as part of a new patient set-up or during conventional ventilation. NIV is intended for use with a mask or similar NIV interface. It is activated from the VENT TYPE button. When NIV is selected, NIV appears in yellow in the alarm display above the waveforms section. In addition, the letter N is displayed next to the mode indicator.

Modes that can be used with NIV include A/C, SIMV, and the spontaneous mode. (NOTE: NIV cannot be used with BiLevel ventilation.) If A/C or SIMV is selected, the mandatory breath type is either VC or PC. (NOTE: VC+ is not available during NIV.) If spontaneous ventilation is selected, the spontaneous breath type can be none (CPAP) or PS. (NOTE: VS is not available with NIV.)

In NIV all breaths are flow triggered. An additional control called *disconnect sensitivity* (DSENS) is available (range, off and 20% to 90%). DSENS sets the amount of delivered volume loss permitted. The default is 75% leak. If the selected value is exceeded, a PATIENT DISCONNECT alarm sounds. The higher the setting, the more returned volume must be lost before the alarm is activated.

A high spontaneous inspiratory time (T_{Ispont}) limit is also provided with either SIMV or the spontaneous mode. When the patient's inspiratory time exceeds the set value, the ventilator ends inspiration. A visual indicator appears ($\uparrow T_{Ispont}$) on the upper screen. Both the inspired and expired V_T are displayed, along with the exhaled minute volume.

Graphics

In the upper screen is a section that displays scalars and loops. This area can display one or two scalars, or one loop. In this same screen, at the top left corner, is a PLOT SET-UP screen button that allows the operator to change the current graphics (see Figure 12-90, top screen). To the right of this screen button is a FREEZE button that freezes the current screen.

Touching the PLOT SET-UP screen button allows the operator to change the graphic display. The subscreen allows selection of Plot 1 (the top graph) and Plot 2 (the bottom graph). Selecting only one graph, using Plot 1, results in an enlarged graph that fills the screen. The control knob is used to change the graph. CONTINUE is then selected on the graphics screen to activate the new waveform. The operator need not press ACCEPT, because ventilator settings are not being changed.

The operator can change the vertical (size) and horizontal (time) scales by using the arrows to the right of the

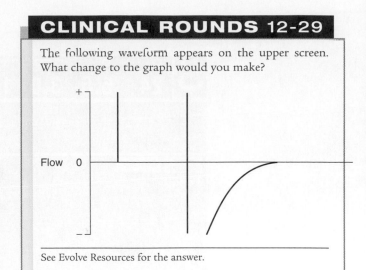

CLINICAL ROUNDS 12-29

The following waveform appears on the upper screen. What change to the graph would you make?

See Evolve Resources for the answer.

waveforms. The FREEZE function actually captures 48 seconds of data. By changing the time line (horizontal scale), the operator can visualize the entire 48 seconds. In this same freeze frame, the graphs can be changed. For example, when a pressure-time scalar is changed to a flow-time scalar, the flow-time scalar appears in the window. This flow-time scalar represents the same time period as the previous pressure-time scalar. Touching UNFREEZE unlocks the waveforms (Clinical Rounds 12-29).

The baseline position of a pressure-volume loop is set automatically at the current PEEP setting. If the PEEP setting is changed, the baseline for the loop resets to the new PEEP level.

The baseline can also be moved manually to another position. To move the baseline, the operator touches the BASELINE PRESSURE button and uses the control knob to position the baseline as desired.

Neonatal Application

The 840 ventilator's NeoMode option can provide ventilation for neonates (IBW range, 0.5 to 7 kg). Additional information on the NeoMode option is available in Chapter 13.

Respiratory Mechanics

The 840 can perform measurements of static compliance, resistance, plateau pressure, total PEEP ($PEEP_{TOT}$), and auto-PEEP or intrinsic PEEP ($PEEP_I$). Static compliance (C_S) is measured when an inspiratory pause maneuver is performed. Airway resistance (R_{aw}) can also be calculated when the constant flow waveform is selected during volume-controlled ventilation. $PEEP_{TOT}$ and $PEEP_I$ are measured when the expiratory pause is activated. Some conditions can interfere with accurate readings of the expiratory pressure, resulting in error messages. These conditions include leaks in the circuit, active patient breathing efforts, and unstable plateau pressure readings. For example, if a patient is actively breathing during an expiratory pause maneuver, the algorithm waits up to 2 minutes for the patient's respiratory rate to decrease so that the ventilator can perform the expiratory phase maneuver.

Rise Time Percent

Rise time percent is the same as sloping or the inspiratory rise time, as described in Chapter 11. The RT % is available with PC, PS, VC+, VS, and BiLevel breaths.

RT % works as follows: During pressure-control breaths (e.g., PC and VC+), the available range of settings is 1% to 100%. A 100% setting allows the ventilator to achieve 95% of the set pressure in about 50 msec (0.05 sec). All other settings (1% to 99%) are based on the set or estimated inspiratory time. For settings less than 100%, the ventilator evaluates the set T_I and RT % and determines the rise in pressure and flow that will be provided at the beginning of inspiration.

For the lowest setting (1%), the ventilator produces a rise in pressure that reaches 95% of the set pressure (set P + PEEP) in 2 seconds or two thirds of the T_I, whichever is shorter. For example, if the T_I is 1 second and the RT % is 1%, the rise to the set pressure will require $2/3 \times 1$ second, or about 669 msec (0.66 second). The ventilator will achieve 95% of the set pressure in 0.66 second when the RT % is set at 1%. One percent is a very low setting and should be used with caution, because it may compromise potential volume delivery for the set pressure.

For values between 1% and 100%, the adjustment to rise creates a curved pressure waveform that is produced from the maximum setting (50 msec at 100%) and the minimum setting ($2/3 \times T_I$ at 1%). For example, if the RT % is 50% and the T_I is 1 second, the time required to rise to the set pressure is 305 msec, based on the following calculation:

$$\begin{aligned}
&\text{Time to 95\% of set pressure} \\
&= [2/3(T_I) - 50 \text{ msec}] \times \text{RT \% as a fraction} \\
&= [(2/3 \times 1) - 50 \text{ msec}] \times 0.5 \\
&= [660 - 50 \text{ msec}] \times 0.5 \\
&= 305 \text{ msec (about 0.3 second)}
\end{aligned}$$

When the RT % is used in PS or VS, the T_I is estimated based on the set IBW. (NOTE: Additional information on the RT % during PS and VS is available from the manufacturer.)

Slowing the rate at which the pressure enters the airways and lungs may be more comfortable for the patient. An appropriately adjusted RT % may reduce WOB and ventilator asynchrony. These adjustments need to be monitored carefully. On the other hand, a quicker rise to the set pressure may give areas of the lungs that have different compliance values (time constants) a better opportunity to inflate more evenly. However, if the rise is too fast, an overshoot of the pressure curve may appear. This is called *chatter*, *ringing*, or *oscillation*.

The RT % screen button appears only when a pressure-targeted mode is selected (i.e., PC, PS, VC+, VS, or BiLevel). Programming of the 840 includes Smart Pressure rise algorithms. Based on evaluation of resistance, compliance, and

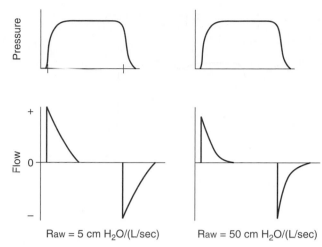

FIGURE 12-95 Using the sloping or rise time feature called *rise time percent (RT %)*, an optimum pressure-time curve is established on the Puritan Bennett 840. The ventilator adjusts flow to achieve the pressure-time curve even when airway resistance (R_{aw}) changes. Compare the right curve to the left curve. Notice how flow delivery is lower in the right curve; this may affect volume delivery. The V_T should be monitored. (See text for further explanation.)

the pressure curve, the ventilator can automatically adjust to achieve an algorithm-driven pressure-time curve (Figure 12-95), or the operator can choose the RT %.

Active Exhalation Valve

The exhalation valve on the 840 is designed so that the set pressure (e.g., in pressure ventilation) not only is delivered through the inspiratory line to the patient, but also powers the exhalation valve. If the pressure in the patient circuit exceeds the set pressure during inspiration, as when a spontaneous breath or cough occurs, the exhalation valve allows either increased flow to the patient for the spontaneous breath or venting of the excess pressure during a cough (Figure 12-96). This helps provide better breath synchrony and prevents the generation of high pressures, which may harm the patient. The active exhalation valve feature is available with pressure breaths (PC and PS) but currently is not available with volume-controlled breaths.

Expiratory Sensitivity

As mentioned in Chapter 11, PS ventilation normally is flow cycled, and some ventilators offer adjustable flow-cycling percentages. On the 840, this feature is called *expiratory sensitivity*. E_{SENS} represents the percent of peak inspiratory flow at which the ventilator cycles in spontaneous breaths (e.g., PSV), and it is adjustable from 1% to 45%. The higher the E_{SENS}, the shorter the T_I. The E_{SENS} needs to be adjusted to match the patient's spontaneous inspiratory phase. If the breath ends too soon, V_T delivery is compromised. If the T_I is too long, the patient may actively exhale, increasing expiratory work and resulting in patient-ventilator dyssynchrony. In PSV, the T_I may also be too long if there is a leak in the system (Figure 12-97).

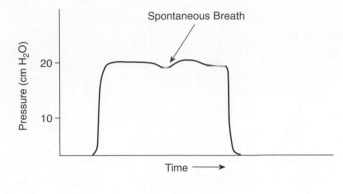

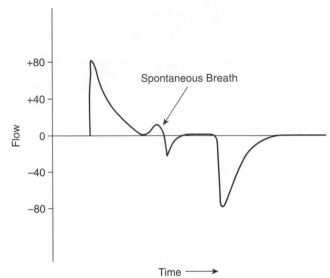

FIGURE 12-96 The active exhalation valve of the Puritan Bennett 840 can accommodate pressure changes in the patient circuit during pressure-targeted breaths. (See text for description.)

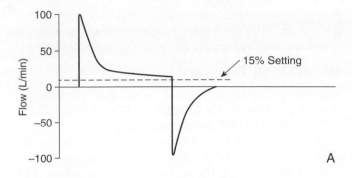

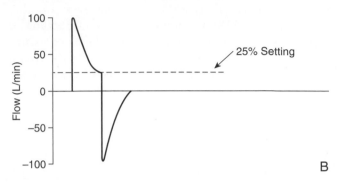

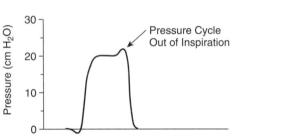

FIGURE 12-97 Puritan Bennett 840 scalars representing PS ventilation. **A,** Flow-time scalar with a prolonged T_I as a result of a leak in the circuit and a low expiratory sensitivity setting of 15%. **B,** Increasing the percent setting to 25% has shortened the T_I to a more reasonable value. **C,** Pressure-time curve in which the pressure rises slightly during P_S because of active exhalation of the patient. This causes pressure cycling out of inspiration.

Tube Compensation

Tube compensation (TC) is a spontaneous breath type that is intended to reduce the work of breathing associated with an ET or tracheostomy (trach) tube. Tube compensation functions in the following manner: When a patient's spontaneous effort is detected, the ventilator provides pressure in proportion to the inspiratory flow and the size of the artificial airway.

Theoretically, TC delivers precisely the amount of pressure required to overcome the resistive load caused by the artificial airway. TC targets pressure for the tracheal level, adjusting delivered pressure at the upper airway to try to maintain the pressure in the trachea at a constant level.[16]

When selecting TC, the operator selects the type of artificial airway (ET tube or trach tube). The ventilator uses the known internal diameter and length of the tube to calculate tube resistance. The operator then selects the percent of support (10% to 100%) to be provided to the patient to overcome the imposed work associated with the artificial airway.

Tube compensation may reduce the work of breathing associated with artificial airways and improve patient comfort.[16]

TROUBLESHOOTING

Operators can easily resolve common alarm errors by reading the alarm messages that provide suggestions about the situation. This provides a rapid method of troubleshooting.

A common problem for individuals just beginning to use the 840 is remembering to press the ACCEPT key. If a parameter has not changed after the value is adjusted, the most likely cause is forgetting to press ACCEPT.

The operator's manual provides an extensive alarm and troubleshooting section, which can help operators solve problems related to operation of the Puritan Bennett 840.

KEY POINTS

▸ The SST should be run when a new circuit or humidifier is added, between patient uses, and at least every 15 days during use.

▸ The internal backup battery that provides power to the BDU and screen is intended as emergency power if the AC power is lost or falls below acceptable levels.

▸ The SandBox allows the operator to view potential changes in ventilation without the changes becoming active until the ACCEPT key is pressed.

▸ The DEVICE ALERT indicates that a background check detects a serious problem. An EST must be run and passed before this alarm will reset.

▸ SAFETY VENTILATION activates whenever a procedure error is detected.

▸ The backup mode, APNEA VENTILATION, is activated when the apnea time interval is exceeded without the ventilator detecting and delivering a breath.

▸ Modes of ventilation on the 840 include assist/control, SIMV, and the spontaneous mode.

▸ Breath delivery types include volume, pressure, and proportional assist ventilation.

▸ The rise time percent is the rate at which the ventilator rises to the set pressure, depending on the set value. It is available with PC and PS breaths.

▸ Expiratory sensitivity is the percent of peak flow at which the ventilator will cycle out of inspiration during PSV.

ASSESSMENT QUESTIONS

See Evolve Resources for answers.

1. The function of the expiratory filter includes which of the following?
   I. Protect the ventilator from contamination with the patient's secretions.
   II. Filter exhaled air to protect clinicians from contamination.
   III. Protect the patient from potential contamination from the ventilator.
   IV. Measure expiratory gas flows for calculating flows and volumes.
   a. II only
   b. I and IV only
   c. I, II, and III only
   d. II, III, and IV only

2. The backup power source will do which of the following when electrical AC power is lost or drops below a minimum level?
   I. Illuminate the battery indicator in the status indicators area of the screen.
   II. Provide backup emergency power to the BDU and screen.
   III. Not power the compressor.
   IV. Not power the humidifier.
   a. I only
   b. II and III only
   c. I and IV only
   d. I, II, III, and IV

3. The respiratory therapist must perform which of the following to begin an SST?
   a. Connect the patient to the ventilator.
   b. Turn off the ventilator.
   c. Press the SST on the touch screen or the test button on the side of the ventilator.
   d. Remove the proximal sensor.

4. During PSV, the E$_{SENS}$ in the 840 is set at 40%. The respiratory therapist notices that the inspiratory time is short and volume delivery is low. What might be the problem?
   a. There may be a leak in the system, and the inspiratory flow never drops to the 40% value.
   b. The patient is actively inhaling from the gas flow.
   c. The patient is making no spontaneous inspiratory effort to begin the next breath.
   d. The E$_{SENS}$ may be set too high for the patient.

5. Which of the following statements is/are true about the volume bar graph?
   I. The volume bar graph shows real-time exhaled volumes.
   II. For low tidal volumes (500 mL or less), the scale is 0 to 2000 mL.
   III. The bar graph on/off control is accessed through the USER SETTING menu.
   IV. The maximum exhaled volume is indicated by moving the LEDs for the last breath.
   a. I only
   b. II and IV
   c. I, III, and IV
   d. I, II, III, and IV

6. The upper screen of the GUI contains which of the following?
   a. The set-up keys
   b. The symbol definition area
   c. The alarm status
   d. The SandBox

7. An indicator in the 840's Status Indicator Panel is blinking rapidly, suggesting a hazardous situation. Which indicator does this describe?
   a. Low priority alarm
   b. Medium priority alarm
   c. High priority alarm
   d. Battery low alarm

ASSESSMENT QUESTIONS—cont'd

8. Which of the following tests is *not* available with the SST?
   a. Leak test
   b. Tubing compliance test
   c. Oxygen sensor calibration
   d. Expiratory filter resistance

9. The on/off power switch for the 840 is located on the:
   a. BDU
   b. GUI
   c. BPS
   d. compressor

10. The FREEZE control on the ventilator graphics screen allows freezing of the last how many seconds of data?
    a. 30
    b. 48
    c. 60
    d. 90

11. PAV+ is best described as a breath delivery method in which:
    a. The greater the patient effort, the higher the pressure delivered
    b. The pressure is set as a percentage of inspiratory effort
    c. The percent of support provided depends on the P0.1 value of the patient
    d. Breaths are time or patient triggered

12. Runaway can occur with PAV+ when which of the following conditions is present?
    I. The % support is set at a high value.
    II. The estimated E exceeds the actual value of E.
    III. The patient's effort exceeds the level of set support.
    IV. The high V_T limit is reached.
    a. I and II
    b. III
    c. I an IV
    d. II and IV

13. The rise time percent is best defined as:
    a. The level of support for a PAV+ breath
    b. The flow at which a PS breath will end
    c. The rate of rise to the set pressure during pressure ventilation
    d. The pressure above $PEEP_H$ when PS is set during BiLevel ventilation

14. What will be the peak inspiratory pressure during BiLevel ventilation when the $PEEP_H$ is set at 20 cm H_2O and the $PEEP_L$ is set at 5 cm H_2O?
    a. 25 cm H_2O
    b. 20 cm H_2O
    c. 15 cm H_2O
    d. 5 cm H_2O

15. During PS, the ventilator goes into apnea ventilation. Under what circumstances will normal ventilation resume?
    a. When the patient takes three consecutive breaths
    b. When the ventilator is switched to a mode that provides mandatory breaths
    c. When the RESET button is pressed
    d. When the ALARM SILENCE button is pressed

16. Safety ventilation begins when which of the following occurs?
    a. When apnea is detected
    b. When a procedure error is detected
    c. When a patient is attached to the ventilator after the set-up is completed
    d. When power is removed from the ventilator for 15 minutes or longer

References

1. Puritan Bennett: Operator's and technical reference manual, 840 ventilator system, part no 4-075609-00, revision C, Boulder, Colo, 1999, Puritan Bennett, a division of Covidien, Mansfield, Mass.

2. Puritan Bennett: User's pocket guide, 840 ventilator system, part no 4-076767-00, revision C, Boulder, Colo, 2000, Puritan Bennett, a division of Covidien, Mansfield, Mass.

3. Puritan Bennett: Learning and mastering the Puritan-Bennett 840 ventilator system, computer-based training, part no A-AA2287-00 revision A, Boulder, Colo, 1999, Puritan Bennett, a division of Covidien, Mansfield, Mass.

4. Milne G, product manager, Puritan Bennett: Personal correspondence, 2007, Boulder, Colo.

5. Habashi NM: Other approaches to open-lung ventilation: airway pressure release ventilation, *Crit Care Med* 33(Suppl 3): S228, 2005.

6. Habashi N, Andrews P: Ventilator strategies for post-traumatic acute respiratory distress syndrome: airway pressure release ventilation and the role of spontaneous breathing in critically ill patients, *Curr Opin Crit Care* 10:337, 2004.

7. Frawley PM, Habashi NM: Airway pressure release ventilation and pediatrics: theory and practice, *Crit Care Nurs Clin North Am* 16:337, 2004.

8. Pilbeam SP, Cairo JM: *Mechanical ventilation: physiological and clinical applications*, ed 4, St Louis, 2006, Mosby-Elsevier.

9. Puritan Bennett: PAV+ option addendum to the 840 ventilator operator's and technical reference manual, part no 10011698, Rev A, Boulder, Colo, 2006, Puritan Bennett, a division of Covidien, Mansfield, Mass.

10. Du HL, Ohtsuji M, Shigeta M et al: Expiratory asynchrony in proportional assist ventilation, *Am J Respir Crit Care Med* 165:972, 2002.
11. Wrigge H, Golisch W, Zinserling J et al: Proportional assist versus pressure support ventilation: effects of breathing pattern and respiratory work of patients with chronic obstructive pulmonary disease, *Intensive Care Med* 25:790, 1999.
12. Giannouli E, Webster K, Roberts D et al: Response of ventilator-dependent patients to different levels of pressure support and proportional assist, *Am J Respir Crit Care Med* 159:1716, 1999.
13. Kondili E, Prinianakis G, Alexopoulou C et al: Respiratory load compensation during mechanical ventilation: proportional assist ventilation with load-adjustable gain factors versus pressure support, *Intensive Care Med* 32:692, 2006.
14. Schulze A, Rieger-Fackeldey E, Gerhardt T et al: Randomized crossover comparison of proportional assist ventilation and patient-triggered ventilation in extremely low birth weight infants with evolving chronic lung disease, *Neonatology* vol. 92:921, 2007.
15. Delaere S, Roeseler J, D'hoore W et al: Respiratory muscle workload in intubated, spontaneously breathing patients with COPD: pressure support versus volume support, *Intensive Care Med* 29:949, 2003.
16. Pilbeam SP: Discontinuation of and weaning from mechanical ventilation. In Pilbeam SP, Cairo JM: *Mechanical ventilation: physiological and clinical applications,* ed 4, St Louis, 2006, Mosby/Elsevier.

Internet Resources

www.puritanbennett.com
www.Covidien.com

PURITAN BENNETT 740

OUTLINE

Power Source
Internal Mechanism
Controls and Alarms
Ventilator Settings
  Mode and Breath Selection Keys
  Support Pressure
Indicators
  Parameter Settings
  Message Window
  Apnea Parameters, 100% O_2, Manual Inspiration, and
    Menu Keys
  User Settings
  PEEP/CPAP, Trigger Sensitivity, and % O_2
  Patient Data Section
  Patient Data Section Alarms

Ventilator Status Section
  Alarm
  Caution
  Normal
  Ventilator Inoperative
  Safety Valve Open
  Internal/External Battery Indicators
  Alarm Silence and Reset
Modes of Ventilation
  Assist/Control
  Synchronized Intermittent Mandatory Ventilation
    (SIMV)
  Spontaneous Mode
  Pressure Support
  Apnea Ventilation
Troubleshooting

OBJECTIVES

Upon completion of this section, you will be able to:
· Name the power source requirements for the Puritan Bennett 740.
· Describe the internal mechanisms involved in breath delivery.
· Explain how ventilator and alarm settings are made.
· Assess an alarm situation and identify the probable cause.
· Identify the messages that appear in the message window.
· Compare the power on self-test (POST) with the short self-test (SST).
· Define the function of the various keys in the ventilator settings and patient status sections.
· Interpret flashing versus constantly lit indicators in the ventilator status section.
· Explain the function of all modes of ventilation available on the 740, including apnea ventilation.
· Identify functions that can be accessed through the menu key.
· Describe the appropriate corrective action when the VENT INOP alarm is activated.

KEY TERMS

Extended self-test (EST)	Linear-drive piston	Safety valve
Galvanic oxygen sensor	Power on self-test (POST)	Short self-test (SST)

The Puritan Bennett 740 ventilator[1,2] is a relatively simple and inexpensive machine that is adaptable for pediatric and adult use in subacute and acute care settings (Figure 12-98). Its lightweight, electrically powered design allows it to be used in patient transport in the hospital. The 740 currently is owned and manufactured by Covidien (Mansfield, Massachusetts).[1-4] (NOTE: In 2007, Covidien separated from Tyco Healthcare, the company that previously owned the Puritan Bennett ventilator line. Puritan Bennett moved with Covidien and has relocated from Pleasanton, California, to Boulder, Colorado.)

The alternative version, the 760, is identical in its platform. The internal mechanical systems, including the **linear-drive piston,** are the same. The basic operating features are also the same. The main difference is that the 760 has a slightly different operating panel (user interface). It also offers pressure-control ventilation (PCV) as an optional mode and has a few added features, which are discussed separately in the section on the 760.

Readers familiar with the Puritan Bennett 7200 ventilator will notice some similarities in this next generation of Puritan Bennett ventilators. The ++ key on the 7200 has been replaced by a menu selection. The self-tests, the **power on self-test (POST), short self-test (SST),** and **extended self-test (EST),** are also available on the 740 and 760. In the 700 series ventilators, to activate new settings and modes, the operator now presses ACCEPT rather than ENTER, as in the 7200.

POWER SOURCE

The 740 is an electrically powered, microprocessor-controlled ventilator that does not require high-pressure gas to function. It normally uses a standard 120-volt AC outlet but can also use the 2.5-hour internal battery or an optional 7-hour external battery. If a fractional inspired oxygen concentration (F_IO_2) above 0.21 is needed, the unit must be connected to a high-pressure oxygen source (40 to 90 psig). The power on/off switch is on the back panel of the machine, and the high pressure connector is on the right side.

When the ventilator is first turned on, the message window shows POST RUNNING . . . and PM DUE: ••. POST checks the essential system functions and must be completed before the unit will operate. The PM DUE message indicates the number of hours until a routine maintenance check is due. The manufacturer recommends letting the unit warm up (run) for 10 minutes after it is turned on before it is connected to a patient so that the flow sensors respond with greater precision.

The SST is a more extensive test that should be run (and alarms should be tested) before the unit is used with a patient (Box 12-76).

When the ventilator is not in use, it is appropriate to store the unit plugged into an AC outlet in the STANDBY

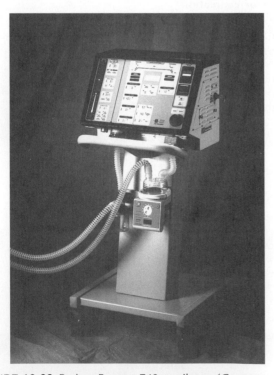

FIGURE 12-98 Puritan Bennett 740 ventilator. (Courtesy Puritan Bennett, a division of Covidien, Mansfield, Mass.)

BOX 12-76	Short Self-Test (SST) on the Puritan Bennett 740

1. Run the SST every 15 days, between patients, and when the patient circuit is changed.
2. Make sure a patient is not connected to the ventilator.
3. Turn the ventilator on (if it is already on, turn it off and then on again).
4. Press MENU and select SST.
5. Follow the instructions as they appear in the message window.
6. The ventilator runs the POST test.
7. When instructed, select the humidifier type: heat and moisture exchanger (HME), dual heated wire (humidifier with heated wire on the expiratory limb or on both the inspiratory and expiratory limbs), or no heated wire (conventional humidifier without a heated wire circuit on the expiratory limb).
8. Select the tubing type (adult or pediatric) when instructed.
9. Select the endotracheal (ET) tube size. Enter the millimeter tube size when instructed. The pressure (flow) rise time is automatically adjusted based on the tube size.
10. When each test run during SST is displayed, press one of the following: ACCEPT, CLEAR (to repeat), RESET (to restart the SST), and ALARM SILENCE (2 minutes) to stop the current test and skip to the end of the SST.
11. When the last test is completed, the message SST FINISHED TESTING is displayed, along with the overall SST result.
12. Unblock the patient Y and press ACCEPT; the ventilator will rerun POST. After this, it is ready for ventilation.

mode. This mode is a waiting state during which the ventilator maintains its settings and the battery charges, which ensures that it will be charged for the next use. Box 12-77 provides instructions on entering the STANDBY mode. (NOTE: The ventilator cannot be put in the STANDBY mode when a patient is connected to it.)

INTERNAL MECHANISM

Information from the control panel is processed by a microprocessor and stored in the ventilator's memory. A second microprocessor responsible for breath delivery uses this information to control and monitor the pattern of gas flow to the patient.

The 740 uses a frictionless, linear-drive piston to provide gas flow to the patient. The piston/cylinder system is designed with a very thin gap (about as thick as a sheet of paper) between the piston and the cylinder wall to reduce friction between the piston and the wall and allow for a faster response than can be obtained with a sealed system. A small amount of gas leaks through the gap between the piston and the cylinder, but the software program compensates for this minimal leak, ensuring accurate volume ventilation. During exhalation, the continuous forward motion of the piston is regulated and maintained to compensate for the leak and maintain set positive end-expiratory pressure (PEEP) levels (Clinical Rounds 12-30).

When inspiration begins, the forward motion of the piston sends the gas past a **galvanic oxygen sensor,** a safety pressure-relief valve, a temperature thermistor, and finally into the patient circuit. (NOTE: The percentage of measured oxygen is displayed in the message window. This O_2 % can be turned on and off using the OXYGEN SENSOR subheading in the MENU listing. The menu is discussed more extensively later.)

BOX 12-77   Entering the Standby Mode (Puritan Bennett 740)

1. Turn on the ventilator (if it is already on, turn it off and then on again).
2. Press MENU and use the control knob to select STANDBY.
3. Press ACCEPT. The message window displays IS PT DISCONNECTED? ACCEPT TO PROCEED.
4. With the patient disconnected, press ACCEPT. The message window displays the confirmation message IN STANDBY MODE. CLEAR TO EXIT.
5. To exit, press CLEAR, and POST will run.

CLINICAL ROUNDS 12-30

Because the 740 uses a linear-drive piston, what waveform or waveforms would you expect it to produce?

See Evolve Resources for the answer.

CONTROLS AND ALARMS

The front panel of the 740 is grouped into three sections (Figure 12-99):
- Ventilator settings section—Allows selection of the mode of ventilation, breath type, oxygen percentage, apnea parameters, and menu functions.
- Patient data section—Displays monitored airway pressure information, breath timing, volumes, and current alarm settings.
- Ventilator status section—Displays the current ventilator parameters and status, including alarms, battery conditions, alarm silence, and alarm reset.

The control knob is located at the lower right corner of the panel. It is used to change the value of a selected parameter and to scroll through menu items when the MENU key is active (Box 12-78).

Just above the control knob are two buttons or keys, CLEAR and ACCEPT. CLEAR cancels recent setting changes and returns the operating panel to the original settings or previously accepted settings. If CLEAR is pressed twice, the ventilator returns to its original operating state. Pressing ACCEPT activates new settings; however, if it is not pressed within 30 seconds of setting a new change, the operating panel returns to its previous settings.

VENTILATOR SETTINGS

Mode and Breath Selection Keys

On the 740, the touch keys for modes are located at the top center of the operating panel. The top left side of this section is labeled MANDATORY, and the right side is labeled SPONTANEOUS. Available ventilator modes include assist-control (A/C), synchronized intermittent mandatory ventilation (SIMV), and spontaneous ventilation (SPONT), which includes pressure-support ventilation (PSV). The area labeled volume-control ventilation (VCV) indicates that A/C and SIMV are volume-targeted mandatory breaths. Pressure-control ventilation (PCV) is available on the 760 but not on the 740. Modes of ventilation and breath delivery are described later.

BOX 12-78   Changing Parameters and Alarm Settings[1] (Puritan Bennett 740)

To change ventilator parameters and alarm settings, perform the following steps:
1. Touch a setting key; the key lights, the selected setting flashes, and the message window shows the current setting.
2. Turn the control knob to adjust the setting.
3. Press ACCEPT to apply the new setting. The key lights go out, and the new settings are displayed. The message window reads SETTING(S) ACCEPTED.

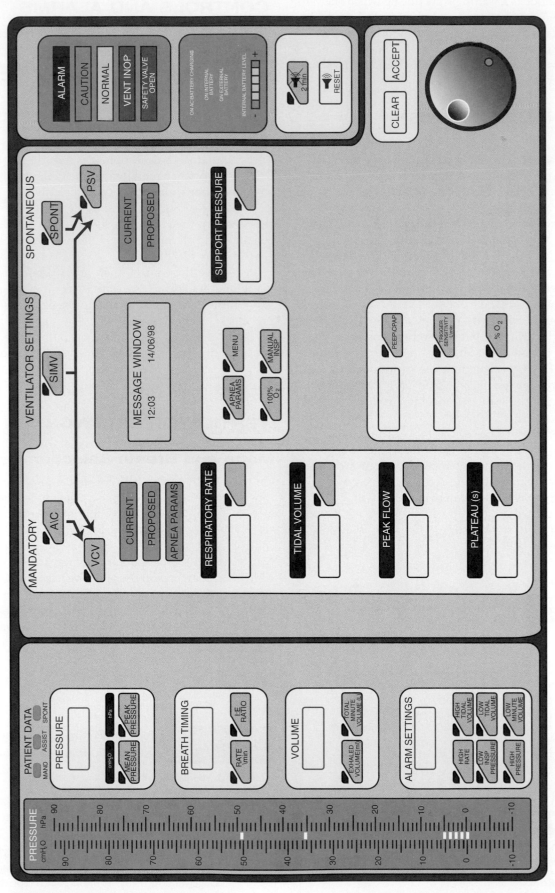

FIGURE 12-99 Front panel of the Puritan Bennett 740 ventilator.

Support Pressure

On the right, just below the CURRENT/PROPOSED indicators, is an active touch key for pressure support. The SUPPORT PRESSURE control sets pressure delivery for spontaneous breaths above the PEEP/CPAP baseline during spontaneous breathing. Support pressure, more commonly called pressure support (PS), can provide up to 70 cm H_2O of pressure. Inspiration ends in PS when the inspiratory flow delivery drops to 25% of the peak flow measured or 10 L/min, whichever is lower. For example, if the peak flow is 100 L/min, then 25 L/min would be the 25% point. Because 10 L/min is less than this, the flow stops at 10 L/min.

Although PS normally is flow cycled out of inspiration, two safety backup features are available to end the breath. If the pressure in the patient circuit exceeds the set PS by 3 cm H_2O, inspiration ends. This could occur if a patient were trying to actively exhale. Inspiratory flow also ends if the inspiratory time (T_I) becomes too long (3.5 seconds for adults, 2.5 seconds for pediatric patients). This could happen if a significant leak were present in the circuit.

INDICATORS

Under the MANDATORY section are three indicator lights: current, proposed, and apnea parameters. CURRENT illuminates when the ventilator is operating using the displayed settings. PROPOSED lights when the operator proposes a mode or breath type but has not yet accepted it. APNEA PARAMS lights when apnea ventilation is active. When apnea is illuminated, the CURRENT indicator also lights, showing the current active apnea settings. When the operator has selected new apnea ventilation settings but has not yet accepted them, the APNEA PARAM and PROPOSED indicators light.

Under the SPONTANEOUS section of the Ventilator Setting panel on the right are two more indicators, CURRENT and PROPOSED, which are active under spontaneous ventilation conditions or when spontaneous ventilation parameters are being set.

Parameter Settings

The ventilator setting section has several parameter keys. The respiratory rate control (3 to 70 breaths/min) sets the respiratory rate in A/C and SIMV. The tidal volume control (40 to 2000 mL) determines mandatory breath delivery in A/C and SIMV. Peak flow (3 to 150 L/min) delivers a peak flow of gas at the set rate during a mandatory breath. The T_I is determined by the tidal volume (V_T), flow, and rate. Plateau (0 to 2 seconds) provides an inspiratory pause at the end of a mandatory breath.

Message Window

At the top center of the operating panel is a window that displays information such as the time and date or the monitored oxygen percent. It can show up to four lines of information.

The first line is reserved for the highest priority alarm when one activates. On the 760, when no alarm is present, this line displays the O_2 % when the sensor is enabled. It can also provide information about the flow pattern during volume ventilation.

The second line provides information about menu functions or settings, the time remaining for an alarm silence, or the current time and date. During normal ventilation, it shows the flow in liters per minute (L/min).

The third and fourth lines are reserved for messages. For each breath the third line shows the peak and end-inspiratory flows. The fourth line shows the end-expiratory flow for PS breaths or pressure-controlled (PC) breaths (760 only) to evaluate for air trapping. The patient needs enough time for expiratory flow to return to zero before another breath begins. If he or she cannot completely exhale, then air trapping is present.

Apnea Parameters, 100% O₂, Manual Inspiration, and Menu Keys

Just below the message window are four more active keys: apnea parameters, 100% O_2, manual inspiration, and menu. The APNEA PARAMS key allows the operator to select settings for apnea ventilation. Apnea ventilation is a backup mode that becomes active when the set apnea time interval (Ta) has elapsed and the ventilator has not detected a patient inspiration. This feature is active in all modes of ventilation. On the 740, the operator designates volume settings for apnea ventilation, such as the V_T, rate, and flow. On the 760, the operator can set either volume-controlled ventilation (VCV) or pressure-controlled ventilation (PCV) parameters. For example, in PCV the operator could select the inspiratory pressure, T_I, or inspiratory to expiratory ratio (I:E) fixed, and so on.

The apnea time interval is not set with the apnea key but with the MENU key. The operator presses the MENU key and uses the control knob to scroll to and highlight USER SETTINGS. Pressing ACCEPT accesses this submenu. The operator then scrolls to APNEA INTERVAL (Ta) and presses ACCEPT to select this option. In the message window, the ventilator displays XX(10-60)S, APNEA INTERVAL. The operator turns the control knob to select the length of the apnea interval (10 to 60 seconds). For example, if 30 seconds is selected, the ventilator will wait 30 seconds to detect a breath. If it does not detect a breath, apnea ventilation begins. Pressing CLEAR eliminates the selection. The new settings are activated by pressing ACCEPT.

To cancel apnea ventilation and return to normal ventilation, the operator presses the ALARM RESET pad on the right side of the control panel in the Ventilator Status section. Apnea ventilation also is canceled if the ventilator detects the patient taking two spontaneous breaths.

The 100% O_2 key switches the delivered oxygen percent to 100% when pressed and gives 2 minutes of 100% O_2. The unit then returns to the original oxygen percent. It takes a

TABLE 12-39

Menu Function Summary—Puritan Bennett 740

Menu Option	Function
More active alarms	Lists other active alarms in order of priority. (The highest priority active alarm is always displayed on the first line of the message window.) Turning the knob displays other active alarms. The alarm reset key clears (erases) this list. Clear returns to menu options.
Autoreset alarms	Lists alarms that have autoreset since alarm reset key was last pressed. Turning the knob lists other autoreset alarms. The alarm reset key clears (erases) this list. Clear returns to menu options.
Self-tests	Begins short self-test (SST) or extended self-test (EST).
User settings	(See text for description.)
Standby mode	Places the ventilator in a nonventilating waiting state.
Battery info	Displays the estimated operational time remaining on the internal and external batteries until they need recharging. (Available only when ventilator is operating on battery power.) Clear returns to menu options.
Software revision	Displays the version of software installed in the ventilator. Clear returns to menu options.
Oxygen sensor	Allows operator to calibrate O_2 sensor, enable or disable O_2 sensor, and enable or disable O_2 display.
Service summary	Allows operator to view estimates of oxygen sensor life remaining, internal battery operational time remaining, and time until the next preventive maintenance is due.
Nebulizer	Allows operator to start, stop, or view the current state of an EasyNebTM nebulizer attached to the ventilator.

From Puritan Bennett, a division of Covidien, Mansfield, Massachusetts.

few breaths to get to the 100% delivery value. (NOTE: The 2-minute interval restarts every time the key is pressed. To stop this maneuver, the operator should wait the 2 minutes or press CLEAR.)

The MANUAL INSP key delivers one mandatory breath to the patient based on the current settings when the A/C or SIMV modes are active. During spontaneous ventilation, pressing the MANUAL INSP key delivers a mandatory breath based on the apnea parameter settings.

The MENU key can be used at any time to view other active alarms and autoreset alarms, run the self-tests, access user settings, enter the STANDBY mode, display battery information, check the software version, control and calibrate the oxygen sensor, obtain a service summary, and use the nebulizer. Table 12-39 summarizes these functions. Menu information is displayed on the second line in the message window. (NOTE: The first line of information in the message window is always reserved for any high priority active or autoreset alarm.)

To access items in the menu, the operator touches MENU, uses the control knob to select the desired item, and presses ACCEPT to enter that particular menu function. To exit the menu, the operator either presses CLEAR, which also cancels the current function or display setting, or presses any ventilator or alarm setting key. These actions cancel any change that was in progress but not completed.

User Settings

Some special menu items are unique to the 740 and 760 and are worth mentioning. These features are found under USER SETTINGS, a subscreen added to the 740 (and 760). To access this screen, the operator touches the MENU key and

uses the control knob to scroll through the choices. When USER SETTINGS is highlighted, the ACCEPT key is pressed. This submenu lists the following:

· Endotracheal tube
· Humidifier type
· Date and time set
· Apnea interval (Ta)
· VCV flow pattern
· Speaking valve set-up
· Alarm volume

Two additional features are available on the 760: PCV timing setting and Volume LED bar (these are described in the section on the 760).

The ENDOTRACHEAL TUBE feature, like other items in this submenu, is selected by using the control knob to scroll to and highlight this line and then pressing ACCEPT. When this feature is selected, an endotracheal (ET) tube size is displayed in the message window. The operator then uses the control knob to dial in the ET tube size the patient is using and presses ACCEPT to activate this setting. This provides additional pressure and flow to the patient in PSV (and in PCV in the 760) to compensate for the work imposed by the resistance of the ET tube.

The HUMIDIFIER setting provides the opportunity to select the type of humidifier being used on the patient. Activating this option corrects calculations for spirometric values when the short self-test (SST) is run. The operator can choose heat and moisture exchanger (HME), dual heated wire patient circuit, or no heated wire.

The date and time setting allows adjustment of the digital display for these values. APNEA INTERVAL (Ta) sets the length of time the ventilator will wait for a breath before beginning apnea ventilation.

CLINICAL ROUNDS 12-31

During volume ventilation, when changing from a square to a ramp flow pattern on the 740 or 760, you change the inspiratory time. For example, suppose you select a square flow (constant flow) pattern to deliver a 50-mL tidal volume at a rate of 20 breaths/min and the peak flow is set at 60 L/min. This flow (60 L/min) is the same as 60 L/60 sec, or 1 L/sec = 1000 mL/sec.

Part I

What are the T_I, T_E, and I:E ratio in this situation?

Part II

If the respiratory therapist switches the flow pattern from square to descending ramp but keeps all the other settings the same, will this affect the inspiratory time?

See Evolve Resources for the answer.

VCV FLOW PATTERN allows the operator to select a square (constant) or descending ramp for a flow pattern during volume ventilation. When this feature is selected, the display screen reads VCV FLOW: SQUARE, T_I = 1.05 s. The square is the current flow pattern, and the T_I is the current inspiratory time in seconds. Turning the knob allows selection of RAMP or SQUARE. Using a descending ramp waveform can lengthen the inspiratory time. The PEAK FLOW is the setting on the control panel (Clinical Rounds 12-31). If the change in flow makes it impossible for the ventilator to deliver the volume in the time set, based on the rate, flow, and volume settings, an error message appears: CHANGE NOT PERMITTED, and the flow needs to be adjusted.

ALARM VOLUME allows for louder or softer audible alarms.

The SPEAKING VALVE SET-UP is a feature that can be used when a special one-way valve that allows the patient to talk is added to the patient circuit (e.g., the Passey Muir valve). Because the patient is exhaling into the room, volumes that normally pass through the exhalation volume measuring device do not do so. In this case, the ventilator actually uses the delivery volume to detect high and low V_T alarms. It turns off the low minute volume and disconnect alarms. Because the ventilator's ability to detect problems is reduced, the operator must be especially vigilant about the patient's safety when a speaking valve is in use and must pay particular attention to the instructions provided by the manufacturer of the valve. To select this feature from the USER SETTINGS menu, the operator highlights it with the control knob and presses accept. The window displays SPEAKING VALVE OFF (assuming that it is off). The operator turns the dial to select SPEAKING VALVE ON and presses ACCEPT. This function must be turned off after the valve is removed from the patient circuit to return the ventilator to normal operation. After the speaking valve function is turned on, the screen lists a set of conditions that must be accepted:

· Volume alarms based on delivered volume
· Alarm DISABLED low minute volume
· Alarm DISABLED disconnect alarm

Accepting each of these statements tells the ventilator that the operator is aware of the changes being made to the ventilator. It is suggested, while proceeding through the subsequent messages, that PEEP be set at zero, the apnea interval be set at 10 seconds, and a low inspiratory pressure be set, which the ventilator can use to detect a disconnect. During normal operation with the speaking valve function on, the message window reads DISCONNECT DISABLED SPEAKING VALVE ON DELIVERED VOLUME ML (740 only). With the 760, using the speaking valve function disables the volume bar graph (more on this graph in the section on the 760). The operator must be sure to return the ventilator to its normal operation when the speaking valve is no longer in use.

PEEP/CPAP, Trigger Sensitivity, and % O₂

At the very bottom center of the Ventilator Settings section of the control panel are three additional function keys: PEEP/CPAP, TRIGGER SENSITIVITY L/MIN, and % O₂. The PEEP/CPAP control sets the baseline between 0 and 35 cm H_2O and establishes the minimum pressure maintained during both inspiration and exhalation.

The 740 and 760 use flow triggering to initiate all breaths. The TRIGGER SENSITIVITY control (1 to 20 L/min) establishes the trigger level. Unlike most ventilators, the 740 and 760 do not require a base flow to measure flow changes to provide flow triggering. The microprocessor monitors flow coming from the piston. When the patient's inspiratory flow exceeds the set flow trigger level, inspiration begins.

The % O₂ key allows the operator to set the percent oxygen delivery to the patient (21% to 100%). After a new setting is selected, it may take several minutes for the O₂ % to stabilize.

Patient Data Section

The Patient Data section of the keyboard allows the operator to view information on pressure, measured volume, rate, and alarm settings. To the far left, a pressure LED bar graph provides immediate readings of the airway pressure. The highest sustained double bar of the pressure graph represents the high pressure limit setting. The next double bar down is the current peak pressure, which is displayed only during exhalation. The last cluster of LEDs on this bar graph rise and fall synchronously with the circuit pressure.

Also in the Patient Data section are monitoring indicators for regular ventilation parameters and common alarms. Table 12-40 lists patient data indicators or keys, along with the function and range of each.

Patient Data Section Alarms

The Patient Data section includes the common alarms for high rate, high and low pressure, low expired minute volume

TABLE 12-40

Patient Data Section with Indicators, Functions, and Ranges—Puritan Bennett 740

Key/Indicator	Function	Range
Pressure		
MEAN PRESSURE	Shows the calculated value of ventilator breathing circuit pressure over an entire respiratory cycle. Updated at the beginning of each breath.	0-99 cm H_2O (0-9.9 kPa) Accuracy: ± (1 + 3% of reading) cm H_2O
PEAK PRESSURE	Shows the pressure measured at the end of inspiration (excluding plateau, if any). Updated at the beginning of each expiratory phase. (Default pressure display.)	0-140 cm H_2O (0-14 kPa) Accuracy: ± (1 + 3% of reading) cm H_2O
Breath Timing		
RATE/MIN	Shows the calculated value of the total respiratory rate, based on the previous 60 sec or 8 breaths (whichever interval is shorter). Updated at the beginning of each breath. (Default breath timing display.) Calculation is reset (and display is blank) when ventilation starts, when apnea ventilation starts or autoresets, and when operator presses the alarm reset key.	3-199 breaths/min Accuracy: ± (0.1 + 1% of reading)/min
I:E RATIO	Shows the ratio of measured inspiratory time to measured expiratory time. Updated at the beginning of each breath.	1:99-9.9:1 Accuracy: ± (0.1 + 2%)
Volume		
EXHALED VOLUME (mL)	Shows the patient's measured expiratory tidal volume for the just-completed breath. Corrected to BTPS and compliance compensated. Updated at the beginning of each inspiration. (Default volume display.)	0-9 L Accuracy: ± (10 mL + 10% of reading)
TOTAL MINUTE VOLUME (L)	Shows the patient's measured expiratory minute volume, based on the previous 60 sec or 8 breaths (whichever interval is shorter). Updated at the beginning of each breath. The calculation is reset when ventilation starts, when apnea ventilation starts or autoresets, and when the operator presses the alarm reset key.	0-99 L Accuracy: ± (10 mL + 10% of reading)
Alarm Settings		
HIGH RATE	Active alarm indicates that the measured respiratory rate is higher than the alarm setting.	3-100 breaths/min Accuracy: ± (0.1 + 1% of setting)/min
LOW INSP PRESSURE	Active alarm indicates that the monitored circuit pressure is below the alarm setting at the end of inspiration. Inactive in spontaneous mode.	3-60 cm H_2O (0.3-6 kPa) Accuracy: ± (1 + 3% of setting)
HIGH PRESSURE	Active alarm indicates that two consecutive breaths were truncated because circuit pressure reached the alarm setting.	10 to 90 cm H_2O (10 to 90 kPa) Accuracy: ± (1 + 3% of setting)
LOW MINUTE VOLUME	Active alarm indicates that monitored minute volume is less than the alarm setting, based on an 8-breath running average.	0-50 L Accuracy: ± (10 mL + 10% of setting)
HIGH TIDAL VOLUME	Active alarm indicates that exhaled volume for 3 out of 4 consecutive breaths was above the alarm setting.	20-9000 mL Accuracy: ± (10 mL + 10% of setting)
LOW TIDAL VOLUME	Active alarm indicates that exhaled volume for 3 of 4 consecutive breaths was below the alarm setting.	0-2000 mL Accuracy: ± (10 mL + 10% of setting)
Other Indicators		
Bar graph	Shows real-time pressures in centimeters of water (cm H_2O) or hectopascals (kPa). LED shows the current high-pressure alarm setting. During exhalation, LEDs show peak pressure of the last breath.	−10-90 cm H_2O (−1-9 kPa) Resolution: 1 cm H_2O (1 kPa)
MAND	Lights at the start of each breath to indicate that a ventilator- or operator-initiated mandatory breath is being delivered.	Not applicable
ASSIST	Lights at the start of each breath to indicate that a patient-initiated mandatory breath is being delivered.	Not applicable
SPONT	Lights at the start of each breath to indicate that a patient-initiated spontaneous breath is being delivered.	Not applicable

From Puritan Bennett, a division of Covidien, Mansfield, Massachusetts.

TABLE 12-41

Clinical Alarm Messages—Puritan Bennett 740

Message	Meaning
Apnea	No patient effort detected for the set apnea interval.
Continuous hi pres	High pressure in circuit has not dropped below high pressure setting (SVO).
Disconnect	Exhaled $V_T \leq 15\%$ of set V_T for 4 breaths; resets if exhaled $V_T > 15\%$.
Hi ex tidal volume	Exhaled $V_T > V_T$ set for 3 of 4 consecutive breaths.
Hi resp rate	Measured rate > high rate alarm set.
High pressure	Circuit pressure > high pressure limit setting for 2 breaths; inspiration ends, and exhalation valve opens for each breath with excessive pressure.
Low ex tidal volume	Measured V_T < low V_T alarm set for 3 of 4 consecutive breaths.
Low ex minute volume	Measured $\dot{V}_E$ < set $\dot{V}_E$ alarm.
Low insp pressure	Circuit pressure < set low pressure alarm during inspiration; active in A/C and SIMV modes only.
O_2% high	Measured O_2% > 10% of set O_2% for ≥30 sec
O_2% low	Measured O_2% < 10% of set O_2% for ≥30 sec
Occlusion	Patient circuit, inspiratory and/or expiratory filters occluded; ventilator detects abnormal differences in measured inspiratory and expiratory pressures; safety valve opens and ventilation is suspended.
Setup time elapsed	Thirty seconds or more have elapsed since operator pressed a key or turned the control knob during power-on.
Partial occlusion	Patient circuit, inspiratory and/or expiratory filters partially occluded. Ventilator detects abnormal differences in measured inspiratory and expiratory pressures. Ventilator continues normal ventilation.

($\dot{V}_E$), and high and low $\dot{V}_T$ (see Table 12-40). The Ventilator Status section uses color indicators to specify the type of alarm occurring (i.e., high or medium priority). If the active alarm is an adjustable alarm, its key light also flashes and the message window is blank. (NOTE: An alarm setting can be changed even while the alarm is active.) The message window also shows additional alarm messages for both clinical and technical alarms. Table 12-41 lists the messages that appear for and the causes of common clinical alarms. Table 12-42 lists the technical alarm messages. When more than one alarm is or has been active, they can be viewed in the message window using the MENU function.

When the alarm condition corrects itself, the alarm autoresets and the alarm or caution indicators light steadily. The alarm condition that occurred is added to the autoreset alarm list.

Pressing ALARM SILENCE stops the audible portion of the alarms for 2 minutes. If a new alarm condition occurs within the 2 minutes, the alarm sounds again. (NOTE: Pressing ALARM SILENCE during normal operation [no alarms] allows 2 minutes to perform bedside procedures without the audible alarm sounding. If an alarm occurs, the alarm or caution indicators flash and the message window displays a message about the alarm.) Pressing the ALARM RESET key clears all alarm indicators and cancels the 2-minute alarm silence.

VENTILATOR STATUS SECTION

At the top right of the front panel is a section showing the current operating conditions of the ventilator.

Alarm

The alarm light flashes red to indicate a high priority alarm and gives an audible signal pattern of three beeps, then two

TABLE 12-42

Technical Alarm Messages—Puritan Bennett 740

Message	Meaning
Air intake absent	Missing air intake filter
Air intake blocked	High resistance on air intake filter
Bat not charging	Battery voltage not increasing
Contact service	Ventilator service required
Deliv gas hi temp	Room air temperature high
Deliv gas low temp	Room air temperature low
Exh cct hi temp	Differential pressure sensor temperature high
Exh cct lo temp	Differential pressure sensor temperature low
Fan failed alert	Fan not operational or fan filter blocked
Hi bbu temp alert	Internal power supply temperature high
Hi sys temp alert	Internal temperature of ventilator high
Loss of AC power	AC power disconnect
Loss of power	AC power lost and batteries are low
Low ext battery	Low external and internal battery power
Low int battery	Low internal battery power
Low O_2 supply	O_2 line pressure low
Replace O_2 sensor	O_2 sensor missing or reading out of range*
Speaker failed	Main alarm speaker failed
Switch int battery	Power source has switched to internal battery

From Puritan Bennett, a division of Covidien, Mansfield, Massachusetts.
*This message will not appear if the O_2 alarm is disabled.

beeps that repeat. The light is lit steadily when an alarm condition existed but has self-corrected (i.e., autoreset). The message window displays the type of alarm that occurred.

Caution

The flashing yellow caution light indicates a medium priority alarm. It repeats a sequence of three beeps and is lit steadily when the condition has corrected itself (autoreset).

Normal

During normal operation, the normal light is constantly green.

Ventilator Inoperative

If a hardware failure or a critical software error occurs that could compromise safe ventilation of the patient, a ventilator inoperative condition occurs. The VENT INOP indicator light illuminates, a high priority alarm sounds, and the **safety valve** opens (SVO; see the following section), allowing a spontaneously breathing patient access to room air. The ventilator must be turned off, and another means of patient ventilation must be established immediately. When the unit is turned on again, a trained individual must run an EST to determine the cause of the problem and correct it.

The ventilator remains in the SVO state until a POST verifies that the power levels to the ventilator are acceptable and that the microprocessors are functioning correctly. The ventilator settings must then be confirmed.

Safety Valve Open

A red indicator shows that the safety valve is open. This may indicate a ventilator inoperative condition or an obstructed patient circuit. If possible, the message window displays the cause and gives the time that has elapsed since the last breath. If the condition is corrected and the VENT INOP indicator is off, the ALARM RESET key can be pressed to resume ventilation.

Internal/External Battery Indicators

The indicator lights for the internal and external batteries are located in the battery charging section of the Ventilator Status panel.

Alarm Silence and Reset

Below the battery indicators are the 2-minute ALARM SILENCE and ALARM RESET touch pads. The 2-minute silence quiets audible alarm sounds for 2 minutes from the most recent time the key was pressed; it also illuminates yellow when the silence is activated. ALARM RESET does three things:

· Clears all alarm indicators
· Cancels the alarm silence period
· Resets the patient data displays

The alarm will reactivate if the condition that caused the alarm is still present. The ALARM RESET key also cancels

APNEA VENTILATION if it is active; it re-establishes previous settings and resumes ventilation. The only exception is a ventilator inoperative condition, which must be treated as a serious condition and the unit taken out of service.

MODES OF VENTILATION

The 740 has three basic modes of ventilation: A/C, SIMV, and the spontaneous (SPONT) mode. Each of these has a touch pad control on the front panel. In the A/C and SIMV modes, mandatory breaths are volume targeted. When either A/C or SIMV is selected, the VCV pad LED lights, indicating that mandatory breaths are volume targeted. Spontaneous breaths can be assisted with PS in the SIMV or SPONT mode.

During ventilation, the active mode key is lit and settings are displayed. To change the mode, the operator follows the same procedure as changing a setting. The mode is selected by pressing the desired key. All of the available settings in that mode flash. For every flashing setting key, the operator must touch the key and adjust the setting with the control knob before the new mode can be applied (Clinical Rounds 12-32). After all entries are completed, pressing ACCEPT activates the new mode.

Assist/Control

In A/C, the ventilator delivers volume-targeted breaths that are labeled as VCV breaths on the control panel. Breaths are patient or time triggered, volume targeted, and volume cycled. The T_I can be extended by adding an inspiratory pause.

Synchronized Intermittent Mandatory Ventilation (SIMV)

In SIMV, mandatory breaths are patient or time triggered, volume targeted, and volume cycled. Spontaneous breaths are flow triggered, pressure targeted, and pressure cycled unless PS is added.

Spontaneous Mode

During spontaneous ventilation, the patient can breathe spontaneously from a zero baseline or from PEEP/CPAP. Breaths are flow triggered, pressure limited, and pressure cycled. In addition, spontaneous breaths may be assisted with PS.

CLINICAL ROUNDS 12-32

The respiratory therapist is setting up the A/C mode for a patient who will be ventilated with the 740. After selecting all the settings she wants to change, she notices that the tidal volume key is flashing. What does this indicate, and what should she do?

See Evolve Resources for the answer.

Pressure Support

With PS selected, patient-triggered spontaneous breaths in either the spontaneous or the SIMV mode receive the set pressure above PEEP/CPAP during inspiration. Breaths are patient triggered, pressure targeted, and flow cycled (see the earlier discussion of support pressure).

Apnea Ventilation

After all the patient parameters have been set and the ventilator has started normal operation, a message appears in the message window: REVIEW TA = 20 S. Ta is the apnea interval, and 20 is the current apnea interval in seconds. At this time the parameters for apnea ventilation should be set.

Apnea backup ventilation is an emergency mode of ventilation available in the spontaneous mode or with mandatory rates set at less than 6 breaths/min. It is triggered when the selected Ta elapses without a patient breath detected. Box 12-79 outlines the procedure for setting apnea ventilation.

TROUBLESHOOTING

The message window and alarm package available with the 740 help in troubleshooting most problems that may occur. The operator's manual provides more detail about the technical and clinical alarm conditions if special problems arise.

As with other microprocessor-operated medical equipment, the Puritan Bennett 740 may be susceptible to certain transmitting devices, such as cellular phones, walkie-talkies, cordless phones, and pagers. The radio frequency emissions from these devices are additive; therefore the ventilator must be located a sufficient distance from them to prevent interruption of operation.

If an abnormal restart alarm occurs when the ventilator is turned on, the unit may be running on AC power, but the battery is low.

Some common errors that respiratory therapists make when using the Puritan Bennett 740 include the following:

· Failing to touch (address) each of the flashing settings buttons during start-up, then connecting the patient and erroneously assuming the ventilator is operating appropriately
· Not setting the low pressure alarm limit appropriately when using the speaking valve mode
· Assuming that the battery will charge when the 740 is plugged in but turned off

As with any ventilator, it is very important that therapists familiarize themselves with all aspects of the safe operation of the 740, according to manufacturer's directions.

BOX 12-79	Setting Apnea Parameters (Puritan Bennett 740)

To set the apnea parameters, perform the following steps:
1. While the ventilator is in the spontaneous mode, or in A/C or SIMV with a rate of fewer than 6 breaths/min, press APNEA PARAMS. The apnea parameter key lights steadily.
2. The following key lights flash for apnea settings: RESPIRATORY RATE, TIDAL VOLUME, and PEAK FLOW. The message window displays APNEA SETUP. SELECT A SETTING.
3. Each flashing light control must be touched. If necessary, adjust the setting as well. For example, touch the TIDAL VOLUME key; it now lights steadily. Use the knob control to change the volume setting if desired, and touch ACCEPT to have the new apnea V_T accepted.
4. Once all settings are set, press ACCEPT again to apply the new apnea settings. The message window will read SETTING(S) ACCEPTED.
5. If CLEAR is pressed before the settings have been accepted, the parameter is not updated. The APNEA PARAMS key flashes, and the message window shows ALL SETUP CANCELED. UPDATE APNEA.

KEY POINTS

▶ Ventilator internal tests include the power on self-test, the short self-test, and the extended self-test.
▶ Gas flow to the patient is provided by a linear-drive piston that can deliver flow in either a constant or a descending waveform.
▶ Modes include assist/control, SIMV, and spontaneous, which can be supported with PS.
▶ Apnea ventilation is available in all modes of ventilation. It becomes active when the set apnea time interval (Ta) has elapsed and the ventilator has not detected a patient inspiration.

▶ The Ta is set by selecting USER SETTINGS under the MENU key.
▶ After a VENT INOP alarm, an alternative method must be found to ventilate the patient and an EST must be performed on the ventilator.
▶ To apply a new mode, the operator must touch and adjust the setting for every setting key that is flashing.
▶ Apnea backup ventilation is an emergency mode of ventilation that operates in the spontaneous mode or with mandatory rates set at less than 6 breaths/min.

ASSESSMENT QUESTIONS

See Evolve Resources for the answers.

1. During ventilation of a patient with the 740, the message window reads O₂% LOW and LOW O₂ SUPPLY. The red alarm indicator is flashing, and an audible pattern of three beeps and then two beeps repeats. Which of the following statements about this situation is/are true?
   - I. The O₂ % setting is higher than 21%.
   - II. The oxygen sensor is malfunctioning.
   - III. The measured O₂ % is at least 10% less than the set O₂ % for 30 seconds or longer.
   - IV. The high-pressure oxygen gas source is not providing adequate pressure.
   - V. This is a medium priority alarm message.
     - a. I only
     - b. III and V only
     - c. II and IV only
     - d. I, III, and IV only

2. After a POST, the 740 ventilator gives the message PM DUE 24, indicating which of the following?
   - a. It is midnight.
   - b. A maintenance check is due in 24 hours.
   - c. The patient's next treatment is in 24 minutes.
   - d. The patient has been on the ventilator for 24 hours.

3. An SST should be run under which of the following conditions?
   - I. Every 15 days
   - II. When a new patient is to be started
   - III. When the patient circuit is changed
   - IV. After any alarm situation
     - a. II only
     - b. I and III only
     - c. I, II, and III only
     - d. I, II, III, and IV

4. Which of the following functions would the respiratory therapist activate before suctioning a patient?
   - I. STANDBY mode
   - II. ALARM SILENCE
   - III. 100% O₂
   - IV. CLEAR
     - a. I only
     - b. II only
     - c. III and IV only
     - d. II and III only

5. The respiratory therapist returns to the bedside of a patient ventilated with the 740 and notices that the alarm indicator is illuminated steadily in red. The message window reads HIGH PRESSURE, and no alarm is sounding. Which of the following statements is true?
   - a. Inspiration has ended because high pressure was reached.
   - b. The inspiratory line is occluded.
   - c. An autoreset of the high pressure alarm has occurred.
   - d. The patient needs suctioning.

6. The modes of ventilation on the 740 include which of the following?
   - I. PSV
   - II. A/C volume ventilation
   - III. PCV
   - IV. SIMV volume ventilation
     - a. II and III only
     - b. III and IV only
     - c. I, II, and IV only
     - d. I, II, III, and IV

7. How should the 740 be maintained when it is not in use?
   - a. The ventilator should be in the STANDBY mode and plugged into an AC power source.
   - b. The ventilator should be plugged into AC power and kept in the off position.
   - c. The ventilator should be plugged into AC power and high-pressure gas sources and kept on STANDBY.
   - d. No special procedure is required when the ventilator is not in use.

8. Which of the following statements are true regarding apnea ventilation?
   - a. Once apnea ventilation is activated, only the operator can return the ventilator to its previous functioning mode.
   - b. Apnea ventilation works in all modes.
   - c. It is active when the mandatory breath rate is less than 6 breaths/min during A/C and SIMV.
   - d. Apnea ventilation is available on the 760 but not on the 740.

9. Patient breath triggering in all modes of ventilation is by what variable?
   - a. Flow triggering
   - b. Volume triggering
   - c. Pressure triggering
   - d. Time triggering

10. Which of the following power sources are required for the 740 to deliver a breath?
    - I. AC electrical outlet
    - II. High-pressure oxygen outlet
    - III. High-pressure air outlet
    - IV. Internal battery power
      - a. I only
      - b. I and II only
      - c. II, III, and IV only
      - d. I, II, III, and IV

11. After completing the mode set-up on a patient who is being switched from A/C to SIMV, the respiratory therapist notices the rate key flashing and the digital display showing 10 breaths/min. Pressing ACCEPT does not initiate the settings she has selected and begin SIMV. The most likely cause of the problem is:
    - a. The rate is set too low for the SIMV mode
    - b. She should have pressed the ACCEPT key after each change in a parameter setting
    - c. She must adjust all parameters in that mode before pressing ACCEPT
    - d. SIMV is not available on the 740 ventilator

References

1. Puritan Bennett: 740 ventilator system operator's manual, G-060143-00 revision B 0697, Pleasanton, Calif, 1997, Puritan Bennett, a division of Covidien, Mansfield, Mass.
2. Puritan Bennett: 740 ventilator system, A-AA2214-00 revision A (02/00), Pleasanton, Calif, 2000, Puritan Bennett, a division of Covidien, Mansfield, Mass.
3. Puritan Bennett: Puritan-Bennett 700 series ventilator system: operator's manual, G-061874-00, revision D, Pleasanton,

Calif, 2000, Puritan Bennett, a division of Covidien, Mansfield, Mass.
4. Milne G, product manager, Puritan Bennett: Personal communication, 2007, Pleasanton, Calif.

Internet Resources
www.puritanbennett.com
www.Covidien.com

PURITAN BENNETT 760[1-2]

OUTLINE

Controls and Alarms
   Ventilator Settings Section
   Patient Data Section
   Ventilator Status Section

Modes of Ventilation

OBJECTIVES

Upon completion of this section, you will be able to:
· List the options and breath types available on the 760 that are not available on the 740.
· Calculate the inspiratory time (T_I), expiratory time (T_E), and inspiratory to expiratory ratio (I:E) when these variables are selected in pressure-controlled ventilation (PCV).
· Explain the setting and function of exhalation sensitivity, rise time factor, and inspiratory and expiratory pause.
· Identify the presence of auto-PEEP using the end-expiratory flow value in the message window.

KEY TERMS

Linear-drive piston   Operating panel   Rise time factor

As with the Puritan Bennett 740, the 760 ventilator is easy to operate but still uses advanced technology (Figure 12-100). The 760 is nearly identical to the 740 in its internal platform. For example, it also uses a **linear-drive piston** and requires only an AC electrical power source to function. It probably is easiest to think of it as a 740 with added options. The primary differences are the operating panel (user interface), the addition of the pressure control breath, and a few features that have been added to the menu.

The reader is assumed to have reviewed the function of the 740 before reading this section, which focuses on the added options and the interface differences in the 760.

CONTROLS AND ALARMS

As with the 740, the **operating panel** of the 760 is divided into three sections: the Ventilator Settings section, the Patient Data section, and the Ventilator Status section (Figure 12-101).

Ventilator Settings Section

The Ventilator Settings section of the 760 has additional controls. Besides A/C and SIMV volume ventilation, it

offers A/C and SIMV with pressure-control ventilation (PCV) for mandatory breaths. The settings and data display for PCV are added to the settings in the left and right columns; these include the inspiratory pressure, inspiratory time (T_I) or inspiratory to expiratory (I:E) ratio setting, **rise time factor,** inspiratory and expiratory pause, and exhalation sensitivity.

INSPIRATORY PRESSURE sets the target pressure for pressure-controlled (PC) breaths and is the pressure above the positive end-expiratory pressure (PEEP) delivered to the patient during inspiration (5 to 80 cm H_2O).

T_I/I:E RATIO displays the T_I and the I:E ratio and is located above the "peak flow" control. Which parameter is constant, T_I or I:E, is determined by the setting the operator uses under the menu section called USER SETTINGS. (More information on this is provided in a later section.) The selected T_I or I:E can be changed at any time during PC. After it is active, the selected value remains constant, even if the respiratory rate is changed (Box 12-80). To help the operator set an appropriate inspiratory time during PCV, the message window displays the peak inspiratory flow, end-inspiratory flow, and end-exhalation flow in liters per minute (L/min). For example, if the operator

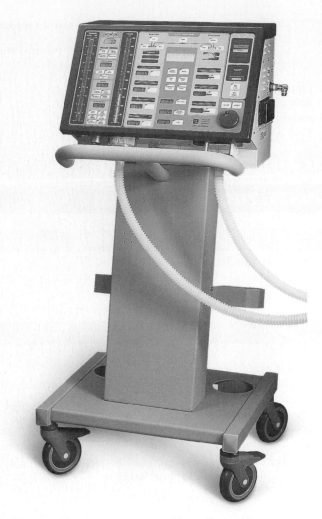

FIGURE 12-100 Puritan Bennett 760 ventilator. (Courtesy Puritan Bennett, a division of Covidien, Mansfield, Mass.)

BOX 12-80	Using Constant T_I and Constant I:E (Puritan Bennett 760)

Suppose pressure-controlled ventilation (PCV) is set with the inspiratory time (T_I) constant and a rate of 12 breaths/min. The total cycle time (TCT) will be 5 seconds. If T_I is set at 1 second, the expiratory time (T_E) is 4 seconds (I:E = 1:4). The T_E can vary and so can the I:E ratio when the rate is changed. Suppose you increase the rate to 15 breaths/min. The TCT now is 4 seconds, the T_I is still 1 second, and the T_E now is 3 seconds (I:E = 1:3).

You can change the selected T_I or I:E ratio, but the setting remains constant when you change the respiratory rate in PCV. Using our previous example, you can still increase the T_I when it is set as a constant. For instance, even with the T_I set as the constant, you can increase it to 2 seconds at the set rate of 15 breaths/min. The new result will be a T_I of 2 seconds, a T_E of 3 seconds, and an I:E ratio of 2:3, or 1:1.5.

Suppose the I:E is held constant at 1:4 with a rate of 12 breaths/min. The T_I is 1 second, and the T_E is 4 seconds. If the rate is increased to 15 breaths/min with a constant I:E of 1:4, then the T_I and T_E vary. The T_I in this case is 0.8 seconds, and the T_E is 3.2 seconds (see Chapter 11 for equations). Again, you can change the I:E, even though it is constant. For example, if the I:E is changed from 1:4 to 1:3 with a rate of 12 breaths/min, the T_I will be 1.25 seconds, and the T_E will be 3.75 seconds.

wants a slight pause at the end of inspiration (no flow period), the T_I can be adjusted so that inspiratory flow ends at zero. To guard against auto-PEEP, the operator must make sure that flow at the end of exhalation is zero.

The 760 has two rise time controls, which allow the rise time for PCV and pressure-support ventilation (PSV) to be adjusted independently. RISE TIME FACTOR for PCV breaths is displayed above the plateau control when PCV is the mandatory breath type. The control for setting the rise time is on the right side of the ventilator panel. *Rise time* is the amount of time it takes for inspiratory pressure to rise from 0 to 95% of the set pressure during PCV. It is adjustable from 5% to 100%. A setting of 100% means that it takes only 100 msec for the pressure to rise to the set pressure. This is a very rapid rise. The set pressure is delivered quickly so that the pressure is in the lungs for a greater part of the inspiratory time. When the rise time is set at 5%, it takes longer (2500 msec or 80% of the T_I, whichever is less) to reach the set pressure. This is a very slow, tapered curve, and the set pressure is in the lungs for a shorter period.

Tapering the rate at which the pressure enters the lungs may be more comfortable for the patient (see the section on sloping or rise time in Chapter 11). When this setting is adjusted, the message window shows the actual time in seconds that it takes to reach 95% of the target pressure.

The center section of the ventilator setting panel has the following items, which also present on the 740: apnea parameters, menu, 100% O_2, manual inspiration, PEEP/CPAP, trigger sensitivity, and % O_2 (these were described in the section on the Puritan Bennett 740). An additional feature with the apnea parameter settings on the 760 is that the operator can select either PCV or volume-controlled ventilation (VCV) in the apnea ventilation (AV) settings. Using PCV in apnea ventilation allows the rate, inspiratory pressure, and I:E or T_I to be set. The 760 fixes the rise time factor in AV at 50%.

The three new items on the 760 control panel are the EXPIRATORY PAUSE key, INSPIRATORY PAUSE key, and EXHALATION SENSITIVITY key. These and the additional menu items are reviewed later.

Menu Items

Two features were added to the 760 menu under USER SETTINGS: a PCV timing variable and a volume LED bar enable/disable function. (NOTE: To enter the menu, the operator presses the MENU key, uses the control knob to scroll to USER SETTINGS, and then presses ACCEPT.)

Pressure-Controlled Ventilation (PCV) Timing Variable. When PCV TIMING VARIABLE is selected, the ventilator displays the currently selected item in the message window.

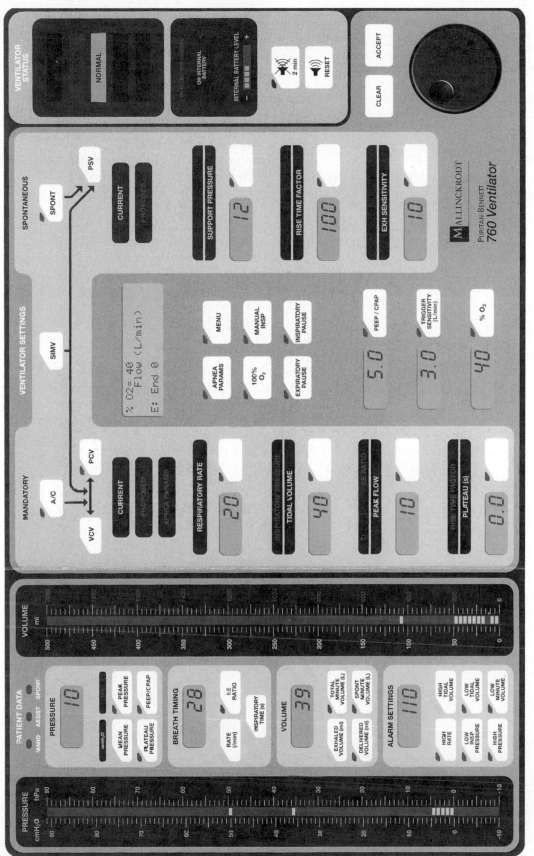

FIGURE 12-101 Graphic user interface (GUI) of the Puritan Bennett 760 ventilator. (Courtesy Puritan Bennett, a division of Covidien, Mansfield, Mass.)

It displays either TIMING VARIABLE = TI or TIMING VARIABLE = I:E. This variable can be changed by turning the control knob to highlight T_I or I:E and pressing the ACCEPT key to activate the change. Pressing CLEAR allows the ventilator to remain with the current setting.

Volume LED. The VOLUME LED BAR menu, also listed under USER SETTINGS, provides two choices: ENABLE LED BAR and DISABLE LED BAR. The VOLUME LED BAR is located in the Patient Data section of the operating panel and is described later.

Expiratory Pause

Using EXPIRATORY PAUSE allows measurement of auto-PEEP. The message window normally shows the end-expiratory flow at the beginning of each breath. If expiratory flow is present when the ventilator delivers the next breath, auto-PEEP is present. At this point it is appropriate to perform an expiratory pause.

It is assumed that the patient is not actively breathing when this measurement is done, because a stable reading cannot be made if the patient is trying to exhale or inhale during the maneuver. When EXPIRATORY PAUSE is activated, the exhalation valve closes at the end of the expiratory phase and the ventilator delays delivery of the next mandatory breath. The pause continues as long as the key is held down (to a maximum of 20 seconds), and it should last only until the expiratory pressure stabilizes. Five circumstances can end the expiratory pause measurement: (1) the operator releases the key, (2) the patient initiates a breath, (3) an alarm occurs, (4) the pause lasts longer than 20 seconds, and (5) the ventilator detects a leak.

After the maneuver, the auto-PEEP and total PEEP values are displayed in the message window for 30 seconds. The expiratory pause cannot be performed if the rate is set at less than 3 breaths/min.

Inspiratory Pause

As its name suggests, the INSPIRATORY PAUSE key is used to provide a pause at the end of inspiration. The ventilator uses the data recorded to calculate lung compliance and airway resistance. These values are displayed in the message window for 30 seconds after the test is performed. As with the end-expiratory pause, the patient cannot be actively breathing if this test is to be performed successfully.

An inspiratory pause can be done in two ways. First, the INSP PAUSE button is pressed once and the ventilator searches for a stable inspiratory plateau pressure reading. This method ends the pause when the plateau stabilizes or at the end of 2 seconds, whichever comes first. With the second method, after pressing the button the first time, the operator presses and holds the button after the pause has begun. The key must be held for at least 2 seconds. The pause can be lengthened for up to 10 seconds. During this maneuver the ventilator closes the expiratory valve. When the button is activated, the ventilator waits until the end of the inspiratory phase of the current breath, or it waits

until the next mandatory breath occurs. At the end of the inspiration, the pause is initiated. If the key is activated during spontaneous ventilation, the ventilator uses a mandatory breath based on the apnea ventilation settings for breath delivery before the pause.

The operator can press CLEAR or release the INSP PAUSE key at any time to cancel the pause maneuver. The occurrence of an alarm also cancels the maneuver.

Exhalation Sensitivity

The EXHALATION SENSITIVITY control adjusts the percent of the peak flow at which inspiratory flow ends during pressure support. Normally, a pressure-support (PS) breath ends when the ventilator determines that the inspiratory flow to the patient has dropped to 25% of the measured peak flow or when the flow is 10 L/min, whichever is less (flow-cycled breath). On the 760, this percent termination point is adjustable from 1% to 80% of peak flow. This applies to spontaneous as well as PS breaths. Exhalation begins when the inspiratory flow is less than the set value. For example, if peak flow during inspiration is 100 L/min and the exhalation sensitivity is set at 50%, exhalation begins when the inspiratory flow drops to 50 L/min (50% of 100 L/min).

To set the EXHALATION SENSITIVITY appropriately, it is important that the operator watch the flow values displayed in the message window and also observe the patient. The patient should not be struggling to exhale, nor should the inspiratory time be too long. (NOTE: It is advisable to check that an SST was run recently. This helps ensure the accuracy of these flows by ensuring that tubing compliance calculations are correct.)

Patient Data Section

As with the 740, the Patient Data section of the 760 has a pressure bar graph and digital windows that display pressure, breath timing, and volume monitored data. It also has an alarm section that displays alarm settings. In addition, the 760 Patient Data section has a volume bar graph.

Plateau pressure and PEEP/CPAP touch pads have been added to the pressure section of the 760 so that these values can be displayed along with the mean and peak pressures. In the timing section, the T_I (in seconds) has been added to the rate and I:E ratio displays of the 740. The operator now can obtain not only the exhaled volume and total minute volume, but the delivered volume and spontaneous minute volume as well. The delivered volume shows the measured inspiratory tidal volume for the last completed PCV or PSV breath.

The alarm section contains the same alarm parameters as the 740: high and low tidal volume, high rate, high and low inspiratory pressure, and low minute volume.

Volume Bar Graph

The volume bar graph (see Figure 12-101) shows real-time exhaled volumes in milliliters (mL). The scale is determined by the high tidal volume alarm setting. For example, for a high tidal volume alarm of less than 500 mL, the scale is 0 to 500 mL with 5 mL resolution. For high tidal volume alarms set at 500 mL or higher, the scale is 0 to 2000 mL with 20 mL resolution.

The volume bar graph can be enabled (turned on) or disabled (turned off) using the USER SETTINGS menu, accessible with the MENU key. LEDs indicate the current high and low tidal volume alarm settings. During exhalation, moving LEDs show the maximum exhaled volume for the last breath.

Ventilator Status Section

The Ventilator Status section on the right side of the operating panel of the 760 is the same as that on the 740, as are the control knob and the CLEAR and ACCEPT keys.

MODES OF VENTILATION

In addition to the modes available on the 740, the 760 includes the PC breath type. It can be selected as the mandatory breath in either assist-control (A/C) or synchronized intermittent mandatory ventilation (SIMV). PC breaths in these two modes are patient or time triggered, pressure targeted (inspiratory pressure setting), and time cycled. After selecting either A/C or SIMV, the operator sets the variables that flash to set up the required parameters for that mode. Remember, as with the 740, the operator must set all of the flashing controls before pressing ACCEPT, which activates the mode. Along with the rate, the operator can select T_I or I:E as constants (PCV TIMING setting). These variables establish the inspiratory time and expiratory time (T_E) and the I:E ratio, which are displayed in the ventilator and data status sections of the operating panel. The operator must be sure to set the desired PCV TIMING SETTING from the USER SETTINGS in the menu. The rise time can be used to taper the beginning of the mandatory PC breath. Clinical Rounds 12-33 presents a problem related to PCV.

When SIMV is selected, the spontaneous breaths occur from the baseline pressure (PEEP/CPAP) and can also be supported with PS. The expiratory sensitivity can be set to adjust the termination point of inspiratory flow.

CLINICAL ROUNDS 12-33

During A/C PCV ventilation with the 760, the respiratory therapist records the following data:

Inspiratory pressure = 18 cm H_2O, PEEP = 5 cm H_2O, V_T exhaled = 350 mL (volume bar graph), rate = 16 breaths/min, T_I constant at 1 second, T_E = 2.75 seconds (I:E 1:2.75), end-inspiratory flow = 5 L/min, end-expiratory flow = 3 L/min.

Do you think the therapist should perform an inspiratory pause? An expiratory pause? What is your opinion of this information?

See Evolve Resources for the answer.

KEY POINTS

▶ The three sections of the operating panel on the Puritan Bennett 760 include the Ventilator Settings section, the Patient Data section, and the Ventilator Status section.

▶ By accessing USER SETTINGS with the MENU key, the operator can set either T_I or the I:E ratio as constant during PCV.

▶ Rise time is the amount of time it takes for inspiratory pressure to rise to 95% of the set pressure during PCV.

▶ When setting up a mode of ventilation, the operator must set all the flashing controls before pressing the ACCEPT key.

ASSESSMENT QUESTIONS

See Evolve Resources for the answers.

1. Which of the following controls adjusts the flow percent at which a pressure-support breath ends on the 760 ventilator?
   a. Expiratory pause
   b. Exhalation sensitivity
   c. Rise time factor
   d. Inspiratory pause
2. Which of the following features is *not* available on the 740 but is available on the 760?
   a. Pressure support
   b. Trigger sensitivity
   c. Volume bar graph
   d. I:E ratio display
3. What is the easiest way to detect the presence of auto-PEEP with the 760?
   a. Observe the end-expiratory pressure
   b. Set the exhalation sensitivity to 100%
   c. Check the flow-time curve on the graphic display
   d. Check the end-expiratory flow in the message window
4. To set the T_I as the constant when PCV is activated, the operator must:
   a. Set it on the control panel using the TI/I:E control
   b. Go to USER SETTINGS in the menu and select TI/I:E
   c. Keep the rate the same at all times
   d. Use another ventilator because the 760 will not allow T_I as a constant
5. Setting the RISE TIME FACTOR to 100% during PCV gives:
   a. The most rapid rise to the set pressure
   b. A flow cycle of 100% of peak flow measured
   c. An inspiratory pause of 0.01 second
   d. The slowest rise to the set pressure

References

1. Puritan Bennett: Puritan Bennett 700 Series ventilator system: operator's manual, G-061874-00, revision D, Pleasanton, Calif, 2000, Puritan Bennett, a division of Tyco Healthcare.
2. Hyde D, product manager, Puritan Bennett: Personal communication, 2000, Pleasanton, Calif.

Internet Resources
www.puritanbennett.com
www.Covidien.com

PURITAN BENNETT 7200

OUTLINE

Power Source
Internal Mechanism
Controls and Alarms
  Self-Test
  Initial Start-Up
  General Setting of Parameters
Ventilator Settings
  Breath Parameter Keys
  Additional Control Parameters
Monitors and Alarms
  Monitors: Patient Data Section
  Setting of Alarms
  Ventilator Status
Modes of Ventilation
  Continuous Mandatory Ventilation (CMV)
  Synchronized Intermittent Mandatory Ventilation (SIMV)

Spontaneous/Continuous Positive Airway Pressure (CPAP)
Pressure-Control Ventilation (PCV)
Pressure-Support Ventilation (PSV)
Special Functions
  Apnea Ventilation
  Back-Up Ventilation
  Disconnect Ventilation
  Respiratory Mechanics
  Flow and Flow-By Triggering
  Ventilator Graphics Waveforms
Troubleshooting

OBJECTIVES

Upon completion of this section, you will be able to:
· Explain the procedure for setting a mode and its parameters.
· Adjust ventilator settings appropriately when the DECR RESP RATE FIRST message appears.
· Identify conditions that activate emergency modes of ventilation.
· Recognize breath delay when switching from continuous mandatory ventilation (CMV) to synchronized intermittent mandatory ventilation (SIMV) and provide an appropriate solution.
· Describe the available flow waveforms and their effect on breath delivery, inspiratory time, and peak flow.
· Recommend appropriate corrections to alarm situations.
· List the weaning measurements available under the respiratory mechanics option.
· Calculate the inspiratory to expiratory (I:E) ratio, inspiratory and expiratory time, and total cycle time during pressure-control ventilation (PCV).
· Recommend an appropriate flow trigger and base flow setting for a patient.
· Compare the functions of the 1.0 version of flow-by on the 7200 with those of the 2.0 version.

KEY TERMS

Antisuffocation (safety) valve   Extended self-test (EST)   Power on self-test (POST)
Backup ventilation   Overpressure-relief valve

The Puritan Bennett 7200[1,2] was one of the first ventilators to provide microprocessor control of its electrical functions (Figure 12-102). It is no longer manufactured (effective January 2002), but Puritan Bennett will support the ventilator with parts and repair until 2012.

The 7200 was released in 1983 and has since gone through a series of upgrades, which included two changes in the front control panel to improve ease of use. The third version of the front panel is described throughout this section. The 7200 is intended for use with pediatric and adult patients in the acute care setting. (NOTE: Readers are advised to check the version and options on the 7200 they are using and to be sure to refer to the operator's manual for instructions.)

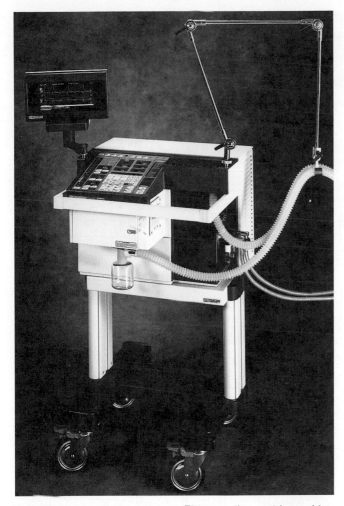

FIGURE 12-102 Puritan Bennett 7200 ventilator with graphics monitor. (Courtesy Puritan Bennett, a division of Covidien, Mansfield, Mass.)

POWER SOURCE

The unit requires both pneumatic and electrical power sources to operate. It normally uses high-pressure air and oxygen sources (35 to 100 psig) for pneumatic functions, but it can also operate from a single gas source or a high-pressure compressor. The latter two options alter oxygen delivery. A standard 115-volt, AC 60 Hz outlet provides the electrical power. (NOTE: If the ventilator is disconnected from the power source, it will stop operating. It does not have an internal battery to power the ventilator.)

INTERNAL MECHANISM

The air and oxygen sources flow through inlet filters to regulators, which reduce and balance pressure to 10 psig (about 700 cm H_2O). The gases are then conducted through flow transducers to electrically operated, microprocessor-controlled proportional solenoid (metering) valves. These valves regulate the amount and pattern of gas flow to the patient based on settings and microprocessor control.

As gas passes from the solenoid valves, it flows through the following:

1. A pressure transducer, which acts as an internal barometer
2. A safety/check valve, which serves two functions:
   · It acts as an **overpressure-relief valve,** which opens at 140 cm H_2O.
   · It serves as an **antisuffocation (safety) valve** (I), which opens during the start-up self-test and if pneumatic or electrical power is lost.

Gas flow to the expiration valve is controlled by a solenoid. During a mandatory breath, the solenoid opens, allowing gas to be directed through the expiratory line and closing the expiratory valve on the patient circuit. During expiration, the expiratory solenoid closes and gas flows from the positive end-expiratory pressure (PEEP) regulator and the PEEP Venturi to the back of the expiratory valve. This produces the set level of PEEP/CPAP during expiration.

The 7200 has two differential pressure transducers. One measures PEEP, and the other measures airway pressure. Exhaled patient air passes through the expiratory flow transducer, which provides information for measuring and calculating the tidal volume (V_T) and expired minute volume ($\dot{V}_E$), as well as monitors and provides some alarm functions.

CONTROLS AND ALARMS

The three front panels designed for the 7200, beginning with its original design in the 1980s and progressing to a more recent version in 1994 (Figure 12-103), are divided into three basic sections:

1. Ventilator settings (controls)
2. Patient data (monitoring information)
3. Ventilator status (alarm information)

Box 12-81 describes the function of each of these sections. Although the positioning of these controls has changed somewhat, the overall design remained consistent. A table on the Evolve Web site for this text lists the specifications for the updated (Enhanced) version of the 7200 (Table 12-43).

Self-Test

When the ventilator is first turned on (the power switch is on the left side), the microprocessor starts the **power on self-test (POST)**. The POST usually lasts about 5 seconds, depending on the version used. Like most microprocessor-controlled ventilators, the 7200 must complete these essential tests before it becomes functional. (NOTE: Neither the **extended self-test [EST]** nor the POST should be run while the ventilator is connected to a patient.)

The POST runs in the following situations:
· When the ventilator is turned on
· When the EST is run
· When power is interrupted
· When ongoing checks detect a system error

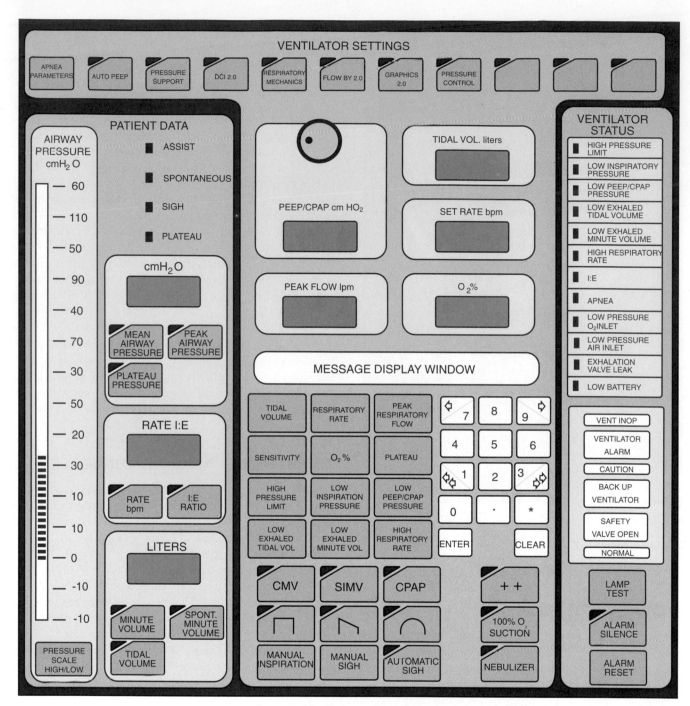

FIGURE 12-103 Third-generation control panel for the Enhanced Plus 7200 ventilator. (Redrawn from Puritan Bennett, a division of Covidien, Mansfield, Mass.)

After the POST, all previous ventilator settings are recalled from memory and activated (Box 12-82). If the POST fails, the **backup ventilation** mode becomes operational. (The discussion of special functions later in this section explains backup ventilation.) In addition, the message window gives all error codes that need to be recorded for the service representative. A replacement ventilator should be provided immediately.

Two additional tests, the quick extended self-test (QUEST) and the total extended self-test (TEST), are also available. QUEST executes 26 tests and takes about 2 minutes. To run QUEST, the operator presses the EST button on the side panel and the ENTER control on the front panel. The operator presses ENTER again when the window reads PAT TUBING OFF–ENTER. (NOTE: This instruction is to ensure that the patient is not being ventilated while the test is run.) The instructions provided in the display window should be followed as they appear. QUEST should be run whenever the patient circuit is changed.

The TEST executes 60 tests and takes about 3 to 5 minutes. It is part of the normal maintenance procedure and is routinely performed by biomedical personnel. As

BOX 12-81	Keyboard Sections (Puritan Bennett 7200)

Patient Data Section
Displays monitored patient information, such as pressure, volume, rate, I:E ratio, and breath type.

Ventilator Settings Section
Contains the keys that allow the operator to set values for specific parameters and alarms. It also contains a message window that displays values for set parameters and allows selection of special functions, such as manual inspiration, manual sigh, and 100% O_2 suction. Use of the key in this section, along with the numeric key pads, provides access to supplemental functions, such as pressure control and flow-by. (NOTE: Some of these functions are also available by pressing the labeled keys at the top of the front panel [see Figure 12-103].)

Ventilator Status Sections
Contains 12 alarm indicators and six status display indicators that notify the operator if an alarm condition exists. In addition, three key pads allow testing of the front panel lights, such as ALARM SILENCING, ALARM RESET, and LAMP TEST.

BOX 12-82	Backup Memory Battery (Puritan Bennett 7200)

The memory that contains previously set parameter values is powered by batteries. This helps prevent loss of information if electrical power is interrupted (e.g., the machine is accidentally unplugged while in use). If the battery fails, the message 1401 ERR indicates that the ventilator is using the default parameters programmed into the read-only memory (ROM) of the microprocessor. The operator should review all settings immediately, according to the following list of default parameters:
· Mode CMV
· Constant flow waveform
· V_T of 0.5 L
· Rate of 12 breaths/min
· Flow of 45 L/min
· Sensitivity of −3 cm H_2O below baseline
· 100% O_2
· High-pressure limit of 20 cm H_2O
· Low-pressure limit of 3 cm H_2O
· Apnea interval of 20 seconds

Functions that are off or disabled include 100% O_2 suction, sigh, nebulizer, low PEEP/CPAP alarm, low V_T alarm, low V_E alarm, and low rate alarm.

TABLE 12-43

++ Key Options and Functions—Puritan Bennett 7200

Number	Function or Option
Function 1	Apnea ventilation*
Function 2	Clock-calendar reset
Function 3	Patient data
Function 4	Auto-PEEP
Option 10	Pressure support
Option 20	Digital communications interface (DCI)
Option 30/40	Respiratory mechanics*
Option 50	Flow-by (flow trigger)*
Option 60	Graphics
Option 80	Pressure-control ventilation
Option 90	Pulse oximetry

From Puritan Bennett, a division of Covidien, Mansfield, Massachusetts.
*Covered in the discussion of special functions in this section.

with QUEST, it is accessed by pressing the EST and ENTER buttons. After the PAT TUBING OFF–ENTER instruction appears, ENTER is pressed, and in response to QUICK EST, the key labeled + + is pressed. Finally, ENTER is pressed again. As with QUEST, the operator then simply follows the instructions sequentially displayed in the window. (NOTE: The explanation for canceling EST and responding to error messages is beyond the scope of this text and is really intended for ventilator maintenance. The reader is referred to the operator's manual if these procedures are required.)

Initial Start-Up

After the machine is turned on and the POST is completed, the message REVIEW APNEA PARAMS appears in the window as a reminder to make sure that the apnea parameters are appropriate for the patient. Then the mode is selected (see the discussion of special functions later in this section).

Automatic sigh parameters also must be checked to ensure that they are set as desired for the new patient; otherwise, old values stored in memory become operational. (The operation of sigh is described in the discussion of additional control parameters in this section.) In addition, it is important that the operator check the PEEP control, because it may have been set for the last patient and not returned to the zero position after use.

General Setting of Parameters

The ventilator is operated with the touch pads on the front panel. Except for the PEEP/CPAP control knob, all parameters are set with these function keys.

To view the set value for any parameter, the operator presses that function key. Some function keys display the parameter value at all times, including the following:
· Tidal volume
· Respiratory rate
· Peak inspiratory flow
· Sensitivity
· O_2 %

The 7200 also has function keys for alarm variables. These are reviewed in the discussion of monitors and alarms.

When the operator presses a key pad, the current set value for that variable appears in the message display window in the central portion of the panel. Changing the value requires several steps, which are outlined in Box 12-83. (NOTE: In addition, see Figure 1 on the Evolve Web site for this text for an algorithm related to changing ventilator parameter values on the Puritan Bennett 7200.)

| BOX 12-83 | Changing a Parameter Value (Puritan Bennett 7200) |

To change the value of any variable (e.g., tidal volume), perform the following steps:
1. Press the key pad labeled with the variable.
2. Press the desired numeric value using the number keys below the message window.
3. Press the ENTER key to place the new value in memory.
4. An acceptable setting is confirmed by two beeps.

If the entry is outside the range of the parameter, four beeps sound and the display screen displays an error message: INVALID ENTRY. For example, a tidal volume of 3 L is outside the range of the unit and therefore invalid. The operator must press CLEAR and try again.

If the change takes longer than about 20 to 30 seconds, the unit reverts to the previous setting. (NOTE: The new setting is not activated until the ENTER key is pressed.)

| BOX 12-84 | DECR RESP RATE FIRST Message (Puritan Bennett 7200) |

The DECR RESP RATE FIRST message appears when a new value for the tidal volume (V_T), peak inspiratory flow, or plateau or flow waveform is selected that results in lengthening of the inspiratory time (T_I) to greater than or equal to 75% of the total cycle time (TCT) based on the rate setting. The ventilator gives preference to T_I to lengthen TCT; therefore it is suggested that the rate be reduced. Other courses of action would be to increase inspiratory flow, alter the plateau time, or change the waveform pattern.

(NOTE: During pressure-controlled ventilation [PCV], the T_I can be greater than or equal to 80% of the TCT to allow for inverse ratios up to 4:1 in this mode.)

VENTILATOR SETTINGS

Establishing appropriate settings includes determining breath parameters and additional control values.

Breath Parameter Keys

The tidal volume (V_T) control is functional in volume-targeted modes (continuous mandatory ventilation [CMV] and synchronized intermittent mandatory ventilation [SIMV]) and provides a range of 0.1 to 2.5 L. The range for the respiratory rate is adjustable from 0.5 to 9.9 breaths/min in increments of 0.1 breaths/min and from 10 to 70 breaths/min in increments of 1 breath/min. The rate control functions in CMV, SIMV, and pressure-controlled ventilation (PCV). The peak inspiratory flow (10 to 120 L/min) operates only during volume ventilation.

Breaths are volume cycled during volume ventilation; that is, a breath ends when the ventilator determines that the flow provided over a specific time has delivered a specific volume (V_T = Flow × Inspiratory time).* If a flow is selected that cannot deliver the set volume within a time that provides an acceptable I:E ratio, a message reads DECR RESP RATE FIRST. The ventilator microprocessor knows that reducing the rate allows a longer inspiratory time (T_I). Of course, increasing the flow also solves the problem and does not change the overall minute ventilation. Box 12-84 provides examples of situations in which this message is displayed. Clinical Rounds 12-34 presents an exercise for calculating the volume, rate, and flow that would result in an error message.

The pressure sensitivity (0.5 to 20 cm H_2O) is adjusted with the key pad and numeric controls. However, flow triggering is also available when the flow-by function is selected. Flow-by and flow triggering in the 7200 are described in the discussion of special functions in this section. The available % O_2 ranges from 21% to 100%. The

*This can also be called *flow cycling;* see Chapter 11.

CLINICAL ROUNDS 12-34

A respiratory therapist selects the following settings on the 7200 ventilator during a laboratory test with the machine: V_T = 1 L (1000 mL), rate = 20 breaths/min, flow = 30 L/min, and flow waveform = constant. Will the DECR RESP RATE FIRST message appear with these settings?

See Evolve Resources for the answer.

7200 does not have a built-in oxygen analyzer to test the delivery of the fractional inspired oxygen concentration (F_IO_2.).

The plateau control closes the inspiratory and expiratory valves at the end of inspiration for the time selected (0 to 2 seconds). An inspiratory plateau is functional only during a volume breath. The inspiratory phase is increased by the time set.

Additional Control Parameters

In addition to the variables and settings already described, three more areas of the front panel (see Figure 12-103) allow functions to be set and settings monitored:
1. The lower central portion of the front panel, below the alarm function keys and the numeric pad
2. A row of controls across the top of the panel
3. A set of display screens that show current settings

The controls at the bottom center of the panel are discussed first. The first three functional keys are used to select CMV, SIMV, and continuous positive airway pressure (CPAP). Pressing the desired key pad and then pressing ENTER activate a new mode (see the discussion of modes of ventilation in this section).

Next are the three function keys that determine the flow waveform in volume-targeted breaths. The available waveforms are constant (rectangular), descending ramp, and sine wave. The amount of flow delivered during each type of waveform is determined by the peak flow setting. For example, if a constant (rectangular) waveform is selected,

BOX 12-85	Sigh Parameters (Puritan Bennett 7200)

After pressing the automatic sigh key, follow the instructions in the message window.

Sigh TV (tidal volume)—0.1 to 2.5 L

Sigh HIPL (high-pressure limit)—10 to 120 cm H_2O

Sigh Events—1 to 15 (corresponds to a sigh every 4 to 60 minutes)

Multiple Sighs—1 to 3 sighs per event

After all new entries are complete, press ENTER when the window message is UPDATE PARAMS–ENTER. This updates the sigh parameters. Finally, press ENTER when the window reads AUTO SIGH ON–ENTER to complete the entries and turn on the automatic sigh function.

To clear the sigh function, press the automatic sigh function key. When AUTO SIGH OFF–ENTER appears in the window, pressing the ENTER key turns off the sigh function.

BOX 12-86	Conditions in Which Nebulizer Function is Suspended (Puritan Bennett 7200)

1. Excessive nebulizer flow, which is checked every eight breaths; NEB DISCONNECT appears in the display window. Excessive flow can be caused by leaks or disconnects in the nebulizer tubing.
2. During apnea and disconnect ventilation.
3. When the RESPIRATORY MECHANICS/MONITORING option is selected.
4. If low oxygen or air inlet pressure alarms sound.
5. If the operator selects any combination of peak flow and O_2 % that yields less than 10 L/min through the solenoid supplying the nebulizer circuit, the microprocessor senses the low flow and deactivates the solenoid supplying the nebulizer. The light on the nebulizer key remains lit.

(NOTE: If FLOW-BY is on, it is turned off when the nebulizer is activated. The operator must be sure to turn FLOW-BY back on when nebulization is complete.)

the flow is constant at the value set on the peak flow control. For a descending ramp, the starting flow is the peak flow setting, and the ending flow is 5 L/min. For a sine curve, the flow begins and ends at 5 L/min and rises to the peak flow setting at the middle of inspiration.

Because breaths are volume cycled in the 7200, changing the peak flow and/or the waveform also changes the I : E ratio. To keep the I : E ratio the same when a waveform is changed from constant to descending, the peak flow is doubled. When changing from constant to sine, the peak flow setting must be increased to 1.5 times the current setting.

The next function pads are manual inspiration, manual sigh, and automatic sigh. Selecting manual inspiration delivers a breath based on the selected parameters. Manual sigh delivers a sigh breath based on the settings selected for automatic sigh. Pressing the AUTOMATIC SIGH function key allows the operator to select sigh parameters. The display window requests entry of sigh parameters, which are described in Box 12-85.

Below the numeric key pads are three more function keys:

- + +
- 100% O_2 suction
- Nebulizer

The + + key allows the operator to select certain functions and options and operates like a computer menu. When it is pressed, the number of the last function selected appears in the window. Table 12-43 lists the available functions and options.

To scroll to the desired option, the operator presses the + + key to go forward or the * key to go backward. Another way to access a specific function is to press the numbers representing the desired option and then ENTER. After an option or function has been selected, the directions in the message window are followed. For example, apnea parameters are Option 1. The message 1 APNEA PARAMETERS appears. Pressing ENTER when that message appears results

in the message APNEA INT XX SEC. The operator uses the numeric keys to set the desired apnea time interval and again presses ENTER. The operator then follows the directions in the next window that appears. This continues until all the necessary parameters have been selected and UPDATE PARAMS–ENTER is displayed. Pressing ENTER updates all the selected apnea parameters and activates them.

Selecting the 100% O_2 suction key causes the ventilator to deliver 100% O_2 for 2 minutes. The message window flashes to indicate that the delivered oxygen percent is different from the set value (as long as the set O_2 is less than 100%). Choosing this option does not deactivate alarms; therefore if the patient is disconnected for suctioning, alarms will activate (e.g., the low pressure alarm).

The nebulization key allows a gas flow at the set O_2 % to exit the nebulizer connector for 30 minutes after it is activated. It automatically turns off the flow-by function and works only during inspiratory flow when the flow is greater than 10 L/min (mandatory or spontaneous breaths).

Box 12-86 lists conditions in which the nebulizer function is suspended. If the nebulizer function is suspended, the nebulizer key's light goes off, and the key does not work. However, the 30-minute clock continues to run. When the condition has been corrected, nebulizer flow resumes.*

The top row of controls in the Ventilator Setting section was added to a more recent version of the 7200 (Enhanced key board) and allows direct access to many of the functions and options listed under the + + key. Pressing one of these keys causes the display window to immediately access that function. The operator simply follows the directions for setting up or operating the selected option, in the same

---

*If flow-by was used before the nebulizer function was activated, the operator must be sure to turn flow-by back on.

way as accessing the function through the + + key. (NOTE: Some of the key selections allow access to more than one function, such as the respiratory mechanics option.) The controls in this row include:

1. Apnea parameters
2. Auto-PEEP
3. Pressure support
4. DCI 2.0
5. Respiratory mechanics
6. Flow-by 2.0
7. Graphics 2.0
8. Pressure control

Items 1, 5, and 6 are covered in the discussion of special functions later in this section. Items 3 and 8 are included in the discussion of modes of ventilation, and item 7 is reviewed in the discussion of ventilator graphics waveforms. Of the remaining keys, two blank touch keys for future upgrades appear on the right, and the two remaining keys, auto-PEEP and DCI 2.0, provide additional special functions.

The auto-PEEP key is function 4 and is currently a standard feature on every Enhanced 7200 ventilator (7200ae, 7200spe, and 7200e). It is used to estimate end-expiratory pressures. The unit measures total PEEP at end-exhalation and estimates auto-PEEP by subtracting the set (extrinsic) PEEP from the total PEEP.

The DCI (digital communications interface) function provides data reports that include data logs, chart summary reports, ventilator status reports, and host reports.

Finally, the top central portion of the Ventilator Setting section has digital display screens for showing the values of the current settings of the following parameters:

1. PEEP/CPAP (in cm H_2O)
2. Tidal volume (in liters)
3. Set rate (in breaths/minute)
4. Peak flow (in liters/minute)
5. O_2 %

MONITORS AND ALARMS

The Puritan Bennett 7200 has two main sections for providing information about monitored values and alarm displays. The monitored values are provided in the Patient Data section of the front panel, and the alarm display is in the Ventilator Status section. Alarms are set using the control pads for the alarms in the lower portion of the Ventilator Setting section, just below the key pads that control breath delivery. The Patient Data section is reviewed first, then the setting of alarms is discussed, and then monitoring of alarm information in the Ventilator Status section is presented.

Monitors: Patient Data Section

The Patient Data section of the front panel includes monitoring displays for the following:

1. Breath type
2. Pressures

3. Rates
4. I : E ratio
5. Volumes

Each of these sections provides calculated or measured patient information that is digitally displayed. All of these displays are blank during a POST. Measured data are obtained from sensors for flow, pressure, and temperature (both inspiratory and expiratory). The microprocessor uses the measurements to calculate and display the information.

Breath Type

Small LEDs at the top right of the Patient Data section light up, depending on the type of breath delivery. There is an LED for a patient assist when the patient triggers a mandatory breath, an LED for a spontaneous breath, one for a sigh breath, and one to indicate that a plateau maneuver is being performed. If a mandatory breath is time triggered, no light illuminates.

Pressures

On the left side of the Patient Data section is a dual scale, pressure reading bar graph that displays the airway pressure in centimeters of water (cm H_2O). The other available selections require pressing the desired variable from the three available, and the value is then displayed in the pressure window. The three available pressures are the mean airway pressure, peak airway pressure, and plateau pressure, along with the measurement for PEEP/CPAP.

Respiratory Rate and I : E Ratio

The operator can select either the measured respiratory rate or the I : E ratio to be displayed. Respiratory rates (in breaths/min) are digitally displayed in the assigned window. Rates are read as the average rate of breathing calculated for a patient's 10 previous breaths (spontaneous or mandatory).

The I : E ratio is only for mandatory breaths and is the actual measured value, displayed as 1 : X.X. For example, an I : E of 1 : 4 is a normal value, whereas a reading of 1 : 0.5 is an inverse ratio of 2 : 1.

Volumes

The digital display in the volume window provides readouts of measured values in liters for V_T, $\dot{V}_E$, and spontaneous $\dot{V}_E$. The operator simply selects the value to be displayed. These values are corrected to body temperature ambient pressure saturated (BTPS), as well as for tubing compliance. (NOTE: This discussion is exclusive to the Enhanced [newest] keyboard and does not apply to the basic keyboard. On the basic keyboard, the exhaled volume is displayed on an analog meter, but this reading is not corrected for BTPS or tubing compliance. As a result, the analog volume reading and the digital volume reading [corrected for both] differ on the basic keyboard.)

The spontaneous V_T is displayed on a breath-by-breath basis. The mandatory breath V_T displayed is usually an

BOX 12-87	Compensation for Compressible Volume (Puritan Bennett 7200)

During an extended self-test (EST), the ventilator determines the compliance of the patient circuit. Whenever a mandatory volume-targeted breath is delivered, the machine measures the peak inspiratory pressure (PIP) and increases or decreases the delivered volume of the next breath to ensure that the set tidal volume (V_T) is the volume that reaches the patient's lungs.

The display of exhaled volume is corrected as well. The microprocessor subtracts the volume added during inspiration from that measured during exhalation at the expiratory valve. Thus the exhaled volume reading shows the amount that theoretically is delivered to the patient's lungs. This amount is theoretical because any leaks in the system affect delivered volumes. Clinical Rounds 12-35 provides a sample problem.

CLINICAL ROUNDS 12-35

A patient is ventilated with the 7200 with a set V_T of 0.6 L (600 mL), a constant (square) flow pattern, and a flow of 60 L/min. The tubing compliance (C_T) was calculated during the last EST as 2 mL/cm H_2O, and the PIP for the last breath was 30 cm H_2O. What amount of volume will be added to the delivered breath? What will the exhaled V_T reading be, assuming that no leaks are present?

See Evolve Resources for the answer.

TABLE 12-44

Key Pad Alarms and Ranges—Puritan Bennett 7200	
Key Pad Alarm	**Range**
High-pressure limit	10-120 cm H_2O
Low inspiratory pressure	3-99 cm H_2O
Low PEEP/CPAP pressure	0-45 cm H_2O
Low exhaled V_T	0-2.5 L
Low exhaled $\dot{V}_E$	0-60 L/min
High respiratory rate	0-70 breaths/min

From Puritan Bennett, a division of Covidien, Mansfield, Massachusetts.

BOX 12-88	Low Battery and I:E Ratio Alarms (Puritan Bennett 7200)

When either a low battery or an I:E condition occurs, the ventilator lights up the corresponding alarm indicator but does not light up the alarm display or provide an audible alarm. Each alarm resets to a normal display when corrected.

CLINICAL ROUNDS 12-36

A patient is ventilated with the 7200 ventilator using volume ventilation. The mode is switched from CMV to SIMV. The mandatory V_T is 0.7 L (700 mL), and the rate is set at 5 breaths/min. The spontaneous rate is 10 breaths/min, and the spontaneous V_T is 0.4 L (400 mL). The low V_T alarm keeps activating even though it is set at 0.6 L (600 mL) and the circuit has no leaks. What is the problem?

See Evolve Resources for the answer.

average of eight breaths. (NOTE: If a breath is 50 mL different than the average volume for the eight mandatory breaths, the digital display shows only that breath, not the average.)

Both mandatory and spontaneous $\dot{V}_E$ are based on an eight-breath projected running average or a 1-minute sample, whichever occurs first.[1] The mandatory and spontaneous $\dot{V}_E$ are calculated separately at the end of each complete breath and are also displayed at the end of a breath.*

Correction for Compressible Volume

The 7200 compensates for volume that is compressed in the patient circuit, so that the amount of air reaching the patient's lungs is very close to the value for V_T set by the operator (Box 12-87 and Clinical Rounds 12-35).

Setting of Alarms

The alarm limits are set in the same manner as the ventilation parameters (see Box 12-83). Table 12-44 provides a list of the key pad alarms and ranges. (NOTE: The low inspiratory pressure alarm parameter applies only to mandatory breaths.)

*When spontaneous $\dot{V}_E$ is used, the type of breath is displayed on the large graphic window.

When alarm limits are violated, three events generally occur:

1. An audible alarm is activated.
2. A visual indicator and the ventilator alarm display in the ventilator status section flash.
3. A message appears in the message window to describe the alarm condition. If the alarm condition is corrected by the next breath, the audible alarm is silenced; however, the caution light is lit continuously, and the appropriate LED indicator changes from flashing to continuous. These are turned off by touching the ALARM RESET key pad. The advantage to this arrangement is if the operator is away from the ventilator when an alarm condition occurs, the data from the event are kept for later reference.

Box 12-88 gives two exceptions to this general condition, and Clinical Rounds 12-36 provides a troubleshooting exercise.

Events that reduce supply gas make the ventilator inoperative or severely compromise its ability to function. For example, if both gas supplies are lost, an audible alarm sounds, safety valve open (SVO) illuminates, and the valve opens. In addition, both the low air and low O_2 LEDs flash. The opening of the safety valve provides a route from which a spontaneously breathing patient can receive room air.

If the microprocessor systems find a major fault that prevents safe ventilator operation, two red alarm indicators flash:

· Ventilator Inoperative
· Safety Valve Open (SVO)

If the gas system is still working but the electronics are not, the red backup ventilator (BUV) indicator flashes and an audible alarm sounds. This provides backup ventilation, as presented in the discussion of special functions in this section. The section on special functions also describes the indicators for the various alarm conditions.

If a ventilator inoperative condition occurs, the microprocessor has determined that the ventilator is not functional because of a system fault. An alternative method ventilation must be obtained for the patient immediately.

Ventilator Status

The ventilator status display has three basic sections: the top provides an LED display of any current or recent alarms; the second section contains the ventilator status display; and the bottom section has three touch pads (LAMP TEST, ALARM SILENCE, and ALARM RESET). (NOTE: For information on the types of alarms, an alarm summary, and the types of events that may occur with the 7200, see Tables 2 and 3 on the Evolve Web site for this text.)

Pressing LAMP TEST and ENTER initiates a test that checks lamps, displays, and meters on the front panel, as well as the audible alarm and the remote alarm if installed. In addition, it cancels the ALARM SILENCE function. The ALARM SILENCE key quiets audible alarms for 2 minutes to allow for undisturbed bedside procedures. It also cancels displays of self-test error messages. The ALARM RESET key clears all alarm indicators, initiates a battery test, and, as does the lamp test, cancels alarm silence.

MODES OF VENTILATION

The 7200 offers three primary modes of ventilation: CMV, SIMV, and CPAP (spontaneous), as well as two optional modes: PCV (assist-control [A/C] or SIMV) and pressure-support ventilation (PSV).

Continuous Mandatory Ventilation (CMV)

CMV is an A/C mode of ventilation in which breaths are patient or time triggered, volume targeted (when PCV is not set), and volume cycled. To set CMV, the operator presses the CMV pad once, then selects the desired V_T, flow, respiratory rate, flow waveform, trigger sensitivity, and alarm thresholds. Pressing the CMV pad a second time activates the new mode.

CLINICAL ROUNDS 12-37

A patient on SIMV plus pressure support has been successfully ventilated for 24 hours at a rate of 2 breaths/min with the 7200 ventilator. Suddenly the patient becomes apneic. How long could the patient remain unventilated?

See Evolve Resources for the answer.

Synchronized Intermittent Mandatory Ventilation (SIMV)

In SIMV, mandatory breaths can be patient or time triggered and are volume targeted or pressure targeted (PCV) and volume or time cycled. Spontaneous breaths are patient triggered (pressure or flow). With the added option of PSV, spontaneous breaths can be assisted with the selected pressure level. Clinical Rounds 12-37 provides an exercise in problem solving related to the SIMV mode.

(NOTE: For additional information on synchronization of mandatory breaths with spontaneous breaths during SIMV, see Box 2 and Figure 2, Puritan Bennett 7200, on the Evolve Web site for this text.)

Spontaneous/Continuous Positive Airway Pressure (CPAP)

The CPAP mode is a purely spontaneous mode. All breaths are patient triggered, pressure limited, and pressure cycled. Breaths can be at a zero baseline or at a positive baseline (CPAP). They can also have PSV added, in which case breaths would become flow cycled.

Pressure-Control Ventilation (PCV)

PCV is an added option (80) that can be accessed in either of the following ways:

· By pressing the PRESSURE CONTROL pad at the top of the front panel
· By activating OPTION 80 under the + + key

PCV provides pressure-targeted mandatory breaths in the CMV and SIMV modes. This option allows selection of either T_I or the I:E ratio as a constant based on the respiratory rate (option 82). Usually when an inverse ratio is desired, a constant I:E is set. With normal I:E ratios, it may be more appropriate to set the T_I as constant. When the respiratory rate is changed, a message appears as a reminder of which parameter (I:E or T_I) is currently constant.

Unlike with other modes of ventilation, during PCV or PCV apnea ventilation, the message window provides a continuous sequence of messages to advise that PCV, not volume-targeted ventilation, is in use. The messages are preceded by an asterisk and, in general, list the following:

1. Mode
2. Pressure
3. T_I
4. I:E ratio

The 7200 provides for pressure-targeted mandatory breaths in apnea ventilation when PCV is the operating mode (see apnea ventilation in the discussion of special functions in this section). Option 81 is the apnea ventilation option for PCV and has parameter ranges similar to those for normal PCV. An apnea interval of 10 to 60 seconds is available, although setting an interval greater than 20 seconds is unusual.

It is important to set the upper pressure limit in PCV. Although the selected inspiratory pressure is the maximum that can be provided by the ventilator, if the patient coughs, the circuit pressure can rise above this value. Just as in volume ventilation, if airway pressure is greater than or equal to the upper pressure limit, inspiration ends.

The plateau function is not operational during PCV. An inspiratory pause can be obtained by increasing the T_I, which results in inspiratory flow returning to zero before the expiratory phase. Sighs are also not operational during PCV. (NOTE: The section on the Puritan Bennett 7200 on the Evolve Web site for this text contains additional information about pressure control.)

Pressure-Support Ventilation (PSV)

PSV (option 10) provides pressure-targeted, spontaneous breaths in the SIMV and CPAP modes. PS breaths are patient triggered, pressure targeted (1 to 70 cm H_2O in the newer version; 1 to 30 cm H_2O in earlier versions), and flow cycled (less than or equal to 5 L/min). As a safety backup feature, PSV also cycles out of inspiration when the airway pressure is 1.5 cm H_2O above PSV + PEEP or if the T_I is 5 seconds or longer.

The pressure setting in PSV is added to the CPAP level. For example, if CPAP is 5 cm H_2O and PSV is 10 cm H_2O, the peak inspiratory pressure (PIP) is 15 cm H_2O. PSV is set by selecting the PRESSURE SUPPORT key pad at the top of the front panel or by selecting OPTION 10 using the + + key and following the instructions in the message window to select the desired settings. (NOTE: PSV cannot be used when older versions of flow-by [option 50] are activated, but it is functional with flow-by version 2.0.)

SPECIAL FUNCTIONS

A wide variety of options and functions are available for the 7200, several of which have already been discussed. A few more important features, including the following, are presented here:

- Three emergency modes of ventilation: apnea ventilation, backup ventilation, and disconnect ventilation
- Respiratory mechanics and flow-by

Whenever certain alarm conditions occur or the ventilator detects certain faults or system errors, the ventilator automatically starts one of the three emergency ventilation modes. When apnea or disconnect ventilation occurs, the ventilator uses the operator-selected parameters for apnea ventilation.

Because the PEEP/CPAP control is not part of the electronics, it is active at its current setting during any emergency mode of ventilation. The displays may not be functioning properly in an emergency situation; therefore the operator should not change the PEEP setting when an emergency mode is active.

Apnea Ventilation

Whenever an apneic period exceeds the set apnea time, the ventilator initiates apnea ventilation using the apnea parameters set by the operator (Table 12-45). These parameters can be set for either volume- or pressure-targeted ventilation. When the unit is in CMV or SIMV, apnea ventilation has no low inspiratory pressure alarm. ALARM illuminates in the alarm summary display, and the message APNEA VENTILATION appears. Only the ALARM SILENCE and ALARM RESET keys are operational. The machine re-establishes ventilation if the patient triggers two consecutive breaths. After ventilation is restored, pressing the RESET key clears the alarm indicators.

Backup Ventilation

Backup ventilation (BUV) occurs whenever POST fails, the ongoing checks detect three system errors within 24 hours, or the AC voltage is less than 90% of the rated value. Audible and visible alarms occur. Under these circumstances, the pneumatic system of the ventilator is controlled by an analog circuit that is separate from the microprocessor systems. BUV uses the following factory-preset parameters to ventilate the patient:

1. Rate = 12 breaths/min
2. V_T = 0.5 L (whether volume or pressure ventilation was previously set)
3. Constant flow delivery at 45 L/min
4. Current PEEP setting
5. 100% O_2 (if available)
6. High-pressure limit about 30 cm H_2O above PEEP

TABLE 12-45	
Parameter Ranges for Volume- and Pressure-Targeted Apnea Ventilation—Puritan Bennett 7200	
Range of Selection	**Default Value**
For Both	
Apnea interval: 10-60 sec	20 sec
Breath rate: 0.5-70 breaths/min	12 breaths/min
Oxygen percentage: 21% to 100%	100%
For Volume Ventilation	
Tidal volume: 0.1-2.5 L	0.5 L
Peak flow: 10-120 L/min	45 L/min
For Pressure Ventilation (Default to Volume Settings)	
Inspiratory pressure: 5-100 cm H_2O	
Inspiratory time: 0.5-50 sec	
I:E ratio: 1:9-3:1 (4:1 in pressure-controlled ventilation [PCV])	

From Puritan Bennett, a division of Covidien, Mansfield, Massachusetts.

The BUV indicator lights in the alarm summary section. All other displays are blank, and all functions except the PEEP/CPAP are nonfunctional. If BUV occurs, another means of ventilating the patient must be provided as soon as possible, and the ventilator must be serviced. With pediatric patients, the patient is protected from excessive volume or pressure provided by BUV by two factors. First, small endotracheal tubes increase resistance to inspiratory flow. Second, the pressure limit of about 30 cm H_2O prevents pressures from rising too high.

Disconnect Ventilation

Whenever the microprocessor detects inconsistencies in airway pressures, PEEP, and gas delivery pressure in the pneumatic system, the disconnect emergency mode activates. Tubing disconnects or plugged tubing can cause these conditions. The machine uses the apnea ventilation setting, but the sensitivity setting is not recognized. When disconnect ventilation activates, the following alarm indicators are turned on:

1. Alarm (in alarm summary display)
2. High peak pressure
3. AIRWAY PRESS DISCONN (in message window)

Only the ALARM RESET and ALARM SILENCE keys are operational. Disconnect ventilation does not automatically reset itself. After the problem that caused the alarm is corrected, pressing RESET restores the ventilator to its previous state.

If something prevents the 7200 from initiating an emergency ventilation mode, the safety valve opens to allow a spontaneously breathing patient access to room air.

Respiratory Mechanics

The 7200 can measure, calculate, and display the following respiratory mechanics when options 30 and 40 have been added:

- Maximum inspiratory pressure (negative inspiratory force)
- Vital capacity
- Airway resistance (static and dynamic)
- Compliance (static and dynamic)
- Peak flow (spontaneous)

The maximum inspiratory pressure (MIP), which is called negative inspiratory pressure (NIP) on the 7200, measures the maximum negative pressure generated by the patient against an occluded airway during a 3-second interval. The maneuver ends when the patient begins to exhale and MIP (NIP) is displayed.

The vital capacity function does not measure forced vital capacity, but rather slow vital capacity. Before the patient begins a maximum inhalation, the message window must read VC MNVR ACTIVE. The maneuver is successful and vital capacity is displayed when the patient begins a breath after the vital capacity–maneuvered breath.

Activation of a static mechanics maneuver causes the ventilator to deliver a volume-targeted breath with a constant flow, followed by a plateau measurement. Calculated

---

BOX 12-89	Static Mechanics Measurements (Puritan Bennett 7200)

If a message followed by an asterisk appears in the display window after a static mechanics measurement (e.g., SM CMP 40* RES 23*), a stable plateau was not obtained during the maneuver. Accuracy of these values depends on whether airway pressure stabilizes during inflation hold and the exhaled values fall to zero (baseline) at the end of the breath cycle.

Blank displays mean that the calculation was out of acceptable range (CMP [compliance], 0 to 500 mL/cm H_2O; RES [resistance], 0 to 100 cm H_2O/L/sec).

---

values for the airway pressure (Raw) and static compliance (C_S) are displayed in the message window at the beginning of the next breath (Box 12-89). The dynamic mechanics for C and Raw measured during active flow delivery are determined by sampling of the instantaneous values for pressure, volume, and flow at numerous intervals during inspiration for a mandatory breath. Using the equation of motion discussed in Chapter 11, the microprocessor determines and calculates the various values.

Peak spontaneous flow (option 41) is measured, calculated, and displayed (in L/min) for spontaneous breaths. The operator can select an eight-breath average or have the most recent breath displayed.

Flow and Flow-By Triggering

Flow-by (version 1.0) was first introduced as a method to provide a continuous flow of air past the upper airway, similar to a continuous-flow IMV circuit. To accomplish mandatory breath triggering with the flow-by feature, the manufacturer had to make the unit flow rather than pressure triggered. In addition, the original version of flow-by (version 1.0) was active in only CPAP and SIMV and only when pressure support was not selected.

It is now known that flow-by actually reduces the work of breathing associated with breath triggering.[3] With continuous flow in the patient circuit, fresh gas is available to the patient as soon as the individual begins to inspire. This reduces the delay between the patient's demand for flow and the beginning of flow from the internal flow valve.

The introduction of flow-by version 2.0 made flow triggering available in all modes of ventilation, including PSV.

To operate flow triggering when flow-by is selected, the operator first selects flow-by using the + + key and selecting option 50 or by pressing the FLOW-BY function key on the top row of controls on the front panel. The message window prompts the operator to set the base flow and the flow-trigger level.

The base flow is the continuous gas flow present in the patient circuit during the expiratory phase. During mandatory inspiration and during inspiration in PSV, the base flow is suspended. At the beginning of exhalation, the base

TABLE 12-46

Recommended Base Flow and Flow Sensitivity Settings—Puritan Bennett 7200

Base Flow Setting	Range of Allowed Flow Sensitivity
5 L/min	1-3 L/min
6-9 L/min	1 L/min to ½ of base flow set
20 L/min	1-15 L/min

From Puritan Bennett, a division of Covidien, Mansfield, Massachusetts.

BOX 12-90   Range of Flow-Trigger Variables (Puritan Bennett 7200)

· In FLOW-BY version 1.0, the flow sensitivity or trigger range is 1 to 10 L/min.
· In FLOW-BY version 2.0, the range is 1 to 15 L/min.
· The minimum base flow for both is 5 L/min, and the maximum is 20 L/min.
· If the base is set too high, it can cause inadvertent PEEP and increase airway pressures.

---

flow is always 5 L/min, regardless of the base flow set. This eliminates resistance to exhalation when it begins. The manufacturer has programmed the 7200 to require base flow to be about twice the flow-trigger or flow sensitivity setting (Table 12-46). For example, if a flow trigger of 4 L/min is selected, a base flow of 8 L/min would be appropriate.

Base flow is monitored by the expiratory flow transducer. When the base flow drops by the trigger flow amount, inspiration begins (Box 12-90). The lower settings for flow sensitivity require less work from the patient to trigger a breath. For example, triggering is easier with a trigger of 1 L/min than it is at a trigger of 3 L/min. The manufacturer recommends the following settings during flow triggering:

· 1 L/min for small patients (those weighing less than 25 kg)
· 2 L/min for patients weighing 25 to 50 kg
· 3 L/min for large patients (those weighing more than 50 kg)

Because flow triggering is so sensitive, the operator needs to watch for autotriggering.

Flow-by is not available during nebulization. The older version of flow-by must be turned off during nebulization and then reactivated after the treatment. With the newer versions (2.0), the unit automatically switches to pressure triggering when nebulization is activated, but the operator must restart flow-by when nebulization is complete.

Ventilator Graphics Waveforms

The graphics 2.0 option allows the operator to select several waveforms to be viewed during ventilation and provides the following monitoring capabilities:

1. Waveforms (function 60), including scalars and loops
2. Trending waveforms (function 61)
3. A cursor for trending curves
4. Freeze/print (function 62) to freeze a waveform on the screen or print it with an attached compatible printer
5. Changing of the patient's number and room (function 3)
6. Plethysmogram, another available waveform that requires option 90 (pulse oximetry)

The waveforms menu allows two waveforms or loops to be displayed at one time (e.g., the scalars for pressure, flow, and volume, and the pressure-volume and flow-volume loops). Selecting the + + key and option 60 accesses the graphics package. Pressing the GRAPHICS 2.0 key at the top of the front panel also accesses graphics. The bottom of the graphics screen allows viewing of graph selections and the directions for selecting those choices.

Option 61 brings up the trending menu on the graphics screen, with appropriate directions for setting up trending plots. About 39 parameters are available for trending, including regularly measured values such as V_T and rate, and added options, including the pulse oximeter and the metabolic monitor.

TROUBLESHOOTING

The alarms and monitors on the 7200 provide a wide variety of methods for solving and detecting problems. In addition, the extensive series of self-tests and the continuous automatic testing verify the functional readiness of every subsystem of the ventilator, including the items listed in Box 12-91.

One problem occasionally encountered by clinicians operating the 7200 is autotriggering. The operator must carefully balance trigger sensitivity with patient effort. On the one hand, the patient must not be required to make an excessive effort to trigger the unit. On the other hand, autotriggering, resulting from leaky circuits or slight dips in pressure when PEEP is set at moderately high levels, is also undesirable.

Another note of caution is indicated when slow SIMV rates are set. First, when switching from CMV to SIMV, the operator should give a manually triggered breath. This

---

BOX 12-91   Systems Evaluated to Verify Proper Functioning (Puritan Bennett 7200)

1. Microprocessor and associated electronics during POST program
2. Pressure and flow transducers
3. Expiratory valve
4. Patient circuit
5. PEEP regulator
6. BUV
7. Safety valve with associated overpressure

prevents any delay that might occur with mandatory breath delivery. It is important to ensure that the apnea time and low V_T alarm limits are set appropriately (see the discussion on SIMV earlier in this section).[1]

As with most medical equipment that is microprocessor controlled, the use of walkie-talkies, cellular phones, and other transmitting devices may interfere with the operation of the 7200 ventilator. Manufacturers are aware of this problem and have begun devising methods to protect against it. However, unless the operator is sure about the equipment, such transmitting devices should not be used near the unit.

KEY POINTS

▶ Self-tests, such as POST, EST, QUEST, and TEST, should never be run while the Puritan Bennett 7200 is connected to a patient.

▶ It is important to check the PEEP control when beginning ventilation on a new patient, because it may have been set for a previous patient and not returned to the zero position.

▶ If the operator selects any combination of peak flow and O_2 % that yields less than 10 L/min through the solenoid supplying the nebulizer circuit, the microprocessor deactivates the solenoid supplying the nebulizer; however, the light on the nebulizer key remains lit.

▶ If both gas supplies are lost, the safety valve opens, allowing a spontaneously breathing patient to receive room air.

▶ Backup ventilation occurs if a serious error is detected, and the gas system is still working but the electronics are not.

▶ The set PEEP/CPAP value is active during any emergency mode of ventilation.

▶ The ventilator initiates apnea ventilation whenever an apneic period exceeds the set apnea time.

▶ If backup ventilation occurs, the operator should provide another means of ventilating the patient as soon as possible.

▶ Disconnect ventilation can be restored to its previous state by pressing the RESET key.

▶ With the 2.0 version of flow-by, the operator must restart flow-by after using the nebulizer function.

ASSESSMENT QUESTIONS

See Evolve Resources for the answers.

1. A respiratory therapist accidentally unplugs the 7200 ventilator being used for a patient in the ICU. Besides activating alarms, the ventilator will:
   a. Continue to ventilate the patient using the current settings and powered by the internal battery
   b. Stop functioning
   c. Continue to ventilate the patient using the default ventilator settings in memory
   d. Continue to ventilate the patient using disconnect parameters

2. A respiratory therapist changes the respiratory rate from 10 to 15 breaths/min during volume ventilation with the 7200. An error message appears in the display window: DECR RESP RATE FIRST. How can the therapist maintain the new $\dot{V}_E$ and correct the error message?
   a. Increase the peak flow setting
   b. Decrease the set V_T
   c. Add a plateau time
   d. Change to pressure-control ventilation

3. A patient is switched from CMV to SIMV with a decrease in rate from 12 to 4 breaths/min. About 30 seconds after the switch, an alarm sounds and apnea ventilation begins. Which of the following is/are true?
   I. The patient did not trigger a mandatory breath.
   II. The apnea period is probably set at 30 seconds.
   III. Switching from CMV to SIMV resulted in a delay in mandatory breath delivery.
   IV. The respiratory therapist should have given a mandatory breath after the switch to prevent the alarm condition.
      a. I only
      b. II only
      c. III and IV only
      d. I, II, III, and IV

4. A respiratory therapist has set a peak flow of 80 L/min and selected the descending flow waveform. At the beginning inspiration, what will be the actual flow delivered to the patient?
   a. 160 L/min
   b. 120 L/min
   c. 100 L/min
   d. 80 L/min

ASSESSMENT QUESTIONS—cont'd

5. When a change is made from a constant (rectangular) to a descending ramp waveform on the 7200, what happens to the T_I?
   a. It increases.
   b. It decreases.
   c. It stays the same.

6. A patient is being ventilated with SIMV at a rate of 3 breaths/min. The set V_T is 0.75 L (750 mL), the spontaneous V_T is 0.35 L (350 mL), and the spontaneous rate is 10 breaths/min. The low V_T alarm is set at 0.65 L (650 mL), and the apnea time is 20 seconds. Based on this information, which alarm is likely to activate?
   a. Apnea alarm
   b. Low V_T alarm
   c. Low pressure alarm
   d. Low rate alarm

7. A respiratory therapist wants to perform weaning measurements using the 7200 ventilator. Which of the following are available under the respiratory mechanics option (options 30 and 40)?
   I. Vital capacity
   II. Maximum inspiratory pressure
   III. Static compliance
   IV. Rapid shallow breathing index
   a. I and II only
   b. II and III only
   c. I, II, and III only
   d. II, III, and IV only

8. The 7200 microprocessor detects inconsistencies in airway pressure, PEEP measurements, and the gas delivery in the pneumatic system. Which of the following will occur?
   a. Apnea ventilation begins.
   b. Backup ventilation begins.
   c. Disconnect ventilation begins.
   d. Alarms activate, but regular ventilation continues.

9. During PCV, the following parameters are set: pressure = 20 cm H_2O; T_I = constant at 1 second; rate = 10 breaths/min; mode = CMV; and PEEP/CPAP = 0 cm H_2O. What will be the I : E ratio if the rate is decreased to 6 breaths/min and the patient does not trigger additional breaths?
   a. 1 : 5
   b. 1 : 6
   c. 1 : 9
   d. It cannot be determined from the information given.

10. With the 7200, what flow trigger and base flow would the therapist set for a 34-kg patient?
    a. Trigger flow would be set at 2 L/min and base flow at 5 L/min, the lowest available setting.
    b. Trigger flow would be set at 4 L/min and base flow at 8 L/min.
    c. Trigger flow would be set at 12 L/min and base flow at 20 L/min, the highest available setting.
    d. Trigger flow would be set at 10 L/min and base flow at 15 L/min.

References

1. Puritan Bennett: 7200 series microprocessor ventilator: operator's manual, Carlsbad, Calif, 1993, Puritan Bennett, a division of Covidien, Mansfield, Mass.

2. Pilbeam SP: Mechanical ventilation. In Burton GG, Hodgkin JE, Ward JJ, editors: Respiratory care: a guide to clinical practice, ed 4, Philadelphia, 1997, JB Lippincott.

3. Pilbeam SP, Cairo JM: Mechanical ventilation: physiological and clinical application, ed 4, St Louis, 2006, Mosby-Elsevier.

RESPIRONICS VENTILATOR

RESPIRONICS ESPRIT VENTILATOR[1]

OUTLINE

Power Source
Internal Mechanism
Controls and Alarms
    Front Panel Indicators
    Front Panel Buttons
    Recessed Controls
    Front Panel Touch Screen Display
    Setting Screens
    Monitor Screen

Alarm Settings
    Active Alarm Conditions
Modes of Ventilation
    Mode Selection
Special Features
Troubleshooting

The Esprit is a microprocessor-controlled ventilator intended for use with adult or pediatric patients (minimum tidal volume, 50 mL) in acute or subacute facilities (Figure 12-104). It can be used for either noninvasive or invasive ventilation.

POWER SOURCE

The Esprit is electrically powered and selects its power source based on the following priority: AC power, external battery (if present), optional backup battery. If the unit is disconnected from AC power, the battery indicator illuminates yellow.

Before turning on the unit, the operator must make sure the main circuit breaker is in the ON position. (NOTE: The manufacturer recommends that when the ventilator is not in use, it should be plugged into AC power and the main circuit breaker should be ON. This helps maintain the expected life of the lead acid backup battery.)

To provide variable oxygen concentrations, the Esprit requires connection to a high-pressure oxygen source (40 to 90 psig).

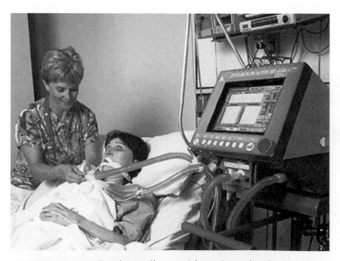

FIGURE 12-104 Esprit ventilator with patient circuit. (Courtesy Respironics, Murrysville, Pa.)

INTERNAL MECHANISM

The internal pneumatic system of the Esprit is based on a three-stage blower capable of providing pressure (100 cm H_2O) and gas flow (minimum, 3 to 140 L/min; maximum, 200 L/min) to the patient. The blower eliminates the need to use an air compressor or high-pressure air source. When the unit is operating and is disconnected from an AC power source (the battery indicator is yellow), the blower continues to operate from the battery, allowing the unit to be used in transport. A fully charged backup battery can power the Esprit for about 30 minutes, depending on the ventilator settings. (NOTE: A change in blower sound occurs, which results from the change in revolutions per minute [RPMs] of the blower [more than 60 cm H_2O Hi Press or less than 60 cm H_2O Hi Press].)

CONTROLS AND ALARMS

All the major operational controls for the Esprit are located on the front panel, which is divided into a top section and a smaller bottom section (Figure 12-105). The top section contains all the indicators, the touch-sensitive display screen, and the controls. The lower section contains the connections for the patient circuit, the heated expiratory valve filter, and the on/off switch.

Front Panel Indicators

Across the top of the ventilator, just above the screen, are the indicators for the operational status and alarm conditions of the Esprit (see Figure 12-105). These LED indicators begin on the left with the NORMAL indicator, which illuminates when the ventilator has been turned on and no active or autoreset alarms are present. The ALARM HIGH indicator, next in line, flashes red during a high priority alarm. The ALARM MED/LOW indicator flashes yellow to indicate a medium alarm and continuously for a low priority alarm. These two alarm indicators show a continuous yellow light if an alarm condition occurred but was corrected (autoreset).

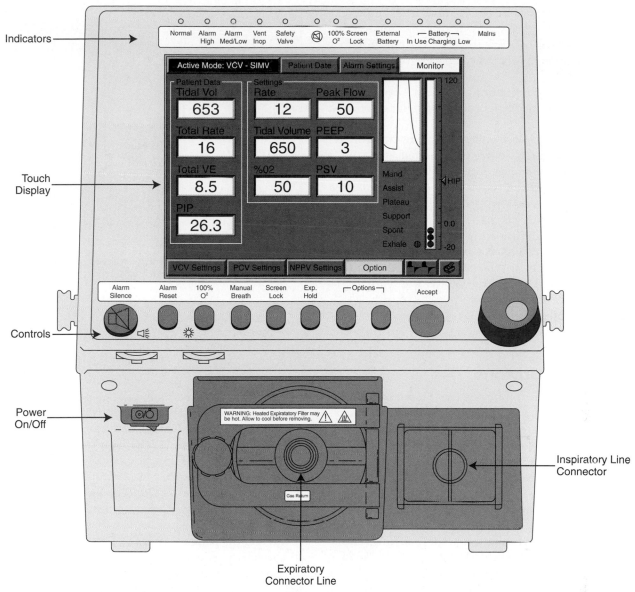

FIGURE 12-105 Diagram of the front panel of the Esprit ventilator, showing *(1)* indicators; *(2)* touch display with monitoring screen; *(3)* controls; *(4)* power on/off switch; *(5)* connector line for exhalation line to heated exhalation filter; and *(6)* inspiratory line connector.

When the ventilator inoperative (VENT INOP) indicator is illuminated, the Esprit has established that a hardware malfunction has been detected and the unit is not capable of supporting ventilation. It should be removed immediately from use and another method should be provided to ventilate the patient.

The SAFETY VALVE open (SVO) alert is illuminated with any of the following conditions:

· An occlusion in the circuit is detected.
· Oxygen and air sources are no longer operable.
· A hardware malfunction is detected, and the ventilator inoperative state (VENT INOP) is activated.

In SVO, the safety valve opens, the exhalation valve remains open, and the air and oxygen valves close. A high priority alarm occurs, the SAFETY VALVE indicator lights,

and the NORMAL indicator is turned off. The ventilator does not provide support to the patient; therefore another method to ventilate the patient must be provided immediately.

The alarm silence icon is yellow when the audible alarm has been disabled. It stays illuminated for 2 minutes when the ALARM SILENCE button (bottom row) is pressed. If a new alarm condition occurs while it is active, the visual alarm function is activated. Pressing the ALARM RESET button in the bottom row of controls clears the alarm silence, and audible alarms can again be heard.

The 100% O_2 indicator is active only when the control button on the front panel labeled 100% O_2 has been pressed and 100% O_2 is being delivered to the patient. The indicator remains illuminated for the 2 minutes of oxygen delivery. The 100% O_2 indicator is not related to the percent oxygen delivery. In other words, if the operator sets the inspired % O_2 setting to 100%, the 100% O_2 indicator does not light. It lights only when the 100% O_2 front panel key has been pressed.

The SCREEN LOCK indicator lights green when active. A screen lock prevents inadvertent changes to the keys on the touch-sensitive screen.

The EXTERNAL BATTERY indicator is intended for use when an external battery source is connected.

BATTERY has three indicator positions. BATTERY IN USE lights yellow to show the ventilator is running from the internal backup battery. BATTERY CHARGING lights yellow when the backup battery is charging; charging can take up to 10 hours. The indicator turns off when the battery is fully charged. BATTERY LOW flashes red when about 5 minutes or less of power remains in the backup battery. The operator must immediately connect the ventilator to an AC power source.

The MAINS indicator illuminates green when the ventilator is connected to an AC power source and the main circuit breaker is on.

Front Panel Buttons

The front panel control buttons (see Figure 12-105) are located just below the screen. Many of these controls correspond to the indicators reviewed previously.

Pressing the ALARM SILENCE button on the far left provides 2 minutes of alarm silence. The alarm silence icon at the top of the unit also illuminates. If an alarm occurs during this time, the appropriate alarm indicator will appear visually, but the silence continues.

ALARM RESET is used to clear the visual indicators for autoreset alarms. It also is used to resume normal ventilation when apnea backup ventilation is present. Pressing this button also ends alarm silence before the 2 minutes expire.

100% O_2 increases the oxygen percent to 100% for 2 minutes. After it is pressed, it cannot be canceled. If an oxygen source is not available and this button is pressed, a low O_2 alarm is active for the duration of the 2 minutes.

Pressing the MANUAL BREATH button results in the delivery of an operator-initiated mandatory breath based on the current ventilator settings. It must be pressed during the expiratory phase of a breath. A manual breath is not permitted during the inspiratory phase of a breath, either mandatory or spontaneous.

The SCREEN LOCK control locks and unlocks the graphics or touch screen. Using the SCREEN LOCK control helps prevent accidental or inadvertent changes in the screen function. When the screen is locked, all screen keys are disabled and the screen lock indicator in the top row illuminates. Only the following controls remain active when the screen lock is on:

· Manual breath
· 100% O_2
· Expiratory hold

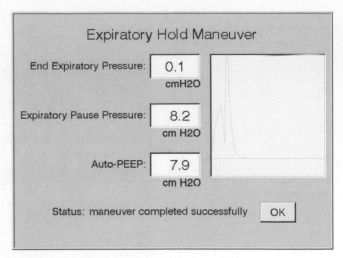

FIGURE 12-106 Expiratory hold maneuver window on the Esprit. (See text for description.) (Courtesy Philips Healthcare, Carlsbad, CA.)

· Alarm reset
· Alarm silence

The expiratory hold (EXP HOLD) button is used to estimate end-expiratory pressure for the determination of auto-PEEP. It is active only at the end of a mandatory breath and is not available in noninvasive positive-pressure ventilation (NPPV) or during emergency ventilation modes. When EXP HOLD is pressed, an exhalation hold function begins after exhalation for the currently active breath, and the EXPIRATORY HOLD MANEUVER subscreen appears on the regular screen (Figure 12-106). The air, O_2, and exhalation valves are closed. No gas flow goes into or out of the patient circuit to allow for equilibration of the pressure in the circuit and the patient's lungs.

The subscreen graphic allows viewing of the pressure-time curve and digitally displays the pressures. After a stable reading is achieved, the unit can calculate and display end-exhalation pressure, exhalation pause pressure, and auto-PEEP. If the button is held continuously and exhalation exceeds 5 seconds, the ventilator automatically ends exhalation and begins a new inspiratory period.

Auto-PEEP is calculated using the following equation: (Auto-PEEP = Exhalation pause pressure − End exhalation pressure). If the auto-PEEP is calculated as a negative number, the auto-PEEP display reads "−." There is also a STATUS: ABORT BY OPERATOR message if the software is not installed.

The OPTIONS buttons are reserved for future use. The ACCEPT button allows the operator to activate selected settings on the touch screen. The control knob to the right of the ACCEPT button is used in conjunction with the touch screen to enter operator-selected values for ventilator settings and alarms.

Recessed Controls

Just below the front panel, in the lower left corner, are two control knobs, the audible alarm volume (icon), and the display brightness (icon). The volume control can lower the audible sound of the alarm volume but cannot turn it off. The brightness control increases or decreases the brightness of the touch screen display.

Front Panel Touch Screen Display

The front operating panel (graphic user interface) is an infrared, touch-sensitive screen. The Esprit has two different categories of screens: ventilator and diagnostic. The former appears when the machine is functioning as a ventilator. The diagnostic screen appears when the Esprit is not functioning as a ventilator and is running self-tests.

Diagnostic Mode

Similar to other ventilators, the Esprit has several diagnostic functions, including a **power on self-test (POST)** that runs when the unit is turned on, a short self-test (SST), and an **extended self-test (EST)**. Diagnostics are available to perform the following:

· Run tests that can be run only when a patient is not attached
· Determine the circuit compliance (enabled or disabled)
· Set the altitude, time, and date
· Perform more detailed service and maintenance functions
· Calibrate the inline oxygen sensor during EST

(NOTE: During the preoperational procedure, if the time is found to be incorrect more than once, the internal battery may need to be replaced.)

Short Self-Test (SST)

The SST usually is run between patient uses and when the circuit is changed. The SST verifies that the patient circuit is free of major leaks. If major leaks are present in the patient circuit, the ventilator will not run. The integrity of the system requires a tight circuit during the SST and EST or these tests will fail. The SST also measures the leak rate and the circuit compliance. It tests critical hardware components, including the safety valve, flow sensors, and the autozero solenoids. If the SST passes, the ventilator and attached components are ready for patient use. A ventilator that has failed the SST must not be used until its operational safety has been verified by other methods. (NOTE: The SST provides a text prompt to remind the clinician to make sure a patient is not connected during the SST, because the high pressures generated to the patient circuit can injure a person.) The SST is run using the diagnostics screen (Box 12-92).

Extended Self-Test (EST)

The EST is a more comprehensive system test that normally is run only by qualified personnel, such as a field service technician, trained in its use. The EST verifies the overall functional integrity of the ventilator by testing all the critical hardware subsystems and components. It is run as part of the regular maintenance of the machine to verify

BOX 12-92	Running the Short Self-Test (SST) (Esprit)

To conduct the SST, perform the following steps:
1. Make sure the patient is disconnected and the ventilator is turned off.
2. Press and hold down the ALARM RESET and 100%O_2 buttons for 5 seconds while turning on the ventilator.
3. The diagnostic screen appears and a message in the center reads: WARNING: ENTERING DIAGNOSTICS MODE. VERIFY THAT THE PATIENT IS DISCONNECTED PRIOR TO PROCEEDING.—OK."
4. Press OK.
5. Press the SST key at the top left corner of the screen, then press START to begin the test.
6. Prompts will appear instructing you to unplug and plug the patient Y.
7. When the test is completed, the calculated patient circuit compliance will appear on the screen.

performance, particularly if the performance of a unit is in question.

As with the SST, the patient should never be connected when the EST is run. Also as with the SST, the EST is accessed through the diagnostics screen. If a ventilator fails to pass the EST, the ventilator must not be used with a patient.

User Configuration Screen and Tubing Compliance

Also available on the diagnostics screen is the user configuration screen. This screen allows the operator to set the date, the time, and the altitude at which the ventilator is operating and to enable or disable the tubing compliance compensation feature. USER CONFIG is pressed to access the user configuration screen, which has a soft pad labeled COMPLIANCE. Circuit compliance is enabled when the COMPLIANCE soft pad has a white background. When COMPLIANCE is active, the exhaled volumes reported by the Esprit are compensated for tubing compliance. Compensation is based on the circuit compliance calculated during the last SST. (NOTE: After completing the SST or EST is completed or the user configuration screen has been used, the ventilator must be turned off to return to a set-up screen.)

Front Panel Touch Screen Display

In the touch screen (see Figure 12-105), menu items appear across the top and bottom of the screen. The center portion of the screen contains the data relevant to the breath type and mode selected. The menus also include PATIENT DATA, ALARM SETTINGS, and MONITOR. Touching one of these labels brings up a new screen.

The elements common to all ventilator screens (nondiagnostic) include a top bar, a bottom bar, and a manometer. The top bar lists the currently active mode and breath type, PATIENT DATA, ALARM SETTINGS, and MONITOR. The bottom bar lists the following:

· VCV SETTINGS—Displays the VCV settings screen, which allows the operator to view and change settings for volume-targeted breath delivery.

· PCV SETTINGS—Displays and allows changes in settings for pressure-targeted breath delivery.

· NPPV SETTINGS—Displays the NPPV settings and allows changes for noninvasive ventilation (SPONT and SPONT/T).

· OPTION—A touch pad for future use.

· Graphics (icon)—Displays the waveforms and loops screen if this option has been installed in the unit. (NOTE: The graphics are available if the waveform picture appears black against a gray background. The graphics are not available if this key is gray on gray.)

When VCV-SIMV is the active mode, ACTIVE MODE: VCV-SIMV (see Figure 12-105, top left) is highlighted. Also visible are the current settings for that mode and centrally located patient data.

The pressure manometer is located on the right side of the screen. The abbreviation HIP, which appears alongside the pressure manometer, marks the high pressure alarm setting. When this value is reached, the inspiratory phase ends. The operator can touch the HIP soft pad and the HIGH PRESSURE subscreen appears. This screen is used to change the high pressure setting. The alarm screen can also be used to set the high pressure limit. When the high pressure is set at a level greater than 60 cm H_2O, the blower motor RPMs increase to provide the necessary pressure. Table 12-47 describes the various symbols used in the bar graph of the manometer to indicate the breath type currently in use.

Setting Screens

In general, the process by which the ventilator is set up for a patient includes selecting the breath type and modes, presetting the parameters and alarms, and activating the changes. During ventilator normal operation, all parameter, mode, and alarm limit settings are selected using the same three-step procedure. First, the parameter is selected by touching the appropriate screen pad. Next a screen

insert appears on the operating screen (Figure 12-107). The current set value appears in the digital window. For example, in Figure 12-107, the value for peak flow is 30 L/min (shown on the screen as LPM). Up and down arrows on the adjacent bar to the right of the value allow the operator to increase or decrease the value. This can also be done with the control knob. A bar graph on the extreme right shows the setting range and current setting. In this case, 3 TO 140 LPM of peak flow is available, and 30 L/min is the current setting. Pressing the ACCEPT pad in the screen insert or pressing the ACCEPT button on the front panel activates the change. Pressing CANCEL returns the ventilator to the previous setting.

The soft pads in the main screen have an active and inactive state. Active settings have a gray background with black letters. Inactive settings have a gray background with gray letters and are not being used by the ventilator to control ventilation or as an alarm limit. Box 12-93 gives an example of an exception.

Selecting Settings for a New Patient

The breath type, whether volume-controlled ventilation (VCV), PCP, or NPPV, is selected and the screen for the selection appears. Specific parameters, such as peak flow in VCV, are then set by touching the parameter soft pad. The subscreen for that parameter allows the desired setting to be adjusted (see Figure 12-107).

TABLE 12-47		
Breath Type Indicators (Esprit)		
Breath	**Symbol**	**Description**
Mand	●	Operator- or ventilator-triggered mandatory breath
Assist	▼	Patient-triggered mandatory breath
Plateau	○	Inspiratory hold, can be set at the end of the inspiratory phase of a VCV breath type
Support	▲	Patient-triggered spontaneous breath with PSV > 0 or IPAP > EPAP
Spont	○	Patient-triggered spontaneous breath, PSV = 0 or IPAP = EPAP
Exhale	⏀	Indicates exhalation phase of any breath

From Respironics, Carlsbad, California.

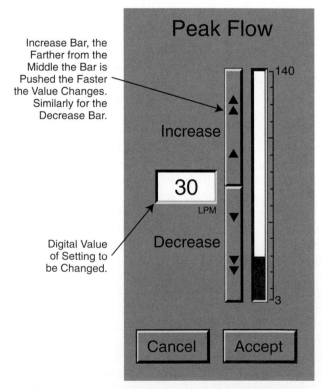

FIGURE 12-107 Subscreen window for setting peak flow on the Esprit ventilator when that parameter has been selected. (See text for description.) (Courtesy Respironics, Murrysville, Pa.)

Some subscreens display not only the selected parameter but also the calculated data based on the setting. For example, during VCV, the rate subscreen displays the calculated minute volume that results from the set rate and volume. In pressure-controlled ventilation (PCV), when the rate is displayed, the calculated value for the I:E ratio is also displayed.

When a new breath type is selected, the mode available for that breath type can also be selected (Box 12-94). Figure 12-108A shows the ventilator currently active in VCV-A/C. The VCV SETTING pad on the bottom menu has been pressed. Some of the parameters are gray lettering on a gray background (PSV, E-trigger, Rise Time) indicating

BOX 12-93	Active Keys Even When They Are Not

Some setting keys appear active even though they are not being used in the current active mode. This happens because the setting of these keys is used in apnea ventilation or when the MANUAL INSPIRATION key is pressed. For example, if CPAP is selected as the active mode, tidal volume (VCV) and inspiratory pressure (PCV) are not active. However, the operator needs to include one or the other, depending on the mode, in case the patient becomes apneic and apnea ventilation begins. A value appropriate for the patient being ventilated needs to be selected for any active key that appears on the screen.

BOX 12-94	Available Breath Types and Ventilator Modes (Esprit)

On the Esprit ventilator, the manufacturer distinguishes between breath type and mode. Breath types are designated:
· VCV (volume control ventilation)
· PCV (pressure control ventilation)
· NPPV (noninvasive positive-pressure ventilation)
VCV and PCV are available in the following mode settings:
· Assist/control (A/C)
· Synchronized intermittent mandatory ventilation (SIMV)
· Continuous positive airway pressure (CPAP)
NPPV is available in two modes:
· Spontaneous (Spont)
· Spontaneous/timed (Spont/T)

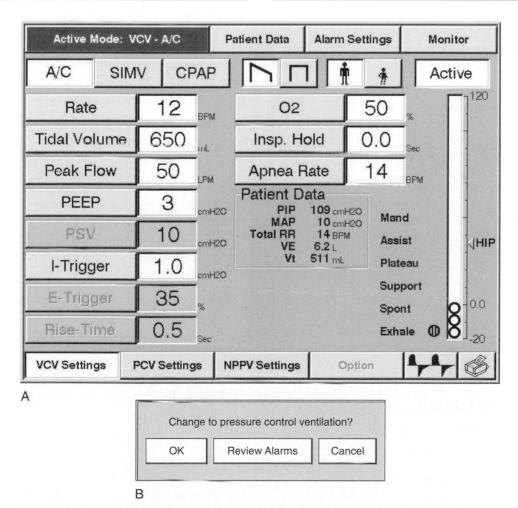

FIGURE 12-108 A, VCV setting screen during the active mode VCV-A/C. **B,** Example of a prompt window when ACTIVATE PCV has been pressed on the setting screen and settings have been selected. (See text for explanation.) (Courtesy Philips Healthcare, Carlsbad, CA.)

TABLE 12-48

Patient Data Parameters and Definitions (Esprit)

Parameter	Description	Range
PIP	Peak inspiratory pressure (maximum pressure during inspiration)	−20-130 cm H_2O
MAP	Mean airway pressure (average airway pressure during the total breath cycle)	−20-130 cm H_2O
Pe End	Pressure at end-expiration (pressure measured at end-expiration)	−20-99.9 cm H_2O
Pi End	Pressure at end-inspiration (pressure measured at end-inspiration or at the end of an inspiratory hold)	−20-130 cm H_2O
Tidal Vol	Exhaled tidal volume (compliance compensated if enabled)	0-999 mL
Spont VE	Spontaneous minute volume	0-99.9 L/min
Total VE	Exhaled minute volume	0-99.9 L/min
%O_2	Delivered O_2 (1-sec average of O_2 readings if O_2 sensor is installed)	0-110%
Spont Rate	Spontaneous respiratory rate	0-150 breaths/min
Rate	Total respiratory rate	0-150 breaths/min
F/Vt	Rapid shallow breathing index (ratio of respiratory rate to exhaled tidal volume for spontaneous breaths)	0-500 breaths/min/L
I : E Ratio	Ratio of inspiratory time to expiratory time	9.9 : 1-1 : 99

that they are not currently active. However, the operator can use the grayed keys to change the settings as needed, such as going into PCV. Table 12-48 lists the available patient data parameters and their definitions.

Pressing the ACTIVATE key at the top right corner of the screen brings up a prompt that asks CHANGE TO CONTROL VENTILATION? Pressing OK in response to this prompt activates the new breath type and all the new settings. Figure 12-108B shows an example of the prompt window when PCV has been selected as the new mode.

Pressing REVIEW ALARMS in the prompt window brings up the subscreen for adjusting the alarms for the new mode (see Alarm section). If CANCEL is pressed, nothing changes and the screen returns to the active mode screen.

Patient Data Section

Touching PATIENT DATA accesses the screen that lists all the current monitored ventilator parameters (see Table 12-48). The format for this screen is the same in VCV, PCV, and NPPV breath types.

Monitor Screen

The monitor screen (see Figure 12-104) is the default screen and automatically displays if the screen has not been touched in 15 minutes. Pressing the MONITOR touch pad also brings it into view. This screen varies, depending on the breath type being delivered.

ALARM SETTINGS

After set-up of the breath type and mode, the alarm settings should be made. Pressing the ALARM SETTINGS touch pad displays the available alarm settings (Figure 12-109). This screen can also be accessed during the process of changing the mode.

To adjust the alarm, the operator touches the pad for that alarm. For example, during VCV, when the operator touches LOW V$_T$ MAND, the subscreen for that alarm appears.

As with setting a parameter, the arrow keys or control knob can be used to increase or decrease the displayed value. Pressing ACCEPT activates the new alarm setting.

The high pressure alarm subscreen can be activated either by this method or by touching the HIP key adjacent to the pressure manometer in PCV or VCV settings. In NPPV the high pressure limit is automatically set at 10 cm H_2O above the inspiratory positive airway pressure (IPAP) setting.

Active Alarm Conditions

In most cases alarms have a visual indicator, an audible sequence of tones, and a screen alert window with a message. Alarms have three priority levels. High urgency alarms illuminate a red indicator and emit a sequence of five tones. These types of alarms require immediate attention. Medium urgency alarms have a yellow flashing indicator with a sequence of three tones. These alarms require a prompt response. Low urgency alarms have a continuous yellow indicator with no audible tone.

The audible alarm for a medium or high level alarm stops when the alarm condition has ended (autoreset). A window in the lower center screen labeled ALERTS lists the current alarms in bold print and autoreset alarms in normal print. The operator must reset the alarms to clear the visual indicators. The ALARM RESET button clears the visual indicators for currently active or autoreset alarms. If the condition occurs again, the visual indicator turns on again. Pressing ALARM SILENCE gives a 2-minute silence.

Only a few alarms cannot be silenced. They are so urgent that they require immediate resolution of the problem to avoid endangering the patient. They include:

- Gas supplies lost—SVO
- Low back-up battery
- Backup battery on (not currently available)

Some alarms cannot be manually reset. The operator must make sure the problem has been resolved rather than trying to reset the alarms. These alarms include:

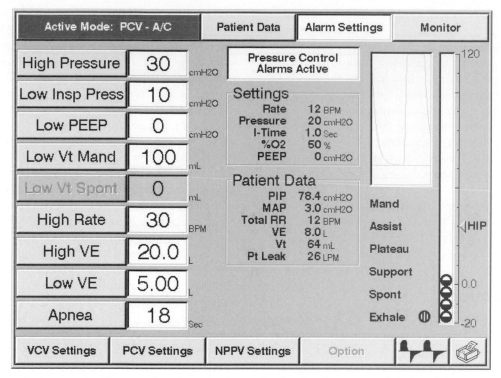

FIGURE 12-109 Alarm setting screen on the Esprit, showing the various alarms available for setting. The active mode is PCV-A/C, and the screen is for setting PCV alarms. (See text for explanation.) (Courtesy Philips Healthcare, Carlsbad, CA.)

· Occlusion—SVO
· Low O₂ (NOTE: The alarm range is ± 6% of the set value. Although the actual percent change in the delivered gas is almost immediate, it takes time for the software to reset the measured value. As a result, a low or high % O₂ alarm occurs after about 30 seconds when the set O₂ % is changed.)
· High O₂
· Low O₂ supply

The Esprit has the same traditional alarms that are present on all ventilators, including high and low inspiratory pressure, low PEEP, high rate, high and low minute volume, low tidal volume (V_T) (spontaneous, mandatory), apnea, high and low O₂, low O₂ supply, gas supplies lost (safety valve open), low backup battery, and battery backup on. Unusual alarms include low expiratory positive airway pressure (EPAP) for NPPV modes, inspiratory time (I-Time) too long, and Occlusion (SVO).

Low EPAP in the NPPV modes indicates that pressure has dropped below the low alarm level during exhalation. A leak may be present in the circuit or the patient interface (mask). An I-Time that is too long is a medium priority alarm indicating that a spontaneous pressure-supported breath has exceeded the maximum time allowed. For adults, the maximum time is 3.5 seconds (averaged over three breaths); for pediatric patients, it is 2.5 seconds (also averaged). A prolonged inspiratory time (T_I) might occur if a leak is present during PSV (Clinical Rounds 12-38).

CLINICAL ROUNDS 12-38

An adult patient is ventilated with the Esprit ventilator in the VCV-SIMV mode at a rate of 4 breaths/min, and PSV is set at 10 cm H₂O. An I-TIME TOO LONG alarm occurs. What condition could have triggered the alarm?

See Evolve Resources for the answer.

If the patient circuit becomes crimped or blocked or the expiratory filter occluded, inspiration ends and the unit goes into exhalation. This results in an OCCLUSION-SVO (safety valve open) alarm. The air and oxygen valves close, and the exhalation and safety valves open. A spontaneously breathing patient can obtain room air through the open valves. The ventilator resumes normal operation when it is determined that the obstruction has been cleared. The operator may need to clear the patient circuit and check the expiratory filter and humidification devices to make sure they are not obstructed or causing too much expiratory flow resistance.

MODES OF VENTILATION

The modes provided by the Esprit for VCV and PCV breath types include assist-control (A/C), synchronized intermittent mandatory ventilation (SIMV), and continuous positive airway pressure (CPAP). These are intended for the intubated patient. NPPV is available for patients using interfaces such as a nasal mask, a full face mask, nasal pillows, or a mouthpiece with a lip seal. NPPV can be spontaneous (SPONT), or it can provide a backup breath rate (spontaneous/timed settings). In addition, the Esprit has a backup mode called *apnea ventilation.*

Before selecting the mode of ventilation, the operator should select the patient size using the ADULT or PEDIATRIC key (Figure 12-108A, top right screen). The one selected adapts the ventilator's breath delivery algorithms to suit the patient type for compliance and resistance. The patient type selected determines the flow output at various rise time settings for pressure-targeted breaths (PCV, PSV, and IPAP). In addition, the I-TIME TOO LONG alarms for spontaneous pressure-supported breaths are set (3.5 seconds for adults and 2.5 seconds for children; averaged over three breaths).

Mode Selection

To select a breath type and mode, the operator needs to make sure the ventilator is in the normal set-up screen. This screen shows the available breath types and the parameters that can be set for that breath type. The breath types appear at the bottom of the operating screen and include VCV, PCV, and noninvasive ventilation (NIV).

After the breath type is selected, the available modes for that breath type appear in the top left portion of the screen. These include A/C, SIMV, and CPAP.

To select a mode, the operator simply touches the mode desired. If NPPV is active, the operator selects SPONT or SPONT/T. The ventilator asks for mode confirmation by bringing up a screen message. For example, it might say, CHANGE MODE TO SIMV? Yes – No.

A/C and SIMV: Volume Control Ventilation (VCV)

If VCV is selected for either A/C (VCV-A/C) or SIMV (SIMV-A/C) modes, the mandatory breaths are either time or patient triggered (pressure or flow), flow limited, and time cycled. (NOTE: This can also be considered volume cycled; that is, flow is delivered over a specific time based on the rate.) In A/C, all breaths are mandatory. In SIMV, the maximum mandatory rate is set and the patient is able to breathe spontaneously between mandatory breaths from the baseline pressure (PEEP/CPAP).

In VCV-A/C or VCV-SIMV, for the mandatory breath the operator can select the rate, tidal volume, peak flow, PEEP, PSV, I-trigger (sensitivity), expiratory trigger, rise time, O$_2$, inspiratory hold, apnea rate, and either a constant (square) or descending (decelerating) ramp for the flow waveform. The selected waveform is highlighted in the set-up screen. Pushing the desired waveform pad activates that flow pattern. (NOTE: The waveform pattern cannot be set in PCV or NPPV modes.) Also available are the % O$_2$, inspiratory hold, and apnea rate.

Machine sensitivity to a patient's inspiratory effort is adjusted using the I-TRIGGER control. Touching the inspi-

ratory trigger (I-TRIGGER) pad in the VCV, PCV or NPPV SETTINGS window brings up the inspiratory trigger subscreen. The operator can select either pressure or flow triggering for PCV and VCV. NPPV is always flow triggered. The trigger works by measuring the drop in either pressure or flow (whichever is active) in the patient circuit. Inspiration begins when the trigger level is detected. A suggested initial setting for pressure is 1 to 3 cm H$_2$O. (NOTE: The operator should monitor for autocycling, particularly if PEEP is increased.) For flow triggering, a flow of 1 to 2 L/min is recommended. The bias flow is automatically set by the ventilator to 3 L/min above the threshold trigger setting. For example, for a trigger of 1 L/min, the bias flow is 4 L/min.

For support of spontaneous breaths in SIMV, PSV can be added. Pressure-supported breaths are patient triggered, pressure limited, and flow cycled. The flow cycling is adjustable from 10% to 45% of the peak flow measured during inspiration. The parameter labeled E-TRIGGER (expiratory trigger) is the control that adjusts the flow-cycling percentage. For example, if the E-trigger is set at 45%, the pressure-support breath ends when the inspiratory flow drops to 45% of the measured peak inspiratory flow. This setting results in a shorter inspiration than does a setting of 10% (see Chapter 11 for additional information on flow cycling in pressure support).

A/C and SIMV: Pressure Control Ventilation (PCV)

When PCV is selected, either A/C or SIMV is available. The mandatory breaths are time or patient triggered (pressure or flow), pressure limited, and time cycled. The parameters set are rate, pressure, inspiratory time (T$_I$ or I-time), PEEP, PSV, I-trigger, E-trigger, rise time, O$_2$ %, and apnea rate (Box 12-95). As with VCV, in A/C all breaths are mandatory and in this case are pressure limited. In SIMV, mandatory breaths are pressure limited, and the patient can breathe spontaneously between these breaths from the established baseline (PEEP/CPAP) and with PS added, if desired.

CPAP Mode

CPAP can be activated during the VCV or PCV breath type. The selection of CPAP assumes a mandatory breath rate of 0 breaths/min. However, the operator must still set a rate

---

BOX 12-95   **Rise Time Percent (Esprit)**

Whenever a breath is pressure targeted, the rise time percent can be set. This parameter is active in pressure-controlled ventilation (PCV), pressure-support ventilation (PSV), and noninvasive positive-pressure ventilation (NPPV). It allows sloping or tapering of the curve during the beginning of inspiration. Rather than rising to the set pressure as rapidly as possible, the ventilator slows delivery of the pressure. It is adjustable from 0.1 to 0.9 second. The shorter the time, the more rapidly the pressure rises to its set value. (See Chapter 11 for more information on sloping or rise time.)

in case apnea occurs. The set rate establishes the breath rate during apnea ventilation. The baseline can be adjusted above zero to 35 cm H_2O. All patient-triggered breaths are spontaneous and can be supported with pressure support. Triggering is based on the I-trigger setting with either pressure or flow selected.

Noninvasive Positive-Pressure Ventilation (NPPV)

In NPPV the operator sets parameters for the spontaneous ventilation mode or the spontaneous/timed ventilation mode. In the spontaneous ventilation mode (SPONT), IPAP and EPAP are set. IPAP must be greater than or equal to EPAP. All breaths are patient triggered using flow triggering (I-trigger). The rise time percent can be used to taper the beginning of the breath. Exhalation (EPAP) begins when the inspiratory flow drops to a percentage of peak flow measured during inspiration. The percentage is determined by the E-trigger setting.

In spontaneous/timed ventilation (SPONT/T), the patient can breathe spontaneously or receive time-triggered breaths from the ventilator, with a set inspiratory time and rate. This minimum rate setting guarantees that the patient receives at least the set number of breaths per minute. In earlier versions of the Esprit, these breaths are synchronized with the patient's inspiratory effort (flow triggered). If no patient effort is detected, time triggering occurs based on the set rate. Again, the high inspiratory pressure (HIP) limit is automatically adjusted by 10 cm H_2O above the current IPAP setting in NPPV.

In rev. 4.0 of the Esprit, some alternations have been made to the SPONT/T mode.[2] It no longer delivers patient-triggered mandatory breaths. The patient either breathes spontaneously or receives ventilator time-triggered breaths. Spontaneous patient-triggered breaths receive the set IPAP level and T_I based on the E-trigger setting. An intrabreath period timer is active and resets with every patient-triggered breath. If the patient does not trigger a spontaneous breath within the time limit, the ventilator begins delivering time-triggered breaths at the set inspiratory time, rate, and IPAP level.

Apnea Ventilation (AV)

As with most ventilators, the operator can set an apnea time interval (10 to 60 seconds). This setting is available on the alarm setting screen. If the ventilator fails to detect a patient breathing effort within this time frame, an alarm occurs and apnea ventilation begins. APNEA appears in the ALERTS window. The Esprit delivers breaths using the A/C mode with either PCV or VCV, depending on which is set. The machine defaults to the settings for VCV or PCV. For example, in VCV it bases AV breath delivery on the set V_T, flow, PEEP, O_2 %, and so on. The breath rate is established by the operator-set apnea rate, which is set in the breath setting screen. There is, however, an exception to this. The set apnea rate cannot be set lower in AV than the rate selected for the normal ventilating mode. If attempts are

made to set it lower, a window appears stating, APNEA RATE MUST BE GREATER THAN OR EQUAL TO SET RATE. The ventilator automatically changes the rate to equal the set rate (Clinical Rounds 12-39).

When AV occurs in NPPV, the ventilator delivers only mandatory breaths at the set apnea rate or in response to patient effort if breathing resumes. The AV settings in NPPV include rate, IPAP, EPAP, I-time, rise time, I-trigger, E-trigger, O_2 %, and apnea rate.

To return to normal ventilation, the operator presses the ALARM RESET button below the screen. Normal ventilation also resumes if the ventilator detects two consecutive inspiratory efforts from the patient.

SPECIAL FEATURES

An optional oxygen sensor may be installed to allow monitoring of inspired oxygen concentrations. O_2 sensor calibration is performed during EST. Sensors are calibrated and replaced as needed based on the manufacturer's specifications. To prevent contamination of the O_2 sensor, it is placed between the ventilator gas output port and the inspiratory bacterial filter before being connected to the main inspiratory line of the patient circuit.

An optional graphics package is also available. This software adds a graphics screen that displays flow-time, pressure-time, and volume-time scalars. In addition, flow-volume and pressure-volume loops are displayed. The graphics screen allows the operator to rescale the graphic, freeze a graphic display, and save and overlay an image. The latter feature can be used for comparisons before and after bronchodilator therapy. The freeze function provides additional scrolling and identification of all parameter-displayed values for both waveforms and loops.

The Flow-Trak option functions during volume-targeted breaths.[3] When activated, it allows the patient to receive as much flow as the person demands, regardless of the flow setting. During volume ventilation with the option active, if a patient's spontaneous effort results in a volume delivery that exceeds the set volume, the ventilator uses 25% of the peak inspiratory flow as the indicator to cycle into exhalation. This helps eliminate breath stacking.

TROUBLESHOOTING

The alarms previously described help point out problems during ventilation. In addition, messages appear on the screen when the operator tries to set up parameters that are outside the available limits of ventilation. For example, in A/C volume ventilation, the I:E ratio is limited to a maximum of 3:1. If a peak flow, tidal volume, inspiratory hold, waveform, or apnea rate setting results in an I:E ratio of greater than 3:1, a message appears that reads, I:E RATIO MUST BE LESS THAN 3:1. CHECK V_T, PEAK FLOW, INSP HOLD (OR APNEA RATE). Also in A/C, the T_I cannot exceed 9 seconds or a similar message appears.

In PCV, the I:E ratio cannot exceed 4:1. A message similar to the one mentioned previously appears if the settings result in an inverse I:E ratio greater than 4:1. The operator needs to check the inspiratory time, apnea rate, and rise time to make sure they are set appropriately. In NPPV, the I:E ratio is also limited to 4:1 or less. In NPPV the operator would adjust the apnea rate, I-time rate, or breath rate to correct an I:E ratio problem.

A common error that operators make when they first begin to use the ventilator is erroneously setting the flow sensitivity. If a flow of 2 L/min is set, the ventilator triggers inspiratory flow when the flow through the circuit at end-exhalation drops by 2 L/min (see Chapter 11, flow triggering). The bias flow is automatically set by the ventilator 3 L/min higher than the trigger flow. For example, with a 2 L/min setting, the bias flow is 5 L/min. If the patient is struggling to trigger the ventilator, the operator needs to check the appropriateness of the I-trigger setting.

Another point that is easy to forget is to press ACTIVATE . . . when the breath type is changed.

The Esprit is not designed for operation near magnetic resonance imaging (MRI) equipment and must be kept away from such equipment.

KEY POINTS

▶ The Respironics Esprit ventilator is electrically powered and can be used for invasive or noninvasive ventilation.

▶ When the Esprit is not in use, it should remain connected to an A/C power source and the circuit breaker should be kept in the ON position.

▶ If a ventilator inoperative condition occurs, another method of ventilating the patient should be provided immediately.

▶ If major leaks are present in the patient circuit, the ventilator will not run.

▶ Some setting keys appear active even though they are not being used in the current active mode. These keys

are used in apnea ventilation or when the manual inspiration key is pressed.

▶ In NPPV the high pressure limit is automatically set at 10 cm H_2O above the IPAP setting.

▶ To select a mode of ventilation, the operator must touch MONITOR or ACTIVE MODE.

▶ In the rev. 4.0 version of the Esprit, during NPPV with the SPONT/T mode, if the patient does not trigger a spontaneous breath within the time limit, the ventilator begins delivering time-triggered breaths at the set inspiratory time, rate, and IPAP level.

ASSESSMENT QUESTIONS

See Evolve Resources for the answers.

1. The respiratory therapist assembles the Esprit for patient use and turns on the main power switch, but nothing happens. What could be the problem?
   I. It is not plugged into an AC outlet.
   II. The backup battery is not charged.
   III. The main circuit breakers are not on.
   IV. The alarms are not set appropriately.
      a. I only
      b. II and III
      c. I, II, and III
      d. III and IV

2. Which of the following statements about the high inspiratory pressure alarm is/are true?
   I. When the pressure during inspiration reaches the high pressure alarm setting, inspiration ends.
   II. The high pressure alarm can only be adjusted by using the alarm setting screen.
   III. During NPPV, the high pressure alarm is automatically set to 10 cm H_2O above IPAP.
   IV. High inspiratory pressure can be adjusted using the HIP icon next to the pressure manometer on the touch-sensitive screen.
      a. I only
      b. II only
      c. II and III only
      d. I, III, and IV only

ASSESSMENT QUESTIONS—cont'd

3. The 100% oxygen indicator above the screen illuminates when:
   a. ALARM SILENCE has been pressed
   b. 100% oxygen has been measured in the patient circuit by the O_2 sensor
   c. The 100% O_2 control button has been pressed
   d. The high-pressure oxygen source has been lost

4. During operation of the Esprit, an audible alarm sounds, the BATTERY LOW indicator is illuminated, and the MAINS indicator is off. These conditions indicate:
   a. Five minutes or less of battery power remains and the main AC power cord is not connected to an electrical source
   b. The external battery is low and is being charged
   c. The unit is now on standby, and the external battery is not available
   d. The unit is off and needs to be connected to a power source to recharge the battery

5. Which of the following statements about the SST and EST is correct?
   a. These are self-tests used to verify system safety and correct operation.
   b. These tests can be run during ventilation of a patient.
   c. These functions are accessible through the normal ventilation screen.
   d. These are alarm conditions indicating that the safety valve is open.

6. Apnea ventilation in the Esprit:
   a. Occurs when 20 seconds have passed without a breath being detected
   b. Is not available on the ventilator
   c. Cannot have an apnea rate set lower than the mandatory rate in A/C and SIMV
   d. Has preset factory parameters for rate, volume, PEEP, flow, and oxygen percent

7. Which of the following statements is/are true about the modes and breath types available on the Esprit?
   a. The available modes depend on the breath type selected.
   b. Breath types include VCV, PCV, and NPPV.
   c. A backup breath rate is available in NPPV-SPONT/T.
   d. PSV is not available for spontaneous breath support.
   (1) I only
   (2) II only
   (3) III and IV only
   (4) I, II, and III only

8. Which of the following is true regarding pressure-targeted breaths in PSV, PCV, and IPAP?
   a. All pressure breaths have volume targeting available.
   b. The rise time percent feature can be used to slope or taper pressure delivery.
   c. Flow-Trak can be used with pressure-targeted breaths.
   d. The upper pressure limit is automatically set at 10 cm H_2O above the set pressure in PSV, PCV, and IPAP.

9. During NPPV-SPONT/T:
   a. IPAP must be set equal to or higher than EPAP
   b. Pressure support can be added to breath delivery
   c. Only pressure triggering is available
   d. All breaths must be patient triggered

10. Expiratory trigger is best defined as:
    a. The variable that triggers inspiration
    b. The baseline pressure setting (PEEP/CPAP)
    c. The flow percentage at which inspiration ends during PSV
    d. The transition during NPPV between IPAP and EPAP

11. The actual breath rate is set at 8 breaths/min in the A/C mode. The apnea rate is set at 6 breaths/min. Which of the following is true?
    a. If apnea ventilation occurs, the rate will be 6 breaths/min.
    b. Apnea ventilation cannot occur because the rate is set higher than 6 breaths/min.
    c. A message will appear on the screen telling the operator that the apnea rate must be greater than or equal to the set rate (defaults to the set rate).
    d. Apnea ventilation is not available in the A/C mode.

12. During NPPV, the IPAP is set at 14 cm H_2O and the EPAP at 4 cm H_2O. The high pressure limit is set:
    a. Based on department policy
    b. 10 to 15 cm H_2O above IPAP
    c. Between 4 and 14 cm H_2O
    d. Automatically at 10 above IPAP

13. If the flow trigger is set at 2 L/min, the bias flow automatically will be set at:
    a. 6 L/min
    b. 3 L/min above the flow trigger
    c. 10 L/min
    d. Twice the set flow

References

1. Respironics: Esprit operator's manual, 580-1000-01F, Murrysville, Pa, Aug 2001, Respironics, Inc.
2. Respironics: Esprit Ventilator 4.0 software release notes, part no 1010639-05/22/02, Murrysville, Pa, 2002, Respironics.
3. Respironics: Respironics Flow-Trak option, PN 1035551, Murrysville, Pa, 2006, Respironics.

Internet Resource
www.respironics.com

CHAPTER SUMMARY

This chapter has presented several mechanical ventilators that represent a broad sample of the types of ventilators available, and those that represent a large part of the ventilator market used by health care facilities.

Because of the competition between companies that manufacture ventilators, the vast majority of the available products have very similar features and modes. However, although marketed modes and features may be similar, frequently the technology driving the devices is very different.

Breath delivery and modes of ventilation have very similar applications, but their names vary widely among companies. For that reason, Appendix 12-1 provides a table that compares common names given to modes and the name given to that mode on each of the ventilators presented in this chapter.

The student of mechanical ventilation should always defer to the manufacturer's operating manual when using a device, because new features can be added and previous features can be changed frequently. Additional material often is available on the manufacturer's Web site.

New ventilators are constantly being developed and released on the market. Therefore keeping up with the most current equipment is a daunting task. Add the fact that companies frequently are being bought and sold, and it makes it difficult for the consumer to keep up-to-date on the changes in medical device development and distribution.

Hopefully, this chapter has provided students of mechanical ventilation with a better grasp of the medical equipment they are using or may be using as they complete their studies.

Comparison of Common Ventilator Mode Names Among Different Manufacturers

Ventilator	Assist/Control CMV-Vol	PCV	SIMV-VC	SIMV-PC	PRVC	SIMV PRVC	PSV/CPAP	APRV	Additional Mode(s) or Feature(s)
Cardinal AVEA	Volume A/C	Pressure A/C	Volume SIMV	Pressure SIMV	PRVC	PRVC SIMV	CPAP-PSV	APRV Biphasic	TCPL-A/C and TCPL-SIMV
Cardinal BEAR 1000	Assist CMV	Pressure control	SIMV/CPAP and PSV	PC-SIMV and CPAP PSV	—	—	PS/CPAP	—	Pressure augment and MMV (operates in SIMV/CPAP and increases rate)
Cardinal VELA	Volume A/C	Pressure A/C	Volume SIMV	Pressure SIMV	PRVC A/C	PRVC and SIMV	CPAP-PSV	APRV and Biphasic	—
Dräger Evita 4	CMV	PCV+	SIMV (vol.) + PSV	SIMV (Press.)+ PSV	AutoFlow™	AutoFlow™ with SIMV (volume)	PSV-CPAP	APRV	MMV & MMV + PS (increase f at set volume)
Dräger EvitaXL	CMV	PCV+ (i.e., BiPAP)	SIMV (vol.) and PSV	SIMV (Press.)+ PSV	AutoFlow™	AutoFlow™ with SIMV (volume)	PSV-CPAP	APRV	MMV & MMV + PS (increase f at set volume)
Hamilton GALILEO Gold (two names: U.S. or U.K.)	S(CMV) or A/C	P-A/C or P-CMV	SIMV	P-SIMV	APVcmv	APVsimv	SPONT (PSV-CPAP)	APRV or DuoPAP	ASV
Hamilton RAPHAEL	S(CMV)+	PCV+	SIMV+	PSIMV+	(S)CMV+	SIMV+	SPONT (PSV-CPAP)	DuoPAP and DuPAP+ (extended I:E)	ASV
Maquet Servo 300	VC	PC	SIMV (Vol. Contr.)	SIMV (Press. Contr.)	PRVC	—	PS/CPAP	—	VS
Maquet Servo[i] and Servo[s]	VC	PC	SIMV (Vol. Contr.)	SIMV (Press. Contr.)	PRVC	SIMV (PRVC)	PSV/CPAP	BiVent	VS, NAVA available on Servo[i]
Newport Medical Instruments Wave E200	A/C (volume)	A/C (pressure)	SIMV (volume)	SIMV (pressure)	—	—	SPONT (PS and CPAP/PEEP)	—	—
Newport e500	A/CMV (volume)	A/CMV (pressure)	SIMV (volume)	SIMV (pressure)	VTPC	SIMV-VTPC	SPONT (PS and VTPS)	—	VTPS
PB 840	Assist/control (volume)	Assist/control (Press.)	SIMV (volume)	SIMV (pressure)	VC+	SIMV VC+	SPONT (PSV-CPAP)	Bilevel	PAV+ VS
PB 740	AC-VCV	—	SIMV-VCV	—	—	—	CPAP and PS	—	—
PB 760	AC-VCV	AC-PCV	SIMV-VCV	SIMV-PCV	—	—	CPAP and PS	—	—
PB 7200	CMV	PCV	SIMV (VC)	SIMV (PC)	—	—	CPAP and PSV	—	—
Respironics Esprit	VCV-A/C	PCV-A/C	VCV-SIMV	PCV-SIMV	—	—	CPAP and PSV	—	NPPV

*See individual sections in this chapter for more information on each ventilator, including a description of the mode and the additional mode(s) or feature(s) listed.

Chapter 13

Infant and Pediatric Ventilators

KENNETH F. WATSON

OUTLINE

*See Evolve Resources for a detailed description of this ventilator.

OUTLINE—cont'd

OBJECTIVES

Upon completion of this chapter, you will be able to:
· Systematically review continuous positive airway pressure (CPAP) delivery devices and infant and pediatric ventilators.
· Name the power sources required for each nasal CPAP device and each infant and pediatric ventilator.
· List the modes of ventilatory support provided by each ventilator.
· When given flow and inspiratory time (T_I), calculate the approximate tidal volume (V_T) delivered by a typical infant ventilator.
· Describe noteworthy internal functions of each infant and pediatric ventilator.
· Explain the location and function of the controls, monitors, alarm, and safety systems for each infant and pediatric ventilator.
· Describe the precautions and key troubleshooting points for each nasal CPAP device or ventilator.

KEY TERMS

accumulator
amplitude
bias flow
circuit positive end-expiratory pressure (PEEP)
demand flow system
dump valve
electromagnetic
expiratory synchrony
hertz (Hz)

high-frequency jet ventilator
hi-lo jet tracheal tube
hot-wire flow sensor
infrared sensor
jet solenoid
leak compensation
message log
oscillator subsystem
piston assembly

pneumatic safety valve
polarity voltage
proportioning valve
pulsation dampener
purge valve
square-wave driver
termination sensitivity
variable-orifice flow pneumotachometer

Treatment of the infant in respiratory failure is an ever-evolving field. Advances in the prevention and treatment of respiratory failure have resulted in reduced mortality and improved outcomes in preterm infants. In spite of these advances, mechanical ventilation remains an essential component in the care of critically ill infants. The basic goal of mechanical ventilation, which is to ensure adequate ventilation and oxygenation, has essentially stayed the same for several decades. However, optimal ventilatory strategies and the devices used to accomplish infant ventilation have most certainly evolved.

In the 1960s we were provided the first published reports of the successful use of neonatal mechanical ventilation.

Since that time, the majority of infants requiring mechanical ventilation have been treated by using the standard time-cycled, pressure-limited (TCPL) ventilation mode. Although there was little scientific evidence to support that infant ventilation using TCPL is superior to volume-control ventilation, there was strong belief that the TCPL mode reduced the risk of barotrauma.[1]

The introduction of positive end-expiratory pressure (PEEP) to restore functional residual capacity and prevent airway collapse resulted in the ability to use lower pressures during ventilation. By the 1970s, CPAP and intermittent mandatory ventilation (IMV) were common modes and neonatal ventilation had changed once again. Along with high-frequency ventilation, surfactant replacement, and *extracorporeal membrane oxygenation* (ECMO), the 1990s brought microprocessor-based mechanical ventilators with the sophisticated transducers that were designed to enable better ventilator-to-patient synchrony.

Further advances in ventilator technology have allowed for more precise patient monitoring and have enabled implementation of additional modes that were previously associated with only adult and pediatric patients. Manufacturers have introduced ventilators with a wide range of modes including both volume-targeted and pressure-targeted modes and modes that allow an element of patient control of the ventilator. These include initiation and termination of inspiration as well as control of flow. Some modes are even hybrids, combining the best features of both the pressure-targeted and volume-targeted modes.

Today, technology has provided not only a variety of modes for ventilation, but also real-time pulmonary function monitoring for these smallest of patients. Neonatal ventilation is no longer solely about adequate gas exchange and oxygenation; it is instead an arena of ventilator-management strategies where the goal is for critically ill infants to receive optimum ventilation with the smallest amount of lung injury.

This chapter will discuss devices that are utilized to both invasively and noninvasively mechanically ventilate the infant patient and the pediatric patient. It is divided into four sections: (1) continuous positive airway pressure (CPAP) devices, (2) infant ventilators, (3) high-frequency jet and oscillatory ventilators, and (3) neonatal and pediatric features of the general-use ventilators discussed in Chapter 12. Although a great deal of care has been taken to ensure that the information within this chapter was accurate at the time of publication, each device is subject to change by the manufacturer. Therefore, the reader is advised to obtain thorough instruction in the proper application before patient use, refer to manufacturer's user manuals, review safety precautions, and remain alert to device updates.

PART I—CONTINUOUS POSITIVE AIRWAY PRESSURE (CPAP) SYSTEMS

Continuous positive airway pressure (CPAP) has been used for many years in the treatment of hypoxia in infants and children. For decades, CPAP has been administered by using a constant flow of a gas mixture adjusted to provide a single pressure level at the airway. One method to accomplish this is for an infant ventilator to serve as the driver for the system. Today, however, free-standing systems are available with interfaces that alter flow characteristics between inspiration and expiration and use drivers with more sophistication. For example, one free-standing system can provide either constant expiratory pressure or biphasic pressure (i.e., pressure on inspiration and expiration). Another system is "bubble CPAP," which has been used in the past and is experiencing a reemergence in popularity. "Bubble CPAP" provides a single pressure and flow, but with minute oscillations around the set pressure level.

In recent years a popular practice has been to fit infant ventilator circuits with noninvasive CPAP interfaces such as nasal prongs. This fitting is accomplished by adding one of the many available interfaces designed for infant nasal CPAP. An example interface is the Argyle CPAP nasal cannula, which connects directly to a standard infant ventilator circuit (Figure 13-1). Some interfaces, such as the Hudson RCI Infant Nasal CPAP System, provide both the integrated ventilator circuit and the nasal-prong interface (Figure 13-2).

Although noninvasive interfaces such as nasal prongs are favored by most clinicians, nasopharyngeal CPAP provides an alternative. Nasopharyngeal CPAP is provided by trimming endotracheal tubes (ETTs) to fit the infant's upper airway (Figure 13-3).[2] Nasopharyngeal CPAP may be used in situations in which nasal appliances and headgear cannot be used because of potential aggravation of a surgical site or skin condition. In addition, nasopharyngeal

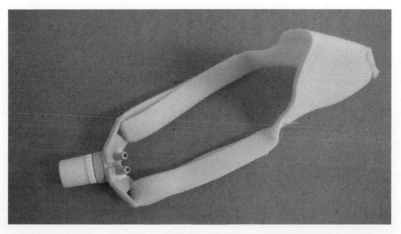

FIGURE 13-1 Photograph of Kendall Health Argyle CPAP nasal prongs and headgear.

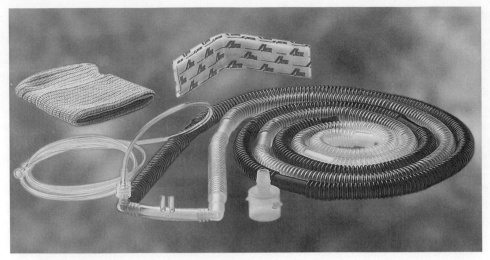

FIGURE 13-2 Photograph of the Hudson RCI Infant Nasal CPAP circuit and patient interface. (Courtesy Telefax Medical, Research Triangle Park, NC.)

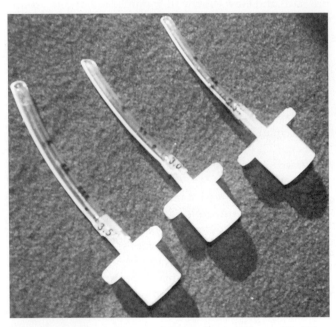

FIGURE 13-3 Nasopharyngeal CPAP. (From Pilbeam SP, Cairo JM: *Mechanical ventilation: physiological and clinical applications,* ed 4, St Louis, 2006, Mosby.)

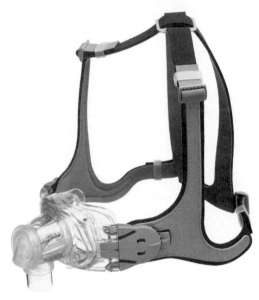

FIGURE 13-4 Mirage Kidsta Mask. (Courtesy © ResMed 2009. Used with permission.)

CPAP may be better tolerated by some patients or its use may simply be the preference of the clinician.

Even though many clinicians lean toward one type of CPAP system and interface over another, no clinical research data are available at this time that conclusively show the superiority of one system or interface type. Moreover, because CPAP is used in the management of several clinical situations, it cannot yet be stated that one type of system or interface is more effective for a certain clinical circumstance than another. Convenience, economics, and staff experience often dictate the type of CPAP system and interface a facility chooses to use.

It is not uncommon for clinicians to use nasal-prong or nasopharyngeal CPAP interfaces in children up to the age of 6 months. For older children, nasal masks have been the preferred device because most available prong sizes are too small. Also, masks and accompanying headgear seem to stay in position better in the older, more active child.

Today, many brands of masks are available for small children. An example, the ResMed Mirage Kidsta mask, is shown in Figure 13-4. Nasal masks are preferred over full-face designs. Although it is known that older children are not obligate nose breathers, most "settle in" to breathing through these masks after becoming accustomed to them. If the patient does not tolerate a nasal mask, it is often because the nasal passages are not fully patent. It is usually a good practice to take measures to clear the nose, if possible, and offer the patient a trial with a nasal mask to evaluate its effectiveness before resorting to a full-face mask.

Although not all clinicians agree, the use of conventional adult CPAP drivers, whether they are ventilators or stand-alone devices, is generally appropriate for providing nasal CPAP to children over 6 months of age.

In this section of the chapter, we will review a few examples of CPAP application devices, including the Cardinal Health Infant Flow Nasal CPAP System, the Cardinal Health Infant Flow synchronized inspiratory positive airway pressure (SiPAP™), the Fisher & Paykel Healthcare Bubble CPAP System, and the Hamilton ARABELLA System.

CARDINAL HEALTH INFANT FLOW NASAL CPAP SYSTEM

Originally, the Cardinal Health Infant Flow Nasal CPAP System was the EME Infant Flow System of Electro Medical Equipment in East Sussex, England. The Infant Flow Nasal CPAP System, as the name implies, is designed to provide nasal CPAP to infants.[3]

The system consists of a driver, a humidifier/hot-wire delivery circuit, an infant flow generator with prongs, and a cap for fitting and stabilizing the prongs in the nasal passages (Figure 13-5). (NOTE: Any humidifier that accommodates standard temperature sensors and heater wire connections can be used with this unit.[3]) A small nasal mask is also available and can be used in lieu of nasal prongs.

Power Source

The CPAP system uses two high-pressure gas sources and an electrical source, which includes a 12-V battery (direct current [DC]) as a backup electrical power source. Compressed air and oxygen from sources of 50 pound-force per square inch gauge (psig) are introduced into the back of the driver.

An on/off power-toggle switch is located on the driver's rear panel. Immediately after the power to the driver is turned on, the system's software version will be displayed in the oxygen ($O_2\%$) window for 2 seconds. The clinician should follow the directions in the operator's manual specific to each driver's software version.

Function of the Flow Generator

Blended gas at a constant flow exits the driver, passes through the humidifier, and is carried to an infant flow generator (Figure 13-6A).

The generator consists of two fluidic jets. The geometric design of the jet delivery ports facilitates the Coanda effect. (For more information, see Fluidics, Chapter 11.) The device operates as follows. An infant's breathing efforts trigger a flip-flop device inside the flow generator. On inspiration, flow from the driver passes through the nasal prongs to the infant. If the infant's inspiratory flow is less than that delivered by the driver, excess flow is diverted away from the prongs. On expiration, pressure from the expiratory gas flow "flips" the direction of flow away from the prongs and through an expiratory port. Diverting flow away from the nasal prongs enables the infant to exhale through a low-resistance system. Only a baseline amount of flow is needed to maintain the set CPAP level.

Patient Interface

The nasal prongs and nasal masks are made from a soft, silicon-based elastomer. The prongs are available in three

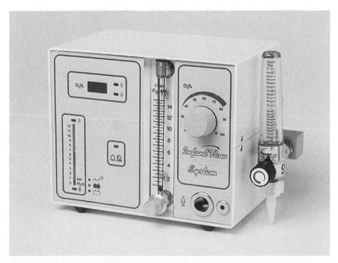

FIGURE 13-5 The EME Infant Flow System. (Courtesy Electro Medical Equipment, East Sussex, England, a Cardinal Health product; Cardinal Health, McGaw Park, Ill.)

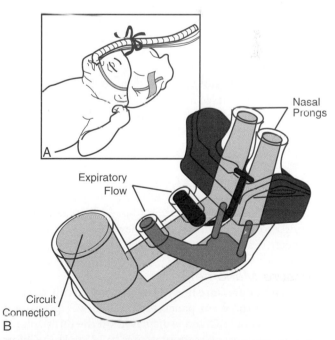

FIGURE 13-6 A, The infant flow generator used with the Infant Flow System. **B,** The mounting system for the infant flow generator.

sizes, and the nasal masks are available in two sizes. A mounting system incorporates a head cap and two positioning straps (Figure 13-6B). The head cap is available in 10 sizes, with each size color-coded. The head cap is attached with straps. The straps connect to the two flanges of the nasal attachment and are inserted into slits along the edge of the head cap. The gas-delivery tube and exhalation tubing are positioned above the patient's head and can be tied to the head cap. The infant can then be repositioned or held while the CPAP prongs remain in position.

Controls, Monitors, and Alarms

The driver contains all the controls. They include the on/off switch, a flowmeter, an oxygen (O_2%) control, and an alarm mute button. A digital pressure manometer provides a dynamic display of airway pressure. Alarm conditions are audible and are visually displayed on the front panel.

O_2%

F_IO_2 is variable from 0.21 to 1.0. The O_2% knob is calibrated in 10% increments, but it will allow adjustment in 1% increments. The set oxygen concentration is according to the knob's position. The digital display, also marked O_2%, is a reading from the unit's built-in oxygen analyzer. This analyzer is calibrated by the clinician before each use by adjusting two potentiometers on the driver's left-side panel, one while the O_2% knob is set at 21% and the other while it is set at 100%.

An oxygen alarm system is incorporated into the analyzer's digital display. The microprocessor sets alarm limits either automatically within 2 minutes of a stable reading or when the alarm keypad is pressed and held for 3 seconds. When the monitored F_IO_2 falls outside of these limits, a red high– or low *light–emitting diode* (LED) will glow and an audible alarm will sound.

Flowmeters

A flowmeter that is not back pressure–compensated, incorporated into the driver, and adjustable to 15 L/min sets the peak flow available to the patient. The flow setting also dictates the CPAP level. A chart is available to guide the clinician in setting the flow for the desired CPAP level. Ideally, if prongs are sized and fitted correctly, a flow of 8 L/min should provide a CPAP level of 5 cm H_2O.

An auxiliary flowmeter is mounted to the side of the driver. This flowmeter, which is adjustable to 15 L/min, is intended to power the accessory devices. Gas exiting this flowmeter is at the same F_IO_2 as the O_2% setting.

Pressure Manometer

The proximal pressure line of the delivery circuit attaches to a port on the front panel. Proximal airway pressure is measured in cm H_2O and is displayed on the multicolored bar graph. This graph reads pressures to 12 cm H_2O. Colors within the bar graph indicate the operational ranges as shown in Table 13-1.

TABLE 13-1

Colors Within Airway Pressure Bar Graph Indicating Operational Ranges for the Cardinal Health Nasal CPAP (nCPAP) Infant Flow System

Color	Pressure (in cm H_2O)
Red	0
Yellow	1-3
Green	4-6
Yellow	7-12

CPAP, Continuous positive airway pressure.

CLINICAL ROUNDS 13-1

A respiratory therapist notices the red light-emitting diodes (LEDs) illuminated above and below the pressure bar on the pressure manometer of the Cardinal Health Infant Flow nasal continuous positive airway pressure (nCPAP) System. What should she do?

See Evolve Resources for the answer.

Red LEDs above and below the bar graph will light when pressure alarm limits are manually set and when pressure alarm limits are violated. If alarm limits are not manually set by pressing the alarm keypad for 3 seconds, the driver's microprocessor will set them automatically within 2 minutes. See Clinical Rounds 13-1 for questions related to the nasal CPAP device.

Alarm Keypad/Alarm Limits

The alarm keypad serves two functions. During an alarm condition, the audible portion may be silenced for 30 seconds by touching the keypad briefly.

The keypad is also used to set alarm limits. After the infant is placed on the desired levels of CPAP and F_IO_2, the clinician should press and hold the keypad for 3 seconds to set alarm limits. A green LED above the keypad will light when alarm limits have been set. Alarm conditions must persist for 15 seconds before alarms are activated.

When limits are set, audiovisual alarms activate when pressures rise more than 3 cm H_2O above or fall below 2 cm H_2O from the baseline CPAP level. Oxygen alarm limits are ±5% of the digitally displayed oxygen concentration.

To protect against excessive system pressures, a solenoid control valve within the driver opens at a pressure of 11 cm H_2O and vents to ambient. An audible alarm also sounds. After 3 seconds, the driver will attempt to restore flow to the patient circuit.

Loss of High-Pressure Gas

Because loss of gas power to the device would be a serious problem, a supply gases failure alarm will activate with a decrease in one source gas pressure to less than 30 psig. Until the alarm condition is corrected, the gas at the higher pressure will be delivered to the patient. This will alter the F_IO_2 delivery. The supply gases failure alarm can be silenced only by correcting the pressure drop or disconnecting both gas sources.

Battery Power

A lead acid battery is contained within the driver. With a full charge, the driver unit will operate for 4 hours on battery power.

Troubleshooting

The prongs should be checked first for fit before adjusting the straps, because this can result in the prongs moving toward the eyes. In general, the straps do not need adjustment if the fit is correct. Obviously some adjustment may be required because not all babies have faces of the same shape. Care should be taken not to pull too tightly on the straps and squash the infant's nose in an effort to get a good seal.

The most common problem seen in the nasal CPAP flow device is leaking at the nose. When leaks are present, the size of the prongs should be checked. Readjusting the straps also improves the fit. Care should be taken, however, not to adjust the straps too tightly to achieve a seal. Doing so will put too much pressure on the nose and will cause patient discomfort and skin breakdown. The prongs or mask should seal gently. Patient agitation occasionally presents a problem to keeping the system tight and delivering the desired level of CPAP.

In the case of oxygen alarms, recalibrating the oxygen analyzer usually resolves the problem. If frequent calibrations are necessary, the oxygen fuel cell may require replacing.

CARDINAL HEALTH AIRLIFE™ NASAL CPAP SYSTEM DRIVER

In addition to the Infant Flow Nasal CPAP System, Cardinal Health has a more recent infant nasal CPAP device called the AirLife™ nCPAP System Driver. Figure 13-7 depicts the AirLife™ nCPAP (Cardinal Health, McGaw Park, Ill.).[4]

Power Source

The AirLife™ nCPAP System Driver requires an electrical power source for operation (120-V alternating current [AC] or internal DC battery) to power the microprocessor system. The on/off switch is located on the back of the unit. There is a built-in battery with an estimated 4 hours of backup power when AC power is not available, such as during transport. In addition to electrical power, air and oxygen high-pressure gas sources are required to provide gas delivery to the patient.

An auxiliary gas port is available that can be used for powering nebulizer treatments, manually ventilating the patient, or for providing a blended gas source through a humidified nasal cannula system.

Because the system is microprocessor-based, when new software becomes available, the AirLife™ nCPAP System Driver can be upgraded.

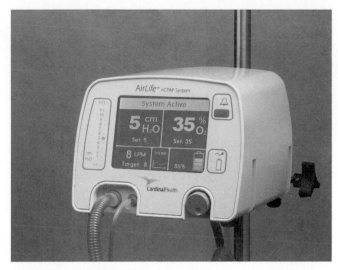

FIGURE 13-7 Photograph of the front panel of the AirLife™ nCPAP System Driver. (Courtesy Cardinal Health, McGaw Park, Ill.)

Flow Delivery

The manufacturer has what it describes as a "comfort-flow feature." The clinician sets the desired nCPAP, then the AirLife™ Infant nCPAP System automatically adjusts the gas flow to achieve the desired pressure levels and to compensate for leaks. A constant level of nCPAP is maintained. This helps the clinician, who might normally have to manually adjust the flow to compensate for leaks in some nasal CPAP systems.

Displayed Values and O₂ Cell

The AirLife™ nCPAP Air Driver has a liquid-crystal display (LCD) that shows the pressure, flow, $O_2\%$, and battery life during normal operation (see Figure 13-7). There is an internal O_2 cell for analysis of F_IO_2 delivery. The system automatically calibrates oxygen blending on start-up.

Controls

Adjustments to ventilation parameters are accomplished by using the interface control knob (lower right-hand corner). The various sections of the screen ($O_2\%$, CPAP, or flow target values) can be highlighted by rotating the knob. Once the desired control is highlighted, pressing the knob selects the parameter. The current setting appears at the top of the screen in the message bar area. Rotating the knob clockwise increases the value of the parameter, and a counterclockwise rotation decreases the value. When the desired value is displayed in the message bar, pressing and releasing the knob activates the new setting.

Alarms

When the practitioner sets the operating parameters, the system automatically adjusts alarms based on the new settings. Alarms are delayed for 120 seconds after entering the main screen in order to allow time for patient set-up. If additional time is required, pressing the alarm mute/reset button provides an additional 120 seconds. In addition, the system can be placed into standby mode (see following section).

Alarms include elevated pressure, low pressure, high pressure, disconnect, O_2% alarms, leak, external power disconnect, battery low, oxygen pressure low, air pressure low, O_2 sensor calibration failure, flow/pressure sensor failure, and software fault. The operating manual for the AirLife™ nCPAP System Driver contains a full description of the alarms and how to correct any problems associated with alarm conditions.

Standby Mode—20-Minute Alarm Silence

The AirLife™ nCPAP System Driver has a standby mode to allow the operator to mute the alarms for up to 20 minutes. The standby mode is activated by pressing and holding the alarm mute/reset button until there is a single audible sound (approximately 3 seconds). The message bar displays "standby mode," and the alarm mute button flashes.

While in standby mode the system will operate normally with all audible alarms muted except for the high-pressure and low-flow alarms. To indicate that the system is in standby mode, there is a single audible alarm burst every 2 minutes.

The operator can exit the standby mode by pressing the alarm mute/reset button. In addition, the alarms will automatically resume normal function after 20 minutes. The driver will automatically exit standby mode if a high-pressure or low-flow alarm occurs.

Trends

The AirLife™ nCPAP System Driver has a trend screen that displays data for the previous 4, 8, 12, or 24 hours. Information stored for the previous patient is automatically removed when the unit is powered up.

Summary

The Cardinal Health AirLife™ nCPAP System Driver provides a more recent alternative to the Cardinal Health Infant Flow nCPAP device, which will probably be completely replaced by the AirLife™ in the near future.

CARDINAL HEALTH INFANT FLOW SiPAP™

The Infant Flow SiPAP™ System from Cardinal Health (previously Viasys Healthcare, Palm Springs, California) is designed to provide noninvasive ventilatory support for infants and pediatric patients (Figure 13-8).[5] The SiPAP™ system is intended to afford a means by which patients can be transitioned from intubation to successful extubation while more support is provided than with traditional noninvasive CPAP. SiPAP™ may provide support efficiently enough that some patients can avoid intubation.

Many infants are placed on noninvasive CPAP systems in an effort to reduce the frequency of apnea periods, such as those seen in apnea of prematurity. With the availability of a bilevel airway pressure device for small infants, it is possible that the problem of spontaneous apnea can be managed better. Moreover, with the capability of providing manual breaths and backup apnea ventilation, an immediate response and resolution to apneic episodes are possible.

Available Configurations

The Infant Flow SiPAP™ System is available in two configurations: the Plus and the Comprehensive. The Plus configuration offers nasal CPAP (nCPAP) and time-triggered biphasic ventilation with breath-rate monitoring. The Comprehensive configuration offers these same features plus patient-triggered biphasic ventilation (called "BiPhasic tr") with backup breath-rate monitoring in the case of apnea. Both configurations deliver blended gas mixtures and incorporate a graphics screen for monitoring and displaying settings, touch-screen technology, patient monitoring, alarm systems, and backup battery power.

In the Comprehensive model, in addition to the patient circuit, an abdominal transducer known as a Grasby capsule is part of the design. This capsule is necessary to the detection of apnea when the "BiPhasic tr" mode is being used.

Power Source

The Infant Flow SiPAP™ Driver connects to 100 AC to 230 AC power and 50-psi O_2 and compressed air. An internal battery can provide up to 2 hours of operating time if the AC power source is lost. The battery requires 16 hours to become fully charged from a discharged state.

When the SiPAP™ driver is powered on, it automatically performs internal electrical and pneumatic checks. Once the set-up screen is visible, the user must calibrate the oxygen sensor and perform the patient circuit leak test and alarms test (see operator's manual).[5]

Once the preuse tests are completed, the clinician can select the desired mode and settings (Box 13-1). As the unit begins operation, monitoring data are displayed on the

---

BOX 13-1	Main Mode Controls on the Infant Flow SiPAP™ (Synchronized Inspiratory Positive Airway Pressure) System

- Nasal continuous positive airway pressure (nCPAP)
- nCPAP with breath-rate monitoring and low breath–rate alarm
- BiPhasic (time-triggered)
- BiPhasic (time-triggered) with breath-rate monitoring and low breath–rate alarm
- BiPhasic tr (time-triggered) with breath-rate monitoring, low breath–rate alarm, and apnea
- Back-up (Comprehensive models only)

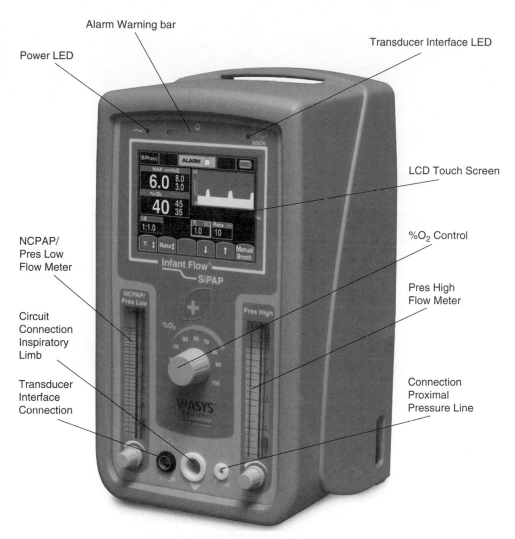

Power LED

Alarm Warning bar

Transducer Interface LED

LCD Touch Screen

NCPAP/
Pres Low
Flow Meter

%O₂ Control

Circuit
Connection
Inspiratory
Limb

Pres High
Flow Meter

Transducer
Interface
Connection

Connection
Proximal
Pressure Line

FIGURE 13-8 The Infant Flow SiPAP™ (Courtesy Cardinal Health, McGaw Park, Ill.)

BOX 13-2	Parameters Monitored by the Infant Flow SiPAP™ System

- Positive end-expiratory pressure (PEEP)
- CPAP
- Mean airway pressure (MAP)
- Peak inspiratory pressure (PIP)
- O₂%
- I : E ratio (ratio of inspiratory time to expiratory time)
- Spontaneous rate (Rsp)
- Battery charge level

driver screen. Box 13-2 lists monitored parameters, and Table 13-2 lists the ranges for monitored parameters.

Mechanism of Operation

The Infant Flow SiPAP™ System consists of a driver, a standard ventilator humidifier, and the patient circuit. The pneumatic components of the Infant Flow SiPAP™ driver consist of two separate flowmeters labeled the "NCPAP/

Pres Low" flowmeter and the "Pres High" flowmeter. The other components are an oxygen/air blending system and a monitoring/alarms system.

A proprietary Infant Flow Generator, which is capable of alternating between two levels of flow and pressure, is incorporated into the patient circuit near the nasal interface. Like its Infant Flow nCPAP predecessor, the Infant Flow SiPAP™ System delivers a humidified flow of gas to produce a targeted level of pressure. However, in the case of the SiPAP™ unit, the generator is capable of alternating between two targeted pressures.

Figure 13-9 shows the relationship of flow and pressure. The low pressure is produced by the "NCPAP/Pres Low" flowmeter from the driver. Flow to the Infant Flow Generator from the "NCPAP/Pres Low" flowmeter is directed toward its expiratory limb (Figure 13-10). This creates an expiratory pressure equal to the targeted CPAP.

When the patient takes a breath, the inspiratory effort diverts gas flow away from the expiratory limb to mix with an existing inspiratory flow (see Figure 13-10). The inspiratory flow is produced by the "Pres High" flowmeter. The

TABLE 13-2

Monitored Parameter Ranges on the SiPAP™

Parameter	Range
Inspiratory time (T$_I$)	0.1-3.0 s
Rate (R)	1-150 breaths/min (Non–U.S. configuration parameters)
	1-54 breaths/min (U.S. configuration parameters)
Apnea interval (T$_{apnea}$)	10-30 s, 5-s intervals (Non–U.S. configuration parameters)
Apnea interval (TLBR)	10-30 s, 5-s intervals (U.S. configuration parameters)
nCPAP/Pres Low flowmeter	0-5 L/min; accuracy ±15% of selected output
Pres High flowmeter	0-15 L/min; accuracy ±15% of selected output
Manual breath	X1
O$_2$%	21-100%

SiPAP, Synchronized inspiratory positive airway pressure.

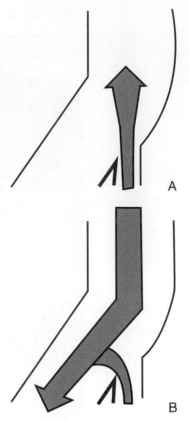

FIGURE 13-10 Twin injector nozzles of the Infant Flow Generator for the SiPAP™ driver. **A,** When the patient makes an inspiratory effort, the flow generator converts the kinetic energy of flow to pressure, to stabilize pressure delivery at the patient interface. **B,** As the patient exhales, the pressure from the exhaled gas causes the flow from the driver to flip around toward the expiratory limb. When expiratory flow stops, the flow from the driver instantly flips back to the inspiratory position (**A**).

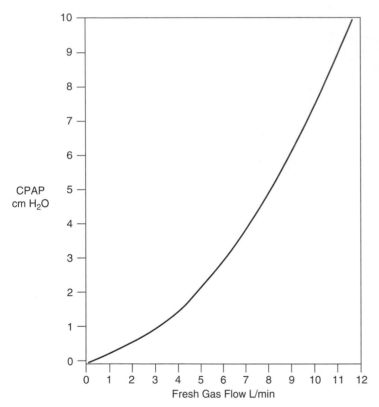

FIGURE 13-9 A graph flow-pressure nomogram for the Cardinal Health SiPAP™ unit showing the CPAP on the Y-axis (cm H$_2$O) and fresh gas flow (L/min) on the X-axis. *Note the exponential rise in fresh gas as the CPAP increases.* (Redrawn from information provided by Cardinal Health, McGaw Park, Ill.)

Patient Interface and Humidification

A variety of patient interfaces are available, including nasal prongs and nasal masks. The circuit/interface is fitted to the patient by using a fabric bonnet, also available in different sizes. A complete guide accompanies the Infant Flow SiPAP™ System to enable the practitioner to select and fit the appropriately sized nasal cannula, nasal mask, and bonnet. It is important to use the sizing templates provided to ensure a good fit. The best performance from the system greatly depends on how well the interface fits the patient.

Once the interface is fitted and the unit operational, the clinician must periodically check the interface for patency and general condition. (NOTE: Any patient interface can become obstructed, misaligned, or dislodged.) In addition, interfaces can cause skin damage if not properly sized or positioned.

The manufacturer does not recommend the use of a specific humidifier. However, the humidifier selected for use must be capable of providing inspired gas temperatures between 36° C and 37° C. A continuous-feed water

sum of the two flows, which is larger than the expiratory flow alone, creates the targeted inspiratory PAP (IPAP). Following inspiration, pressure from the patient's expiratory flow diverts gas to the expiratory limb to return to the expiratory baseline flow and expiratory PAP (EPAP). The inspiratory-to-expiratory function uses fluidics. (See Chapter 11 for additional information on fluidics.)

source for the humidifier chamber is strongly recommended to maintain stable circuit compliance.

Control Settings

Once the SiPAP™ is powered on, the default parameter settings are displayed. The front panel of the Infant Flow SiPAP™ driver is shown in Figure 13-8. All parameter controls on the Infant Flow SiPAP™ driver are accessed through its touch-screen design. Box 13-1 lists the main controls.

When a parameter is touched, it becomes highlighted and *increase* and *decrease* buttons appear. After the parameter is selected and changed, the button is touched once again to confirm the new setting. If the setting is not confirmed within 15 seconds, the highlighted parameter will return automatically to its last keystroke and the screen will return to its prior configuration.

If no control is touched for 120 seconds, the screen panel automatically locks to prevent inadvertent changes. The "screen lock" button must be touched to unlock the controls. However, if a high-priority alarm is activated, the screen immediately unlocks to allow parameter changes.

If a setting is changed that is incompatible with other parameters, the driver software will automatically adjust other settings to bring them back into compatibility. If the clinician returns the adjusted parameter back to its original setting within 15 seconds, the automatically adjusted parameter(s) will return to their original settings.

One of the parameters available is time-triggering. Timed triggering from EPAP to IPAP can be controlled by selecting an inspiratory time (T_I) on the touch screen. In addition, breath frequency can be set. This is a backup setting, however, and is operational only when the patient does not actively cycle respirations. (NOTE: In the Comprehensive configuration, an apnea backup rate, time interval, and apnea alarm can be set.)

By using the two flowmeters, the clinician can set both an inspiratory and an expiratory pressure. If just CPAP is desired, only the "NCPAP/Pres Low" flowmeter is set to deliver flow. The "Pres High" flowmeter is turned off unless it is desirable to deliver a manual breath, in which case the "Pres High" flowmeter is set. (NOTE: When operating the system in the NCPAP mode and the "Pres High" flowmeter is set, "biphasic" manual breaths can be delivered by pressing the manual breath button.)

The actual pressure for a given flow (as shown in Figure 13-9) can fall outside of the predicted value by as much as 10%. The predicted flow-to-pressure relationship increases to more than 10% when flows are decreased to achieve low pressures (e.g., 2 cm H_2O). For this reason, it is recommended that the SiPAP™ system not be used to deliver pressures of 2 cm H_2O or less.

Alarms

The driver automatically sets some alarm limits based on the parameter settings that have been selected. Other alarms are preset. Alarms and conditions that trigger

TABLE 13-3

Alarms and Conditions That Trigger Alarms on the SiPAP™

Alarm	Trigger
Supply gases failure	Activates with a ±20-psi pressure change in either gas line
High airway pressure	Activates with a pressure rise 3 cm H_2O over set pressure
Airway overpressure limit	Activates at 11 cm H_2O in nCPAP and BiPhasic Activates at 15 cm H_2O in "BiPhasic tr" mode
Low airway pressure	Activates if pressure falls 2 cm H_2O below set pressure
High and low %	Activates if measured oxygen concentration is greater than ±5% of set value
Low battery charge	Activates if battery charge falls below 40%
Low battery voltage	Activates if battery voltage falls below 10 V

alarms are listed in Table 13-3. By pressing the alarm mute/reset button, the clinician can silence alarm conditions for 30 seconds. If the button is pressed and held for 3 seconds, alarms are reset.

Modes of Ventilation

Available modes for the SiPAP™ are listed in Box 13-1. The Infant Flow SiPAP™ System provides two basic modes: CPAP and BiPhasic. The other mode choices are simply additional features for these two basic modes.

Summary

Noninvasive bilevel airway pressure has been an effective tool in adult and pediatric patients for many years. As is the case with mechanical ventilators, a practical device to provide the same type of support to the smallest of infants has been a technical challenge. In the meantime, a gap between CPAP and mechanical ventilation has persisted in neonatal critical care settings. This gap has led to many extubation failures and untold additional ventilator days for patients. The Infant Flow SiPAP™ System is the first practical infant bilevel application that may effectively bridge that gap and provide a real alternative to more invasive care.

FISHER & PAYKEL HEALTHCARE BUBBLE CPAP SYSTEM

The Fisher & Paykel Healthcare Bubble CPAP System (Fisher & Paykel Healthcare, Auckland, New Zealand) was introduced to provide clinicians with a commercially available free-standing CPAP delivery device that takes advantage of the "high-frequency," or "bubbling," effect that is reported to be unique to this system. The application of bubble CPAP has been associated with reduced incidence of chronic lung disease (CLD) in premature infants.[6] However, no randomized trials have been published that compare this method with the more conventional forms of CPAP delivery.

The Fisher & Paykel Healthcare Bubble CPAP System consists of two components: a delivery system and a patient interface. These components can be used together as a single system or can be employed separately as parts of clinician-designed hybrid systems.

Delivery System

The Fisher & Paykel Healthcare Bubble CPAP System is shown in Figure 13-11. The manufacturer recommends the use of a Fisher & Paykel Healthcare MR290 humidifier chamber (Figure 13-12), which is designed to operate with either the MR850 or the MR730 humidifier unit. If the MR850 is used, it is set to the "invasive" mode. If the MR730 is used, the temperature control is initially set at 40° C and the chamber control at −3. Fine adjustments to these settings may be necessary once the system is in use.

A continuous-feed sterile water system keeps a constant water level within the chamber.

The system also depends upon a standard air/oxygen blender, a 0 L/min to 15 L/min flowmeter, and standard oxygen tubing to deliver inspiratory gas flow to the unit. Flow enters the system by way of a plastic manifold (Figure 13-13), which is connected to the inlet of the humidifier chamber. This manifold system incorporates a safety pressure vent, as well as optional ports, to place an oxygen analyzer sensor and a pressure-monitoring device or alarm.

The hot-wire inspiratory limb of the patient circuit is connected to the humidifier outlet. Two temperature probes in the circuit provide servo feedback to the humidifier unit. Humidified gas with a minimum of condensation flows to the patient interface, which is described later in this section. Gas exiting the patient interface flows to the CPAP generator (Figure 13-14).

The generator, which is usually mounted on the same stand as the humidifier, consists of a clear plastic container

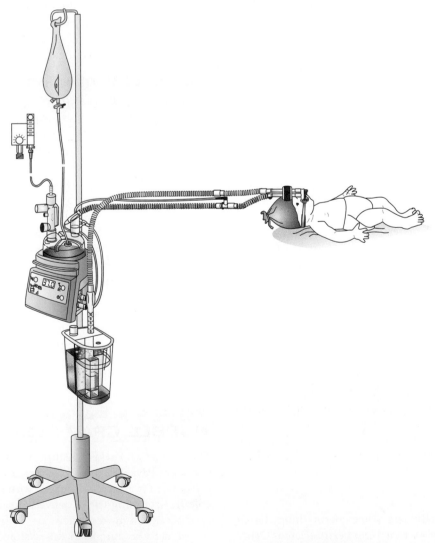

FIGURE 13-11 Fisher & Paykel Healthcare Bubble CPAP System.

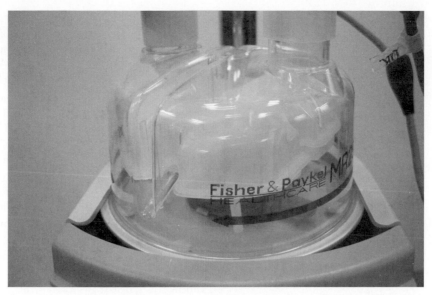

FIGURE 13-12 Fisher & Paykel Healthcare MR290 humidifier for the Bubble CPAP System.

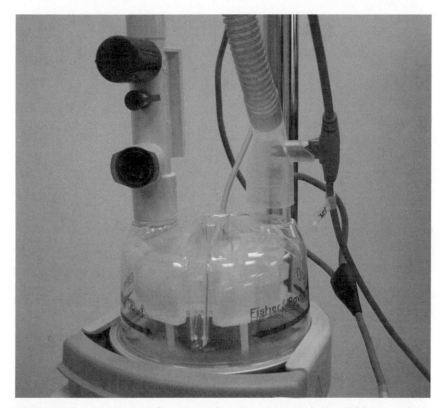

FIGURE 13-13 The attachment of an oxygen line (*top center*) to the humidifier manifold system for the Fisher & Paykel Healthcare Bubble CPAP System. This manifold integrates a safety pressure vent, as well as optional ports, to place an oxygen analyzer sensor and a pressure-monitoring device or alarm. Two temperature probes in the circuit provide servo feedback to the humidifier unit (*right side*).

made up of two compartments. With the plastic funnel provided, the clinician fills the main compartment of the humidifier with either sterile water or a weak acetic acid solution. The main compartment is filled until it begins to overflow into the other compartment. The desired CPAP level is set by adjusting the CPAP probe, which is a tube with numbers exactly embedded at 1-cm increments in the plastic. The number that is positioned directly above the lid is the CPAP setting. A CPAP range from 3 cm H_2O to 10 cm H_2O is available.

The manufacturer recommends a system test for leaks. Instructions for this test are included with the circuit packaging. The manufacturer packages the manifold, humidifier chamber, and circuit limbs together as a convenience.

Patient Interface

The patient interface consists of a choice of 3 lengths of nasal tubing, 4 sizes of head bonnets, 3 sizes of head straps (called *headgear*), 11 sizes of nasal prongs, and 4 sizes of chin straps. In part because of so many different component sizes, the Fisher & Paykel Healthcare patient interface system is one of the most complex of all CPAP application devices on the market today. Appropriate sizes of prongs, head straps or bonnets, and nasal tubing have to be chosen. The clinician must be skilled at fitting and adjusting the various mounting straps. If proper emphasis is not given to both sizing and proper fitting, CPAP delivery may be ineffective and patient stress caused by discomfort may be excessive.

The method by which the interface is applied is to first measure the patient's head circumference and choose the head strap or bonnet whose range corresponds with the measurement. Bonnets are usually chosen for premature infants because they offer more stability and provide some aid in preserving core temperature.

The next step is to select the proper size of nasal prongs (Figure 13-15). To assist with this, the manufacturer recommends its sizing guide, which consists of templates used to match nare opening sizes and septum gap. Generally, it is recommended that the clinician choose the largest prong size that occupies the entire nare opening, but that does not stretch the skin. The prong set that meets those criteria, but with the narrowest septum gap, should be tried. However, the clinician often must move up or down one size after a brief trial period with the system.

Once prongs are sized, the nasal tubing must be selected. From the three available sizes, the clinician selects the size in which the clear tubing extends from the patient's nares to just before the top of the head. The clinician should also see that the accompanying foam block allows the tubing to lie parallel to the patient's face. Foam strips can be peeled away one at a time to adjust the foam block. Figure 13-16 shows the prongs, nasal tubing, and foam strips.

With the nasal tubing selected and sized, the nasal-prong set is then attached to its end. The patient circuit is then attached and a flow of 6 L/min to 8 L/min is set. The prongs can then be inserted into the nares and the nasal tubing secured by using the velcro strap at the patient's forehead. Finally, the glider clips are secured in such a way that a slight bend is seen. Box 13-3 describes the key steps

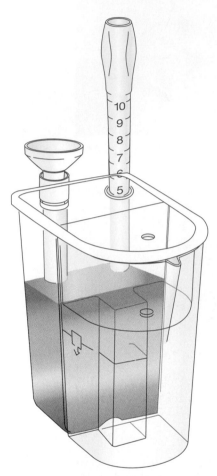

FIGURE 13-14 The CPAP probe for the Fisher & Paykel Healthcare Bubble CPAP System. The desired CPAP level is set by adjusting the CPAP probe. The number that is positioned directly above the lid is the CPAP setting (3 to 10 cm H₂O).

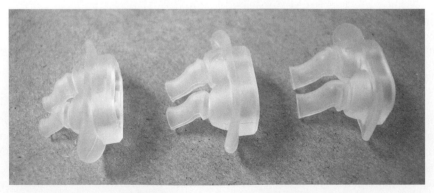

FIGURE 13-15 Infant nasal prongs.

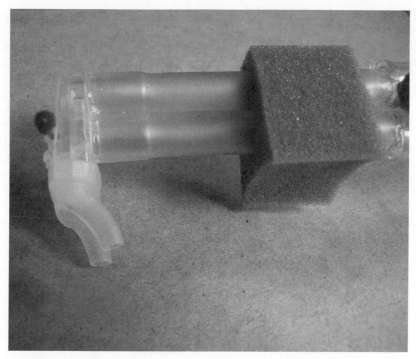

FIGURE 13-16 The prongs, nasal tubing, and foam strips (*left side*) with the nasal prong attached to the far-left end. The patient circuit is then attached (*right side*). The prongs can then be inserted into the nares and the nasal tubing secured by using the velcro strap at the patient's forehead. (See text for additional information.)

BOX 13-3	Bubble CPAP: Key Steps to Set-up and Use

- Attach oxygen tubing to flowmeter and connect to humidifier inlet. Adjust flow to 5-10 L/min. This flow will provide sufficient CPAP.
- Verify system tightness by observing bubbling of water in CPAP generator. Look for a gentle, continuous bubbling Vigorous bubbling is not recommended.
- Set required F_IO_2 on air/oxygen blender.
- Fill bubble chamber with sterile water (or weak acetic acid solution) up to fill mark, and set CPAP tubing to desired level. Depth of the tubing under the water controls the amount of positive pressure in system.
- Choose appropriately sized nasal tubing.
- Choose the appropriately sized nasal prongs by using the size guide included in the nasal tubing packaging. Prongs should fit the nares snugly without pinching the nasal septum. If prongs are too small, there will be an increase in airway pressure and gas will leak from the system, making it difficult to maintain the desired positive pressure.

- Patient's mouth, nose, and pharynx should be thoroughly suctioned before the nasal prongs are inserted.
- Prongs can be moistened with saline, sterile water, or small amounts of water-soluble lubricant before they are placed curve-side down into the infant's nose. Long-term use of prongs may necessitate use of a hydrocolloid dressing to protect nasal openings.
- Nasal prongs should fill nasal opening completely without stretching the skin or putting undue pressure on the nares. Blanching around rim of nostrils suggests that prongs are too large.
- Correct positioning reduces the risk of trauma and ensures effective delivery of CPAP.
- If the infant's mouth is open, this can cause a significant decrease in airway pressure. This situation should be prevented or corrected by placing a pacifier in the infant's mouth. Mouth-breathing will usually stop once the infant adjusts to the system. Chin straps, although available, are not recommended and should be used only as a last resort.

---

in setting up the Bubble CPAP device (see also Clinical Rounds 13-2).

Some clinicians have used the Fisher & Paykel Healthcare patient interface with other CPAP systems and with ventilators that provide CPAP. Also, the Fisher & Paykel Healthcare CPAP delivery system has found its way into other types of applications, such as in the delivery of high-flow oxygen by nasal cannula and in helium/oxygen mixtures.

The Fisher & Paykel Healthcare Bubble CPAP System offers the clinician a convenient and inexpensive means of providing noninvasive ventilatory support to infants, especially those who are premature or who cannot tolerate conventional face masks.

HAMILTON ARABELLA SYSTEM

The Hamilton ARABELLA (Hamilton Medical, Inc., Reno, Nev.) is an integrated noninvasive CPAP system similar in design to the EME Infant Flow. The ARABELLA system consists of a universal generator set with interchangeable silicone nasal prongs, a hot-wire delivery circuit, the ARABELLA cap, and the monitoring gas mixer.

Prongs for the ARABELLA come in four sizes. A guide is provided with printed silhouettes that can be matched to the infant's nares. This facilitates the choice of an appropriate size. Caps are available in five color-coded sizes.[7]

The major difference between the ARABELLA and the Cardinal Health Infant Flow Nasal CPAP System lies in the design of their flow generators. In the ARABELLA, the jets delivering expiratory flow extend part of the way into a single common chamber within the generator housing. In the Infant Flow Nasal CPAP System, the jet nozzles are positioned flush with the housing wall and each set serves a separate chamber. The cavity of the ARABELLA's generator is slightly larger and the geometric angles for guiding flows are arranged differently. Also, unlike the Infant Flow Nasal CPAP device, the ARABELLA's jets protrude into a single common chamber. Because of the ARABELLA's flow generator design, the difference in functional characteristics is that the flow of gas from the jet is more stable than that in the Infant Flow Nasal CPAP. A more-stable jet flow seems to require a more substantial patient expiratory flow to cause the device to switch into expiration. The additional flow that is required for the ARABELLA suggests that a patient must work harder to breathe when this system is used.

The ARABELLA's Monitoring Gas Mixer and the Infant Flow Driver, although labeled differently, are essentially the same device. Both are set up and operated in exactly the same way. The ARABELLA device is not available with an internal battery.

PART II—THE INFANT VENTILATOR

For more than three decades, infants have been ventilated primarily in the TCPL mode. The reason for this probably relates to the historical evolution of infant ventilators. Although no scientific evidence confirms TCPL as being superior to volume control in infants, many clinicians have believed that this mode reduces the risk of barotrauma.[1] As a result, until recently, infant ventilators were designed to provide TCPL and CPAP exclusively. These devices were simple in design and incorporated many similar features.

Today, however, more-precise monitoring and patient sensing have made it possible to apply additional modes of ventilation in infants. These modes were associated only with adult and pediatric patients. Manufacturers have introduced more-sophisticated models with unique features. Although these infant ventilators have retained the basic design that enables them to provide TCPL and CPAP, many now offer additional options. Volume-limited ventilation and pressure support are available on many models, for example.

Most infant ventilators have been designed to provide a continuous flow of an air/oxygen mixture into the ventilator circuit (Figure 13-17A).[8] In this design, a positive pres-

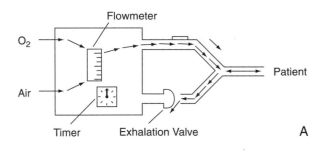

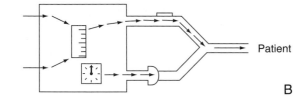

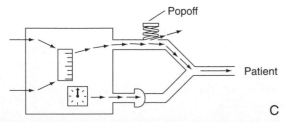

FIGURE 13-17 The typical continuous-flow ventilator circuit designed for *time-triggered, pressure-limited, time-cycled* ventilation (TPTV). **A,** Spontaneous phase; **B,** inspiratory phase; **C,** pressure-limiting phase. (From Koff PB, Eitzman D, Neu J: *Neonatal and pediatric respiratory care,* ed 2, St Louis, 1993, Mosby.)

sure breath results when the machine's exhalation valve closes, permitting the gas mixture to flow to the patient (Figure 13-17B). During the inspiratory phase when a preset pressure limit is reached, pressure is maintained until the ventilator time-cycles into expiration (Figure 13-17C). When the exhalation valve opens, the expiratory phase begins. As long as the exhalation valve remains open, a constant flow of the gas mixture passes through the patient's airway and is available for spontaneous breaths.

If the pressure limit is reached in this type of ventilator, tidal volume will depend on flow, pressure limit, and inspiratory time (see calculation, Box 13-4). However, alterations in the patient's compliance and airway resistance can affect the tidal volume. For example, consider the patient whose compliance improves over a few hours. If the ventilator settings are not modified, the patient's lungs will accommodate flow from the ventilator over a longer period during the inspiratory phase. Peak pressure will be reached later in the inspiratory phase. Therefore, a larger-than-desired tidal volume may be delivered by the ventilator. Inspiratory time and flow are set and digitally displayed on most TCPL ventilators. The calculation shown in Box 13-4 can be used to estimate the available tidal volume if the pressure limit is reached. However, if the pressure limit is reached early in the inspiratory phase, tidal volume could be substantially less than calculated.

Some ventilators use a **demand flow system** to provide inspiratory gas for spontaneous breaths. This type of system delivers flow at a variable rate proportional to patient inspiratory flow. The ventilator matches the patient's inspiratory flow. Demand flow is believed by some clinicians to be advantageous to operator-selected continuous-flow systems, because continuous-flow systems tend to produce resistance to expiration at the airway, commonly known as **circuit PEEP**. For patients whose ventilatory needs include high-inspiratory flows but low end-expiratory pressure, the demand system eliminates the need to set a high continuous flow. Some patients may present with highly variable ventilatory patterns. The use of a demand system may ensure sufficient flow to meet transiently high inspiratory flow needs.

In a typical demand system, a minimal preset continuous flow is delivered by the ventilator. On spontaneous inspiration this flow will increase to maintain the baseline pressure. When the ventilator delivers a mandatory breath, the flow increases to the value set with the flow rate control knob.

With the development of improved flow-sensing capability, newer ventilator models can now enable the clinician to distinguish between the patient's inspiratory flow and machine-generated flow even in very tiny patients. This allows the clinician to select the TCPL mode and adjust the ventilator to deliver patient-triggered mandatory breaths. This type of continuous-flow synchronized intermittent mandatory ventilation (SIMV) is possible even with small ETT leaks. Flow-sensing capability has led to other advances, many of which are unique to a specific ventilator model. The ways in which flow-sensing applications have been developed will be discussed with each ventilator that uses this technology.

The same flow-sensing technology that provides better ventilator/patient synchrony has enabled clinicians to return to volume modes of ventilation in infants. By closely monitoring inspired and expired tidal volume, ventilatory pressures, and waveforms, clinicians can better adjust ventilator settings according to physiologic changes. Compliance and airway resistance measurements are now possible. Providing the appropriate level of support, responding to physiologic changes more quickly, and weaning infants from the ventilator more effectively are greatly facilitated by some of the latest developments in infant ventilators.

As pressure-limited, volume-targeted modes of ventilation (e.g., pressure-regulated volume control [PRVC]) increasingly have been used in adults, their application in infants and pediatric patients has been growing as well. (See Chapter 11 for more information on these modes.) Clinicians working with adults have long recognized that pressure control and pressure support modes are desirable in many clinical situations, primarily because of their decelerating waveforms. With the addition of a volume-targeting capability to these modes, a patient receives a more-consistent tidal volume in spite of compliance or airway resistance changes. In infants, rapid and sometimes dramatic changes are often seen in compliance after surfactant replacement therapy.[9] In many pediatric patients, marked compliance or airway resistance changes can occur very rapidly because of the progression of a disease process or after an intervention. Therefore, a ventilator that is capable of delivering consistent tidal volumes with pressure ventilation (e.g., PRVC and volume support) while providing decelerating flow can be very useful in both the neonatal and the pediatric setting.

In small infants, such as those weighing less than 1000 g, use of pressure-limited, volume-targeted breath delivery has not yet won widespread acceptance. The tried and proven TCPL mode, with its simplicity and safety, continues to be the most widely used in premature and very low-birth-weight infants.

With infants, some clinicians continue to prefer to use mechanical ventilators that were designed exclusively for infants and small children. Part II of this chapter provides information on ventilators specifically designed for infants and children. However, manufacturers are beginning to design models that are suitable for any size of patient.

BOX 13-4	Calculation of Maximum Available Tidal Volume for *Time*-Triggered, *Pressure*-Limited, *Time*-Cycled Ventilation (TPTV)

$$V_T = \frac{\text{Inspiratory time (seconds)} \times \text{Flow (L/min)}}{60}$$

Features such as flow-triggering and flow-cycling, short response times, volume monitoring, and low internal compressible volume are being incorporated into most new ventilator designs. Part IV of this chapter will look specifically at the neonatal and pediatric application of general-purpose ventilators.

Today, some hospitals have chosen a single ventilator model that can be used with adult, pediatric, and neonatal patients. However, extra care must be used when these ventilators are used in very small patients, especially with uncuffed artificial airways. It is good practice to monitor tidal volume at the infant's airway when using these ventilators; this measure will enable a more-precise determination of ventilator function. The use of calculations to correct for compressible volume does not take artificial airway leak into account. Moreover, in situations in which compliance is markedly low or airway resistance is markedly high, volume loss in the patient/circuit system can be greater than that calculated.

This following section reviews some of the ventilators specifically designed for the ventilation of infants and children.

CARDINAL HEALTH—BEAR CUB VENTILATORS

As mentioned previously, Cardinal Health purchased Viasys Healthcare Systems (2008). Viasys owned all Bear ventilator products. Information on the Bear Cub ventilators—including the Bear Cub BP-200 and BP-2001, the Bear Cub 750vs, and the Bear Cub 750psv ventilator—is available at Evolve Resources.

CARDINAL HEALTH V.I.P. BIRD INFANT-PEDIATRIC VENTILATOR

The V.I.P. Bird ventilator (Cardinal Health, which owns Viasys Healthcare, Critical Care Division, Palm Springs, Calif.) mechanically supports neonatal, infant, and pediatric patients with the most common ventilator modes (Figure 13-18). It is electrically powered with 110-V AC and pneumatically powered by external compressed air and oxygen at 40 psig to 75 psig. DC power operation from an external power source is possible.

The V.I.P. Bird is microprocessor-controlled by three processors. Flow-triggering and flow-cycling can be accomplished by using the Bird Partner IIi Volume Monitor and infant flow sensor. An oxygen blender auxiliary output flowmeter (0 to15 L/min) is located on the side of the ventilator for use with a nebulizer or handheld resuscitator.[10]

Noteworthy Internal Functions

The microblender mixes the two gases according to the set oxygen percentage. The blended gas then enters the 1.1-L **accumulator**. The accumulator reserves pressurized gas during the expiratory phase to meet high inspiratory flow

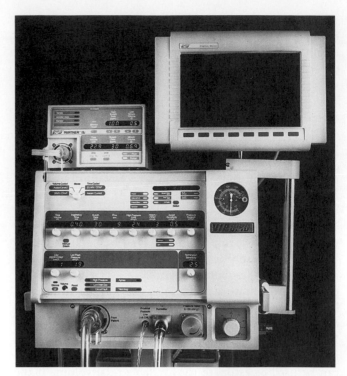

FIGURE 13-18 The V.I.P. Bird Ventilator. (Courtesy Cardinal Health, McGaw Park, Ill., which owns Viasys Healthcare, Critical Care Division, Palm Springs, Calif.)

demands of the patient with maximum flow capabilities up to 120 L/min. The gas exits the accumulator and enters a pneumatic regulator that adjusts the flow-control valve, driving pressure to 25 psig. A **pulsation dampener** is located between the regulator and the flow-control valve and is used to stabilize pressure and maintain driving pressure to the flow control valve.

Gas flow is delivered to the patient by means of an electromechanical **proportioning valve** and an **electromagnetic** exhalation valve. (See Chapter 11 for a description of these valves.) Delivered flow rates are determined by the system driving pressure and the diameter of the valve opening. Flow rates are unaffected by downstream patient circuit pressures of up to 350 cm H_2O with a system pressure of 25 psig.

Because of the possibility of inadvertent PEEP developing from the continuous flow present in the expiratory limb of the patient circuit during TCPL ventilation, a jet Venturi is incorporated into the exhalation manifold. The **jet solenoid** controls the driving pressure to the exhalation valve jet Venturi and is controlled by the microprocessor. It is active when the flow rate control is set at 5 L/min or greater with a PEEP of 0 cm H_2O to 5 cm H_2O or when PEEP is set at 0 and flow at any setting.

A pneumatically driven safety valve is activated when a ventilator-inoperative event or electrical power failure occurs. This allows the spontaneously breathing patient to breath room air.

If a pressure difference of 20 psig occurs between the air and oxygen sources, the gas source with the highest pressure will be used by the ventilator. This will result in a delivered oxygen concentration of either 21% or 100%.

Control and Alarm Panel

Figure 13-19 provides a diagram of the control and alarm panel. The mode selector knob is located on the front top-left panel and has two groups of modes. The volume-cycled (VC) modes are assist/control (A/C) and SIMV/CPAP. The time-cycled (TC) modes are assist/control (A/C) and (S)IMV/CPAP.

The front-panel control settings are tidal volume, inspiratory time, rate, flow, high pressure (Box 13-5), PEEP/CPAP, assist sensitivity, and pressure support. Table 13-4 lists parameter specifications and their available ranges for the V.I.P. Bird Infant-Pediatric Ventilator. The manual breath-control button is located on the control panel and is a single, operator-initiated controlled breath that is available in all modes.

Illumination of displays highlights the controls that are functional for that specific mode. Dimmed displays are controls that are not functional in a certain mode. For example, tidal volume will have a dimmed display when the ventilator is operating in a TCPL mode. During CPAP the inspiratory time and peak inspiratory pressure displays remain illuminated and are functional during manual ventilation.

Directly below the control section is the alarm section, which includes the following knobs: low PEEP/CPAP (-9 to 24 cm H_2O), low peak pressure (off, 3 to 120 cm H_2O), high pressure, low inlet gas, circuit fault, apnea (inactive with continuous flow), vent inop (inoperative), alarm silence (60 seconds), and reset. An additional safety feature is the mechanical pressure-relief knob, which is located next to the oxygen concentration dial and can be adjusted between 0 cm H_2O and 130 cm H_2O in all modes. Turning the pressure-relief knob clockwise increases the value and counterclockwise decreases the value. The high-pressure limit is normally set below the overpressure-relief valve setting for the high-pressure limit to be activated (see Box 13-5).

When the power switch located on the rear top-left panel is turned off, the ventilator inoperable alarm can be silenced by depressing the alarm silence button. The alarm silence button is located on the front bottom-left panel. It will silence the alarm for 60 seconds, unless the reset button located on the right is depressed.

Front-panel digital displays are listed in Table 13-5. There are some additional displays worth mentioning. The patient effort LED will flash when the patient's inspiratory effort exceeds the assist sensitivity setting. The demand LED will flash when the demand flow system is triggered by spontaneous efforts decreasing airway pressure 1 cm H_2O below the baseline pressure during TC IMV. Airway pressures are displayed on a pressure gauge. In the IMV mode, only the mandatory breaths are shown in the breath-rate display. The I:E ratio LED flashes when an inverse I:E ratio is present.

Modes of Ventilation

Two basic types of breath delivery or modes are provided by the V.I.P. Bird: VC and TC.

BOX 13-5	Function of the High-Pressure Control

The high-pressure limit controls the set peak inspiratory pressure in the time-cycled, pressure-limited (TCPL) modes. Its function in the volume-cycled (VC) modes is a high-pressure limit.

TABLE 13-4

Specifications for V.I.P. Bird Infant-Pediatric Ventilator

Tidal volume	20-995 mL
Inspiratory time	0.1-3.0 s
Rate	0-150 breaths/min
Flow (TC modes)	3-40 L/min
Flow (VC modes)	3-120 L/min
Peak inspiratory pressure	0-80 cm H_2O
(TC modes)	
High-pressure limit	0-120 cm H_2O
(VC modes)	
PEEP/CPAP	0-24 cm H_2O
Assist sensitivity	Off, 0.1-5.0 L/min
(TC modes)	
Assist sensitivity	Off, 1-20 cm H_2O
(VC modes)	
Pressure support	0-50 cm H_2O
Trigger mechanism	Pressure (VC)/Flow (TC)
Alarms	Low PEEP/CPAP, low peak pressure, high pressure, low inlet pressure, circuit fault, apnea, ventilator inoperative

TC, Time-cycled; *VC,* volume-cycled; *PEEP,* positive end-expiratory pressure.

TABLE 13-5

Digital Displays on the V.I.P. Bird Ventilator

Parameter	Range
Breath rate	0-250 breaths/min
Inspiratory time	0.05-60 s
I:E ratio	1:0.1 to 1:60
PIP	0-130 cm H_2O
MAP	0-120 cm H_2O
Power	Illuminates when power is on
External DC	Illuminates when external DC power source is being used
Patient effort	Illuminates when assist sensitivity is met
Demand	Illuminates when demand system is triggered

PIP, Peak inspiratory pressure; *MAP,* mean airway pressure; *DC,* direct current.

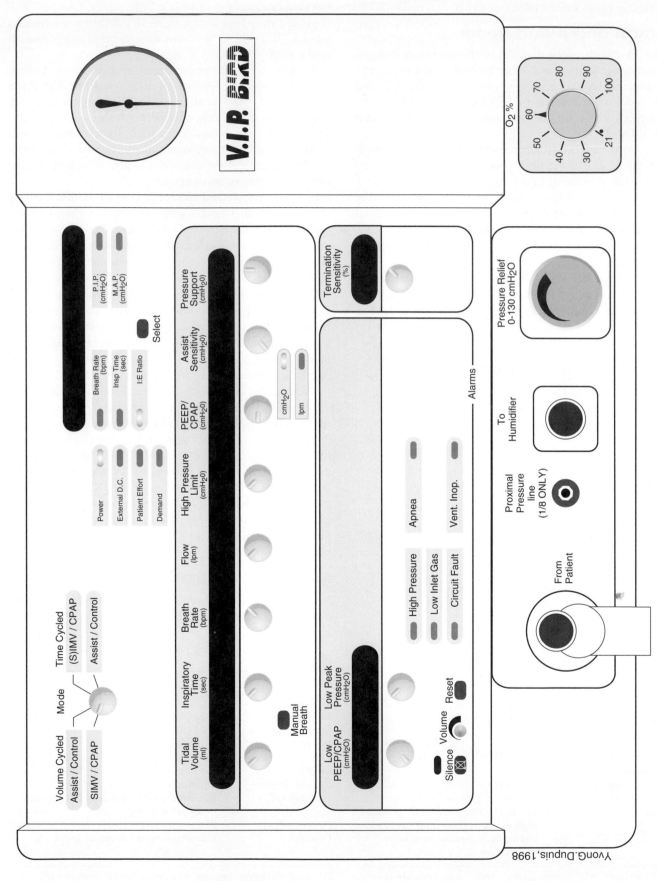

FIGURE 13-19 The V.I.P. Bird Ventilator control and alarm panel. (Courtesy Yvon Dupuis.)

Volume-Cycled (VC) Modes

In the assist/control (A/C) VC mode, inspiration is time-triggered or pressure-triggered, volume-targeted, flow-limited, and volume-cycled. Inspiration can be pressure-cycled if the airway pressure reaches the set high-pressure alarm setting. The operator sets the following parameters: tidal volume, breath rate, flow, high-pressure limit, PEEP/CPAP, and assist sensitivity.

In the SIMV/CPAP VC mode, mandatory breaths are time-triggered or pressure-triggered, volume-targeted, flow-limited, and volume-cycled. Inspiration can be pressure-cycled if the airway pressure reaches the set high-pressure alarm setting. Spontaneous respiratory efforts between mandatory breaths are pressure-triggered, pressure-targeted, and time-cycled. Pressure support can be added to spontaneous efforts and are pressure-triggered, pressure-limited, and flow-cycled. (NOTE: The maximum demand flow available is 120 L/min for spontaneous and pressure-supported breaths.) The operator sets the following parameters: tidal volume, inspiratory time (pressure support time limit), breath rate, flow, high-pressure limit, PEEP/CPAP, assist sensitivity, and pressure support (if desired).

Pressure support termination criteria are set up differently with the V.I.P. Bird ventilator because of the varied patient population that can be ventilated with this device. For example, if the unit fails to flow-cycle at 25% of peak flow because of an air leak around the artificial airway, this may result in excessive inspiratory times (some units will time-cycle at 2 to 3 seconds). The termination criteria for the V.I.P. Bird are based on delivered tidal volume ranges (Box 13-6). The pressure-support display will flash when the breath is time-cycled.

Time-Cycled (TC) Modes

In the IMV TC mode, mandatory breaths are time-triggered, pressure-targeted, and time-cycled. In IMV the operator sets the following parameters: breath rate, inspiratory time, flow, high-pressure limit (peak inspiratory pressure [PIP] desired), and PEEP/CPAP. The continuous-flow and demand flow systems support spontaneous efforts. Continuous flow is determined by the flow knob setting (range: 0 to 15 L/min). Demand flow is available when spontaneous inspiration decreases the airway pressure 1 cm H_2O below the baseline pressure. The maximum level of demand flow is 120 L/min. Sensitivity is set at 1 cm H_2O below

baseline pressure in the IMV/CPAP mode. CPAP is activated when the breath-rate setting is 0.

In (S)IMV/CPAP (with the Bird Partner IIi Volume Monitor and infant flow sensor), the mandatory breath is flow-triggered or time-triggered, pressure-targeted, and time-cycled. CPAP is activated when the breath-rate setting is 0. In SIMV the operator sets the following parameters: breath rate, inspiratory time, flow, high-pressure limit, PEEP/CPAP, and assist sensitivity (L/min).

In the A/C mode, inspiration is flow-triggered or time-triggered, pressure-targeted, and flow-cycled or time-cycled. The patient receives the set pressure with every spontaneous respiratory effort. The breath-rate setting acts as a backup rate in the event of decreased respiratory effort. The operator sets the following parameters: breath rate, inspiratory time, flow, high-pressure limit, PEEP/CPAP, assist sensitivity (L/min), and **termination sensitivity**.

The termination sensitivity control is an additional feature that adjusts the flow termination point of the breath, preventing air-trapping and an inverse I:E ratio, thus providing **expiratory synchrony**. It is only used in the assist/control (A/C) TC mode. Termination sensitivity ranges are off, and they are 5% to 25% of peak flow. For example, a setting of 25% means that the breath will be terminated when the inspiratory flow (measured at the proximal airway) decreases to 25% of measured peak inspiratory flow. If the flow fails to decrease to the percentage set, which might occur with a low percentage setting and the presence of an air leak around the artificial airway, the breath is time-cycled. The termination percentage setting will flash to indicate that the breath is time-cycled. Airway graphics are helpful in evaluating patient/ventilator synchrony, and their use is strongly recommended with this mode of ventilation (Box 13-7).

The assist sensitivity control is adjustable from 0.2 L/min to 5 L/min with the use of the infant flow sensor. By pressing the continuous flow button on the Bird Partner IIi monitor, the real-time flow signal can be evaluated by observing the continuous flow readout at end exhalation. If the digital readout returns to 0, the operator should set the assist sensitivity value at 0.2 L/min to provide optimal patient-triggering capabilities. If there is a leak (flow readout does not return to 0), the assist sensitivity should be adjusted to 0.2 L/min above the digital readout. Adjusting the sensitivity to a level above the leak helps prevent autocycling and requires the patient to generate only the flow difference between the leak and the assist sensitivity setting.

BOX 13-6	Breath Termination Ranges According to Tidal Volume

- For delivered tidal volume (V_T) of 0 mL to 50 mL, the flow-cycle value is 5% of peak flow.
- For delivered V_T 50 mL to 200 mL, the flow-cycle value is a range of 5%-25% of peak flow.
- For delivered V_T greater than 200 mL, the flow-cycle value is 25% of peak flow.

BOX 13-7	Important Clinical Note About the Terminal Sensitivity and Mode

If the patient is unable to self-regulate ventilation (e.g., because of hiccups), the termination sensitivity should be turned off or the mode of ventilation should be changed until the situation resolves.

Graphics Displays

Airway graphics are an invaluable tool that allows the clinician to monitor and adjust ventilatory strategies for each patient. Graphical analysis also provides real-time and trend assessment of ventilator parameters and of patient/ventilator interactions. The Bird Graphics Monitor is designed for use with the V.I.P. Bird and Bird 8400STi ventilators (see Figure 13-18). It requires use of the Bird Partner or Bird Partner IIi monitor (see the following section on the Partner IIi monitor). The graphics monitor is easily moved between ventilators. A communication port is available for connection to a printer. Compatible printers include the HP (Hewlett-Packard Company; Palo Alto, Calif.) ThinkJet and Epson FX-850 (Epson America, Inc., Long Beach, Calif.).

The graphics monitor displays real-time scalar waveforms for pressure, flow, and volume (vertical axis) plotted over time (horizontal axis). The waveform-select screen allows the clinician to select two waveforms at a time. Positive values (above 0 on the vertical axis) relate to the inspiratory phase and negative values to the expiratory phase of ventilation.

Pressure/volume and flow/volume loops are also available, along with reference loop storage. The pressure/volume graphic loop displays tidal volume on the vertical axis and airway pressure on the horizontal axis. The flow/volume graphic loop displays flow on the vertical axis and tidal volume on the horizontal axis. The freeze screen provides movable target and reference cursors that allow the clinician to hold and evaluate significant events. The trend feature has 10 selectable parameters and can be set for 15 minutes or 1-, 2-, 4-, 8-, or 24-hour windows.[11]

Special Features of the V.I.P. Ventilator

One of the notable special features with the V.I.P. Bird is **leak compensation.** Leak compensation is used to stabilize baseline pressure, prevent autocycling, and optimize assist sensitivity in the presence of leaks. It is recommended for use only with leaks around artificial airways. It is not recommended for those patients with minimal respiratory effort and no leak, because some patients are unable to trigger appropriately with leak compensation active. Leak compensation is functional only in the VC modes.

When pressure decreases 0.25 cm H_2O below baseline pressure, the leak-compensation feature introduces small amounts of flow into the circuit, an attempt to reestablish baseline pressure. The amount of leak compensation needed is learned by the exhalation valve pressure transducer so that the flow control valve returns to the determined value after each breath. The amount of flow is reevaluated every 8 milliseconds. The maximum amount of flow available is either 5 L/min with assist sensitivity set at −1 cm H_2O or 10 L/min with assist sensitivity set at −2 cm H_2O to −5 cm H_2O. The default setting after any power-up is "leak compensation on." The leak compensation is turned on or off by pressing the select button until the desired feature is displayed in the digital window (top-left digital display).

Bird Partner IIi Monitor

The Bird Partner IIi monitor is a microprocessor-controlled volume monitor with a variable-orifice, differential-pressure, flow-measuring device that is placed in the patient circuit near the upper airway. (See Chapter 8 for a description of the variable orifice differential pressure transducer.) The flow-measuring device does the following:

- Measures effective inspiratory and expiratory volumes
- Displays digital measured values (tidal volume, breath rate, minute ventilation, and the real-time flow signal-only with infant sensor)
- Displays digital alarm parameters (high rate, low minute ventilation)
- Provides an adjustable apnea alarm (10 to 60 seconds in 5-second increments)

Alarm limits can be set by using the monitor's touch pad controls. The apnea button (red) is located on the rear panel of the monitor. The clinician can visualize the current apnea setting by depressing the red button and observing the displayed value in the tidal volume window. Repeated depression of the button will allow the clinician to adjust the apnea setting.

The monitor can be used with the infant sensor or the pediatric sensor. The infant sensor is placed at the proximal airway and circuit Y-connector. It can be used only with artificial airways having an internal diameter (ID) of 4.5 mm or less (Figure 13-20). The sensor (*B*) is placed with the arrow pointing toward the patient (*A*) and the monitoring tubes (*C*) facing upward to prevent condensation or secretion accumulation within the lines. Box 13-8 contains important information about cleaning the infant sensor.

The gas inlet on the back of the ventilator connects to a 50-psig source and is used to inject 12 mL/min of gas through the pressure line to prevent obstructions within the line and to prevent water from entering the differential pressure transducer. The gas flow is synchronized with the expiratory phase so no additional volume is delivered to the patient during inspiration. The tidal volume readout is the effective tidal volume, because the sensor placement is at the patient's airway. Box 13-9 explains the use of a capnograph with an infant flow sensor.

If a continuous artificial airway leak is present, the "CONT V" function can be used to determine the liter flow of the leak. By pressing and holding the "CONT V" on the touch pad, a real-time flow through the infant sensor is displayed. The clinician can use the baseline leak or the flow displayed between breaths to determine the best trigger sensitivity setting and to prevent autotriggering. Generally, trigger sensitivity is set 0.2 L/min to 0.4 L/min above the baseline leak flow. Measurement of artificial airway leak is possible only with use of the infant sensor.

The pediatric sensor (Figure 13-21B) is placed just before the expiratory valve with the arrow pointing

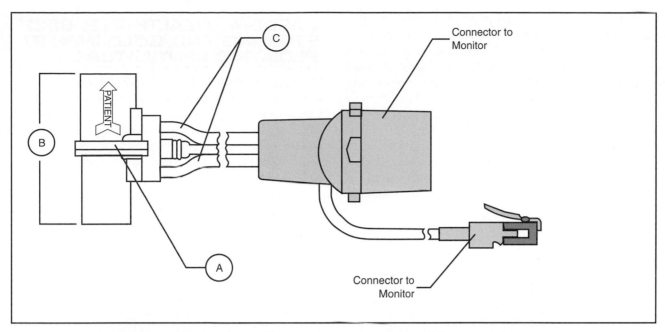

FIGURE 13-20 Infant sensor used with the Partner IIi monitor and the V.I.P. Bird. (Courtesy Cardinal Health, McGaw Park, Ill., which owns Viasys Healthcare, Critical Care Division, Palm Springs, Calif.)

BOX 13-8	Important Clinical Note Regarding the Flow Sensor

The infant flow sensor should be cleaned every 24 hours to maintain accurate tidal volume measurements and flow-triggering capabilities. The sensor can be sterilized in a cold solution or gas-sterilized. Steam autoclave or pasteurization cannot be used because the high temperatures will damage the flow element.

BOX 13-9	Use of a Capnograph with an Inline Sensor

When performing capnographic monitoring, place the end-tidal CO_2 sensor between the infant sensor and the patient circuit Y-sensor to provide optimal flow-triggering capabilities. There are special connectors available to facilitate the additional monitoring. The infant sensor has less than 1 mm of dead space.

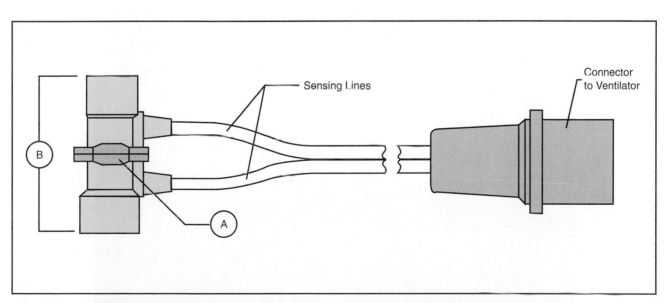

FIGURE 13-21 Pediatric sensor used with Partner IIi monitor and V.I.P. Bird. (Courtesy Cardinal Health, McGaw Park, Ill., which owns Viasys Healthcare, Critical Care Division, Palm Springs, Calif.)

toward the direction of gas flow. The tidal volume readout includes compressible volume and effective tidal volume. Tidal volume measurements are derived from the measurement of flow. As flow passes through the sensor and past the variable-orifice flow element (*A*), which is located between two chambers, the flow element bends in the direction of flow, creating a small pressure difference between the two chambers. The differential pressure transducer measures the pressure differences between the two chambers, then sends an analog signal that is read by the microprocessor, which compares the signal to a calibration curve and translates the value to a volume.[10,11]

CARDINAL HEALTH V.I.P. BIRD STERLING AND GOLD INFANT/ PEDIATRIC VENTILATORS

The V.I.P. Sterling and Gold Infant/Pediatric ventilators (Cardinal Health, which owns Viasys Healthcare, Critical Care Division, Palm Springs, Calif.) are improved models of the original V.I.P. (see Figure 13-18). The internal design and most of the controls, alarms, and specifications are identical to the original. Therefore, only the changes and new features will be presented here.

The most noteworthy differences are in two areas. First, both ventilators use redesigned flow sensors called the

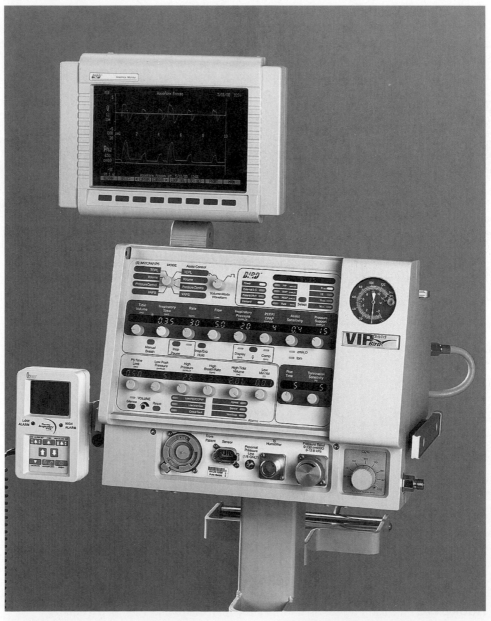

FIGURE 13-22 The V.I.P. Bird Gold Infant Ventilator. (Courtesy Cardinal Health, McGaw Park, Ill., which owns Viasys Healthcare, Critical Care Division, Palm Springs, Calif.)

Infant "Smart" Flow Sensor and the *Pediatric "Smart" Flow Sensor*. The other major change is the incorporation of the functions of the Partner IIi monitor into the main ventilator housing. Some expanded setting limits and some new features have also been added. Volume-assured pressure support (VAPS), a dual-control mode, is a key addition on the V.I.P. Gold. It is described later in this section.

The heart of the redesigned flow sensors for both the Sterling and the Gold is a stainless steel flap that replaces the former plastic design. A variable-orifice differential pressure transducer, similar to that in the original sensors, is used to measure flow. With the new design, the Infant "Smart" Flow Sensor can be used with artificial airway sizes up to 5.5-mm ID. For larger ETTs, the Pediatric "Smart" Flow Sensor is necessary. This sensor is placed at the exhalation valve rather than at the artificial airway.[12]

The ventilator's microprocessor is able to determine which flow sensor is in use. When the Infant "Smart" Flow Sensor is in use, a **bias flow** of 3 L/min is present unless the ventilator is operating in the TCPL mode. In the TCPL mode, flow is set by the operator. When the Pediatric "Smart" Flow Sensor is in use, bias flow can be turned on or off by pressing the bias flow control. Bias flow operates at a fixed 5 L/min with the pediatric sensor when turned on.

Changes in Controls/Alarms

Although many of the controls, indicators, and alarms on the Sterling and Gold models are identical to those of the original V.I.P., some additions and changes have been made. The front panel of the V.I.P. Bird Gold is shown in Figure 13-23. The layout of controls and indicators is very similar to that of the original. As in the original model, push buttons are used to activate functions, visualize certain parameter settings, or turn functions on or off. A single selector switch is used to change modes. Dials are used to adjust parameters and alarm limits.

Ventilator Modes and the Mode Select Switch

The mode select switch, located in the upper-left portion of the front control panel, is a multiposition dial. The position of the switch sets either the mode or the breath type. As is the case in the original V.I.P., some controls are deactivated when certain modes are selected. Displays for deactivated controls remain illuminated but dimmed.

The A/C modes for both the Sterling and Gold models are grouped in a mode category column to the right of the control dial. The TCPL mode and the volume-limited

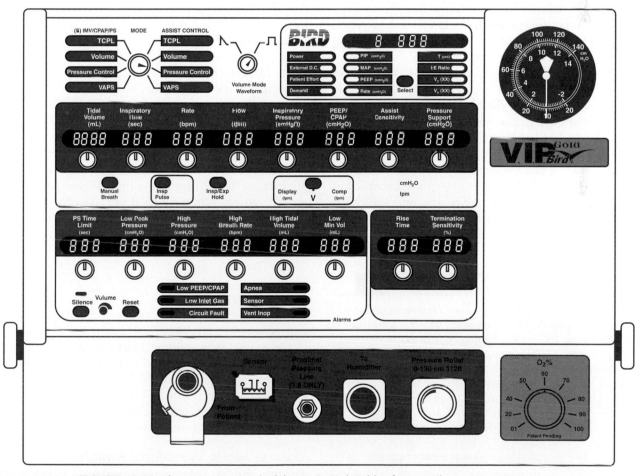

FIGURE 13-23 The operating panel of the V.I.P. Bird Gold Infant Ventilator. (Courtesy Cardinal Health, McGaw Park, Ill., which owns Viasys Healthcare, Critical Care Division, Palm Springs, Calif.)

mode are the only A/C modes available on the Sterling in this mode category. Two additional assist/control modes are available on the Gold model: pressure control and VAPS (described later). The left column of both models lists the (S)IMV/CPAP/PS (pressure support) modes. On the Sterling, only TCPL and volume modes are available in this mode category. CPAP can be provided in either of these modes, and pressure support can be added to non-mandatory breaths. In addition to the two (S)IMV/CPAP/PS modes that are included on the Sterling, the Gold also provides pressure control and VAPS in this mode category. When adding PS to spontaneous breaths, the level can be adjusted with a separate control allowing separate inspiratory pressures for mandatory and pressure-supported, spontaneous breaths.

The VAPS mode is available only on the V.I.P. Bird Gold model. It is a dual-control mode that guarantees that a pressure-control breath, a pressure-supported breath, or a TCPL breath will reach a preset volume. During a VAPS breath, tidal volume (V_T) may be augmented by extending the inspiratory phase at the set flow for a segment of time beyond the point that flow would otherwise terminate. An example of how the ventilator augments a breath is represented by waveforms in Figure 13-24. **Breath A** is a pressure-supported breath that terminates at a set flow. In this breath, the desired tidal volume (V_T) is reached within the set inspiratory time. In contrast, **Breath B** represents a breath in which delivery of the set tidal volume (V_T) is not achieved during the allotted inspiratory time. When the ventilator determines that the delivered volume is too low, it allows flow to decelerate to its minimum set point. However, rather than terminating, the set flow continues over a slightly lengthened inspiratory time, causing the peak inspiratory pressure to rise. The breath is therefore augmented to the desired tidal volume (V_T). An augmented breath essentially transitions from a pressure-control or TCPL breath to a volume-control breath. With VAPS, electronic extension of the inspiratory phase occurs only if the microprocessor determines that the pressure settings alone cannot deliver the preset tidal volume (Clinical Rounds 13-3).

CLINICAL ROUNDS 13-3

A respiratory therapist (RT) is setting up volume-assured pressure support (VAPS) for a patient who has spontaneous breathing efforts. The ventilator is in assist/control (A/C) volume ventilation mode with positive end-expiratory pressure (PEEP) = 3 cm H_2O, flow = 15 L/min, tidal volume (V_T) set at 50 mL, and a pressure limit of 20 cm H_2O. The RT observes that the flow-time curve rises rapidly at the beginning of inspiration and then tapers off until it finally reaches 0 at the end of inspiration. Actual delivered V_T is 60 mL.

What is the cycling variable that ends inspiration in this example?

See Evolve Resources for the answer.

VAPS can be selected from either the (S)IMV/CPAP/PS column or the assist/control column of the mode select switch. When selected from the (S)IMV/CPAP/PS column, mandatory pressure-control breaths are delivered at a guaranteed volume. The clinician must set tidal volume (V_T), inspiratory pressure, rate, and flow. Nonmandatory breaths in this form of VAPS will be unsupported if no pressure support level is present. When the clinician sets a PS level and a PS/VAPS time limit, both pressure support breaths and mandatory pressure-control breaths will be delivered at a guaranteed volume. The PS level and the PS/VAPS time limit controls must be set by the clinician.

When VAPS is selected from the assist/control column, breaths delivered to the patient are either patient-triggered or mandatory TCPL breaths. In this version of VAPS, the clinician sets inspiratory pressure as well as tidal volume (V_T), flow, PS/VAPS time limit, and rate.

Pressure Support/VAPS Time Limit Control
This control is active only in the PS mode on both the Sterling and Gold and in the VAPS mode on the Gold. It is automatically activated when these modes are selected. This control sets a time limit for the inspiratory phase in case of a leak or any other condition in which inspiratory flow does not drop to the termination level. Adjustable from 0.1 second to 3.0 seconds, the PS/VAPS Time Limit is displayed in a window above the control.

Rise Time Control
Available on the Gold model only, the rise time control allows the inspiratory pressure rise time to be adjusted. This control is active only in the pressure control, VAPS, and PS modes. The control is adjustable from a setting of 1 to 7. At a setting of 1, the fastest rise time, the set peak inspiratory pressure is reached quickly and is held for the duration of the set inspiratory time (Figure 13-25). At the slowest setting, 7, inspiratory flow is decreased to allow a gradual rise to set peak inspiratory pressure. The selected setting is displayed in a window above the control knob. The inspiratory time and the breath cycle are not affected by this control.

Tidal Volume Control
Tidal volume for both the Sterling and Gold models is set and adjusted in the same way as for the original V.I.P. However, the tidal volume limit has been increased to 1200 mL. On the Gold model in the VAPS mode, the tidal volume control setting establishes a target volume. This volume is not necessarily delivered if the set tidal volume, measured on exhalation, is achieved by the effects of inspiratory pressure settings alone.

Volume Mode Waveform Switch
The two-position volume mode waveform switch is active only when volume-controlled breaths are delivered. The left position sets a decelerating (descending) flow wave-

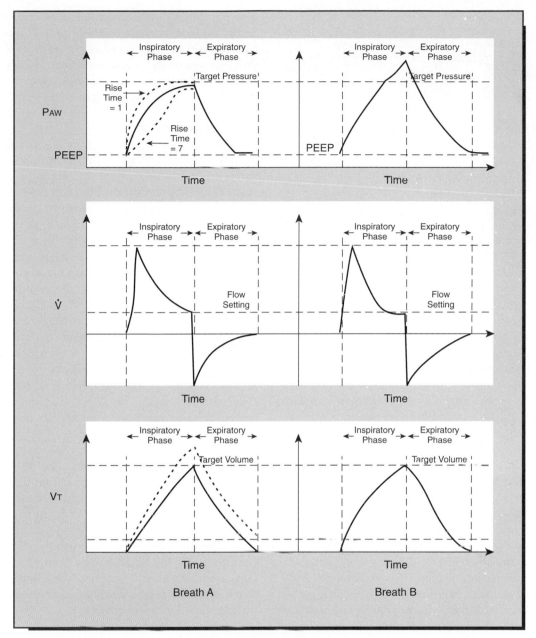

FIGURE 13-24 Volume-assured pressure support (VAPS) breath delivery with V.I.P. Bird Sterling and Gold Infant ventilators. **Breath A** (*left column*) depicts breaths that flow-cycle at the set flow after the minimum tidal volume has been delivered. (NOTE: The target pressure is delivered. Flow decelerates to the flow setting. V_T has met or exceeded the set V_T. The breath cycles out of inspiration at the set flow.) **Breath B** (*right column*) shows a transition from a pressure supported breath to a volume-assured breath. Transition occurs when flow drops to the set peak flow and the set V_T has not been delivered. (NOTE: The target pressure is delivered. Flow decelerates to the flow setting. V_T has not met the set V_T. Flow remains constant at the set peak flow until the set V_T is achieved. Peak pressure continues to rise and T_I increases until V_T is delivered.) (Courtesy Cardinal Health, McGaw Park, Ill., which owns Viasys Healthcare, Critical Care Division, Palm Springs, Calif.)

form during the inspiratory phase. The right position sets a square (constant) waveform.

Apnea Indicator and Apnea Interval Switch

A period of apnea equal to the set apnea interval will trigger an audible alarm and a flashing visual indicator. The audible alarm can be silenced with the alarm silence button, or it will silence itself once the alarm condition is corrected. The visual indicator will continue to flash until the reset button is pressed.

The apnea interval is set by the operator and is adjustable from 10 seconds to 60 seconds. The current apnea interval can be determined by pressing and holding the select button for 2 seconds. The interval will appear in the

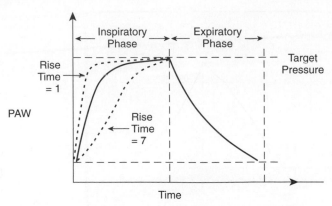

FIGURE 13-25 The rise time control available on the Gold model tapers pressure delivery at the beginning of inspiration. See text for a description. (Courtesy Cardinal Health, McGaw Park, Ill., which owns Viasys Healthcare, Critical Care Division, Palm Springs, Calif.)

monitor display window. The apnea interval is also displayed when the apnea interval switch is pressed. This switch is a push button located on the rear panel of the ventilator. Upon pressing the button one time, the current apnea interval is displayed in the monitor display window for 3 seconds. Each push of the button after the first time will increase the apnea interval by 5-second increments up to a maximum of 60 seconds. After the operator toggles to the 60-second maximum, pressing the button again returns the interval to 10 seconds.

Bias Flow, Assist Sensitivity, and Triggering

The purpose of bias flow within the patient circuit is to provide a reference flow for the sensors in order to put flow-triggering into operation. When the infant sensor is in use, the bias flow is automatically on and delivering 3 L/min. With the infant sensor, the bias flow status will not appear in the monitor display window. When the pediatric sensor is used, the bias flow level runs at a preset 5 L/min. However, with the pediatric sensor, the bias flow status can be viewed in the monitor display window by using the select button. Repeatedly pressing the select button enables you to scroll through all monitored parameters. After the final parameter is scanned, the message "BF ON" or "BF OFF" will be displayed. At this point, the operator can turn the bias flow on or off by pressing and holding the select button for 2 seconds. When no flow sensor is used, no bias flow is delivered.

Both the V.I.P. Bird Sterling and Gold ventilators provide either flow-triggering or pressure-triggering in all modes. The assist sensitivity control sets either the flow or pressure necessary to trigger the ventilator into inspiration, depending upon the type of triggering that is active. An indicator for each type of triggering illuminates when active. Triggering can be locked out completely by turning the assist sensitivity control to the off position. When using the infant flow sensor, only flow-triggering is active and is adjustable from 0.1 L/min to 3.0 L/min through the assist sensitivity control. When the pediatric flow sensor is

in use and bias flow is turned on, flow-triggering is active and is adjustable from 2.2 L/min to 5.0 L/min. When the bias flow is turned on, pressure-triggering is active with the pediatric sensor and is adjustable from 1 cm H_2O to 20 cm H_2O. If no flow sensor is used, both models automatically default to pressure-triggering in all modes.

Flow Display/Comp

The "Flow Display Comp" button on both the Sterling and Gold models replaces the "Cont V" button on the original Partner IIi monitor. This control serves the same function as the Cont V button when the infant flow sensor is in use. When the Flow Display Comp button is pressed, the display indicator to the left will illuminate. Flow values will then be displayed in the ventilator's monitor display window. The operator can then use the select button to toggle between inspiratory and expiratory real-time flows. This function is particularly useful in determining the amount of baseline leak at the artificial airway and adjusting the assist sensitivity to eliminate autotriggering. The clinician can toggle to the inspiratory flow, note the amount of baseline leak, and set the assist sensitivity control at least 0.2 L/min above the detected leak.

With the use of the pediatric flow sensor, the Flow Display Comp button serves another function. With this sensor, pressing the button establishes a 0 point for the volume monitor based on the set level of continuous flow. This function is called *flow compensation*. To accurately monitor volumes, flow compensation is activated each time the flow setting is changed. When the Flow Display Comp button with the pediatric sensor connected is pressed, the "Comp" indicator to the right will illuminate for 3 seconds and the level of flow compensation will appear in the monitor display window. To disable flow compensation, the Flow Display Comp function must be pressed and held for 2 seconds. The Flow Display Comp function is not available when the ventilator is operated without either of the flow sensors.

Inspiratory/Expiratory Hold

An inspiratory/expiratory hold function is available on the V.I.P. Bird Gold model only. When the "Insp/Exp Hold" button is pressed once, an "I/E Hold" prompt will appear in the monitor display window. If the Select button is pressed once while this message is displayed, it will toggle to the "I Hold" message. To attain an inspiratory hold for up to 3 seconds, the Insp/Exp Hold button is pressed and held. When the button is released, the inspiratory plateau pressure appears in the monitor display window.

An expiratory hold can be performed by first pressing the Insp/Exp Hold button to bring up the I/E Hold prompt in the monitor display window. The select button is then pressed two times to display the "E Hold" message. To attain an expiratory hold for up to 3 seconds, the Insp/Exp Hold button is pressed and held. When the button is released, the expiratory plateau pressure appears in the monitor display window.

Inspiratory Pause

An inspiratory pause control is available only on the V.I.P. Bird Gold. This control allows an inspiratory pause time to be set when operating the ventilator in either volume-targeted or VAPS modes. When the "Insp Pause" button is pressed once, the current setting, if any has been selected, is shown in the display monitor window. The window will first show IP followed by the current pause setting. While the pause time is being displayed, the value can be changed by pressing the select button. Each time the select button is pressed, the inspiratory pause time will increase by 0.1 second up to a maximum of 2 seconds. If the clinician holds the button, this action will also allow the pause time to increase. To reset the pause time to 0, the clinician must press the reset button.

Leak Compensation Control

Leak compensation has been changed on the Sterling and Gold models. This function is no longer available with the infant flow sensor. It can be activated only when using the pediatric sensor with the bias flow turned off or when using the ventilator without a flow sensor. Leak compensation can be activated on the V.I.P. Bird Sterling only when in a volume mode or on the V.I.P. Bird Gold when in a volume mode or in pressure control or VAPS.

Leak compensation can be activated by scrolling through the displayed parameters using the select button until the current leak compensation message appears in the monitor display window. This message will be either "LK ON" or "LK OFF." Pressing and holding the select button will enable you to toggle between the "LK ON" and "LK OFF" settings.

Leak compensation is used when artificial airway leak prevents the ventilator from otherwise maintaining the PEEP level. Small increments of flow are introduced into the circuit to provide back pressure compensation for the leak. When you use leak compensation, you must be aware that the patient's ability to trigger may be diminished. Careful attention to the assist sensitivity setting is necessary. In some cases, removal of the source of the leak is preferable to the use of the leak compensation function (Clinical Rounds 13-4).

Specifications for the V.I.P. Bird Gold and Sterling ventilators are listed in Table 13-6.

CLINICAL ROUNDS 13-4

A respiratory therapist is assessing a patient being ventilated with the V.I.P. Bird Gold ventilator. The therapist notices the patient using accessory muscles to inspire. The patient's efforts do not trigger a ventilator breath even though the trigger sensitivity seems to be at an appropriate setting. What is a possible cause of the problem?

See Evolve Resources for the answer.

TABLE 13-6

Specifications for V.I.P. Bird Gold and Sterling Ventilators

Controls	Available Settings and Ranges
Mode select	
Waveform select	Square wave/decelerating flow
Tidal volume	10-1200 mL
Inspiratory time	0.10-3.0 s
Breath rate	0-150 breaths/min
Flow	3-120 L/min—volume modes and VAPS (Gold only)
	3-40 L/min—TCPL, inspiratory flow
	3-15 L/min—TCPL, expiratory bias flow
Inspiratory pressure	3-80 cm H_2O
PEEP/CPAP	0-24 cm H_2O
Assist sensitivity	Pressure-triggered: 1-29 cm H_2O
	Flow-triggered—Infant "Smart" Flow Sensor: 0.02-3 L/M
	Flow-triggered—Pediatric "Smart" Flow Sensor: 1-5 L/min
Pressure support	1-50 cm H_2O
Termination sensitivity	5, 10, 15, 20, and 25% of peak flow
Rise time	1-7 (1, fastest; 7, slowest)
Manual breath	
Inspiratory pause	0-2 s
Inspiratory/expiratory hold	3 s (maximum)
Flow display/comp	
Alarm silence	
Alarm reset	
Monitor display select	
Apnea switch	10-60 s
Alarm intensity	Minimum 66 dB
O_2 concentration	21-100%
Monitors and Indicators	
Peak inspiratory pressure	0-130 cm H_2O
Airway pressure manometer	−20 to 140 cm H_2O
Inspiratory time	0.05-60 s
Mean airway pressure	0-120 cm H_2O
I : E ratio	1 : 0.1 to 1 : 60
Minute volume	0.0-99.9 L (with flow sensor)
PEEP	0-24 cm H_2O
Tidal volume	0-9999 mL (with flow sensor)
Respiratory rate	0-250 breaths/min
Alarms	Low peak pressure
	High pressure
	Low PEEP/CPAP
	Pressure support/VAPS time limit
	High tidal volume
	Low minute volume
	High breath-rate
	High/prolonged pressure
	Low inlet gas pressure
	Blender input gas
	Circuit fault
	Apnea
	Sensor
	Ventilator inoperative

VAPS, Volume-assured pressure support; *TCPL,* time-cycled, pressure-limited; *I : E ratio,* ratio of inspiratory time to expiratory time.

DRÄGER BABYLOG 8000 INFANT VENTILATOR

The Dräger Babylog 8000 Infant Ventilator (Dräger Medical AG & Co., Lübeck, Germany) (Figure 13-26) is used to mechanically ventilate premature babies and infants. The weight limit use for the ventilator is 20 kg. It is electrically and pneumatically powered, microprocessor-controlled, and pneumatically controlled. A proximal flow sensor, which is a hot-wire anemometer, is placed at the patient's Y-connector. It allows the Babylog to monitor flow and detect patient effort at the ETT level, thereby providing improved patient/ventilator synchrony[13] (Clinical Rounds 13-5).

Noteworthy Internal Functions

The compressed air and oxygen sources pass through a filter and nonreturn valve before entering the pressure

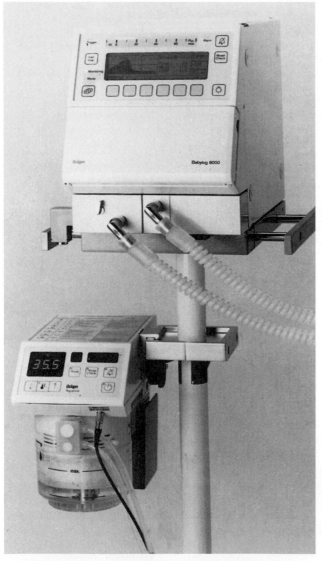

FIGURE 13-26 The Dräger Babylog 8000 Infant Ventilator. (Courtesy Dräger Medical AG & Co., Lübeck, Germany.)

CLINICAL ROUNDS 13-5

An infant is being ventilated on the Dräger Babylog 8000 in the synchronized intermittent mandatory ventilation (SIMV) mode with volume guarantee. A proximal flow sensor alarm activates and the airway pressure increases to 30 cm H_2O, although average pressures for breath delivery have been 19 cm H_2O. The infant appears to be breathing out of synchrony with the ventilator. A nurse silences the alarm and notifies the respiratory therapist. What might have caused the pressure to rise to 30 cm H_2O in this situation?

See Evolve Resources for the answer.

regulators. The two gas sources then enter the solenoid valves and flow adjusters, which blend and control the gas flowing through the inspiratory limb of the patient circuit. In the event of a gas supply or electrical failure, the patient can spontaneously breathe room air through a filter and nonreturn valve. Expiratory gas flow from the patient circuit is regulated by a pneumatic exhalation valve. The **pneumatic safety valve** directs excessive pressure buildup within the ventilator system through the exhalation valve.

Control and Alarm Panel

Figure 13-27 provides an illustration of the control and alarm panel of the Babylog 8000plus, which is almost identical to the 8000 (see following section on the 8000plus). In the 8000plus the continuous mandatory ventilation (CMV) soft-key pad of the 8000 is replaced with "Vent. Options." The CPAP pad of the 8000 is replaced with the vent mode.

The panel contains a rotary dial panel and a display/soft-key panel. The dial panel contains buttons for the operating modes (CPAP and IPPV) and rotary dials for ventilator parameters. Activated modes are indicated by an illuminated LED located within the button. The button must be depressed until the green LED is continuously illuminated for the mode to be activated. This is a safety feature that is in place to prevent accidental mode changes. Illuminated green LEDs indicate mandatory parameters to be set for that particular mode of ventilation. If a parameter has been internally limited or needs attention, the green LED will flash.

The rotary dial panel contains six dials: "OXYGEN CONCENTRATION %," "INSPIRATORY TIME," "EXPIRATORY TIME," "INSPIRATORY FLOW," "INSPIRATORY PRESSURE LIMIT," and PEEP/CPAP. Table 13-7 provides parameter specifications for the Dräger Babylog 8000 Ventilator.

The screen and soft-key panel that are located on the top of the ventilator serve various functions. The waveform display window displays either pressure or flow scalar waveforms over time. The measured values window digitally displays minute ventilation, oxygen concentration,

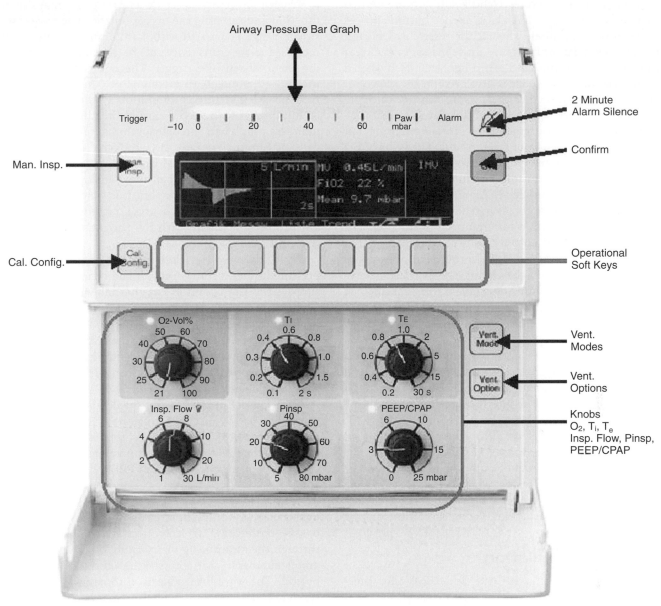

Airway Pressure Bar Graph

2 Minute
Alarm Silence

Confirm

Man. Insp.

Cal. Config.

Trigger   −10   0   20   40   60   Paw   Alarm
mbar

Operational
Soft Keys

Vent.
Modes

Vent.
Options

Knobs
O_2, T_i, T_e
Insp. Flow, Pinsp,
PEEP/CPAP

O2-Vol%   Ti   TE
Insp. Flow   Pinsp   PEEP/CPAP

FIGURE 13-27 The control and alarm panel of the Babylog 8000plus Infant Ventilator (see text for further information). (Courtesy Dräger Medical AG & Co., Lübeck, Germany.)

<table>
<tr><td colspan="2">TABLE 13-7</td></tr>
<tr><td colspan="2">Specifications for Dräger Babylog 8000 Infant Ventilator</td></tr>
<tr><td>Inspiratory time</td><td>0.1-2.0 s</td></tr>
<tr><td>Expiratory time</td><td>0.2-30 s</td></tr>
<tr><td>Inspiratory flow</td><td>1-30 L/min</td></tr>
<tr><td>Expiratory flow</td><td>1-30 L/min</td></tr>
<tr><td>Peak inspiratory
pressure</td><td>10-80 cm H_2O</td></tr>
<tr><td>PEEP/CPAP</td><td>0-15 cm H_2O</td></tr>
<tr><td>O_2 concentration</td><td>21-100%</td></tr>
<tr><td>Rate</td><td>2-150 breaths/min</td></tr>
<tr><td>Trigger mechanism</td><td>Flow/volume trigger</td></tr>
<tr><td>Alarms</td><td>Loss of PEEP/CPAP, high pressure,
high minute ventilation, low
minute ventilation, minute-
ventilation delay, and apnea</td></tr>
</table>

peak inspiratory pressure, mean airway pressure, and PEEP. The current mode of ventilation and other pertinent information are displayed on the far right in the status window.

The soft keys are used to select ventilation modes and ventilator functions, as well as to access other windows. The menu keys are located on the bottom of the screen. The screen functions are selected from the monitoring and functions menu with their respective submenus. Green LED illuminating lights will indicate whether monitoring or functions has been selected. The manual soft key is located above the monitoring LED and activates a manual breath or an *extension* of an existing breath in progress. The maximum inspiratory time available is 5 seconds. Text messages are displayed as pop-up windows at the top of any current screen.

The alarm silence and reset/check soft keys are located on the top-right panel. The alarm silence button silences the alarm for 2 minutes, whereas the reset/check button allows the clinician to recognize those messages and clear them from the screen. A red alarm light will flash when a warning or caution message is displayed on the screen.

Inspiratory and expiratory pressure sensors calculate the airway pressure, which is then displayed as real-time airway pressure measurements on an illuminating bar graph located on the top of the monitor. The yellow LED is illuminated when inspiration is triggered.

The oxygen concentration alarm limits are set internally at ±4%. The alarm limits for PEEP and Pinsp are also set internally by the microprocessor. The loss of PEEP/CPAP limit is −4 cm H_2O with a minimum of −2 cm H_2O. The high-pressure alarm is automatically set to Pinsp +10 cm H_2O or PEEP/CPAP +4 cm H_2O. In the event of excessive pressure buildup within the circuit, the exhalation valve opens, allowing exhalation. Adjustable alarm limits include high minute ventilation, low minute ventilation, minute ventilation delay (0 to 30 seconds), and apnea (5 to 20 seconds).

The ventilator alarms are arranged in order of importance. The alarms are grouped into advisory, warning, and alarm messages that are digitally displayed on the ventilator screen, eliminating the guesswork of troubleshooting alarm conditions. Incidents such as obstructed ETT, kinked circuit, and apnea are clearly identified on the ventilator screen. Each alarm level has a distinctive audible tone that indicates its level of importance. Every message is recorded in the **message log**, which is capable of storing the 100 most-recent entries. The log records the time of occurrence, displayed text, and information on the response.

Modes of Ventilation

The mandatory breaths in A/C and SIMV are time-triggered or patient-triggered, pressure-targeted, and time-cycled. The operator sets the following parameters: inspiratory time, expiratory time, inspiratory flow, inspiratory pressure, PEEP, and trigger sensitivity. Mandatory breaths are volume-triggered when a patient's spontaneous inspiratory volume is equal to or greater than the set trigger volume (set value of 2 or greater); otherwise the mandatory breath is time-triggered.

Continuous flow supports spontaneous respiratory efforts between the mandatory breaths in the CPAP mode. The amount of continuous flow available is determined by either the inspiratory flow control or the VIVE (variable inspiratory, variable expiratory) flow option.

The VIVE operating mode allows the clinician to adjust the flow during the expiratory phase to match the patient's needs during mandatory and spontaneous breaths. The inspiratory flow rate is displayed on the left bar graph, and adjustments can be made with the rotary dial. The expiratory flow rate is displayed on the right bar graph and can be adjusted with the up and down menu buttons.

Trigger sensitivity is set by accessing the main menu function and selecting the trigger button. The trigger sensitivity range is 1 to 10 with 1 (minimum) representing increased trigger sensitivity and 10 (maximum) representing the least-sensitive trigger. The trigger threshold of 1 to 10 corresponds with a volume of 0 mL to 3 mL. The recommended setting is minimum; a yellow trigger LED is illuminated with each triggered breath. A setting of 1 indicates that when the Babylog measures a flow change of 0.25 L/min (straight flow-trigger), the mandatory breath is then synchronized with the patient's effort. Settings above 1 indicate that the Babylog is evaluating the system for flow changes, but it is waiting until a particular volume moves across the flow sensor, then it will synchronize the breath with the patient's negative effort (Figure 13-28).

The IMV breath is time-triggered, pressure-targeted, pressure-limited or flow-limited, and time-cycled or pressure-cycled. The operator sets the following parameters: oxygen concentration, inspiratory time, expiratory time, inspiratory flow, inspiratory pressure, and PEEP. The mandatory rate is calculated by adding the inspiratory time and expiratory time that are set and dividing the sum into 60 seconds. The mandatory breath is time-triggered based on the rate calculation.

Nasal CPAP can be used, but the flow measurement has to be disabled by disconnecting the connector from the proximal flow sensor and pressing the reset/check button. The operator sets the following parameters: oxygen concentration, inspiratory flow, and PEEP.

Graphics Displays

Real-time pressure and flow scalar waveforms are displayed on the monitoring screen. The waveforms are accessed through the monitoring main menu; one must select the graph submenu then press either the "P–aw" or flow button. The waveform scale is automatically set by the ventilator. The displayed flow scalar waveform indicates the inspiratory flow pattern above the baseline and expiratory flow below. Freeze and trend options are also available if desired. The trend feature stores a 24-hour window.

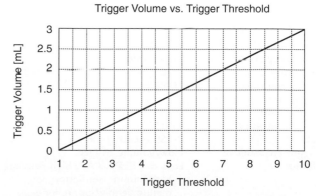

FIGURE 13-28 The trigger sensitivity setting on the Babylog 8000 Infant Ventilator (see text for further information).

Special Features

The ventilator performs an automatic calibration of the oxygen analyzer every 24 hours. Calibration can also be done manually under the function menu and the "cal sub-menu" (calibration submenu). The calibration takes approximately 5 minutes to complete. The flow sensor calibration is accessed through the function menu and calibration submenu. To calibrate the flow sensor, the operator simply follows the instructions given on the screen. The monitoring of minute ventilation and apnea is made possible only with a calibrated flow sensor. It is recommended that calibration of the flow sensor be performed every time the ventilator is turned on, after sensor assembly, and after sensor replacement.

DRÄGER BABYLOG 8000plus INFANT VENTILATOR

The Dräger Babylog 8000 has had several upgrades. Software version 4 is the original. The next two upgrades were version 5 and 6. The company then added "plus" to the unit's name, a term that is probably best defined as indicative of (1) extra monitoring, (2) pressure support, and (3) the addition of a volume guarantee. (NOTE: Some individuals do not consider pressure support to be part of the "plus" package.)

The Dräger Babylog 8000plus is an updated version of the original 8000 model. In this newer model, additional monitoring parameters have been added. A pressure support ventilation mode and volume guarantee are available as options. A high-frequency feature capable of rates from 5 Hz to 20 Hz is another option with this model, but this feature is not available in the United States.

Additional monitoring includes measurement of lung mechanics. These parameters are accessible from the monitoring menu and include airway resistance, dynamic compliance, time constant, C20/C, and r, which is the correlation coefficient of linear regression. A low tidal volume alarm is also available.

The pressure support ventilation mode is provided as a spontaneous-only mode. It cannot be combined with other modes or used with mandatory breaths. However, if apnea is detected, the ventilator will begin delivering mandatory breaths according to the set pressure and inspiratory and expiratory times. Pressure support breaths are flow-triggered and either flow-cycled or time-cycled. When inspiratory flow drops to a fixed 15% of peak flow, inspiration terminates. Flow termination is not adjustable. Time cycling will occur if the set T_I is reached.

Volume guarantee is a dual-mode feature that can be used in all patient-triggered modes. As its name implies, a tidal volume can be set by the clinician. However, the ventilator will continue to provide characteristic waveforms of pressure-targeted ventilation. In other words, volume guarantee is pressure-limited ventilation with a volume target. The clinician continues to have control over the delivered peak pressure, but she also can select a tidal volume target. The volume guarantee feature can be utilized only when the airway flow sensor is in use.

When volume guarantee is activated, the ventilator software continuously measures and compares inspired and expired tidal volume. Each following breath uses the comparisons from the previous breath to make adjustments to the peak inspiratory pressure so that a tidal volume as close as possible to the preset value can be delivered. The lowest inspiratory pressure that can result in delivery of the target tidal volume is then administered.

When activating the volume guarantee, the clinician sets the maximum peak inspiratory pressure. This setting becomes an inspiratory pressure limit. Over the next six to eight breaths, the ventilator determines the appropriate inspiratory pressure and begins to achieve and maintain the target tidal volume. If the patient's inspiratory effort adds to the tidal volume, the ventilator peak inspiratory pressure (PIP) will immediately decrease. If the total inspiratory tidal volume exceeds the set target volume by 130%, the expiratory valve will open and no additional ventilator-driven gas will be delivered to the patient.

The clinician needs to exercise care when using the volume guarantee and closely monitor patient-ventilator interaction. Because the patient is breathing spontaneously, an increase in metabolic demand or change in pulmonary compliance can dramatically affect the patient's ventilatory pattern. An appropriate target tidal volume must be selected based on the patient's weight. A clinically safe peak inspiratory pressure must be set as must an appropriate value for the low V_T alarm. Frequent patient assessment and careful monitoring are essential. The volume guarantee is potentially hazardous in the face of significant continuous or positional ETT leak. Its use is discouraged under these conditions.

INFRASONICS INFANT STAR VENTILATORS

Infrasonics Infant Star ventilators were owned by Puritan Bennett, a division of Tyco Healthcare. Then Tyco split its medical division, and Puritan Bennett became a part of Covidien. Information on Infrasonics Infant Star ventilator products—including the Infant Star 500, Infant Star Synch, Infant Star 100 Neonatal Ventilator, and the Infant Star 200 Neonatal-Pediatric Ventilator—is available on the Evolve Resources site for this text.

SECHRIST IV200 Savi™ INFANT/ PEDIATRIC VENTILATOR WITH TOTAL SYNCHRONY™ SYSTEM

The Sechrist IV200 Infant/Pediatric ventilator is a pressure-limited, time-cycled, continuous-flow ventilator. It is capable of providing TCPL ventilation. Additional information on the Sechrist IV200 is available on the Evolve Resources site for this text.

PART III—HIGH-FREQUENCY VENTILATORS

High-frequency ventilation (HFV) is an alternative method of ventilation in infants, children, and adults. The two HFV instruments currently used are high-frequency jet ventilation (HFJV) and high-frequency oscillation (HFO) devices. These have been used most frequently in infants, but one oscillator, the SensorMedics Model 3100B, is available for use in the adult population. These high-frequency devices will be reviewed. The theory behind how HFV achieves gas exchange is described elsewhere.[2]

BUNNELL LIFE PULSE HIGH-FREQUENCY JET VENTILATOR

The Bunnell Life Pulse High-Frequency Jet Ventilator (Bunnell Incorporated, Salt Lake City, Utah) is indicated for patients with severe respiratory distress syndrome complicated by pulmonary air leak that has been untreatable with conventional mechanical ventilation strategies (Figure 13-29). The Bunnell HFJV system is a microprocessor-controlled, pressure-limited, time-cycled, constant-flow, **high-frequency jet ventilator** that works in conjunction with a conventional ventilator. The conventional ventilator provides background conventional ventilation (if desired), supplies entrained gas, and regulates the PEEP level.[14]

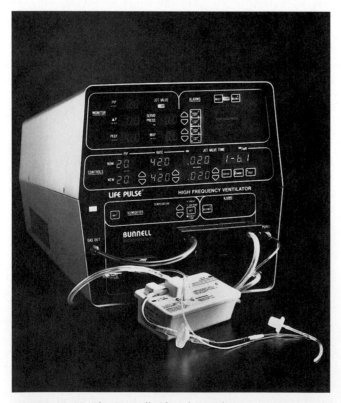

FIGURE 13-29 The Bunnell Life Pulse High-Frequency Jet Ventilator. (Courtesy Bunnell Incorporated, Salt Lake City, Utah.)

Control and Alarm Panel

The on/off switch is located midway on the front left panel. If you press the button once, this powers the ventilator on (displays green light); pressing the button again turns the ventilator off (no light). Figure 13-30 provides a diagram of the seven components of the ventilator. The ventilator consists of the following seven sections: monitoring; alarms; controls; patient box; disposable cartridge/circuit; rear panel; and humidifier monitor, alarms, and controls.

Monitoring Display

The ventilator monitoring displays provide pertinent information on the patient and on ventilator performance and are located on the front top-left panel of the control panel. These displays are PIP, DELTA P (PIP-PEEP), PEEP, SERVO PRESSURE, AND PAW. The four patient pressures are sensed at the distal end of the hi-lo jet tube (if used) and measured by the transducer in the patient box. The displays are averages calculated over a short period and are not reflective of alveolar pressures. Mean airway pressure can be increased by increasing peak inspiratory pressure, increasing PEEP, and increasing the rate and tidal volume of the sigh breaths. The PEEP level is controlled by the conventional ventilator even though it displayed on the Bunnell's control panel.

The servo pressure measurement (0 to 20 psig) is the amount of internal pressure required to generate the PIP displayed in the NOW (current requirement) display and is a clinical indicator of improved lung status or acute changes (e.g., tension pneumothorax, ETT leak, atelectasis). For example, a decrease in lung compliance may result in a decrease in servo pressure, because less gas is required to meet the set PIP. Increases in lung compliance or the development of a pneumothorax may result in elevated servo pressures (Clinical Rounds 13-6).

The pinch valve on/off lights located on the front top-left panel (monitor panel) indicate the communication between the ventilator and pinch valve (located on patient box). The illuminated on light indicates the valve is signaled to open for inspiration. The illuminated off light indicates the valve is signaled to close for expiration. The light will alternate rapidly between the on and off displays.

CLINICAL ROUNDS 13-6

An infant with acute respiratory distress syndrome is receiving high-frequency ventilation with the Bunnell Life Pulse High-Frequency Jet Ventilator. Breath sounds and arterial blood gases have been improving over the past 24 hours. The servo pressure has been slowly increasing over several hours. The increase in servo pressure might indicate what change in the patient?

See Evolve Resources for the answer.

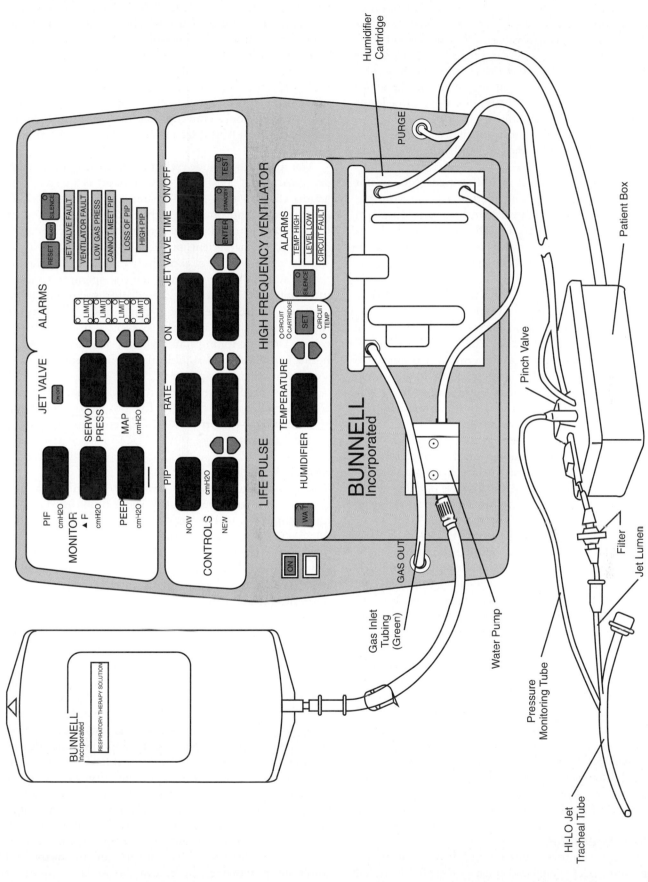

FIGURE 13-30 Seven components of the Bunnell Life Pulse High-frequency Jet Ventilator (see text for further information). (Courtesy Bunnell Incorporated, Salt Lake City, Utah.)

Alarm Display

The ventilator alarm displays are located on the front top-right panel and consist of the following: A SERVO PRESSURE button (+1 cm H_2O present value), a PAW button (+1.5 cm H_2O), a high PIP button (i.e., greater than 5 cm H_2O PIP for 2 seconds or greater than 10 cm H_2O for 30 seconds), and LOSS OF PIP button (i.e., less than 25% PIP). The MEAN AIRWAY PRESSURE and SERVO PRESSURE upper and lower limits can be adjusted manually.

The high PIP, jet valve fault, ventilator fault, low gas pressure, cannot meet PIP, and loss of PIP alarms are back-lighted displays. The jet valve fault alarm alerts the clinician that the pinch valve in the patient box is not functioning appropriately. The microprocessor is continuously monitoring the pinch valve and activates the alarm when malfunctions are detected. The Life Pulse continues to operate even if the pinch valve is not cycling. The ventilator fault alarm alerts the clinician that a problem is present within the Life Pulse's electronics or valves. A numeric code will be displayed in the jet valve on/off time window to indicate the type of failure.

The low gas pressure alarm alerts the clinician that the gas supply is less than 30 psig. The "cannot meet PIP" alarm warns the clinician that the ventilator is unable to deliver the pressures within a set range while the servo pressure has increased to the maximum level available. The alarm can be a result of a leak in the humidifier cartridge/patient circuit; incomplete connection of the circuit to the jet tube; a defective or damaged jet tube (e.g., a kinked tube, improper positioning, occlusion, or leak); the present settings being insufficient to ventilate larger patient; a patient fighting the Life Pulse; or the pinch valve opening action is not effective, resulting in higher servo pressures being necessary to meet current settings.

The reset, ready light, and alarm silence (60 seconds) buttons are located above the ventilator alarm displays. The reset button has the machine recalculate automatic upper and lower limits for the SERVO PRESSURE, PIP, and MEAN AIRWAY PRESSURE (MEAN PAW) parameters. It is recommended for use when changes are made on the conventional side of ventilation and manual adjustments are not made. When the reset button is pressed, the ready light turns off and alarm indicators are inactive. The Life Pulse calculates new alarm limits; after this is accomplished, the ready light will illuminate and all alarms are reactivated. The ready light indicates that the machine is ready for operation and has stabilized after start-up or reset, calculated alarm limits, and is ready for operation. The silence button will silence audible alarms for 60 seconds. The alarm will resume after this period of time if the condition has not resolved. A red light will illuminate in the corner of the silence button when the silence function is in effect.

Control Parameters

The ventilator control parameters and displays are located on the front middle panel and consist of the following: PIP (8 to 50 cm H_2O), RATE (240 to 660 insufflations/minute),

JET ON TIME (inspiratory time; .02 to 0.034 second), and ON/OFF RATIO (1:1.2 to 1:12). The "NOW" displays indicate current operating settings. The "NEW" display and control area allows the operator to adjust set parameters and visualize the change before entering new parameters. Some hospitals interrupt HFJV by setting the sigh breath peak pressure (on a conventional ventilator) higher than it is set with HFJV, whereas others adjust the sigh breath peak pressure (on a conventional ventilator) to equal or less than the HFJV PIP setting (i.e., HFJV breaths are not interrupted).

The operating mode selection buttons are ENTER, STANDBY, and TEST. If the enter button is pressed, this action changes the "NOW" parameters to the "NEW" parameters. Inappropriately high servo pressure may occur if the enter button is pressed before the patient circuit is connected to the patient, possibly resulting in high pressures and the delivery of excessively high tidal volumes.

The standby mode is used when the operator wants to interrupt HFJV temporarily (i.e., during suctioning or to monitor the effectiveness of conventional ventilation). Alarms are inactive while the system is in the standby mode. The functioning standby mode is indicated by red lights, and a 5-second audible alarm and is automatically set up with ventilator power-up.

The test mode is an automatic test that checks the ventilator systems and circuitry for proper function and should **NOT** be performed with a patient connected to the jet ventilator.

Humidification

The disposable humidifier cartridge/patient breathing circuit is a closed system that provides humidity, heating, and monitoring of the gas exiting the ventilator (Figure 13-31). The humidifier cartridge heats and humidifies the gas before patient delivery. The cartridge receptacle holds the humidifier cartridge in place by securing the latch in place. The water in the cartridge is warmed by the anodized aluminum heater plate.

The "gas-out" and "purge pneumatic" connectors located on the front panel are of different sizes in order to prevent improper connections. The short, green gas-inlet tube connects the gas flow from the ventilator to the cartridge. The clear water-inlet tube transfers water from the pump when the water-level sensors detect a decrease in the water level, thus filling the humidifier cartridge. Water is transferred from a nonpressurized source (i.e., solution bag or bottle) to the pressurized humidifier cartridge by the water pump. The water level is regulated by the water-level sensor pins in the cartridge. The purge port supplies gas to the **purge valve**, which is located in the patient box. The gas is used to provide a moisture-free environment in the monitoring line of the hi-lo jet tube. The small, clear, second lumen of the patient circuit connects to this port.

The "humidifier wait" button turns off the heater and water pump, allowing easy removal and replacement of the cartridge/circuit. A red light in the corner of the button

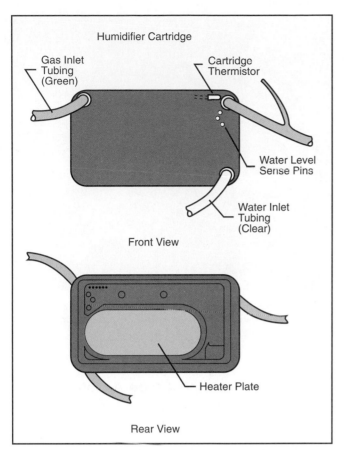

FIGURE 13-31 The humidifier cartridge/patient breathing circuit of the Bunnell Life Pulse High-Frequency Jet Ventilator.

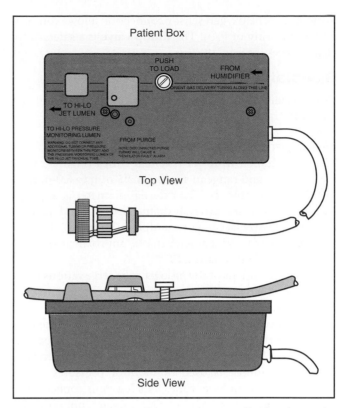

FIGURE 13-32 The patient box on the Bunnell Life Pulse High-Frequency Jet Ventilator.

will flash to indicate activation of the wait feature. To resume normal function, simply depress the button again.

A thermistor is located at the patient breathing circuit and cartridge connection; this device ensures adequate gas temperature delivery to the patient. The available temperature range is 32° C to 42° C.

The temperature is displayed in three separate windows, which are labeled *circuit (desired)*, *cartridge (desired)*, and *circuit temperature (actual temperature)*. The set button allows the clinician to select the temperature setting/measurement to be displayed. The window display will automatically return to the circuit temperature display reading. The humidifier system has a separate "silence" button (separate from the ventilator's alarm silence button) and various back-lighted alarm messages. The messages warn the clinician of any temperature/water level changes and electrical problems within the cartridge/circuit.

Patient Box and Pinch Valve

The patient box is a satellite component that contains the pinch valve, purge valve, and pressure transducer (Figure 13-32). It is designed for placement near the patient's head to ensure accurate pressure monitoring and delivery of jet bursts.

The patient box electrical cable connects to the rear panel of the ventilator. An **electromagnetic** solenoid activates the pinch valve. The pinch valve breaks the flow of pressurized gas into small bursts with the pinch-and-release action on the silicone tube of the patient breathing circuit. The "push to load" button opens the valve to allow for correct placement of the silicone tube within the patient box and to facilitate repositioning of the silicone tube. The silicone tube should be moved 2 mm every 8 hours to prevent areas of wear and to prevent tearing.

A bacterial filter is present downstream from the pinch valve to provide particle filtration. A millimeter measuring guide is printed on the patient box for visual use. The purge valve maintains a moisture-free, pressure-monitoring line of the ETT by allowing pressurized gas from the ventilator to pass through the line. A 10-millisecond burst of gas is introduced through the monitoring line. The pressure transducer measures tracheal pressure and sends the information to the microprocessor.

Rear Panel

The rear panel contains the mixed-gas input connection, oxygen sensor connection, hour meter, circuit breaker, alarm volume control, patient box connector, analog output, and **dump valve** outlet. The gas-input fitting connects the ventilator to an oxygen blender to provide varied oxygen concentrations. A 30-psig to 100-psig supply source is required. The oxygen sensor connection allows continuous monitoring of F_IO_2. The **dump valve** is a safety valve that releases internal pressure.

Special Features

Two special-function devices worth noting are the hi-lo jet ETT and the LifePort™ Endotracheal Tube Adapter.

Hi-Lo Jet Endotracheal Tube

The triple-lumen **hi-lo jet tracheal tubes** (Figure 13-33) are uncuffed and range in size from 2.5-mm to 6.0-mm ID in 0.5-mm increments. The external diameter is approximately equal to the external diameter of a standard ETT that is a half-size larger. For example, a 3.0-mm ID hi-lo jet tube has an external diameter that is approximately equal to a 3.5-mm ID standard ETT.[14]

The three lumens of the hi-lo jet tube serve various functions. The main lumen contains a 15-mm connector that provides the connection point for the conventional ventilator circuit Y-connector. The jet lumen provides the connection to the patient breathing circuit from the patient box. The jet bursts are delivered through this lumen. The monitoring lumen is used to monitor pressures at the distal end of the hi-lo jet tube. This lumen is connected to the "To Hi-Lo Pressure Monitoring Lumen" connection on the patient box.

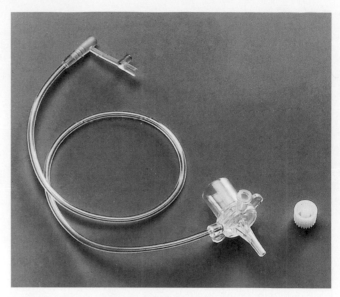

FIGURE 13-34 Bunnell LifePort™ Endotracheal Tube Adapter for use in high-frequency jet ventilation. (Courtesy Bunnell Incorporated, Salt Lake City, Utah.)

LifePort™ Endotracheal Tube Adapter

The development of the LifePort™ Endotracheal Tube Adapter (Figure 13-34) has nullified the requirement of intubating/reintubating patients with the specialized jet tube prior to the initiation of HFJV. With the use of the double-port ETT adapter and a conventional single-lumen ETT, HFJV can be implemented easily and quickly. The adapters are available with ID sizes of 2.5 mm, 3.5 mm, and 4.5 mm. To initiate HFJV, the operator simply replaces the 15-mm standard ETT adapter with the 15-mm connection of the jet tube adapter. The jet port facilitates the entry of gas from the jet ventilator. The inspired gas is redirected through a nozzle, which increases the gas's velocity. The momentum of the gas is converted to pressure as the gas exits from the nozzle.

Bunnell Incorporated suggests that, when using the 2.5-mm ID LifePort™ adapter, the HFJV PIP must be adjusted to equal that of the conventional PIP. When the larger adapters are used, the clinician should set up the initial HFJV PIP at 90% of the conventional PIP.

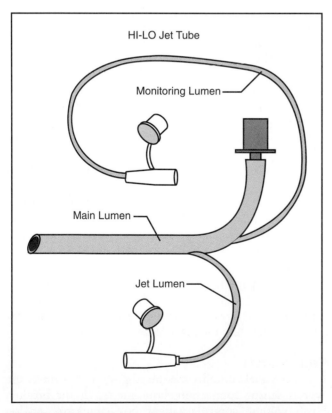

HI-LO Jet Tube

Monitoring Lumen

Main Lumen

Jet Lumen

FIGURE 13-33 Triple-lumen hi-lo jet tracheal tubes for use in high-frequency jet ventilation. (Courtesy Puritan Bennett, a division of Tyco Healthcare. As of 2008, Tyco is now part of Covidien; Covidien Ltd., Hamilton, Bermuda.)

SensorMedics 3100 AND 3100A HIGH-FREQUENCY OSCILLATORY VENTILATORS

The SensorMedics model 3100 high-frequency oscillator was the first of two high-frequency oscillators for use with neonates, originally introduced by the SensorMedics Corporation of Yorba Linda, Calif. An improved model, the 3100A, replaced the 3100 (Figure 13-35). Both of these models have been used extensively in the treatment of acute respiratory failure in infants. The 3100A is also being used in older pediatric patients and adults. (NOTE: Sensor-Medics Corporation was purchased by Viasys Healthcare,

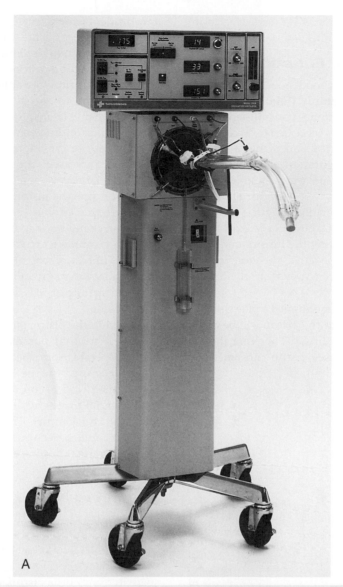

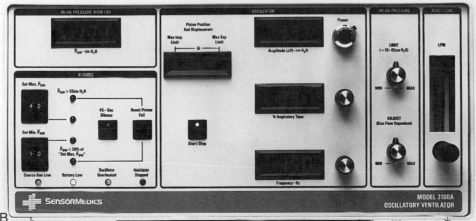

FIGURE 13-35 A, SensorMedics Model 3100A High-Frequency Oscillator. **B**, Control panel of the 3100A. (Courtesy Cardinal Health, McGaw Park, Ill., which was Viasys Healthcare, Critical Care Division, Palm Springs, Calif.)

Palm Springs, Calif. Then, in June 2008, Viasys Healthcare was purchased by Cardinal Health.)

Noteworthy Internal Functions

The heart of the SensorMedics models is the **oscillator subsystem**, or the **piston assembly** (Figure 13-36). The system incorporates an electronic control circuit, or **square-wave driver**, which powers a linear-drive motor. The motor consists of an electrical coil within a magnet, which is similar to the configuration of a permanent magnet speaker. When positive polarity is applied to the square-wave driver, the coil is driven forward. The coil is attached to a rubber bellows, or diaphragm, to create a piston. When the coil moves forward, the piston moves toward the patient airway, creating the inspiratory phase. When the polarity changes to negative, the electrical coil and the attached piston are driven away from the patient, creating an active expiration.[15]

The amount of **polarity voltage** applied to the electrical coil determines the distance that the piston will be driven toward or away from the patient airway. Therefore, increasing the polarity voltage increases piston movement, or

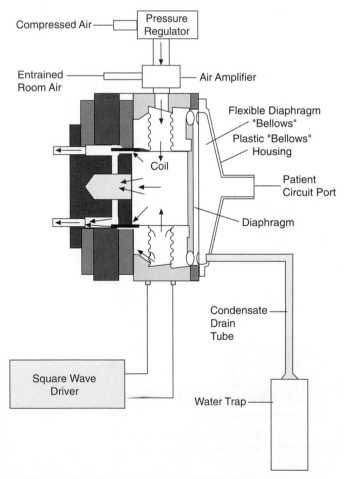

FIGURE 13-36 The piston assembly of the SensorMedics Model 3100A High-Frequency Oscillator. (Courtesy Cardinal Health, McGaw Park, Ill., which owns Viasys Healthcare, Critical Care Division, Palm Springs, Calif.)

amplitude. Piston excursion is limited, however, by resistance from the pressure within the patient circuit. The oscillator subsystem also limits the piston stroke to 365 mL. The total time for a piston stroke is a few milliseconds.

When oscillations are at low frequencies, the piston has sufficient time to travel the available excursion length during either the inspiratory or expiratory phase and remain at maximum position until it begins its movement in the opposite direction. Conversely, as oscillating frequency is increased, the excursion time of the piston becomes a larger percentage of the breath phase. The percentage of time the piston remains completely forward or backward decreases. At very high frequencies, the polarity to the coil changes so rapidly that the piston does not have time for a complete excursion and arrival to its maximum position. In fact, it may only travel a fraction of its potential distance before changing direction. Therefore, volume delivered by the piston is decreased as oscillatory frequency is increased.

Although the piston subsystem is designed to produce as little friction as possible, the rapid movement of the piston generates some heat. Therefore, a Venturi-type air amplifier is used on the 3100A to introduce cooling air around the electrical coil. A separate compressed air source of at least 30 psig serves this system, which consists of a regulator and Venturi. The regulator reduces airflow to 15 L/min, and the Venturi entrains 45 L/min of room air. This provides 60 L/min of cooling air for the subsystem.

Circuit Design

Figure 13-37 shows the basic circuit of the 3100A. After exiting the back panel of the ventilator and passing through a humidifier, blended gas enters the patient circuit at the **bias flow** inlet. Flow is set by using the bias flow control on the front panel (see Figure 13-35B). The gas mixture fills the space in front of the piston, then flows past the limit valve and on toward the ETT connection. Gas then passes the dump valve and exits through either the control valve or a small restricted orifice next to the control valve housing. The oscillating piston moves the circuit gas in a forward and backward direction toward the airway. The rate of bias flow, the pressure maintained at the airway, and the speed and excursion of the piston are all set by the clinician.

Any standard humidifier can be used with the 3100 and 3100A. Circuits are designed to accommodate heater sensors to provide servo-controlled temperature at the airway. Hot-wire circuits are available to reduce water condensation. All circuits incorporate a water outlet, tubing, and water trap that permit water condensate to drain away from the piston.

Controls

See Figure 13-35B.

On/Off Switch

The ventilator's on/off switch is located on the front of the unit below the piston and to the right (see Figure 13-35A).

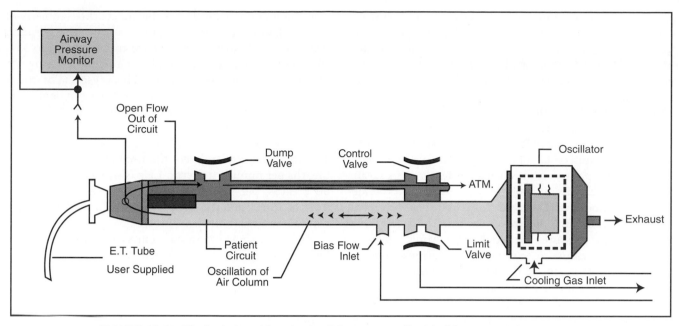

FIGURE 13-37 The basic breathing circuit of the SensorMedics Model 3100A High-Frequency Oscillator. (Courtesy Cardinal Health, McGaw Park, Ill., which owns Viasys Healthcare, Critical Care Division, Palm Springs, Calif.)

If power to the unit is turned off or electrical power is interrupted while the ventilator is in operation, an audible alarm will sound and the red "power failure" LED on the front control panel will be illuminated. This alarm can only be silenced by depressing the reset button on the front panel. With any interruption in ventilator operation, pressurization of the circuit's three mushroom valves stops immediately, allowing the circuit to vent to the atmosphere. This venting allows the patient to breathe room air. The proximity of the vented dump valve close to the airway enables the spontaneously breathing patient to breathe room air with minimal resistance from the ventilator circuit.

Piston Centering

The piston's forward and backward excursions are limited by two mechanical stops. If time and amplitude allow the piston to encounter one of the stops, it will remain stationary for the duration of the inspiratory or expiratory time and then change direction. An **infrared sensor** is used to track the movement of the piston between the mechanical stops. Piston movement is displayed by a bar graph on the control panel. The left end of the bar graph is labeled *MIN INSP LIMIT* and the right, *MAX INSP LIMIT*. The dot represents the piston's center position.

The piston centering control knob (see Figure 13-35A, beneath and to the left of the diaphragm) adjusts an electrical counterforce to the piston. This counterforce acts in opposition to the Paw on the front side of the piston. The result of this opposing counterforce is a centering effect on the piston. At a constant Paw, as the piston centering control knob is turned clockwise, the piston will move toward the "MAX INSP LIMIT," one of the mechanical

stops. The oscillator should not be operated so that the piston is driven against a mechanical stop for an extended period of time. The piston needs to be maintained in the center of the bar graph to maintain piston efficiency and to maximize the life of the oscillator mechanism.

Adjusting other controls, such as the mean pressure adjust control or the power control, will change the piston position. The clinician should regularly check and adjust piston centering after making changes in other settings.

Bias Flow

The bias flow control sets the rate of continuous flow through the patient circuit. Adjusting this control counterclockwise increases flow to an internal limit of 40 L/min. Gas flow is indicated by a ball float that is located within a glass tube. The tube is graduated in 5-L/min increments.

F_IO_2

A standard air/oxygen blender is used to provide blended gas to the ventilator. A minimum pressure of 30 psig is required. The gas mixture should be adjusted to the desired F_IO_2 before it enters the ventilator.

Mean Pressure Adjust

The mean pressure adjust control knob adjusts the Paw. This control varies the resistance placed on the control valve, the mushroom valve in the patient circuit at the end of the expiratory limb. Paw is digitally displayed in the mean pressure monitor window. Although the mean pressure adjust control is the primary determinant of Paw, other controls will also affect it. For example, increasing bias flow will increase Paw. Changes to the power, frequency, inspiratory time, and piston centering controls will also change the Paw. Therefore, if a change in Paw occurs because another control has been adjusted, the mean pressure adjust control knob should be used to return the Paw to the desired level.

Mean Pressure Limit

The mean pressure limit control knob is normally used to set a limit above which the Paw cannot be exceeded. Adjustable to a maximum of 45 cm H_2O, this control can be used to protect the patient from an inadvertent rise in mean airway pressure. This control sets a pressure in the limit valve, a mushroom valve located close to the bias flow inlet of the patient circuit. If the pressure within the circuit were to exceed this pressure, the limit valve would open to permit excess pressure to be vented to the atmosphere.

An alternative use of the mean pressure limit control is to set it above the mean airway pressure that would otherwise exist when the clinician uses only the mean pressure adjust control. Using the control in this way assures the clinician that Paw will not exceed that prescribed, regardless of changes made in bias flow, percent inspiratory time, or frequency. However, the clinician should be aware that changes made to controls that result in an uncentered piston can still change Paw, regardless of where the mean pressure limit control is set. Increasing the power, or amplitude, also can increase Paw.

Power/ΔP

The power control determines the amount of polarity voltage applied to the oscillator's subsystem electrical coil. Adjusting this control clockwise increases the forward and backward displacement of the piston, thereby increasing oscillatory pressure (ΔP), which is also called amplitude, and delivered volume. Pressure is adjustable from approximately 7 cm H_2O to 90 cm H_2O.

The extent to which the ΔP increases depends on the resistance to forward movement the piston encounters. For example, when the oscillator is used with a patient with extremely low pulmonary or chest wall compliance, the piston will meet a high resistance in the inspiratory phase. Increasing the power setting will increase ΔP, but not in the same proportion as the amount of resistance the piston encounters from the Paw. Therefore, if a low level of Paw is present, ΔP adjustments for the same change in power will be greater than if a high level of Paw is present.

Percentage of Inspiratory Time

The fraction of time that the piston is in the inspiratory position is determined by the "% Inspiratory Time" control. For example, if the control is set at 33%, the piston will spend 33% of the breath cycle in the inspiratory position and the remaining 67% in the expiratory position. The control is adjustable from 30% to 50%. The setting is digitally displayed in the window to the left of the control knob.

Changing the inspiratory time affects the symmetry of the oscillator waveform. If, for example, the clinician decreases the % inspiratory time control from 50% to 33%, the amount of time for the piston to travel during the inspiratory phase may be limited. This is especially true at high frequencies. Therefore, the ΔP and Paw can be affected by changes in the percentage of inspiratory time.

Frequency

The frequency control sets the oscillatory frequency, or breaths per minute, in **hertz**; 1 Hz is equal to 60 cycles, or 60 breaths, per minute. The control is adjustable from 3 Hz to 15 Hz, and the setting is digitally displayed in the window to the left of the control.

As frequency is increased, excursion of the piston will be limited by the time allotted for each breath cycle. Changes in the frequency will affect mean airway pressure (Paw) and ΔP (Boxes 13-10 and 13-11).

Start/Stop

The start/stop control button either enables or disables oscillator operation. Pressing this start/stop button will light the green LED labeled *OSCILLATOR STOPPED* if the ventilator's microprocessor determines that the unit is safe to operate. This control allows the oscillator to begin operation only if the start-up procedure was properly performed.

Reset

The reset button sets or resets the unit's safety alarms and the power failure alarm. Conditions triggering an alarm

---

BOX 13-10	Clinical Example of Changing Frequency with the 3100A

A patient is on the SensorMedics 3100A at a frequency of 15 Hz. The clinician decides to lower the frequency to 10 Hz. Doing so allows the piston more travel time. This results in greater piston displacement, or more delivered volume to the patient. The exact amount of the volume increase is unknown. In some patients, an inadvertent (and unknown) increase in tidal volume may contribute to volutrauma. Therefore, the clinician should always use caution when lowering the oscillatory frequency.

BOX 13-11	Effect of Control Changes on Mean Airway Pressure

Many of the controls on the 3100 affect more than one parameter. For example, when adjusting the amplitude with the power control, the alteration in piston thrust will change the level of mean airway pressure. When the frequency is adjusted, changes in amplitude, piston position, and mean airway pressure will occur. Therefore, the clinician should use caution when making a setting change and carefully readjust other settings that might also change.

must be corrected before resetting can occur. This button does not function unless the ventilator has been activated with the start/stop button.

Certain alarm conditions, such as the "PAW < 20% SET MAX PAW" alarm, cause the circuit dump valve to immediately deflate. When the clinician depresses the reset button, the dump valve will reinflate. It is necessary to press the reset button until the airway pressure exceeds 20% of that on the "SET MAX PAW" thumb wheel. Otherwise, reset may not occur.

The reset button also is used to silence the ventilator's battery powered audible power failure alarm if the unit is turned off or if electrical power is interrupted.

Alarms

45-Second Silence

For most alarm conditions, the audible portion can be silenced for 45 seconds by pressing the "45-SEC SILENCE" button. When activated, the button's yellow LED will light until the silence period lapses.

When the oscillator is turned off at the power switch or the oscillator stops because of a power interruption, the audible alarm can be silenced only by pressing the reset button.

Set Maximum and Minimum Paw

The "SET MAX PAW" and "SET MIN PAW" thumb wheel switches enable the clinician to set maximum and minimum limits for Paw. Because some drifting of Paw may be attributable to ETT leaks or spontaneous breathing, a safety range needs to be set. When either limit is reached, a red LED next to the corresponding thumb wheel will light and an audible alarm will sound. The ventilator continues to operate, but the alarm condition will persist until the mean pressure adjust control is readjusted or new alarm limits are set.

PAW < 20% SET MAX PAW

Conditions causing a sharp drop in Paw to a level less than 20% of the value set on the "SET MAX PAW" thumb wheel will result in an alarm condition. The thumb wheel will trigger a "PAW < 20% SET MAX PAW" alarm. When this alarm is triggered, the oscillator stops, the red LED lights to indicate this alarm condition, and the audible alarm sounds. Bias flow will continue to be delivered to permit spontaneous ventilation.

PAW > 50 cm H₂O

The "PAW > 50 cm H_2O" alarm is activated if mean airway pressure rises above 50 cm H_2O for any reason. When this alarm is activated, the dump valve opens, causing the oscillator to stop. The red LED lights up to indicate this alarm condition, and an audible alarm sounds. Although the audible alarm can be silenced with the "45-SEC SILENCE" button, the oscillator will not resume operating until the reset button is pressed and held until mean airway pressure

exceeds 20% of that set with the "SET MAX PAW" thumb wheel.

Power Failure

The battery-powered power failure alarm is activated if the power switch to the ventilator is turned off or if electrical power is interrupted. If the unit's main circuit breaker is tripped or the main power supply fails, this alarm condition also occurs. The power failure LED lights up, and the audible alarm sounds. Both can be extinguished by pressing the reset button.

When power is restored to the ventilator, the circuit must be occluded and the reset button pressed and held until mean airway pressure exceeds 20% of that set with the "SET MAX PAW" thumb wheel. Only then will oscillations resume (Box 13-12).

Battery Low

The yellow "battery low" LED lights up when the battery serving the power failure alarm is low. No audible alarm is activated.

Source Gas Low

The yellow "source gas low" LED lights up whenever gas pressure from the blender falls below 30 psig. This LED also lights up if the pressure drops below 30 psig in the separate compressed-air source for cooling the piston subsystem. The most common cause of this alarm condition is obstruction of the inlet filter cartridge with dirt. If this problem is not corrected, the piston subsystem is likely to overheat, resulting in piston failure.

Oscillator Overheated

The yellow "OSCILLATOR OVERHEATED" LED lights when the oscillator coil temperature reaches 175° C. No audible alarm sounds. If this problem is not corrected, piston failure can result.

Troubleshooting

The array of visual and audible alarms assists the clinician in troubleshooting specific problems with the Sensor-

BOX 13-12	Returning the Oscillator to Operation After Disconnect

When alarm conditions occur, especially those that shut down the oscillator, the clinician should immediately remove the patient from the circuit and provide manual ventilation. After the cause of the alarm condition is corrected, the airway connector should be plugged and oscillations restarted by using the reset button. Plugging the circuit and restarting oscillations are necessary to confirm safe operation. When that is done, the plug is then removed and the connection is immediately occluded by hand. Next, the circuit is quickly reconnected to the patient's airway.

Medics oscillator. The instruction manual also provides a troubleshooting guide.

Circuit leaks are most likely to occur at the many connection points. For example, the pressure line going from the airway Y-connector to the front of the unit may be loose. Lines going from the front to each of the mushroom valves can be the source of leaks. All of these lines have Luer-Lok connections that need to be tight. Although it occurs only rarely, any of the mushroom valves can rupture, which will cause the unit to stop oscillating and will activate the alarm.

When a circuit not equipped with heater wires is used, pooling of water can occur at any low point in the circuit. If the patient is positioned lower than the circuit, excessive condensate can run into the patient's airway. Therefore, care must be taken to keep water drained from the circuit.

If the SensorMedics is operated for long periods of time at very low frequencies, the piston can begin to fail. If the piston housing is not connected to a compressed-air source or if the unit is operated without sufficient piston centering, the piston will wear out more rapidly than normal. Piston failure is usually indicated by a knocking sound and by drifting in the mean airway pressure and amplitude levels.

Every clinician who uses the SensorMedics oscillators needs to be capable of performing a system calibration and check. An outline of this procedure is printed on the left side and top of the unit. If a clinician notes problems in maintaining the desired settings, the patient must be removed from the ventilator and provided with another means of ventilation support. Then the clinician should perform a system calibration and check. Doing so often reveals the source of the problem.

SensorMedics 3100B HIGH-FREQUENCY OSCILLATORY VENTILATOR

The SensorMedics 3100B High-Frequency Oscillatory Ventilator, a different version of the model 3100A, is intended to be used with adult patients. Appropriate for the patient with a weight greater than 35 kg, the model 3100B (Figure 13-38A) is designed with greater power, flow, and pressure capabilities than the 3100A. Because the design and controls of the two models are very similar, only the differences between the two will be discussed here.

Overview of Differences Between 3100A and 3100B Models

Power and mean airway pressure controls for the 3100B are identical to those for the 3100A. Although the power control remains a graduated 10-turn locking dial, the ΔP is adjustable to greater than 90 cm H_2O of the maximum amplitude of the proximal airway pressure. Mean airway pressure is adjustable to approximately 55 cm H_2O. Piston-centering is performed automatically by updated electronic

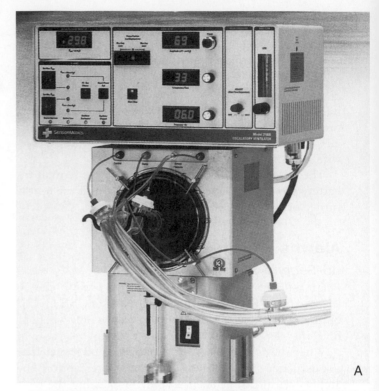

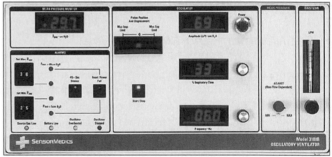

FIGURE 13-38 A, The SensorMedics Model 3100B High-Frequency Oscillator. **B,** The control panel of the 3100B. (Courtesy Cardinal Health, McGaw Park, Ill., which owns Viasys Healthcare, Critical Care Division, Palm Springs, Calif.)

sensors. Therefore, the center piston control has been eliminated from this model.[16]

The mean pressure limit control has also been eliminated. The "SET MAX PAW" is the only adjustable control that prevents inadvertent increases in mean airway pressure. The limit controls are discussed next.

The bias flow capability of the 3100B has been expanded to an internal limit of 60 L/min. The rotameter glass tube, which indicates flow, is graduated from 0 L/min to 60 L/min in 5-L/min increments (Figure 13-38B).

The frequency control and digital display, which operate identically to the same controls on the 3100A, permit the operator to adjust the frequency from 3 Hz to 15 Hz. These are the same limits that are used on the 3100A. The inspiratory time control is also identical, with limits from 30% to 50%.

The alarm panel on the model 3100B is arranged identically to that on the 3100A. However, there are several differences in alarm limits and function. A major difference is in the set maximum Paw control. The maximum setting for this control is 59 cm H_2O. When the ventilator is operating and the set pressure limit is reached or exceeded by the proximal pressure, the unit no longer shuts down entirely. The audible and visual alarm will activate, but instead of shutting down, the ventilator will depressurize the limit valve seat until the mean airway pressure falls to a level of 12 cm H_2O ($\pm$3 cm H_2O) below the set mean. After the pressure drops to this point, the limit valve will allow the circuit to repressurize and rise again and the audible and visual alarms will be deactivated. If the proximal pressure rises again to meet or exceed the limit setting, the same cycle of events will repeat until the alarm condition is resolved.

The "PAW > 60 cm H_2O" red LED and audible alarm operate the same as the "PAW > 50 cm H_2O" LED on the 3100A, with the only difference being the higher pressure required to trigger the alarm condition. The "PAW < 5 cm H_2O" red LED and alarm operate identically to the "PAW < 20% OF SET MAX PAW" button, except that a mean airway pressure less than 5 cm H_2O will trigger the alarm.

PART IV—PEDIATRIC AND NEONATAL APPLICATION OF GENERAL-USE VENTILATORS

Many of the newer-generation ventilators are capable of ventilating patients of all sizes, from small infants to large adults. Chapter 12 of this text provides information on the adult application of many of these ventilators. This section will review the neonatal and pediatric application of five of these ventilators: the Cardinal Health AVEA, the Dräger EvitaXL, the Hamilton GALILEO Gold, the Maquet Servo[i], and the Puritan Bennett 840™.

CARDINAL HEALTH AVEA VENTILATOR—INFANT/ PEDIATRIC USE

The AVEA ventilator, like many fourth-generation ventilators, is designed for use in adult, pediatric, and neonatal patients, including very low-birth-weight (VLBW) infants.[17,18] A complete description of the AVEA ventilator appears in Chapter 12 of this text (see also Figure 12-1). This section reviews application of the AVEA in infant and pediatric patients.

The AVEA is available in three models: the Standard, the Plus, and the Comprehensive. All three models are designed to provide a hot-wire proximal airway flow sensor for ventilation in infant and pediatric settings. The Plus and Comprehensive models also offer a variable-orifice flow sensor and proximal airway monitoring. Heliox (helium/oxygen) delivery is available in the Comprehensive model or can be added as an option in the other two models. In addition, the Comprehensive model is also capable of tandem connection for independent lung ventilation.

Patient Circuit and Flow Sensor

For patients weighing 5 kg or less, an infant circuit is recommended. The circuit available from AVEA has a compressible volume of approximately 1 mL/cm H_2O. For patients in the 5-kg to 20-kg weight range, a pediatric circuit can be used. The compressible volume of this circuit is approximately 2 mL/cm H_2O.

A proximal airway flow sensor is recommended when the AVEA is used with infants weighing less than 5 kg.[17,18] The ventilator's internal inspiratory and expiratory flow sensors are not accurate for volume monitoring in these patients. Moreover, circuit compliance is not factored into volume measurement when the infant patient's size range is selected. The ventilator's accompanying **hot-wire flow sensor** (Figure 13-39) is compatible in applications in which a maximum flow rate is less than 30 L/min. Another accompanying sensor, a **variable-orifice flow pneumotachometer** called the VarFlex, is available in two sizes: Neonatal and Pediatric/Adult. The Neonatal VarFlex (Figure 13-40) is recommended for applications in which maximum flow is less than 30 L/min. The Pediatric/Adult size is designed for flows between 1.2 L/min and 180 L/min.

Both the hot-wire and Neonatal VarFlex flow sensors are reliable proximal airway monitors. Dead space volume for the hot-wire sensor and the Neonatal VarFlex sensor is 0.7 mL and 0.8 mL, respectively. The Pediatric/Adult VarFlex has a dead space volume of 9.6 mL, making it less useful in smaller pediatric patients.

When heliox delivery is needed, the AVEA's monitoring data and graphics adjust automatically for gas density if the ventilator's VarFlex flow sensors or internal inspiratory and expiratory flow sensors are used. The hot-wire flow sensor will not function with heliox mixtures.

Because of the importance of monitoring end-tidal CO_2 during infant ventilation, some clinicians use a capnographic monitoring device, such as the Novametrix Cosmo Plus monitor. Capnography is described in Chapter 8. The Cosmo Plus uses a single sensor at the proximal airway to provide simultaneous monitoring of flow/time (i.e., volume) and end-tidal CO_2. This minimizes the mechanical dead space volume and eliminates the need for more than one airway-monitoring device. This also provides the clinician with additional information, including CO_2 elimination and dead space measurements. Two possible concerns exist when the Cosmo Plus is used. One is the weight of the sensor on an artificial airway. Another is the tendency for readings to be "blanked out" when water condensation accumulates in the device.

For patients weighing more than 5 kg, the AVEA's internal inspiratory and expiratory flow sensors are reliable for flow and volume-monitoring. A proximal airway sensor is not necessary for larger patients unless volumetric CO_2 monitoring is desired. When the clinician ventilates patients in this larger (pediatric) size range, the ventilator's compressible volume compensation needs to be active.

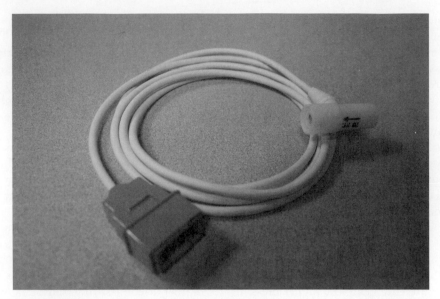

FIGURE 13-39 Hot-wire flow sensor for the AVEA Infant Circuit. (Courtesy Cardinal Health, McGaw Park, Ill., which owns Viasys Healthcare, Critical Care Division, Palm Springs, Calif.)

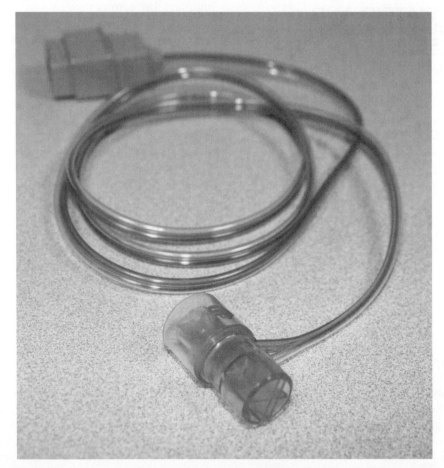

FIGURE 13-40 Photograph of the Neonatal VarFlex variable-orifice flow sensor recommended for applications in which maximum flow is less than 30 L/min. (Courtesy Cardinal Health, McGaw Park, Ill., which owns Viasys Healthcare, Critical Care Division, Palm Springs, Calif.)

Patient Size Selection

The infant patient size range is used for patients weighing 5 kg or less. Most clinicians select the pediatric patient size range for patients greater than 5 kg but less than 20 kg.

The ventilator is designed to provide flow and volume limits that are greater than the average-size patient (i.e., an infant or pediatric patient) requires. For example, a patient who weighs 7 kg can be ventilated by means of the infant patient size range with TCPL ventilation, because the flow and pressure available from the ventilator are adequate for this patient's size. As another example, if the pressure-control mode is desired, the operator can select either the infant or pediatric patient size and the ventilator will provide adequate flow and pressure to support ventilation. Box 13-13 lists the ranges for rate, volume, pressure, and flow based on patient size.

Modes of Ventilation

One of the advantages to using the AVEA in the neonatal/pediatric setting is the availability of modes not offered by most ventilators that are specifically designed for infant/pediatric use. Although most infants can be effectively managed in the TCPL mode, those with more complex problems may benefit from features such as descending-flow pattern available with pressure-control ventilation or from a combination of pressure control and pressure-support breaths (e.g., SIMV-PC plus pressure-support ventilation [PSV]). In some cases, better results may be attained with a pressure-limited, volume-targeted mode, such as PRVC (See Chapter 11 for additional information on PRVC.) These modes are available with the AVEA.

In the pediatric patient size range with the AVEA, the clinician can select pressure-targeted and volume-targeted modes as well as PRVC (delivered by SIMV) or CMV. Spontaneous breaths in SIMV can be pressure-supported, or pressure support can be selected as a separate mode. CPAP is also available. These options offer the clinician flexibility in achieving optimal ventilator settings for a variety of patients, including those with highly irregular spontaneous breathing patterns.

Another mode available in the pediatric patient size range—airway pressure release ventilation (APRV), which is also called biphasic—is available. In APRV (biphasic), the ventilator permits spontaneous breaths to be pressure-supported, if desired. (See Chapter 11 for additional information on APRV.)

TCPL is available in either CMV or SIMV when the infant patient size range is needed. The same modes offered in the pediatric patient size range are also available in the infant range, with the exception of APRV. In addition, the option to add sigh breaths is not available when the infant patient size range is selected.

Settings for the TCPL mode with the AVEA are very similar to those of other ventilators. The tidal volume delivered to the patient is a function of flow and set inspiratory pressure level (PIP) over the selected inspiratory

time. As in other pressure modes, the actual peak pressure achieved for each breath is a combination of the set inspiratory pressure level and the PEEP.

Experience with infants who have high physiologic dead space has led to the use of pressure-controlled ventilation (PCV) in its assist/control (A/C) form. Examples of patients who benefit from this strategy are those with congenital diaphragmatic hernia, hypoplastic lung syndromes, or congenital cystic adenomatoid malformation. Many of these patients require a high level of minute ventilation. Because of high ventilation/perfusion relationships, patients may be permitted to spontaneously breathe with minimum pharmacologic suppression of the ventilatory effort. Many of these patients breathe at spontaneous rates as high as 100 breaths/min.

BOX 13-13   Rate, Volume, Pressure, and Flow Ranges According to Patient Size Selection for the AVEA Ventilator

Displayed Control
Infant
Pediatric
Adult

Rate
1-150 breaths/min
1-150 breaths/min
1-120 breaths/min

Tidal Volume
2.0-300 mL
25-500 mL
0.10-2.5 L

Volume Limit (Pressure-Limited Breaths)
2.0-300 mL
2.0-750 mL
0.10 to 2.5 L

Machine Volume (Mach Vol)
2.0-300 mL
25-500 mL
0.10-2.5 L

Inspiratory Pressure
0-80 cm H_2O
0-90 cm H_2O
0-90 cm H_2O

Peak Flow
0.4-30 L/min
1-75 L/min
3-150 L/min

Maximum Flow
≤50 L/min
≤120 L/min
>200 L/min

Inspiratory Time (in seconds)
0.15-3 s
0.2-5 s
0.2-5 s

Pressure Support
0-80 cm H_2O
0-90 cm H_2O
0-90 cm H_2O

To effectively use PCV, set a safe minimum breath rate as a backup. The set rate is below the patient's baseline spontaneous rate. Inspiratory time can also be set as a backup, because actual inspiratory time can be determined through analysis of the patient's spontaneous pattern. For example, by viewing the patient's graphics of flow and pressure and monitoring the patient's actual inspiratory time, one can adjust a flow-cycle control to allow the patient to flow-terminate each breath, rather than time-terminate the breath.

Because appropriate patient-triggering is essential, the flow trigger control is set to be as sensitive as possible to patient effort, while still preventing autotriggering of the ventilator.

Summary

The AVEA is capable of ventilating adults and pediatric or neonatal patients. With this range of patient capabilities, the AVEA offers flexibility in use. It is advised that the user of the infant and pediatric applications with the Cardinal Health AVEA follow the operating manual for the ventilator they are using and check the ventilator itself to be sure what options are available.

DRÄGER EvitaXL VENTILATOR— INFANT/PEDIATRIC USE

The Dräger EvitaXL is designed for patients with a body weight of at least 3 kg (6.6 lb); furthermore, with the Neo-Flow™ option added, it can be used to ventilate infants weighing less than 3 kg. A complete description of the EvitaXL ventilator appears in Chapter 12 (see Figure 12-33). The EvitaXL can be used in infants and children as either an invasive or a noninvasive ventilator. Noninvasive support requires the use of manufacturer-provided nasal and facial masks in sizes suitable for infants and pediatric patients.[19]

Patient Circuit and Humidification

Disposable pediatric patient circuits having a compressible volume of approximately 2 mL/cm H_2O are recommended for patients in the 5-kg to 20-kg weight range. An infant circuit, typically with a compressible volume of 1 mL/cm H_2O or less, is recommended for patients weighing less than 6 kg.

The manufacturer recommends installing the Fisher & Paykel Healthcare MR850 humidifier on any EvitaXL that is to be used with infants or small children. This humidifier's heating chamber has a lower compliance than do most standard units.

Other than the aforementioned circuit modifications, pediatric patients weighing 6 kg or more can be ventilated with the EvitaXL by selecting all modes and settings that are used in adults. (See Chapter 12, the section on the EvitaXL, for further information.)

Beginning Ventilation

When the ventilator is first switched on and the start screen is displayed (see Figure 12-36), the clinician may choose "Previous Patient" to start ventilation using the most recent settings. Alternately, the clinician can choose "New Patient" and select either the "Adult" or "Ped." range. Once the range is selected, the patient's ideal body weight (IBW) is set by using the touch control on the right of the screen. At the bottom of the screen, initial default settings are displayed. These are the settings at which the ventilator will operate if no setting adjustments are made.

NeoFlow™

With patients weighing less than 6 kg, the NeoFlow™ option is essential. As is the case in the adult/pediatric setting, with the NeoFlow™ option, both invasive and noninvasive applications are available.

NeoFlow™ requires the placement of a flow sensor between the artificial airway and the Y-connector of the patient circuit. The flow sensor's cable is connected to the back of the ventilator unit. Before the flow sensor is positioned at the artificial airway, it must be calibrated at 0 flow. This calibration is performed at set-up as part of the preuse check and then at least once every 24 hours (see the operator's manual). If the flow sensor is removed for cleaning or is exchanged, recalibration is also required.

When the NeoFlow™ sensor and cable are connected to the ventilator, the clinician can select either "Ped" or "Neo." from the start screen.

Once NeoFlow™ is activated, a continuous base flow of 6 L/min of bias flow is maintained in the patient circuit. In addition to a continuous base flow of 6 L/min, the infant may obtain additional flow on demand. As soon as the patient begins inspiration, the unit delivers additional flow to maintain the 6 L/min baseline, thus keeping flow compatible with the patient's needs.

NeoFlow™ Sensor Function

The NeoFlow™ sensor enables flow triggering and pressure monitoring at the proximal airway, as well as monitoring of the artificial airway for leaks.

The NeoFlow™ sensor detects the patient's inspiratory effort and is responsible for triggering any assisted breaths or any patient-initiated gas flow from the ventilator. To prevent inappropriate triggering due to leaks around the ETT, the ventilator takes into account the flow sensor signal (inspiratory flow) plus the calculated leak flow (minute ventilation leak [MVleak]), if any. A trigger range of 0.3 L/min to 3 L/min is recommended for neonatal and pediatric ventilation. Rise time is adjustable with the flow sensor in place.

If the sensor detects an excessive amount of gas leak or if it becomes partially occluded with water or secretions, it will cease operation and trigger audible and visual alarms. When this occurs the ventilator will continue to operate in the pressure-control mode. The pressure applied is the last peak pressure measured during a mandatory breath. Inspiratory time, breath frequency, F_IO_2, and PEEP remain the same as the set values. However, volume, pressure, leak monitoring, and patient triggering will be interrupted.

The leaks that normally occur around uncuffed infant ETTs can be monitored with the NeoFlow™ sensor. The displayed value for an MVleak represents the difference between inspiratory and expiratory flow averaged over time and is displayed as a percentage of the delivered inspired minute volume on the ventilator monitor screen. The unit assumes that any gas that does not flow back through the sensor from the patient must have escaped through a leak around the ETT and out through the patient's upper airway. The unit automatically corrects V_T (inspiratory and expiratory) and flow values based on its calculation of the leak.

Modes of Ventilation with NeoFlow™

The modes and features specific to NeoFlow™ include volume ventilation with either CMV, mandatory minute ventilation (MMV), or SIMV; AutoFlow™; and PSV (i.e., assisted spontaneous breathing [ASB]). Pressure support is available in combination with mandatory breaths or as a separate mode, with apnea backup ventilation. (See Chapter 12 for information on modes of ventilation with the EvitaXL.) Box 13-14 contains important information about volume ventilation with pediatric patients.

Because its use with the NeoFlow™ sensor is slightly different, AutoFlow™ will be reviewed here. AutoFlow™ is a self-regulating mode of ventilation where breaths are pressure-limited and volume-targeted to the set volume. (See Chapter 11 for further information.) With the sensor in place, AutoFlow™ functions in CMV, SIMV, and MMV modes. When any of these modes is selected, AutoFlow™ allows the patient to breathe spontaneously at any time. Without the sensor, the ventilator cannot provide volume targeted ventilation, although pressure-targeted, time-cycled ventilation is available. As is the case when Auto-Flow™ is used in the adult, it is important to set the upper Paw alarm limit so that if the patient's lung characteristics change or there is a sudden change in airway leak, the patient will be protected from high pressures. (See Chapter 12, the section on the Dräger EvitaXL, for information on AutoFlow™ use in the adult patient.)

When AutoFlow™ is initiated in neonates with the flow sensor attached, the unit provides two test breaths, first with a pressure of 5 cm H_2O and then with a pressure equal to 75% of that required to deliver the set volume. The third breath is at a pressure determined to be appropriate to achieve the set V_T. The ventilator automatically adjusts the pressure up and down in order to maintain the target volume. The maximum ventilating pressure is the high-pressure limit −5 cm H_2O, and the lowest ventilating pressure is the PEEP or baseline pressure setting.

Backup Ventilation

As is the case in adult and pediatric ventilation, the EvitaXL will provide backup ventilation for spontaneous modes when operating in the "Neo." setting. However, unlike the "Adult" or "Peds." setting, apnea ventilation in the "Neo." setting defaults to pressure control. The clinician selects apnea frequency (f_{apnea}) and pressure above PEEP (P_{apnea}). The I:E ratio is fixed.

Nebulizer Operation

When administering aerosolized medications to infants and pediatric patients through the ventilator circuit, a removable nebulizer should be used. The nebulizer is placed inline for medication delivery and then removed when the treatment is completed. Use of the EvitaXL's nebulizer in the "Neo." setting increases the base flow from 6 L/min to 9 L/min. Delivered oxygen concentrations drop slightly from the level set. The amount of drop is less than 4% at breath rates greater than 12 per minute. When operating at mandatory breath rates of less that 12 per minute, the nebulizer should **NOT** be used, because of the potential significant drop in oxygen concentration.

Summary

The EvitaXL is fully capable of ventilating the pediatric or neonatal patient. With its range of features designed specifically for use in every size of patient, routine applications can be effectively managed. It is advised that the user of the infant and pediatric applications with the Dräger EvitaXL follow the operating manual for the ventilator they are using and check the ventilator to be sure what options are available.

HAMILTON GALILEO GOLD— INFANT AND PEDIATRIC APPLICATIONS*

The GALILEO Gold features options for the ventilation of infants and children as well as for adult patients.[20] Infant and pediatric applications are accessible from the set-up screen. Once the ventilator is powered on, the set-up screen appears. In the lower right-hand corner of the set-up screen is a standard set-up box where the appropriate application may be chosen (see Figure 12-46). If you highlight and

---

BOX 13-14	Volume Ventilation in Pediatric Patients

It is important to note that volume delivery in volume-targeted modes in the "Ped." size range are accurate only to ±10% of the set tidal volume, or 10 mL, whichever is greater. Because of this, some clinicians prefer to use the NeoFlow™ sensor with smaller pediatric patients. Alternatively, with these patients, some clinicians prefer to select a pressure-targeted mode when the EvitaXL is in use. They then monitor tidal volume delivery using the Novametrix Cosmo Plus or a similar monitoring device.

---

*A special thanks to Melissa Turner, Application Specialist for Hamilton Medical, for her assistance with this section.

select either the infant or the pediatric application, then that selection becomes active.

The pediatric application is used for patients who weigh between 3 kg and 42 kg (IBW). The infant application is intended for patients who weigh up to 10 kg (IBW). If a patient application must be changed after ventilation has started, the operator can do so by selecting "MODES," then "PATIENT," and, finally, the desired application.

Patient Circuit and Flow Sensor

The pediatric circuit size may be either 15-mm ID or 22-mm ID depending on the patient's size. The circuit used for the infant application is a 10-mm ID circuit.

As is the case in the adult application, a proximal flow sensor is used for monitoring (see Figure 12-47). The use of the flow sensor enables measurement of all parameters directly at the patient airway. The flow sensor needs to be calibrated before placing the ventilator on the patient. The flow sensor used for pediatric patients is the same one used for adult patients. The infant-size flow sensor must be used in the infant application.

Parameter Settings

The monitored parameters and alarms that are available for use with the pediatric population are the same as those for use with the adult population.

Parameter values in the pediatric population are limited to specific patient sizes. For example, in the adult application, the set range for tidal volume is 100 mL to 2000 mL, whereas in the pediatric application, the tidal volume range is only 20 mL to 300 mL.

In infant use, parameter values are limited to ranges that are safe for infant application. A list of all the available parameters and their ranges is found in the operator's manual.[20] Monitored parameter and alarm availability is identical to that available for use in the adult application. Setting the parameters is described in Chapter 12. The special consideration required in the selection of trigger sensitivity, expiratory trigger sensitivity, and T_I Max (maximum inspiratory time) will be reviewed here.

The default trigger type for infants is flow. If the leak flow around the ETT becomes higher than the flow trigger, autocycling will occur. For example, if the flow trigger is set to 0.5 L/min and the leak around the ETT is 2 L/min, the ventilator will begin autocycling. In this example, the operator needs to raise the flow-trigger setting to 2.5 L/min to prevent autocycling. The patient then actually triggers breaths at 0.5 L/min, because 2.5 L/min −2.0 L/min is 0.5 L/min. The flow trigger needs to be assessed and adjusted from time to time, because the leak may vary according to the patient's position.

The expiratory trigger sensitivity (ETS) control is used in all applications (i.e., infant, pediatric, and adult) to end inspiration. (See Chapter 12, GALILEO, for a description of ETS.) However, if gas leakage around the ETT is significant, the ETS criteria may never be reached. Because uncuffed ETTs are used for infants, there may be signifi-

cant leaks and the function of the ETS control may be affected. The "T_I Max" control is set for spontaneous breaths in modes that allow for spontaneous breathing. This would include P-SIMV, adaptive pressure ventilation SIMV (APVsimv), DuoPAP, APRV, and SPONT. T_I Max provides a backup, so inspiration can be terminated. Once T_I Max is reached, the GALILEO will switch over to exhalation.

Modes of Ventilation

In the pediatric application, the modes available are identical to those used in the adult application. (See Modes of Ventilation for the GALILEO in Chapter 12 for definitions and descriptions of modes.)

The modes available in the infant application are listed in Box 13-15. APVcmv and APVsimv are recommended for use with infants who weigh from 2 kg to 10 kg, because the lowest tidal volume that may be set for these modes is 10 mL. (NOTE: Tidal volume settings to 2 mL are currently pending U.S. Food and Drug Administration approval.) All other modes may be used with infants who weigh less than 2 kg and up to 10 kg.

The adaptive support ventilation (ASV) mode, which is described in Chapter 12, is not available in the infant application, although it may be used for patients weighing more than 3 kg. If ASV is used, the pediatric application must be selected to access this mode.

Special Considerations

The integrated nebulizer available with the GALILEO Gold is not recommended in the infant application if the nebulizer volume is greater than 50% of the total delivered volume. For example, if the tidal volume is 6 mL and the nebulizer volume if 5 mL, use of the nebulizer is not recommended. (NOTE: The nebulizer can generally be selected for use anytime, because its function will automatically be suppressed if the nebulizer volume condition is met.)

The maximum inspiratory or expiratory hold time is 3 seconds in the infant modes as opposed to the 10-second maximum in the adult or pediatric modes.

BOX 13-15	Infant Modes on the GALILEO Gold

P-A/C / P-CMV (Pressure Control),
P-SIMV,
APVcmv,
APVsimv,
DuoPAP,
APRV, and
SPONT.

P-A/C, Pressure–*assist*/control ventilation; **P-CMV,** *pressure–continuous mandatory ventilation;* **P-SIMV,** *pressure–synchronized intermittent mandatory ventilation;* **APVcmv,** adaptive pressure ventilation, continuous mandatory ventilation; **APVsimv,** adaptive pressure ventilation, synchronized intermittent mandatory ventilation; **APRV,** airway pressure-release ventilation; **SPONT.,** spontaneous breathing.

Summary

The GALILEO Gold is available for neonatal, pediatric, and adult use and provides a variety of available modes for these applications. It is advised that the users of the infant and pediatric applications with the GALILEO Gold follow the operator's manual for the correct version of the ventilator they are using and check the ventilator to be sure what options have been added.

MAQUET Servo[i] VENTILATOR—NEONATAL AND PEDIATRIC APPLICATIONS*

The Maquet Servo[i] Ventilator, described in Chapter 12, has two patient categories: adult and infant.[21,22] The adult category has adequate parameter ranges to include both pediatric and adult patients. For example, the tidal volume range in the adult mode is 100 mL to 4000 mL, which allows for the ventilation of children and adults. The infant tidal volume ranges from 2 mL to 350 mL, which allows for the ventilation of very small infants.

Neonatal Application

The Servo[i] can be factory-set to fit the specific sizes of patients with whom it will be used. Optional designs consist of universal (infant to adult), adult only, or infant only.

From the standby screen the operator selects the appropriate patient category. The standby screen appears when the ventilator is turned on. When the infant option is selected, an icon of a pink baby will appear in the upper left-hand corner of the operating screen. (NOTE: This icon changes to a blue adult when in the adult option.) (See Chapter 12, the section on the Maquet Servo[i] ventilator, for more information.) In the neonatal option, the maximum available flow is 33 L/min, with a circulating bias flow of 0.5 L/min.

Patient Circuit and Proximal Airway Sensor Monitoring

It is recommended that a low-compliance infant circuit be used for infants and a low-compliance pediatric circuit be used for pediatric patients. (NOTE: The user is not required to use a patient circuit provided by the company, Maquet, Inc.) For safety reasons, the maximum available flow for the infant application is 33 L/min. For this reason, an infant circuit is recommended when ventilating an infant.

The Servo[i] has an airway sensor (differential pressure transducer) that can be positioned at the upper airway. The dead space of the sensor is less than 0.45 mL. The airway sensor monitors pressure and flow measurements. The

flow-measuring rate is 0.125 L/min to 40 L/min (2 to 667 mL/s). When the airway sensor is in place, the measured parameters from the sensor are displayed on the user interface (main screen). The message "Y-sensor" is visible at the top-left corner of each waveform graph. A Y-sensor test is part of the preuse check/patient circuit test. (NOTE: Use of the airway sensor during neonatal ventilation is optional.)

During ventilation, if the Y-sensor becomes compromised because of secretions, water, or surfactant accumulating in the sensor or sensor lines, the ventilator will automatically disable the Y-sensor measurements and revert to the internal measurements and will display these values. The ventilator gives an audible signal and displays a message to indicate that the Y-sensor has been disabled and an assessment of the equipment must be performed. If the sensor becomes inactive, this does not affect patient-triggering or the mode of ventilation. In response to a patient's inspiratory effort, the ventilator is sufficiently rapid to provide quick breath delivery without relying on a proximal sensing device to do so.

A circuit compliance feature is available in the infant volume ventilation modes. This feature can be used in combination with the Y-sensor. When it is used, the ventilator automatically compensates for volume loss in the selected patient circuit and delivers the selected volumes to the patient. (See Chapter 11 for additional information on compressible volume/tubing compliance.)

Any device placed inline with the patient circuit can have an impact on the compressible volume. Consequently, all of the parts that will be included in the patient circuit need to be placed inline before a patient circuit test is performed. This test checks the circuit for leaks and also determines the circuit's compressible volume. For example, if a heated humidifier will be placed in the circuit, it is recommended that the humidifier be filled with water to the recommended level before a patient circuit test is performed. Otherwise, if the humidifier is filled after it is connected to the patient, this will affect the compressible volume and volume delivery.

Controls and Alarms

The parameter controls are used the same way in the infant mode as they are in the adult mode. These were described in the section on the Maquet Servo[i] ventilator in Chapter 12. Alarm parameters in the infant category are the same as in the adult/pediatric configuration, but with different ranges appropriate for infants. Alarms are adjusted by using the alarm profile key in the upper right-hand corner of the user interface (fixed key) (Box 13-16).

Modes of Ventilation

The infant configuration of the Servo[i] ventilator comes standard with the following modes of ventilation available: pressure control, SIMV pressure, and pressure support/CPAP. In addition, other modes of ventilation can be added, including volume control, SIMV volume, volume

---

*A special thanks to Carla Terlaje and Christian Joseph, Clinical Application. Specialists, Maquet, Inc., for their assistance with this section.

support, PRVC, and BiVent (airway pressure-release ventilation). (NOTE: Because PRVC and volume support are closed-loop modes, they are not recommended for use when there is a leak, such as around the ETT.) Chapter 12 provides a description of the available modes available with the Servo[i]. The ventilator also has noninvasive modes available for infants. These include nasal CPAP (nCPAP), NIV pressure support, and NIV pressure control.

It is worth mentioning a few special situations that can occur when a clinician is setting up various modes of ventilation.

During pressure-targeted ventilation, if the patient tries to exhale during inspiration, this will result in a pressure increase. When the pressure increases to 3 cm H_2O above the set inspiratory pressure, the exhalation valve opens and regulates the pressure down to the set level. If the patient coughs and the pressure increases to the upper pressure-limit setting, the expiratory valve will open and inspiration will end. (NOTE: Reaching the upper pressure limit during inspiration in any mode will end inspiration.)

PS modes (patient-triggered, pressure-limited, flow-cycled) include both pressure-support (PS) and volume-support (VS) modes. The latter (VS) not only meets the other criteria for a PS breath, but it is also volume-targeted.

In a PS mode, inspiration ends when a specific flow is detected (flow-cycled). (See Chapter 11 for more information about flow-cycling.) It is important to set the flow-cycling value appropriately. If it is set at too high of a percent, it may shorten the patient's inspiratory phase and tidal volume delivery may be too short. On the other hand, if it is set too low, inspiration may be prolonged and the patient may try to actively exhale. Consequently, the practitioner needs to monitor the patient and ventilation parameters when adjusting inspiratory flow cycle.

Apnea backup ventilation is available for modes such as PSV or VS, in which spontaneous ventilation is possible. For example, during PSV, the clinician can set a backup ventilating pressure that the infant will receive if apnea occurs. In the VS mode the clinician can select a backup volume. (NOTE: Backup is not applicable in NIV nasal CPAP. This mode is selected only for patients who are capable of sustaining spontaneous ventilation.)

During backup ventilation, the ventilator uses default settings for the I:E ratio (1:2), respiratory rate (30 breaths/

min for infants), and inspiratory rise time (5%). On the alarm-profile screen the clinician can also select the amount of time he wants to elapse before apnea ventilation becomes activated. In the infant the time range is 5 seconds to 45 seconds.

When apnea backup ventilation begins, an audible and visual high-priority alarm occurs. A message appears on the window that states "Ventilating in Back-up Mode. Change mode or go back to support mode!" The clinician responds on the basis of the situation. If the patient is still capable of supporting spontaneous ventilation, the support mode selection is chosen. However, if the patient is no longer capable of supporting spontaneous breathing, "Change mode" is selected and then the practitioner can select the appropriate mode and parameters for the patient.

Patient Monitoring

Monitoring of patient-measured values is done by viewing the column on the right-hand side of the user interface (see Figure 12-72). Using the "Additional Values" soft key, the clinician can scroll through additional monitoring options. "Additional Values" includes a third page that displays calculated values. These mechanics require an inspiratory or expiratory hold, or both. Care should be taken when performing these measurements with uncuffed ETTs, because this can yield erroneous results.

Special Considerations

A few special situations that might occur with the Servo[i] in the infant category will be discussed here.

Trigger Sensitivity

Flow triggering in the infant setting during invasive ventilation provides the sensing mechanism for patient triggering. If a leak occurs, it is important that the trigger sensitivity be set appropriately to prevent autotriggering. It may be necessary to set the trigger sensitivity to a pressure trigger, depending on the amount of leakage.

Noninvasive Ventilation—Nasal CPAP

General use of NIV with the Servo[i] is described in Chapter 12. However, nasal CPAP as an NIV option will be briefly reviewed in this chapter.

Nasal CPAP is a NIV option for infants weighing from 500 g to 10 kg. When NIV nCPAP is started, the ventilator begins a "waiting" period. During this time a window appears on the screen with the words "Time in waiting position." All patient-related alarms, except O_2, are inactivated. This provides the clinician enough time to get the patient set up on the device. In the waiting position, the ventilator will not deliver a massive flow of air, which prevents patient discomfort. Once the patient is connected and initiates an inspiratory effort, the ventilator will provide flow. (NOTE: The user can also press the "Start ventilation" soft key to start flow to the patient.)

During nCPAP, the ventilator provides enough flow to maintain the pressure set (range: 2 to 20 cm H_2O). If a leak occurs around the prongs, the ventilator will automatically and immediately increase the flow to maintain the pressure. The amount of flow available to the infant is 33 L/min.

Leaks during nCPAP therapy can change considerably. To reduce the frequency of nuisance alarms, the user has the option of turning off the audio portion of the following alarms:

·   High and Low Minute Volume
·   High and Low Respiratory Rate
·   High and Low CPAP

If a leak exceeds 10 L/min (in the infant mode) or if the patient is disconnected, a high-priority alarm occurs and the available bias flow drops to 7.5 L/min. This helps prevent excessive flow from being accidentally directed into an infant's eyes. The practitioner needs to evaluate the cause of the excessive leak and reposition or change the size of the nasal prongs.

Summary

The Servo^i ventilator has the ability to ventilate small infants to adult-sized patients, with appropriate parameter ranges and flows available to all categories. It is advised that the users of the infant or adult applications with the Servo^i follow the operator's manual for the Servo^i ventilator they are using and check the unit to be sure what options have been included for use.

PURITAN BENNETT 840™ VENTILATOR—INFANT/ PEDIATRIC USE

A complete description of the Puritan Bennett 840™ ventilator appears in Chapter 12 (see Figure 12-89). The Puritan Bennett 840™ is designed for use in adult and pediatric patients of at least 7-kg IBW or approximately 15-lb IBW. With the "NeoMode" option, this ventilator can also be used in infants who weigh as little as 0.5-kg IBW (1.1-lb IBW).[23]

Noninvasive support for infants and pediatric patients is also available with the use of nasal and facial masks and nasal prongs. Box 13-17 gives examples of some interfaces that work well with the 840 in NIV.

BOX 13-17	Noninvasive Interfaces for Infant and Pediatric Use with the PB840

Some examples of full-face masks that work well for pediatric patients are the ResMed nonvented Mirage (ResMed, Poway, Calif.) and the Puritan Bennett Full Face Mask. Examples of nasal masks that work well with the Puritan Bennett 840 are the various sizes of the nonvented ResMed Ultra Mirage™. The infant nasal-prong interfaces that work well with the 840 include the Sherwood Davis & Geck Argyle and the Hudson RCI CPAP cannulas.

Pediatric Use

The following section includes information appropriate for setting the PB840 for use with pediatric patients.

Circuit, Humidification, and Preuse Test

It is recommended that disposable circuits having a compressible volume of approximately 2 mL/cm H_2O be used for patients in the 7- to 24-kg weight range. (NOTE: For patients who weigh less than 7 kg, infant circuits with a compressible volume of 1 mL/cm H_2O should be used.)

For humidification, the manufacturer recommends installing a Fisher & Paykel Healthcare humidifier or a unit with similar features. The humidifier must have a heating chamber with low compliance that is suitable for pediatric/neonatal use.

Pediatric patients weighing more than 7 kg can be ventilated with the 840, but the operator must be careful to select the same modes and settings that are used in adults with respect to the appropriate humidifier, patient circuit, and inspiratory and expiratory filters.

When the ventilator is first switched on, the system conducts the POST (power-on self-test) and then displays the ventilator start-up screen. On this screen the user must select "Same Patient," "New Patient," or "SST" (short self-test). If SST is chosen, a 10-minute warm-up or stabilization period is recommended. During the SST, the user will be asked to select neonatal, pediatric, or adult patient. The ventilator will measure the compressible volume of the circuit during this test. After the SST the clinician will be asked to enter the IBW, which will result in default settings that are weight-based.

Aside from circuit and humidifier considerations, no modifications to the 840 are necessary for pediatric (i.e., nonneonatal) use. Both volume-targeted and pressure-targeted modes are available. However, some clinicians prefer to monitor tidal volume and other parameters at the upper airway by using an adjunct monitor such as the Novametrix Cosmo Plus. The VC+ mode (dual–pressure/volume delivery mode) or proportional assist ventilation (PAV) also can be used with pediatric patients.

Neonatal Use of the PB840

The 840 can be equipped with optional NeoMode software designed to make the ventilator capable of ventilating neonates weighing 0.5 kg to 7 kg. This software permits the controlled delivery of tidal volume as low as 5 mL and extends the maximum mandatory breath rate up to 150 breaths/min. The software also adds flow sensitivity from 0.1 L/min to 10 L/min to enable breath triggering and to compensate for leaks (Table 13-8). Pressure triggering is not available. In addition to the software, the ventilator must be fitted with a neonatal expiratory block and filter.

The 840 NeoMode option also provides heightened rise-time adjustment sensitivity and greater flow-termination adjustment than is available with the adult version.

TABLE 13-8

Specifications for NeoMode Software in the Puritan-Bennett 840™ Ventilator

Parameter	Range
Expiratory sensitivity	1-80%
Flow pattern	Square or descending ramp
Flow sensitivity	0.1-10 L/min
Ideal body weight	0.5-7 kg
Inspiratory time	0.2-8.0 s
Mandatory breath type	Volume-controlled or pressure-controlled
Peak flow	1.0-30 L/min
Respiratory rate	1-150 breaths/min
Spontaneous breath type	Pressure-supported or not pressure-supported (none)
Tidal volume	5-315 mL
Trigger type	Flow only
Interface type	Neonatal nasal CPAP prongs

NIV with CPAP nasal prongs is also easily accomplished by using this software modification.

CHAPTER SUMMARY

The ventilators discussed in this chapter represent those that are widely used in the infant and pediatric settings. In many clinical settings, mechanical ventilation is provided to patients of all ages and sizes by staff members who also work with this wide range of patients. In such settings, a ventilator that is easily adapted to fit any need presents a cost savings and time savings in terms of staff technical training. General-purpose ventilators that were originally designed to be used with adults have been found to be easily adapted to pediatric applications and, in some cases, to neonatal applications.

Infant and pediatric ventilators will continue to be developed, particularly to provide better monitoring capabilities. Additional developments in specialized applications unique to the neonatal/pediatric population are certain, including ventilatory support to spontaneously breathing patients and high-frequency technology. In addition, some clinicians have shown interest in ventilators capable of delivering subambient oxygen concentrations. Others have envisioned systems capable of providing specialty gases, such as nitric oxide and heliox. In the planning stages for years, prototype closed-loop systems that monitor arterial blood and expired gases and adjust their own ventilator settings are now being tested.

As with all technology, necessity drives the scope and the direction of advancement. As clinical problems present themselves, technical innovation will provide more-sophisticated solutions. Factors such as medical advances, economics, demographics, and even ideology will continue to affect the infant/pediatric ventilator market.

KEY POINTS

▶ The Cardinal Health Infant Flow generator consists of two fluidic jets, which on inspiration direct flow through the nasal prongs; on expiration, pressure from the expiratory gas flow "flips" the direction of flow away from the prongs and through an expiratory port.

▶ With the Cardinal Health AirLife™ Infant nCPAP System, the clinician sets the desired nCPAP and the AirLife™ Infant nCPAP System adjusts the flow to achieve the desired pressure levels and to compensate for leaks, which helps to maintain a constant level of nCPAP.

▶ When using the Cardinal Health Infant Flow SiPAP™, the clinician can set both an inspiratory and an expiratory pressure by adjusting the two flowmeters.

▶ Because of the flow generator's design in the Hamilton ARABELLA noninvasive CPAP system, the flow of gas from the jet is very stable, which seems to require a more substantial patient expiratory flow to cause the device to switch into expiration.

▶ Bubble CPAP, such as the Fisher & Paykel Healthcare Bubble CPAP System, provides a single pressure and flow, but with minute oscillations around the set pressure level and has been associated with reduced incidence of chronic lung disease (CLD) in premature infants.

▶ With the Cardinal Health V.I.P. Bird, flow triggering and flow cycling are accomplished by using the Bird Partner IIi volume monitor and the Infant "Smart" Flow Sensor.

▶ The termination sensitivity control on the V.I.P. Bird allows adjustment of the flow-termination point of the breath and is used only in the assist/control (A/C) time-cycled mode.

▶ Leak compensation available with volume-cycled modes on the V.I.P. Bird is recommended for use only with leaks around artificial airways and is not for use with patients who have minimal inspiratory effort and no leakage.

▶ In the V.I.P. Bird Sterling and Gold ventilators, the functions of the Partner IIi Volume Monitor have been directly incorporated into the main ventilator housing.

▶ VAPS, available on the V.I.P. Bird Gold, is a dual-control mode that begins as a pressure-targeted breath (descending flow) but switches to constant-flow delivery with a volume-target, if the *set* volume has not been achieved during the breath.

▶ With the Dräger Babylog 8000, the high-pressure alarm is automatically set to a pressure of 10 cm H_2O or a PEEP/CPAP of +4 cm H_2O. In the event of excessive pressure buildup within the circuit, the exhalation valve opens, allowing exhalation.

▶ During IMV with the Dräger Babylog 8000, the mandatory breath is time-triggered based on the rate calculation.

▶ The application of nasal CPAP with the Dräger Babylog 8000 requires disabling of the flow measurement by disconnecting the attachment from the proximal flow sensor and pressing the reset/check button.

KEY POINTS—cont'd

▶ The volume guarantee feature on the Dräger Babylog 8000plus provides pressure-limited ventilation with a volume target (a dual-control mode) and can be used only when the airway flow sensor is in use.

▶ The Bunnell Life Pulse High-Frequency Jet Ventilator is a microprocessor-controlled, pressure-limited, TC, constant-flow, high-frequency jet ventilator that works in conjunction with a conventional ventilator.

▶ On the Bunnell High-Frequency Jet Ventilator, an electromagnetic solenoid activates the pinch valve, which interrupts the flow of pressurized gas and gives small bursts of air to the patient's airway.

▶ The Bunnell HFJV system is indicated for patients with severe respiratory distress syndrome complicated by pulmonary air leak that has been untreatable with conventional mechanical ventilation strategies.

▶ With the SensorMedics HFO system, volume delivered by the piston is decreased as oscillatory frequency is increased.

▶ Any interruption of ventilator operation on the SensorMedics HFO system causes immediately pressurization of the circuit's three mushroom valves, allowing the circuit to open to the atmosphere.

▶ When using the SensorMedics HFO system, the mean pressure adjust control is the primary determinant of Paw, although increasing bias flow will increase Paw and changes to the power, frequency, inspiratory time, and piston-centering controls will also alter the Paw.

▶ When the SensorMedics HFO system is turned off at the power switch or the oscillator stops because of a power interruption, the audible alarm can be silenced only by pressing the reset button.

▶ Many general-use ICU ventilators now have optional neonatal software and monitoring for ventilation of very small infants.

▶ In the Cardinal Health AVEA, the Dräger EvitaXL, the Hamilton GALILEO, and the Servo[i], a proximal flow sensor is used for measuring ventilation parameters directly at the patient airway.

▶ A proximal airway flow sensor is typically recommended when a general-purpose ventilator is used for small infants (approximate weight range: 0.5 to 5 kg).

▶ When general-purpose ventilators are used on infants intubated with uncuffed ETTs, the sensitivity parameter should be set to be as sensitive as possible while still preventing autotriggering of the ventilator.

ASSESSMENT QUESTIONS

See Evolve Resources for the answers.

1. One of the most common modes of ventilation used in infants for more than 30 years is:
   a. Volume ventilation
   b. SIMV with pressure support
   c. Time-triggered, pressure-limited, time-cycled ventilation
   d. VAPS

2. Better ventilator-to-patient synchrony has been developed in infant ventilation because of the technologic advancement of which of the following devices?
   a. Floating expiratory valves
   b. Flow-sensing devices
   c. Volume-measuring devices
   d. Rapid-response pressure monitors

3. In children up to the age of 6 months, the interface most often used to provide nasal CPAP is the:
   a. Nasal prong
   b. Nasopharyngeal CPAP interface
   c. Nasal mask
   d. Nasal trumpet

4. Which of the following power sources can be used to power the Cardinal Health Infant Flow Nasal CPAP System?
   I. High-pressure air source
   II. High-pressure oxygen source
   III. An electrical source
   IV. A 12-V battery
   　a. III
   　b. I and II
   　c. III and IV
   　d. I, II, III, and IV

5. When the Cardinal Health AirLife™ nCPAP System Driver is in the standby mode, which of the following statements are true?
   I. The standby mode is activated by pressing and holding the alarm mute/reset button until a single audible sound is heard.
   II. Alarms are muted for up to 20 minutes.
   III. The high-pressure and low-flow alarms remain active. To indicate that the system is in standby mode, there is a single audible alarm burst every 2 minutes.
   IV. The operator must press the alarm mute/reset button to exit the standby mode.
   　a. I and III
   　b. II and IV
   　c. I, II, and III
   　d. I, II, III, and IV

6. When the patient takes a breath from the Cardinal Health SiPAP™, the inspiratory effort results in which of the following?
   a. Gas flow is diverted away from the expiratory limb to mix with existing inspiratory flow.
   b. The inspiratory flow is produced by the "Pres Low" flowmeter.
   c. The targeted IPAP is the "Pres High" flowmeter alone.
   d. Pressure from the patient's inspiratory flow draws gas from the expiratory limb.

ASSESSMENT QUESTIONS—cont'd

7. The Fisher & Paykel Healthcare Bubble CPAP System requires which of the following components?
   I. A humidifier chamber with a continuous-feed sterile water system
   II. A standard air/oxygen blender with standard oxygen tubing
   III. A hot-wire inspiratory limb of the patient circuit
   IV. A CPAP generator
   a. IV
   b. II and IV
   c. I, II, and III
   d. I, II, III, and IV

8. When the Bubble CPAP System is in use, the desired CPAP level is set by:
   a. Increasing the flow from the gas source
   b. Adjusting the position of the CPAP probe
   c. Increasing the generator's pressure
   d. Increasing the CPAP setting

9. When the Fisher & Paykel Healthcare MR730 humidifier is used with the Bubble CPAP System, what should the temperature control and chamber control be set for?
   a. Temperature control at 37° C and chamber control at −1
   b. Temperature control at 39° C and chamber control at +3
   c. Temperature control at 42° C and chamber control at −2
   d. Temperature control at 40° C and chamber control at −3

10. The Cardinal Health Infant Nasal CPAP System incorporates an alarm system for which of the following conditions?
    a. Spontaneous respiratory rate falling outside of set parameters
    b. F_IO_2 reading different from set F_IO_2
    c. Apnea
    d. Spontaneous minute volume falling outside of set parameters

11. Termination sensitivity is an added feature on the V.I.P. Bird ventilator that:
    a. Allows the clinician to adjust the flow-termination point of the breath
    b. Operates in all modes
    c. Can be adjusted from 0% to 55% in increments of 10%
    d. Sets the breath trigger sensitivity to patient effort

12. On the V.I.P. Bird, the termination sensitivity setting flashes when the:
    a. Breath is terminated at the set value
    b. Breath is TC
    c. Breath is both flow-triggered and flow-cycled
    d. Expiratory time is deemed too short by the ventilator's microprocessor

13. On the V.I.P. Bird, leak compensation is:
    I. Available in all modes
    II. Only available in VC modes
    III. Used to stabilize baseline pressure in the presence of leaks
    IV. Available in pressure control and PS
    a. I
    b. II
    c. IV
    d. II and III

14. The flow sensor in the Sterling and Gold versions of the V.I.P. Bird differs from the original because it:
    a. Incorporates a hot-wire anemometer
    b. Contains a stainless steel flap in the variable-orifice differential pressure transducer
    c. Uses an ultrasonic wave–detection monitor
    d. Incorporates a laser beam–splitter

15. In the Dräger Babylog 8000 infant ventilator, all **EXCEPT** which of the following are automatically set by the microprocessor?
    a. Oxygen concentration alarms
    b. PEEP alarm limits
    c. Low V_T alarm
    d. Inspiratory pressure alarm

16. When the V.I.P. Gold ventilator rise-time control is set at 1:
    a. A rapid rise to set pressure occurs
    b. Only volume breaths are affected
    c. The inspiratory time increases
    d. The respiratory rate increases

17. When the V.I.P. Bird mode switch is set at TC SIMV, what are the breath variables for mandatory breaths?
    I. Time-triggering or patient-triggering
    II. Volume-targeted breaths
    III. Pressure-targeted breaths
    IV. TC
    a. III only
    b. I and II only
    c. I, III, and IV only
    d. I, II, and IV only

18. The Bunnell Life Pulse High-Frequency Jet Ventilator:
    I. Operates in tandem with a conventional ventilator
    II. Requires the use of the hi-lo jet tube
    III. Delivers rates of 240 insufflations/minute to 660 insufflations/minute
    IV. Operates independently with the use of another device
    a. I and II
    b. II and IV
    c. I and III
    d. III and IV

19. The triple-lumen hi-lo jet tube:
    a. Is the only type of ETT that can be used with the Bunnell Life Pulse High-Frequency Jet Ventilator
    b. Ranges in size from 2.5-mm ID to 6.0-mm ID
    c. Must be replaced with a standard ETT when the patient is switched to conventional ventilation
    d. All of the aforementioned

ASSESSMENT QUESTIONS—cont'd

20. The Dräger Babylog 8000 infant ventilator:
    a. Is used to ventilate premature and term infants
    b. Has a weight limit of 10 kg
    c. Has a built-in battery
    d. All of the aforementioned

21. Which of the following statements are true regarding the use of the activated volume guarantee feature of the Dräger Babylog 8000plus?
    I. The proximal flow sensor must be attached when this feature is used.
    II. The clinician sets the maximum peak inspiratory pressure.
    III. The maximum peak inspiratory pressure becomes an inspiratory pressure limit.
    IV. Over six to eight breaths, the ventilator determines the appropriate inspiratory pressure and begins to achieve and maintain the target tidal volume.
    a. I
    b. III
    c. I and II
    d. I, II, III, and IV

22. During volume guarantee on the Dräger Babylog 8000plus, the volume is set at 5 mL, but the patient's inspiratory effort results in a 7-mL volume demand. How will the ventilator respond?
    a. The ventilator's PIP will immediately decrease.
    b. If the total inspiratory tidal volume exceeds the set target volume by 200%, the expiratory valve will open and no additional ventilator-driven gas will be delivered to the patient.
    c. The 7-mL volume will be given and displayed without a ventilator response.
    d. A high tidal volume alarm will activate.

23. The power control on the SensorMedics 3100A is primarily used to change the:
    a. Mean airway pressure
    b. Frequency
    c. Bias flow
    d. Amplitude

24. If the frequency on the SensorMedics 3100A is increased from 10 Hz to 15 Hz and no other settings are changed, which of the following will occur?
    a. Inspiratory time will increase.
    b. Volume delivered by the piston will decrease.
    c. Amplitude will increase.
    d. None of the aforementioned

25. Mean airway pressure in the SensorMedics 3100A high-frequency oscillator can be affected by which of the following?
    I. Bias flow
    II. Frequency setting
    III. % T_I
    IV. Piston-centering
    V. Mean airway adjustment control
    a. V only
    b. I and III only
    c. II, IV, and V only
    d. I, II, III, IV, and V

26. A new feature of the SensorMedics 3100B oscillator compared with the 3100A is the:
    a. Frequency control
    b. Inspiratory time control
    c. Automatic piston-centering
    d. Mean airway pressure control

27. Which of the following statements is(are) true regarding proximal flow sensors with the Cardinal Health AVEA ventilator when used in infants?
    I. A proximal airway flow sensor is recommended when the ventilator is used with infants weighing less than 5 kg.
    II. The ventilator's internal inspiratory and expiratory flow sensors are accurate for volume monitoring in infants.
    III. The AVEA's hot-wire flow sensor can be used in flow rates greater than 30 L/min.
    IV. The variable-orifice flow sensor, called the Neonatal VarFlex, is recommended for applications in which maximum flow is less than 30 L/min.
    a. I only
    b. II only
    c. I and IV
    d. II and IV

28. When the AVEA is in use, which of the following is **NOT** available in the infant patient size range?
    I. TCPL
    II. APRV
    III. Sigh breaths
    IV. PRVC
    a. I and III
    b. II and III
    c. III and IV
    d. I, II, and IV

29. A newborn weighing 2 kg is going to be ventilated with the Dräger EvitaXL. Before its use, the therapist must be sure that:
    a. A heat and moisture exchanger is in place
    b. A facial mask is available to use as an interface
    c. The NeoFlow™ option is available on the ventilator
    d. The graphics display is working

30. An infant is being ventilated with the GALILEO ventilator in the P-SIMV mode. The infant has a spontaneous breath rate of 30 breaths/min. ETS is set at 50%. What additional control needs to be set to provide a backup inspiratory time termination criterion?
    a. Volume limit
    b. I : E ratio constant
    c. T_I Max
    d. Flow trigger

ASSESSMENT QUESTIONS—cont'd

31. During ventilation of a premature infant using the Servo[i] ventilator, the proximal flow sensor lines become blocked with secretions. Which of the following would occur in this situation?
   I. An audible and visual signal will activate.
   II. The sensor will be deactivated.
   III. The ventilator will revert to using the internal measurements and displaying these values.
   IV. The ventilator will be unable to detect a patient trigger.
   a. I only
   b. II and IV
   c. I, II, and III
   d. II, III, and IV

32. Use of the NeoMode option with the Puritan Bennett 840™ ventilator provides which of the following features?
   a. Low tidal volume setting of 2 mL
   b. The ability to ventilate an infant weighing 0.5 kg
   c. A respiratory rate up to 100 breaths/min
   d. A proximal sensor for monitoring tidal volumes and flows

References

1. Chatburn RL: Principles and practices of neonatal and pediatric ventilation, *Respir Care* 36:573, 1991.
2. Watson K: Neonatal and pediatric mechanical ventilation. In Pilbeam SP, Cairo JM: *Mechanical ventilation—physiological and clinical application,* St Louis, 2006, Elsevier.
3. Electro Medical Equipment, Ltd: *Instruction manual, EME Infant Flow System,* Brighton, East Sussex, England, 2000, Electro Medical Equipment, Ltd.
4. Cardinal Health: *Operator's & Routine Maintenance Manual,* Driver Model 006900, Firmware Version 2.02, part number 36-5031 Rev C, 2006, McGaw Park, Ill, Cardinal Health.
5. Cardinal Health: Operator's Manual, Infant Flow SiPAP, 675:101-101.
6. de Klerk AM, de Klerk RK: Use of continuous positive airway pressure in preterm infants: comments and experience from New Zealand, *Pediatrics* 108:761-763, 2001.
7. Hamilton Medical, Inc: *Instruction manual, ARABELLA System,* Reno, Nev, 2001, Hamilton Medical, Inc.
8. Betit P, Thompson JE, Benjamin PK: Mechanical ventilation. In Koff PB, Eitzman D, Neu J, editors: *Neonatal and pediatric respiratory care,* ed 2, St Louis, 1993, Mosby.
9. Thompson MA: Early nasal CPAP and prophylactic surfactant for neonates at risk of RDS: the IFDAS trial, presented at the European Society for Paediatric Research, annual meeting, Helsinki, Finland, August 2001.
10. *Instruction manual: V.I.P. Bird Infant-Pediatric Ventilator,* Palm Springs, Calif, 1991, Viasys Healthcare Systems, Critical Care Division.
11. *Instruction manual: V.I.P. Graphics instruction manual,* Palm Springs, Calif, 1991, Viasys Healthcare Systems, Critical Care Division.
12. *Operator's manual: V.I.P. Bird Gold and Sterling Ventilator Systems,* Palm Springs, Calif, 2000, Viasys Healthcare Systems, Critical Care Division.
13. Dräger Medical AG & Co: *Operator's manual: Dräger Babylog 8000,* 1st U.S. edition, Lübeck, Germany, 1993, Dräger Inc.
14. Bunnell Incorporated: *Operator's manual: Life Pulse High-Frequency Jet Ventilator,* Salt Lake City, Utah, 1991, Bunnell Incorporated.
15. *Operator's manual: 3100A High-Frequency Oscillatory Ventilator,* form P/N 767124, Palm Springs, Calif, 1991, Viasys Healthcare Systems, Critical Care Division.
16. *Operator's manual: 3100B High-Frequency Oscillatory Ventilator,* form P/N 767164, rev. J, Palm Springs, Calif, 2001, Viasys Healthcare Systems, Critical Care Division.
17. AVEA Ventilator Systems: *Operator's Manual (revision A), L1523,* Palm Springs, Calif, March 2005, Cardinal Health.
18. Clinical Education Materials, Monographs and Presentations, L1490 revision A, software disc, Palm Springs, Calif, 2002, Viasys Healthcare, Critical Care Division.
19. *EvitaXL: Intensive care ventilator Software 6.1n Operating Instructions.* ed 1; Nov 2005, 90 38 733—GA 5664.660 enUS © Dräger Medical AG & Co. KG; Lübeck, Germany, Dräger, Inc, Drägerwerk AG.
20. *GALILEO operator's manual,* May 2004, 610862/01, Software version 3. Manufacturer: Hamilton Medical AG, Bonaduz, Switzerland.
21. *User's manual, ventilator systems Servo[i] V3.1, critical care,* Maquet, Inc., Solna, Sweden, Part No. 66 00 261.
22. *Pocket guide, ventilation Servo[i] V3.0, ventilation of neonates & pediatrics,* Maquet Critical Care, Maquet, Inc., Solna, Sweden, Part No. 66 71 225.
23. *Puritan Bennett operator's and technical reference manual, 840 Ventilator system,* part no 4-075609-00, revision C, Boulder, Col, Nov 1999, Puritan Bennett, a division of Covidien.

Internet Resources

Cardinal Health: http://www.CardinalHealth.com
Dräger Inc: http://www.draeger.com
Hamilton Medical, Inc: http://www.Hamilton-Medical.com
Maquet, Inc: http://www.Maquetusa.com
Puritan Bennett, a division of Covidien Medical: http://www.puritanbennett.com
VentWorld, a ventilator Web site: http://www.VentWorld.com
Viasys Healthcare, which is now part of Cardinal Health: http://http://www.viasyshealthcare.com

Chapter 14

Transport, Home Care, and Alternative Ventilatory Devices

STEVEN E. SITTIG

OUTLINE

OBJECTIVES

Upon completion of this chapter, you will be able to:
· Give the value in liters per minute of the logic flow for the patient-disconnect feature when the pNeuton model A ventilator is in use.
· Determine the length of time that elapses between a low-battery event and a ventilator-inoperative event with the Crossvent ventilator when there is a power loss.
· State the value for the gas supply pressure that will result in a low source-pressure alarm when the Crossvent 3+ is in use.
· Describe the operating features, alarms, and parameter ranges of the following ventilators: Bio-Med MVP 10, Impact Uni-Vent 750, Pulmonetic Systems LTV 1200, Puritan Bennett LP10, Newport Medical Instruments HT50, and the Pulmonetic Systems LTV 950.
· Compare the alarm functions on the Dräger Oxylog 2000 with those on the Dräger Oxylog 3000.

*See Evolve Resources for further information.

OBJECTIVES—cont'd

- Describe the affect of the oxygen flow on oxygen delivery in the Oxylog 3000.
- Explain the function of the apnea alarm on the Uni-Vent 750.
- Provide the value for logic gas consumption on the Impact Uni-Vent Eagle™ 754.
- State the liter flow required to operate the internal logic of the Percussionaire Bronchotron TXP Ventilator.
- Review the function of the low-pressure "eyeball" alarm in the Smiths Medical Pneupac™ ventiPAC Ventilator.
- State the method of delivery (i.e., invasive or noninvasive) available with the Dräger Carina™*home* ventilator.
- Give the value for the maximum oxygen bleed in the Dräger Carina™*home* ventilator.
- Discuss the ability of the Newport HT50 to provide enriched oxygen delivery.
- Describe the adjustment of the positive end-expiratory pressure/continuous positive airway pressure (PEEP/CPAP) control on the HT50 ventilator.
- Tell how long the internal ventilator battery will operate on the Pulmonetic Systems LTV 800.
- Name the two operator-adjustable alarms on the Respironics BiPAP Focus™.
- Explain the possible cause of a discrepancy between the set fractional inspired oxygen (F_IO_2) and the delivered F_IO_2 for the Respironics BiPAP Vision.
- Give the patient size limit for the Respironics Synchrony ventilator.
- List the alarms available on the Puritan Bennett GoodKnight 425.

KEY TERMS

accumulator/silencer	external positive end-expiratory	rocking bed
chest cuirass	pressure (PEEP) valve	synchronized minimum
expiratory positive	internal regulator	mandatory ventilation
airway pressure	iron lung	(SMMV)
(EPAP)	pressure-relief valve	

Previous chapters in this text related to mechanical ventilation focused primarily on ventilators that are used in the intensive care unit (ICU). But the use of ventilators also extends into other areas, including patient transport and home care. This chapter provides a review of ventilators used in these two areas. In addition, this chapter includes examples of related devices such as bilevel airway pressure equipment and continuous positive airway pressure (CPAP) machines, noninvasive ventilators, and adjunct ventilating devices such as negative-pressure ventilators.

PART I: TRANSPORT VENTILATORS

There are few procedures that require greater care and skill than does the transportation of a critically ill patient. Advancements in technology and the ability of diagnostic tests to render information critical to treatment of the patient have created a gray area between risk and benefit. Some literature suggests that physiologic changes that occur during patient relocation are not a result of the transport, but of the gravity of the patient's condition.[1] The statement can then be made that the likelihood of changes in heart rate, respiratory rate, blood pressure, and oxygen saturation developing during transport is no greater than if the patient remained in the ICU. However, transport of a patient is not without the risk of complica-

tions. Loss of an intravenous line; changes in body temperature; hyperventilation or hypoventilation, which can perpetuate arrhythmias; and equipment malfunction are all perceivable problems resulting from the relocation of the patient. In addition, manual ventilation during transport has been reported as a cause for episodic hypotension, hyperventilation, and ventilation asynchrony.[2,3] Therefore, every attempt should be made to ensure that monitoring, ventilation, oxygenation, and patient care remain constant during movement and that protocols and policies are put in place to guide the decision to transport and serve as a checklist for the transport team. The movement of a patient from one location to another should never be considered routine. Preparation and communication are vital components to a successful transport.

The attributes commonly shared among transport ventilators are compact size, light weight, and an ability to be maintained by a reliable power source. The power source must allow the ventilator to operate from an internal battery or a gas source to permit mobility. Durability and ease of use are two added features that make for a good transport ventilator. The incorporation of microprocessors and the miniaturization of components have increased the capabilities and functionality of modern transport ventilators, which has extended to improvements in monitoring and available alarms. Today's transport ventilator has features once associated only with costly intensive care ventilators; these attributes are flow-triggering, pressure support, and even high-frequency ventilation.[4,5] Newer transport ventilators can provide a variety of alarms and modes of ventilation to rival the ICU ventilators.

The respiratory therapist (RT) must understand the ventilator's capabilites and limitations and be able to apply the needed patient support during the transport process. Although the use of a transport ventilator can reduce the risks associated with manual ventilation, a well-qualified operator is mandatory to ensure the proper application of the equipment.

Transport ventilators must be capable of working in extreme conditions that include temperature extremes, vibrations, and altitude changes. They should contain sufficient shielding to protect the ventilator's internal mechanisms from electromagnetic energy.

In addition to durability, the device should remain simple to operate. This does not imply that the machine should be basic in operation; it suggests only that the user controls should be easy to recognize and easy to adjust. The volume, rate, and pressure controls should be large and easy to find, and all displays should be clearly visible in both the daytime and nighttime to reduce the chance of mistakes caused by missed or misread information.

The American Association for Respiratory Care (AARC) has developed a clinical practice guideline specifically addressing the purpose, indications, methods of providing, and complications associated with transporting mechanically ventilated patients, which is a valuable resource to practitioners interested in transport ventilation (Clinical Practice Guideline 14-1).[3]

In-Hospital Transport of the Mechanically Ventilated Patient

Clinical Practice Guideline 14-1

■ DEFINITION/DESCRIPTION

Transportation of mechanically ventilated patients for diagnostic or therapeutic procedures is always associated with a degree of risk. Every attempt should be made to ensure monitoring, ventilation, oxygenation, and patient care remain constant during movement. Patient transport includes preparation, movement to and from, and time spent at the destination.

■ INDICATIONS

Transportation of mechanically ventilated patients should only be undertaken following a careful evaluation of the risk-to-benefit ratio.

■ CONTRAINDICATIONS

Contraindications include the inability to do the following: maintain an airway, provide adequate oxygenation and ventilation, maintain acceptable hemodynamic performance, and adequately monitor cardiopulmonary signs during transport.

■ PRECAUTIONS AND COMPLICATIONS

The potential hazards and complications of transport include the following:
· Hyperventilation during manual ventilation, resulting in respiratory alkalosis, cardiac dysrhythmias, and hypotension
· Loss of positive end-expiratory pressure/continuous positive airway pressure (PEEP/CPAP), resulting in hypoxemia
· Position changes that result in hypotension, hypercarbia, and hypoxemia
· Dysrhythmias resulting from relocation of the patient
· Equipment failure, which causes inaccurate data or loss of monitoring capabilities
· Inadvertent disconnection of intravenous pharmacologic agents, which results in hemodynamic instability
· Accidental extubation
· Accidental removal of vascular access
· Loss of oxygen supply, resulting in hypoxemia

■ LIMITATIONS

The literature suggests that nearly two thirds of all transports for diagnostic studies fail to yield results that affect patient care.

■ MONITORING

Monitoring provided during transport should be maintained at the level of stationary care.

For complete guidelines, see Chang DW, American Association for Respiratory Care: Clinical practice guideline: in-hospital transport of the mechanically ventilated patient—2002 revision & update, Resp Care 47:721-723, 2002.

Today's transport ventilators have, in general, become very sophisticated and reliable. Many are now comparable to contemporary ICU ventilators. However, it remains the responsibility of the operator to ensure the comfort and safety of the patient.

AIRON pNeuton

The pNeuton (Airon Corporation, Melbourne, Fla.) is a small transport ventilator that is designed for use with pediatric and adult patients who weigh 23 kg and more (Figure 14-1).[6] It is totally pneumatically operated and controlled. The modes of operation offered are intermittent mandatory ventilation (IMV) and CPAP, and this unit also includes a pressure-limiting feature. The pNeuton can be used for invasive and noninvasive ventilation. It measures $5 \text{ in} \times 10 \text{ in} \times 7 \text{ in}$, weighs 6.5 lb, and is magnetic resonance imaging (MRI)–compatible up to a 3-T static field. Table 14-1 provides a summary of some of the specifications of the pNeuton transport ventilator.

Power Source

The pNeuton is a pneumatically powered ventilator and requires a 55-psi (±15 psi) gas source to operate. It has no battery backup or alternating current (AC) power option. The pNeuton comes in two models: the A model and the S model. The internal system of the model A with the patient-disconnect alarm uses 4 L/min for operation. The model S without the disconnect alarm uses 3 L/min for operation of the internal logic system.

Internal Mechanism/Oxygen Source

The pNeuton typically operates from a 55-psi oxygen source. The operator can select either the 100% or the 65% oxygen setting, with the lower setting entraining room air to lower the oxygen concentration. A low-oxygen inlet alarm is standard on both models and activates if the gas source pressure drops below 30 psi. The pNeuton will operate normally up to an altitude of 15,000 feet. Altitude will not affect pressure settings. However, tidal volume will increase and respiratory rate will decrease with increases in

TABLE 14-1	
Specifications for the pNeuton Ventilator	
Control Settings	**Range**
Modes	Nonsynchronized IMV, CPAP
Power source	Pneumatic-powered
Rate	3-50 breaths/min
Noninvasive ventilation mode	Yes
Peak pressure	15-75 cm H_2O
Tidal volume	360-1500 mL
Inspiratory time	Auto set
PEEP/CPAP	0-20 cm H_2O
Oxygen percent	65%-100% oxygen
Pressure support	N/A
Monitors/displays	Analog pressure gauge: 0-120 cm H_2O
Dimensions	5 in × 10 in × 7 in; 6.5 lb
Gas consumption	4 L/min
Alarms	Low oxygen inlet pressure alarm; patient disconnect alarm
Battery duration	N/A

IMV, Intermittent mandatory ventilation; *CPAP,* continuous positive airway pressure; *PEEP,* positive end-expiratory pressure; *N/A,* not applicable.

altitude. This is because the ventilator's internal calibration is for sea level. It is recommended that an external respirometer be used to check the accuracy of tidal volume (V_T) delivery at higher altitudes.

Controls and Alarms

The pNeuton contains several front-panel controls for setting ventilator parameters and for monitoring patient data and alarms (see Figure 14-1).

PEEP/CPAP

The positive end-expiratory pressure/CPAP (PEEP/CPAP) is built-in and adjustable between 0 cm H_2O and 20 cm H_2O. The trigger sensitivity does not need to be readjusted with increases in PEEP/CPAP, because this is done automatically by the ventilator.

Peak Pressure

Peak pressure control is adjustable from 15 cm H_2O to 75 cm H_2O, and pressure is displayed on an analog pressure manometer. When peak pressures are set at more than 50 cm H_2O, the control pointer will be in the red bar area, indicating that the set pressure is high.

Tidal Volume

V_T is set by a knob in the lower left-hand corner. The range available is 360 mL to 1500 mL. For ease of use there are V_T markings at 360, 750, 1200, and 1500 mL.

Respiratory Rate

The respiratory rate is set with a control knob located in the lower left-hand corner of the control panel near the pressure gauge. It is adjustable from 3 breaths/min to 50 breaths/min in the IMV mode.

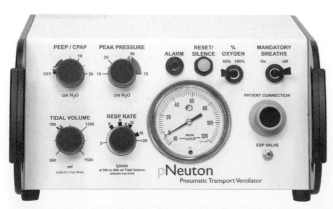

FIGURE 14-1 The Airon pNeuton transport ventilator. (Courtesy Airon Corporation, Melbourne, Fla.)

Percentage Oxygen

This function is controlled by a two-position switch located in the upper right-hand corner of the control panel. The available options are 65% and 100% O_2.

Mandatory Breaths Control

This function is controlled by a two-position (on/off) switch located in the upper right-hand corner of the control panel next to the percentage oxygen switch. This control determines whether the pNeuton is operating in IMV or CPAP mode and thus represents the mode control for the ventilator.

Pressure Gauge

The pNeuton has an analog pressure gauge located in the center of the control panel. It displays delivered peak pressures and PEEP/CPAP levels in a range from 0 cm H_2O to 120 cm H_2O.

Alarms

The pNeuton has a totally pneumatically powered alarm system and has two functional alarms that are always active. A low-oxygen inlet pressure alarm will activate when the pressure falls below 30 psi, and a patient-disconnect alarm will sound when a disconnect situation is sensed by the ventilator. Clinical Rounds 14-1 provides an example of this potential situation. For the patient-disconnect alarm, the ventilator is always looking for a specific pressure to be reached within 22 seconds. In the IMV mode this target pressure is a minimum of 15 cm H_2O, while in CPAP mode, it is a minimum pressure of 5 cm H_2O. If the pressure is not reached, the patient-disconnect alarm will sound. Alarms automatically reset once the alarm condition resolves.

There is also a 1-minute silence/reset button located on the control panel directly above the pressure gauge, which silences alarms for 1 minute. An output for a remote alarm is also provided on the front panel of the pNeuton.

Modes of Operation

The pNeuton offers nonsynchronized volume-controlled IMV or pressure-controlled IMV along with CPAP/PEEP modes. These two modes can be easily used as noninvasive modes, if desired, when an appropriate face mask or other interface is used.

During PEEP/CPAP when no rate is set, the pneumatic system provides a continuous flow of gas through the circuit of approximately 10 L/min to meet the inspiratory demand during spontaneous breaths. As the spontaneously breathing patient inhales, the ventilator detects a drop in bias flow and increases inspiratory flow up to 140 L/min. The flow sensitivity is preset and not adjustable.

BIO-MED CROSSVENT

The Crossvent ventilator (Bio-Med Devices, Inc, Guilford, Conn.) is a compact ventilator that can be used for transport and also in the intensive care unit (Figure 14-2).[7] It is an electronically controlled, pneumatically powered ventilator. It can be time-triggered or patient-triggered, volume-limited or pressure-limited, and time-cycled.

The Crossvent ventilator comes in several models; a comparison of model features is provided in Table 14-2. The Crossvent ventilator is capable of ventilating newborns through adult-sized patients, depending on which model is selected. The following discussion will focus on the Crossvent 3+ model.

The Crossvent 3 is designed to provide ventilatory support from pediatric through adult patients. The available ventilation modes include assist/control (A/C), syn-

---

CLINICAL ROUNDS 14-1

You are a respiratory therapist who has been dispatched via helicopter to tranport a 43-year-old female with severe acute respiratory distress syndrome (ARDS). Upon arrival to the scene you place the patient on the pNeuton ventilator settings as follows: intermittent mandatory ventilation (IMV) rate = 20 breaths/min; tidal volume (V_T), 700 mL; positive end-expiratory pressure (PEEP) = 15 cm H_2O; and fractional inspired oxygen (F_IO_2) = 1.0. Oxygen saturations are 92%, with a total respiratory rate of 30 breaths/min. Peak airway pressures are 38 cm H_2O. End-tidal CO_2 is 44 mm Hg.

Transfer to the helicopter is uneventful, but shortly after liftoff the patient begins fighting the ventilator and saturations drop into the 70% range. You then note the low oxygen inlet alarm is activated. What is the likely cause, and what would you do?

See Evolve Resources for the answers.

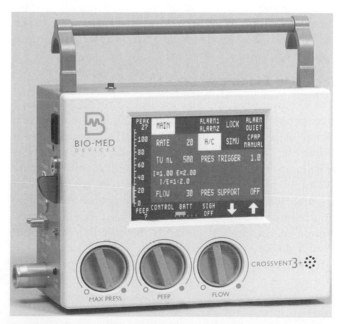

FIGURE 14-2 The Bio-Med Crossvent ventilator. (Courtesy Bio-Med Devices, Inc, Guilford, Conn.)

TABLE 14-2

Table Showing the Comparisons Between the Available Features of the Crossvent Models CV-4, CV-3+, CV-2+, and the CV-2i+

Display	CV-4	CV-3+	CV-2+	CV-2i+
C, Color display; M, monochrome display	M	C	C	C

Modes	CV-4	CV-3+	CV-2+	CV-2i+
Adult	√	√		
Pediatric	√	√	√	
Neonatal	√		√	√
Assist control	√	√	√	√
IMV	√		√	√
SIMV	√	√	√	√
CPAP	√	√	√	√
PEEP	√	√	√	√
Sigh	√	√		
Pressure support	√	√	√	√
Pressure limit	√	√	√	√

Monitors/alarms	CV-4	CV-3+	CV-2+	CV-2i+
Pressure	√	√	√	√
Rate	√	√	√	√
Oxygen %	√	√	√	√
Temperature	√			
Mean pressure	√	√	√	√
PEEP	√	√	√	√
Exhale tidal volume	√	√	√	√
Exhale minute volume	√	√	√	√
PWI (pressure wave index)	√			
Low battery	√	√	√	√
Low supply pressure		√	√	
Apnea	√	*	*	*

SIMV, Synchronized intermittent mandatory ventilation.

TABLE 14-3

Specifications for the Bio-Med Crossvent 3+

Control Settings	Range
Modes	Assist control, SIMV, pressure support, CPAP
Power sources	AC power; internal DC battery
Rate	Assist/control mode: 5-150 breaths/min SIMV mode: 0.6-50 breaths/min
Noninvasive ventilation mode	N/A
Peak pressure	0-120 cm H_2O
Tidal volume	5-2500 mL
Inspiratory time	0.1-3 seconds
PEEP/CPAP	0-35 cm H_2O
Oxygen percent	21-100%
Pressure support	0-50 cm H_2O
Monitors/displays	Integrated LCD screen
Dimensions	10 in × 11 in × 5.5 in; 10.5 lb
Gas consumption	4 L/min
Alarms	Peak pressure, high respiratory rate, exhaled tidal volume and exhaled minute volume, PEEP/CPAP, high and low mean airway pressure, high and low oxygen percentage, low battery alarm
Battery duration	6 hours when fully charged

AC, Alternating current; *DC*, direct current; *LCD*, liquid-crystal display.

chronized intermittent mandatory ventilation (SIMV), and pressure-support ventilation (PSV). The Crossvent 3 weighs 10.5 lb and is 10 in × 11 in × 5.5 in. Table 14-3 outlines specific features.

Power Source

The Crossvent requires an electrical power source to function properly. It can use either a standard AC electrical outlet or its internal direct current (DC) battery power. When the Crossvent is connected to an AC power outlet, it will automatically default to the AC as its power source. When AC power is not available, the Crossvent switches to its internal DC battery. The battery operational time is approximately 6 hours when fully charged. The Crossvent's source of operational power is displayed in the liquid-crystal display (LCD) screen and displayed on the lower left-hand corner. When the battery is within approximately 20 minutes of remaining power, the alarm menu will flash "Low Battery, Connect External Power" on the LCD screen and sound an alarm. The ventilator must be connected to AC power to continue operation. When AC power is detected, the Crossvent will then switch to AC power as its primary source and the internal battery will begin to recharge.

Internal Mechanism/Oxygen Source

The Crossvent requires a compressed-gas source of 31 psi to 75 psi to ensure adequate gas flow to a patient. If the supply pressure falls below the minimum 31 psi, a low source pressure alarm will activate.

A gas blender can be used to deliver precise fractional inspired oxygen (F_IO_2). The output of the blender is connected to the Crossvent's supply inlet connection. For optimum performance, the gas sources to the blender should provide 45 to 75 psi of pressure. The Crossvent then delivers the oxygen concentration set on the blender. An optional Air Entrainment module can be used instead of a blender. This module offers the ability to deliver 100% oxygen or 50% oxygen to the patient.

Controls and Alarms

The main controls for the Crossvent are located on the front panel of the ventilator (see Figure 14-2). The operator can either use the touch screen LCD controls or the three control knobs located below the LCD screen.

Flow-Control Knob

The flow-control knob is located on the lower right side of the Crossvent 3+. Adjusting the flow-control knob sets the inspiratory gas flow from 0 L/min to 120 L/min. The set value is displayed on the ventilator's LCD screen.

PEEP Knob

The PEEP control is located to the left of the flow control. Adjusting the PEEP control sets the amount of PEEP or CPAP applied to the exhalation valve. The PEEP level is internally controlled in the Crossvent, which can deliver a PEEP range of 0 cm H_2O to 35 cm H_2O. The sensitivity control automatically compensates for the set level of PEEP, so sensitivity does not have to be readjusted when the PEEP/CPAP level is changed. ([NOTE: When the Crossvent is connected to an active gas source and not in use, the PEEP control should be turned fully counterclockwise to conserve gas supply [Clinical Rounds 14-2]).

Maximum Pressure Knob

The maximum pressure control knob is located to the left of the PEEP control. Adjusting this knob sets the pressure applied to the exhalation valve and to an internal adjustable **pressure-relief valve**. The set pressure determines the maximum amount of pressure delivered during patient-triggered or time-triggered mandatory breaths. Pressure is adjustable from 0 cm H_2O to 120 cm H_2O. The maximum pressure knob should always be set higher than the set PEEP level to ensure the correct PEEP level is delivered.

Display Interface and Menus

The Crossvent's main display and control-setting functions are located on the LCD screen. Several menus can be found on the LCD and are listed in Box 14-1. A menu item or parameter is selected by touching the desired variable or parameter on the LCD screen, as seen in Figure 14-3. Once

---

CLINICAL ROUNDS 14-2

A respiratory therapist uses the Crossvent 3+ to transport a patient to the radiology department. Once in the radiology department, the patient is switched to another ventilator and the Crossvent 3+ is placed in the hallway for the return transport back to the intensive care unit (ICU).

The therapist returns to transport the patient 1 hour later, but he finds that the oxygen cylinder that was originally used is completely empty. What is one possible cause for this problem?

See Evolve Resources for the answer.

BOX 14-1	Crossvent Menus Available on the Liquid Crystal Display (LCD) Screen

Main menu
Functions menu
Primary alarms menu
Secondary alarms menu
Set-up menu

---

the parameter is selected, it is highlighted in yellow for 30 seconds. If no change is made, the highlighted area deactivates. Changes in parameters are accomplished by touching the up (↑) and down (↓) arrows located on the lower right-hand side of the screen. It is not necessary to use on-screen arrows to select a menu or mode. These can also be adjusted by simply pressing the desired key—for example, the SIMV mode key.

The value for flow is displayed in the flow key itself, but it can only be adjusted by using the flow-control knob.

The I:E ratio (the ratio of inspiratory time to expiratory time) is a displayed value only. The I:E is calculated from the set rate, tidal volume V_T, and flow.

On the left side of the screen is a digital display of delivered airway pressures. The top and bottom keys are always available for use unless the set-up screen is activated. As shown in Figure 14-3, the top row of touch-screen keys allow the user to move between menus, as well as silence the alarm and lock the touch screen. The bottom row provides information on the type of breath that is delivered, be it mandatory or spontaneous; operating power source; application of sigh breaths; and the set-up screen key.

The LCD has a backlit screen for visibility. The default setting ensures that this backlight is always on, but it can be turned off to save battery life. When the backlight is not active, the LCD screen is not viewable.

Alarms

The Crossvent has three alarm menu screens; alarm menu 1 and 2 are accessed by pressing the corresponding top-row keys on the LCD screen, which is depicted in Figure 14-3. The third alarm menu screen appears only with a specific alarm situation such as a low battery alarm or a ventilator failure alarm.

- **Alarm 1 screen** (Figure 14-4) monitors standard alarms such as peak pressure and high respiratory rate. Alarms for exhaled tidal volume (V_T) and exhaled minute volume are also available in this alarm section, but they can be disabled if desired.

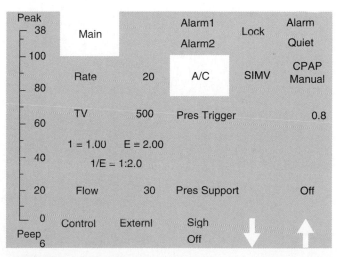

FIGURE 14-3 The Bio-Med Crossvent's main display screen.

- **Alarm 2 screen** (Figure 14-5) monitors such parameters as PEEP and CPAP, high and low mean airway pressure, and high- and low-oxygen percentage. The mean airway pressure alarm and the oxygen alarm can be disabled if desired. An alarm overview with ranges and set limits is shown in Table 14-4.

Modes

The Crossvent provides five modes of operation. The modes available are control, assist control (A/C), SIMV, CPAP, and manual ventilation and are also listed in Box 14-2.

Assist/Control (A/C)

The A/C mode provides either patient-triggered or time-triggered mandatory breaths. The breaths may be either volume-targeted or pressure-targeted as set by the operator. (See Chapter 11 for additional information on assist/control ventilation.) The set respiratory rate range in the A/C mode is from 5 breaths/min to 150 breaths/min.

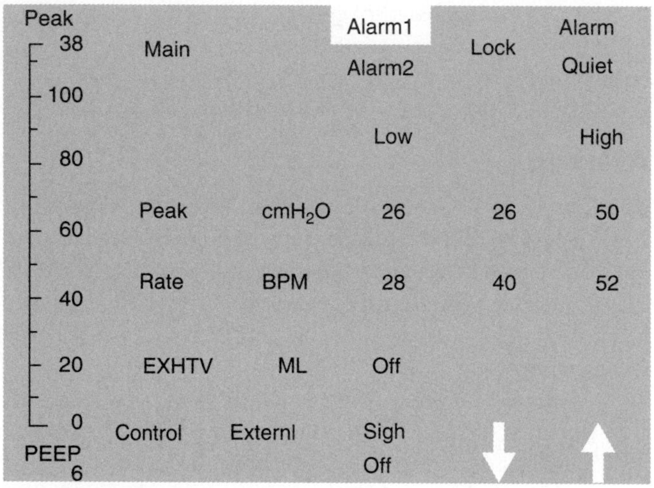

TABLE 14-4

Crossvent Alarm Parameter Ranges and Alarm Limits

Parameter (Range)	Display (Range)	Set Limits	
		Low	High
Peak pressure (cm H_2O)	0-125	3-124	4-125
Rate (breaths/min)	0-199	4-159	5-160
Exhaled tidal volume (mL)	50-4000	50-3199	51-3200
Exhaled minute volume (L)	0-200	0-99	1-100
PEEP/CPAP (cm H_2O)	0-99	−1-99	0-100
Mean airway pressure (cm H_2O)	0-125	0-124	1-125
Oxygen %	0-100	18-100	19-105

BOX 14-2   Crossvent Modes of Operation

Control
Assist control
Synchronized intermittent mandatory ventilation (SIMV)
Continuous positive airway pressure (CPAP)
Manual ventilation

FIGURE 14-4 The Bio-Med Crossvent's alarm 1 screen.

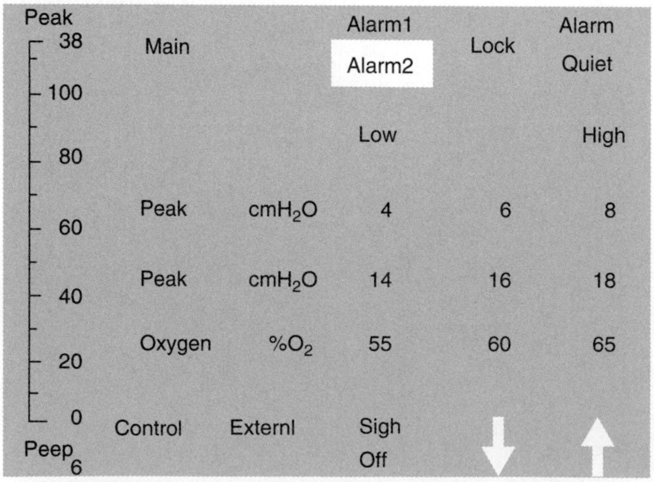

FIGURE 14-5 The Bio-Med Crossvent's alarm 2 screen.

SIMV

As is the case with the A/C mode, in the SIMV mode, mandatory breaths are patient-triggered or time-triggered and volume-targeted or pressure-targeted as desired. However, with SIMV, only the set mandatory breaths are delivered at set parameters, whereas the patient's spontaneous effort between mandatory breaths is met by a fresh supply of gas. The set rate range in the SIMV mode is 0.6 breaths/min to 50 breaths/min. The sigh breath option is available in the volume-targeted SIMV mode and operates as described below on the sigh section.

Sigh Breaths

A sigh breath option is available in the volume-targeted A/C and in the volume-targeted SIMV mode. Once the sigh key is activated through the LCD screen, beginning with the next breath, 1 sigh breath is provided every 100 breaths or 1 every 7 minutes, whichever occurs first. The tidal volume (V_T) for the sigh breath is equal to 1.5 times the normal set tidal volume (V_T). This is accomplished by increasing the inspiratory time for that breath. There is a tidal volume (V_T) maximum of 2500 mL and an inspiratory time limit of 3 seconds for these sigh breaths. The expiratory time for a sigh breath is also increased to maintain the same I:E ratio for a set ventilator breath.

CPAP/Manual Mode

In the CPAP/manual mode gas flow is provided for spontaneous breaths at the set PEEP/CPAP level or atmospheric pressure when PEEP/CPAP is set at 0. The manual breath key will initiate 1 controlled breath each time the key is pressed, delivering the set tidal volume and inspiratory time set on the backup rate control. This mode also offers an apnea backup rate. If the patient has a significant apnea episode, the ventilator will switch to a selected rate, V_T, inspiratory time, and F_IO_2.

Pressure Support

The Crossvent also can provide set levels of pressure support in the SIMV and CPAP modes (range: 1 to 50 cm H_2O). When pressure support is selected, the Crossvent provides the set pressure support level for the spontaneous breaths.

BIO-MED IC-2A

Information about the Bio-Med IC-2A ventilator (Bio-Med Devices, Inc, Guilford, Conn.) is now available on Evolve Resources for this text.

BIO-MED MVP 10

The Bio-Med MVP 10 is available from Bio-Med Devices, Inc (Guilford, Conn.). It is gas-powered and fluidically controlled. Breath delivery is time-cycled and pressure-limited. The MVP 10 was designed for respiratory support of neonatal and pediatric patients, both during transport and in the hospital.[8] It is designed for all applications, ranging up to a 400-mL V_T. It is a continuous-flow ventilator that can operate in IMV or CPAP modes or provide continuous-flow oxygen. It is portable and lightweight, at 5 lb 2 oz and 8 in × 9 in × 3 in (Figure 14-6). The MVP 10 also comes in an MRI-compatible version. Table 14-5 lists important specifications of the MVP 10.

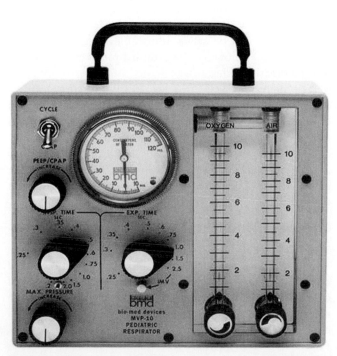

FIGURE 14-6 The Bio-Med MVP 10. (Courtesy Bio-Med Devices, Inc, Guilford, Conn.)

TABLE 14-5	
Specifications for the Bio-Med MVP 10	
Control Settings	**Range**
Modes	IMV, CPAP, or continuous flow oxygen
Power source	Completely pneumatically powered
Rate	0-120 breaths/min
Noninvasive ventilation mode	N/A
Peak pressure	0-120 cm H_2O
Tidal volume	Up to 400 mL
Inspiratory time	0.2-2.0 s
PEEP/CPAP	0-18 cm H_2O at a flow of 6 L/min
Oxygen percent	21-100%
Pressure support	N/A
Monitors/displays	8 in × 9 in × 3 in; 5 lb 2 oz
Gas consumption	4 L/min
Alarms	N/A
Battery duration	N/A

Power Source

The fluidic system of the MVP 10 requires medical-grade oxygen and compressed air at 50 psi (±50 psi). The gas sources may be a cylinder or a wall outlet with a Diameter Index Safety System (DISS) connector. The fluidic logic circuits are normally powered by oxygen. If only one source gas is used, it must be connected to the oxygen power line connector in order for the fluidic logic circuits to receive pressurized gas. If compressed air is used in the oxygen power line, the set time intervals are approximately 10% less than if powered by 100% oxygen because of the difference in gas density.

A blender may be connected to the oxygen power line. If both oxygen and air from a blender are used, a *biomedical device* (BMD) Y-adapter would be needed.

The fluidic logic consumes approximately 4 L/min of gas supply and needs to be included in gas-supply calculations. Clinical Rounds 14-3 illustrates some examples of calculating oxygen cylinder duration. As seen with other uncompensated transport ventilators, such as the IC-2A, the set inspiratory and expiratory time may also be affected during air transport because of the changes in barometric pressure that occur at different altitudes.

Controls and Alarms

Figure 14-6 shows the front panel of the MVP 10 and its controls. The primary controls are the mode switch, PEEP/CPAP dial, inspiratory time control, expiratory time control, maximum pressure dial, and the built-in air/oxygen blender. The MVP 10 has no built-in alarms.

Mode Switch

The cycle/CPAP switch is a two-position switch that enables the selection of either a time-cycled mode or the CPAP position. The ventilator allows a noncycling flow of gas with or without a continuous PEEP. Clinical Rounds 14-4 presents a scenario based on this control.

CLINICAL ROUNDS 14-3

You are transporting an infant of 34 weeks' gestation who is connected to an MVP 10 unit. You are on 60% F_IO_2, and IMV rate of 30 breaths/min. Peak pressure is 25 cm H_2O, and PEEP is 5 cm H_2O. To obtain the desired peak pressure and 60% F_IO_2, you need 2 L/min of oxygen and 2 L/min of air. The MVP 10 requires 4 L/min of oxygen for logic flow to operate and an additional 2 L/min of oxygen to deliver the desired F_IO_2 (total oxygen flow required = 6 L/min).

To estimate how long a cylinder of oxygen will last for the MVP 10 in the IMV mode, use the following formula:

Pressure of gas supply = tank pressure × conversion factor

For example:
2200 psig = tank pressure
0.28 = conversion factor for an E cylinder
volume of gas supply = (2200 psig) (0.28) = 622 L

You can now calculate cylinder duration one of two ways:

First, you can calculate minutes by dividing the 622 L in the cylinder by the required 6 L/min.

Answer: 622 L ÷ 6 L/min = approximately 103 minutes.

To calculate hourly duration, multiply the 6 L/min consumption by 60 min/h, for an hourly consumption of 360 L.

How much time (hours) will it take before the oxygen cylinder is completely empty?

Answer: 622 L ÷ 360 L/h = 1.73 hours.

Problem

Assume the ventilator is now operating at 100% oxygen. It requires 4 L/min of oxygen. To provide the desired peak pressure and F_IO_2, a flow of 4 L/min is needed. The E cylinder of oxygen has 1800 psi displayed on the gauge. How long will the cylinder last until it is completely empty?

See Evolve Resources for the answer.

CLINICAL ROUNDS 14-4

You are transporting a term newborn who is connected to the MVP 10 by air with settings of 60% oxygen, an IMV rate of 30 breaths/min, peak pressure of 25 cm H_2O, and a PEEP of 5 cm H_2O. The transporter is loaded in the aircraft.

While securing yourself in the aircraft, you notice that the ventilator is suddenly not cycling. However, the PEEP level is being maintained at 5 cm H_2O. The flowmeters show gas flow from both oxygen and compressed-air sources. What is a likely cause of the malfunction?

See Evolve Resources for the answer.

PEEP/CPAP Dial

In adjusting the PEEP/CPAP dial, a positive pressure will be maintained in the patient's ventilator circuit during expiration in either the time-cycled IMV mode or in the CPAP mode. Adjustment of this control places a controlled pressure on the expiration valve while maintaining the set pressure in the patient's circuit during exhalation. The PEEP/CPAP range is variable up to 16 cm H_2O (±4 cm H_2O) at a flow of 6 L/min. The levels of PEEP/CPAP are affected by flow. When flow to the built-in blender is increased, the set pressures may increase somewhat. These changes can be noted on the pressure gauge and readjusted accordingly.

Inspiratory and Expiratory Time Controls

The IMV rate is set on the MVP 10 by the controlled interaction of the inspiratory and expiratory time controls. The inspiratory time control is adjustable from 0.2 seconds to 2.0 seconds, whereas the expiratory time control is adjustable from 0.25 seconds to 2.5 seconds. The inspiratory and expiratory time controls determine the respiratory rate (variable from 0 to 120 breaths/min). The pneumatic logic circuit controls the opening and closing of the expiratory valve, cycling the ventilator into inspiration and expiration. Adjustment of the inspiratory and expiratory time controls determines how quickly the gas pressure builds in the pneumatic logic controller and switches from inspiration to expiration and back to inspiration.

Maximum Pressure Control and Pressure Gauge

The maximum pressure control is used to set the maximum peak pressure to be delivered in the patient circuit during inspiration. This control is located on the back panel of the MVP 10 and is shown in Figure 14-7. The maximum pressure that can be set is adjustable up to 70 cm H_2O (±10 cm H_2O), allowing the establishment of a pressure-limited breath mode.

The delivered peak and set PEEP pressures can be observed on the analog pressure gauge, which is designed to show pressure in the patient circuit of −10 cm H_2O to +120 cm H_2O. The MVP 10 is typically used as a pressure-control ventilator. In certain cases in which set inspiratory flow and inspiratory time are not sufficient for the set peak pressure to be delivered, the MVP 10 becomes a flow-controller.

Oxygen and Air Flowmeters

The MVP 10 has two built-in Thorpe tube flowmeters. They are both designed to be set from 0 L/min to 10 L/min. The air and oxygen flowmeters control the level of continuous flow through the patient circuit, in addition to the oxygen concentration. Manipulation of the air and oxygen flowmeters together delivers an approximate F_IO_2. Figure 14-8 shows a chart that helps to estimate the F_IO_2 delivery in relation to the set air and oxygen flow rates. For example, a ratio of 1:1 (air-to-oxygen) is equal to an F_IO_2

of approximately 0.6. The MVP 10 has no built-in oxygen analyzer, so it is recommended that the operator carefully measure the amount of delivered gas.

Modes

The MVP 10 has two optional modes of ventilation. The first is nonsynchronized IMV, in which the ventilator will time-trigger a pressure-targeted mandatory breath based on the set inspiratory time and rate. For this mode to be activated, the mode switch needs to be in the cycle position.

The second operational mode is the CPAP mode, in which a continuous supply of gas is provided through the patient circuit at the set level of CPAP.

BIRD AVIAN

The Bird Avian transport ventilator was described in the 7th edition of this text. This material is now available on Evolve Resources.

DRÄGER MICROVENT

The Dräger Microvent transport ventilator was described in the 7th edition of this text. This material is now available on Evolve Resources.

DRÄGER OXYLOG 2000

The Oxylog 2000 (Figure 14-9) is a time-triggered or patient-triggered, volume-targeted ventilator used primarily for emergencies and transporting adults; however, it can be used for pediatric patients who weigh at least 33 lb.[9] The Oxylog can function in three modes: control, SIMV, and CPAP. It is lightweight (9.5 lb) and portable (8.5 in × 4.7 in × 8.1 in) (Dräger Medical AG & Co, Lübeck, Germany). Additional important specifications for the Oxylog 2000 are listed in Table 14-6.

Power Source

The Dräger Oxylog requires an electrical and a pneumatic source to properly function. The electronic system can use the following three separate power sources:

- An AC outlet
- An external 12-V battery
- An internal rechargeable or nonrechargeable battery

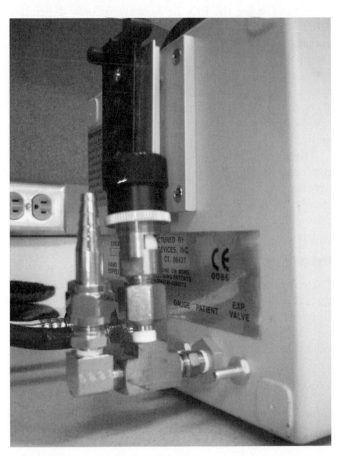

FIGURE 14-7 Bio-Med MVP 10; maximum pressure control.

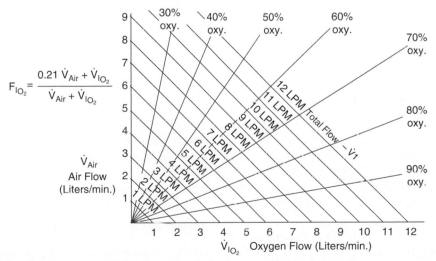

$$F_{IO_2} = \frac{0.21\,\dot{V}_{Air} + \dot{V}_{IO_2}}{\dot{V}_{Air} + \dot{V}_{IO_2}}$$

FIGURE 14-8 Bio-Med MVP 10 air-oxygen-mixing ratio chart. (Redrawn from information provided by Bio-Med Devices, Inc, Guilford, Conn.)

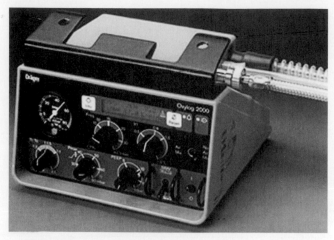

FIGURE 14-9 The Dräger Oxylog 2000 ventilator. (Courtesy Dräger Medical AG & Co, Lübeck, Germany.)

TABLE 14-6	
Specifications for the Dräger Oxylog 2000	
Control Settings	Range
Modes	Control, SIMV, and CPAP
Power source	AC, external 12-V battery, internal battery
Rate	5 breaths/min
Noninvasive ventilation mode	N/A
Peak pressure	20-60 cm H_2O
Tidal volume	100-1500 mL
Inspiratory time	5-12 breaths/min = 2 s 12-40 breaths/min = 1 s
PEEP/CPAP	1-15 cm H_2O
Oxygen percent	60% or 100%
Pressure support	N/A
Monitors/displays	Analog pressure gauge, LCD
Dimensions	8.5 in × 4.8 in × 8.2 in; 9.5 lb
Gas consumption	1 L/min
Alarms	Low supply pressure, high peak airway pressure, low airway pressure, leakage, apnea, high-frequency
Battery duration	6 h maximum

When the ventilator is connected to one of the two external power sources, the green "power connected" status light goes on and the rechargeable internal battery pack starts charging regardless of whether the ventilator is on or off. This internal battery is essential to the operation of the machine. It has a functional lifespan of approximately 6 hours when fully charged and requires approximately 8 hours to recharge to maximum capacity. When approximately 10 minutes of operation is left, a message in the display window reads: "Charge NiCd," where *NiCd* denotes nickel-cadmium.

The pneumatic component requires a high-pressure medical-grade gas (oxygen or air) supplied in a range of 38 psi to 84 psi. The source may be a cylinder, wall outlet, or oxygen/air blender with a DISS connector.

BOX 14-3	Dräger Oxylog 2000 Air/Mix Injector

When the air/mix switch is on, the gas source passes through the internal injector, which draws ambient air from the room to dilute the mixture to 60%. This conserves gas use by 50% and allows for prolonged transport when a limited source gas is used.

In the Oxylog the F_IO_2 delivery is not only dependent on the gas source being used, but also on the air/mix switch and the mode selected for use. The air/mix switch allows the operator to choose from 1.0 to 0.60 F_IO_2 when oxygen is the gas source. The air/mix function is only operational for mandatory breaths. All spontaneous breaths receive 100% of the source gas. Attaching an air/oxygen blender to regulate F_IO_2 gives the operator more control over oxygen delivery.

The internal pneumatic components of the ventilator consume 1 L/min of gas to support their functions. It is necessary to include this factor in the calculation for cylinder duration when a cylinder is used to power the unit during transport. The Oxylog is also equipped with an oxygen-conserving device, an air/mix injector (Box 14-3).

Internal Mechanism

The gas source enters through the inlet port at the rear of the machine and is immediately filtered and reduced to a constant working pressure by a regulator. From the regulator, the flow is diverted to prime the PEEP and exhalation valves; from these valves, the flow makes its way to the inspiratory/expiratory (I/E) valve. The I/E valve regulates the release of inspiratory flow in a time-cycled fashion.

Next, the gas flow passes through an electronically controlled pressure regulator, which governs the rate and pattern of flow before it passes through one of the following two valves:
1. A pneumatic control valve that supplies the patient with a 100% gas source
2. An injector that supplies the patient with a 60% gas source

The route is determined by the position of the air/mix switch (see Box 14-3). After its route through the pneumatic valve or the injector, the gas flows to the patient circuit.

To initiate a spontaneous breath, the patient must open the demand valve by generating a minimum pressure change of −1 cm H_2O. During a spontaneous breath, gas from the demand valve bypasses the injector that is regulated by the air/mix switch. As a result, all spontaneous breaths are provided at 100% source gas. The maximum flow for a spontaneous breath is 120 L/min.

Controls and Alarms

The controls and alarms on the Oxylog 2000 are easy to operate (Figure 14-10) and are described in the following section.

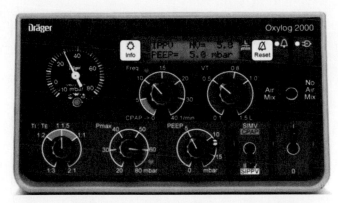

FIGURE 14-10 The Dräger Oxylog 2000 ventilator's control panel. (Courtesy Dräger Medical AG & Co, Lübeck, Germany.)

TABLE 14-7

Dräger Oxylog 2000 and Oxylog 3000: Color-Coded Settings for Patient Size, Minute Ventilation, and Rate

Color	Patient Size Range (kg)	Minute Ventilation	Ventilator Rate
Green	Infants: 10-20 kg	0.1-0.3 L	30-40 breaths/min
Blue	Children: 20-40 kg	0.3-0.8 L	20-30 breaths/min
Brown	Adults: >40 kg	0.8-1.5 L	5-20 breaths/min

Courtesy of Dräger Medical AG & Co, Lübeck, Germany.

Pressure-Monitoring Gauge

The pressure gauge is on the top-left part of the control panel and provides continuous measurements of airway pressure in centimeters of water.

Control Parameters

The control parameters include the following: V_T, rate, I:E RATIO, and PEEP. The V_T knob regulates the volume delivered to the patient during each mandatory breath (100 to 1500 mL). The V_T is also color-coded for quick set-up. The Oxylog has three tidal ranges from which the operator can choose. The green range is for infants who weigh from 10 kg to 20 kg and have a respiratory rate of 30 breaths/min to 40 breaths/min. The blue range is for children who weigh from 20 kg to 40 kg and have a respiratory rate of 20 breaths/min to 30 breaths/min. The final range is the brown range for adults who weigh more than 40 kg and who have a respiratory rate of 5 breaths/min to 20 breaths/min. (See the discussion in this section and Table 14-7 for further information.)

The rate knob is to the left of the volume setting and functions to regulate the set number of mandatory breaths in the control mode and the minimum number of mandatory breaths in SIMV. The ventilator has an adjustable range of 5 breaths/min to 60 breaths/min in the control and SIMV modes. When the mode selector is placed in SIMV mode and the rate is less than 5 breaths/min, the ventilator switches to CPAP.

The I:E knob is at the bottom left of the control panel and has an operational range of 1:3 to 2:1 (±5%). The

---

TABLE 14-8

I:E Ratio in the SIMV Mode for the Dräger Oxylog 2000

Frequency Setting	Effect
0	No ventilator breaths (CPAP)
5-12 breaths/min	Fixed T_I (2 s)
12-40 breaths/min	Fixed T_I (1 s)
	I:E = 1:1.5

Courtesy of Dräger Medical AG & Co, Lübeck, Germany.
I:E, Inspiratory/expiratory (ratio); T_I, inspiratory time.

Oxylog allows for inverse-ratio ventilation (IRV) in the control mode, which is not a common feature in transport ventilators. In the SIMV mode, the I:E ratio is determined by the rate setting (Table 14-8).

The PEEP control is located on the lower-middle part of the control panel and has an operational range of 0 cm H_2O to 15 cm H_2O. The PEEP control is functional in all modes.

Alarms and Alarm Reset

The Oxylog provides high and low airway pressure alarms, high and low minute ventilation alarms, and power source alarms.

High-Pressure Alarm

The high-pressure alarm labeled "P_{max}" is in the lower-left section of the control panel and has an adjustable range of 20 cm H_2O to 60 cm H_2O. When airway pressures exceed the P_{max} (maximum pressure) setting, a red alarm status light starts blinking and an intermittent audible alarm is triggered. Simultaneously, the inspiratory flow stops and the exhalation valve opens. When the problem is corrected, the audible alarm is silenced, but the visual display must be manually reset with the alarm reset button at the top right of the control panel. The alarm reset button can also be used to silence audible alarms for 2 minutes. If the problem is corrected, the alarm reset button clears the display screen.

Low-Pressure Alarms

The low-pressure alarm does not have a control knob. It is activated when the pressure in the patient circuit does not reach at least 10 cm H_2O within 20 seconds of the previous mandatory breath. An audiovisual alarm is activated that is not functional in the CPAP mode.

High and Low Minute Ventilation Alarms

Minute ventilation is an additional parameter that is monitored by the Oxylog. The Oxylog monitors expired minute ventilation through the flow sensor near the expiratory valve and ensures that the patient is being properly ventilated. The current reading is shown in the display window. A fluctuation outside of set parameters may activate the audiovisual alarm. If the expiratory minute volume falls below 40% of the inspiratory minute volume, the alarm is activated. Tubing and connections should be checked for any possible problems, because a leak is suggested.

Apnea Alarm

The apnea alarm is functional only in the CPAP mode. When the patient does not make sufficient effort to open the demand valve within 15 seconds, an audiovisual alarm is activated.

Power System Alarm

The pneumatic system has an O_2 "pressure low" alarm that is activated when the gas inlet pressure falls below 28 psi. This indicates that the gas source is not providing sufficient pressure for proper ventilator function. The electronic system has a power-failure alarm and a "Charge NiCd" alarm that are activated when the external power supply fails or the internal battery has less than 10 minutes of power left.

Modes of Ventilation

The Dräger Oxylog 2000 offers control, SIMV, and CPAP modes. In the control mode, the ventilator requires that the V_T, rate, and I:E ratio be set. The unit is then time-triggered. To trigger a mandatory breath, the machine requires the patient to initiate a 4 L/min change in flow. To receive gas flow for a spontaneous breath in the SIMV mode, the patient must generate a pressure change of −2 cm H_2O below baseline to open the demand valve. As in the control mode, V_T and rate are set and active in SIMV, but the I:E ratio is not; it is determined by the rate setting (see Table 14-8).

The third option of ventilation is CPAP. In CPAP, only the PEEP control is set. As with spontaneous breaths in SIMV, to trigger gas flow in this mode, the patient must generate a pressure change of −2 cm H_2O below baseline. The air/mix switch is nonfunctional because all breaths come from the demand valve, which bypasses the air/mix injector.

DRÄGER OXYLOG 3000

The Oxylog 3000 (Dräger Medical AG & Co, Lübeck, Germany) is another of the Dräger ventilators used for transport (Figure 14-11). The Oxylog 3000 is a time-triggered or patient-triggered, volume-controlled or pressure controlled, time-cycled ventilator for patients requiring V_T of 50 mL to 2000 mL. The basic dimensions excluding the handle are 11.10 in × 7.24 in × 6.89 in. It weighs 11.9 lb, including the internal battery.[10] Table 14-9 provides some of the available parameters and features of the Oxylog 3000.

There are several differences between the Oxylog 2000 and the Oxylog 3000. The most notable feature on the Oxylog 3000 is the electroluminescence screen, which displays flow graphics, ventilation mode, expired V_T, minute volume, calculated F_IO_2, trigger sensitivity, PEEP level, a battery-power indicator, and the amount of gas consump-

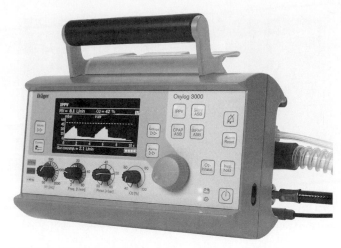

FIGURE 14-11 The Dräger Oxylog 3000 ventilator. (Courtesy Dräger Medical AG & Co, Lübeck, Germany.)

TABLE 14-9	
Specifications of the Dräger Oxylog 3000	
Control Settings	**Range**
Modes	CMV, SIMV/PS, CPAP/PS, PCV/PS, BiPAP
Power source	AC power, external 10-V to 32-V power source, internal rechargeable battery
Rate	2-60 breaths/min
Noninvasive ventilation mode	Yes
Peak pressure	20-100 cm H_2O
Tidal volume	50-2000 mL
Inspiratory time	0.2-10 s
PEEP/CPAP	0-20 cm H_2O
Oxygen percent	40-100%
Pressure support	0-35 cm H_2O
Monitors/displays	Electroluminescence screen
Dimensions	11.10 in × 7.24 in × 6.89 in; 11.9 lb
Gas consumption	0.1-0.5 L/min
Alarms	Low supply pressure, high peak airway pressure, low airway pressure, leakage, apnea, high-frequency
Battery duration	3 h with nickel–metal hydride battery 4 h with lithium ion battery

PS, Pressure support; *CMV,* continuous mandatory ventilation; *PCV,* pressure-controlled ventilation; *BiPAP,* bilevel positive airway pressure.

tion. The Oxylog 3000 also allows for noninvasive (mask) ventilation with enhanced ventilatory control with functions such as pressure support and pressure-controlled ventilation plus (PCV+, or BiPAP). The Oxylog 3000 also automatically compensates for changes in altitude.

Power Source

The Dräger Oxylog 3000 requires both an electrical and a pneumatic power source to properly function. The electronic system can use the following three separate power sources:

- An AC outlet (100- to 240-V AC power)
- An external 10- to 32-V power source via an optional DC/DC converter
- An internal rechargeable lithium ion or nickel metal-hydride battery

When the ventilator is connected to one of the two external power sources, the green "power connected" status light goes on and the rechargeable internal battery pack starts charging regardless of whether the ventilator is on or off. This internal battery is essential to the operation of the machine. It has a functional lifespan of approximately 4 hours with the lithium ion battery and 3 hours with the nickel–metal hydride battery when fully charged and requires approximately 5 hours to recharge. The lithium ion battery requires approximately 5 hours to recharge, and the nickel–metal hydride battery requires approximately 4 hours to recharge. The battery pack can be "hot-swapped," which means that it can be replaced by a charged battery within a few seconds without having to restart the ventilator.

The pneumatic component requires a high-pressure medical-grade gas (oxygen or air) supplied in a range of 39 psi to 87 psi. The source may be a cylinder, wall outlet, or oxygen/air blender with a DISS connector.

Internal Mechanism

High-pressure oxygen enters through the inlet port at the right side of the Oxylog, and it is immediately filtered and reduced to a constant working pressure by a regulator. Next, the gas source passes into an electronically controlled pressure regulator, which governs the rate and pattern of flow of the gas. The gas then enters the pneumatic connection block, which internally controls PEEP during exhalation and with the ventilation accessories provides the interface with the patient.

The incoming oxygen supply is also routed to the metering block, which entrains room air through a patented Venturi principle, blending it to the desired F_IO_2 (range: 0.4 to 1.0).

Oxygen

In the Oxylog 3000, the F_IO_2 delivery is controlled by the metering block. In flow ranges of 9 L/min to 35 L/min, an oxygen concentration of 40% to 100% can be delivered. If the flows are less than 9 L/min or greater than 35 L/min, the minimum concentration of 40% can no longer be guaranteed. The internal pneumatic components of the ventilator consume only 0.1 L/min to 0.5 L/min of gas to support their functions, so the bulk of oxygen used is for patient ventilation.

Controls

The control panel of the Oxylog 3000 is shown in Figure 14-12.

Start/Standby Key and LED Indicators

The Start/Standby soft key is located in the lower right-hand corner of the control surface. Pressing this soft key

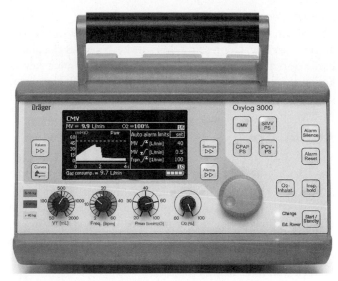

FIGURE 14-12 The Dräger Oxylog 3000 ventilator's control panel. (Courtesy Dräger Medical AG & Co, Lübeck, Germany.)

will power up the Oxylog 3000. To the immediate left of the start/standby soft key are two light-emitting diode (LED) indicators. The "Ext Power" indicator will illuminate if the ventilator is operating on external power—either AC or external DC power. Just above the Ext Power LED is the charge indicator, which is illuminated in orange when the battery is charging and in green when the battery is fully charged.

Inspiratory Hold

The inspiratory hold soft key is located directly above the start/standby soft key. Once the inspiratory hold key is depressed, the Oxylog 3000 will either extend the momentary ventilation breath or start a new inspiratory breath and hold it for a maximum of 15 seconds.

O₂ Inhalation

To help reduce the risk of hypoxia during bronchial suctioning, a 100% O_2 support function is available. The O_2 inhalation soft key is located to the left of the inspiratory hold soft key. Depressing this soft key will increase the F_IO_2 to 100% for 3 minutes regardless of the preset F_IO_2. A green LED on the soft key is illuminated when this feature is active. The set F_IO_2 will be resumed at the end of the 3-minute period or when the 100% O_2 key is pressed again. When medical air is used as the drive gas, the 100% O_2 function will not deliver pure oxygen. This soft key is to help oxygenate before suctioning or intubation in non-invasive ventilation.

Alarm Reset

The alarm reset soft key is located just above the inspiratory hold soft key. Once pressed, it will reset all alarms to their set limits and clear the display of any alarm messages.

Alarm Silence

The alarm silence soft key is located directly above the alarm reset key. Depressing this soft key silences the alarm condition for 2 minutes. Once the alarm silence key is active, it is indicated by an LED on the soft key. If the alarm condition has not been remedied, the alarm will sound again.

Mode Keys

The Oxylog 3000 has four mode soft keys located just above the control dial. Modes are CMV, SIMV/PS, CPAP/PS, and PCV + PS. The desired default ventilation mode can be set in the "user configuration" menu, so that the Oxylog 3000 will begin ventilation in the mode of choice. Activating the soft key for any of the modes of ventilation enables that mode to become operational. The modes will be reviewed later in this section.

Rotary Selection Dial/Settings Key/Alarms Key

This control dial is located below the mode soft keys. Used in conjunction with the settings and alarm soft keys, the operator can select desired operating parameters using a process of "select-change-confirm." The operator can select any function or value displayed in the settings or alarm menu by rotating the button until the desired value is highlighted; then by pushing the button to select the desired value; by rotating the button to change the value or function; and, finally, by pushing the button to confirm the new setting. Requiring an active confirmation of a setting helps support patient safety.

Additional Controls

The O_2 % control dial is located to the left of the rotary selection dial. This dial allows adjustment of F_IO_2 from 0.4 to 1.0. The Oxylog 3000 blends room air through the Venturi system to achieve the selected F_IO_2. The F_IO_2 is displayed on the screen.

The P_{max} control is located to the left of the oxygen control. It allows the operator to set a maximum pressure limit (adjustable range: 20 to 100 cm H_2O).

The frequency control is adjustable from 2 breaths/min to 60 breaths/min, and it is color-coded to assist the operator in setting a respiratory rate appropriate for the patient's size (see Table 14-7). The green range is for infants who weigh from 10 kg to 20 kg (respiratory rate range: 30 to 40 breaths/min). The blue range is for children 20 kg to 40 kg (respiratory rate range: 20 to 30 breaths/min). The brown range is for adults who weigh more than 40 kg (respiratory rate range: 5 to 20 breaths/min).

The V_T control is also color-coded in a manner similar to the frequency control. The V_T is adjustable from 50 mL to 2000 mL. The Oxylog 3000 measures V_T at body temperature and pressure-saturated (BTPS) conditions. The Oxylog 3000 can automatically compensate for V_T delivery when altitude changes.

Curves/Volumes

The soft keys for curves and volumes are located to the left of the electroluminescence display screen. These soft keys allow the operator to change displayed waveforms to either flow/time or pressure/time. They also allow for changes in displayed volumes, including the following: minute volume, set frequency, exhaled V_T, PEEP, peak pressure, mean airway pressure, plateau pressure, spontaneous minute volume, spontaneous respiratory rate, and oxygen percentage.

Alarms

The Oxylog 3000 has multiple built-in alarms and has three distinct levels of alarm conditions. Each alarm condition has its own display and audible alert. This information is detailed in Box 14-4.

The Oxylog 3000 also has an auto alarm function to help support quick start-up of the ventilator. Once initial ventilation has been set up, the auto alarm function can be activated in the settings menu. The function "auto alarm limits" sets the alarm limits on the ventilator based on the actual measured values at the time of activation:

Minute ventilation high alarm (MVhigh)
= measured minute ventilation + 2 L/min
Minute ventilation low alarm (MVlow)
= measured minute ventilation − 2 L/min
Spontaneous frequency alarm (fspn)
= measured spontaneous frequency + 5 breaths/min

BOX 14-4	**Dräger Oxylog 3000 Alarm Conditions**

In the event of an alarm, the red or yellow alarm light-emitting diode (LED) flashes. The alarm message appears on the right of the top line on the screen.

The Oxylog 3000 assigns corresponding priority to the alarm message, highlights the text with the appropriate number of exclamation marks (as follows), and generates different tone sequences for the respective alarms:

!!! = Warning
!! = Caution
! = Advisory

Warning
A warning is an alarm with top priority. The red alarm LED flashes. Warnings are highlighted by 3 exclamation marks and displayed in inverted form. The Oxylog 3000 generates a sequence of 5 tones that sound twice and repeat every 7.5 seconds.

Caution
A caution is an alarm of medium priority. The yellow alarm LED flashes. Caution messages are highlighted by 2 exclamation marks. The Oxylog 3000 generates a 3-tone sequence that is repeated every 20 seconds.

Advisory
An advisory is a low-priority alarm. The yellow alarm LED lights up. Advisory messages are identified by 1 exclamation mark. The Oxylog 3000 generates a 2-tone alarm sequence that only sounds once.

Supply Pressure Low

This alarm is activated when the supply pressure of the source gas is below 39 psi. Audible and visual alarm indicators are active with this condition.

High Peak Airway Pressure

This alarm is activated when the delivered peak airway pressure exceeds the operator-set limit. The peak airway pressure is adjustable from 20 cm H_2O to 100 cm H_2O and is set with the P_{max} control dial, which was described earlier in this chapter. Audible and visual alarm indicators are active with this condition.

Low Airway Pressure

This alarm is activated when the pressure difference between the delivered peak airway pressure and the expiratory pressure is less than 5 cm H_2O or when the set peak airway pressure is not attained. Audible and visual alarm indicators are active with this condition.

Apnea Alarm

An apnea alarm condition is activated when no respiratory activity is detected. This alarm response time is adjustable from 15 seconds to 60 seconds. Audible and visual alarm indicators are active with this condition.

Leakage

A leakage alarm activates when the measured expired V_T is approximately 40% lower than the measured inspired V_T. This alarm is not available in the noninvasive mode.

High Frequency

The high-frequency alarm is activated when the total respiratory rate exceeds the set high respiratory rate limit set by the operator. The adjustable range of the high-frequency alarm is from 2 breaths/min to 60 breaths/min.

Modes of Ventilation

The modes of ventilation available on the Oxylog 3000 are listed in Box 14-5. An apnea backup rate is available on the Oxylog 3000 with an adjustable apnea delay activation time from 15 seconds to 60 seconds. When the apnea ventilation activation time (T_{apnea}) is selected, the Dräger 3000 will then ask the operator to select a desired apnea rate and V_T to be applied during an apneic event. This means that once set, apnea ventilation will remain unchanged until the values (rate and volume) are changed in the menu.

The selected maximum airway pressure (P_{max}) must be adjusted high enough to allow pressure to build up for the volume-controlled ventilation breath. The I : E ratio during apnea ventilation is automatically preset at a 1 : 1.5 ratio. To deactivate the apnea backup ventilation mode, the operator needs to once again enter the menu and turn T_{apnea} to the off position.

The Oxylog 3000 also has the capability to provide noninvasive ventilatory support via an appropriate mask interface.

CMV/CMV_assist

The CMV mode provides breaths that are patient- or time-triggered, volume-targeted, and time-cycled. The controls for respiratory rate (range: 5 to 60 breaths/min) and V_T (range: 50 to 2000 mL) establish a baseline minute ventilation. All breaths deliver the set V_T.

CMV_assist is used for patients who have some spontaneous effort. Adjustment of the trigger sensitivity is necessary to synchronize with the patient's breathing efforts. Trigger sensitivity is accessed through the settings menu.

SIMV/PS

The SIMV mode provides a maximum number of mandatory breaths and allows the patient to breathe spontaneously between the mandatory breaths. Mandatory breaths can be either time-triggered or patient-triggered, volume-targeted or pressure-targeted, and time-cycled. Spontaneous breaths can be supplemented with pressure support (PS). PS breaths are patient-triggered, pressure-limited, and flow-cycled.

Selecting the SIMV/PS mode soft key allows the operator to set an SIMV rate ranging from 2 breaths/min to 60 breaths/min and a V_T of 50 mL to 2000 mL. Pressure support (PS) is available in this mode from 0 cm H_2O to 35 cm H_2O above baseline (set PEEP). Both PEEP and PS levels can be changed through accessing the settings menu on the display screen. PEEP levels greater than 10 cm H_2O have to be confirmed with an additional step for patient safety (Clinical Rounds 14-5).

BOX 14-5	Oxylog 3000 Modes of Operation

CMV/CMV_assist (continuous mandatory ventilation/CMV assistance)
SIMV/PS (pressure support)
PCV+/PS (pressure-controlled ventilation plus/pressure support)
CPAP/PS
Apnea backup

CLINICAL ROUNDS 14-5

You are transporting a 43-year-old patient to receive a computed tomography (CT) scan; the patient is connected to the Dräger Oxylog 3000. The patient is on an F_IO_2 of 70%, synchronized IMV (SIMV) rate of 14 breaths/min, and a tidal volume (V_T) of 900 mL. PEEP is 12 cm H_2O. You enter the patient's settings in the Oxylog 3000 and connect the patient to the unit. Then an alarm sounds and a message appears in the display window: "PEEP > 10 mbar?" What must you do to clear this alarm message?

See Evolve Resources for the answer.

PCV+/PS

PCV is a mode in which the patient can breathe spontaneously at any time, even during the inspiratory inflation cycle. This mode is described in detail in Chapter 12 in the section on the Dräger Evita 4. It is sometimes referred to as *bilevel positive pressure ventilation* by the manufacturer. Mandatory breaths are time-triggered or patient-triggered, pressure-targeted, and time-cycled. This mode is similar to that found in a high-flow CPAP device because of the presence of an open expiratory valve system.

In PCV+ the operator sets the minimum respiratory rate, inspiratory pressure above PEEP, and the flow trigger. The PCV+ mode in this ventilator is always SIMV-based because the patient can breathe spontaneously during the expiratory time. A patient's spontaneous breaths independent of the set mandatory breaths can be assisted with PS. The delivered V_T and minute ventilation may vary, so the operator needs to carefully set minute ventilation alarm limits.

Activating the PCV + PS soft key allows the operator to set a rate from 2 breaths/min to 60 breaths/min with an adjustable set inspiratory control pressure value ranging from PEEP 3 cm H_2O to 55 cm H_2O.

CPAP/PS

The CPAP mode is used for spontaneously breathing patients who may only require a set level of PEEP to restore their functional residual capacity and possibly reduce work of breathing. The operator sets the desired PEEP level and F_IO_2. PS can also be added.

The apnea backup function is operational in this mode and should be set to provide adequate ventilation if apnea should occur.

Touching the CPAP/PS soft key allows the operator to set a CPAP level from 0 cm H_2O to 20 cm H_2O. The maximum inspiratory flow for spontaneous breaths is 100 L/min, which includes leakage. The PS level is adjustable, as described earlier, from 0 cm H_2O to 35 cm H_2O relative to the set PEEP level.

HAMILTON MEDICAL MAX

The Hamilton Medical MAX is used to transport pediatric or adult patients requiring ventilation. Further information on the MAX is available on Evolve Resources.

IMPACT UNI-VENT 750

The Uni-Vent 750 (Impact Instrumentation, Inc, West Caldwell, New Jersey) is a pressure-triggered or time-triggered, volume-targeted, pressure-cycled or time-cycled, microprocessor-controlled ventilator used primarily for patient transport.[11] It is 9 in × 11.5 in × 4.5 in and weighs approximately 12.5 lb (Figure 14-13). This ventilator can provide control, A/C, and SIMV modes of ventilation. Table 14-10 illustrates important features of the Impact Uni-Vent 750.

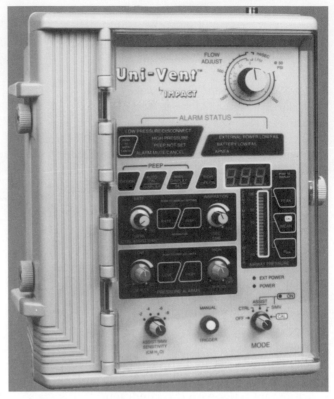

FIGURE 14-13 The Impact Uni-Vent 750 ventilator. (Courtesy Impact Instrumentation, Inc, West Caldwell, New Jersey)

TABLE 14-10	
Specifications for the Impact Uni-Vent 750	
Control Settings	**Range**
Modes	A/C and SIMV
Power source	Pneumatic and electric power internal DC battery, external DC battery or 120-VAC outlet (with a converter)
Rate	1-150 breaths/min
Noninvasive ventilation mode	N/A
Peak pressure	100 cm H_2O
Tidal volume	0-3000 mL
Inspiratory time	0.1-3 s
PEEP/CPAP	0-20 cm H_2O external valve
Oxygen percent	100% unless blended
Pressure support	N/A
Monitors/displays	Alphanumeric display and digital bar graph
Dimensions	9 in × 11.5 in × 4.5 in; approximately 12.5 lb
Gas consumption	N/A
Alarms	High- and low-pressure/disconnect, PEEP not set, inverse I : E, and apnea
Battery duration	Estimated life of 9 h

A/C, Assist/control.

Power Source

The Uni-Vent 750 requires pneumatic and electric power supplies to perform properly. The electronic system requires one of the following three sources to power the microprocessor and its electrical components:

· An internal DC battery
· An external DC battery
· A 120-V AC outlet (with a converter)

The internal battery has an estimated life of 9 hours.

The pneumatic system requires a high-pressure source gas at 50 psi to 100 psi to properly perform. The source may be a cylinder, wall outlet, or oxygen/air blender. Because the Uni-Vent operates exclusively from one gas source, the oxygen percentage depends on the gas powering the ventilator. To precisely regulate the F_IO_2, the operator should connect the unit to an air/oxygen blender. There is no entrainment feature on this ventilator.

Internal Mechanism

The pneumatic system receives the source gas from the oxygen inlet on the rear panel and routes the gas through an **internal regulator** that precisely adjusts the pressure to 50 psi. After passing the regulator, the gas flow is guided through two parallel circuits. The first circuit, which contains two main inspiratory flow valves, is used during control and A/C modes. If one valve does not close when the machine cycles into expiration, the second valve stops gas flow to the patient and prevents overinflation. This is a safety feature of the system. During a patient-triggered or time-triggered breath, the inspiratory flow solenoid opens and gas passes the flow-control valve and is directed to the patient. The Uni-Vent has no V_T setting. The volume delivered to the patient depends on the set inspiratory time (T_I) and flow.

When spontaneous breaths are initiated, the flow through the system is directed to the pneumatically controlled demand valve. The demand valve has an opening pressure of −1 cm H_2O below baseline. After the demand valve is opened, the gas source passes through a fixed orifice, which limits the peak flow for spontaneous breaths to the patient to 60 L/min.

When disposable patient circuits are used, a separate antiasphyxia valve must be attached at the patient connection to allow for spontaneous breaths in case of valve failure. The nondisposable circuits have a patient valve instead of an exhalation valve (Figure 14-14). The patient valve in the nondisposable units serves the function of the exhalation valve and also contains the antiasphyxia valve.

The Uni-Vent 750 requires that an **external PEEP valve** be attached to the exhalation valve. The ventilator compensates for added PEEP with one of two mechanisms: automatic or manual. In the automatic mode, the microprocessor analyzes the patient circuit's pressure waveforms over three consecutive breaths to determine the level of PEEP. This process of updating the PEEP in the patient circuit is a continuous one. The manual process requires

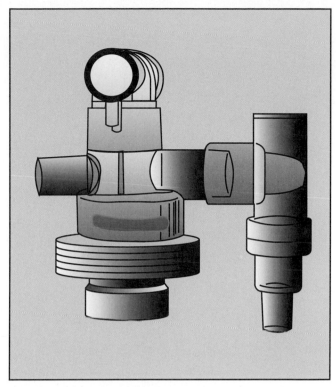

FIGURE 14-14 The Impact Uni-Vent 750 ventilator's patient valve. (Courtesy Impact Instrumentation, Inc, West Caldwell, New Jersey.)

the operator to enter the PEEP value directly into the microprocessor using the keypad. When the operator chooses to use the manual method, the "PEEP not set" alarm is inactivated.

Controls and Alarms

The Uni-Vent contains several controls for setting and monitoring parameters and alarms. The controls are sequentially numbered for operator ease of use (Figure 14-15).

Rate

The respiratory rate control is active in control, A/C, and SIMV modes of ventilation and time-triggers a mandatory breath in each of these modes. It has an adjustable range of 1 breath/min to 150 breaths/min. The set rate, in combination with the set T_I, controls the I:E ratio of the ventilator.

Flow Adjust

The flow adjust control allows for adjustable flow rates from 50 mL/s to 1500 mL/s (3 to 90 L/min). If the flow setting is insufficient for the inspiratory demands of the patient, then the antiasphyxia valve allows room air to be entrained for additional flow. When air entrainment occurs, the valve creates a whistling sound, alerting the operator to the problem. (NOTE: Opening of the antiasphyxia valve and entrainment of room air can alter the F_IO_2 delivered to the patient.) (See also Clinical Rounds 14-6.)

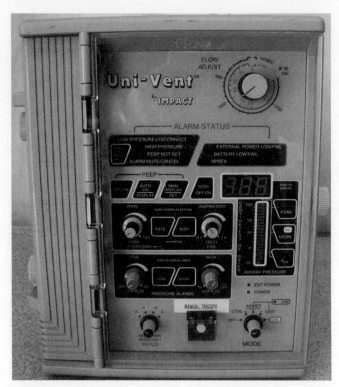

FIGURE 14-15 The Impact Uni-Vent 750 ventilator's control panel. (Courtesy Impact Instrumentation, Inc, West Caldwell, N.J.)

CLINICAL ROUNDS 14-6

You are asked to transport a trauma patient from the emergency department to the ICU. You quickly apply the ventilator settings reported to you. Once you attach the patient to the circuit and begin to ventilate, you note a whistling sound coming from the ventilator. The patient continues to be ventilated, but what is the likely cause of this sound and how can you remedy the situation?

See Evolve Resources for the answer.

Manual Breath

The manual breath button can be used to deliver a positive pressure breath whenever the operator considers it appropriate. The manual breath function is operational in all modes. When activated, the ventilator delivers a breath at the set flow for as long as the operator holds the button. This control is designed to be operational if there is a central processing unit (CPU) or electronics failure. The breath timer is reset after a full exhalation period elapses, thereby preventing the stacking of a time-delivered breath.

Airway Pressure Alarms

There are two airway pressure alarms on the 750 that can be adjusted and monitored. They are the high-pressure and the low–pressure/disconnect alarms. The high-pressure alarm is activated when the airway pressure exceeds the set

high-pressure alarm for 2 seconds during a single breath. It also acts as a pressure relief for the ventilator. If the high-pressure setting is surpassed, the ventilator vents the excess flow to the atmosphere and allows the set T_I to complete its cycle. The adjustable range of this function is 15 cm H_2O to 100 cm H_2O.

The low–pressure/disconnect alarm detects leaks and disconnections in the patient circuit and has an adjustable range of 0 cm H_2O to 50 cm H_2O. If the patient fails to meet the low-pressure setting or if the airway pressure fails to reach +1 cm H_2O at the time of the next mandatory breath, the alarm is activated.

Additional Alarms

Three additional alarms on the Uni-Vent 750 are the apnea, the PEEP not set, and the inverse I:E alarms. The apnea alarm is activated when the patient fails to trigger a spontaneous or mandatory breath within 19 seconds (nonadjustable). The ventilator defaults to a backup rate of 12 breaths/min and uses the currently set V_T. The apnea alarm is operational only in the assist and SIMV modes.

The PEEP not set alarm is activated when the end-expiratory pressure fails to return to the set value by +2 to −1 cm H_2O for three consecutive breaths. This alarm is inactivated when the manual instead of the automatic mode is used to set PEEP.

The Uni-Vent 750 does not allow for IRV. Any combination of rate and T_I that creates a longer inspiratory than expiratory period activates the inverse I:E alarm. The ventilator defaults to exhalation and elicits an audiovisual alarm that cannot be deactivated until the problem is corrected.

Power Alarms

The Uni-Vent 750 has two power alarms: external power low/fail and battery low/fail. The external power low/fail alerts the operator when the external power source is disconnected or fails. The battery low/fail alarm is set off when the internal battery voltage falls below 11 V; when the battery is defective; or when the battery will not recharge.

Modes of Ventilation

The Uni-Vent 750 offers three modes of ventilation: control, A/C, and SIMV. In the control mode, the machine delivers time-triggered, volume-targeted breaths based on the set rate, T_I, and flow. If necessary, the patient can breathe spontaneously between the mandatory breaths through the antiasphyxia valve (see Figure 14-14). In a sense, this is like an IMV mode.

The A/C mode lets the patient initiate mandatory breaths and ultimately control the total rate of the ventilator (time-triggered and patient-triggered). All other functions that were set in the control mode are still active in A/C mode with the addition of assist sensitivity. Breaths are patient-triggered or time-triggered, volume-targeted, and time-cycled.

BOX 14-6	Control and SIMV Modes on the Uni-Vent 750

With the unit in the control mode, the patient receives time-triggered mandatory breaths. Between these breaths, the patient can breathe spontaneously from the antiasphyxia valve in the patient circuit.

In the SIMV mode, the mandatory breaths are patient-triggered or time-triggered. Between mandatory breaths, the patient breathes spontaneously from the internal demand valve.

In the control mode, spontaneous breaths are at room air (fractional inspired oxygen [F_IO_2] = 0.21). In the SIMV mode, spontaneous breaths receive the F_IO_2 provided by the gas source.

When the SIMV mode is used, the patient can breathe spontaneously through the internal demand valve and receive mandatory breaths through the main inspiratory valve. All controls set in the A/C mode are set for the mandatory breaths in SIMV. The patient's spontaneous efforts must generate a pressure change of at least −1 cm H_2O to open the internal demand valve and obtain flow (Box 14-6).

IMPACT UNI-VENT EAGLE™ 754

The Uni-Vent Eagle™ 754 (Figure 14-16) is an upgraded version of Impact's Uni-Vent 750 (Impact Instrumentation, Inc, West Caldwell, N.J.). Additions include a direct V_T setting and an alarm package that features scroll knobs that allow high-pressure and low-pressure alarms to be set directly on the digital bar graph. The Eagle™ 754 also includes a backup ventilation mode that is activated during apneic periods.[11] The 754 ventilators are sequentially numbered for ease of set-up and operation as seen in Figure 14-17.

In addition, the Eagle™ 754 allows the operator the option of pressure plateau ventilation. In this mode, the ventilator limits the pressure allowed in the circuit and airways but does not end inspiration until the desired V_T is delivered. If the pressure in the airways reaches the set pressure limit before the entire V_T is delivered, a pressure plateau occurs, venting the excess flow until the ventilator delivers the entire V_T.

The Eagle 754™ also has an LCD display that lets the operator view all settings continuously along with real-time pressure waveforms, a built-in compressor with a blender, an F_IO_2 display, an interactive operator demonstration mode, and an internally calibrated and adjustable PEEP control.

Table 14-11 lists modes, ventilation parameters, and other features of the Uni-Vent 754. The Uni-Vent 754 is currently included in the Strategic National Stockpile for deployment in any human-made or natural disaster.

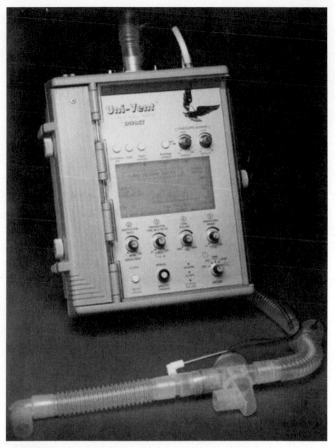

FIGURE 14-16 The Uni-Vent Eagle™ 754 ventilator. (Courtesy Impact Instrumentation, Inc, West Caldwell, N.J.)

NEWPORT MEDICAL INSTRUMENTS E100I

The Newport E100i (Newport Medical Instruments, Costa Mesa, Calif.) was originally presented in the sixth edition (1999) of this text. The information regarding that ventilator has been moved to Evolve Resources.

NEWPORT MEDICAL INSTRUMENTS E100M

The Newport E100M was originally presented in the sixth edition (1999) of this text. The information regarding that ventilator has been moved to Evolve Resources.

PERCUSSIONAIRE BRONCHOTRON TXP VENTILATOR

The Percussionaire Bronchotron TXP Ventilator (Percussionaire Corporation, Sand Point, Idaho) (Figure 14-18) is a pneumatically powered, pressure-limited, time-cycled, high-frequency flow-interrupter ventilator. It is capable of providing conventional IMV ventilation and high-frequency ventilation (HFV) for the transport of critically ill patients (Box 14-7).[12] The Bronchotron's dimensions are

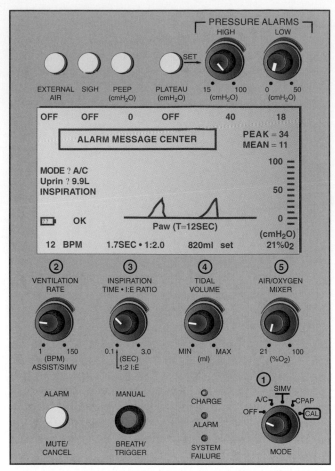

FIGURE 14-17 The Uni-Vent Eagle™ 754 ventilator's control panel.

12 in × 8 in × 6 in, and it weighs 5 lb. Table 14-12 lists some of the features of the Bronchotron TXP Ventilator.

Power Source

The Bronchotron is pneumatically powered (30 psi for conventional; 40 psi for HFV). It is usually delivered from the factory preset at 40 psi to 45 psi, so all modes of ventilation are operational. The Bronchotron TXP requires 8 L/min to 12 L/min logic flow to operate. This factor must be taken into account when calculating needed gas supply for transport. The Bronchotron also requires 4 AA batteries for the frequency counter, as well as a 9-V battery for the low-pressure alarm.

Internal Mechanism

The compressed gas enters the Bronchotron in the rear of the unit and is then routed through the mode-control manifold. Depending on the mode chosen, source gas is diverted to either the HFV or conventional CMV regulator. Gas then enters its specific logic cell cartridge and associ-

BOX 14-7	Examples of Respiratory Conditions for which the Percussionaire Bronchotron TXP May be Used in Transport

· Acute respiratory distress syndrome
· Hyaline membrane disease
· Inhalation injuries
· Pneumothoraces
· Persistent pulmonary hypertension
· Meconium aspiration syndrome
· Pneumonia
· Obstructive airway disease

TABLE 14-11

Specifications for Impact Uni-Vent Eagle™ 754

Control Settings	Range
Modes	A/C, CMV, SIMV, and CPAP
Power source	Pneumatic and electric power internal DC battery, external DC battery or 120-V AC outlet (with a converter)
Rate	1-150 breaths/min
Noninvasive ventilation mode	N/A
Peak pressure	100 cm H_2O
Tidal volume	0-3000 mL
Inspiratory time	0.1-3 s
PEEP/CPAP	1-20 cm H_2O
Oxygen percent	21-100%
Pressure support	N/A
Monitors/displays	Alphanumeric display and digital bar graph
Dimensions	9 in × 11.5 in × 4.5 in; approximately 12.5 lb
Gas consumption	N/A
Alarms	High- and Low-pressure/disconnect, PEEP not set, inverse I:E, and apnea
Battery duration	Estimated life of 9 h

TABLE 14-12

Specifications for the Percussionaire Bronchotron TXP Ventilator

Control Settings	Range
Modes	IMV, high-frequency
Power source	Pneumatic
Rate	IMV rates of 8-60 breaths/min unsynchronized. High-frequency: 185-700 breaths/min
Noninvasive ventilation mode	N/A
Peak pressure	60 cm H_2O
Tidal volume	N/A
Inspiratory time	0.25-3 s
PEEP/CPAP	0-20 cm H_2O
Oxygen percent	100 % or blended
Pressure support	N/A
Monitors/displays	Analog pressure gauge, digital frequency counter
Dimensions	12 in × 8 in × 6 in; 5 lb
Logic gas consumption	8-12 L/min
Alarms	Low-pressure alarm
Battery duration	N/A

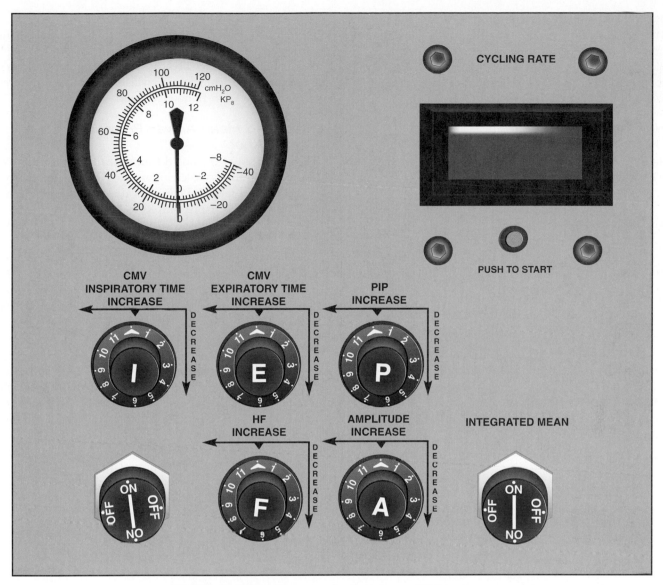

FIGURE 14-18 The Percussionaire Bronchotron TXP Ventilator.

ated timing circuitry. Source gas from the logic cell is then metered for flow by clinician adjustment of the PIP (peak inspiratory pressure) control knob or amplitude control knob, depending on the mode selected before entering the Phasitron (the mechanical interface of the ventilator).

Oxygen Source

An external blender can be added so the user can titrate the proper F_IO_2. Oxygen delivery is affected, in part, by a component called the Phasitron. In the Phasitron there is a sliding Venturi. This Venturi acts as both an inhalation and an exhalation valve. Exhalation is passive. The pulsated gas that is entered through the jet orifice entrains humidified and blended gases. There are two types of Venturi: green and red. The difference is the size of the Venturi orifice. The green Venturi has a larger "opening" compared with the red Venturi, resulting in a lower driving pressure and mean airway pressure (MAP).

During the air entrainment phase of ventilation, the entrainment port, or one-way valve, opens as the pulse or breath occurs. The smaller the diameter distal to the patient connection, the less the ambient gas is entrained. This will allow 100% oxygen delivery, if connected to an O_2 gas source. When equipped with an air/oxygen blender, it can be used to control the F_IO_2.

Controls

The Bronchotron has six controls to deliver the desired mode of ventilation: inspiratory time (T_I), expiratory time, peak pressure, high-frequency rate, and amplitude (see Figure 14-18). There are operator-controlled parameters and variable-controlled parameters. These are listed in Box 14-8.

Conventional Ventilation

The CMV inspiratory time knob controls the inspiratory time of a conventional breath (range: 0.25 to 3 seconds).

At the 12 o'clock position, inspiratory time is 0.35 second. The CMV expiratory time knob controls the expiratory time of a conventional breath (range: 0.5 to 4 seconds). The PIP knob controls the peak inspiratory pressure during a conventional breath. By increasing the PIP, you are actually increasing the flow delivery.

High-Frequency Controls

The HF knob controls the high-frequency rate (range: 200 to 700 breaths/min) with an automatically set I:E ratio. I:E ratios are as follows:
- Rate: 185-250 breaths/min; I:E = 1:2
- Rate: 250-400 breaths/min; I:E = 1:1.5
- Rate: >400 breaths/min; I:E = 1:1

The ventilator will not deliver an inverse I:E.

The amplitude knob determines the amplitude of the high-frequency breaths. Increasing the amplitude will normally increase the removal of CO_2.

PEEP Valve

The PEEP valve controls MAP during both HFV and conventional ventilation. The operational range of PEEP on the Bronchotron is 0 cm H_2O to 20 cm H_2O.

Mode-Control Knob

The mode-control knob (lower left-hand corner) is a two-position control used to select either a high-frequency mode or a conventional ventilation mode on the Bronchotron TXP.

BOX 14-8	Bronchotron Operator Set and Variable Parameters

Operator-Set Parameters
PIP/amplitude (peak inspiratory pressure)
CMV/high-frequency rate
F_iO_2
Mean airway pressure (MAP)

Variable Parameters
Flow
Tidal volume

Frequency Counter

The frequency counter is located on the upper right-hand corner of the control panel and is labeled *cycling rate*. It counts high-frequency breaths. When the power button is pressed, the frequency counter will remain on for 5 minutes, displaying the high-frequency breath rate.

Integrated Mean Airway Pressure Control Knob

The integrated MAP knob displays breath-by-breath proximal airway pressures when in the "on" position. It is located on the lower right-hand corner of the control panel. In the "off" position, it displays integrated MAP.

Alarms

The Bronchotron has one main alarm. The one internal alarm is the low-pressure alarm, which is powered by a 9-V battery. The activation of the alarm is controlled by a pressure drop. The time delay for this alarm is set by the user.

Modes of Ventilation

The Bronchotron provides conventional IMV and HFV. During IMV, breaths are nonsynchronized IMV breaths (range: 8 to 60 breaths/min). V_T delivered is dependent on the pressure setting and the patient's lung characteristics, because there is no control for setting a specific V_T.

The high-frequency mode is accomplished by using a high-frequency flow interruptor. Unlike high-frequency oscillation, where both inspiration and expiration are active, only inspiration is active with the Bronchotron. The exhalation phase is totally passive. The high-frequency rate is controlled by the high-frequency control knob. An example of the breathing pattern during HFV is shown in Figure 14-19.

PULMONETIC SYSTEMS LTV 1000 VENTILATOR

The Pulmonetic Systems LTV (lap top ventilator; Pulmonetic Systems, Inc, Minneapolis) currently comes in five models: the LTV 1200, 1000, 950, 900, and 800.[13-18] The

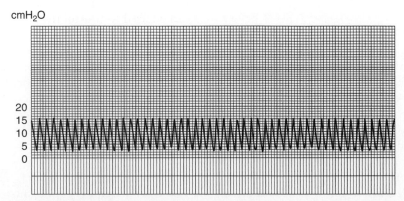

FIGURE 14-19 The Percussionaire Bronchotron TXP Ventilator's breathing pattern.

LTV 1200 and 1000 ventilators are primarily used in the transport and hospital settings, whereas the 950, 900, and 800 are mainly used in the home care setting. Box 14-9 lists the basic differences among the 1000, 950, 900, and 800. The LTV 950, 900, and 800 will be discussed in the home care section of this chapter. The 1200 will also be reviewed later. Table 14-13 lists important features of the LTV 1000 and 1200. However, this section's discussion will be restricted to the LTV 1000.

The LTV 1000 (Figure 14-20) is an electrically powered unit that uses an internal rotary compressor to generate gas flow to the patient. On the left side of the unit are the connecting ports for the ventilator (Figure 14-21). These

consist of (1) a power cord connector, (2) a patient assist call cable or a remote alarm port, (3) a communications port, and (4) an oxygen hose connector. On the same side are two vents. The ventilator uses room air and oxygen to provide gas flow to the patient. The room air enters the ventilator through a large opening covered by a filter (5).

BOX 14-9	The Basic Differences in the LTV 1000, 950, 900, and 800 Ventilators

The 1000 has a built-in oxygen blender and can provide PCV. The 950 does not have a built-in blender, but it does provide PCV. The 900 has flow-triggering, volume ventilation, and pressure support, but neither the blender nor PCV. The LTV 800 and 900 models have only volume-targeted mandatory breaths. The 800 is strictly a pressure-triggered, volume-controlled ventilator without PSV. The low-pressure O_2 source button is on the LTV 1200 and 1000, but this function is not available with the 800, 900, or 950 models.

TABLE 14-13	
Specifications for the Pulmonetic Systems LTV 1000 and 1200	
Control Settings	**Range**
Modes	Control, A/C, SIMV, CPAP, NPPV, apnea back-up
Power source	AC power, internal DC power, external DC power
Rate	1-80 breaths/min
Noninvasive ventilation mode	Yes
Peak pressure	120 cm H_2O
Tidal volume	50-2000 mL
Inspiratory time	0.3-9.9 s
PEEP/CPAP	0-20 cm H_2O
Oxygen percent	21-100%
Pressure support	1-60 cm H_2O
Monitors/displays	Digital airway pressure gauge, LED display window
Dimensions	10 in × 12 in × 3 in; 13.4 lb
Gas consumption	N/A
Alarms*	Apnea interval, high respiratory rate, high PEEP, low PEEP, high-pressure limit, high/low oxygen pressure, low minute ventilation, low-pressure
Battery duration	Approximately 6 h with external DC battery. 2 h with internal battery

NPPV, Noninvasive positive-pressure ventilation; *LED,* light-emitting diode.
*Additional alarms are detailed in the LTV 1200 manual and in the section on the LTV 1000.

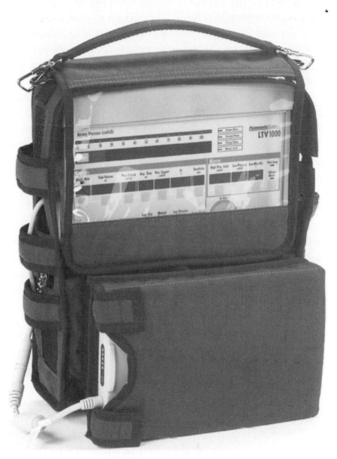

FIGURE 14-20 The Pulmonetic Systems LTV 1000 ventilator. (Courtesy Pulmonetic Systems, Inc, Minneapolis; Pulmonetic Systems is a division of Cardinal Health, McGaw Park, Ill.)

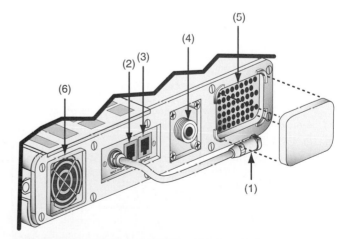

FIGURE 14-21 The left side of the Pulmonetic Systems LTV 1000 ventilator. (Courtesy Pulmonetic Systems, Inc, Minneapolis; Pulmonetic Systems is a division of Cardinal Health, McGaw Park, Ill.)

This opening must not be blocked or flow to the patient will be restricted. The second smaller opening allows air to be drawn in to cool the internal components of the unit (6). It also must be kept unblocked.

The oxygen-connecting port can be attached to either a high-pressure or a low-pressure oxygen source. An example of a high-pressure source is wall oxygen (40 to 70 psig). For low-pressure oxygen sources such as an oxygen concentrator, a female DISS oxygen adapter is available that allows connection to regular oxygen tubing. Other low-pressure O_2 sources might include an O_2 flowmeter attached to a wall outlet or an O_2 cylinder with a regulator and flowmeter attached. (NOTE: The internal oxygen blender is available only on the LTV 1000 and 1200.) Oxygen enters the ventilator and blends with room air in the mixing chamber, which is called an **accumulator/silencer**. This chamber both blends the gas and acts as an acoustic silencer to reduce compressor noise.

Power Source

The LTV series units are designed to run on AC or DC (12-V) power. Although the unit normally uses an AC power cord adapter, more recently released LTV models have a 6-in pigtail adapter located on the left side of the ventilator (see Figure 14-20). When connected to an AC power outlet, the internal battery is continuously charged.

For DC power, the LTV can use either its own internal battery or one of two available external DC batteries. The internal battery can last approximately 60 minutes when fully charged (Box 14-10). The fully charged large external battery can provide up to approximately 8 hours of power; the smaller battery, approximately 3 to 4 hours. It takes up to 8 hours to recharge the large external battery when it is completely depleted. (NOTE: An optional auto lighter adapter is also available for LTV use while in a car.)

Patient Circuit

On the right side of the ventilator are the connections for the patient circuit and a small opening for the alarm sound

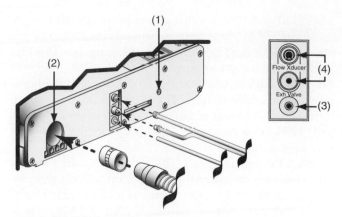

FIGURE 14-22 The right side of the Pulmonetic Systems LTV 1000 ventilator. (See text for additional information.) (Courtesy Pulmonetic Systems, Inc, Minneapolis; Pulmonetic Systems is a division of Cardinal Health, McGaw Park, Ill.)

(Figure 14-22, #1). This alarm opening should not be covered or the alarm volume will be reduced. There is a 22-mm connector for the main inspiratory flow line (Figure 14-22, #2) and a small connector for the exhalation valve line (#3) that powers the external exhalation valve.

There are also two flow transducer connectors located on the right side (Figure 14-22, #4). Two small-gauge gas lines are attached to these connectors and to the two connectors located on the patient Y-adapter. The transducer located by the patient Y-connector is used for flow, volume, and pressure-monitoring. A pulse of gas is sent through these lines with each breath during the first minute of ventilation and then once a minute thereafter. This helps keep the lines clear of moisture.

In addition to closing the patient circuit during inspiration, the exhalation valve of the LTV also controls the PEEP levels. This is done by pushing the PEEP valve lock with one hand and rotating the valve with the other to increase and decrease PEEP levels (Figure 14-23, patient circuit, *detail A*).

Controls and Alarms

The commonly used controls are located on the front panel of the LTV. As with many of the newer ventilators that use built-in microprocessors, some controls are menu-driven and are not located on the panel itself but are pulled up on the display window when needed.

Front-Panel Controls

The front panel (Figure 14-24) contains controls, alarm, and monitoring displays. The controls are divided into two rows. The bottom row contains main function buttons or touch pads, and the upper row contains parameter-setting buttons.

Above the row of parameter controls is a display window that has two main functions. It displays current ventilator data and provides access to additional control functions. To the right of the controls, alarm-setting keys are located. Just below the alarm keys is a set value knob.

BOX 14-10	Internal Battery—Alternating Current (AC) Power Not Connected, LTV Series

When the internal battery is operational, the battery level indicator illuminates. The color code provides information about available charge time remaining.

LED Color	Internal Battery Level	Battery Time*
Green	Acceptable	60 minutes
Yellow	Low	30 minutes
Red	Critically low	7 minutes

*Approximate value.

Available time depends on currently active ventilator settings. To conserve power, the other screen displays go blank. Only the pressure manometer remains illuminated.

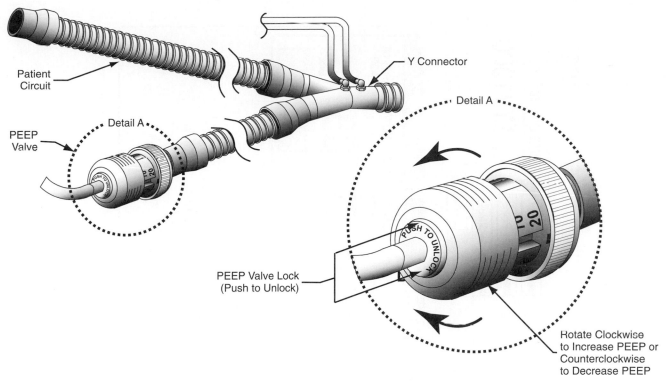

FIGURE 14-23 The Pulmonetic Systems LTV 1000 ventilator's patient circuit. (See text for additional information.) (Courtesy Pulmonetic Systems, Inc, Minneapolis; Pulmonetic Systems is a division of Cardinal Health, McGaw Park, Ill.)

BOX 14-11	The Warm-Up Period for the LTV 1000

When the ventilator is first turned on, the transducers need 60 seconds to warm up to ensure normal function. During this period the message "WARMUP XX" appears in the display window. This message is removed after the warm-up period. The leak test and calibration should not be run during this period.

The on/standby button turns the ventilator on and illuminates the LED above it (Box 14-11). The ventilator automatically begins to ventilate the patient by using the last settings. To place the ventilator into standby, the operator presses and holds the button for 3 seconds. As long as the unit is plugged into an AC outlet and placed in standby, the internal battery will be charged.

The select (volume/pressure) button allows the operator to choose either volume-targeted or pressure-targeted breaths. Pressing the button toggles between the two choices. The currently active breath type is continuously illuminated. Pressing the button causes the new selection to flash. A change in breath type is confirmed by pressing the button again. If the button is not pressed to confirm the change, the ventilator simply remains in the current breath type. (NOTE: The LTV 800 and 900 models have only volume-targeted mandatory breaths.)

Between the breath-type button and the mode button is an indicator labeled *NPPV*, for noninvasive positive pressure ventilation. This illuminates when the NPPV mode has been selected from the extended features menu. A noninvasive interface, such as a mask, can be used to connect a patient to the LTV during any mode of ventilation. However, when NPPV is enabled, some of the alarms are deactivated. (See "Modes of Ventilation.")

The mode-control select provides the options of A/C or SIMV/CPAP. To select a mode, the operator presses the select button. The flashing LED indicates that the mode that is selected will become active if the select key is pressed again.

The "Insp/Exp Hold" (inspiratory/expiratory hold) button allows the operator to perform either of these two functions. The operator presses the button and reads the display window (monitoring screen), which will show one of the following: INSP HOLD or EXP HOLD. Pressing the Insp/Exp Hold button scrolls through the choices on the screen. Following the screen prompts will guide the operator through the desired procedure.

The next control is the manual breath button. When this button is pressed, a manual breath based on current volume or pressure settings is delivered to the patient. In addition, a bolus of air purges the flow sensor line.

The low-pressure O_2 source is a feature available only for the LTV 1200 and LTV 1000. Certain changes in alarm features occur when oxygen is supplied from a

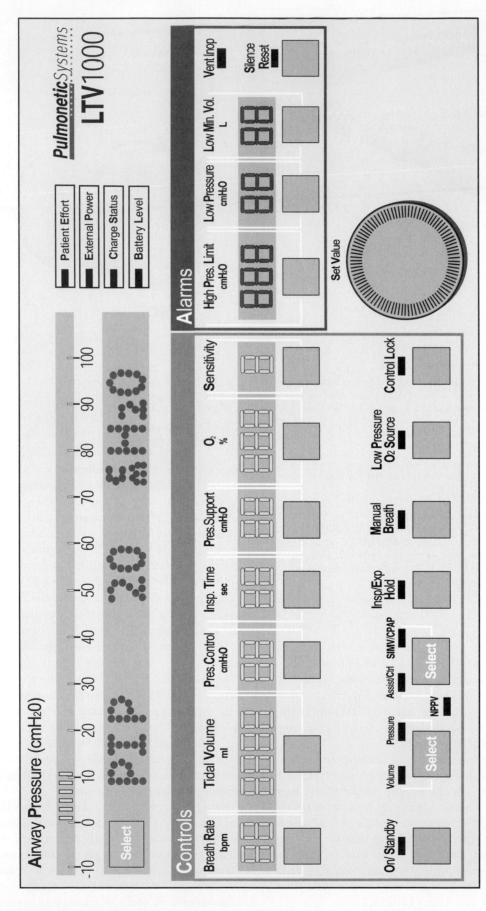

FIGURE 14-24 The Pulmonetic Systems LTV 1000 ventilator's control panel. (See text for additional information.) (Courtesy Pulmonetic Systems, Inc, Minneapolis; Pulmonetic Systems is a division of Cardinal Health, McGaw Park, Ill.)

BOX 14-12	Low-Pressure O₂ Source—Not Installed or Installed (LTV 1000 & 1200)

O_2 *Blending Option* **NOT** *Installed*

Oxygen may still be provided from a low-pressure O_2 source through the low-flow inlet, but the following are inactive:
- Low-pressure O_2 source button
- O_2% control
- Oxygen inlet pressure alarms (high and low)

O_2 *Blending Option Installed*

The low-pressure O_2 source button is active only when the oxygen-blending option is installed. To activate this option, the operator pushes the low-pressure O_2 source button until it is on and its LED illuminated. While it is on:
- The O_2 inlet pressure low alarm is **NOT** active.
- The O_2 pressure high alarm activates when the O_2 source is more than 10 psi.
- The O_2% display shows only dimmed dashes, and the O_2% cannot be set.
- The O_2 inlet flow must be set to obtain the desired O_2%.
- O_2% delivery varies with the input O_2 flow (L/min) and the minute volume based on the figure below.

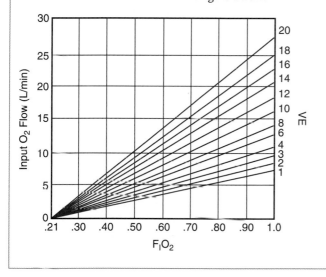

BOX 14-13	Conditions In Which Displays Will Flash on the LTV 1000

1. When the limit has been reached for a value as the operator is adjusting that value, the display will flash. For example, when setting tidal volume, if the V_T is set too high for the available peak flow based on the set inspiratory time (T_I), the V_T display will flash.
2. A flashing display results when alarm conditions are occurring or an alarm has just occurred.
3. If a control display flashes, a special condition has occurred. For example, pressure-support (PS) breaths are normally flow-cycled. If a time-cycled PS breath occurs, the pressure support indicator will flash.
4. The message "Locked" will flash in the display window if someone has tried to change the controls when the panel is locked. It will flash for 3 seconds.

low-pressure/low-flow O_2 source and the low-pressure O_2 feature is activated (Box 14-12). When the low-pressure/O_2 source is **NOT** on, a high-pressure oxygen source is expected and gas-blending is done within the ventilator. The delivered O_2 concentration is determined by the O_2% setting on the ventilator's front panel. (NOTE: The ventilator does not have a built-in O_2 analyzer.)

The control lock button allows the screen to be locked so that the settings cannot be accidentally changed. Pushing once turns the lock on. The LED above the control lock illuminates (which means the panel is locked). If the operator tries to change a setting when the panel is locked, the display window reads "LOCKED" and the LED flashes. Pressing the "control lock" button again unlocks the screen.

The **HARD** method of locking should be used when children or others may have access to the ventilator, such as in the patient's home. The operator selects "CTRL UNLOCK" from the extended features menu (reviewed later in this section). If **HARD** lock has been selected in this menu, the operator must press the "control lock" button for 3 seconds to unlock the control panel.

The upper row of controls contains the parameter settings such as rate and tidal volume. The procedure for changing the variables in this row, and in the alarms, is basically the same. The parameter button is touched to make a change. This action brightly illuminates the set value for the parameter and dulls the displays for all other parameters. The "set value" knob is rotated until the desired value appears in the display above the parameter button. The change is immediately active if the "set value" knob is pressed again or after 5 seconds.

The number in the window above each parameter represents the value set for that parameter. Numbers appear bright when the parameter is active in the current mode and breath type. They appear dim when they are not. A parameter's digital display will also brighten if it is selected for changing. All others then dim. Three parameters—sensitivity, pressure support, and respiratory rate—can be turned off. The respective display for any of those three parameters will be blank ("- -") when it is turned off.

When the LTV is being powered by the internal battery, after 60 seconds all the digital displays turn off, if no button has been pushed or any controls changed. The displays can be reilluminated by pushing any button or turning the set value knob. Flashing displays will also occur (Box 14-13).

The breath rate control sets the minimum mandatory breath rate (breaths/minute). It can be turned off ("- -"). The rate range is 1 breath/min to 80 breaths/min. The tidal volume button controls volume delivery during volume-targeted ventilation (range: 50 to 2000 mL). The inspiratory time (T_I) button sets the length of inspiration for volume-targeted and pressure-targeted breaths (range: 0.3 to 9.9 seconds). Inspiration cannot be shorter than 300 milliseconds. When V_T or T_I is being adjusted, the calculated flow ($\dot{V}$ calc) is shown in the display window. The peak flow is based on the setting of T_I and V_T (Box 14-14).

<table>
<tr><td>**BOX 14-14**</td><td>**Flow Pattern and Peak Flow in the LTV 1000**</td></tr>
</table>

The flow pattern is automatically set as a descending ramp for all volume-targeted breaths. The peak flow at the beginning of inspiration is calculated by the ventilator so that the tidal volume can be delivered during the set T_I and inspiration ends when flow drops to 50% of the peak, or 10 L/min, whichever is highest. The range of available flow is 10 L/min to 100 L/min for a mandatory breath.

PCV is a feature available in the LTV 1200, 1000, and 950 models. The "Press. Control" button establishes the inspiratory pressure for pressure-targeted breaths. The operator pushes the Press. Control button and uses the set value knob to change to the desired inspiratory pressure (range: 1 to 99 cm H_2O). This pressure is not added to the baseline PEEP. PEEP/CPAP is set mechanically by using the expiratory/PEEP valve.

Press support establishes the target pressure above 0 baseline for pressure-supported spontaneous breaths (range: off ["- -"], or 1 to 60 cm H_2O). PS is available for spontaneous breaths with SIMV in either pressure- or volume-targeted ventilation and for CPAP breaths (see "Modes of Ventilation").

The O_2% button establishes the percent O_2 delivery when it is on and a high-pressure oxygen source is available. (NOTE: The low-pressure O_2 button must be in the off position.)

The sensitivity button is used to set the flow-trigger sensitivity level for assisted or spontaneous breaths. The range is off ("- -") and 1 L/min to 9 L/min. The most-sensitive setting is 1 L/min. The base flow is preset at 10 L/min and requires no setting by the operator. When a trigger is detected, the patient effort LED illuminates.

There are only a few clinical circumstances in which turning off the sensitivity might be appropriate. For example, if a patient has a large air leak through a bronchopleural fistula (BPF); for example, if the leak resulting from the BPF is more than 15 L/min, even with the sensitivity at 9 L/min (least sensitivity) and leak compensation available (newer models compensate at 6 L/min leak), air may still leak from the system. Large air leaks can prolong inspiration and also result in accidental early triggering of a breath during exhalation (autotriggering). The leak is falsely seen as a patient effort. In this case it may be appropriate to set a mandatory breath rate and turn the sensitivity off.

In addition to flow-triggering, there is a backup pressure-sensing trigger that will pressure-trigger a breath in the following circumstances:

· When sensitivity is set between 1 L/min and 9 L/min
· The ventilator is in exhalation
· A minimum expiratory time has elapsed (300 milliseconds)
· The airway pressure drops below −3 cm H_2O

The leak-compensation feature in newer versions is constantly measuring for leaks and adjusting the baseline of the ventilator in order to compensate for leaks (up to 6 L/min). For example, if the operator sets the flow sensitivity to 2 L, the ventilator would normally trigger a breath when a 2-L change in baseline (bias flow) was detected during expiration. Suppose a 4 L/min leak exists with a 2 L/min sensitivity setting. The ventilator identifies the 4 L/min leak and adjusts the baseline flow so that the required patient effort is still only 2 L/min to trigger a breath and autotriggering is prevented.

In earlier versions of the LTV 1000, which do not have leak compensation, the sensitivity is usually set higher than the leak measurement. The operator can check the current leak measurement by going into the "RT XDCR DATA" menu and selecting the "LEAK" measurement displayed. For example, if the leak is measured at 2.38 L/min, an appropriate sensitivity setting would be 3 L/min. The difference would represent the trigger ($3 - 2.38 = 0.62$). An effort of 0.62 L/min would have to be inhaled by the patient from the bias flow to trigger the next breath.

Alarms

The alarm controls and settings are to the right of the parameter controls. The first alarm is the "High Press. Limit" (cm H_2O). This control establishes the maximum pressure allowed in the patient circuit. If the set value is reached, an audible alarm sounds, the display window reads "HIGH PRES," inspiration ends, and the exhalation valve opens. If a high-pressure condition continues for more than 3 seconds, the internal turbine stops rotating and circuit pressure empties to the atmosphere. The audible alarm automatically stops when the pressure drops to the high-pressure limit −5 cm H_2O or drops to a circuit pressure of 25 cm H_2O, whichever is less. To set the high-pressure limit, the button is pressed and the set value knob rotated to the desired value (range: 5 to 100 cm H_2O).

To set the low-pressure alarm value (cm H_2O), the operator pushes the low-pressure button and rotates the set value knob. The actual value appears in the display window. The knob is rotated until the desired value is seen (range: 1 to 60 cm H_2O). The low-pressure alarm has two possible functions. The LTV can apply the low-pressure alarm to all breaths, both spontaneous and mandatory ("ALL BREATHS" selection) or to mandatory breaths only ("VC/PC ONLY" selection). The mandatory breaths can be pressure-targeted or volume-targeted.

The operator accesses the extended menu functions (discussed later in this section) to set the low-pressure alarm for either all breaths or for mandatory breaths only (Box 14-15). When the LPPS (low peak pressure *spontaneous*) alarm is turned off, the message "LPPS OFF" appears in the display window. Spontaneous breaths have no low-pressure alarm. This is an informational message only. (NOTE: The operator can remove the LPPS Off message from the screen by activating the scroll feature of the display window [Box 14-16].)

BOX 14-15	LTV 1000—Low-Pressure Alarm Settings: All Breaths Versus Mandatory Breaths

Assume the ventilator is set with the inspiratory pressure at 25 cm H_2O in SIMV pressure-targeted ventilation with a pressure support of 15 cm H_2O.

If **ALL** breaths are monitored for low pressure, the operator would set the low-pressure alarm to a value lower than the PS level. In this case it might be approximately 10 cm H_2O. If the circuit pressure does not rise to 10 cm H_2O for any breath, the alarm will sound.

If only mandatory breaths were monitored, the operator might set the low-pressure alarm at approximately 20 cm H_2O. The alarm would occur only if a mandatory breath's pressure dropped below 20 cm H_2O. The alarm would not be active for spontaneous breaths.

BOX 14-16	The Scroll Feature for the LTV

Double clicking (pressing twice) on the select button adjacent to the display window results in a scrolling through of ventilator parameters in the window. For example, peak airway pressure, positive end-expiratory pressure (PEEP), respiratory rate, and other ventilator parameters appear consecutively in the window. Each parameter remains in the window with the current measured value for 2 seconds, and then the next parameter appears.

When scrolling is active, the "LPPS off" message also appears for 2 seconds, notifying the operator that LPPS (low peak pressure spontaneous) is off.

If the operator wants to stop the scrolling to freeze a particular parameter in the window, he or she would press the select button once when the desired parameter is in the window. This allows continuous monitoring of a specific parameter such as respiratory rate.

To reactivate scrolling, simply press the select button twice.

When scrolling is active and the low minute volume alarm is off, the "LMV Alarm off" message appears in the message window in the sequence of ventilator parameters.

The "Low Min. Vol." alarm sets the minimum expected exhaled $\dot{V}_E$ (range: Off ["- -"] or 0.1 L to 99 L). If $\dot{V}_E$ drops below the set value, an audible alarm sounds and the message "LOW MIN VOL" appears in the message window. If the low $\dot{V}_E$ alarm is turned to the off ("- -") position, a message will appear saying "LMV-off alarm off" in the display window after 60 seconds. It is an informational message only. The operator can resume scrolling of parameters by pressing the select button twice (see Box 14-16). (NOTE: The LMV alarm is not active in the NPPV mode.)

The message "LMV LPPS OFF" appears in the window when both the low $\dot{V}_E$ and low peak pressure for spontaneous breath alarms are off (Clinical Rounds 14-7). The message appears in the window after the disabling of the alarm(s) as a safety feature and at all times, unless scrolling

CLINICAL ROUNDS 14-7

A respiratory therapist turns the LTV 1000 on to begin ventilating a new patient. The patient is to receive CPAP at 10 cm H_2O and 90% O_2. The therapist notices the following message in the display window: "LMV LPPS OFF." What does the message mean, and what should the therapist do?

See Evolve Resources for the answer.

is active. If scrolling is active, the message becomes one of the scrolled parameters.

The "Vent Inop" indicator just right of the alarm controls is illuminated only when the ventilator is in the inoperative state. This occurs under the following conditions:

1. The ventilator has been put into standby (i.e., the on/standby button is held for 3 seconds).
2. The power sources, either internal or external, are insufficient to operate the ventilator.
3. The ventilator has been turned off.
4. A condition exists that renders the ventilator unable to provide patient ventilation and is unsafe.

When a ventilator inoperative alarm occurs, the inspiratory flow stops; the exhalation valve opens, allowing the patient to breathe spontaneously from room air; the oxygen blender solenoids close; the "INOP" LED is red; and an audible alarm sounds continuously. Another mode of ventilating must be provided for the patient immediately.

The silence/reset button is used to silence an alarm for 60 seconds. This button can also be used to start a 60-second alarm silence period—for example, before disconnecting the patient for some procedure or when the ventilator is placed in standby. After an alarm condition has been resolved, this button can also be used to clear the visual alarm displays. The silence/reset button also silences the Vent Inop audible alarm, but the Vent Inop LED will remain lit for at least 5 minutes.

In addition to the alarms described, additional alarm conditions may occur and present an alarm message in the display window.

The Set Value Knob

This knob allows adjustment of the numerical values of the ventilator parameters and alarms, and it scrolls through menu items that appear in the display window.

Airway Pressure Bar Graph and Display Window

At the very top of the operating panel is the airway pressure display. This horizontal bar graph displays the pressure in the patient circuit (range: −10 to +108 cm H_2O).

The display window shows monitored data, alarm messages, and the extended features menu. During normal operation, the monitored data are presented sequentially.

TABLE 14-14

LTV 1000 (and 1200) Monitored Data

Parameter	Description
PIP	Peak inspiratory pressure (cm H_2O). Greatest pressure measured during inspiration and the first 300 ms of exhalation.
MAP	Mean airway pressure (cm H_2O). Calculation of mean airway pressure for the last 60 s, displayed in 10-s intervals.
PEEP	Positive end-expiratory pressure (cm H_2O). The measured pressure at the end of exhalation.
f	Total respiratory rate per minute based on the last 8 breaths. Updated every 20 s. Includes all breath types.
V_{TE}	Measured exhaled tidal volume. Measured and displayed at the end of each exhalation.
V_E	Minute volume monitor displays the exhaled tidal volume for the last 60 s as calculated from the last 8 breaths. Recalculated and displayed every 20 s or at the completion of every exhalation, whichever occurs first.
I : E	Displays the calculated ratio inspiration to expiration with the smaller of the two reduced to a value of 1. Displays regular and inverse ratios.
$\dot{V}$ calc	The calculated peak flow, which occurs at the beginning of the breath for a volume-targeted breath (not included with pressure ventilation). The calculation is based on set V_T, T_I, and a predetermined minimum flow at the end of inspiration. Flow normally drops in a descending ramp fashion to 50% of the calculated peak or 10 L/min, whichever is greater.

Table 14-14 shows the sequence of monitored data and how the values are calculated. Each item is displayed for 3 seconds.

The Select Button—Display Screen

The select button to the left of the display screen has several functions. It is used to stop the normal scrolling of monitored ventilator parameters. Pushing the button once while the normal data scan is active halts the screen with the current parameter data showing. Each time the button is pushed after that, the next data item in the list is displayed. Scanning can be resumed by pressing the button twice within 3 seconds.

The extended features menu is selected by pushing the select button for 3 seconds. The first menu item is displayed in the window (see the "extended features" section, which follows the next section).

Front-Panel Indicators

To the right of the pressure manometer are four indicators. The patient effort indicator illuminates when the ventilator detects a patient's inspiratory effort based on the sensitivity setting. The external power illuminates when the unit is operating from an external power source. This can be an AC power source or an external battery. The adjacent LED is green when power is adequate and yellow when external power is low. Table 14-15 and Box 14-10 provide information on the battery-charging status and related indicator colors.

Extended Features

Other than the alarms available on the operating panel, the extended features menu accesses additional alarm controls. Several other functions are available through this menu, including oxygen cylinder duration calculation. The extended features menu is accessed by pushing the select button for 3 seconds. The first menu item is displayed in the window. While scrolling through the features menu,

TABLE 14-15

Battery Charge Status and LED Color Indicators (Charge Status LED) for the LTV 1000

LED Color	Charge Status
Flashing yellow	The ventilator is performing precharge qualification testing of the internal battery before beginning the charging procedure. Occurs when the external power is first applied to the unit. Takes from a few seconds to an hour on a very depleted battery.
Green	Internal battery fully charged.
Yellow	Internal battery is being charged but has not reached a full charge level.
Red	The internal battery cannot be charged. The ventilator has detected a charge fault or internal battery fault. Remove from service and contact a certified service technician.

the operator will come to a useful tool for transport operation. The LTV 1200 and 1000 have built-in oxygen cylinder duration calculators. The operator only needs to select the cylinder size and pressure in the cylinder in pounds per square inch (psi) and the cylinder duration will be calculated with the current settings. Users are advised to follow the ventilator maintenance procedures outlined in the operator's manual provided by the manufacturer for viewing the following: transducer Autozero, real-time transducer data, event trace, and ventilator maintenance.

Breath Types

As with other ventilators, the LTV series distinguishes between breath type and mode. For example, breaths can be volume-targeted or pressure-targeted. Each of these breath types is available in the A/C mode or SIMV mode.

There are four breath types in the LTV unit: volume control, pressure control, pressure support, and spontaneous. To select volume or pressure breaths, the operator toggles the select—volume (or) pressure button to establish breath type (bottom row of controls).

Volume-controlled breaths are patient-triggered (flow or pressure), time-triggered, or manually triggered. The limiting value is the set V_T. Flow is delivered in a descending ramp waveform. The cycling method is inspiratory time (T_I). The operator can also set breath rate, O_2%, and sensitivity.

Pressure-controlled breaths are also patient-triggered, time-triggered, or manually triggered. (NOTE: The LTV 900 and 800 do not have pressure control.) The target inspiratory pressure is set with the "Press. Control" button (cm H_2O). The target pressure is the maximum pressure delivered by the ventilator during inspiration and is **NOT** additive to PEEP.

PEEP is set by the mechanical PEEP valve located on the expiratory valve. For example, if the pressure control is set to 25 cm H_2O and the PEEP is at 5 cm H_2O, the normal pressure reached during inspiration will be 25 cm H_2O. Baseline pressure will be 5 cm H_2O. The usual cycle mechanism for a pressure-control breath is time. Breath rate, T_I, O_2%, and sensitivity are also set.

If desired, the operator can select flow-cycling for pressure-controlled breaths rather than time-cycling by activating the flow-termination percent feature through the extended features menu. Flow-cycling percent can be adjusted from 10% to 40% of peak flow. The default setting is 25%. For example, if the peak flow during inspiration is 50 L/min and the flow-cycling setting is 25%, inspiratory flow ends when the flow drops to 12.5 L/min (25% of 50 L/min). A pressure-controlled breath will time-cycle unless the flow-termination setting occurs before the set inspiratory time elapses. If a long T_I is set, such as 1.5 seconds, it is more likely that the flow will drop to the set flow-termination point before 1.5 seconds have elapsed.

A rise-time profile can also be set with pressure control to taper pressure and flow delivery at the beginning of inspiration. This is also selected by using the extended features menu. The default setting for rise time is profile no. 4. (NOTE: The fastest rise-time setting is no. 1, and the slowest is no. 9.)

Pressure-support breaths are patient-triggered, pressure-limited, and flow-cycled. As with pressure-control breaths, pressure support assumes a 0 baseline, so the set value is not added to the PEEP pressure as in most other ventilators. Flow-cycling can be adjusted by using the flow-termination feature described earlier. A default of 3 L/min is preset so that inspiratory flow cannot drop lower than 3 L/min (Clinical Rounds 14-8).

Pressure-support breaths are time-cycled if T_I exceeds the time termination limit (range: 0.3 to 3 seconds), which is set through the extended features menu. PS breaths will also time-cycle if T_I exceeds the length of two breath periods. The "Press. Support" display will flash briefly when a breath is time-cycled. As with pressure control, the rise-time profile may be selected from the extended features menu for PSV.

Spontaneous breaths are designed to meet patient demand and maintain the circuit pressure at the measured PEEP value from the previous breath. The breath is cycled when the flow drops below 10% of the maximum flow measured during inspiration or 2 L/min, whichever occurs first. Spontaneous breaths will also time-cycle if the breath time exceeds 2 breath periods.

Modes of Ventilation

The LTV series ventilator provides the following modes of ventilation: control, assist/control, SIMV, CPAP, apnea backup ventilation, and noninvasive positive pressure ventilation (NPPV).

Control and assist/control are available when the "Assist/Ctrl" LED is illuminated near the mode SELECT button. The manufacturer considers control to be active when the sensitivity is set to off ("–"). However, there is seldom a good reason to make a ventilator insensitive to the patient (see previous discussion on sensitivity setting).

Assist/control is considered active when a value greater than 0 sensitivity is set. The breath type is established by the breath-type select button (volume-targeted or pressure-targeted). The minimum rate is set by the breath rate control. The patient can trigger additional mandatory breaths.

The SIMV mode is active when the "SIMV/CPAP" LED is illuminated near the mode-select button. The breath rate (1 to 80 breaths/min) establishes the maximum mandatory breath rate. Patients can spontaneously breathe between mandatory breaths. Spontaneous breaths can be from the set baseline pressure (0 or PEEP) and can also be supported with pressure support.

CPAP is considered the active mode if the "SIMV/CPAP" LED is illuminated and the Breath Rate is off (" "). In CPAP, spontaneous breaths can be from the baseline pressure and can also be given pressure support (Clinical Rounds 14-9).

CLINICAL ROUNDS 14-8

You are transporting a patient who is connected to the LTV 1000 and who has an SIMV/pressure-support (PS) rate of 6 breaths/min. The peak flow measured by the ventilator is 25 L/min. The flow-termination level is set at 10%. At what flow will inspiratory flow end?

See Evolve Resources for the answer.

CLINICAL ROUNDS 14-9

A physician wants her patient weaned from mandatory breaths and orders a pressure support of 12 cm H_2O plus a PEEP of 3 cm H_2O, for a total inspiratory pressure of 15 cm H_2O. How would the therapist adjust these values on the LTV?

See Evolve Resources for the answer.

Apnea backup ventilation is available should the patient become apneic. The apnea interval is set by using the extended features menu. The ventilator begins apnea backup ventilation in the assist/control mode based on the current settings. The active controls are displayed at full intensity, and others are dimmed. If the set breath rate is greater than or equal to 12 breaths/min, the apnea breath rate is the set breath rate. If the set breath rate is less than 12 breaths/min and the breath rate is not limited by other control settings, the apnea breath rate is 12 breaths/min. If the set breath rate is limited to less than 12 breaths/min, because of tidal volume, flow, and T_I settings, the apnea breath rate is the highest allowed rate. Normal ventilation resumes when two consecutive patient-triggered breaths occur or when the operator resets the apnea alarm using the silence/reset control.

NPPV is provided as a secondary mode that may be selected in addition to the primary ventilation mode. NPPV is selected through the extended features menu and specific alarms are available (Box 14-17). When activated, ventilation is delivered according to the selected mode and breath type that are currently active. The NPPV LED is lit when it is on. The number of alarms in NPPV is limited when it is active.

BOX 14-17	Alarms Available During Noninvasive Positive-Pressure Ventilation (NPPV) with the LTV 1000*

High pressure
Internal battery low
Apnea alarm and Apnea back-up
Internal battery empty ventilation
Sense line disconnected
Vent Inop (ventilator inoperative)
External power low
Defaults

*All other alarms are disabled. The displays for low minute volume and low peak pressure are set to dimmed dashes showing they are not active.

Special Features

One of the optional features of the LTV series is a monitor screen that provides several display windows including scalars, loops, and data. Figure 14-25 shows the waveform screen with scalars for pressure-time, flow-time, and volume-time displayed. The screen can be frozen to view an event or scaled to size the waveforms. Another screen provides pressure-volume and flow-volume loops.

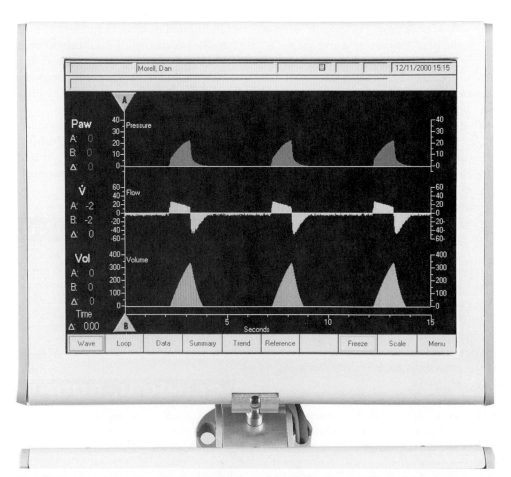

FIGURE 14-25 The Pulmonetic Systems LTV 1000 ventilator's monitor screen. (Courtesy Pulmonetic Systems, Inc, Minneapolis; Pulmonetic Systems is a division of Cardinal Health, McGaw Park, Ill.)

The data screen displays information normally scrolled in the display window of the operating panel. The data include PIP, PEEP, Vte (exhaled tidal volume), MAP (mean airway pressure), f (respiratory rate), $\dot{V}_E$, I:E, Vcalc, and peak flow. The right side of the data screen lists information on current parameter and alarm settings and also settings of the items available in the special features menu such as flow termination and rise time. The advantage of having a monitoring screen is the easy and immediate access to information, including trends.

Troubleshooting

To prevent difficulties in ventilator operation, it is appropriate to run the ventilator checkout tests before the LTV is used on a new patient and following a circuit change. Before running the checkout tests, the patient circuit and all related components should be attached. The patient should be disconnected from the unit during any testing.

General Troubleshooting

The exhalation valve is cleaned during regular maintenance. This valve is delicate and needs to be handled carefully. If apparent leak problems occur and the circuit does not pass the leak test, the operator should be sure the exhalation valve diaphragm is correctly seated.

The operator's manual contains a section on troubleshooting that is symptom-based. For example, suppose a control does not operate. The manual explains that the control may not be active in the current mode or breath type. Or the controls could be locked. Or perhaps the control has not been "selected" by pushing the associated button. The user is advised to review the suggestions listed in the troubleshooting section of the operator's manual for more detail.

PULMONETIC SYSTEMS LTV 1200

The LTV 1200 is similar to the LTV 1000 ventilator. It also features an electromechanical pneumatic turbine system under the control of a microprocessor, which delivers patient ventilation. The turbine technology allows the ventilator to operate without a compressed-gas source. This section will focus on the LTV 1200 and will illustrate differences between it and the LTV 1000.

The LTV 1200 ventilator (Figure 14-26) is designed for use on adults and pediatric patients who weigh a minimum of 5 kg (11 lb) and who need either invasive or noninvasive ventilation. The dimensions of the LTV 1200 are 10 in × 12 in × 3 in, and it weighs 13.4 lb.

The internal mechanisms, operating controls, modes, alarms, and features are similar to those found on the LTV 1000 ventilator. Currently, the LTV 1200 has a method to present ventilator settings for rapid patient set-up that is not available on other models of the LTV. (See also the operations section that follows shortly.)

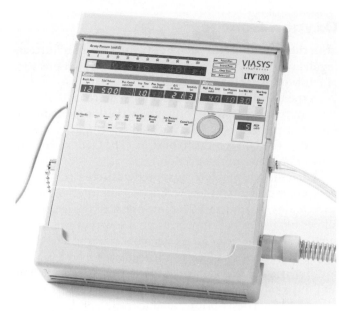

FIGURE 14-26 The Pulmonetic Systems LTV 1200 ventilator. (Courtesy Pulmonetic Systems, Inc, Minneapolis; Pulmonetic Systems is a division of Cardinal Health, McGaw Park, Ill.)

Power Source

Like the LTV 1000, the LTV 1200 ventilator is designed to run on an 110-V or 220-V AC power source or an 11-V to 15-V DC power source. This may be an external battery or a DC power system. When connected to an AC power outlet, the internal battery is continuously charged.

For DC power, the LTV can use either its own internal battery or one of many available external DC batteries. The internal battery can last approximately 60 minutes when fully charged. An external lithium ion battery is available for transport and hospital that lasts 3 hours each and the UPS (universal power supply) that lasts 4 hours fully charged. There is also an optional auto lighter adapter that enables the use of the LTV unit while in a car.

Internal Mechanism

The internal mechanism of operation is similar to that of the LTV 1000. Room air is drawn into the LTV unit from a flexible foam inlet filter on the side of the LTV unit. Once past the filter, the air then enters an accumulator/silencer, where it mixes with oxygen supplied from the oxygen blender.

The gas flow then enters a rotary compressor, where the gas is pressurized to deliver the correct flow rate and pressure needed to meet the set parameters. Unlike the case with the LTV 1000, the PEEP control is internal in the LTV 1200. A PEEP transducer is used in conjunction with the airway pressure transducer and monitored by the LTV's software to deliver the set PEEP level. The PEEP on the LTV 1200 is adjusted on the front panel of the unit.

Oxygen Source

Both the LTV 1200 and 1000 have a dual means of increasing delivered oxygen percentage via either a high-pressure or a low-pressure oxygen source.

In the LTV 1200, oxygen blending requires a high-pressure source and is active only when the low-pressure O_2 source is not selected. The high-pressure system is controlled by the O_2% (O_2 flush) button. (The O_2 flush control is described later in this section.)

When the low-pressure O_2 source is selected, the oxygen percentage display window will display dimmed dashes (–) and cannot be adjusted. The low-pressure oxygen source allows oxygen to be supplied from a low-pressure source such as a flowmeter or an oxygen concentrator. The delivered percentage of oxygen is not regulated by the ventilator, but it is instead dependent on the oxygen inlet flow and the total minute ventilation set on the ventilator. See Box 14-12 for a description and illustration of the approximate delivered F_IO_2 based on the set minute ventilation and the oxygen flow. As with any bleed-in system, it is recommended that a calibrated oxygen analyzer be used to determine the exact delivered F_IO_2.

Operations

To turn on the LTV 1200, the operator presses the on/standby button. The front panel (Figure 14-27) will illuminate and an audible alarm will activate for 1 second. If the "patient query" function is active, the message "SAME PATIENT" is displayed in the LED window. If this is the same patient, a press of the select button will begin ventilation with the settings used during the last power-down.

If this is a new patient, the operator should turn the set value knob until "NEW PATIENT" is displayed, then press the select button. A new query will then be displayed in the LED window, asking the operator if this patient is an adult, pediatric patient, or infant. The operator should then turn the set value knob until the desired patient type is displayed. Pressing the select button again will cause the ventilator to begin ventilating with appropriate preset settings for the selected patient type. If the patient query function is turned off, the ventilator will begin to immediately ventilate the patient with the settings set during the last power-down.

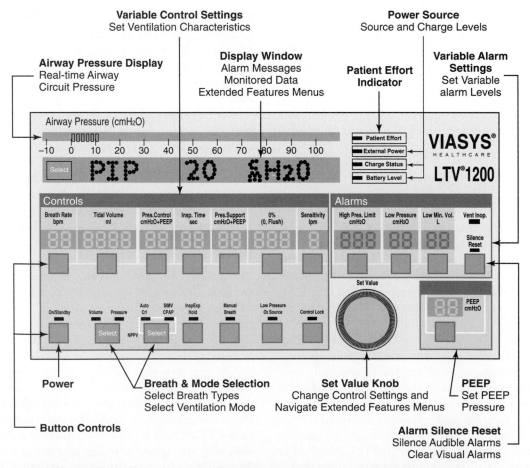

FIGURE 14-27 The Pulmonetic Systems LTV 1200 ventilator's control panel. (Courtesy Pulmonetic Systems, Inc, Minneapolis; Pulmonetic Systems is a division of Cardinal Health, McGaw Park, Ill.)

TABLE 14-16	
Five Types of Controls on the LTV 1200 Ventilator	
Types of Controls	Description
Variable controls	Controls and alarms that have front-panel displays
Buttons	Push buttons that select an option or perform a function
Set value knob	Used to set control values and navigate extended features menus
Extended features	Ventilation options that do not have front-panel controls, but are available through a special menu
Mechanical controls	Controls (e.g., overpressure relief) that are hardware-regulated and are not operator-adjustable

Controls and Alarms

The commonly used controls are located on the front panel of the LTV. As with many of the newer ventilators that use built-in microprocessors, some controls are menu-driven and are not located on the panel itself, but are pulled up on the display window when needed.

Front-Panel Controls

The front-panel diagram (see Figure 14-27) shows how the controls and displays are arranged. The controls are divided into two rows. The bottom row contains main function buttons or touch pads, and the upper row contains parameter-setting buttons.

Above the row of parameter controls is a display window, which has two main functions. It displays current ventilator data and provides access to additional control functions. To the right of the controls, alarm setting keys are located. Just below the alarm keys is a set value knob. Table 14-16 lists the five types of controls available with the LTV 1200 ventilator.

Select (Volume/Pressure) Button

As in the LTV 1000, this control allows the operator to choose either volume-targeted or pressure-targeted breaths. (See the section "Front-Panel Controls" in the LTV 1000 section for more information on this control.)

Select Mode Control

The mode control select provides the options of assist/control or SIMV/CPAP and NPPV. It is similar in function to the same control on the LTV 1000 with the following differences. Each press of the button advances or confirms your selection as follows:

- One press selects the first mode in the series (assist/control) and the associated LED flashes. A second press confirms the selection and the associated LED lights solid green.
- If you press the button again, the SIMV/CPAP LED flashes. Pressing again confirms and causes the SIMV/CPAP LED to light solid green.
- Press once more to select NPPV mode and the NPPV LED flashes. To confirm NPPV mode, you must press the button again, but be aware that the NPPV LED will continue to flash until the inspiratory positive airway pressure (IPAP) and **expiratory positive airway pressure (EPAP)** values have been set.

- Note: The LTV 1000 toggles only between AC and SIMV. NPPV is selected from the menu function.

Insp/Exp Hold Button

The inspiratory/expiratory hold button allows the operator to perform either of these two functions. The operator presses the button and reads the display window (monitoring screen), which will show one of the following: "INSP HOLD" or "EXP HOLD." If the operator presses the Insp/Exp Hold button, this allows her to scroll through the choices on the screen.

Manual Breath Button

When the manual breath button is pressed, a manual breath with volume and pressure based on current settings is delivered to the patient. In addition, a bolus of air purges the flow sensor line.

Low-Pressure O_2 Source Button

When selected, this option allows oxygen to be supplied from a low-pressure/low-flow oxygen source, such as an oxygen concentrator or a line-mounted flowmeter. Oxygen from the low-pressure source is mixed with air inside the ventilator. The O_2 percent delivered to the patient is determined by the O_2 inlet flow and the total minute volume and is not regulated by the ventilator.

When the low-pressure O_2 source option is selected and a high O_2 pressure source is attached to the ventilator, an automatic high O_2 switchover safety response generates a "HIGH O_2 PRES" alarm; switches the ventilator to high-pressure O_2 source mode; and sets the percentage of oxygen to be delivered in the gas flow to 21%. When the low-pressure O_2 source option is not selected, a high-pressure oxygen source is expected and oxygen blending is done within the ventilator. The ventilator expects an oxygen source with a pressure of 40 psi to 80 psi. The O_2 percent delivered to the patient is determined by the O_2% setting on the ventilator's front panel.

Low-Pressure O_2 Source

To select this option, you push and hold the "Low-Pressure O_2 Source" button for 3 seconds. As the low-pressure O_2 source is being selected, the associated LED will be flashing. Once the low-pressure O_2 source has been selected, the associated LED will remain on continually.

While the low-pressure O_2 source is on, the O_2 inlet pressure low alarm is inactive, but the O_2 pressure high alarm is set to activate at more than 10 psi. The O_2 % (O_2 flush) display will display dimmed dashes and O_2% cannot be set. To set the desired oxygen percentage, the flow of oxygen inlet must be adjusted.

O_2% (O_2 Flush)

The O_2% (O_2 flush) button is a dual-function control (O_2% **AND** O_2 Flush). When being used to set the percentage of oxygen delivered by the ventilator through the oxygen-blending system (O_2%), push and release the O_2% (O_2 flush) button, and change the setting with the set value knob. When being used to elevate the F_1O_2 to 100% for a preset period of time (O_2 flush), push and hold the O_2% (O_2 flush) button for 3 seconds.

The O_2% control establishes the percentage of oxygen to be delivered through the oxygen-blending system.

PEEP Control

Adjustment of the PEEP on the LTV 1200 is different from adjustment of the externally mounted PEEP valve on the LTV 1000. On the LTV 1200, the operator pushes the PEEP control button, which highlights the PEEP LED window. Adjustment of the PEEP level is accomplished by turning the set value knob to the desired level and then confirming by pressing the PEEP control button. The adjustable range of PEEP is 0 cm H_2O to 20 cm H_2O. The LTV 1200 has PEEP-compensated pressure support and pressure control.

Upper-Row Parameters

The upper row of controls contains the parameter settings such as rate and tidal volume. The procedure for changing the variables in this row, and in the alarms, is basically the same as for the lower row. The parameter button is touched to make a change. This action brightly illuminates the set value for the parameter and dulls the displays for all other parameters. The set value knob is rotated until the value desired appears in the display above the parameter button. The change is immediately active when the desired parameter button is pressed again or after 5 seconds.

The number in the window above each parameter represents the value set for that parameter. Numbers appear bright when the parameter is active in the current mode and breath type. They appear dim when they are not. A parameter's digital display will also brighten if it is selected for changing. All others then dim.

Three parameters—sensitivity, pressure support, and respiratory rate—can be turned off. The respective display for any of those three parameters will be blank ("- -") when it is turned off.

When the LTV is being powered by the internal battery, after 60 seconds all the digital displays turn off if no button has been pushed or any control changed. The displays can be reilluminated by pushing any button or turning the set value knob. Flashing displays will also occur.

Breath Rate

The breath rate control sets the minimum mandatory breath rate (in breaths/minute). It can be turned off, so that the breaths LED display will show dashes ("- -"). The rate range is 1 breath/min to 80 breaths/min. The process for selecting the desired rate is similar to that described with the PEEP control on the LTV 1200. Pressing the breath rate button will brighten the breaths LED. The operator turns the select value knob to the desired rate, then confirms by pressing the breath rate button again.

Tidal Volume

The tidal volume button controls volume delivery during volume-targeted ventilation. The adjustable tidal volume (V_T) range is from 50 mL to 2000 mL. Pressing the tidal volume button will brighten the tidal volume display LED. Turn the select value knob until the desired tidal volume is displayed, then confirm by pressing the tidal volume button again.

Pressure Control Button

The "Press. Control" button establishes the inspiratory pressure for pressure-targeted breaths. The operator pushes the "Press. Control" button and uses the set value knob to change to the desired inspiratory pressure (range: 1 to 99 cm H_2O). With the LTV 1000, this pressure is not added to the baseline PEEP. PEEP/CPAP is set mechanically by using the expiratory/PEEP valve. However, in the LTV 1200, pressure is automatically set above the PEEP level.

Inspiratory Time (T_I)

The "Insp Time" control sets the length of inspiration for volume-targeted and pressure-targeted breaths (range: 0.3 to 9.9 seconds). Inspiration cannot be shorter than 300 milliseconds. When V_T or T_I is being adjusted, the calculated flow ($\dot{V}$calc) is shown in the display window. The peak flow is based on the setting of T_I and V_T.

Pressure Support

The "Press. Support" button control establishes the target pressure above baseline for pressure-supported spontaneous breaths (range: off ("- -") or 1 to 60 cm H_2O). For the LTV 1000 unit, the baseline will always be 0, whereas for the LTV 1200 the pressure support level will be above PEEP level. PS is available for spontaneous breaths with SIMV in either pressure-targeted or volume-targeted ventilation and for CPAP breaths (see "Modes of Ventilation").

O_2% Button

The O_2% button establishes the percentage of O_2 delivery when it is on and a high-pressure oxygen source is available. If the operator presses the O_2 button, this will highlight the LED window; he must then rotate the set value knob to the desired percentage. Pressing the O_2 button again will confirm the new setting. The LED display will return to the normal intensity as will all other active parameters. (NOTE: The low-pressure O_2 button must be in the off position.)

Sensitivity

The sensitivity button is used to set the flow-trigger sensitivity level for assisted or spontaneous breaths. The range goes from off ("- -") up to 1 L/min to 9 L/min. The most-sensitive setting is 1 L/min. The base flow is preset at 10 L/min and requires no setting by the operator. When a trigger is detected, the patient effort LED illuminates. (See the section on the LTV 1000 for additional information on sensitivity.)

Leak Compensation

The leak-compensation feature enables constant monitoring for leaks and adjustment of the baseline of the ventilator in order to compensate for leaks (up to 6 L/min). This feature is described in the same section as is the LTV 1000 ventilator.

Alarms

The alarm controls and settings are to the right of the parameter controls. These alarms are similar to those described with the LTV 1000 ventilator in the preceding section.

Airway Pressure Bar Graph and Display Window

At the very top of the operating panel is the airway pressure display. This horizontal bar graph displays the pressure in the patient circuit (range: −10 to +108 cm H_2O).

The display window displays monitored data, alarm messages, and the extended features menu. During normal operation, the monitored data are presented sequentially. Each item is displayed for 3 seconds. See Table 14-14 for a complete list of displayed items.

Select Button—Display Screen

As is the case with the LTV 1000, the select button to the left of the display screen has several functions. It is used to stop the normal scrolling of monitored ventilator parameters. If the button is pushed once while the normal data scan is active, this halts the screen with the current parameter data showing. Each time the button is pushed after that, the next data item in the list is displayed. Scanning can be resumed by pressing the button twice within 3 seconds.

Breath Types and Modes of Ventilation

As with the LTV 1000, the LTV 1200 has specific breath types and modes. The reader is directed to the preceding section on the LTV 1000 to learn about these two features. Only the differences will be reviewed here.

If desired, the operator can select flow-cycling for pressure-controlled (PC) breaths rather than time-cycling by activating the flow termination percent feature using the extended features menu. The flow-cycling percent can be adjusted from 10% to 40% of peak flow. With the LTV 1200, the default setting is made in terms of the patient type selected (i.e., adult, pediatric, or infant) when the machine is powered on or it can be adjusted in the extended features menu.

Additional Features

Two additional features are accessed through the extended features mode. The extended features menu is selected by pushing the select button for 3 seconds. The first menu item is displayed in the window. Scrolling through the features menu, the operator will find a useful tool for transport operation. The LTV 1200 and 1000 have built-in oxygen cylinder duration calculators. The operator needs to select only the cylinder size and pressure in psi and the cylinder duration will be calculated with the current settings. As is the case with any procedure, the readers are directed to consult the manufacturer's manual for the particular ventilator they are using.

With the LTV 1200, an additional feature found in the extended menu is a spontaneous breathing trial (SBT) mode. With the SBT option you can temporarily minimize ventilatory support and perform clinical assessments of a patient's dependence on, or ability to be removed from, positive pressure ventilation. The SBT mode should be used only when a respiratory therapist or other properly trained and qualified personnel are present.

Modes of Ventilation

The LTV series ventilator provides the following modes of ventilation: control, assist/control (A/C), SIMV, CPAP, apnea backup ventilation, and NPPV. These modes are described in the preceding section on the LTV 1000 ventilator.

On the LTV 1200 unit, NPPV can be easily set up on the front panel as discussed earlier with the LTV 1000. With NPPV used in the LTV 1000 and 1200, masks must be ***nonvented*** to operate correctly and not consume excess gas supply.

SMITHS MEDICAL Pneupac™ ventiPAC VENTILATOR

The ventiPAC (Smiths Medical, Watford, United Kingdom) is a portable, time-cycled, volume ventilator that is designed for adults and for children who weigh more than 11 lb (5 kg). It is totally pneumatically operated and is MRI-compatible. The ventiPAC's dimensions are 3.7 in × 8.7 in × 6.4 in, and it weighs 6.6 lb (3 kg) without integrated alarms (6.8 lb [3.1 kg] with integrated alarms) (Figure 14-28). Table 14-17 lists modes, ventilator parameters, and other features of the Smiths Medical Pneupac™ ventiPAC.[19]

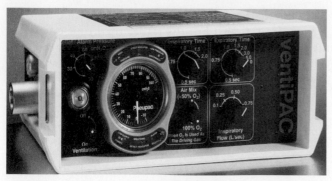

FIGURE 14-28 The Smiths Medical Pneupac™ ventiPAC Ventilator. (Courtesy Smiths Medical, Watford, United Kingdom.)

TABLE 14-17

Specifications for the Smiths Medical Pneupac™ ventiPAC

Control Settings	Range
Modes	SMMV, demand/CPAP
Power source	Pneumatic
Rate	7-60 breaths/min
Noninvasive ventilation mode	Yes
Peak pressure	80 cm H_2O
Tidal volume	50-1500 mL
Inspiratory time	0.5-2.0 s
PEEP/CPAP	Optional 0-20 cm H_2O
Oxygen percent	50% or 100%
Pressure support	NA
Monitors/displays	Analog airway pressure gauge, low-pressure display
Dimensions	3.7 in × 8.7 in × 6.4 in; 6.5 lbs
Logic gas consumption	Not specified
Alarms	High-pressure, low-pressure disconnect, low gas supply
Battery duration	N/A

SMMV, Synchronized minimum mandatory ventilation.

Power Source

The ventiPAC unit is totally pneumatically powered with medical-grade oxygen at 45 psi to 70 psi. The ventiPAC unit has no battery backup or AC power option.

Internal Mechanism

A compressed-gas source enters the ventiPAC through a DISS connection in the rear of the unit. The gas source is then filtered and directed to the internal flow-control mechanism. The ventiPAC does not incorporate an internal PEEP control. A disposable PEEP valve must be added to the circuit and adjusted as indicated.

Oxygen Source

The ventiPAC has two options for supplied F_IO_2 to the patient. Either 50% or 100% oxygen may be selected by adjusting the air mix selector. (Air mix will be discussed in greater detail later in this chapter.)

Controls

The ventiPAC has six individual controls to select the desired settings required by the patient. Figure 14-28 shows the controls on the front of the unit. The on ventilation/off ventilation switch is in the lower left-hand corner. The ventiPAC has an analog pressure gauge to display delivered pressures to the patient as measured at the ventilator outlet. The range of this gauge is −10 cm H_2O to +100 cm H_2O.

The ventiPAC does not have an internal PEEP mechanism. PEEP is generated via an external PEEP valve incorporated into the patient circuit. The adjustable range of this valve is from 0 cm H_2O to 20 cm H_2O. The PEEP pressure value (in cm H_2O) will only be displayed if the optional PEEP valve is attached to the ventilator circuit. The external PEEP valve is MRI-compliant.

Respiratory Rate

Respiratory rate is set by manipulation of the inspiratory and expiratory time control knobs located on the upper-right side of the control panel. Inspiratory time is adjustable from 0.5 second to 2 seconds. Expiratory time is adjustable from 0.6 second to 6 seconds. The deliverable respiratory rate is from 7 breaths/min to 60 breaths/min.

Tidal Volume

Deliverable tidal volume (V_T) is a product of the set T_I and the inspiratory flow, which is adjustable from 6 L/min to 60 L/min. The V_T range of the ventiPAC is 50 mL to 1500 mL. V_T is calculated by multiplying the inspiratory flow in liters per second by the set inspiratory time in seconds (T_I). The following formula illustrates this concept.

$$\frac{\text{Inspiratory flow}}{\text{(L/second)}} \times \frac{\text{Inspiratory Time}}{\text{(T_I, seconds)}} = \frac{\text{Tidal volume}}{\text{(L)}}$$

(See also Clinical Rounds 14-10.)

Air Mix Control

The position control is a two-position rotary switch—air/mix or 100% O_2. When in the air mix position, ambient air mixes with the drive gas to a ratio of 2:1 via a Venturi system. This will result in 45% O_2 being delivered to the

CLINICAL ROUNDS 14-10

A respiratory therapist is asked to transport a 60-year-old male patient who recently suffered a cardiac arrest. Upon arrival to the local referral facility, the therapist finds the patient is on the Pneupac™ ventiPAC Ventilator, which is using a 100% oxygen cylinder. The inspiratory time (T_I) is set at 1 second, and the expiratory time (T_E) is set at 4 seconds. The inspiratory flow is set at 0.5 L/s. What is the set respiratory rate and the tidal volume delivery?

See Evolve Resources for the answer.

patient when 100% oxygen is used as the drive gas. The air mix position is more efficient, providing an approximate 70% savings in drive-gas consumption when it is selected.

When the air mix switch is in the 100% O_2 position, the supply gas will be delivered to the patient. This could be 21% or 100% oxygen depending on whether air or an oxygen source is being used.

Pressure Relief

This control is located in the upper left-hand corner of the control panel and is adjustable from 20 cm H_2O to 80 cm H_2O. This rotary control knob allows continuous adjustment of the maximum patient inflation pressure through the setting of the spring-loaded relief valve. An audible alarm sounds when the set limit is reached.

Alarms

The ventiPAC has incorporated visual and audible alarms into a display ring surrounding the pressure gauge. The alarms consist of a high-pressure alarm, low pressure/disconnect, and other safety features. A visual eyeball type of indicator is used to warn the user of a low gas supply, and an audible and visual alarm is used to warn of low battery level. The battery provides power to the alarms.

High-Pressure Alarm

The high-pressure alarm is a pneumatically operated alarm with an electronically generated audible and visual indicator on the alarm monitor. The high-pressure alarm activates after the set high-pressure alarm has been maintained for a period of 1 second.

Low Inflation Pressure (Disconnect) Alarm

An audible and visual alarm warns the operator if the inflation pressure does not rise above the set level of 10 cm H_2O at least once in a 10-second period. This is not affected by PEEP applications.

Breathing Detector

The breathing detector illuminates when a spontaneous breathing effort has been detected and the low inflation pressure is reset.

Low Battery Alarm

A yellow visual indicator illuminates when the internal battery is at a reduced voltage. The rate at which the yellow indicator flashes gives the user an idea of how low the voltage level is. When the flash rate increases to twice a second, an audible alarm will sound for the remainder of the battery life.

Low Gas Supply Indicator

Directly below the relief/alarm pressure control is a visual indicator relaying to the operator when the operating gas supply is nearly exhausted. When the supply gas pressure is adequate, the gas-supply indicator will show white. When the supply pressure is low enough to not allow the

ventilator to operate properly, the indicator will turn red. At 45 psi the indicator will begin to change color from white to red. Any visible red in the indicator means that the gas supply is inadequate. In most cases the display will oscillate between white and red as the supply pressure falls. This visual indication will be accompanied by an electronically generated medium-priority audible alarm. If this alarm is ignored for more than 60 seconds, the alarm will shut itself off to conserve battery power.

Synchronized Minimum Mandatory Ventilation (SMMV)/Demand

This control has two positions. First is the ventilation off (demand), in which only the internal demand valve is powered by the gas supply. Any spontaneous breathing effort by the patient is met by flow from the demand valve. This position allows the operator to provide 100% oxygen therapy.

In the ventilation on position, the ventiPAC offers a mode of ventilation called **synchronized minimum mandatory ventilation (SMMV)**. SMMV allows the patient to breathe spontaneously without the risk of stacking mandatory breaths on top of spontaneous breaths.

If an adult patient has an adequate ventilation level, mandatory cycling by the ventiPAC will not occur. This is true as long as the minute ventilation is maintained. If the spontaneous rate becomes inadequate, the set rate and tidal volume (V_T) will be delivered. This SMMV feature applies only to V_T of more than 400 mL.

For a spontaneous V_T between 150 mL and 400 mL during SMMV, the mandatory breath is inhibited until spontaneous exhalation is completed and the expiratory time is proportionally extended, as long as the set minute ventilation is maintained.

With a spontaneous V_T of less than 150 mL, the ventilator will deliver a mandatory breath.

SUMMARY OF TRANSPORT VENTILATORS

The ideal transport ventilator is small, lightweight, and able to withstand the rigors of transport in a variety of environmental extremes, while providing adequate, safe ventilation to the patient at all times. For this reason, facilities looking to purchase a ventilator for transport should first determine the conditions in which they will be used.

When transporting patients, particular care must be taken to ensure optimal monitoring of patient status, ventilation, oxygenation, and patient safety.[20] Choosing and using the right equipment are part of the respiratory therapist's responsibilities.

Operating features available with a particular ventilator may be changed frequently by the manufacturers. For example, a new range for trigger sensitivity may be added or a new alarm added to a ventilator. For this and patient safety reasons, the user should always refer to the operating manual and information from the manufacturer when operating a ventilator.

Transport ventilators are becoming increasingly popular, not only for their intended purpose of transporting patients, but for use as ventilators in response to both natural and human-made disasters. Many states are now purchasing transport ventilators to help meet any potential catastrophic event.

PART II: HOME CARE VENTILATORS

Home care began in the United States more than 100 years ago.[1] Individuals discharged from the hospital who still required routine care were the primary candidates for this emerging sector of medicine. Today it is one of the fastest-growing areas of health care. With the continued rise in the cost of caring for patients in the acute or extended care environment, home care is a realistic alternative for individuals battling primarily chronic diseases. Conditions that might meet the indications for home ventilatory support are not limited to the following: ventilatory muscle disorders, alveolar hypoventilation syndrome, primary respiratory disorders, obstructive lung diseases, restrictive lung diseases, and cardiac disorders, including congenital anomalies. The goals of home invasive mechanical ventilation are as follows[21]:

· To sustain and extend life
· To enhance the quality of life
· To reduce morbidity
· To improve or sustain physical and psychological function of all patients needing ventilator assistance and to enhance growth and development in the pediatric patients who need ventilator assistance
· To provide cost-effective care

The following section focuses on the technical aspects of the equipment available for home care ventilation. The supportive measures include primarily positive-pressure ventilators, which are the most commonly used, and noninvasive positive-pressure ventilators.[22]

ACHIEVA, ACHIEVA PS, AND ACHIEVA PSO₂ VENTILATORS

The Achieva ventilators were described in the 7th edition of this text. This material is now available on Evolve Resources.

DRÄGER Carina™*home*

The Dräger Carina™*home* ventilator (Dräger Medical AG & Co, Lübeck, Germany) is a newly designed home care ventilator (Figure 14-29). The Carina™*home* ventilator provides both invasive and noninvasive ventilation with both pressure-targeted and volume-targeted modes.[23] The minimum tidal volume recommended is 100 mL. It is designed to be used for pediatric and adult patients. The

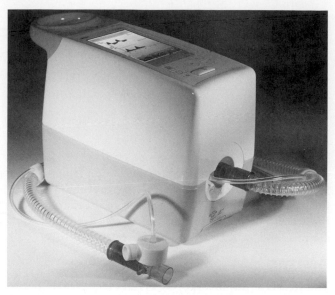

FIGURE 14-29 The Dräger Carina™*home* ventilator. (Courtesy Dräger Medical AG & Co, Lübeck, Germany.)

Carina's dimensions are 38.5 in × 17.5 in × 27.5 in, and it weighs 10.6 lb (4.9 kg).

Power Source

The Carina ventilator has two sources of external power. The primary power source is 100-V or 240-V AC, and a secondary power source is a 12-V to 24-V DC battery power. The internal battery is rated for a minimum of 2 hours under normal conditions. The Carina also has an optional external battery pack that offers an additional 10 hours of operation when fully charged.

Internal Mechanism

The Carina is electrically powered and microprocessor-controlled. Room air is drawn into the unit through the air inlet HEPA filter. The internal blower generates the pressure or flow delivered to the patient according to the set parameters. A control circuit measures the ventilation pressure and flow and adjusts the pressure as needed.

Patient safety devices are provided, for example, in order to prevent excessive pressure at the patient side or in the event of a total device failure. In the event of a failure, the ventilator enters the rescue mode and will allow the patient to continue breathing room air through a safety valve inlet.

Oxygen Source

The Carina™*home* ventilator operates by using room air under normal conditions, but it can be modified to increase the F_IO_2. The Carina has an oxygen low-pressure input port, where supplemental oxygen can be bled in to a maximum of 10 L/min. The Carina has two optional valves that dictate the oxygen percentage delivered. As with any supplemental system in which a blender is not used, the percentage of oxygen delivered should be analyzed periodically with a calibrated oxygen analyzer.

Operations of the Ventilator

Pressing the power switch located on the bottom rear panel of the ventilator powers on the machine. After a 6-second self-test, the ventilator is ready to begin ventilation with the last mode that was programmed. The current settings are shown on the display panel, and the clinician is able to make changes to these settings while the machine is in standby mode. This allows for the correct settings to be entered before the patient is connected. After the ventilator

has been checked and the correct settings entered, the start/standby key flashes until the clinician activates the ventilator by depressing the start key.

Controls and Display Panel

As with most newer microprocessor-controlled units, the controls are incorporated in a menu-driven program rather than by individual controls. Figure 14-30 shows the Carina's control panel and display screen.

Similar to the situation with other Dräger microprocessor-controlled ventilators, the operator uses the principle of "Select, Change, and Confirm" to make changes

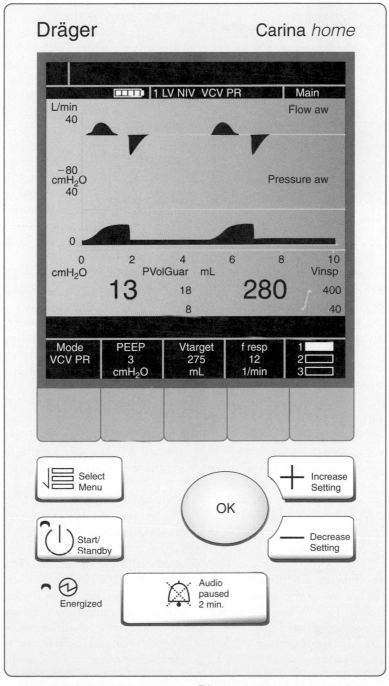

FIGURE 14-30 The Dräger Carina™*home* ventilator's control panel.

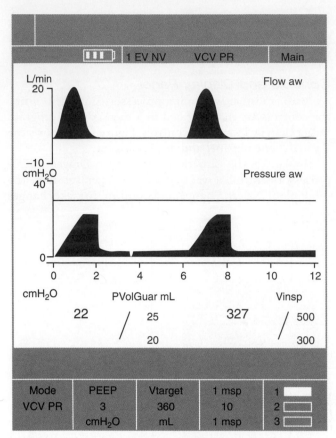

FIGURE 14-31 The Carina™*home* ventilator's liquid-crystal display (LCD) screen.

to parameters in the Carina ventilator. The operator selects a function using the soft keys on the control panel. The operator then uses the (+) or (−) keys to adjust the parameter up or down, respectively. The final step is to press the "OK" key to confirm the new setting.

Display Screen
The Carina's LCD display screen (Figure 14-31) has multiple functions dependent on the mode chosen. The display screen will automatically dim after 2 minutes. Following are the parameters that may be displayed:

· Inspired tidal volume, including volume range
· Actual inspiratory pressure, including pressure range
· Respiratory rate
· Battery capacity
· Airway pressure curve (P_{aw})
· Flow curve

Mode Selection
The Carina™*home* ventilator offers several different modes that can be applied with either invasive or noninvasive ventilation. The modes are CPAP, PSV, PCV+, and volume control ventilation plus/pressure-regulated plus (VCV-PR+). These modes are set by pressing the mode soft key. The operator can then use the (+) and (−) keys to select the desired mode. Pressing the "OK" key confirms mode selection. All modes will be detailed later in this section.

Tidal Volume
To select the desired V_T, the operator follows the procedure described earlier. The V_T soft key is pressed first, then the (+) or (−) keys are used to set the desired V_T. This newly selected value must be confirmed by pressing the OK key.

The adjustable range of tidal volume for the Carina ventilator is 100 mL to 2000 mL. The V_T value is delivered at the BTPS value. This is accomplished by the ventilator comparing measured ambient pressure with the current pressure level measured at the airway and compensating the delivered V_T for any changes in ambient pressure such as higher or changing altitudes.

Respiratory Rate
To adjust the respiratory rate, one follows the same procedure as with adjusting the V_T. The respiratory rate range in the PCV(+), VCV-PR(+) and in apnea ventilation is 5 breaths/min to 50 breaths/min.

Trigger Sensitivity
The "normal" trigger sensitivity level is recommended with patients who have relatively healthy lungs. For patients with obstructive or restrictive lung disease, the SyncPlus trigger level is recommended. The Carina™*home* uses an algorithm for SyncPlus triggering. The algorithm was designed to do the following:
1. Optimize synchronicity of the ventilator with the patient
2. Minimize autotriggering
3. Enhance ventilator responsiveness while lowering the work of breathing

It is a learning algorithm, which means that it will "learn" and adapt to the optimal sensitivity for each patient by looking back at previous breaths, anticipating upcoming breaths, and adjusting the trigger sensitivity accordingly.

PEEP
PEEP is controlled internally on the Carina™*home* ventilator and is adjustable from 3 to 20 cm H_2O through the parameter setting process described above.

Inspiratory Time
Inspiratory time is adjustable within a range of 0.3 second to 8.0 seconds.

Inspiratory Pressure (Pinsp)
The adjustable range of deliverable peak pressure on the Carina™*home* ventilator is dependent on which of two available circuits is used and whether a controlled expiration valve or a Silentflow valve is incorporated into the circuit. Deliverable pressures with the controlled expiration valve range from 5 cm H_2O to 50 cm H_2O. If the Silentflow valve is incorporated, the deliverable range is 5 cm H_2O to 40 cm H_2O.

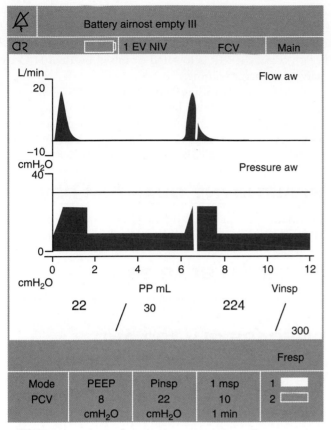

FIGURE 14-32 The Carina™*home* ventilator LCD alarms screen.

Alarms

The Carina™*home* ventilator has an extensive alarm package to accurately monitor patients, whether they are being supported invasively or noninvasively. Some alarms are automatic, whereas others are adjustable and require the operator to enter a desired value to an alarm setting.

The adjustable alarms are high peak airway pressure, disconnect, tidal volume, high respiratory rate, and apnea response time. Figure 14-32 shows a battery alarm message, which would be accompanied by an audible alarm.

High Peak Airway Pressure Alarm
The high peak airway pressure alarm is adjustable from 10 cm H_2O to 55 cm H_2O. When this alarm is triggered, both an audible and a visual alarm become active, with a specific high-pressure alarm message displayed in the LCD display.

Disconnect Time Alarm
The disconnect time alarm has two time settings because of the Carina's ability to provide both invasive and noninvasive support. For invasive support, the disconnect time is adjustable from 0 second to 60 seconds, whereas for noninvasive support the disconnect alarm is adjustable from 0 second to 120 seconds.

Tidal Volume Alarms
The high V_T alarm limits are from 130 mL to 2000 mL, whereas the low V_T alarm range is 40 mL to 1200 mL. When either alarm is triggered, both an audible and a visual alarm is activated, with a specific alarm message displayed in the LCD display.

High-Frequency Alarm
The high respiratory rate (high-frequency) alarm is adjustable from 10 breaths/min to 70 breaths/min. As with all adjustable alarms, it is signaled by both an audible alarm and a visual message in the alarm window portion of the LCD display.

Alarm Intensity Level
The alarm-monitoring system of the Carina also has the capability of four levels of alarms dependent on the severity of the situation. The lowest-priority alarm is a level 0 alarm, in which the alarm situation is displayed only in the alarm message window of the LCD display window.

The second alarm level is a level 1 (low) alarm, in which the error message is displayed in the alarm message window and the alarm key lights up (yellow) on the control panel. An audible beep is activated at 1-minute intervals until the situation is remedied.

A level 2 (medium) alarm indicates a serious error, and the alarm is identified in the alarm message window of the display LCD while the alarm key flashes yellow. This is accompanied by an audible 3-tone alarm sequence at repeated intervals. If the remote alarm (nurse call) is connected, this alarm is also activated.

The final alarm level is a level 3 (high) alarm situation, which indicates a serious alarm situation. An alarm message is displayed while the alarm key flashes red. A twofold, 5-tone audible alarm sequence is activated as well, which requires the immediate attention of the caregiver.

Modes of Ventilation
As a home care ventilator, the Carina™*home* offers a variety of modes that will be reviewed here.

CPAP. CPAP is used for spontaneously breathing patients who may require only a set level of PEEP/CPAP to decrease work of breathing, to increase their functional residual capacity, or to treat problems such as obstructive sleep apnea. The adjustable range of CPAP is 3 cm H_2O to 20 cm H_2O. This mode is truly a spontaneous mode, relying entirely on the patient to maintain his or her own minute ventilation.

Apnea backup ventilation is available in this mode. Appropriate settings are instituted by the clinician if apnea ventilation is considered necessary based on the patient's presentation and history.

PSV. In the PSV mode, the ventilator provides inspiratory assistance through the use of a set pressure (P_{insp}). The ventilator detects inspiration by the patient (patient-triggered) and supplies the set pressure during inspiration (pressure-limited). Inspiration is flow-cycled. The amount of assist pressure can be varied. Expiratory pressure is determined by the PEEP setting.

The Carina™*home* ventilator has a special feature (dual-control mode) that can be activated during called volume guarantee. (See Chapter 11 for additional information on dual-control modes.) Volume guarantee can be selected by using the support soft key. When this mode is activated, the user is asked to set a target V_T and a pressure range. In volume guarantee, the Carina will vary the PIP within the selected pressure range. It will deliver the target V_T by raising or lowering the PIP within the set pressure range (Pvg min and Pvg max) by 1 cm H_2O per breath. Should the patient's airway resistance or lung compliance change, this feature will adapt to the new requirements within a few breaths and adjust the PIP to deliver the targeted volume. Volume guarantee should be used to optimize ventilator synchrony under changing situations.

Apnea backup ventilation can be set in PSV, in case the patient becomes apneic. Once in the backup mode, the ventilator will resume PSV as soon as a spontaneous breathing effort is detected. Apnea backup ventilation is the Carina™*home* ventilator's alternative to SIMV with PS. Recall that in SIMV/PS, the pattern of patient-triggered PS breaths is periodically interrupted by a mandatory volume breath. By moving the mandatory breathing to the background (apnea ventilation set), the patient can breathe with PS or volume-targeted PS (with volume guarantee) without the periodic interruption of a mandatory breath.

PCV$_{assist}$ or PCV+. With PCV$_{assist}$, also know as PCV+, the patient can breathe spontaneously at any time, even during the inspiratory inflation cycle. This mode is described in detail in Chapter 12 with the Dräger Evita 4 (and Evita 2 Dura). PCV+ is sometimes referred to as *bilevel positive pressure ventilation* by the manufacturer. In PCV+, mandatory breaths are time-triggered or patient-triggered, pressure-targeted, and time-cycled. This mode is similar to that found on a high-flow CPAP device, because it uses an open expiratory valve system.

In PCV+, the operator sets the minimum respiratory rate, inspiratory pressure above PEEP, slope time (or Auto-Slope), and inspiratory time (or I:E ratio). Setting the trigger to normal or sensitive makes this an assist mode. The PCV+ mode in this ventilator is an assist mode, because the patient can breathe spontaneously during the expiratory time and between mandatory breaths. The patient can breathe spontaneously at any time, independent of the set mandatory breaths.

Volume-Controlled Ventilation, Pressure-Regulated (VCV-PR+). Volume-controlled ventilation can be used both as a control mode and as an assist mode by switching off or on the triggering. If the ventilation is set up as an assist mode, this is indicated as VCV-PR+.

In VCV-PR+, the Carina™*home* delivers volume breaths at a set target volume and a set rate. This volume-control mode is pressure-regulated, and, therefore, it allows the user to control the pressure with which these volume breaths are delivered. Quite similar to the procedure with volume guarantee in the PSV mode, the clinician sets an appropriate pressure range in which the Carina™*home* ventilator will deliver the set target volume. On a breath-to-breath basis, the PIP is lowered or raised by 1 cm H_2O to deliver the target volume.

If used as a control mode (trigger set to "NONE"), the minute volume is defined by the control rate. If used as an assist mode (VCV-PR+), the minute volume depends on the spontaneous rate of the patient. Appropriate alarms must be set. VCV-PR+ can also be used as an alternative to SIMV.

HEALTHDYNE QUANTUM PSV

Information on the Healthdyne Quantum PSV noninvasive ventilator is now available on Evolve Resources.

INTERMED BEAR 33

The Intermed Bear 33 is reviewed on Evolve Resources.

LIFECARE PLV-100 AND PLV-102 VENTILATORS

The Lifecare PLV ventilators were described in the 7th edition of this text. This material is now available on Evolve Resources.

NEWPORT HT50

The Newport HT50 (Newport Medical Instruments, Costa Mesa, Calif.) is a portable ventilator designed for home care, subacute care, transport use, and hospital use (Figure 14-33). It is a microprocessor-controlled ventilator that may be used for adult or pediatric patients (who weigh ≥10 kg).[24]

The device functions in three modes: assist/control mode ventilation (A/CMV), SIMV, and spontaneous ventilation (spont). It is lightweight (15 lb without a humidifier) and compact (10.6 in × 7.87 in × 10.24 in).

Power Source

The HT50 is electrically powered and requires no gas sources to properly perform all of its operations. Oxygen enrichment is available through a 50-psi entrainment (0 bleed) mixer or a low flow blending bag kit. The electronic system can use three possible power sources:

- A standard AC outlet (100 to 240 V)
- An external DC battery (12 to 30 V)
- An internal DC battery

Indicators on the top-right section of the front provide information about the current power source (Ext. Power/Charging Int. Battery, Int. Battery [Push to Test]).

The internal battery can sustain ventilator operation for up to 10 hours and requires 8 hours to fully recharge from any AC or DC power source, even while the ventilation is in operation. Newport recommends charging the battery for a minimum of 5 hours after the battery

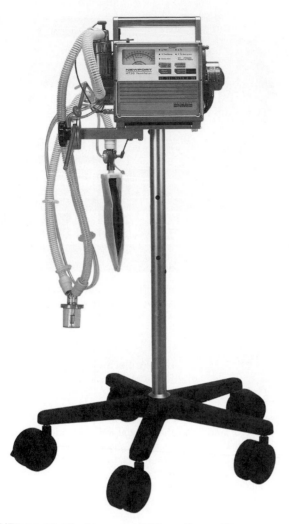

FIGURE 14-33 The Newport HT50 ventilator. (Courtesy Newport Medical Instruments, Costa Mesa, Calif.)

empty alarm, and "No ext. power" (a power switchover alarm).

When the "battery low" message appears in the message display window, an audible, intermittent 3-pulse cautionary beep sounds and a visible alert (i.e., the LED blinks red adjacent to "Int. Battery") is activated. This alarm indicates that the internal battery is in use and less than 1 hour of battery charge remains. Pressing the silence/reset button can silence the audible alarm, but the visual alarm will remain illuminated until the ventilator is plugged into an AC outlet or an external battery is connected.

The battery empty message is activated when less than 30 minutes of power remains in the internal battery. It is accompanied by an audible, intermittent 3-pulse cautionary alarm and a visible alert (LED blinks red adjacent to "Int. Battery").

The power switchover alarm notifies the clinician that the external power source has failed and the internal battery is now in use. It occurs when a switch from an external battery to the internal battery has occurred because of disconnection from the power cord or a power interruption. The message "No Ext. Power" appears in the message window, the LED next to the "Int Battery" blinks red, and the red LED next to the "Ext.Power/Charging Int. Battery" message is constantly lit. This alarm can be silenced by pressing the silence/reset button or by plugging the ventilator into a working outlet.

The internal pneumatic circuit does not require external compressed air but does require a medical-grade high-pressure oxygen gas source capable of delivering 35 psi to 90 psi of low-flow oxygen. The 35-psi to 90-psi oxygen source may be a cylinder or wall outlet. The low-flow source may be a flowmeter from a cylinder, wall outlet, liquid system, or concentrator.

Internal Mechanism

All gas enters the HT50 through an opening in the filter cover located on the right side of the machine. If neither oxygen accessory is connected, the ventilator delivers room air to the patient. For oxygen enrichment, either the air-oxygen entrainment mixer or oxygen-blending bag kit is inserted into the opening (see oxygen source below). This ventilator uses a dual-micropiston delivery system that allows the ventilator to operate without an external air compressor.

The respiratory rate, trigger sensitivity, pressure control or tidal volume, PEEP, and pressure support set by the clinician determine the stroke rate and stroke speed of the pistons.

Oxygen Source

The HT50 comes with two oxygen-delivery options: (1) an optional air-oxygen entrainment mixer or (2) an oxygen-blending bag kit. The air-oxygen entrainment mixer attaches to the fresh gas intake valve on the right side of the ventilator and allows for the attachment of a high-pressure oxygen gas source. This device allows the clinician

has been completely depleted (approximately 80% of a full charge).

The HT50 has a universal power entry module. This module allows the clinician to use the same port for connecting the plug for AC as it does for an external DC. To use external DC, the source must be capable of delivering a minimum of 12 V and a maximum of 30 V to be compatible with the ventilator. The auto DC power connector allows for powering the HT50 from the cigarette lighter in an automobile.

The HT50 comes equipped with several battery indicators and alarms that monitor the status of the power supply to the ventilator. The indicators are located in the upper right section of the front panel. The button, labeled "Int Battery (Push to Test)," allows you to read the battery charge level in the pressure gauge window when operating from the internal battery. When the LED adjacent to this control is amber, the internal battery is partially to fully charged. When red, the battery is low.

The message display window in the center of the front panel will provide written messages of battery conditions. They include the following: battery low alarm, battery to control the oxygen percentage delivered to the patient from 21% to 100% oxygen with a knob located on the blender itself. It is a unique high-pressure ambient mixing system that uses no bleed.

The oxygen-blending bag kit also attaches to the fresh gas intake valve on the right side of the ventilator and allows for the attachment of a low-flow oxygen gas source. This device allows the clinician to control the oxygen percentage delivered to the patient by varying the flow set on a flowmeter attached to the blending bag kit. Two charts (one for use with PEEP and one for use without PEEP) assist the clinician in setting proper flow rates to achieve a given F_IO_2.

Humidifier

The HT50 offers a humidifier option. When the humidifier is attached (left side of machine), it is only functional if the ventilator is powered by an external AC power source.

The humidifier is activated by a button located on the front right of the control panel, which allows the operator to activate the humidifier and set a temperature ranging from 19°C to 39°C. The operator presses the humidifier button to adjust the temperature and uses the up and down arrows in the center of the front panel to increase and decrease the temperature setting. During ventilation, the displayed temperature is measured at the patient connector. The displayed temperature is measured at the humidifier bottle outlet. To turn off the humidifier, the operator presses and holds the button for 3 seconds.

If the message "Check Humidifier" appears in the message display window and the LED adjacent to the humidifier control blinks red, a malfunction has been detected. The humidifier shuts down. One of five possible messages is displayed. The user is advised to see the operating manual for instructions.

Patient Circuit

The connections for the patient circuit are located on the left side of the ventilator. They include a temperature plug when the humidifier is attached, a proximal pressure line with filter, a drive line for the externally mounted exhalation valve, and the main inspiratory line.

Control Panel and Alarms

The front panel of the HT50 contains several controls for setting parameters and monitoring patient data and alarms, as well as for powering up the ventilator (Figure 14-34). The on/standby selector is located at the bottom right of the front panel. It allows the user to select one of three operating conditions by pressing the on/standby button.

In the first condition, the ventilator is in the off/standby mode. Standby means that the ventilator is plugged into an external power supply and the internal battery is charging.

The second condition (button pressed once) is the settings feature. The settings feature allows the clinician to program the ventilator settings before turning the machine on and connecting it to a patient. It is also the condition

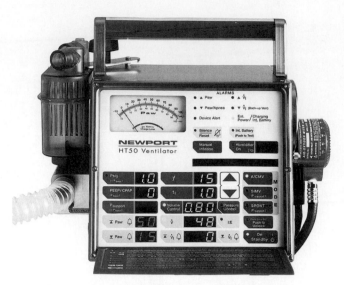

FIGURE 14-34 The Newport HT50 ventilator's control panel. (See text for further information.). (Courtesy Newport Medical Instruments, Costa Mesa, Calif.)

BOX 14-18	Use of the Settings Feature to Calibrate the Expiration Valve in the HT50

To perform this procedure, occlude the patient circuit connector and press the manual inflation button twice. The ventilator performs a leak check on the breathing circuit and also provides a linearization curve for the ventilator pressure management in conjunction with the exhalation valve in use.

during which an exhalation valve calibration is performed (Box 14-18). This simple procedure (occlude the circuit and press the manual inflation button twice) performs a leak check on the breathing circuit and also provides a linearization curve for the ventilator pressure management in conjunction with the exhalation valve in use. When operating in settings, the parameter values that are entered (e.g., tidal volume, respiratory rate) do not have to be confirmed by pressing the key a second time, as they do during normal operation (Box 14-19).

To begin ventilation, the third condition, the on/standby button, is pressed again. Two safety features help prevent any accidental changes in the set parameters from occurring. The first is a panel cover, which blocks the control settings from view and must be opened to gain front-panel access. The second is the panel lock feature located at the bottom right of the ventilator, just above the on/standby selector. When activated, it locks all settings on the ventilator and prevents someone from inadvertently changing the parameters.

Control Parameters

The front panel is divided into roughly three sections: the central panel containing parameter controls and modes,

BOX 14-19	Setting Ventilator Parameters in the Settings Position and in the "on" Position on the Newport HT50

In the settings position, if the mode is changed or breath control switched from volume control to pressure control and vice versa, the change is implemented without further action on the part of the user. On the other hand, if the ventilator had been in the on position, the clinician would have had to confirm the mode or breath control change by depressing the button for the newly selected parameter a second time. If the parameter change is not confirmed when the ventilator is in the on position, then it will return to the previous setting.

TABLE 14-18

Setting Limitation Messages on the Newport Medical Instruments HT50

Messages	Meaning
Reached max $\dot{V}$	Maximum flow setting reached
Reached min $\dot{V}$	Minimum flow setting reached
Inverse I:E	An inverse I:E ratio has been set
Reached max I:E	The maximum inverse ratio of 3:1 has been reached
$\dot{V}$ unavailable	Flow value cannot be displayed during pressure ventilation
PEEP + PS too high	Maximum limit of PEEP + PS is 60 cm H_2O
PC−PEEP too low	PC/PEEP is less than 5 cm H_2O
↑ PEEP too low	High P_{limit}−PEEP is <5 cm H_2O
Reminder Messages	
Panel lock	Operator has tried to change a parameter with the panel lock activated
Press again	Pressing the same button is required to confirm and activate the parameter change requested

the bottom section of alarms, and the top section of monitored data and alarm indicators (Figure 14-34).

As a general rule, when changing parameter values, the operator first presses the desired parameter button, uses the up or down arrow to change the displayed setting, and then presses the parameter button again to confirm and activate the change. Alarms are set in the same way. A setting limitation message will appear in the message display window when the operator adjusts a parameter to its limits. Table 14-18 lists setting limitation messages.

The first control parameter displayed is trigger sensitivity (PTRIG; 0 to −9.9 cm H_2O). The sensitivity is automatically PEEP-compensated. For example, if PEEP is 5 cm H_2O and the sensitivity is −0.5 cm H_2O, the breath triggers when an inspiratory effort drops the airway pressure to 4.5 cm H_2O. The PTRIG LED indicator light illuminates every time a spontaneous breath is detected, allowing the clinician to track the patient's breathing pattern.

The PEEP/CPAP (0 to 30 cm H_2O) control governs the baseline pressure. PEEP/CPAP cannot be set higher than the pressure-control target setting of −5 cm H_2O. This is to ensure that the ventilator is able to deliver a breath during pressure ventilation, even if it is just 5 cm H_2O (i.e., the difference between set pressure target and PEEP).

Pressure support (PS) has an available range of 0 cm H_2O to 60 cm H_2O. The ventilator will not allow the combined value of PEEP/CPAP plus pressure support to be greater than 60 cm H_2O.

The available mandatory respiratory rate (f) range is 1 breath/min to 99 breaths/min. Inspiratory time (T_I) is adjustable from 0.1 second to 3.0 seconds. The next control is the volume control (100 to 2200 mL)/pressure control (5 to 60 cm H_2O). This allows the operator to select either volume-targeted or pressure-targeted breaths and set the desired parameter value—that is, volume in liters or pressure in cm H_2O.

Mode controls include A/CMV, SIMV, and SPONT (see section on Modes of Ventilation). To activate the mode the operator presses the desired mode once and then a second time to activate it. However, before confirming a mode, all the appropriate parameter settings for that mode should be set and checked.

The lower section of the panel includes the high- and low-pressure alarm controls (P_{aw}), inspiratory flow display, and I:E ratio display, minute volume display, and the high and low minute volume alarm controls ($\dot{V}_I$). The alarms will be reviewed later in this section.

The inspiratory flow ($\dot{V}$) and I:E ratio LCD display allow the clinician to select viewing either one or the other in the adjacent display window by touching the desired parameter control. To the left is the flow display.

When operating in volume control ventilation, the flow delivered to the patient is determined by the inspiratory time and the tidal volume setting.

$$V_T(L) = T_I \text{ (seconds)} \times \text{Flow (liters/second)}$$

The calculated flow value is displayed in an LCD panel in the bottom middle of the front panel as $\dot{V}$. (NOTE: If the T_I allows the flow to reach a maximum- or minimum-range level [range is 6 to 100 L/min], adjustment of T_I stops and a beep sounds. A setting limitation message appears in the message display window.) The flow display is not available during pressure control or spontaneous ventilation.

The I:E ratio is determined by the frequency and the inspiratory time settings (range, 1:99 up to 3:1). When the entered parameters generate an inverse I:E ratio, the ventilator briefly alarms, making the clinician aware of the changes, but continues with ventilation. The I:E ratio cannot exceed 3:1.

The upper portion of the control panel contains a pressure gauge (−10 to 100 cm H_2O or mBar) that monitors real-time airway pressure. This section of the front panel also includes a manual inflation control (3 seconds maximum) and the humidifier control described previously.

The manual inflation feature is only active in the A/CMV and SIMV modes. It allows the clinician to control the amount of the V_T for the manual breath by controlling the inspiratory time. The flow is determined by the variables of V_T and T_I set in volume-targeted A/CMV and SIMV. In pressure control, the set pressure is delivered. A manual breath is terminated under three conditions:

1. When the clinician stops pressing the control.
2. The set high-pressure alarm limit is reached.
3. Three seconds have elapsed.

A backup safety feature will not allow the clinician to deliver a manual breath while the patient is in inspiration or if the airway pressure is greater than 5 cm H_2O above PEEP.

Just below the manual inflation control is the message display window discussed previously. When the display is blank, the operator can view monitored parameters by using the up and down arrows on the front panel. Monitored values that appear include V_T, $\dot{V}_I$, f, or Paw (peak, mean and base). These are updated every 10 seconds or at the end of each breath, allowing the operator to record current values.

Airway Pressure and Minute Ventilation Alarms

The high airway pressure alarm control is located on the lower left portion of the control panel and has an adjustable range of 4 cm H_2O to 99 cm H_2O. When the set high-pressure level is reached, audiovisual alarms are activated and the machine cycles into exhalation. The visual indicator is in the top section of the front panel. (NOTE: The high peak pressure alarm cannot be set below the PEEP setting.)

The low airway pressure alarm control is below the high airway pressure alarm control. Its operating range is 3 cm H_2O to 98 cm H_2O. The low airway pressure alarm is active only during mandatory breaths in the A/CMV and SIMV modes. It activates when the rise in pressure does not exceed the alarm setting during the inspiratory phase for two consecutive patient-triggered or time-triggered mandatory breaths. The visual indicator is in the top section of the front panel.

The high and low minute ventilation alarm controls are also located on the lower panel. The high $\dot{V}_I$ (high inspiratory minute volume) alarm has a setting range of 1.1 L to 50 L. The low $\dot{V}_I$ (low inspiratory minute volume) has a setting range of 0.3 L to 49 L. If the measured minute volume falls outside of the set limits, the appropriate alarm becomes active, producing both an audible and a visible alert. The visual indicator is in the upper section of the front panel. (NOTE: The alarm measures the volume delivered from the ventilator and not what is exhaled by the patient.) If at any time the minute ventilation falls below the "low minute ventilation" alarm value, the backup ventilation (BUV) feature is activated and the $\dot{V}_I$ ("Back-up Vent.") indicator illuminates. This feature is active in all modes and is described in the section on modes of ventilation.

Additional Alarms

Additional alarms that are monitored and have messages that appear in the message display window include the following: high baseline pressure, occlusion, low baseline pressure, check proximal line, apnea, PC cannot be reached, and device alerts.

High Baseline Pressure Alarm

The high baseline pressure alarm occurs when the baseline pressure is greater than the low airway pressure alarm setting at the beginning of a time-triggered mandatory breath. The alarm message will display "HIGH Pbase." The alarm will reset when airway pressure drops to within 5 cm H_2O of the PEEP/CPAP level.

Occlusion Alarm

The occlusion alarm activates when the airway pressure remains +15 cm H_2O above the PEEP setting for 3 seconds after exhalation has begun or at the end of exhalation, whichever comes first. It is corrected if airway pressure falls to within 5 cm H_2O of baseline.

If this alarm occurs, no additional mandatory breaths are delivered until it is corrected. The device alert indicator blinks and the ventilator attempts to release pressure through the redundant safety system. The safety system allows the patient to draw ambient air into the breathing circuit through an emergency intake valve when no other flow is available. The patient effort required to open this valve is approximately 2 cm H_2O.

Low Baseline Pressure Alarm

The low baseline pressure alarm ("LOW Pbase") indicates an unstable baseline. For example, this could occur with a large leak in the patient circuit (pressure ≥2 cm H_2O below baseline for 3 seconds). In addition to the message displayed, the low Paw indicator blinks. The alarm resets when the baseline pressure difference is less than 2 cm H_2O (Clinical Rounds 14-11).

Check Proximal Line Alarm

The check proximal line ("CHECK PROX LINE") alarm occurs during inspiration when the proximal pressure measured is significantly different from the internal backup pressure sensor measurement taken inside the ventilator. In addition to the message, the low Paw/Apnea indicator blinks red. Causes include disconnections, kinking of the circuit, and a water-filled proximal sensor line. Ventilation continues during this condition by using the pressure monitored by the internal pressure transducer.

CLINICAL ROUNDS 14-11

A patient's nurse calls you to an intermediate care area to troubleshoot a reported alarm on the HT50 unit. You arrive to find the following message on the ventilator's message window: "LOW Pbase." What is the meaning of the alarm message?

See Evolve Resources for the answer.

Apnea Alarm

When a patient breath goes undetected for 30 seconds, an apnea alarm occurs ("APNEA").

PCV Not Reached Alarm

"PCV not reached" signals to the operator that the maximum inspiratory pressure measured is less than 50% of the set pressure during PCV. The operator should check the patient to be sure he or she is being adequately ventilated and then check the circuit for leaks.

Device Alert

When the device alert LED illuminates, a steady red and an internal beep occur. This indicates that the ventilator has detected one of four message conditions:

· OCCL Shutdown
· Motor Fault
· 10 V SHUTDOWN
· SYSTEM ERROR

With the exception of an occlusion alert, in all these conditions the ventilator will stop ventilating. Another method must be found to ventilate the patient, and the HT50 should be taken out of service and not used on patients until it is checked by a qualified technician.

Alarm/Silence-Reset

The alarm/silence-reset button is in the upper alarm indicator section on the control panel. When it is activated, this control silences the alarm for 60 seconds. It is also used to clear "latched" alarms that are no longer active, including alarm messages in the message window.

Modes of Ventilation

The mode settings located on the right front panel of the HT50 are A/CMV, SIMV and "Spont.," or spontaneous. (NOTE: When selecting a mode after the ventilator has been turned on, the operator must press the button twice to confirm the selection. If the button is not pressed a second time within 5 seconds, the selection is cancelled.)

When operating in the A/CMV or SIMV mode, the ventilator can be programmed for either VC or PC ventilation for the mandatory breaths. This control was described previously. When VC ventilation is chosen, the LED display allows the clinician to determine the tidal volume delivered. If PC is the desired option, then the LED display allows the clinician to determine the pressure target delivered to the patient.

In A/CMV VC mode, the clinician sets the V_T, frequency (minimum respiratory rate), inspiratory time, and trigger sensitivity. PEEP can also be set. All breaths have the same V_T delivered, regardless of whether they are patient-triggered or time-triggered.

The SIMV VC mode lets the patient breath spontaneously between mandatory breaths without receiving the set V_T. The operator sets V_T, breath rate, T_I, pressure support for spontaneous breaths, PEEP, and trigger sensitivity.

For PC mandatory breaths, the operator selects the PC option and adjusts the pressure to the desired target value. Mandatory breaths in either A/CMV or SIMV then become pressure-targeted rather than volume-targeted.

When the spontaneous mode is used to ventilate, all breaths become patient-triggered and pressure-targeted. Pressure support may be used in addition to PEEP/CPAP to aid the spontaneous breaths. (NOTE: When a patient circuit is disconnected during PC or pressure support, flow may increase through the circuit to compensate for the low pressure. After reconnecting the patient circuit, the operator should press the PC or pressure support button twice to quickly readjust the flow to a lower level.)

BUV is a safety feature that becomes active, as noted, when the low $\dot{V}_I$ alarm is violated. It is available in all modes. During BUV the message "Low $\dot{V}_I$ (BUV)" is displayed. When the HT50 is operating in the spontaneous mode and BUV becomes active, the ventilator delivers a pressure-targeted breath. The pressure delivered to the patient is 15 cm H_2O above the PEEP setting, and it is maintained for 1 second at a respiratory rate of 15 breaths/min.

The BUV feature is deactivated if there is a recorded rise in minute ventilation to 10% above the set low $\dot{V}_I$ alarm value. It is important to note that the "low minute ventilation" alarm responds to the volume delivered from the ventilator, not the volume exhaled from the patient. If there is a leak or the circuit becomes disconnected, the alarm will not sound and BUV will not be activated. A high minute volume is usually the indicator of an increase in leak or disconnection.

PULMONETIC SYSTEMS LTV 800 VENTILATOR

The LTV 800 ventilator (Figure 14-35) is the base model of the LTV series and is designed for use in the home or skilled nursing facility for patients requiring ventilatory support. The LTV 800 is designed to ventilate adult through pediatric patients who are 11 lb (5 kg) or larger.[25] Its dimensions are 12 in × 10 in × 3 in, and it weighs 12 lb. In general, the 800, 900, and 950 are used in the home care and skilled nursing facilities. A previous section in this chapter focused on the LTV 1000 and 1200. This section will focus on the LTV 800 and point out some differences among the 800, the 900, and the 950. For a detailed comparison of these models, the reader is directed to the Pulmonetic Systems Web site at: http://www.pulmonetic.com/catalog/catalog_homecare.aspx.

Power Source

The LTV series ventilators are designed to run on AC or DC (12-V) power. Although the unit normally uses an AC power cord adapter, when connected to an AC power outlet, the internal battery is continuously charged via a pigtail adapter. For DC power, the LTV 800 can use either its own internal battery or one of two available external DC batteries. The internal battery can last approximately 60 minutes

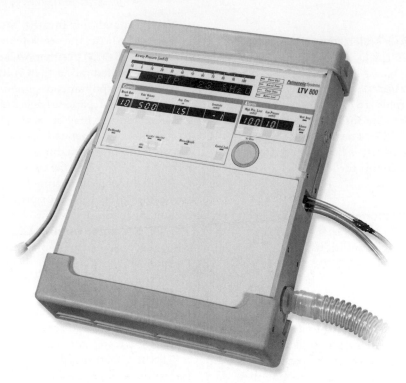

FIGURE 14-35 The Pulmonetic Systems LTV 800 ventilator. (Courtesy Pulmonetic Systems, Inc, Minneapolis; Pulmonetic Systems is a division of Cardinal Health, McGaw Park, Ill.)

when fully charged. The fully charged large external battery can provide up to 8 hours of power, whereas the smaller battery, approximately 3 to 4 hours. It takes up to 8 hours to recharge the large external battery when it is completely depleted. (NOTE: An optional auto lighter adapter is also available for use of the LTV unit while in a car.)

Internal Mechanism

The LTV 800 ventilator is electrically powered with an internal rotary compressor to generate gas flow to the patient. Air is entrained into the LTV through the air inlet port on the left side of the ventilator. The microprocessor then controls the inspiratory flow to deliver the desired tidal volume and respiratory rate.

The LTV 800 is strictly a pressure-triggered, volume-controlled ventilator. Low-pressure oxygen enters the ventilator from either a flowmeter, oxygen cylinder, or concentrator and blends with room air in the mixing chamber, which is called an accumulator/silencer. This chamber both blends the gas and acts as an acoustic silencer to reduce compressor noise. The 800, 900, and 950 have no internal blender and require a low-pressure oxygen source to enrich the delivered gas supply to the patient. The use of the oxygen analyzer is recommended to determine the exact F_IO_2.

Controls/Displays

The most commonly used controls are located on the front panel of the LTV 800. As with many of the newer ventilators that use built-in microprocessors, some controls are

menu-driven and are not located on the panel itself but are pulled up on the display window when needed. The front panel of the LTV 800 (Figure 14-36) contains controls, alarm, and monitoring displays. The controls are divided into two rows. The bottom row contains main function buttons or touch pads, and the upper row contains parameter-setting buttons.

Above the row of parameter controls is a display window, which has two main functions. It displays current ventilator data and provides access to additional control functions. Alarm-setting keys are located to the right of the controls. Just below the alarm keys is a set value knob.

On/Standby

The on/standby button turns the ventilator on and illuminates the LED above it. The ventilator automatically begins to ventilate the patient by using the last settings. To place the ventilator into standby, the operator presses and holds the button for 3 seconds.

Mode-Selection Key

This button allows the operator to chose the desired delivery mode. The operator may choose A/C, SIMV/CPAP, or noninvasive modes. Pushing the mode-selection button will cause the desired mode LED to flash for 5 seconds. Once the desired mode has been highlighted, the operator must press the mode button a second time to confirm the mode selected. The ventilator will now begin to operate in the selected mode.

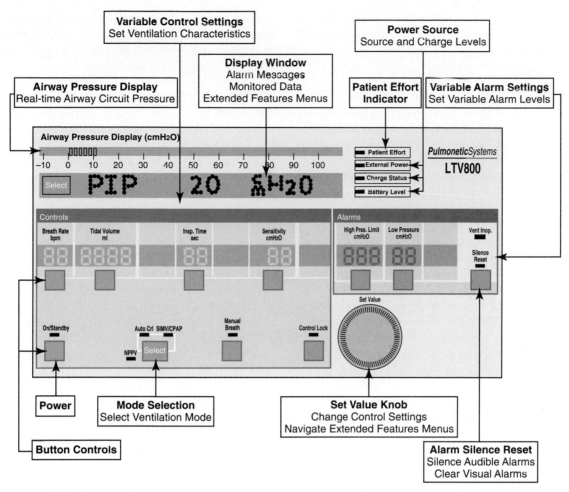

FIGURE 14-36 The control panel of the Pulmonetic Systems LTV 800 ventilator. (Courtesy Pulmonetic Systems, Inc, Minneapolis; Pulmonetic Systems is a division of Cardinal Health, McGaw Park, Ill.)

Control Lock

The control lock button allows the screen to be locked so that the settings cannot be accidentally changed. Pushing once turns the lock on. The LED above the control lock illuminates (i.e., the panel is locked). If the operator tries to change a setting when the panel is locked, the display window reads "LOCKED" and the LED flashes. Pressing the control lock button again unlocks the screen.

The Set Value Knob

The set value knob is located to the right of the control lock soft key. This knob allows adjustment of the numerical values of the ventilator parameters and alarms, and it scrolls through menu items that appear in the display window.

Parameter Controls

The upper row of controls contains the parameter settings such as rate and tidal volume. The procedure for changing the variables in this row, and in the alarms, is basically the same. The parameter button is touched to make a change. This action brightly illuminates the set value for the parameter and dulls the displays for all other parameters. The set value knob is rotated until the value desired appears in the display above the parameter button. The change is immediately active when the parameter button is pressed again or after 5 seconds.

The number in the window above each parameter represents the value set for that parameter. Numbers appear bright when the parameter is active in the current mode and breath type. They appear dim when they are not. A parameter's digital display will also brighten if it is selected for changing. All others then dim. Three parameters—sensitivity, pressure support, and respiratory rate—can be turned off. The corresponding display for each of those three parameters will be blank ("- -") when it is turned off.

Respiratory Rate

The breath rate control sets the minimum mandatory breath rate (breaths/minute). It can be turned off ("- -"). The adjustable rate range is 0 breath/min to 80 breaths/min. Pressing the button below the respiratory rate LED display will highlight that parameter. The operator turns the set value control to attain the desired value on the respiratory rate LED. Pressing the rate button again will activate the new setting.

Tidal Volume

The tidal volume soft key controls volume delivery during volume-targeted ventilation. The adjustable tidal volume range is 50 mL to 2000 mL. Pressing the soft key below the tidal volume LED display will highlight that parameter. With the set value knob, the operator can attain the desired value on the tidal volume LED. Pressing the tidal volume button will activate the new setting.

Inspiratory Time (T_I)

Inspiratory time sets the length of inspiration for volume-targeted and pressure-targeted breaths (range: 0.3 to 9.9 seconds). Inspiration cannot be shorter than 300 milliseconds. When V_T or T_I is being adjusted, the calculated flow ($\dot{V}$ calc) is shown in the display window. The peak flow is based on the setting of T_I and V_T. The procedure for setting the inspiratory time is the same as that described earlier for setting the respiratory rate and tidal volume.

Sensitivity

The sensitivity soft key is used to set the pressure trigger sensitivity level for assisted or spontaneous breaths. The range is from off ("- -") up to −2 to +20 cm H_2O. When a trigger is detected, the patient effort LED illuminates. The LTV 950 has flow-triggering with an adjustable range of 1 L/min to 9 L/min.

Leak Compensation

A leak-compensation feature is available on both the 900 and 950 (not in the 800); this feature constantly measures for leaks and adjusts the baseline of the ventilator in order to compensate for leaks of up to 6 L/min. In earlier models of the LTV that do not have leak compensation, the sensitivity is usually set higher than the leak measurement.

PEEP/CPAP

In the LTV 800, 900, 950, and 1000 ventilators, PEEP is not internally controlled. An external PEEP valve is required as part of the ventilator circuit and is illustrated in Figure 14-23 (detail A). The adjustable range for PEEP/CPAP is 0 cm H_2O to 20 cm H_2O. The operator can adjust PEEP by pushing the PEEP valve lock with one hand and rotating the valve with the other. It is important to note that the PEEP level is not compensated on the LTV 800, 900, and 950, so sensitivity must be readjusted when PEEP is added.

Airway Pressure Bar Graph and Display Window

At the very top of the operating panel is the airway pressure display. This horizontal bar graph displays the pressure in the patient circuit (range: −10 to +108 cm H_2O). The

display window shows monitored data, alarm messages, and the extended features menu. During normal operation, the monitored data are presented sequentially. Each item is displayed for 3 seconds.

The Select Button—Display Screen

The select button to the left of the display screen has several functions. It is used to stop the normal scrolling of monitored ventilator parameters. Pushing the button once while the normal data scan is active halts the screen with the current parameter data showing. Each time the button is pushed after that, the next data item in the list is displayed. Scanning can be resumed by pressing the button twice within 3 seconds.

Front-Panel Indicators

To the right of the pressure manometer are four indicators. The patient effort indicator illuminates when the ventilator detects a patient's inspiratory effort based on the sensitivity setting. The external power illuminates when the unit is operating from an external power source. This can be an AC power source or an external battery. The adjacent LED is green when power is adequate and yellow when external power is low.

Alarms

The alarm controls and settings are to the right of the parameter controls. The first alarm is the "High Press. Limit" alarm (in cm H_2O). This control establishes the maximum pressure allowed in the patient circuit. If the set value is reached, an audible alarm sounds, the display window reads "HIGH PRES," inspiration ends, and the exhalation valve opens. If a high-pressure condition continues for more than 3 seconds, the internal turbine stops rotating and circuit pressure empties to the atmosphere. The audible alarm automatically stops when the pressure drops to the high-pressure limit −5 cm H_2O or drops to a circuit pressure of 25 cm H_2O, whichever is less. To set the high-pressure limit, the soft key is pressed and the set value knob is rotated to the desired value (range: 5 to 100 cm H_2O).

To set the low-pressure alarm value (cm H_2O), the operator pushes the low pressure soft key and rotates the set value knob. The actual value appears in the display window. The knob is rotated until the desired value is seen (range: from "off" up to 1 to 60 cm H_2O).

Vent Inop Display

The "Vent Inop" indicator just right of the alarm controls is illuminated only when the ventilator is in the inoperative state. This occurs under the following conditions:

1. The ventilator has been put into standby (on/standby button held for 3 seconds).
2. The power sources, either internal or external, are insufficient to operate the ventilator.
3. The ventilator has been turned off.

4. A condition exists that renders the ventilator unable to provide patient ventilation and unsafe to use.

When a ventilator inoperative alarm occurs, the inspiratory flow stops; the exhalation valve opens, allowing the patient to breathe spontaneously from room air; the oxygen blender solenoids close; the "INOP" LED is red; and an audible alarm sounds continuously. The patient needs to be removed from the ventilator, and another mode of ventilating must be provided for the patient immediately.

Alarm Silence

The silence/reset button is located to the right of the pressure alarm LED display and is used to silence an alarm for 60 seconds. This button can also be used to start a 60-second alarm-silence period, for example, before disconnecting the patient for some procedure or when the ventilator is placed in standby. After an alarm condition has been resolved, this button can also be used to clear the visual alarm displays. The silence/reset button also silences the audible ventilator inoperative alarm, but the ventilator inoperative LED will remain lit for at least 5 minutes.

Modes of Ventilation

The LTV 800 series ventilator provides the following modes of ventilation: control, A/C, SIMV, CPAP, apnea BUV, and NPPV. Only the LTV 800 and 900 provide volume-controlled ventilation breaths, whereas the LTV 950 can provide both volume-controlled and pressure-controlled breaths.

Control and Assist/Control

Control and A/C are available when the "Assist/Ctrl" LED is illuminated near the mode select button. Control is considered active, by the manufacturer, when the sensitivity is set to off ("--"). If using the control mode, one must consider the patient's effort to breathe over the set rate, because this could be very uncomfortable for the patient and lead to patient/ventilator dysynchrony.

Assist Control

A/C is considered active when a value greater than zero sensitivity is set. The breath type is established by the breath-type select button (volume-targeted or pressure-targeted, in the 950 unit only). The rate is set by the breath rate control. In the A/C mode, the set rate can be the minimum rate setting. The patient can trigger additional mandatory breaths as desired.

SIMV

The SIMV mode is active when the "SIMV/CPAP" LED is illuminated near the mode select button. The breath rate (1 to 80 breaths/min) establishes the minimum mandatory breath rate. Patients can spontaneously breathe between mandatory breaths. Spontaneous breaths can be from the set baseline pressure (0 or PEEP) and can also be supported with pressure support with the LTV 950.

CPAP

The CPAP mode is considered the active mode if the SIMV/CPAP LED is illuminated and the breath rate is off ("- -"). In CPAP, spontaneous breaths can be from the baseline pressure and can also be pressure-supported with the LTV 900 and 950.

Pressure Support

The LTV 800 does not offer a pressure-support mode, but the LTV 900 and 950 both offer pressure support. The adjustable range goes from off up to 1 cm H_2O to 60 cm H_2O.

Apnea Backup

Apnea backup ventilation is available should the patient become apneic. The apnea interval is set by using the extended features menu. The ventilator begins apnea BUV in the A/C mode based on the current settings.

The active controls are displayed at full intensity, and others are dimmed. If the set breath rate is ≥12 breaths/min, the apnea breath rate is the set breath rate. If the set breath rate is <12 breaths/min and the breath rate is not limited by other control settings, the apnea breath rate is 12 breaths/min. If the set breath rate is limited to <12 breaths/min, because of tidal volume, flow, and T_I settings, the apnea breath rate is the highest allowed rate. Normal ventilation resumes when two consecutive patient-triggered breaths occur or when the operator resets the apnea alarm using the silence/reset control.

NPPV

NPPV is provided as a secondary mode that may be selected in addition to the primary ventilation mode. NPPV is selected by using the extended features menu. When activated, ventilation is delivered according to the selected mode and breath type that are currently active by way of a full mask or other noninvasive interface. The NPPV LED is lit when it is on. The number of alarms in NPPV is limited when it is active and is similar to those on the LTV 1000 (see Box 14-17). Again, the operator must remember that only the LTV 800 and 900 can support volume-targeted ventilation and the LTV 950 can supply both volume and pressure ventilation.

Summary of the LTV 800, 900, 950, 1000, and 1200

The LTV 800, 900, and 950 ventilators are primarily designed for home care and skilled nursing facilities. The LTV 1000 and 1200 are primarily designed for transport and acute care.

PURITAN BENNETT COMPANION 2801

The Puritan Bennett Companion 2801 home care ventilator is presented in the Evolve Resources.

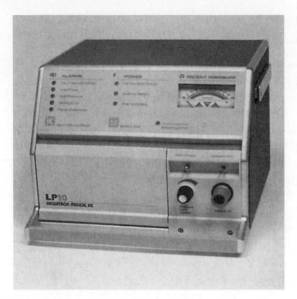

FIGURE 14-37 The Puritan Bennett LP10 ventilator. (Courtesy Puritan Bennett, Boulder, Colo.; Puritan Bennett is a division of Covidien Ltd, Hamilton, Bermuda.)

PURITAN BENNETT LP10

The LP10 is a microprocessor-controlled, volume-targeted ventilator primarily used for home care ventilation (Puritan Bennett, Boulder, Colo.; PB is now owned by Covidien Ltd, Hamilton, Bermuda).* The LP10's dimensions are 9.25 in × 13.5 in × 12.5 in, and it weighs 33 lb. It can be used for pediatric and adult patients (Figure 14-37).[26]

Power Source

The LP10 normally operates on a standard 110-V or 220-V electrical outlet. If there is a power failure or an inability to use an AC outlet, the following alternative power sources are available:

- An external 12-V battery
- An internal 12-V battery

The internal 12-V battery is intended as an emergency backup only and is able to supply power for 30 to 60 minutes when fully charged. A power light display on the front panel enables the operator to see which power source is currently in use. When the AC light is green, the ventilator is using an AC outlet while charging the internal battery. A constant amber light indicates that an external power source is in use, and a flashing amber light signifies that the internal battery is in use. When the internal battery is in use, an audible alarm sounds every 5 minutes to remind the operator that the battery is in use. When approximately 5 minutes of energy are left, the low-power alarm rings continuously, signaling the need to change power sources. After the internal battery has been used, it is imperative to recharge it for at least 3 hours.

*The LP6 is identical to the LP10 except for the pressure-limit control, which gives the operator the option of PCV with the LP10.

Internal Mechanism

The LP10 uses a rotary drive piston, which delivers a sinusoidal flow waveform to the patient. The piston draws gas into the housing through the inlet filter port during a downward stroke of the piston. The gas passes a one-way check valve before entering the piston chamber. On the upstroke, the compressed gas moves through another one-way valve and out to the patient circuit and exhalation valve, passing the pressure transducer. The pressure transducer monitors airway pressures and relays the information to the microprocessor.

Oxygen Source

The LP10 can deliver oxygen concentrations greater than 21% by two methods. It bleeds oxygen directly into the patient circuit and can deliver F_IO_2 up to 0.4 with this method, but it is important to remember that additional volume is being added to the circuit, too. Be sure to consider this when setting the volume control. The second method of increasing F_IO_2 is by delivering oxygen directly into the rear-panel air inlet port. This method can provide an F_IO_2 of 1.0.

When delivering additional oxygen to the LP10, the F_IO_2 must be measured as close to the patient as possible with the aid of an oxygen analyzer. The machine does not provide a means of measuring F_IO_2.

Control Panel and Alarms

The front panel of the LP10 (Figure 14-38) contains several controls for setting parameters and monitoring patient data and alarms.

Tidal Volume

The tidal volume (V_T) control is on the bottom left of the control panel. It has an operational range of 100 mL to 2200 mL that is adjustable in 100-mL increments.

Rate

The rate control (1 to 38 breaths/min) is on the bottom-left part of the control panel and sets the minimum number of mandatory breaths in A/C and the maximum number of mandatory breaths in SIMV.

Inspiratory Time

The inspiratory time control is at the bottom middle of the control panel (0.5 to 5.5 seconds). The T_I and rate are responsible for the T_E and the I:E ratio. The machine does not allow an inverse I:E ratio to be set. If the operator uses inappropriate settings that create an inverse I:E ratio, an alarm sounds and the ventilator delivers the set number of breaths at an I:E ratio of 1:1 (Clinical Rounds 14-12).

Breathing Effort (Trigger Sensitivity)

The function of this control is to set the threshold pressure required for the patient to trigger a mandatory breath. It has an operational range of −10 cm H_2O to +10 cm H_2O.

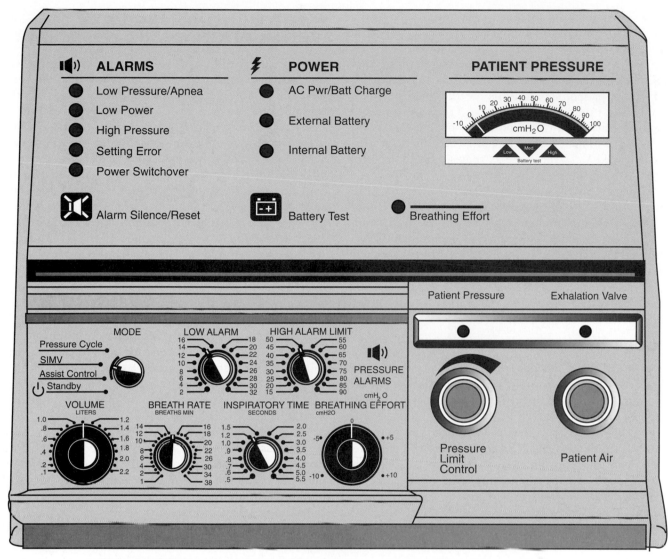

FIGURE 14-38 The control panel of the Puritan Bennett LP10 ventilator. (Courtesy Puritan Bennett, Boulder, Colo.; Puritan Bennett is a division of Covidien Ltd, Hamilton, Bermuda.)

CLINICAL ROUNDS 14-12

The respiratory therapist is using an LP10 unit to ventilate a home care patient. The set rate is 15 breaths/min; the T_I is 2.5 seconds; and the V_T is 700 mL. Will the patient receive the full 2.5 seconds of inspiration?

See Evolve Resources for the answer.

The breathing effort should be adjusted for increased levels of PEEP to prevent any unnecessary increase in the patient's work of breathing because the sensitivity is not PEEP-compensated.

PEEP

The LP10 does not have an internal PEEP control, but an external valve can be attached to the exhalation manifold. The ventilator allows for PEEP compensation for mandatory breaths by adjusting the trigger sensitivity up to +10 cm H_2O. If the trigger sensitivity is set above the PEEP setting, autocycling may occur. For example, if PEEP is +6 cm H_2O and sensitivity is +7 cm H_2O, the unit may autocycle.[27]

Alarms

The LP10 monitors several parameters. When the parameters fall outside their acceptable ranges, the ventilator alarms go off to alert the operator to the specific problem. The first of these alarms is the high alarm/limit, which is active only when the ventilator is working in a volume-targeted mode without the pressure-limit control function. When the ventilator is in the pressure-limit control mode, the alarm sounds only if the pressure-limit valve fails to open.

During pressure-targeted ventilation, the high alarm/limit is used to determine the desired pressure level. It only warns if the set pressure level is exceeded by 10 cm H_2O or more in this mode.

The low-pressure control is at the top middle of the control panel and has an adjustable range of 2 cm H_2O to 32 cm H_2O. When this alarm is activated, the low-pressure/apnea light illuminates. The problems most commonly associated with this alarm are leaks in the circuit and lack of patient spontaneous breathing efforts. If the set rate is less than 6 breaths/min and the patient fails to trigger a breath within 10 seconds, the low-pressure/apnea alarm sounds, and a backup rate of 10 breaths/min starts. The delivered V_T is the same as that set on the control panel.

There are two basic alarms that monitor the LP10 power sources: the low-power alarm and the power switchover alarm. The low-power alarm, which is a continuous audible alarm, is activated when approximately 5 minutes of power are left in the internal battery. The power switchover alarm is activated when the ventilator switches from an AC outlet or an external DC source to the internal battery. Both features are in the alarms section of the control panel.

Modes of Ventilation

When using the A/C mode, the operator sets V_T, breath rate, T_I, and trigger sensitivity. In this mode, the patient can initiate mandatory breaths at or above the set rate, but every breath is at the set V_T.

The A/C mode also offers the ability to use pressure-targeted, time-cycled breaths (PCV). When the pressure-limit control function is active, it alters the pressure waveform of the ventilator, allowing for a plateau to occur during inspiration when the set pressure level is achieved. The ventilator vents the excess pressure for the remainder of the inspiratory cycle. The pressure-limit control is not calibrated. It uses a spring-loaded valve for its operation.

Before the parameters are set, the patient should be disconnected. The operator then occludes the patient Y-connector and rotates the dial until the desired pressure is achieved. After the patient has been reconnected, it is important to closely monitor the pressure because there may be a fall in the set pressure. Further adjustment of the pressure-limit control may be necessary if this occurs.

The volume-targeted SIMV mode lets the patient breathe spontaneously between mandatory breaths. The operator sets V_T, breath rate, T_I, and breathing effort (trigger sensitivity). When the ventilator is operating in the SIMV mode, the operator can also use the pressure-limit control, which operates the same in SIMV as in A/C.

The pressure-cycled mode operates by limiting the maximum pressure allowed in the patient circuit during inspiration. The ventilator assists or controls the patient-triggered or time-triggered breaths. When the set pressure determined by the high alarm limit is achieved, inspiration stops. There is no plateau phase. A high-pressure alarm sounds only if the pressure in the airway exceeds the pressure setting by more than 10 cm H_2O.

PART III: NONINVASIVE VENTILATION

The first successful use of NPPV was recorded as early as the mid-eighteenth century. The following 200 years involved improvements in the equipment used and the testing of this mode of ventilation as a possible form of treatment. During this period there were a number of pioneers. Dräger, one of the earliest supporters of NPPV, used a mask and a compressed gas source to manage the airway of drowning victims as early as 1911.[28] The experiments with PPV continued in the late 1930s when Barach and colleagues used intermittent positive pressure ventilation (IPPV) to treat patients with pulmonary edema and in the 1950s with **Motely** and colleagues for the treatment of acute respiratory failure.[28] However, the mainstay of ventilatory support in the United States until the 1960s was the **iron lung**, with IPPB being relegated mainly to the administration of aerosolized medication.

During the 1960s, invasive ventilation by way of endotracheal tubes progressively became more popular than noninvasive ventilation by iron lung. Cuffed endotracheal tubes provided better protection to the airway, and PPV provided superior ventilatory support. These two factors significantly decreased interest in noninvasive ventilation for a number of years.

Then, in the 1980s, improved patient interfaces (masks) and success with the treatment of obstructive sleep apnea through mask ventilation led to the resurrection of noninvasive ventilation as a more-popular mode.[29] Soon it began to be viewed again as a possible alternative to traditional invasive ventilation.

In the last 20 years, NPPV has gained widespread approval for use in the hospital and home care environments. The increased interest can be attributed to many factors (Box 14-20), with the most recent being the advent of portable and safe ventilators, user-friendly interfaces, and a better understanding of respiratory muscle function.[1,30] Physicians and clinicians are beginning to aggressively use NPPV for a variety of disease states that were previously managed with conventional mechanical ventilation.[31] The use of noninvasive ventilation in addition to

BOX 14-20	Factors Contributing to NPPV Interest

- Success in the treatment of obstructive sleep apnea[1]
- Improved patient interfaces[1]
- Does not inhibit natural pulmonary defense mechanisms
- Allows the patient to eat, drink, and talk
- Allows the patient to expectorate secretions
- Less costly than conventional mechanical ventilation
- Possibility of use in acute and chronic ventilatory failure
- Prevention of complications of intubation and tracheostomy[1]
- Able to be used when patients resist intubation[1]

modern medical therapy is now considered the standard of care for a select population of patients with acute respiratory failure caused by severe exacerbations of chronic obstructive pulmonary disease.[30,32]

There are ongoing clinical trials evaluating the effectiveness of NPPV for patients with neuromuscular disease, chronic obstructive pulmonary disease necessitating nighttime respiratory muscle rest, and acute respiratory failure, as well as for postoperative support and the facilitation of weaning. Randomized, controlled trials indicate that noninvasive ventilation is associated with lower rates of endotracheal intubation, lower intensive care and hospital mortality rates, and a decreased number of admission days in the intensive care unit and hospital.[32]

The remainder of this chapter will focus on the various patient interfaces and a description of many of the noninvasive positive pressure ventilators that are available.

THE PATIENT INTERFACE

When applying NPPV, it is critical to use a properly fitting mask that combines minimal air leakage with maximum comfort.[30] It does not matter how successful the device may be at alleviating the medical problem if the person is not comfortable. Poor comfort leads to poor compliance, resulting in less use and a deterioration of the condition. The interfaces that are presently being used are nasal mask, nasal pillows, oronasal mask, total face mask, and mouthpiece.

Selecting the correct mask size, particularly nasal mask size, may be the most challenging job for the respiratory therapist. The nasal mask is the most commonly used mask and often the most difficult to properly apply to the patient (Figure 14-39). The most-common mistake associated with the device is the use of a larger-than-necessary mask. It is the patient's nose, not the face, that needs to be covered. The top of the mask should lie at the junction of the nasal bone and the frontal bone and be fitted to cover the nares snugly. The sizes most frequently used for adult patients are small and medium. It is not uncommon for the maker of a nasal mask to provide a gauging device that guides the clinician in estimating the proper size. However, these devices are manufactured specifically for the home ventilator or CPAP device in use and should not be used with other equipment.

Nasal pillows are a second form of nasal NPPV and are often used as an alternative to the nasal mask (Figure 14-40). The interface consists of two cushions that are inserted into the nares of the patient that allow for ventilation. There is no pressure applied to the bridge of the nose as with the nasal mask, thereby reducing the risk of pressure sores. It is not uncommon to alternate between the nasal mask and nasal pillow interfaces to reduce the risk of developing pressure sores.

The oronasal mask is slightly larger than the nasal mask (Figure 14-41). Fitting the mask starts with placement

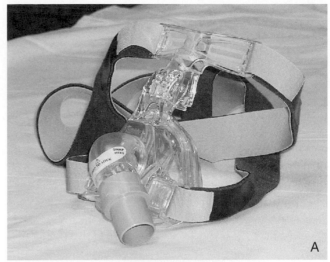

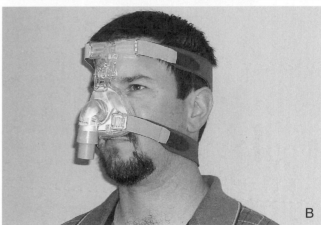

FIGURE 14-39 An example of a nasal mask.

above the junction of the nasal bone and frontal bone and includes the mouth and the nose. The bottom of the mask should rest just under the bottom lip. When first fitting the mask, it is not unusual to have large air leaks around the mouth. A period of adjustment is usually required that allows the patient to acclimate to the oronasal mask. This adjustment generally results in a reduction in the amount of leak. Nonetheless, leaks are inevitable. On the other hand, if a mask fits so tightly that no volume is lost, the pressure generated from the mask may cause the patient to be uncomfortable and place the person at increased risk for pressure necrosis.

The NPPV machines that are used with these devices are designed to compensate for leaks and the subsequent loss of volume. A large, uncontrolled leak, however, is not acceptable. A chin strap may be effective at alleviating the problem if an excessive leak persists. Chin straps are most commonly used with nasal masks or pillows.

Another alternative mask for patients who experience claustrophobia or who cannot tolerate nasal or oronasal masks may be the full-face mask. The total face mask is a clear, lightweight plastic faceplate surrounded by a soft,

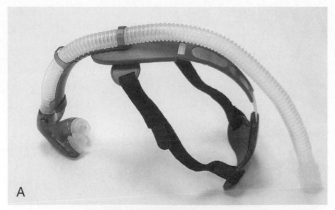

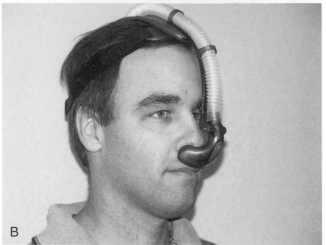

FIGURE 14-40 An example of nasal pillows.

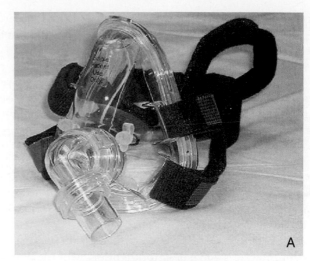

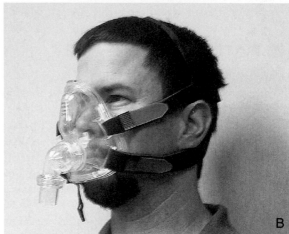

FIGURE 14-41 An example of an oronasal mask.

inflatable cushion that seals the perimeter of the face (Figure 14-42). The tendency for pressure sores lessens with the total face mask, because the mask seals the entire face.

The final type of interface that can be used for NPPV is the oral mask. An oral mask allows intermittent positive pressure ventilation when patients have trouble tolerating or achieving a seal with other conventional mask options. The Oracle™ Mask (Figure 14-43) which was designed and manufactured by Fisher & Paykel Healthcare in 2000 was the first Oral mask available for CPAP/bilevel therapy. The actual device uses a soft Silicone oblong design that seals through the interaction of two silicone flanges which fit against the inside and outside of the patient's mouth. A benefit of the mouth seal is that it rarely contributes to the development of pressure sores. In addition, it is easy to use.

The equipment used to attach the masks to the client is often overlooked. Securing the various interfaces is just as important as selecting the appropriate size. The apparatus most commonly used consists of cloth straps and Velcro headgear (see Figure 14-41B). It is customary to have three points of attachment (prongs or slots) on the oronasal and nasal mask that allow the straps to fasten to the headgear. These prongs or slots for straps are often found on the outer edge of the mask and allow the clini-

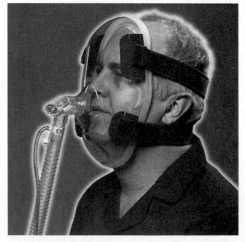

FIGURE 14-42 A full-face mask. (Courtesy Philips Respironics, Murrysville, Pa.)

cian to evenly distribute the pressure on the face, thereby reducing leaks. The slots for the Velcro straps or the plastic prongs are positioned to evenly distribute the mask on the face of the user. It is easiest if the clinician makes all strap attachments before placing the mask on the client.

VENTILATORS

Home care NPPV ventilators and other support devices may have any of the following features:

·   The ability to provide full ventilatory support
·   The ability to ventilate at night only
·   BiPAP support or CPAP
·   Low-pressure or disconnect alarms

Controls that are common to noninvasive positive pressure ventilators include the following: A/C, SIMV, PSV,

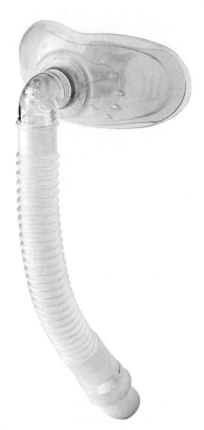

FIGURE 14-43 An oral continuous positive airway pressure (CPAP) device. (Courtesy Fisher & Paykel Healthcare, Auckland, New Zealand.)

bilevel pressure ventilation modes, volume ventilation, respiratory rate, inspiratory time, PEEP, F_IO_2, and humidification. Following is information about several NPPV modes that are commonly used today.

RESPIRONICS BiPAP S/T

The Respironics BiPAP S/T was originally presented in the sixth edition (1999) of this text. The information regarding that ventilator has been moved to Evolve Resources for the text.

RESPIRONICS BiPAP FOCUS™

The BiPAP Focus™ noninvasive ventilator (Respironics, Inc, Murrysville, Pa.) provides noninvasive breathing support for adult patients who weigh 30 kg (65 lb) or more and is used for the treatment of respiratory insufficiency, respiratory distress, and obstructive sleep apnea (Figure 14-44).[33] The Focus™ is microprocessor-controlled and offers two modes of support. The BiPAP Focus™ features CPAP and spontaneous/timed (S/T) modes to provide needed nonivasive support. The unit weighs 10 lb (4.5 kg), and its dimensions are 5.5 in × 11.4 in × 14 in. The BiPAP Focus™ is contraindicated for the conditions listed in Box 14-21.

Power Source

The BiPAP Focus™ is designed to operate on 100-V AC/230-V AC and 50/60 Hz via a DC power converter. The unit also has an internal battery as a backup power source. This internal battery is designed to operate the unit for 45 minutes. The internal battery will be charged when the unit is connected to the AC power and the on/off switch in the back of the unit is in the on position, which is denoted by an illuminated charging LED. The battery charge time is typically less than 5 hours, but it can be longer because of environmental conditions such as lower temperatures. The battery is intended only as a backup power source and for use during intrahospital transport.

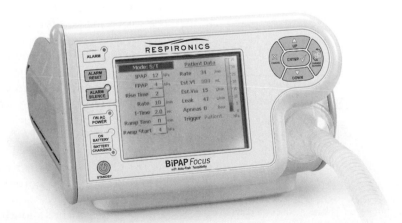

FIGURE 14-44 Respironics BiPAP Focus. (Courtesy Philips Respironics, Murrysville, Pa.)

The manufactuer warns that the BiPAP Focus™ will not operate without a functioning battery installed in the unit. Estimated internal battery life is illustrated in Table 14-19.

Internal Mechanism

The ventilator uses a blower-driven, sleeve valve–controlled system that is able to deliver and maintain pressures from 0 cm H_2O to 40 cm H_2O at one constant level (CPAP) or at two levels (IPAP and EPAP) or bilevel ventilation. The delivery of a breath begins with room air that is entrained through an inlet filter at the rear of the ventilator and then pressurized by the internal blower. The entrained air moves from the blower to the pressure valve assembly (PVA), which regulates the desired inspiratory, expiratory, or continuous pressures that are selected for the patient.

In line after the PVA and just before the machine outlet is the airflow module. This device monitors total gas flow and patient pressures. This information is sent to the main control system of the Focus™, where it is processed and used to maintain set pressure levels and trigger and cycle thresholds.

Oxygen Source

The BiPAP Focus™ is designed to provide noninvasive support, primarily at room air concentrations. Supplemental oxygen may be added by placing a Respironics oxygen-enrichment adapter and an oxygen safety valve in line with the patient circuit immediately after the bacteria filter on the breathing circuit connector on the front of the unit. The potential range of supplemental oxygen concentration is dependent on factors such as given tidal volume, pressures used, and flow of supplemental oxygen into the

---

BOX 14-21	BiPAP Focus™ Contraindications

- Lack of spontaneous respiratory drive
- Inability to maintain a patent airway or adequately clear secretions
- At risk for aspiration of gastric contents
- Acute sinusitis or otitis media
- Hypotension

TABLE 14-19

BiPAP Focus™ Internal Battery Life Expectancy

CPAP or IPAP Setting	Approximate Battery Life*
10 cm H_2O	60 min
15 cm H_2O	50 min
20 cm H_2O	40 min
25 cm H_2O	30 min
30 cm H_2O	20 min

IPAP, Inspiratory positive airway pressure.

***Warning**: When a ventilator is running on its battery, the high flows that occur during a patient disconnect will cause the battery to deplete in as little as 2 minutes. Connect to AC power as soon as the battery depletion alarm sounds to prevent total loss of power.

---

enrichment adapter. The use of a calibrated oxygen analyzer is recommended, and that oxygen flow into the enrichment adapter should not exceed 15 L/min.

Leak Compensation

Leaks are inherent to user interfaces and patient circuits in NPPV machines. These leaks can affect the device's ability to trigger and cycle a breath effectively. In addition, the estimation of a leak is important for proper analysis of the signal in order to ensure patient-ventilator synchrony. Therefore, monitoring and compensating for changes in leaks are critical for maintaining the appropriate trigger and cycle levels for the ventilator.

The BiPAP Focus™ uses a digital trigger-sensitivity system called digital Auto-Trak™ sensitivity that features a combination of different mechanisms to identify and modify baseline values in response to leaks. It also automatically adjusts its variable trigger and cycle threshold to maintain performance in the presence of leaks.

The built-in microprocessor governs the digital signal process. It does this by modeling the patient's flow patterns. In this process it analyzes and estimates leak rates in order to provide triggering sensitivity. The ventilator works to synchronize the transition between inhalation and exhalation.

The expiratory flow rate adjustment primarily works to make course adjustments in baseline values. When the ventilator is initially turned on, it measures the total flow through the circuit before it is connected to the patient. This includes the intentional leak created by the exhalation port. The BiPAP Focus™ is then attached to the patient, and the expiratory flow through the circuit is measured after the machine has cycled into expiration. Through measurement and calculation, the ventilator is able to determine the intentional and unintentional leak of the system. This allows the ventilator to establish and monitor the baseline pressure, which allows the trigger and cycle values to be set.

Triggering to inspiration (IPAP) occurs by two methods. The first is by volume-triggering. When 6 mL of volume from patient effort is inhaled from the circuit, the ventilator will volume-trigger to IPAP.

The second method for triggering to IPAP is the shape signal. The shape signal is actually a shadow image of the patient's actual flow/time waveform that is "redrawn" by the microprocessor to overlap the actual signal (Figure 14-45). The shape signal is part of the digital Auto-Trak™ sensitivity. When the patient flow intersects the shadow flow from the shape signal, the ventilator triggers to IPAP.

Cycling to exhalation (EPAP) occurs when the patient's flow intersects the shape signal flow. A second method of cycling to EPAP occurs when the microprocessor's electronic signal rises in proportion to the inspiratory flow waveform.

Sometimes a patient's mouth will open at the end of inspiration during BiPAP ventilation. This results in a rise in flow from the ventilator to maintain the set IPAP pres-

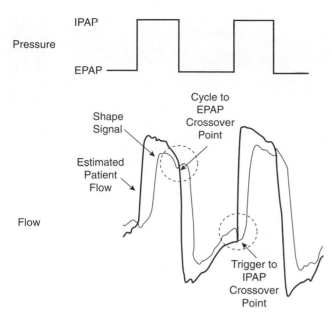

FIGURE 14-45 The shape signal of the Respironics BiPAP Focus™ unit. (Located at the bottom of the figures.)

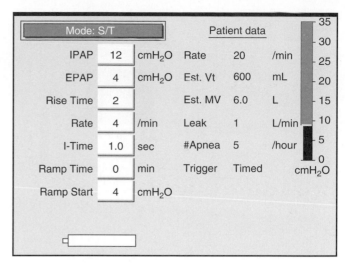

FIGURE 14-46 The patient data screen on the BiPAP Focus™.

sure. The sudden rush of flow through the upper airway and sinuses can arouse the patient and adversely affect cycling. When this occurs with the Focus™, the Digital Auto-Trak™ system recognizes the rapid increase in flow at end inspiration as a result of a leak and immediately cycles to EPAP in order to maintain patient-ventilator synchrony.

Tidal Volume Estimation

Although the BiPAP Focus™ does not directly measure volume, it is able to estimate inspiratory and expiratory tidal volumes based on the patient flow and the time spent in inspiration and expiration. Differences that occur between the inspiratory and expiratory tidal volumes are then assumed to be the result of a change in the amount of intentional leak and are accounted for by an adjustment in baseline for the next breath. This feature allows the ventilator to adjust the baseline on a breath-to-breath basis, thereby reducing large corrections.

Controls and Displays

The BiPAP Focus™ is powered up by pressing the on/off switch located on the back of the unit, followed by pressing the standby button on the front of the unit in the lower left-hand corner. It is recommended that a preoperational check be completed before the unit is connected to the patient.

The front panel of the BiPAP Focus™ consists of three sections. On the left-hand side of the unit, you will find a standby key, a battery charging/on battery indicator, AC power indicators, an alarm silence key, alarm reset, and an alarm indicator.

The second section consists of the navigation LCD screen, which provides three different screen options for

the operator to view. The option screen allows the operator to view or change mode and settings. This screen can also display real-time patient data (Figure 14-46). The patient data screen will display the total respiratory rate, estimated tidal volume, estimated minute volume, percent leak, number of apneic events, and trigger, whether patient-initiated or time-triggered by the ventilator. A pressure bar graph is located on the right side of the patient data screen.

The second screen option is the alarm settings screen. In this screen, the operator can view or adjust needed alarms and these will be detailed under the alarms section below. The third screen option allows the operator to change the unit's audio and visual settings such as alarm volume, contrast, brightness, and display units. In any of the three option screens, real-time patient data are displayed.

Accessing the LCD screen is accomplished through an adjustable control shown in the upper-right corner of Figure 14-46. For the purpose of this discussion, this control is referred to as the mode and operations selector switch (MOSS).

To change modes or settings, the operator needs only to use the arrow keys to highlight the desired parameter on the LCD screen and press the enter key. A pop-up window for the setting will then appear (Figure 14-47). Using the up or down arrow keys, the operator can apply a new setting. Pressing the the enter key again confirms the new setting; pressing the cancel key allows the user to exit the pop-up screen without changing the setting.

Parameters that can be adjusted in the CPAP mode screen include the CPAP level, ramp time, and ramp pressure initation level. Adjustable parameters in the S/T mode screen include IPAP, EPAP, rise time, respiratory rate, inspiratory time, ramp time, and ramp pressure start.

Alarms

The BiPAP Focus™ alarm system has two types of alarms: autoresettable and nonresettable. Autoresettable

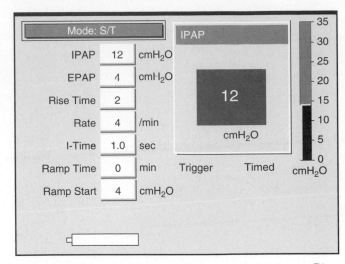

FIGURE 14-47 The pop-up window on the BiPAP Focus™.

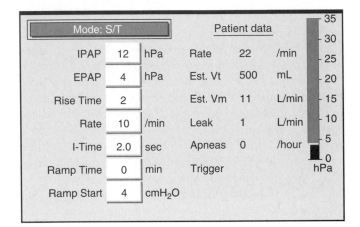

FIGURE 14-48 The alarm-message screen on the BiPAP Focus™.

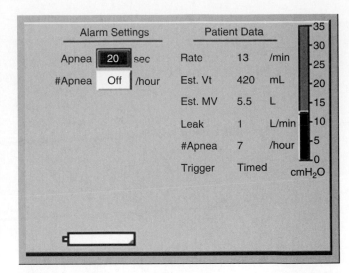

FIGURE 14-49 The apnea alarm-settings screen on the BiPAP Focus™.

TABLE 14-20

The Adjustable Parameters for the BiPAP Focus™ in the S/T Mode*

Parameter	Range
Rate	1-30 breaths/min
IPAP	4-30 cm H_2O
EPAP	4-25 cm H_2O
Inspiratory time	0.5-3 s
Rise time	1-6, where 1 = 0.1 s and 6 = 0.6 s
Ramp time	0-45 min
Ramp pressure initiation level	4 cm H_2O EPAP

S/T, Spontaneous/timed; *EPAP*, expiratory positive airway pressure.
*In the CPAP mode the adjustable parameters are CPAP level, ramp time, and ramp start (with a default level of 4 cm H_2O).

alarms automatically reset after an alarm situation occurs and is corrected. Nonresettable alarms must be manually reset.

When an alarm is activated, the alarm indicator flashes, an alarm message is diplayed in the lower right-hand corner on the LCD screen (Figure 14-48), and the Focus™ sounds a repeated sequence of beeps. Most of the alarms found on the BiPAP Focus™ are preset from the manufacturer; only the apnea detection time and number of apnea events in an hour are adjustable by the operator and are illustrated in Figure 14-49. The apnea period is defined by the Focus™ as the amount of time with no spontaneous patient breathing effort. The number of apnea events is the second programmable alarm on the BiPAP Focus. This alarm will count the number of apnea events lasting 10 seconds or more in the previous hour of operation. The operator must note that in the first hour of operation, this value is only estimated. Major preset alarms include high- or low-pressure alarm, apnea, patient disconnect, low power, or loss of main power.

Modes of Ventilation

The BiPAP Focus™ system has two modes available: CPAP and spontaneous timed (S/T) modes. In the CPAP mode the adjustable parameters are CPAP level, ramp time, and ramp start, which has a default level of 4 cm H_2O.

The S/T mode's adjustable settings are listed in Table 14-20. The S/T breaths may be flow-triggered by the patient or time-triggered dependent on the set rate. In the S/T mode, the rate control does not guarantee a set number of mandatory breaths. Instead, it gives a set number of breaths regardless of whether they are patient-triggered or time-triggered by the machine.

RESPIRONICS BiPAP VISION

The Respironics BiPAP Vision (Respironics, Inc, Murrysville, Pa.) is a microprocessor-controlled ventilator that is capable of operating in CPAP mode or pressure support (S/T) mode (Figure 14-50). The BiPAP Vision is generally thought of as a noninvasive system; however, it may be the audible alarm system and a lithium cell that maintains the data-retention functions.

If at any time the system were to be disconnected from the electrical outlet, the ventilator would cease to function. The NiCd or lithium battery would not be able to support the operations of the machine; their purpose is strictly for adjunct functions. For example, the NiCd battery powers the audible ventilator inoperative alarm and the lithium battery maintains the internal clock.

Internal Mechanism

The ventilator uses a blower-driven, dual-valve–controlled system that is able to deliver and maintain pressures from 0 cm H_2O to 40 cm H_2O. The delivery of a breath begins with room air that is entrained through an inlet filter at the rear of the ventilator and then pressurized by the internal blower.

The entrained air moves from the blower to the PVA, which regulates the desired inspiratory, expiratory, or continuous pressures that are selected for the patient. The first valve in the PVA adjusts for the IPAP pressure to be delivered, and a second valve works as an exhaust, modifying the pressure during the transition from IPAP to EPAP.

In line after the PVA and just before the machine outlet is the airflow module. This device monitors total gas flow and pressure being delivered to the patient and the pressure at the proximal pressure line. This information is sent to the main control system of the Vision, where it is processed and used to maintain set pressure levels and trigger and cycle thresholds.

Oxygen Source

The BiPAP Vision allows the clinician to deliver an F_IO_2 greater than 0.21 (range: 0.21 to 1.0) to the patient by attaching a high-pressure gas source to the oxygen module found at the rear of the machine (Figure 14-51). The oxygen control located on the front control panel allows the

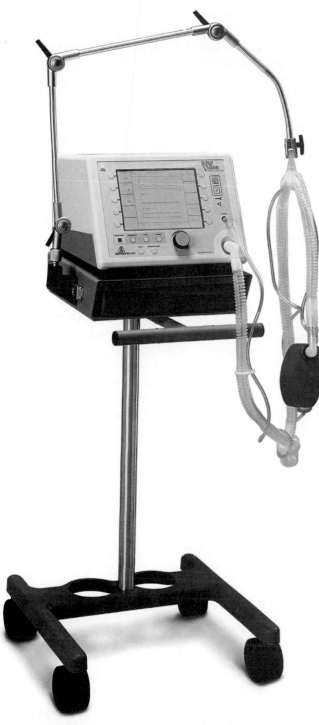

FIGURE 14-50 The Respironics BiPAP Vision. (Courtesy Respironics, Inc, Murrysville, Pa.)

used to provide bilevel PPV to intubated patients. The specific guidelines set forth by the manufacturer in the operating manual should be closely followed.[34]

Power Source

A standard 120-V AC electrical outlet powers the main operations of the BiPAP Vision, in combination with a rechargeable NiCd (nickel-cadmium) battery that drives

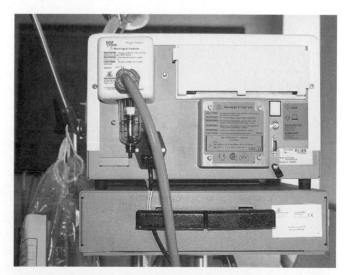

FIGURE 14-51 The rear panel of the Respironics BiPAP Vision. (Courtesy Philips Respironics, Murrysville, Pa.)

clinician to regulate the amount of oxygen delivered to the blower. (NOTE: The accuracy of this device is ±3% at concentrations of 30% or less and may vary by as much as ±10% as the F_IO_2 approaches 100%.)

Leak Compensation

Leaks are inherent to user interfaces and patient circuits in NPPV machines. Therefore, monitoring and compensating for changes in unintentional leaks are critical to maintaining the appropriate trigger and cycle levels for the ventilator. The BiPAP Vision has a system called Auto-Trak™ sensitivity that uses a combination of two mechanisms to identify and modify baseline values in response to leaks. These are expiratory flow rate and tidal volume adjustments.

The expiratory flow rate adjustment primarily works to make course adjustments in baseline values. When the ventilator is initially turned on, it measures the total flow through the circuit before it is connected to the patient. This includes the intentional leak created by the exhalation port. The BiPAP Vision is then attached to the patient, and the expiratory flow through the circuit is measured after the machine has cycled into expiration for 5 seconds. Through measurement and calculation, the ventilator is able to determine the intentional and unintentional leak of the system. This allows the ventilator to establish and monitor the baseline pressure, which allows the trigger and cycle values to be set.

The tidal volume adjustment is used for fine-tuning of the baseline pressure on a breath-to-breath basis. Although the BiPAP Vision does not directly measure volume, it is able to estimate inspiratory and expiratory tidal volumes based on the patient flow and the time spent in inspiration and expiration. Differences that occur between the inspiratory and expiratory tidal volumes are then assumed to be the result of a change in the amount of intentional leak and are accounted for by an adjustment in baseline for the next breath. This feature allows the ventilator to adjust the baseline on a breath-to-breath basis, thereby reducing large corrections.

Controls and Displays

The control panel of the BiPAP Vision contains eight hard keys or controls, soft keys, and an adjustment knob used to set ventilator parameters (Figure 14-52). The hard keys are as follows: monitoring, parameters, mode, alarms, scale, freeze/unfreeze, alarm silence, and alarm reset. The soft keys are located to the left and right of the display panel. Soft keys change in accordance with the hard key activated. For example, if the hard key "parameters" was activated, the soft-key options along the right and left side of the display panel would be IPAP, EPAP, Rate, Time Inspiration, %O$_2$, and IPAP rise time. Depressing the soft key of choice and using the adjustment knob allow the clinician to change the value of the selected parameter.

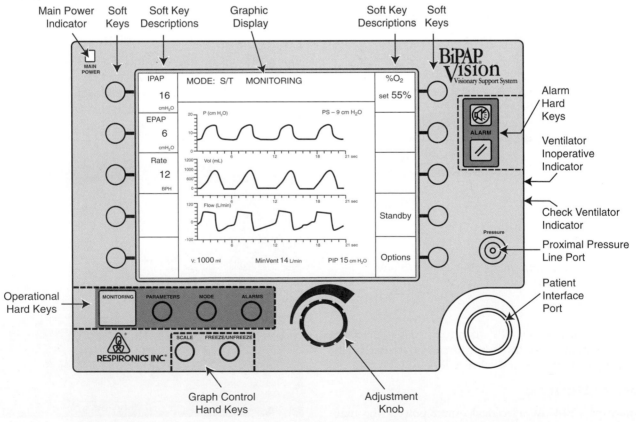

FIGURE 14-52 The control panel of the Respironics BiPAP Vision. (Courtesy Respironics, Inc, Murrysville, Pa.)

Monitoring

The monitoring screen is also called the home screen. This screen displays graphic waveforms, calculated parameters, and measured parameters and is the default screen when the machine is in operation. However, none of the displayed values can be changed. This screen is strictly for viewing the patient's current conditions. Information that can be found on the home screen is as follows: CPAP or IPAP, EPAP, rate (i.e., the total respiratory rate), V_T, minute ventilation, and peak inspiratory pressure.

Parameters

The parameters key displays the settings that are able to be modified in the current operating mode. These settings are IPAP, EPAP, F_IO_2, inspiratory time, and rate (if in the S/T mode). Additional information is displayed on the parameters screen that cannot be changed, but that may be useful to the clinician. This includes patient leak (unintentional leak), inspiratory time/total cycle time, and % of patient-triggered breaths.

Mode Key

The mode key displays the mode screen. This allows the clinician to view the current mode or change to a new operating mode. Whenever the clinician changes the mode of ventilation or any parameters within that mode, it is important that she confirms the new changes by depressing the soft key a second time. If the new settings are not confirmed, the ventilator will return to the previous values.

The BiPAP Vision operates in two modes: CPAP or the pressure support mode (S/T). (Refer to the "Modes of Ventilation" section on p. 770 for additional details.)

Alarms

The alarm hard key allows the clinician to view all current alarm settings and make any changes if necessary (see the Alarm Controls section for details).

Scale and Freeze/Unfreeze

The scale and freeze/unfreeze hard keys are self-explanatory. Scale allows the operator to increase or decrease the graph scales. The freeze/unfreeze key allows the operator to freeze and unfreeze the real-time graphic display on the front panel.

Alarm Silence and Alarm Reset

The alarm silence key, when activated, turns off all audible alarms for 2 minutes. However, this does not prevent the ventilator from displaying a visual alarm. If an alarm limit is violated, a visual alarm will appear in the message box on the front panel. Once the 2 minutes has expired, any additional violations will result in audible and visual alarms.

The alarm reset function cancels the alarm silence and any alarm message displayed on the front panel. If another parameter were to exceed its alarm limits, the ventilator would display a visual and audible alarm.

Sensitivity

Because of the constant fluctuations in the amount of unintentional leak, the BiPAP Vision uses a series of algorithms to minimize the work to cycle the ventilator from IPAP to EPAP. The Vision uses specific threshold values above and below the base flow to determine when the patient is initiating inspiration and then beginning expiration. The clinician does not set the sensitivity. (NOTE: For information on how baseline values are obtained, refer to the discussion on leak compensation.)

Alarm Controls

With the option of the newer-generation noninvasive ventilators to ventilate intubated patients, it has become increasingly important for the manufacturer to provide an extensive alarm system. The BiPAP Vision does just that. The available alarms are high-pressure, low-pressure, low-pressure delay, apnea, low minute volume, low rate and high rate, and a ventilator inoperative alarm.

High Pressure

The high-pressure alarm (range: 5 to 50 cm H_2O) is set above the IPAP value. An audiovisual alarm is activated when the airway pressure exceeds the high-pressure alarm limit for more than 0.5 second. When this occurs, the machine immediately cycles from IPAP to EPAP.

Low-Pressure and Low-Pressure Delay

The low-pressure alarm (range: 0 to 40 cm H_2O) and low-pressure delay alarm work together as a unit. The low-pressure alarm is set below the IPAP value and above the EPAP value. The low-pressure delay is set for the maximum amount of time that the patient is allowed between breaths. If a breath is not triggered in this time frame, then the airway pressure does not rise above the low-pressure alarm value. The low-pressure alarm activates, indicating the ventilator or the patient has failed to cycle into inspiration. This alarm is active in both modes of ventilation. This may be indicative of a leak, insufficient rise time for the patient, or apnea.

Apnea

The apnea alarm monitors only spontaneous breaths. It is an adjustable alarm that can be turned off or set at 20-, 30-, or 40-second intervals. If a spontaneous breath is not triggered within the set time frame, an audio and visual alarm will be activated.

Low Minute Volume

The low minute volume alarm (range: 0 to 99 L/min) monitors the patient's exhaled volumes, calculated from patient flow and inspiratory time. The alarm activates if the measured minute volume does not meet the minimum setting.

Low Rate/High Rate

The BiPAP Vision is equipped with two alarm features that continuously compare the total respiratory rate of the patient with an adjustable maximal and minimal respiratory rate. If at any time the total respiratory rate goes above the high rate alarm level or below the low rate alarm level, audible and visual indicators are activated. The alarms automatically reset when the total respiratory rate returns to acceptable limits.

Vent Inop

If at any time the internal mechanisms of the machine were to fail or the AC power source were to fail, a red icon in the shape of a wrench would appear in the display window, and it would be accompanied by a continuous audible alarm that cannot be silenced. These conditions indicate a ventilator inoperative alarm. As a safety feature, all system valves would open and the patient would be able to breathe room air. However, depending on the patient's respiratory pattern, it is very possible that he or she may experience rebreathing of exhaled gases because of the length of the circuit. In the event this alarm is activated, the clinician must disconnect the patient from the machine and provide another means of ventilation.

Modes of Ventilation

As previously mentioned in the controls and display section, the BiPAP Vision offers two modes of ventilation: CPAP and the S/T mode. The CPAP mode delivers CPAP to the patient circuit and requires that the patient trigger each breath. If the patient is not breathing spontaneously, then it is recommended that the clinician immediately change to the S/T mode.

During operation the monitoring screen displays the respiratory rate of the patient, the CPAP pressure that is delivered, and the F_1O_2. At the bottom of the screen the ventilator also tracks estimated exhaled tidal volume, minute ventilation, and PIP. When the ventilator is operating in CPAP mode, all alarms can be set to function.

The active S/T mode allows the clinician to set an IPAP (4 to 40 cm H_2O), EPAP (4 to 20 cm H_2O), respiratory rate (4 to 40 breaths/min), inspiratory time (0.5 to 3.0 sec), and IPAP rise time (Box 14-22). The S/T mode, unlike the CPAP, guarantees that the ventilator will cycle into IPAP a set number of times a minute based on the T_I setting. The rate setting and the inspiratory time setting are coupled so

that the ventilator never allows an inverse ratio in the I : E ratio. If at any time this were to occur, the ventilator will reduce the inspiratory time to ensure a 1:1 ratio. The pressure settings and rate setting will be unaffected.

There are two important points to note in regard to the IPAP and EPAP values. The EPAP setting can never be set higher than the IPAP value. If this were to occur, the ventilator would sound an alarm and prevent any further increase in the pressure. If the EPAP is equal to the IPAP, then the mode has essentially been changed to CPAP. Also, at very low EPAP values, the flow through the exhalation port may be insufficient to clear the expired tidal volume, which could result in a rise in the CO_2 levels of the patient. Clinical Rounds 14-13 provides some examples of these potential situations.

To reduce the sudden pressure change from EPAP to IPAP, the BiPAP Vision allows the clinician to set an IPAP rise time when the ventilator is in the active S/T mode. The ventilator allows the clinician to select a set amount of time that this pressure change is to occur: 0.05, 0.1, 0.2, or 0.4 second.

PART IV: HOME BILEVEL DEVICES

The ever-increasing understanding of sleep medicine and the ability to have smaller bilevel airway pressure units designed for home and institutional use have led to an expanding portion of noninvasive support for patients with obstructive sleep apnea (OSA) or treatment of respiratory insufficiency. There are many devices on the market today to help treat these patients. We will look at a few models of these kinds of devices. The theory of operation in these models is similar to that used in all units.

RESPIRONICS SYNCHRONY

The BiPAP Synchrony (Figure 14-53) is designed to provide noninvasive ventilatory assistance to adult patients (those who weigh >30 kg [66 lb or more]) for the treatment of respiratory insufficiency or OSA. The Synchrony is designed for use with nasal masks and full masks as recommended

---

BOX 14-22	BiPAP Vision Inspiratory Positive Airway Pressure (IPAP) Rise Time

The IPAP rise time is not a hard key, but it is an important soft-key parameter in the mode display. It functions to adjust the rate of pressure change when the machine cycles from expiratory positive airway pressure (EPAP) to IPAP. This value can be adjusted in increments of 0.05, 0.1, 0.2, and 0.4 second. The purpose of IPAP rise time is to gradually deliver the higher IPAP pressure to the patient to provide more comfortable breath delivery and improve patient-ventilator synchrony.

CLINICAL ROUNDS 14-13

A respiratory therapist who is accustomed to using the Respironics BiPAP S/T unit is adjusting the pressure levels for a patient during noninvasive positive-pressure ventilation (NPPV). The mode is set at spontaneous/timed (S/T). Inspiratory positive airway pressure (IPAP) is set at +10 cm H_2O, and expiratory positive airway pressure (EPAP) is set at +12 cm H_2O. Suddenly an alarm occurs. Pressures do not go to the +12 cm H_2O setting. What should the respiratory therapist do to correct this situation?

See Evolve Resources for the answer.

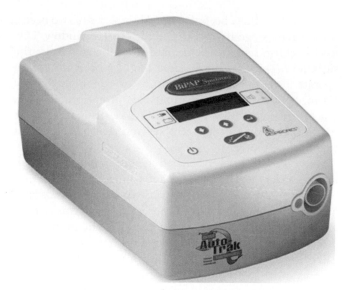

FIGURE 14-53 The Respironics BiPAP Synchrony. (Courtesy Philips Healthcare, Carlsbad, Calif.)

by the manufacturer (Respironics, Inc, Murrysville, Pa.). The Synchrony is 12 in × 7 in × 6 in and weighs approximately 6 lb.[35]

Power Source

The BiPAP Synchrony has two power options available for operation. The primary power source is 100-V to 240-V AC power or 12-V DC.

Internal Mechanism

Air is drawn into the Synchrony unit through the air inlet located in the back of the unit. The air is then directed to the microprocessor-controlled blower, where the set IPAP, EPAP, and rate control are located.

Oxygen Source

The BiPAP Synchrony is designed to operate primarily with room air, but it can be supplemented with an oxygen source. To provide enriched oxygen, the BiPAP Synchrony must be equipped with an optional oxygen valve, which would be located on the right side of the unit. The oxygen source cannot exceed 15 L/min in flow or more than 50 psi.

Supplemental oxygen can also be added to the mask port of the patient's interface. As with any blended system, it is recommended that the delivered gas be periodically analyzed with an oxygen analyzer.

Operations/Controls

The control panel for the Synchrony BiPAP is located on the top of the unit and illustrated in Figure 14-54. Once the Synchrony is connected to a power source, the operator needs to press the standby button. The Synchrony will then sound two beeps and briefly illuminate the alarm indicators and display the start-up screen, followed by the self-test screen. The available controls are listed in Box 14-23.

Display Screen

The display screen has two different windows—the Control screen or the Monitoring screen. Figure 14-55 illustrates the monitoring screen with the displayed parameters. The activity indicator (●) is shown next to the IPAP icon and will alternate between the IPAP icon and the EPAP icon as the unit cycles the breath. The activity indicator is also present when an alarm is activated, alerting the operator to the alarm message. The selection symbol (►) indicates a

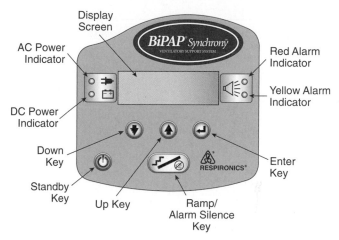

FIGURE 14-54 The control panel of the Respironics BiPAP Synchrony. (Courtesy Philips Respironics, Murrysville, Pa.)

BOX 14-23   BiPAP Synchrony™ Controls

The following controls are available:
- AC Power indicator: A green LED is lit when AC power is present to operate the unit.
- DC power indicator: A green LED is lit when direct current power is present to operate the unit.
- Standby key: The standby key starts and stops the Synchrony unit.
- Control keys (up, down, enter): These keys allow the operator to change menu screens and adjust modes of operation and set parameters.
- Ramp/alarm silence key: The ramp/alarm silence key is a dual-function key. In a nonalarm situation, pressing this key will activate the ramp feature, in which the Synchrony unit begins pressure at the EPAP level and gradually increases the IPAP level slowly at each breath until the set IPAP level is achieved.
- Yellow alarm indicator: When the yellow indicator light is flashing, this indicates the presence of a medium-priority alarm. If the yellow indicator light is continuously illuminated, this denotes a silenced medium alarm condition or a low-priority alarm.
- Red alarm indicator: When the red indicator light is flashing, this indicates the presence of a high-priority alarm. If the red indicator light is continuously illuminated, this denotes a loss of power or silenced alarm condition.

parameter that can be adjusted (Figure 14-56). Navigation symbol (↕) (shown here as up and down arrows) illustrates a parameter or screen that can be changed (Figure 14-57).

Alarms

The Synchrony has three levels of alarms, each with a distinct audio tone and an illuminating LED on the alarm soft key located on the right side of the unit. To silence or reset the alarm, the operator need only press the ramp/silence key located on the bottom-middle portion of the control panel.

The first level of alarms is the high-priority level, which is announced by a flashing red LED on the alarm display

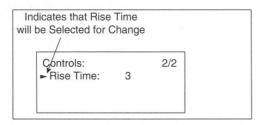

Mode:	S		1/2 ▲▼
IPAP ●		10	cm	H₂O
EPAP		5	cm	H₂O
RR		20	BPM

FIGURE 14-55 The monitoring screen of the Respironics BiPAP Synchrony.

Indicates that Rise Time will be Selected for Change

| Controls: | | 2/2 |
| ►Rise Time: | 3 |

FIGURE 14-56 The parameter-adjustment screen of the Respironics BiPAP Synchrony.

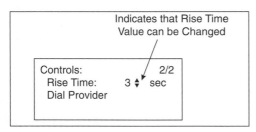

Indicates that Rise Time Value can be Changed

| Controls: | | 2/2 |
| Rise Time: | 3 ↕ sec |
| Dial Provider |

FIGURE 14-57 The navigation screen of the Respironics BiPAP Synchrony.

and a series of three beeps followed by a series of two beeps. An alarm message also appears in the display window. This level of alarm requires immediate attention to correct the situation. The Synchrony unit might not continue to operate depending on the nature of the high-priority alarm, hence the need for immediate attention. There is one priority alarm condition that will result in a constant red LED display on the alarm key and that occurs with a total loss of power.

The second level of alarm is the medium-priority alarm, which is signaled by a flashing yellow LED in the alarm key, then a series of three beeps sounds and an alarm message is displayed. Second-level alarms require a prompt response to assess the nature of the problem.

Low-priority alarms are announced by a steady yellow LED light on the alarm key, then a series of two beeps sounds and an alarm message or error code is displayed on the screen. The Synchrony unit will continue to function during medium- and low-level alarms. Table 14-21 shows the alarm levels and their associated alarm conditions.

Modes

The BiPAP Synchrony has four modes of operation: CPAP, spontaneous, S/T (upgrade), timed (upgrade), and pressure-controlled (upgrade). The modes listed with an upgrade symbol (upgrade) are optional modes.

CPAP

During CPAP the unit maintains the pressure set at the EPAP set level throughout inspiration and expiration. There is no apnea backup rate available.

Spontaneous Ventilation

Spontaneous ventilation is a bilevel mode that responds to the patient's inspiration and expiration by increasing pressure during inhalation and decreasing the delivered pressure during exhalation. There is no mandatory rate in this mode.

Spontaneous/Timed (S/T)

S/T is an optional bilevel mode that responds to both the patient's inspiration and expiration effort by increasing the delivered pressure during inhalation and decreasing

---

TABLE 14-21
Alarm Levels of the BiPAP Synchrony

High (Red Flashing)	Medium (Yellow Flashing)	Low (Yellow/Constant)
Apnea	Battery voltage too high	Battery in use
Low pressure support	Low Battery	Call for service
High pressure		Momentary loss of power
Low minute ventilation		Power failure (battery in use)
Invalid prescription		
Low pressure		
Patient disconnect		
Ventilator failure		
Battery failure		

the delivered pressure when exhalation is detected. If the patient does not initiate a breath within a set time period, the Synchrony will initiate a breath. During these timed breaths, the Synchrony controls the time of inhalation and decreases the delivered pressure for exhalation within a set time period.

Timed (T) Mode

The timed (T) mode of ventilation is also an optional bilevel mode in which the Synchrony controls both the inspiration and exhalation components (time, pressure) of the delivered breath independent of the patient's spontaneous effort.

Pressure-Controlled (PC)

PC is a bilevel mode that responds to the patient's inspiratory effort by increasing the delivered pressure. The length of the inspiration is controlled by the Synchrony. As in the S/T mode, if the patient does not initiate a breath within a set time period, the Synchrony will automatically initiate a breath.

PURITAN BENNETT
GoodKnight 425

The Puritan Bennett GoodKnight 425 is a bilevel positive airway pressure device designed for use in treating OSA in spontaneously breathing patients who weigh more than 66 lb (30 kg) (Figure 14-58). The GoodKnight 425 can be used in the home or hospital setting. It is not intended for invasive ventilation. The GoodKnight's dimensions are 5.6 in × 2.9 in × 7.7 in, and it weighs 1.5 lb without the power supply.[36]

Power Supply

The GoodKnight 425 is primarily powered by a 100-V or 240-V AC power source and can also be powered by an optional 12-V automotive battery. DC operation is possi-

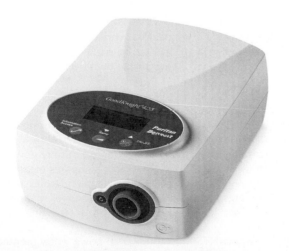

FIGURE 14-58 The Puritan Bennett GoodKnight 425 ventilator. (Courtesy Puritan Bennett, Boulder, Colo.; Puritan Bennett is a division of Covidien Ltd, Hamilton, Bermuda.)

ble without a DC/AC inverter by using an optional cable and adapter. An additional adapter may be needed to plug the unit into a wall outlet if the user is outside the United States.

Oxygen

The GoodKnight deleivers room air under normal conditions but can be supplemented with oxygen added by using an oxygen adapter placed just past the unit's patient circuit outlet connector. The supplemental oxygen may also be added to the mask port of the patient's interface. The maximum recommended supplemental bleed is 10 L/min. The F_IO_2 delivered to the patient will depend on factors such as pressure settings, patient breathing pattern, interface selection, leak rate, and flow of the oxygen source. It is recommended that the oxygen concentration from the unit be periodically analyzed.

Internal Mechanism

The GoodKnight 425 is powered by a microprocessor blower that entrains room air through the air inlet located in the rear of the unit. The microprocessor-controlled blower then develops the set IPAP, EPAP, and rate set by the operator.

Operations/Controls

The main controls of the GoodKnight unit are located on the top panel. To power-up the unit, the operator need only push the on/off soft key located in the lower right-hand corner of the control panel. To access all settings, the operator must press and hold the "hidden button" located under the word *GoodKnight* and simultaneously press the information-access button located in the lower left-hand corner of the control panel.

Alarms

The GoodKnight 425 has no built-in alarms.

Modes

The GoodKnight 425 has two modes of operation: CPAP and spontaneous bilevel. There is no apnea backup rate on the GoodKnight 425. However, the GoodKnight 425 S/T model does have an apnea backup rate option.

CPAP

The CPAP mode delivers CPAP to the patient circuit and requires that the patient trigger each breath. The range of CPAP available on the GoodKnight 425 is 4 cm H_2O to 25 cm H_2O.

Spontaneous Mode

This bilevel mode is not a timed mode, but rather a strictly spontaneous mode. The pressure settings available on the GoodKnght 425 are an IPAP of 4 cm H_2O to 25 cm H_2O and an EPAP setting of 4 cm H_2O to 25 cm H_2O. If apneic events are a significant issue, the patient should be placed on the 425 S/T to ensure adequate ventilation.

PART V: OTHER NONINVASIVE SUPPORT DEVICES

The 6th edition of this text discussed the **rocking bed** and **pneumobelt** as optional noninvasive respiratory support devices. The 7th edition included such negative-pressure devices as the body respirator, the **chest cuirass**, and the pneumosuit. These devices will be reviewed on Evolve Resources for this text.

SUMMARY OF HOME CARE EQUIPMENT

With increasing life expectancy of the adult population in America and our ability to support diseases once thought to be untreatable, home care has become a viable alternative to hospital care for the ventilator-dependent patient. In addition, there are a growing number of children who also require continuous mechanical respiratory support for chronic conditions. Home care provides an option for these children as well.[30,37]

In addition to the diagnosis of chronic pulmonary disease, there has been a shift in diagnoses to neurogenic respiratory insufficiency. This shift has resulted in implications for both hospital and community-based providers in extending services to the home setting.[38-40]

A study by Luján et al[38] compared the effectiveness and efficiency of an initiation protocol for *noninvasive home* mechanical *ventilation* (NIHMV) carried out at a pulmonary outpatient clinic with the standard in-hospital model. The NIHMV model reduced costs by 50%. Indihar did a cost-based study comparing five different sites of chronic ventilator care.[39] In a comparison of the step-down unit in a hospital with home care supported by the family, it was found that the costs were reduced by approximately one third. Cost is not the only reason for home care ventilation, but it is a major reason why home mechanical ventilation is so aggressively pursued.

The estimate of health-related quality of life (HRQOL) needs to be included in the assessment of costs and benefits of modern treatment modalities such as home mechanical ventilation. The level of HRQOL is dependent on the type of disease process involved.[40]

When choosing among positive-pressure ventilators, invasive or noninvasive techniques, negative-pressure ventilators, or supportive aids, it is important that the patient and family be well-educated about the operations of the equipment. They should be aware of the possible problems that might arise and how to identify them. When looking at supportive devices for the home, the clinician should choose one that is simple and operator-friendly, with clear alarms to alert the user of any malfunctions. It is important to remember that the primary operators of home care devices are nonmedical personnel. Operators should refer to the manufacturer's instructions to accomplish correct operation of any life support device.

KEY POINTS

- The pNeuton transport ventilator has no battery backup or AC power option and operates strictly from pneumatic power.
- With the Crossvent ventilator the alarm menu will flash "Low Battery, Connect External Power" on the LCG screen and sound an alarm when operating from the internal battery with only 20 minutes of remaining power. At this point the ventilator must be connected to AC power to continue operation.
- When the Crossvent is connected to an active gas source and not in use, the PEEP control should be turned fully counterclockwise to conserve gas supply.
- The Bio-Med MVP 10 has no alarms, so it should not be left to operate unattended.
- With the Dräger Oxylog 2000, all spontaneous breaths are provided at 100% source gas with a maximum flow for a spontaneous breath of 120 L/min.
- When the mode selector switch on the Oxylog 2000 is placed in SIMV position and the rate is set at less than 5 breaths/min, the ventilator switches to CPAP.
- The Percussionaire Bronchotron provides conventional IMV and HFV during patient transport.
- During conventional ventilation with the Bronchotron, tidal volume is dependent on the pressure setting and the patient's lung characteristics.

- The hard method of locking the LTV 1000 ventilator should be used when children or others may have access to the ventilator, such as in the patient's home.
- The flow pattern for the LTV 1200 ventilator is automatically set as a descending ramp for all volume-targeted breaths and occurs naturally in all pressure-targeted breaths.
- The select button on the LTV 1200 is used to stop the normal scrolling of monitored ventilator parameters.
- The extended features menu of the LTV 1000 and 1200 ventilators is selected by pressing the select button for 3 seconds.
- A visual indication on the Smiths Medical Pneupac™ ventiPAC Ventilator will begin to turn red and sound an audible alarm when the gas supply source is losing pressure. If this alarm is ignored for more than 60 seconds, the alarm will shut itself off to conserve battery power.
- The Dräger Carina™*home* ventilator compares measured ambient pressure with the current ventilating pressure and compensates the delivered V_T for any changes in ambient pressure, such as that which occurs with changing altitudes.
- The Newport HT50 has a universal power entry module that allows the same port to be used for connecting to an AC or external DC power source.

KEY POINTS—cont'd

▶ The BiPAP Focus™ will not operate without a functioning battery installed in the unit.

▶ The BiPAP Vision never allows an inverse ratio in the I : E ratio. If the operator attempts to set an I : E greater than 1:1, the ventilator will reduce the inspiratory time to ensure a 1:1 ratio. The pressure settings and rate setting are unaffected.

▶ To provide enriched oxygen, the BiPAP Synchrony must be equipped with an optional oxygen valve.

▶ The GoodKnight 425 CPAP device has two modes of operation: CPAP and spontaneous Bi-level and includes no built-in alarms.

ASSESSMENT QUESTIONS

See Evolve Resources for the answers.

1. The logic flow for the pNeuton model A with the patient-disconnect feature is how many liters per minute?
   a. 3 L/min
   b. 4 L/min
   c. 6 L/min
   d. 10 L/min

2. When the Crossvent sounds an alarm for low battery, approximately how long will you have power before the vent becomes inoperative?
   a. 10 minutes
   b. 15 minutes
   c. 20 minutes
   d. 40 minutes

3. What level does the supply pressure fall below for the Crossvent 3+ to activate the low source pressure alarm?
   a. 40 psi
   b. 30 psi
   c. 31 psi
   d. 44 psi

4. The approximate upper delivered tidal volume for the MVP 10 is:
   a. 300 mL
   b. 150 mL
   c. 600 mL
   d. 400 mL

5. The MVP 10 can be made MRI-compatible. True or False?
   a. True
   b. False

6. The apnea alarm on the Oxylog 2000 is:
   a. Adjustable from 10 to 30 seconds
   b. Constant at 15 seconds
   c. Constant at 20 seconds
   d. Based on the rate setting

7. On the Oxylog 3000, at what flow rates can the minimum oxygen concentration of 40% no longer be guaranteed?
   a. Less than 12 or greater than 30 L/min
   b. Less than 9 or greater than 35 L/min
   c. Less than 9 or greater than 25 L/min
   d. There is no minimum or maximum flow.

8. Which of the following features does the Uni-Vent 750 **NOT** have?
   a. Internal PEEP valve
   b. Internal compresser
   c. Altitude compensation
   d. Automatic PEEP compensation
   (1) I and IV
   (2) I and III
   (3) II and IV
   (4) I and II

9. If the apnea alarm on the Uni-Vent 750 is activated, which of the following is(are) true?
   a. An apnea period of 15 seconds has been detected.
   b. The ventilator is in either the A/C mode or the SIMV mode.
   c. A backup rate of 12 breaths/min at the current settings for V_T delivery starts.
   d. The antiasphyxia valve opens, letting the patient breathe spontaneously from room air.
   (1) IV only
   (2) I and IV only
   (3) II and III only
   (4) I, II, and IV

10. What is the logic gas consumption on the Uni-Vent Eagle™ 754 ventilator?
    a. 4 L/min
    b. 2 L/min
    c. 10 L/min
    d. None

11. The Percussonaire Bronchotron TXP requires how much liter flow to operate the internal logic?
    a. 4 to 6 L/min
    b. 8 to 14 L/min
    c. 8 to 12 L/min
    d. 4 to 10 L/min

12. Apnea ventilation on the LTV 1000 will terminate when how many consecutive patient-triggered breaths are detected?
    a. 1
    b. 3
    c. 4
    d. 2

ASSESSMENT QUESTIONS—cont'd

13. The Pulmonetic Systems LTV 1200 offers which of the following features?
    I. Noninvasive ventilation mode
    II. External PEEP valve
    III. Cylinder duration calculator
    IV. High-frequency ventilation
    a. II and III
    b. I and IV
    c. III and IV
    d. I and III

14. What type of mask needs to be used in order for the LTV 1000 and 1200 to operate correctly in the non-invasive mode?
    a. Vented masks
    b. Partial vented mask
    c. Nonvented masks
    d. All of the above

15. At what psi will the Smiths Medical Pneupac™ ventiPAC low-pressure "eyeball" alarm begin to change from white to red, indicating a low gas supply pressure?
    a. 40 psi
    b. 25 psi
    c. 45 psi
    d. 30 psi

16. What is the maximum oxygen bleed-in with the Dräger Carina™home ventilator?
    a. 8 L/min
    b. 10 L/min
    c. 12 L/min
    d. 15 L/min

17. The Dräger Carina™home ventilator internal battery is rated for a minimum of how many minutes?
    a. 120 minutes
    b. 240 minutes
    c. 60 minutes
    d. 180 minutes

18. The Newport HT50 can provide enriched oxygen delivery by which of the following methods?
    I. An optional oxygen blender through a high-pressure oxygen gas source
    II. An oxygen-blending bag for providing additional oxygen for spontaneous breaths
    III. By using the two high-pressure gas sources required for powering the device
    IV. By bleeding oxygen into the patient circuit
    a. III only
    b. IV only
    c. I and II
    d. I and IV only

19. A respiratory therapist is increasing the PEEP/CPAP control on the HT50 from 5 cm H_2O to 10 cm H_2O. The patient's pressure setting is 10 cm H_2O. The ventilator does not allow the increase in PEEP. The most likely reason is:
    a. The therapist must toggle past a safety switch to increase PEEP above 9 cm H_2O
    b. The high-pressure alarm is set at 20 cm H_2O, and the settings would cause this alarm to activate
    c. The PEEP/CPAP level cannot be set higher than the pressure setting—5 cm H_2O
    d. The low-pressure alarm must be readjusted before the change in PEEP can occur

20. The internal ventilator battery on the LTV 800 is rated for how long?
    a. 45 minutes
    b. 120 minutes
    c. 60 minutes
    d. 30 minutes

21. The leak compensation on the LTV 900 and LTV 950 can compensate for leaks up to how many liters per minute?
    a. 6 L/min
    b. 3 L/min
    c. 1 L/min
    d. 8 L/min

22. A constant amber light is illuminated on the front panel of the LP10, indicating:
    a. An external power source is in use
    b. PEEP is active
    c. The sensitivity is turned off
    d. The internal battery voltage is adequate

23. The Respironics BiPAP Focus™ has two operator-adjustable alarms in which combination?
    a. High-pressure and apnea detection time
    b. High respiratory rate and low-pressure
    c. Apnea detection time and number of apneic events in 1 hour
    d. Number of apneic events in 1 hour and low tidal volume

24. The BiPAP Vision is connected to an oxygen source. The F_IO_2 is set at 0.8 on a patient in the intensive care unit. The respiratory therapist measures the F_IO_2 as 0.9. A possible cause of this discrepancy is:
    a. The internal concentrator is out of calibration
    b. The setting control for O_2 is out of calibration
    c. The Vision has a 10% error range for oxygen values approaching 100%
    d. The air source has failed

25. The BiPAP Vision apnea alarms cannot be be set to:
    a. 20 seconds
    b. 40 seconds
    c. 0 seconds
    d. 45 seconds

ASSESSMENT QUESTIONS—cont'd

26. The Repironics Synchrony is designed to be used on patients who weigh more than:
   - a. 20 kg
   - b. 30 kg
   - c. 20 kg
   - d. 35 kg

27. The GoodKnight 425 alarms include the following:
   - a. High pressure
   - b. Apnea alarm
   - c. Low pressure
   - d. No alarm

References

1. Pierson JD: Noninvasive positive pressure ventilation: history and terminology, *Respir Care* 42:370, 1996.

2. Miyoshi E, Fujino Y, Mashimo T, Nishimura M: Performance of transport ventilator with patient-triggered ventilation, *Chest* 118:1109-1115, 2000.

3. Chang DW, American Association for Respiratory Care: Clinical practice guideline: in-hospital transport of the mechanically ventilated patient—2002 revision and update, *Respir Care* 47:721-723, 2002.

4. Anonymous: Evaluation of portable transport ventilators, *Health Devices* 11:381-398, 2004.

5. Austin PN, Campbell RS, Johannigman JA, Branson RD: Transport ventilators, *Respir Care Clin N Am* 8:119-150, 2002.

6. Airon Corporation: *pNeuton Transport Ventilator Operators Manual, Part no. 58501 rev. 2A*, Melbourne, Fla, 2007, Airon Corporation.

7. Bio-Med Devices, Inc: *Crossvent 3+ Operator's Manual*, Guilford, Conn, 2005, Bio-Med Devices, Inc.

8. Bio-Med Devices, Inc: *Bio-Med MVP 10 Operator's Manual*, Guilford, Conn, 1990, Bio-Med Devices, Inc.

9. Dräger Medical AG & Co: *Oxylog 2000 Operator's Instruction Manual*, Lübeck, Germany 1995, Dräger Medical AG & Co.

10. Dräger Medical AG & Co: *Oxylog 3000 Operator's Manual*, Lübeck, Germany, 2006, Dräger Medical AG & Co.

11. Impact Instrumentation, Inc: *Uni-Vent 750/754 operator's manual, Rev B*, West Caldwell, NJ, 1991, Impact Instrumentation, Inc.

12. Percussionaire Corporation: *Percussionaire Bronchotron TXP Ventilator Operating Manual*, Sandpoint, Idaho, 2004, Percussionaire Corporation.

13. Pulmonetic Systems, Inc: *LTV Series Ventilator Operator's Manual, part no. 10664, revision J*, Minneapolis, 2000, Pulmonetic Systems, Inc, a division of Viasys Healthcare.

14. Pulmonetic Systems, Inc: *LTV Series Caregiver Video, part no. 11522, revision A*, Minneapolis, 2001, Pulmonetic Systems, Inc, a division of Viasys Healthcare.

15. Pulmonetic Systems, Inc: *LTV Series In-Service Video, part no. 11462, revision B*, Minneapolis, 2000, Pulmonetic Systems, Inc, a division of Viasys Healthcare.

16. Pulmonetic Systems, Inc: *Produce Simulator for the LTV 1000 Ventilator, LTV 1000 Series Software CD, part no. 11600, version 1.03*, Minneapolis, 2000, Pulmonetic Systems, Inc, a division of Viasys Healthcare.

17. Pulmonetic Systems, Inc: *LTV 1200 Operator's Manual, part no. 18247-001*, Minneapolis, 2000, Pulmonetic Systems, Inc, a division of Viasys Healthcare.

18. Pulmonetic Systems, Inc: *LTV 1200 Operator's Manual, part no. 18247-001*, Minneapolis, 2000, Pulmonetic Systems, Inc, a division of Viasys Healthcare.

19. Smiths Medical: *Pneupac™ ventiPAC. Operator's Manual*, Watford, United Kingdom, 2005, Smiths Medical.

20. Chipman DW, Caramez MP, Miyoshi E, Kratohvil JP, Kacmarek RM: Performance comparison of 15 transport ventilators, *Respir Care* 52:740-751, 2007.

21. AARC; Respiratory Home Care Focus Group: AARC clinical practice guideline. Long-term invasive mechanical ventilation in the home—2007 revision & update, *Respir Care* 52:1056-1062, 2007.

22. Dunne PJ, McInturff SL: *Respiratory home care: the essentials*, Philadelphia, 1998, FA Davis.

23. Dräger Medical AG & Co: *Dräger Carina™home Ventilator Operating Manual*, Lübeck, Germany, 2004, Dräger Medical AG & Co.

24. Newport Medical Instruments: *Newport HT50 operator's manual*, Costa Mesa, Calif, 2002, Newport Medical Instruments.

25. Pulmonetic Systems, Inc: *LTV 800 Operator's Manual*, Minneapolis, 2003, Pulmonetic Systems, Inc, a division of Viasys Healthcare.

26. Aequitron Medical: *LP10 Operator's Manual*, 1994, Aequitron Medical.

27. Gietzen JW, Lund JA, Swegarden JL: Effect of PEEP-valve placement on function of a home care ventilator, *Respir Care* 36:1093-1098, 1991.

28. Bach JR: A historical perspective on the use of noninvasive ventilatory support alternatives, *Respir Care Clin N Am* 2:161-181, 1996.

29. Sullivan CE, Berthon-Jones M, Issa FG, Eves L: Reversal of obstructive sleep apnoea by continuous positive airway pressure applied through the nares, *Lancet* 1:862-865, 1981.

30. Gramlich T: Basic concepts of noninvasive positive pressure ventilation. In: Pilbeam SP, Cairo JM: *Mechanical ventilation—physiological and clinical application*, ed 4, St Louis, 2006, Mosby/Elsevier.

31. Barreiro TJ, Gemmel DJ: Noninvasive ventilation, *Crit Care Clin* 23:201-222, 2007.

32. Sinuff T, Kahnamoui K, Cook DJ, Giacomini M: Practice guidelines as multipurpose tools: a qualitative study of noninvasive ventilation, *Crit Care Med* 35:776-782, 2007.

33. Respironics, Inc: *Respironics BiPAP Focus™ Clinical Manual*, Murrysville, Pa, 2006, Respironics, Inc.

34. Respironics, Inc: *Respironics Vision Clinical Manual*, Murrysville, Pa, 2000, Respironics, Inc.

35. Respironics, Inc: *Respironics Synchrony Operating Manual*, Murrysville, Pa, 2006, Respironics, Inc.

36. Puritan Bennett: *Puritan Bennett GoodKnight 425 Operator's Manual*, Boulder, Colo, 2005, Puritan Bennett Inc, a division of Covidien Ltd.

37. Graham RJ, Fleegler EW, Robinson WM: Chronic ventilator need in the community: a 2005 pediatric census of Massachusetts, *Pediatrics* 119:e1280-1287:2007.

38. Luján M, Moreno A, Veigas C, Montón C, Pomares X, Domingo C: Noninvasive home mechanical ventilation: effectiveness and efficiency of an outpatient initiation protocol compared with the standard in-hospital model, *Respir Med* 101:1177-1182, 2007.

39. Indihar SF: Cost of comparison care for chronic ventilator patients, *Chest* 99:260, 1991.

40. Windisch W, Criée CP: Quality of life in patients with home mechanical ventilation, *Pneumologie* 60:539-546, 2006.

Internet Resources

Airon Corporation: http://www.pneuton.com/
Bio-Med Devices, Inc: http://www.biomeddevices.com/
Dräger Medical AG & Co: http://www.draeger.com/
Impact Instrumentation, Inc: http://www.impactii.com/
Newport Medical Instruments: http://www.ventilators.com/
Percussionaire Corporation: http://www1.ivenue.com/percussionaire/

Pulmonetic Systems: http://www.pulmonetic.com/
Puritan Bennett: http://www.mallinckrodt.com/
Respironics, Inc: http://www.respironics.com/
Smiths Medical: http://www.smiths-medical.com/
VentWorld, a ventilator Web site: http://www.ventworld.com/
Viasys Healthcare: http://www.viasyshealthcare.com/default.aspx

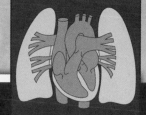

Chapter 15

Sleep Diagnostics

J.M. CAIRO

OUTLINE

OBJECTIVES

Upon completion of this chapter, you will be able to:
· Describe the various stages of sleep in adults and children.
· Discuss the physiologic effects of sleep on cardiopulmonary function in healthy individuals.
· List the measurements most commonly recorded during polysomnography.
· Summarize the clinical and laboratory criteria used to diagnose obstructive, central, and mixed apnea.
· Describe various strategies that can be used to monitor arterial oxygen saturation, nasal-oral airflow, and respiratory effort of patients with obstructive sleep apnea syndrome.
· Explain the physiologic consequences of obstructive sleep apnea.
· Name several common diseases associated with central sleep apnea.

KEY TERMS

alpha waves
apnea/hypopnea index (AHI)
apnea index (AI)
arousal response
beta waves
central sleep apnea
Cheyne-Stokes respiration
circadian cycle

collodion
delta waves
Holter monitoring
International 10-20 EEG system
K-complexes
mixed sleep apnea
non–rapid eye movement (non–REM) sleep

obstructive sleep apnea (OSA)
polysomnography
relatively low-voltage, mixed-frequency (RLVMF) waves
REM sleep
sleep spindles
theta waves

The effect of sleep on breathing has received considerable attention in the past 30 years. Much of this attention relates to an increased awareness of sleep-related disorders and improved technology for assessing neurologic and cardiopulmonary functions during sleep. The physiologic effect of sleep on breathing is normally of little consequence in healthy individuals. Its effect on patients with altered respiratory function (i.e., those afflicted with chronic pulmonary diseases) can be profound, however, and lead to significant consequences.

PHYSIOLOGY OF SLEEP

Sleep is part of a cyclic phenomenon (i.e., the **circadian cycle**) controlled by an endogenous pacemaker that remains active even in an isolated environment free of time cues.[1] Sleep in itself is a nonhomogenous phenomenon consisting of two distinct states: **non–rapid eye movement (non-REM) sleep** and rapid eye movement **(REM) sleep**. As seen in Table 15-1, these states can be defined by electrographic and behavioral criteria such as brain wave

TABLE 15-1

Behavioral and Electrographic Characteristics of Sleep-Awake States

	SLEEP-WAKE STATE		
Characteristic	Wake	Non–REM Sleep	REM Sleep
Eyelids	Open or closed	Closed	Closed
Eye movements	Slow or rapid	Slow or absent	Rapid
Responsiveness to external stimuli	Simple or complex	Simple	Often absent
Electroencephalogram	Low-voltage, high-frequency	High-voltage, low-frequency	Low-voltage, high-frequency
Electromyogram	High-level tonic activity	Lower-level tonic activity	Absence of tonic activity
Electro-oculogram	Slow or rapid movements	Slow or rapid movements	Rapid movements

From Phillipson EA: Sleep disorders. In Murray JF, Nadel JA: *Textbook of respiratory medicine*, ed 3, Philadelphia, 1994, WB Saunders.
REM, Rapid eye movement.

activity, oculomotor activity, responsiveness to external stimuli, and muscle tone.[2,3]

Non-REM sleep, or quiet sleep, consists of four stages that are thought to represent progressively deeper levels of sleep. At sleep onset (non-REM stage 1), normal sleepers can be easily aroused because they alternate between wakefulness and sleep. The electroencephalogram (EEG) shows **alpha waves** and **beta waves**, which are present during wakefulness and diminish as the sleeper's EEG converts to **relatively low-voltage, mixed-frequency (RLVMF) waves** (Figure 15-1A). (NOTE: Alpha waves are rhythmic waves that occur at a frequency of 8 to 13 cycles per second, whereas beta waves occur at frequencies of 14 to 80 cycles per second.[4]) Skeletal muscle tone changes only slightly from waking levels; eye movements throughout non-REM sleep are slow, rolling, pendulous, and disconjugate.[5]

Stage 1 sleep lasts for only a brief time and is followed by a transition to stage 2 non-REM sleep, which is identified by the appearance of **sleep spindles** and **K-complexes** on the sleeper's EEG (Figure 15-1B). Sleep spindles are waveforms with waxing and waning amplitude that occur at a frequency of 9 to 13 cycles per second. K-complexes are large, vertical, slow waves that have an amplitude of at least 75 μV, with an initial negative deflection.[5] Arousal thresholds (i.e., the level of stimuli required to change to a "lighter" stage of sleep or wakefulness) are higher in stage 2 than those in stage 1.

The deepest stages of non-REM sleep (stages 3 and 4) are referred to as *slow-wave sleep* because of the presence of large **delta waves** that appear when the sleeper enters these stages (Figure 15-1C). Delta waves include all electroencephalographic waves with a frequency of less than 3.5 cycles per second.[5] The distinction between stage 3 and stage 4 is somewhat arbitrary because both appear almost identical on EEGs. For example, most clinicians define the beginning of stage 3 as the period in which slow waves constitute from 20% to 50% of the electroencephalographic recording. Stage 4, on the other hand, is identified by the presence of slow waves for at least 50% of the electroencephalographic recording.[2,5] The arousal threshold during stages 3 and 4 is considerably higher than that during stages 1 and 2 of non-REM sleep.

After approximately 70 to 100 minutes of non-REM sleep, the normal sleeper enters REM sleep. During this phase of sleep, there is an increase in cerebral activity, as evidenced by the presence of an RLVMF pattern on the EEG, with a burst of **theta waves** (see Figure 15-1D). Theta waves have a sawtooth appearance and occur at a frequency of 4 to 7 cycles per second.[4,5] It is generally accepted that dreaming occurs during REM sleep because sleepers who awaken after dreaming during REM sleep can recall their dreams. Although dreaming does occur during non-REM sleep, those dreams are usually not remembered. Eye movements during REM sleep are rapid, and conjugate eye movements are present. The arousal threshold (i.e., skeletal muscle tone) during REM sleep varies and may actually be absent. (It is interesting that if the arousal stimulus is incorporated into the dream content, arousal is less likely.[5])

During a typical night of sleep, a normal adult sleeper cycles between non-REM sleep and REM sleep approximately every 90 to 120 minutes.[1] Slow-wave sleep (non-REM stages 3 and 4) is most prominent during the first half of the night and decreases as the night progresses. REM sleep, on the other hand, becomes longer and more intense throughout the sleep period, with the longest and most-intense REM sleep occurring in the early morning hours.

Figure 15-2 illustrates the average amount of time that a healthy adult spends in each sleep state. Normally, 4 to 6 cycles of sleep stages occur per night. Although there are variations among sleepers, these averages are a good approximation of the time distribution of non-REM sleep, REM sleep, and wakefulness during a typical night of sleep (Box 15-1).

The classic states of non-REM sleep and REM sleep are not easily identified at birth by means of standard electroencephalographic, electromyographic (EMG), and electro-oculographic (EOG) analysis. Although similarities exist between the sleep states that occur in newborns and those in adults, sleep stages during the neonatal period are generally categorized as active sleep, quiet sleep, and intermediate sleep. Active sleep is comparable to REM sleep; quiet and intermediate sleep states have many of the same characteristics of non-REM. It is worth noting that infants

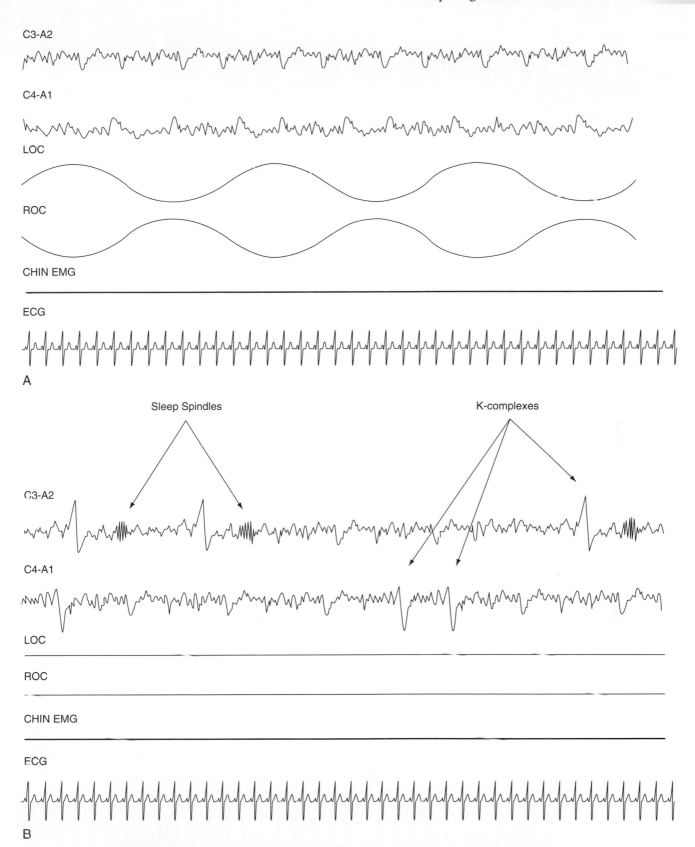

C3-A2

C4-A1

LOC

ROC

CHIN EMG

ECG

A

Sleep Spindles

K-complexes

C3-A2

C4-A1

LOC

ROC

CHIN EMG

ECG

B

FIGURE 15-1 A, Stage 1 sleep. Stage 1 is characterized by relatively low-voltage, mixed-frequency electroencephalographic (EEG) results; slow, rolling eye movements (*LOC* and *ROC* relate to eye movements that are left of center and right of center, respectively); and tonic electromyographic (EMG) activity. **B,** Stage 2 sleep. Stage 2 is characterized by relatively low-voltage background EEG activity; sleep spindles and K-complexes; absence of eye movements; and tonic EMG activity.   *Continued*

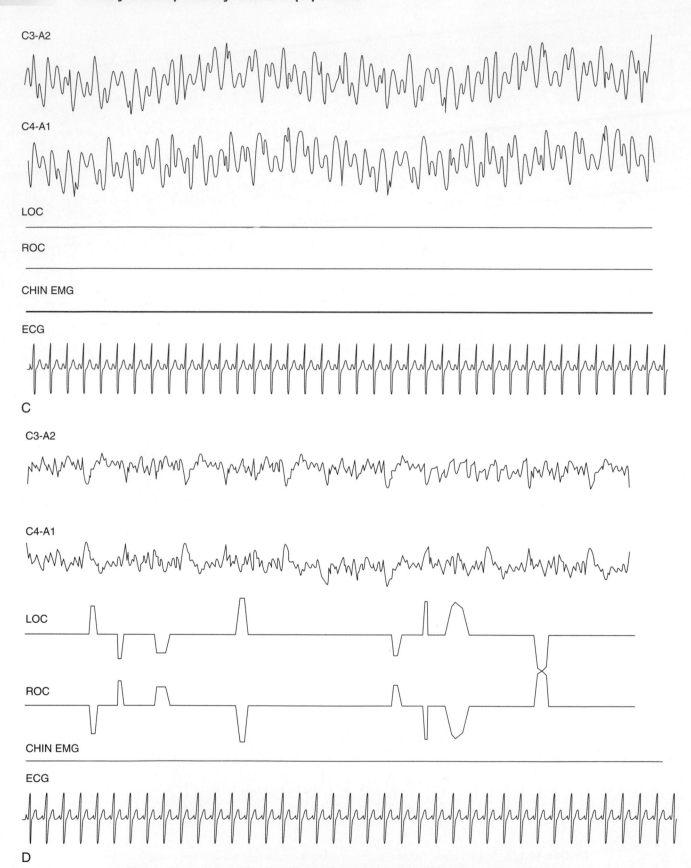

C3-A2

C4-A1

LOC

ROC

CHIN EMG

ECG

C

C3-A2

C4-A1

LOC

ROC

CHIN EMG

ECG

D

FIGURE 15-1, cont'd C, Stage 4 sleep. Stage 4 is characterized by high-voltage, slow-wave EEG activity; absence of eye movements; and tonic EMG activity. **D,** Rapid eye movement (REM) sleep. REM sleep is characterized by relatively low-voltage, mixed-frequency background EEG activity, with a burst of notched theta waves; rapid, saccadic, conjugate eye movements; chin muscle tone significantly decreased from that found with waking; and non–rapid eye movement (NREM) sleep level. (Redrawn from Sheldon SH, Spire JP, Levy HB: *Pediatric sleep medicine,* Philadelphia, 1992, WB Saunders.)

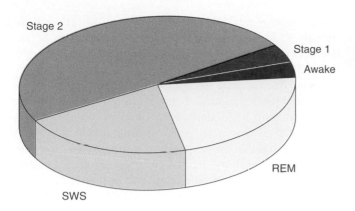

Stage	Percent of Total Recording Time
Wake After Sleep Onset	Less Than 5%
Stage 1	2% to 5%
Stage 2	45% to 55%
Slow-Wave Sleep (SWS)	13% to 23%
REM	20% to 25%

FIGURE 15-2 Sleep-stage distribution in normal healthy adults. (Redrawn from Sheldon SH, Spire JP, Levy HB: *Pediatric sleep medicine*, Philadelphia, 1992, WB Saunders.)

BOX 15-1	How Much Sleep Do We Need?

It is generally accepted that the amount of sleep that an individual requires is influenced by their age. Infants typically require approximately 16 hours per day, and teenagers need 8 or 9 hours per night on average. For most adults, 7 to 8 hours per night seems to be sufficient, although some people require only approximately 5 hours per day and others require as much as 10 hours of sleep each day. As they get older (i.e., over 60 years of age), people tend to sleep more lightly and for shorter periods. What may not be obvious is that we continue to need approximately the same amount of sleep that we require in early adulthood.

Certain conditions can also influence the amount of sleep that we require. That is, we have an increased need for sleep while recovering from an acute illness, such as a cold or the flu. Women in their first trimester of pregnancy often need several more hours of sleep than usual. The amount of sleep a person needs also increases when there has been a deprivation of sleep in previous days. Getting too little sleep creates a "sleep debt" that ultimately must be repaid. Although we may think that we can adapt to getting less sleep than we need, sleep deprivation can severely alter our judgment, reaction time, and other neurologic functions.

See the Web site for the National Institute of Neurological Disorders and Stroke http://www.ninds.nih.gov for more information.

TABLE 15-2			
Physiologic Effects of Sleep on Respiration			
Feature	**Sleep Stages 1 and 2**	**Sleep Stages 3 and 4**	**REM Sleep**
Pattern of breathing	Periodic	Stable	Irregular
Apneas	Short, central	Rare	Short, central
PaCO₂	Variable	↑ 2-8 mm Hg above wakefulness	Variable, similar to stages 3, 4
Rib cage muscles	Active	Active	Inhibited
Diaphragm	Active	Active	Active
Upper airway muscles	Active	Active	Inhibited
Chemoresponsiveness	↓ Compared with wakefulness	↓ Compared with stages 1, 2	↓ Compared with stages 3, 4
Arousability to respiratory stimuli	Low thresholds	Low thresholds	High thresholds

From Phillipson EA: Sleep disorders. In Murray JF, Nadel JF: *Textbook of respiratory medicine*, Philadelphia, 1994, WB Saunders.
PaCO₂, Partial pressure of arterial carbon dioxide.

---

enter active sleep first instead of entering into quiet sleep as adults do. Between 6 and 8 weeks of age, infant sleep becomes more predictable, and, by 12 weeks of age, the various stages of non-REM sleep and REM sleep are recognizable. By 12 months of age, infants exhibit the classic sleep stages seen in adults. As mentioned previously, sleep-state distribution for healthy adult sleepers during a typical 8-hour period of sleep usually involves both non-REM sleep and REM sleep states alternating cyclically every 90 to 120 minutes, with periods of REM sleep lasting from 10 to 30 minutes. In contrast, infants spend considerably more time in REM sleep than do adult sleepers (i.e., during various stages in development, infants may spend as much as 75% of their sleep in REM).[1,5]

Effect of Sleep on Breathing

The effects of sleep on breathing are summarized in Table 15-2. As the sleeper passes through the various stages of non-REM sleep, there is a progressive reduction in chemosensitivity and respiratory drive. The reduction in respiratory drive that occurs during the early stages of non-REM sleep (stages 1 and 2) predisposes the person to apneic periods (i.e., **Cheyne-Stokes respiration**) when fluctuating between being awake and asleep. With the establishment of non-REM slow-wave sleep (stages 3 and 4), nonrespiratory inputs are minimized and minute ventilation is regulated by metabolic control. Minute ventilation decreases by 1 L/min to 2 L/min when compared with wakefulness. As a consequence, the partial pressure of arterial carbon dioxide ($PaCO_2$) rises by 2 mm Hg to 8 mm Hg, and the partial pressure of oxygen in the arteries (PaO_2) decreases by 5 mm Hg to 10 mm Hg.

As the sleeper enters into REM sleep, breathing becomes irregular as the ventilatory response to chemical and mechanical respiratory stimuli is further reduced and even transiently abolished. Skeletal muscle activity, along with activity in the intercostal and accessory muscles of respiration, is decreased, and the upper airway muscles are inhibited. This inhibition leads to an increase in upper airway resistance, whereas inhibition of the intercostal and accessory muscles is associated with diminished thoracoabdominal coupling and short periods of central apnea for durations of 10 seconds to 20 seconds. $PaCO_2$ and PaO_2 levels are variable, but they are generally similar to those in the latter stages of non-REM sleep.

Effect of Sleep on Cardiovascular Function

The effects of sleep on cardiovascular function are shown in Figure 15-3. In most individuals, both heart rate and blood pressure are generally reduced during sleep. Reductions in heart rate average approximately 5 to 10 beats/ minute during non-REM sleep and up to 15 beats/minute during REM sleep. Blood pressure shows a moderate decrease of 10 to 15 mm Hg during non-REM sleep and up to 25 mm Hg during REM sleep. Alterations in heart rate seen during sleep seem to parallel sleep-related alterations in blood pressure. These variations are especially evident during REM sleep, when arterial blood pressure varies to a greater extent than it does during non-REM sleep.[5] Changes in blood pressure during REM sleep are characterized as sharp increases in mean arterial pressure that are superimposed on a relatively hypotensive state.

Cardiac output is usually only slightly reduced during non-REM sleep when compared with the waking state. The reduction in cardiac output, however, is more pronounced during REM sleep (i.e., an approximately 10% reduction).[5] Changes in cardiac output that are seen during sleep are not accompanied by changes in stroke volume, which tend to remain similar to values measured while the person is in a quiet, awake state.[5]

DIAGNOSIS OF SLEEP APNEA

The ability to wake from sleep or to rouse to a lighter stage of sleep requires the activation of higher neurologic centers

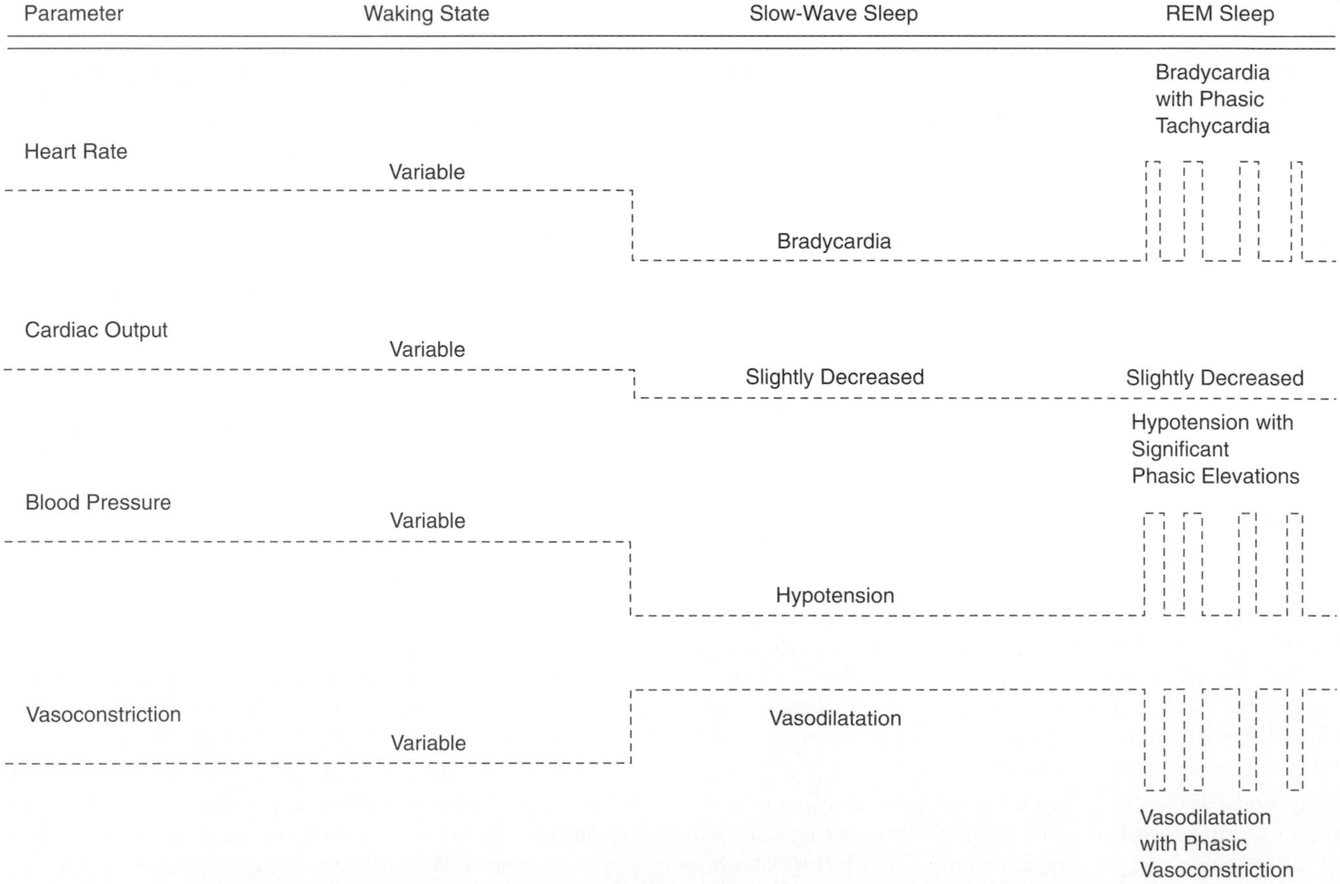

FIGURE 15-3 The effects of sleep on cardiovascular function in awake and sleep states. (Redrawn from Sheldon SH, Spire JP, Levy HB: *Pediatric sleep medicine,* Philadelphia, 1992, WB Saunders.)

(i.e., the reticular activating system and cortex).[2] Such activation results in an immediate increase in respiratory drive, activation of the upper airway muscles, stimulation of the cough reflex, and initiation of behavioral responses—specifically, increases in skeletal muscle tone.[2,4] If these **arousal responses** do not occur, sleep apnea or alveolar hypoventilation can result.

Diagnosis of sleep apnea is based on information derived from a patient history, a physical examination, and from laboratory studies that focus on sleep structure and cardiorespiratory function. The medical history and physical examination provide information that can be used to determine whether patients are at risk for sleep apnea and whether they demonstrate the common symptoms and signs associated with various sleep-related disorders. Laboratory studies range from simple overnight monitoring of arterial blood gases with pulse oximetry and transcutaneous monitoring to analyzing cardiopulmonary and neuromuscular function with **polysomnography**.

Polysomnography

Although a patient history and a physical examination can provide evidence that a patient may be afflicted with sleep apnea, the data may be equivocal and thus lead the clinician to underestimate or overestimate the severity of the patient's sleep-disordered breathing. For this reason, laboratory assessment of patients suspected to have sleep apnea should be performed to ensure a definitive diagnosis.

Table 15-3 summarizes the various laboratory procedures that can be used to investigate physiologic function during sleep. Although screening tests can provide valuable information about cardiopulmonary function during sleep, they do not allow for sleep staging and quantification of patient arousal or awakening during the course of the study. It is generally accepted that polysomnography

is the gold standard for identifying the type and severity of sleep apnea. Polysomnography usually includes all-night audio/video monitoring of the patient, as well as recordings of electrocardiograms (ECGs), respiratory activity, EEGs, electro-oculograms, and electromyograms.[6] (Clinical Practice Guideline 15-1 summarizes the American Association for Respiratory Care [AARC] Clinical Practice Guideline for Polysomnography.) Besides being used to determine whether a patient demonstrates sleep apnea or hypopnea, polysomnography can also provide valuable information about the most-effective means of treating these patients.

Electrocardiography

Cardiac activity, including heart rate and rhythm, is usually monitored with at least two electrocardiographic leads (e.g., lead II and a modified chest lead). It is important to recognize that monitoring two electrocardiographic leads can provide only limited information about the electrical activity of the heart. If more information about the patient's ECG is required, a 12-lead ECG or **Holter monitoring** may be indicated.

Electroencephalography

An EEG is a recording of fluctuations in the electric potentials of cortical neurons. These electric potentials are transmitted from the cortex through the coverings of the brain to the scalp, where electrodes placed at various points on the scalp are used to sense the sum of the potentials in the underlying cortex. EEGs provide valuable information on the integrity of the central nervous system and form the basis for identifying the various sleep stages that the patient enters during the sleep study.

To ensure that the information is meaningful and can be compared with that of different laboratories, a stan-

TABLE 15-3		
Types of Laboratory Investigation of Respiratory Disturbances During Sleep		
Type of Test	**Variable Measured**	**Technique**
Screening	SaO$_2$	Ear oximeter
	PCO$_2$	Transcutaneous sensor
	Heart rate, rhythm	Holter monitoring
Standard polysomnography	EEG	Surface electrodes
	EOG	Surface electrodes
	Submental EMG	Surface electrodes
	Tibialis EMG	Surface electrodes
	Breathing pattern	Surface electrodes
	SaO$_2$, PCO$_2$	Ear oximeter, transcutaneous sensor
	Electrocardiogram	Standard electrodes
Special procedures	Intrapleural pressure	Esophageal catheter
	Diaphragm EMG	Esophageal or surface electrodes
	Esophageal pH	Esophageal electrodes
	Arterial blood gases	Arterial catheter
	Pulmonary arterial pressure	Swan-Ganz catheter
	Systemic blood pressure	Arterial catheter

From Phillipson EA: Sleep disorders. In Murray JF, Nadel JF: *Textbook of respiratory medicine*, Philadelphia, 1994, WB Saunders.
SaO$_2$, Hemoximetry oxygen saturation; *PCO$_2$*, partial pressure of carbon dioxide; *EEG*, electroencephalogram; *EOG*, electro-oculogram; *EMG*, electromyogram.

Polysomnography

Clinical Practice Guideline 15-1

■ INDICATIONS

Polysomnography may be indicated for patients with any of the following conditions:

· Chronic obstructive pulmonary disease with an awake partial pressure of arterial oxygen (PaO_2) > 55 mm Hg; the illness is complicated by pulmonary hypertension, right ventricle failure, polycythemia, or excessive daytime sleepiness.

· Restrictive ventilatory impairment secondary to chest wall and neuromuscular disturbances; the illness is complicated by chronic hypoventilation, polycythemia, pulmonary hypertension, disturbed sleep, morning headaches, or daytime somnolence and fatigue.

· Disturbances of respiratory control with an awake partial pressure of arterial carbon dioxide ($PaCO_2$) > 45 mm Hg; the illness is complicated by pulmonary hypertension, polycythemia, disturbed sleep, morning headaches, or daytime somnolence and fatigue.

· Nocturnal cyclic bradyarrhythmias or tachyarrhythmias, nocturnal abnormalities of atrioventricular conduction, or ventricular ectopy that appears to increase in frequency during sleep.

· Excessive daytime sleepiness or insomnia.

· Snoring, which is associated with observed apneas or excessive daytime sleepiness.

■ CONTRAINDICATIONS

There are no absolute contraindications to polysomnography when indications are clearly established. Risk/benefit ratios should be assessed, however, if medically unstable inpatients are to be transferred from the clinical setting to a sleep laboratory for overnight polysomnography.

■ PRECAUTIONS/COMPLICATIONS:

· Skin irritation may occur as a result of the adhesive used to attach electrodes to the patient.

· At the conclusion of the study, adhesive remover is used to dissolve adhesive on the patient's skin. Adhesive removers (e.g., acetone) should be used only in well-ventilated areas.

· Engineering (or qualified biomedical) personnel must certify the integrity of the polysomnographic equipment's electrical isolation.

· The adhesive used to attach electroencephalographic electrodes (e.g., collodion) should not be used to attach electrodes near the patient's eyes and should always be used in well-ventilated areas.

· Because of the high flammability of collodion and acetone, they should be used with caution, especially with patients requiring supplemental oxygen.

· Collodion should be used with caution in infants and in patients with reactive airway disease.

· Patients with parasomnias or seizures may be at risk for injury related to movements during sleep. Institution-specific policies and guidelines describing personnel responsibilities and appropriate responses should be developed.

■ ASSESSMENT OF NEED

Polysomnography should be used to assess oxygenation, cardiac status, and sleep continuity in those patients who are suspected of having sleep-related respiratory disturbances, periodic limb-movement disorders, or any of the sleep disorders described in *The International Classification of Sleep Disorders: Diagnostic and Coding Manual.*

■ ASSESSMENT OF TEST QUALITY

· Polysomnography should either confirm or eliminate a diagnosis of a sleep-related respiratory disturbance.

· Documentation of findings, suggested therapeutic intervention, or other clinical decisions resulting from polysomnography should be noted on the patient's chart.

· Each laboratory should devise and implement indicators of quality assurance for equipment calibration and maintenance, patient preparation and monitoring, scoring methodology, and scoring variances among technicians.

For a complete copy of this guideline, see AARC-APT (American Association of Respiratory Care–Association of Polysomnography Technologists) clinical practice guideline. Polysomnography, Respir Care 40:1336-1343, 1995.

dardized system for electrode placement is used to record EEGs during sleep studies. The standard electroencephalographic montage used for polysomnography is based on the **International 10-20 EEG system** (Figure 15-4).[5,7] Note that modified electroencephalographic recordings that are typically used to determine sleep stages may not enable the identification of seizure disorders; therefore, in cases in which seizures are suspected, more elaborate electroencephalographic recordings, as well as a neurologic consultation, may be necessary.

To place electrodes properly, one should first mark where they will be placed on the scalp. It is important to

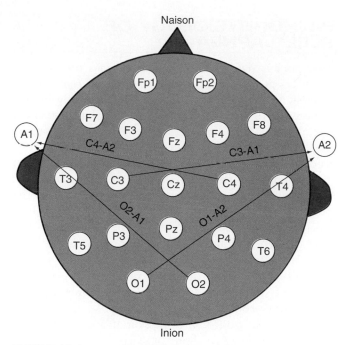

FIGURE 15-4 A standard polysomnographic EEG montage. (Redrawn from Sheldon SH, Spire JP, Levy HB: *Pediatric sleep medicine,* Philadelphia, 1992, WB Saunders.)

recognize that improper placement of these electrodes can severely affect the validity of the sleep study and lead to erroneous data. The scalp should be cleaned with alcohol to minimize electrical impedance. The cup-shaped electrodes are filled with conductive paste or jelly and affixed to the scalp with cotton or gauze. The electrodes can be affixed to the scalp with tape or glue, or they can be anchored to the scalp by placing a piece of gauze soaked in **collodion** over the electrode (notice that the gauze can be dried with compressed air after it has been positioned over the electrode). After the electrodes are affixed to the patient, the electrode wires are then plugged into a junction box, which is coupled to the polygraph recorder.

Respiratory Activity

Assessment of respiratory activity during sleep usually involves measuring oxygen saturation, nasal-oral airflow, and respiratory effort. Oxygen saturation can be easily assessed by using pulse oximetry or transcutaneous monitoring. (See Chapter 10 for a detailed discussion of noninvasive blood gas monitoring.) The pulse oximeter probe is placed on an earlobe, finger, or toe. Although transcutaneous monitoring can be used to assess oxygenation during sleep, the transcutaneous probe must be repositioned intermittently (every 2 to 4 hours) and may therefore interfere with the patient's sleep and lead to inadvertent arousal during the study. Indwelling arterial catheters can also be used to assess arterial blood gases, but the risks outweigh the benefits of using this approach and may lead to unnecessary complications.

Nasal-oral airflow is typically measured by a thermistor or thermocouple device at the airway opening. The most-

common problems with these devices relate to probe position (i.e., the technician may have to reposition the probe frequently and adjust the amplifier sensitivity, thus disturbing the patient's sleep and reducing the validity of the study).

Respiratory effort can be measured by recording rib cage and abdominal movements, by measuring intrapleural pressure changes, or by measuring airflow at the airway opening with a pneumotachograph. A variety of devices and techniques are available for measuring rib cage and abdominal movements, including strain gauge or piezoelectric belts placed around the chest or abdomen; respiratory inductance plethysmography; and impedance pneumography. Intrapleural pressure changes can be measured with an esophageal balloon catheter positioned in the upper third of the esophagus that is connected to a standard strain gauge pressure transducer.

Remember that although all of these techniques can provide measurements of respiratory effort, techniques that restrict patient movement can compromise test results. Techniques that make the patient uncomfortable can ultimately decrease patient compliance during the study.

Electromyography

EMG recording of various skeletal muscles can be accomplished during sleep by using surface electrodes similar to those used for ECGs. EMG signals can provide information about the patient's sleep-wake behavior; such monitoring also allows arousal responses and sleep movements to be quantified. EMG signals recorded from the intercostal muscles can also be used to assess respiratory movements, which is a rather cumbersome technique considering the alternative methods of measuring respiratory activity that were discussed in the previous section.

Three electrodes are typically affixed to the chin with tape. Two of these electrodes are placed between the tip of the chin and the hyoid bone, lateral to each other and 2 cm apart; a third electrode is placed in the center of the chin. The submental EMG signal recorded from these electrodes is used to detect activation of the muscles that expand the upper airways (e.g., the genioglossus and the geniohyoid).[8] When leg movements are to be assessed, two surface electrodes are taped approximately 3 cm to 5 cm apart on each leg over the tibialis anterior muscle.

Electro-oculography

The recording of eye movements during sleep allows the clinician to differentiate non-REM sleep states from REM sleep states. Electrodes are placed on the skin surface in the periorbital region, specifically about 1 cm lateral to the outer canthi of the eyes and offset from the horizontal plane (i.e., 1 cm above the horizontal plane on one side and 1 cm below the horizontal plane on the other side). With this configuration, the horizontal, vertical, and oblique movements of the eye can be detected. Figure 15-5 shows how these movements are recorded. Note that the height or depth of the deflection depends on the move-

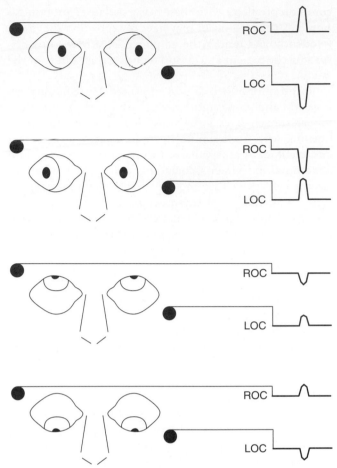

FIGURE 15-5 Electro-oculogram electrode placement. *ROC* indicates eye movement to the right of center; *LOC* indicates eye movement to the left of center. (Redrawn from Sheldon SH, Spire JP, Levy HB: *Pediatric sleep medicine,* Philadelphia, 1992, WB Saunders.)

ment of the eyes relative to the fixed electrodes and is described as being either *right-of-center* (ROC) or *left-of-center* (LOC).[5]

Calibration of Polysomnography Signals

An initial calibration of the polysomnography equipment should be performed before the electrodes are placed on the patient; for accurate calibration, the manufacturer's recommendations should be followed closely. (NOTE: Check the user's manual for details on calibrating various channels.) After the electrodes and sensors are affixed to the patient, a presleep calibration should be performed. This calibration lets the technician determine whether all of the electrodes and sensors are positioned properly, whether the amplifier settings are appropriate for retrieving meaningful data, and whether there are any recording device malfunctions (e.g., the chart recorder is functioning improperly). Calibration also provides a series of baseline references for awake measurements. Documenting all calibrations is essential because if calibration is performed inadequately, the test results are ultimately invalid.

PATHOPHYSIOLOGY OF SLEEP APNEA

Sleep apnea is defined as repeated episodes of complete airflow cessation for longer than 10 seconds.[9] *Hypopnea*, in contrast, is usually defined as a reduction in airflow by 50% or more for 10 seconds, with some residual airflow and a physiologic consequence (e.g., arterial oxygen desaturation).[10,11] To compare the frequency of apnea with that of hypopnea during a sleep study, an **apnea index (AI)** or an **apnea/hypopnea index (AHI)** is usually calculated. The AI is the number of apneic periods observed divided by the total number of hours of sleep; the AHI consists of both apneic and hypopneic episodes for the total number of hours of sleep. Normative data on asymptomatic individuals from the study by Guilleminault and Dement[12] suggest that males average approximately seven apneic episodes per 8 hours of sleep, whereas females average only approximately two episodes per 8 hours of sleep.

Sleep apnea syndrome is present if apnea occurs in excess of five times per hour of sleep.[10,11] As such, three types of sleep apnea are generally described: **obstructive sleep apnea (OSA)**, **central sleep apnea**, and **mixed sleep apnea**. OSA is characterized by the lack of airflow resulting from occlusion of the upper airways despite continued respiratory efforts. Central sleep apnea is characterized by the absence of airflow and respiratory efforts. Mixed sleep apnea has characteristics of both central and obstructive sleep apnea, with the central event usually preceding the obstructive event.

Obstructive Sleep Apnea

In OSA, airflow at the airway opening ceases because of complete occlusion of the upper airway. Occlusion of the upper airway may occur with posterior movements of the tongue and palate. As these structures move posteriorly, they come into apposition with the posterior pharyngeal wall, resulting in occlusion of the nasopharynx and the oropharynx.[2] Figure 15-6 shows the sequence of events that typically occur in OSA. Notice that obstruction of the upper airways initiates the primary sequence of events. Then apnea and progressive asphyxia develop until there is arousal from sleep, restoration of upper airway patency, and resumption of airflow. With relief from the asphyxia, the person quickly returns to sleep—only to have the sequence of events repeat itself over and over. In fact, the sequence can repeat itself several hundred times per night.[13]

As seen in Figure 15-7, OSA is associated with several physiologic consequences and clinical features.[14] The physiologic consequences of OSA include the development of cardiac arrhythmias, pulmonary and systemic hypertension, acute hypercapnia, cerebral dysfunction, loss of deep sleep, sleep fragmentation, and excessive motor activity. These physiologic alterations can in turn result in restless sleep, excessive daytime sleepiness, personality and behavioral changes, intellectual deterioration, right heart failure, and unexplained nocturnal death.[2]

Underlying Mechanisms   Primary Events

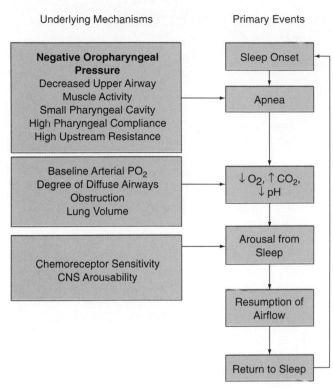

FIGURE 15-6 The primary sequence of events in obstructive sleep apnea (OSA), along with the pathogenic mechanisms that contribute to these events. (Redrawn from Bradley TD, Phillipson EA: Pathogenesis and pathophysiology of the obstructive sleep apnea syndrome, *Med Clin North Am* 69:1169-1185, 1985.)

The symptoms most commonly associated with OSA in adult patients include chronic loud snoring, gasping or choking episodes during sleep, excessive daytime sleepiness, morning headaches, and personality and cognitive deterioration related to fatigue from lack of sleep. Box 15-2 contains the standard definition of OSA, which was published by the American Sleep Disorders Association.[15] Patients at the greatest risk of developing OSA are those who are obese (particularly those with nuchal obesity [i.e., neck size >17 inches for men and >16 inches for women] and nasopharyngeal narrowing). Systemic hypertension also adds to the risk of OSA. The symptoms of OSA may be worse when patients ingest central nervous system depressants (e.g., sedatives, hypnotics) or consume alcohol, especially when it is ingested close to bedtime. Partial sleep deprivation, which can occur with shift work, may also affect patients with moderate OSA symptoms. Respiratory allergies and environmental factors such as smoking and ascent to altitude can augment the symptoms of patients with mild OSA.

Figure 15-8 shows the key polysomnographic events that occur during the apneic episode of a patient with OSA. Although there is a cessation of airflow, the patient's respiratory efforts continue, as evidenced by movement of the rib cage and the abdomen. During the apneic episode, there is a fall in oxygen saturation. Clinical Rounds 15-1 presents the case of a patient with OSA.

BOX 15-2   Standard Definition of Obstructive Sleep Apnea

1. A patient reports excessive sleepiness or insomnia. Occasionally, patients are unaware of the clinical features observed by others.
2. A patient experiences frequent episodes of obstructed breathing during sleep.
3. Associated features include loud snoring, morning headaches, a dry mouth upon awakening, and chest retraction during sleep in younger children.
4. Polysomnographic monitoring reveals more than five obstructive apneas, each of 10 seconds' duration, per hour of sleep, and one or more of the following:
   · Frequent arousal from sleep, a condition associated with apneas
   · Bradytachycardia
   · Arterial oxygen desaturation in association with the apneic episode—with or without a multi–sleep latency period of less than 10 minutes
5. OSA can be associated with other medical disorders (e.g., tonsillar enlargement).
6. Other sleep disorders can be present (e.g., periodic limb-movement disorder or narcolepsy).

From American Sleep Disorders Association, Diagnostic Steering Committee: *The international classification of sleep disorders: diagnostic and coding manual*, ed 2, Lawrence, Kansas, 1997, Allen Press.

CLINICAL ROUNDS 15-1

Mr. H. is a 62-year-old automobile mechanic with a 60 pack-per-year history of smoking cigarettes. He was referred to the sleep laboratory after he was involved in an automobile accident when he reportedly fell asleep while driving home from work. He is unaware of any chronic abnormalities with his sleep pattern, but he does acknowledge that he has experienced excessive daytime sleepiness. His wife reports that she has noticed that he snores throughout the night and his sleep has become increasingly restless during the past 6 months. In fact, his wife reports that his snoring has become loud enough to disturb her sleep and she jokes that if his snoring gets any louder, the neighbor may begin to complain. She also reports that his snoring episodes are more frequent and considerably louder if he has a nightcap (i.e., consumes an alcoholic drink) before going to sleep.

Does this patient demonstrate any history and physical findings that suggest the presence of obstructive sleep apnea? Briefly describe a diagnostic strategy to properly diagnose his condition.

See Evolve Resources for the answer.

The criteria for defining OSA in children are not as well established as those in adults.[10] In children, OSA is best identified by combining phasic oxygen desaturation, hypercarbia, and intermittent paradoxical respiratory efforts. (NOTE: Oxygen desaturation of less than 92% is generally considered abnormal in children, depending on their baseline oxygen saturation. Brief oxygen desaturations of >4% occur infrequently in children and thus should be

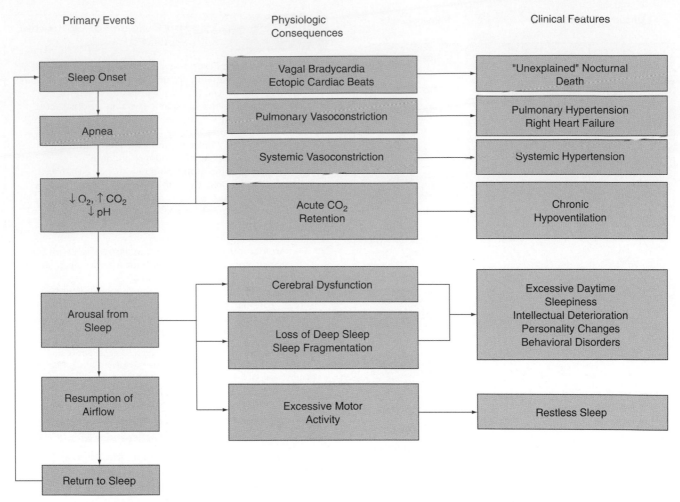

Primary Events   Physiologic   Clinical Features
                          Consequences

FIGURE 15-7 The physiologic response and clinical features that result from sleep apnea. (Redrawn from Phillipson EA: Sleep apnea, *Med Clin North Am* 23:2314-2323, 1982.)

considered abnormal. Measurements of end-tidal partial pressure of carbon dioxide [$P_{ET}CO_2$] can also provide evidence of sleep-disordered breathing in children. It has been suggested that $P_{ET}CO_2$ values of >45 mm Hg for at least 60% of the total sleep time or $P_{ET}CO_2$ values >13 mm Hg above baseline values indicate sleep-disordered breathing.)[10] Other criteria that should be noted when diagnosing sleep apnea in children are snoring, frequent arousal, and difficulty breathing while asleep, as well as failure to thrive, cor pulmonale, or neurobehavioral disturbances.[16]

Central Sleep Apnea

Central sleep apnea includes several disorders associated with the cessation of respiratory drive and a complete loss of EMG activity in the respiratory muscles. Several mechanisms that have been proposed to account for these alterations involve defects in respiratory control or muscle function, transient fluctuation in respiratory drive, and reflex inhibition of the central respiratory drive.[2] Central sleep apnea is associated with central alveolar hypoventilation, neuromuscular diseases involving the respiratory muscles, and central nervous system diseases, but it can occur secondary to hyperventilation when a person ascends

to high altitudes. Central sleep apnea is also a common finding in patients who experience esophageal reflux or upper airway collapse. It is important to mention that only approximately 10% of patients with apnea who are seen in most sleep laboratories have central sleep apnea; thus, our knowledge of this disorder is somewhat limited when compared with the information available about OSA.[17]

Patients with central sleep apnea typically report gasping for air and shortness of breath upon awakening from a central sleep apneic episode. Depression, as assessed both subjectively and by formal testing, is a common finding among patients with central sleep apnea. It is interesting to note that patients with central sleep apnea do not normally report insomnia and hypersomnolence as do those with OSA. Patients with central sleep apnea typically have a normal body habitus, although obese patients may also exhibit this form of sleep apnea.

Figure 15-9 shows an example of a polysomnographic tracing for a patient with central sleep apnea. As with OSA, there is a complete cessation of airflow that lasts for 10 seconds or longer. However, in contrast to OSA, airflow cessation is associated with a cessation in respiratory effort and thus no movement of the rib cage or abdomen.

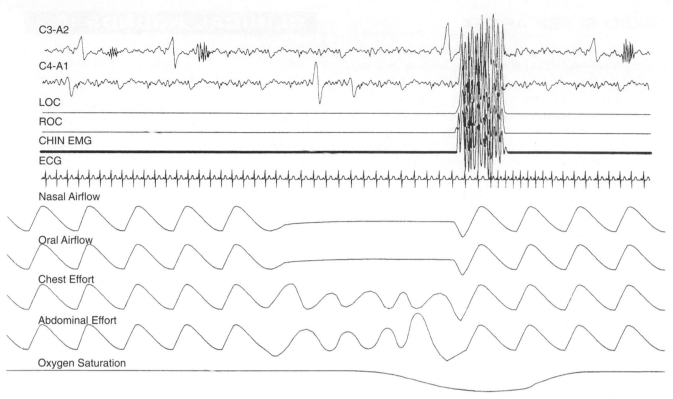

FIGURE 15-8 Polysomnographic tracings of a patient exhibiting OSA during REM sleep. The patient exhibited constant loud snoring, paradoxical movement of the chest and abdomen, and recurrent complete airway obstructions, leading to oxygen desaturation. (Redrawn from Sheldon SH, Spire JP, Levy HB: *Pediatric sleep medicine,* Philadelphia, 1992, WB Saunders.)

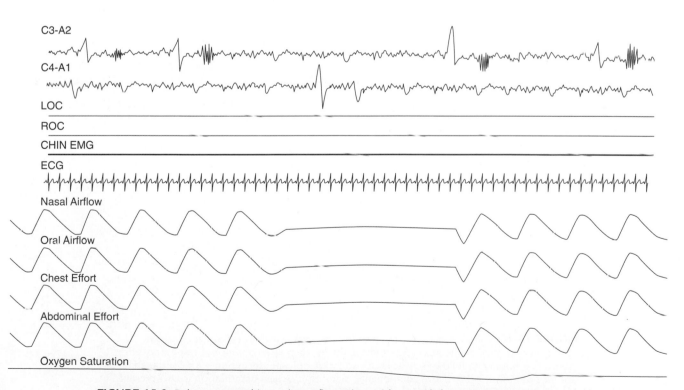

FIGURE 15-9 Polysomnographic tracings of a patient with central sleep apnea. Note that during the apneic episode there is complete cessation of nasal and oral airflow with concomitant absence of respiratory effort (i.e., no movements of chest or abdomen). (Redrawn from Sheldon SH, Spire JP, Levy HB: *Pediatric sleep medicine,* Philadelphia, 1992, WB Saunders.)

MIXED SLEEP APNEA

Most patients who experience central sleep apnea also demonstrate evidence of OSA. In fact, because these two types of apnea typically coexist, most authors define *central sleep apnea* as a condition occurring in individuals in whom more than 55% of the apneic episodes are central in origin. The exact cause of mixed apnea is unclear at this time; nonetheless, it has been suggested that the mechanisms responsible for central and obstructive sleep apnea may be related, because several studies have shown that the upper airway muscles behave like respiratory muscles. That is, the upper airway muscles contract and dilate the pharynx when the diaphragm is stimulated.[18,19]

Polysomnography provides clear evidence of the presence of mixed apnea. As Figure 15-10 shows, airflow cessation is preceded by a central apneic event (i.e., no movement of the rib cage or abdomen). The obstructive component can be ascertained by observing that there is a resumption of respiratory effort, although there is still a cessation of airflow. With arousal from sleep, the apneic event ends and airflow resumes as the airway opens (Clinical Rounds 15-2).

CLINICAL ROUNDS 15-2

The following polysomnogram was obtained from a 45-year-old patient who had been treated for polio and who was later referred to the sleep laboratory for diagnosis of possible sleep apnea. She reports restless sleep, morning headaches, chronic fatigue, and daytime sleepiness. Interpret these findings.

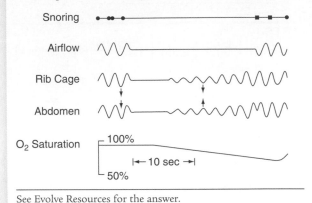

See Evolve Resources for the answer.

FIGURE 15-10 Polysomnographic tracings from a patient with mixed apnea. There is cessation of airflow at the nose and mouth. Initially, there is an absence of respiratory effort (central component), followed by at least two cycles of respiratory effort with continued absence of airflow (obstructive component). Significant oxygen desaturation is also present. Note that the EEG, electro-oculographic, and EMG signals are obscured by motion artifacts. (Redrawn from Sheldon SH, Spire JP, Levy HB: *Pediatric sleep medicine*, Philadelphia, 1992, WB Saunders.)

KEY POINTS

▶ The physiologic effects of sleep on breathing are normally of little consequence in healthy individuals. In patients with altered respiratory function, however, sleep can have profound effects on physiologic function that—if left untreated—can lead to dire consequences.

▶ Recent advances in our understanding of sleep structure and the ability to assess cardiopulmonary and neuromuscular function during sleep have greatly improved our ability to recognize and treat sleep-related disorders.

▶ Three types of sleep apnea have been described: obstructive, central, and mixed.

▶ OSA is characterized by airflow cessation at the airway opening, even though the patient continues to make respiratory efforts.

▶ Central sleep apnea involves a complete cessation of respiratory efforts and airflow, and mixed apnea includes characteristics of both obstructive apnea and central apnea.

▶ Patients with mixed apnea typically experience a central apneic component before the obstructive event occurs.

▶ Diagnosis of sleep apnea is based on clinical findings, including patient history and physical examination, along with the data from laboratory studies.

▶ Obtaining a complete history and the results of a physical examination is the first step in identifying whether an individual is at risk for sleep apnea.

▶ Overnight monitoring of arterial blood gases with pulse oximetry or transcutaneous electrodes or polysomnography is then performed to make a definitive diagnosis of sleep apnea.

▶ Although there is some controversy about the best strategy to use when attempting to diagnose sleep apnea, it is generally agreed that polysomnography is the gold standard for evaluating the presence and severity of sleep apnea.

▶ Polysomnography involves recording various electrogenic potentials (e.g., ECGs, EEGs, respiratory activity, and electrooculograms) and can also be used to select the most effective management strategy after sleep apnea is identified in a patient.

ASSESSMENT QUESTIONS

See Evolve Resources for answers.

1. Which of the following are characteristic findings of stage 2 non-REM sleep?
   I. Sleep spindles and K-complexes are seen on an EEG.
   II. Slow, pendulous, and disconjugate movements of the eyes.
   III. A relatively low threshold for arousal from sleep.
   IV. Adult patients typically enter this stage of sleep after approximately 90 minutes of non-REM sleep.
   a. I and II only
   b. II and IV only
   c. I, II, and III only
   d. II, III, and IV only

2. The classic states of non-REM sleep and REM sleep are not easily identified at birth with the use of standard polysomnography. Briefly describe the structure of sleep for a 2-week-old neonate.

3. Describe the impact of sleep on breathing in a healthy adult.

4. Which of the following changes in cardiovascular function occurs during sleep?
   a. Heart rate increases by approximately 5 to 10 beats/min during non-REM sleep.
   b. Blood pressure decreases by as much as 25 mm Hg during REM sleep.
   c. Cardiac output increases only slightly during non-REM sleep.
   d. Stroke volume remains constant during non-REM sleep and REM sleep.

5. It is suggested that when performing polysomnography, the technician monitor a minimum of at least two modified electrocardiographic leads. True or False?

6. Sleep apnea is present if the person experiences at least how many apneic events per hour of sleep?
   a. 3
   b. 5
   c. 8
   d. 10

7. List three variables that should be monitored to assess respiratory activity during polysomnography.

8. Which of the following are typical history and physical findings in patients with OSA?
   I. Chronic loud snoring
   II. Excessive daytime sleepiness
   III. Personality changes
   IV. Obesity
   a. I and III only
   b. II and IV only
   c. I, II, and III only
   d. I, II, III, and IV

9. Describe the physiologic consequences of OSA.

10. Which of the following are associated with central sleep apnea?
    I. Alveolar hypoventilation
    II. Myasthenia gravis
    III. Stroke
    IV. Angina pectoris
    a. I and II only
    b. II and III only
    c. I, II, and III only
    d. I, III, and IV only

ASSESSMENT QUESTIONS—cont'd

11. Which of the following conditions will a patient experience during periods of mixed apnea with hypoxemia?
    a. Systemic hypotension
    b. Increased cardiac output
    c. Decreased heart rate
    d. Pulmonary hypertension

12. Which of the following are characteristic findings in children with obstructive sleep apnea?
    I. Phasic oxygen desaturation
    II. Hypercarbia
    III. Intermittent paradoxical respiratory efforts
    IV. Sinus tachycardia
    a. I and III only
    b. II and IV only
    c. I, II, and III only
    d. I, II, III, and IV

13. Which of the following are typical findings for patients with central sleep apnea?
    I. These patients rarely report insomnia.
    II. The patient reports gasping for air upon awakening after an apneic event.
    III. Depression is a common finding in these patients.
    IV. Most of these patients are grossly overweight.
    a. I and II only
    b. II and III only
    c. I, II, and III only
    d. II, III, and IV only

14. Define the apnea/hypopnea index, and describe how normative data for male subjects differ from those for female subjects.

15. Which of the following drugs increase the incidence of obstructive sleep apnea?
    I. Ethanol
    II. Sedatives
    III. Tricyclic antidepressants
    IV. Hypnotics
    a. II and III only
    b. I, II, and III only
    c. I, II, and IV only
    d. I, III, and IV only

References

1. Guilleminault C, Dement WC: General physiology of sleep. In Crystal RG, West JB, editors: *The lung: scientific foundations*, New York, 1991, Raven Press, Ltd.
2. Bradley TD, Phillipson EA: Sleep disorders. In Murray JF, Nadel JA, editors: *Respiratory medicine*, ed 3, Philadelphia, 1994, WB Saunders.
3. Aserinsky E, Kleitman N: Regularly occurring periods of eye motility, and concomitant phenomena, during sleep, *Science* 118:273-274, 1953.
4. Guyton AC, Hall JE: *Human physiology and mechanisms of disease*, ed 6, Philadelphia, 1996, WB Saunders.
5. Sheldon SH, Spire JP, Levy HB: *Pediatric sleep medicine*, Philadelphia, 1992, WB Saunders.
6. AARC-APT (American Association of Respiratory Care-Association of Polysomnography Technologists) clinical practice guideline. Polysomnography, *Respir Care* 40:1336-1343, 1995.
7. Jasper HH: The ten-twenty system of the International Federation, *Electroencephalogr Clin Neurophysiol* 10:371, 1958.
8. Funsten AW, Suratt PM: Evaluation of respiratory disorders during sleep, *Clin Chest Med* 10:265-276, 1989.
9. Strollo PJ, Fernandez KS: Disorders of sleep. In Scanlan CL, Wilkins RL, Stoller JK, editors: *Egan's fundamentals of respiratory care*, ed 7, St Louis, 1998, Mosby.
10. Phillips BA, Anstead MI, Gottlieb DJ: Monitoring sleep and breathing: methodology. Part I: Monitoring breathing, *Clin Chest Med* 19:203-212, 1998.
11. Arand DL, Bonnet MH: Sleep-disordered breathing. In Burton GC, Hodgkin JE, Ward JJ: *Respiratory care: a guide to clinical practice*, ed 4, Philadelphia, 1997, Lippincott Williams & Wilkins.
12. Guilleminault C, Dement WC: Sleep apnea syndromes and related sleep disorders. In Williams RL, Karacan I, editors: *Sleep disorders: diagnosis and treatment*, New York, 1978, Wiley & Sons.
13. McNicholas WT, Phillipson EA: *Breathing disorders in sleep*, Philadelphia, 2002, WB Saunders.
14. Phillipson EA: Sleep apnea, *Med Clin North Am* 23:2314, 1982.
15. American Sleep Disorders Association, Diagnostic Steering Committee: *The international classification of sleep disorders: diagnostic and coding manual*, ed 2, Lawrence, Kan, 1997, Allen Press.
16. Dyson M, Beckerman RC, Brouillette RT: Obstructive sleep apnea syndrome. In Beckerman RC, Brouillette RT, Hunt CE, editors: *Respiratory control disorders in infants and children*, Baltimore, 1992, Williams & Wilkins.
17. Guilleminault C, van den Hoed J, Mitler MM: Clinical overview of the sleep apnea syndromes. In Guilleminault C, Dement WC, editors: *Sleep apnea syndromes*, New York, 1978, Alan R. Liss.
18. Onal E, Lopata M, O'Connor T: Pathogenesis of apneas in hypersomnia–sleep apnea syndrome, *Am Rev Respir Dis* 125:167-174, 1982.
19. Dement WC, Vaughan C: *The promise of sleep*, New York, 1999, Delacorte Press/Random House.

Internet Resources

American Association for Respiratory Care: http://www.aarc.org

American Sleep Apnea Association: http://www.sleepapnea.org

American Thoracic Society: http://www.thoracic.org

The American Association of Sleep Technologists (formerly The Association of Polysomnographic Technologists, at http://www.aptweb.org): http://www.aastweb.org/

National Heart, Lung, and Blood Institute: http://www.nhlbi.nih.gov/

National Institute of Neurological Disorders and Stroke: http://www.ninds.nih.gov

National Jewish Health™ (formerly National Jewish Medical and Research Center, at http://www.njc.org): http://www.nationaljewish.org/

Sleepnet: http://www.sleepnet.com

Glossary

100% O₂ suction A control on the Puritan Bennett 7200 ventilator that enables the ventilator to deliver 100% O_2 for 2 minutes. Intended for use before suctioning the patient.

absolute humidity The actual mass or content of water in a measured volume of air. It is usually expressed in grams per cubic meter or pounds.

absolute zero The temperature at which no molecular motion occurs: $-273°$ C, or $0°$ K.

absorbance sensor An apparatus designed to react to physical stimuli from light or other radiant energy.

accelerating waveform A pressure-time or flow-time tracing that indicates upward or increasing movement (acceleration) of the pressure or flow value over time.

accumulator A device that allows a volume of gas to be held for a period of time and then releases the gas at a preset rate. Used as a timing or limiting mechanism.

accuracy The state or quality of being precise or exact.

acid-fast bacteria Of, or pertaining to, certain bacteria (especially *Mycobacteria* spp.) that retain red dyes after an acid wash.

acoustics The science of sounds.

action potential An electrical impulse consisting of a self-propagating series of polarizations and depolarizations transmitted across the plasma membrane of nerve and muscle cells.

actual bicarbonate The concentration of HCO_3^- that is present in the plasma of anaerobically drawn blood. It is derived from measurements of pH and partial pressure of arterial carbon dioxide ($PaCO_2$) with the Henderson-Hasselbalch equation.

adaptive pressure ventilation (APV) A closed-loop (servo-controlled) mode of ventilation available on the Hamilton GALILEO ventilator that provides pressure-targeted ventilation with a volume guarantee.

adaptive support ventilation (ASV) A closed-loop mode of ventilation available on the Hamilton GALILEO that uses pressure-targeted ventilation to ensure a certain minute volume. The ventilator enables prediction of tidal volume and respiratory rate based on the patient information entered by the operator, constantly monitors patient and ventilator parameters, and adjusts breath delivery to establish the least amount of work possible for the patient.

adhesion The physical property by which unlike substances are attracted and hold together; also refers to the abnormal formation of fibrous tissues (resulting from inflammation or injury) that bind together body structures that are normally separate.

adjustable reducing valve See *adjustable regulator*.

adjustable regulator A valve that allows the user to determine (adjust) pressure limits.

adjustable restrictor A mechanism that governs flow or pressure with a series of variable-sized orifices.

aerobe A microorganism that lives and grows in the presence of free oxygen.

aerosol A suspension of solid or liquid particles in a gas.

aerosol mask A device covering both the nose and mouth that is used to deliver aerosols in respiratory care.

air dilution Adding air to a primary gas to reduce the oxygen concentration of the primary gas.

air-dilution control A mechanism that allows the user to set the amount of air dilution in a device.

air-entrainment mask An oxygen mask that uses a Venturi or Pitot type of device to provide precise concentrations of high-flow oxygen to a patient.

air foil A device that acts like an airplane wing in the generation of pressure differences by creating areas of high and low resistance in an airstream.

air inlet regulator A regulator that determines the inlet pressure on a gas system or ventilator.

air-mix control Another name for an air-dilution control. Used in the Bird Mark and Bennett TV and PR series respirators.

airborne Carried in the air via aerosol droplets, droplet nuclei, or dust particles.

airborne precautions Safeguards designed to reduce the risk of airborne transmission of infectious agents.

airway pressure Pressure achieved in the patient airway.

airway pressure-release ventilation (APRV) A mode of ventilation during which the patient breathes spontaneously at an elevated baseline but the airway is periodically "released" to allow expiration.

airway resistance (R_{aw}) A measure of the impedance to ventilation caused by gas movement through the airways. It is computed as the change in pressure along a tube, divided by the gas flow through the tube.

alarm A signal that is a warning of danger, such as a high-pressure or apnea alarm.

alarm silence A control button that silences audible alarms for approximately 60 seconds or until it is pressed a second time.

Allen's test A test for the patency of the ulnar or radial artery. The patient's hand is formed into a fist while the therapist compresses the ulnar or radial arteries. Compression continues while the fist is flexed. If blood perfusion through the ulnar artery is adequate, the hand should flush and resume normal (pink) coloration when the ulnar artery compression is released.

alpha wave One of the four types of brain waves, characterized by a relatively high voltage or amplitude and a frequency of 8 to 13 Hertz. Alpha waves are the "relaxed waves" of the brain and are the majority of the waves recorded by electroencephalograms. Compare this term with *beta wave*, *delta wave*, and *theta wave*.

alternating current (AC) An electric current that reverses direction according to a consistent sinusoidal pattern. Compare this with *direct current*.

alternating supply system A gas-supply system that has two supplies of compressed gas (primary and secondary). The secondary system is used when the primary system fails.

alveolar ventilation (AV) The volume of air that ventilates all the perfused alveoli, measured as minute volume in liters per minute. This figure is also the difference between total ventilation and dead space ventilation. The normal average is from 4 to 5 L/min.

ambient compartment In the Bird Mark ventilator series, the portion of the ventilator casing that is open to the environment and hence to ambient pressures.

ambient inlet filter A portion of an air entrainment device that removes dust particles and other debris from the entrained air before it enters the gas circuit.

AMBU (air-mask-bag-unit) A type of manual resuscitator consisting of a pliable bag, a one-way valve system, and either a mask or an artificial airway connector.

American Standard Indexing A type of safety system for high-pressure gas connections. American Standard connections are noninterchangeable to prevent the interchange of regulator equipment among gases. American Standard Indexing has separate systems for large and small cylinders.

ammeter An instrument for measuring the strength of an electric current in terms of amperes.

amorphous solids A solid, such as glass or margarine, in which the constituent atoms and molecules are arranged in a fashion that is not rigid. In contrast, the constituent particles of crystalline solids are more rigidly arranged.

amperometric Refers to measuring an electric current at a single applied potential.

amplitude The height of a waveform; usually indicative of intensity.

anaerobe A microorganism that grows and lives in the absence of oxygen.

analog pressure manometer A backup method of verifying digitally displayed pressure values (peak, mean, and plateau pressure).

analyte Any substance that is measured; usually applied to a component of blood or other body fluid.

AND/NAND gate A monostable fluidic element with two control ports and two outlet ports.

anemometer A gauge for determining the force or speed and sometimes the direction of the wind or air.

aneroid barometer See *aneroid manometer.*

aneroid manometer A pressure-measuring device that compares a reference pressure to an observed pressure (by using one of several methods).

aneroid manometer assist indicator (cycle indicator) A light that signals a pressure change in an aneroid manometer indicating that the patient has generated a negative pressure (assist effort).

antisuffocation valve An internal, subambient relief valve on a ventilator that opens if the ventilator cannot provide a breath to the patient. The patient can then inhale, open the valve, and receive room air.

AP series A Bennett ventilator series used for intermittent positive pressure breathing (IPPB) administration. *AP* stands for *air-compressor-powered.*

apnea alarm A system that warns that the patient is not breathing or is not being ventilated.

apneic period A reference to a setting that is adjustable from 2 to 60 seconds to warn that a patient is not breathing.

apneic ventilation Emergency backup ventilation triggered when no patient breath is detected for a certain period of time.

apneustic flow time A reference to a control on the old Bird Mark series ventilators that limited the length of apnea or no flow allowed by the ventilator.

Archimedes' principle States that when an object is submerged in a fluid, it will be buoyed up by a force equal to the weight of the fluid that is displaced by the object.

arousal response A response to sensory stimulation to induce active wakefulness.

artificial nose See *heat and moisture exchanger.*

assist A mode of ventilation in which every breath is patient triggered.

assist and sensitivity mechanism A device that sets the maximum effort a patient must make (sensitivity) before the ventilator triggers (assists).

assist/control (A/C) mode Continuous mandatory ventilation (CMV) in which the minimum breathing rate is predetermined, but the patient can initiate ventilation at an increased rate with a set tidal volume or pressure.

assist/control pressure-targeted A mode of ventilation in which the operator selects a pressure for inspiration. Breaths can be patient triggered or time triggered.

assisted breaths Breaths in which the patient begins inspiration, but the ventilator controls the inspiratory phase and ends inspiration.

assistor A ventilator that lets the patient initiate inspiration.

assistor/controller A ventilator that can function as an assistor or as a controller.

atmospheric barometric pressure The force exerted by the air column extending from the measuring site to the edge of space (i.e., 760 mm Hg at sea level). Sometimes called *ambient pressure.*

atmospheric-to-subatmospheric pressure gradient The difference in the force exerted by the ambient pressure and that exerted in a negative-pressure system. May be called *driving pressure.*

atom The smallest division of an element that exhibits all the properties and characteristics of that element, including neutrons, electrons, and protons. The number of protons in the nucleus of every atom of a given element is the same and is called its *atomic number.*

atomic theory The concept that all matter is composed of submicroscopic atoms that are in turn composed of protons, electrons, and neutrons. A chemical element is identified by the number of protons in its atoms.

atrial diastole A period of rest of the atria of the heart.

atrial fibrillation A cardiac rhythm characterized by disorganized electrical activity in the atria accompanied by an irregular ventricular response that is usually rapid.

atrial flutter A type of atrial tachycardia with rates greater than 230 beats per minute. The atria lose their ability to contract normally and typically appear to quiver.

atrial premature depolarization An atrial beat that occurs earlier than expected. Also known as *premature atrial beat.*

atrial systole The contraction of the atria of the heart, which precedes ventricular contraction by a fraction of a second.

autoclave An apparatus that uses steam under pressure to sterilize articles and equipment.

autoflow A dual mode of ventilation that provides pressure-targeted breaths with volume guarantee whenever *volume ventilation* (CMV, synchronized intermittent mandatory ventilation [SIMV], or mandatory minute ventilation [MMV]) is simultaneously selected in the Dräger E-4 ventilator. It also alters the function of the inspiratory and expiratory valves, allowing patients to receive whatever inspiratory flow they demand—up to 180 L/min in any volume mode—regardless of the volume settings.

automaticity The property of the heart to initiate an action potential in the absence of external stimuli.

automode A ventilator feature (available on the Servo 300A) designed to switch from a control to a support mode of ventilation if the patient triggers two consecutive breaths. The ventilator remains in the support mode as long as the patient keeps triggering breaths.

auto-PEEP (positive end-expiratory pressure) Abnormal and usually undetected residual pressure above atmospheric pressure remaining in the alveoli at end-exhalation caused by dynamic air trapping. Also called *intrinsic PEEP*.

B

Babington/hydrosphere nebulizer A type of nebulizer in which a thin film of water flows over a hollow glass sphere with a slit in it, through which a high-flow gas stream is passed, creating a high-density aerosol.

bacilli Aerobic or facultatively aerobic, spore-bearing, rod-shaped microorganisms of *Bacillaceae* spp.

back pressure A reduction in the pressure gradient secondary to downflow resistance.

back-pressure compensation Any method that allows accurate pressures and flows to be read.

back-pressure switch A fluidic element with one control port that has a loop with a built-in restriction and two outlet ports.

backup rate A control rate set on a ventilator to take over if a patient's assisted ventilation falls below the desired rate.

backup ventilation (BUV) A mode of volume ventilation (available on the Puritan Bennett 7200 ventilators) with a minimum breath rate that goes into effect if the patient becomes apneic.

bacteria filter A device designed to remove particles and bacteria from the system. Usually rated in pore size or in microns.

bactericide Any drug or other agent that kills bacteria.

baffle Any obstruction in an aerosol's path that breaks the aerosol into smaller particles.

base excess/deficit The number of millimoles of strong acid or base required to titrate a blood sample to a pH of 7.4, a partial pressure of carbon dioxide (PCO_2) of 40 mm Hg, and a temperature of 37° C.

base flow The flow added to the circuit during exhalation to provide flow-triggering; see also *bias flow*.

baseline pressure The pressure level at which inspiration begins and ends.

beam deflection The change in the direction of a beam or jet of gas when it is hit with another jet of gas moving through a fluid device.

Bell factor In a water-sealed spirometer, the number of milliliters of gas that must be displaced to cause a kymographic pen to move 1 mm.

bellows accumulator A device used to store a volume of gas that will be pressurized for delivery to the patient. Usually a bag or bellows.

bellows chamber The inside of a bellows containing a volume of gas.

bellows potentiometer A mechanism that senses the volume displacement of a bellows and releases the contents at a preset value, usually through an electrical signal.

Bennett Cascade A specialized, heated passover humidifier that makes use of a water-air froth as a humidifying technique.

Bennett circuit The patient gas-delivery tubing that includes all of the tubing and ancillary devices from the machine to the patient and back.

Bennett MA-1 (Mechanical Assistor-1) ventilator A mechanical volume ventilator previously manufactured by the Puritan Bennett Corporation.

Bennett PR ventilators Bennett Pressure Respirator series (1 and 2) pneumatically powered assistor/controllers. No longer produced.

Bennett valve A drumlike device with pressure/flow–sensitive vanes that controls gas pressure and flow in the Bennett PR and AP series respirators.

Berman airway An upper airway device (oropharyngeal airway) used to provide air passage distal to the tongue by keeping the base of the tongue away from the back of the throat.

beta wave One of the four types of brain waves, characterized by relatively low voltage and a frequency of more than 13 Hertz. Beta waves are the "busy waves" of the brain. Compare this term with *alpha wave*, *delta wave*, and *theta wave*.

bias alert A message provided on the Bird T-Bird AVS ventilator that informs the operator of the bias flow setting after self-testing at start-up.

bias flow Flow in the circuit during the expiratory phase of mechanical ventilation that makes fresh gas immediately available when the patient inhales. Bias flow also reduces the ventilator's response time for triggering a breath.

bilevel positive airway pressure (BiPAP) A variant of continuous positive airway pressure in which both inspiratory and expiratory pressures are set by the operator.

bilevel positive airway pressure (BiPAP) A spontaneous breath mode of ventilatory support that allows separate regulation of the inspiratory and expiratory pressures. Also called *bilevel pressure assist* or *bilevel pressure support*.

BiPAP Abbreviation for *bilevel positive airway pressure*.

bistable A special type of fluidic control unit that acts as a switch mechanism.

bleed hole A small hole in the center body of the Bird Mark series respirators that allows pressure equalization across the center body or a small hole in an accumulator device that allows the measured escape of gas to "dump" the accumulator's contents.

bleed regulator An adjustable bleed hole.

blower A mechanical device sometimes used to control volume delivery in a mechanical ventilator (e.g., a rotating vane that produces a flow of gas).

body humidity The absolute humidity in a volume of gas saturated at a body temperature of 37° C; equivalent to 43.8 mg/L.

body plethysmography A method of studying alveolar pressures, lung volumes, and airway resistance. The patient sits or reclines in an airtight compartment and breathes normally. The pressure changes in the alveoli are reciprocated in the compartment and recorded automatically by the body plethysmograph.

body tank respirator An iron lung; a type of negative-pressure ventilator.

boiling point The temperature at which a liquid begins to turn to a gas. For water at 1 atm: 100° C, 212° F, or 373° K Absolute.

Boothby-Lovelace-Bulbulian (BLB) mask An apparatus for administering oxygen; consists of a mask fitted with an inspiratory-expiratory valve and a rebreathing bag.

Bourdon flowmeter A flowmeter that incorporates a Bourdon gauge.

Bourdon gauge A device that indicates pressure measurements from the use of a hollow, coiled tube that attempts to straighten in response to increased pressure.

Bourdon regulator A regulator that incorporates a Bourdon gauge.

bpm (breaths per minute) respiratory rate Usually a digital or analog indicator on the ventilator control panel.

brownian movement The random movement of molecules/particles caused by the molecules being struck by other molecules/particles.

BTPS Abbreviation for *body temperature, ambient pressure, saturated* (with water vapor).

bubble humidifier A device that increases the water content of a gas by passing it through a volume of water.

buffer base The total blood buffer capable of binding hydrogen ions. Normal buffer base (NBB) ranges from 48 to 52 mEq/L.

C

calorimetry A method of determining energy expenditure by using the measurements of the amount of heat radiated and absorbed by an organism.

capillary blood gases (CBGs) Gases dissolved in the blood that are obtained from a capillary sample. Results include pH, PCO_2, and partial pressure of oxygen (PO_2) values, which may differ from arterial blood gas values.

capillary mesh A netlike web with small openings that are used to measure flow and resistance in monitoring devices.

capillary system Microscopic tubes that connect arteries and veins and provide perfusion to tissues and cells.

capnogram A tracing that shows the proportion of carbon dioxide in exhaled air.

capnograph A device that measures and provides a graphic representation of the amount of carbon dioxide in a gas sample. A mainstream capnograph analyzes gas at the airway. With a sidestream capnograph, however, the gas to be analyzed is aspirated from the airway through a narrow-bore polyethylene tube and transferred to a sample chamber.

cardiac cycle The pressure, volume, and flow events that occur in the heart and great vessels during a typical heartbeat.

cardiac work The product of pressure and volume measurements that accompany ventricular contraction.

cardiopulmonary resuscitation (CPR) A basic emergency procedure for life support involving artificial respiration and manual external cardiac massage.

cascade humidifier A bubble humidifier in which gases travel down a tower and pass through a grid into a chamber of heated water. The displaced water rises above the grid, forming a liquid film that is converted to froth as the gas also rises from the chamber through the grid. The process results in an airflow that can have a relative humidity of up to 100%. See also *Bennett Cascade*.

caudad Toward the tail or end of the body; away from the head.

Celsius (C) Temperature scale in which 0° is the freezing point of water and 100° is the boiling point of water at sea level.

center body The metallic divider in the midportion of the Bird Mark series that was a site for gas channels and control devices.

central processing unit (CPU) The component of a computer that controls the encoding and execution of instructions. Mainly consists of an arithmetic unit, which performs arithmetic functions, and an internal memory, which controls the sequencing of operations. Also called a *processor*.

centrifugal nebulizer A humidification device in which a spinning disk with vanes on it breaks water into particles.

central sleep apnea Absence of breathing as the result of medullary depression, which inhibits respiratory movement; becomes more pronounced during sleep. Compare this term with *mixed sleep apnea* and *obstructive sleep apnea*.

cephalad Toward the head.

ceramic switch Part of the Bird Mark series ventilators that controls flow through the gas channels. Consists of a ceramic tube with offset grooves and holes that selectively match up with gas channel inlets in the center body.

chamber An accessory to enhance aerosol deposition from a metered-dose inhaler.

check valve A device usually consisting of a one-way valve that prevents back or retrograde gas flow.

chemical analyzer A device that enables measurement of the amount of a specific gas in a system by assessing the results of chemical reactions.

chemical potential energy Potential energy stored in a chemical bond, such as petroleum reserves of coal, gas, or oil.

chemical sterilant Any chemical agent that destroys all living organisms, including viruses, in a material.

chemiluminescent monitoring A type of nitrogen oxide monitoring system routinely used during nitric oxide administration. It involves the quantification of gas-specific photoemission. See also *electrochemical monitoring*.

chest cuirass The shell-like part of a negative-pressure ventilator.

chest shell piece The rigid portion of a cuirass type of negative-pressure ventilator that covers the thorax.

Cheyne-Stokes respiration An abnormal, repeating pattern of breathing characterized by progressive hypopnea alternating with hyperpnea and ending in a brief apnea.

child adult mist (CAM) tent An environmental enclosure that controls oxygen concentration, humidity, and temperature.

CIRC alarm circuit-integrity warning Denotes a leak or disconnection in the patient circuit.

circadian rhythm A pattern based on a 24-hour cycle, especially the repetition of certain physiologic phenomena, such as sleeping and eating.

Clark electrode The electrode most commonly used to measure the partial pressure of oxygen.

cleaning The removal of all foreign material, especially organic matter (e.g., blood, serum, pus, and fecal matter), from objects by using hot water, soaps, detergents, and enzymatic products.

closed-circuit calorimeter See *indirect calorimeter*.

closed-loop system A hardware/software combination that controls a mechanical or electronic process without user input.

clutch plate In the Bird Mark series, the steel plates that are connected by a wire shaft and suspended between two magnets. The clutch plates act as on/off switches for gas flow.

Coanda effect A term in fluidics that refers to the sidewall attachment phenomenon of gas streams.

cocci Bacteria that are round, spherical, or oval, such as gonococci, pneumococci, staphylococci, and streptococci.

cohesion The attractive force between like molecules.

collodion A clear or slightly opaque, highly inflammable liquid composed of pyroxylin, ether, and alcohol. It dries to a strong, transparent film that is used as a surgical dressing.

combined-power ventilator A ventilator that requires both pneumatic and electric sources for operation. The electric source often powers a microprocessor.

combined-pressure device A ventilator that makes use of both positive and negative pressure during breath delivery. For example, a high-frequency oscillator delivers positive pressure on inspiration and negative pressure on expiration.

combined-pressure gradient The additive pressure difference in a multipart system, such as the combined air-to-arterial-to-cell pressure difference.

Combitube A double-lumen device designed to provide a patent upper airway when inserted blindly after failed intubation or in a comatose patient with airway difficulties.

compensated leak alarm A warning that activates when the leak-compensation mechanism is engaged.

compensator valve A system designed to provide additional flow or volume to overcome the effects of leaks in a pressurized system.

compound A substance composed of two or more elements, chemically combined in definite proportions, that cannot be separated by physical means.

compressibility factor A mathematical expression of the reduction of volume delivery in a ventilator setting in response to increased pressure in the system.

compressor A machine that uses electrical power to move a piston, fan, or bellows and that in turn reduces the volume of air and increases its pressure.

compressor-driven unit A mechanical ventilator that is powered by an air compressor.

concentration gradient In open or communicating systems, the difference between the amount of a substance in part of the system and the amount of the same substance in another part of the system.

condensation Change of state from gas to liquid, such as with water vapor condensation.

conductivity The property of cardiac muscle to propagate an impulse throughout the heart.

constant positive airway pressure See *continuous positive airway pressure (CPAP)*.

constant positive-pressure breathing (CPPB) A mode of ventilation in which the ventilating pressures are always elevated above 0.

contact precautions Safeguards designed to reduce the risk of transmission of epidemiologically important microorganisms by direct or indirect contact.

continuous flow CPAP system A continuous positive airway pressure (CPAP) system incorporating a constant flow of gas.

continuous-flow IMV system A volume ventilator with the addition of an intermittent mandatory ventilation circuit that incorporates a constant flow of gas. The one-way valve going toward the patient circuit is kept open by the continuous flow and does not have to be opened by the patient. Also called a *closed-circuit IMV system*.

continuous-flow ventilation (CFV) A mode of ventilation in which a gas stream constantly passes through the airway and is hence continually available.

continuous mandatory ventilation (CMV) A mode of ventilation that provides control or assist/control ventilation. Breaths are time-triggered or patient-triggered, volume-targeted or pressure-targeted, and volume-cycled or time-cycled.

continuous nebulizer A nebulizer that runs during the entire ventilatory cycle.

continuous positive airway pressure (CPAP) A method of providing positive pressure without mechanical assistance (i.e.,

mandatory breath delivery) for spontaneously breathing patients. A technique for increasing functional residual capacity and arterial oxygenation.

continuous supply system A mechanism that delivers a gas or an aerosol throughout the ventilatory cycle.

control mode A type of CMV in which the breathing frequency is determined by the ventilator, without patient initiation, according to a preset cycling pattern (time-triggered ventilatory support).

control panel The user interface, with the controls for the operator to set desired parameters.

control pneumatic logic circuit A fluidic circuit that controls the operation of other circuits.

control pressure manometer A gauge that indicates the maximum or control pressure in a ventilator system.

control variables Four elements of breath delivery: flow, volume, pressure, and time. The elements are controlled or limited by the ventilator. The operator sets the numeric values for each element on the front panel of the ventilator.

controlled expiratory time A system that controls rate or end-expiration by limiting expiratory time.

controller A type of ventilator that will not allow spontaneous breathing.

convoluted tube A tube that has many bends and turns.

counterweight A weight used to offset the effects of pressure on a system.

coupling chamber In an ultrasonic nebulizer, the water-filled space between the ultrasonic source and the solution to be nebulized. It transmits the ultrasonic waves from the transducer to the medication chamber.

CPAP Abbreviation for *continuous positive airway pressure*. A method of pressurized gas delivery whereby the patient breathes spontaneously without mechanical assistance at pressures above ambient pressure.

critical pressure The pressure above which a material cannot exist as a gas.

critical temperature The temperature below which a material cannot exist as a gas.

cryogenic Producing extremely low temperatures.

cuirass The shell-like part of a negative-pressure ventilator.

cupped-disk valve A type of valve that looks like a shallow bowl. The convex side of the disk fits into an orifice, sealing it to end inspiration and inspiratory flow delivery and to begin the expiratory phase during mechanical ventilation.

cyber knob The term given by Dräger for the icons on the monitor screen of the Dräger E-4 ventilator that are shaped like knobs and used to control the unit.

cyber pad The term given by Dräger for the icons on the monitor screen of the Dräger E-4 ventilator that are shaped like touch pads and used to control the unit.

cycle rate control The part of the ventilator that determines the length of the ventilatory cycle.

cycle variable The phase variable that is measured and used to end inspiration; the element of breath delivery that determines the end of inspiration. See also *control variables*.

D

dead space ventilation Ventilation characterized by respired gas volume that does not participate in gas exchange. Alveolar dead space is characterized by alveoli that are ventilated but not perfused.

dead space volume (V_D) The amount of volume during ventilation that is not involved in gas exchange because of lack of pulmonary perfusion to the area.

decelerating taper (ramp) A flow curve in which the flow gradually decreases over time.

decelerating waveform See *decelerating taper* (ramp).

decompression port A gas channel that relieves pressure in part of the gas circuit.

decontamination The process whereby contaminants are removed from objects, usually by simple physical means (e.g., washing).

default Failure to do something when it is required or expected.

delay time control A device that controls the back-up rate on a ventilator by setting a maximum time between cycles.

delta wave The slowest of the four types of brain waves, characterized by a frequency of less than 3.5 Hertz and a relatively high voltage. Delta waves are "deep-sleep waves" associated with a dreamless state from which an individual is not easily aroused. Compare this term with *alpha wave*, *beta wave*, and *theta wave*.

demand-flow accelerator servo An automatic device that increases patient gas flow in response to patient effort.

demand-flow CPAP system A CPAP system in which the patient must open a one-way valve to receive gas flow from a warmed and humidified blended gas source.

demand-flow IMV system An intermittent mandatory ventilation system in which the patient is required to perform the work of opening a one-way valve. Also called a *parallel-flow IMV* or *open-circuit IMV*.

demand sensitivity system A subsystem that sets the level of inspiratory effort needed to trigger a ventilator into the inspiratory phase.

demand valve A mechanism that provides pressurized gas when the patient makes an inspiratory effort.

density An expression of the amount of mass per unit of volume a substance possesses.

Diameter Index Safety System (DISS) A safety system for compressed gas fittings. The DISS is used in respiratory care when equipment is connected to a low-pressure gas source ($\leq$200 psi).

diameter restrictor A device that controls or reduces flow by reducing the diameter of the flow path.

diaphragm compressor A gas-delivery system that operates to reduce gas volume by increasing pressure via movement of a flexible diaphragm.

diaphragm/leaf valves Comparatively thin, flat valves that have many applications in respiratory care. They may separate high- and low-pressure areas as one-way valves or as backflow-prevention devices.

diaphragm valve See *diaphragm/leaf valves*.

diastasis A longer period of reduced filling that typically follows the rapid filling period during the beginning third of ventricular filling.

diastolic depolarization A phenomenon in which cardiac nodal tissue (i.e., nodal tissue) gradually becomes depolarized during phase 4 of its action potential.

differential area gas-blending valve A gas-mixing device that changes the proportions of a gas mixture by varying the size of each gas inlet port.

differential output The difference between the output of O_1 and O_2 in a fluidic element.

diffuser A device used to mix or dissipate gases. Also a device to muffle the sound of a loud turbine or compressor.

diffuser humidifier A device that forces gas flow through a porous material submerged in water, causing the gas to form many bubbles that rise to the surface of the gas.

diffusion The physical process whereby atoms or molecules tend to move from an area of higher concentration or pressure to an area of lower concentration or pressure.

Digital Communications Interface (DCI) A function on the Puritan Bennett 7200 ventilator that provides data reports including data logs, chart summary reports, ventilator status reports, and host reports.

digital flowmeter A flowmeter on the panel of the Newport Breeze E150 that displays and controls the flow during spontaneous breaths and is used to stabilize baseline pressure between mandatory breaths in assist/control.

diluter regulator A mechanism that controls the entrained air in an oxygen diluter system.

diode A high-vacuum type of electron tube with a cold anode and a heated cathode that is used as a rectifier of alternating current.

diplobacilli Bacilli that occur in pairs.

diplococcus A member of the *Coccaceae* family that occurs in pairs because of incomplete cell division. Diplococci are often found as parasites of saprophytes. Also used to describe bacteria of the *Coccaceae* family that occur as pairs of cocci.

dipole-dipole interaction The interaction of equal and opposite electrical charges.

direct-acting valve A device that provides volume or flow by direct action from a control knob or device, such as the valve connected to a water faucet. As the faucet is turned, the valve opens or closes.

direct contact Mutual touching of two individuals or organisms. Many communicable diseases may be spread by direct contact between infected and healthy persons.

direct current (DC) Current flowing in one direction. Compare this term with *alternating current*.

direct-drive piston A piston whose movement is governed by linear (straight line) movement of a shaft that is connected to the piston head. Also called a *linear drive piston*. Compare with the term *rotary drive piston*.

direct-drive piston ventilator A ventilator that incorporates a linear drive piston.

disconnect ventilation An emergency mode of ventilation available on the Puritan Bennett 7200 ventilator that activates when the microprocessor detects inconsistencies in airway pressures, PEEP, and the gas-delivery pressure in the pneumatic system, which can occur in conditions such as tubing disconnects or plugged tubing.

disinfection The process of destroying at least the vegetative phase of pathogenic microorganisms by physical or chemical means.

display window A monitoring screen on the front panel of a ventilator that displays ventilator parameters.

DISS See *Diameter Index Safety System*.

Doppler effect The apparent change in frequency of sound or light waves emitted by a source as it moves away from or toward an observer. The frequency increases as the source moves toward the observer and decreases as it moves away (e.g., the rising pitch of an approaching train and the falling pitch of a departing train). The Doppler effect is also observed in electromagnetic radiation (e.g., light and radio waves).

double circuit A type of ventilator with two distinct gas flows, one of which provides power to deliver a breath, and the other is the actual flow delivered to the patient's airway.

double-lumen endotracheal tube (DLET) A specialized endotracheal tube that allows the right and left lungs to be ventilated separately (i.e., independent lung ventilation).

double-stage reducing valve A pressure-control device that lowers line pressure to working pressure in two steps. Generally, from 2200 pound-force per square inch gauge (psig) to 750 psig to 50 psig.

drag turbine The name of the flow-control device in the Bird T-Bird AVS ventilator.

drive mechanism Refers to the method by which gas flow to the patient is achieved with a mechanical ventilator.

droplet precautions Safeguards designed to reduce the risk of transmitting infectious agents by droplet.

drum vane The air foils on the Bennett valve in the PR, TV, and AP series respirators, which act as sensitivity and flow-cycling mechanisms.

dry-powder inhaler A type of metered dose inhaler that delivers a drug as a powder rather than as a liquid aerosol.

dry-rolling seal spirometer A type of device measuring volume changes in the airway opening. Consists of a canister containing a piston sealed to it with a rolling diaphragm-like seal.

dual modes of ventilation A phrase used to describe pressure-targeted ventilation that also guarantees delivery of a set volume.

duckbill/diaphragm/fishmouth valves Valves made of elastic materials that have a slit in the middle; the slit opens when pressurized to allow gas flow.

dump port A mechanism that allows expired gas to exit the ventilator. May be part of the expiration valve.

E

effective refractory period A period after firing of an impulse during which cardiac tissue is unable to propagate the impulse.

EGTA See *esophageal gastric tube airway*.

elastic potential energy The potential energy stored in a compressed spring that will be converted into kinetic energy when the spring is allowed to uncoil.

electrical analyzer A type of gas analyzer that enables the detection of changes in electrical current in response to varying gas concentrations.

electrical impedance The total opposition offered by an electric circuit to the flow of an alternating current of electrons. Impedance is a combination of the effects of electrical resistance and reactance.

electrically powered Energy supplied by the activity of electrons or other subatomic particles in motion. Also said of a mechanical device or ventilator requiring electricity to operate.

electricity A form of energy expressed by the activity of electrons and other subatomic particles in motion—as in dynamic electricity—or at rest, as in static electricity. Electricity can be produced by heat; generated by a voltaic cell; or produced by induction, rubbing on nonconductors with dry materials, or chemical activity.

electrochemical Pertains to the electrical effects that accompany chemical action and the chemical activity produced by electrical influence.

electrochemical monitoring A type of monitoring system routinely used when oxygen or nitric oxide is administered. Gases diffusing across a semipermeable membrane react with an electrolyte solution, generating a current flow between two polarized electrodes as electrons are liberated or consumed. See also *chemiluminescent monitoring*.

electrochemical sensor An apparatus designed to react to physical stimuli that accompany chemical activity produced by electrical influence.

electrode A contact for the induction or detection of electrical activity. Also a medium for conducting an electrical current from the body to physiologic monitoring equipment.

electromagnetic frequency interference (EFI) The disruption of the operation of a device caused by electromagnetic waves in the vicinity.

electromechanical transducer A mechanical device that is activated by electricity and capable of converting one form of energy into another. Commonly used to measure physical events.

electromechanical valve A mechanical valve system that responds to an electrical signal; also called an *electrically powered mechanical valve*.

electromotive force (EMF) The electrical potential, or the ability of electric energy to perform work. Usually measured in joules per coulomb or volts. Any device, such as a storage battery, that converts some form of energy into electricity is a source of EMF.

electronic capacitance transducer An electronic component that changes one form of energy to another based on the strength of the electrical charge stored in the unit.

electronic logic In the Bear 3 ventilator, this is the term applied to the control mechanism that governs ventilator operation.

electronically controlled PEEP valve A PEEP valve whose pressure limits are maintained by electrically operated valves.

element One of more than 100 primary, simple substances that cannot be broken down into any other substance by chemical means. Each atom of any element contains a specific number of protons in the nucleus and an equal number of electrons outside the nucleus. The nucleus contains a variable number of neutrons. An element with a disproportionate number of neutrons may be unstable, in which case the nucleus undergoes radioactive decay into a more stable elemental form.

endotracheal tube A type of artificial airway inserted through the mouth or nose and the larynx into the trachea.

energy expenditure The metabolic cost (in calories or kilojoules) of various forms of physical activity.

entrainment device A device designed to add ambient gas into a primary gas stream. Usually a jet Venturi device.

entrainment nebulizer A nebulizer designed to entrain gas or liquids into the primary gas stream. See also *entrainment device*.

entrainment reservoir The part of an entrainment nebulizer that contains the substance to be entrained and nebulized.

EOA See *esophageal obturator airway*.

esophageal gastric tube airway (EGTA) A type of artificial airway that consists of a double-lumen tube that passes through a tight-fitting face mask and extends through the mouth into the esophagus (this portion has an inflatable cuff above the distal opening). The oral portion of the airway has a ventilation tube with holes through which gas from a resuscitation device ventilates the lungs.

esophageal obturator airway (EOA) A type of artificial airway used in emergency situations. Consists of a blind tube that passes through a tight-fitting face mask and extends through the mouth into the esophagus (this portion has an inflatable cuff). The oral portion of the airway has holes through which gas from a resuscitation device is forced into the lungs.

EST See *extended self-test*.

eukaryotic Of or pertaining to cells with true nuclei bounded by a nuclear membrane and capable of mitosis.

evaporation The process by which liquids change into the vapor state. This occurs because of changes in temperature, pressure, and vapor pressure gradients.

excitability The ability of the heart to respond to a stimulus by producing an action potential.

exhalation timer A control that determines the length of the expiratory portion of the respiratory cycle.

exhalation valve A one-way valve system through which exhaled gases exit the ventilator and its circuit.

exhalation valve leak alarm A device that warns that the integrity of the exhalation valve has failed.

exhausted fuel cell alarm A warning that the sensing mechanism in a fuel cell gas analyzer is not functional.

expiratory flow cartridge In the Bird Mark series, an accumulator cartridge that used an adjustable and controlled leak to vary expiratory time.

expiratory flow gradient control A device that allows the adjustment of expiration by manipulation of back pressure and expiratory pressure gradients.

expiratory hold A mechanical ventilator control that delays mandatory breath delivery when it is pressed during the end of exhalation, used for measuring auto-PEEP.

expiratory hold (end-expiratory pause) The time at the end of exhalation after a mandatory breath during which the ventilator delays delivery of another mandatory breath for the purpose of measuring end-expiratory pressure. Usually performed to check for auto-PEEP.

expiratory pause See *expiratory hold*.

expiratory positive airway pressure (EPAP) The pressure measured in a patient circuit during exhalation. A parameter that can be set during BiPAP ventilation that governs pressure delivery during exhalation.

expiratory resistance control An adjustable device that allows back pressure to increase forces opposing expiratory flow.

expiratory retard A device or control designed to increase the resistance to exhaled gas flow, which increases the pressure maintained in the circuit during exhalation and can increase expiratory time.

expiratory servo valve The device that controls the expiratory scissor valve in the Siemens 900 series ventilators.

expiratory tidal volume The volume from a normal inspiration to a normal expiration measured from a patient's exhaled air.

expiratory time The length of time of the expiratory portion of a breath. From the end of inspiration to the beginning of the next inspiration.

expiratory time accumulator See *expiratory flow cartridge*.

expiratory time control See *expiratory flow cartridge*.

expiratory timer See *expiratory flow cartridge*.

expiratory trigger sensitivity (ETS) The adjustable control available on the Hamilton GALILEO ventilator used to establish the percentage of peak flow at which pressure support or spontaneous breaths will cycle out of inspiration.

extended self-test (EST) A series of tests that are part of the normal maintenance procedure for the Puritan Bennett 7200 ventilator and that trained personnel perform between patient uses.

external battery A DC power source sometimes used by ventilators as an alternative power supply when the normal electrical power source is not available.

external circuit The portion of the pneumatic circuit consisting of tubing from a ventilator to a patient. Also called a *patient circuit* or a *ventilator circuit*.

external IMV reservoir A reservoir bag or tubing that provides a volume of gas at a predetermined fractional inspired oxygen (F_IO_2) in a sufficient amount to accommodate the patient's volume.

external IMV system A reservoir, tubing, gas source, and valve system attached to the outside of a ventilator. Sometimes referred to as an *H-valve assembly* because of its design.

external PEEP valve A threshold or flow resistor added to the exhalation valve assembly of a ventilator or breathing device (e.g., resuscitation valve) to provide positive pressure during exhalation.

extreme extension See *sniffer's position*.

F

facultative Not obligatory; having the ability to adapt to more than one condition (e.g., a facultative anaerobe that can live with or without oxygen).

Fahrenheit (F) A temperature scale in which the boiling point of water is 212° F and the freezing point of water is 32° F at sea level.

fail-safe baseline metering orifice A variable metering device whose orifice opens during failure of power or pressure.

fail-safe valve A safety measure designed to provide a way for the patient to breathe if the gas delivery devices fail.

feedback channel In pneumatic or fluid devices, a mechanism that provides a signal or flow to a control device.

feedback line See *feedback channel*.

fenestrated tracheotomy tube A tracheotomy tube with a hole or "window" (*fenestra* in Latin) on the posterior wall of the outer cannula above the cuff. This allows the patient to speak when the inner cannula is removed, the cuff is deflated, and the tracheostomy tube is occluded at the connector. Fenestrated tubes aid in weaning patients from the artificial airway.

fetal hemoglobin (HbF) A hemoglobin variant that has a greater affinity for oxygen than adult hemoglobin. HbF is gradually replaced over the first year of life by HbA (adult hemoglobin).

F_IO_2 (fraction of inspired oxygen) The ratio (amount) of oxygen to the total volume of a gas mixture; expressed as a decimal.

fishmouth valve See *duckbill/diaphragm/fishmouth valves*.

fixed orifice A hole in a device that has a specific, unchanging size.

fixed-performance oxygen-delivery system Oxygen therapy equipment that supplies inspired gases at a consistent preset oxygen concentration. Also called a *high-flow system*.

fixed restrictor A device that is designed to produce a set back pressure (resistance) that inhibits forward flow.

flap vane In the Puritan Bennett PR, AP, and TV series ventilators, the winglike protrusions extending from the Bennett valve's internal cylinder that react to the force of airflow to cycle the device.

flapper A type of valve system that uses a lightweight diaphragm to occlude an orifice.

Fleisch pneumotachometer A device that operates on the principle that the flow of gas through the device is proportional to the pressure drop that occurs as the gas flows across a known resistance (a bundle of brass capillary tubes arranged in parallel).

flip-flop device See *flip-flop unit*.

flip-flop unit A fluidic element that contains two outlets and two control ports. The main flow switches flow from one outlet to the other when a signal gas pulse acts on the main flow.

floating electrode Electrocardiographic (ECG) electrodes, which consist of a silver–silver chloride electrode that is encased within a plastic housing. The surface of the electrode is covered with a conductive gel or paste. The entire electrode assembly can be attached to the skin with a double-sided ring, which adheres to the patient's skin and to the plastic housing of the electrode. These electrodes are referred to as "floating" electrodes because the only conductive path between the electrode and the patient's skin is the electrolyte gel or paste.

floating-island nebulizer A type of aerosol production device in which the jet assembly floats underneath a pontoon assembly in a reservoir of water. Also called a *Win-Liz nebulizer* after the wives of the inventors.

flow acceleration cartridge In the Bird Mark series, a pneumatic device designed to increase inspiratory flow.

flow- and volume-augmented breaths in the Bear 1000 A function that provides additional flow or volume when the patient's inspiratory effort drops pressure below the set baseline pressure.

flow control See *flow control valve*.

flow-control valve A device that controls and adjusts inspiratory flow on a ventilator, thus affecting respiratory rate and volume.

flow-dependent incentive spirometer A device that encourages a patient to take slow, deep breaths. The patient is encouraged to achieve a specific airflow during inspiration by using a visual cue that indicates airflow.

flow-dependent valve A device that responds to low flow by halting inspiration, the operating principle of the Bennett valve in the AP, PR, and TV series Puritan Bennett respirators. A flow-dependent valve measures and displays the inspiratory flow that the patient achieves during a maximum sustained inspiratory effort.

flow rate control See *flow control* valve.

flow resistor See *flow restrictor*.

flow restrictor A device that reduces the flow of a fluid/gas out of a system by providing an in-stream obstruction, usually in the form of an orifice of reduced size, thus causing back pressure in the system. Increases or decreases in gas flow result in increases or decreases in the back pressure created by the restrictor.

flow restrictor/regulator See *flow restrictor*.

flow sensor A mechanism that detects the movement of a volume of gas.

flow transducer An electronic device that changes one type of signal to another type proportionate to the flow that passes through it.

flow trigger The amount the flow must drop from the base flow value to trigger a breath during mechanical ventilation.

flow-triggering When the ventilator detects a drop in gas flow, then inspiration is set to occur.

flow waveforms The graphic pattern produced when flow is plotted against time.

flowby option A feature available on the Puritan Bennett 7200 ventilator that provides continuous flow during the expiratory phase to provide fresh gas at the beginning of inspiration and reduce the ventilator response time to patient inspiratory effort (also see *bias flow* and *base flow*).

flowmeter A device that controls and measures a flow of gas or liquid. Usually stated in volume per unit of time.

fluid logic A method for delivering gas flow that uses fluidic elements that do not require moving parts. See also *fluidic*.

fluidic Referring to hydrodynamic principles used to direct gas flow through circuits, resulting in switching of flow directions and signal amplification. Also used in pressure-sensing and flow-sensing.

fluidic-breathing assistor A device that uses the principles of fluidics to augment the patient's ventilatory efforts.

fluidic drive A type of pneumatically powered ventilator or device that uses fluidic principles (elements). A mechanism to provide the primary power source for gas delivery with fluidics.

fluorescent sensor An optical blood gas sensor that uses dyes that fluoresce when struck by light in the ultraviolet or near-ultraviolet visible range. The pH, PCO_2, or PO_2 of arterial blood can be determined by using these devices.

flutter valve A mucus clearance device that consists of a pipe-shaped apparatus with a steel ball in a bowl covered with a perforated cap. The flutter valve uses the principles associated with positive expiratory pressure and high-frequency airway oscillations.

fomite Nonliving material, such as bed linens or equipment, that may transmit pathogenic organisms.

fractional distillation of liquid air A method of reducing air to its component gases using pressure and temperature changes. See also *Joule-Kelvin-Thompson method*.

fractional hemoglobin saturation The amount of oxyhemoglobin measured divided by the amount of all four types of hemoglobin (Hb) present, written as follows:

$$\text{Fractional } O_2Hb = O_2Hb \div (HHb + O_2Hb + COHb + MetHb)$$

FRC See *functional residual capacity*.

freezing point The temperature at which a liquid becomes a solid.

French scale A measurement scale commonly used to delineate the external diameter of catheters; 1 French unit equals approximately 0.33 mm.

French sizes See *French scale*.

froth A mixture of liquid and gas that forms a dense layer of bubbles, increasing the gas/liquid surface area.

functional hemoglobin saturation The oxyhemoglobin concentration divided by the concentration of hemoglobin capable of carrying oxygen, written as follows:

$$\text{Functional } O_2Hb = O_2Hb \div (HHb + O_2Hb)$$

functional residual capacity (FRC) The total amount of gas left in the lungs after a normal, quiet exhalation.

fungicide An agent that is destructive to fungi.

fusible plug A type of pressure-relief mechanism made of a metal alloy that melts when the temperature of the gas in the tank exceeds a predetermined temperature. Fusible plugs operate on the principle that as the pressure in a tank increases, the temperature of the gas increases, which causes the plug to melt. The melting of the plug releases excess pressure.

G

galvanic analyzer An electric analyzer that determines gas concentrations by measuring the change in resistance of electric current in both reference and sampling circuits.

gas A fluid state of matter with the least organization and definition.

gas-collector exhalation valve A device that allows expired gases to be collected through a one-directional port.

gas streaming Asymmetric velocity profiles that occur when gas flows in both directions through a conductive airway (tube) at the same time that exhaled gas travels on the outside of the tube and inspired gas moves down the center.

geometric standard deviation (GSD) A measure of the variability of particle diameters within an aerosol. The higher the GSD, the more (larger and smaller) particles are present.

germicide A drug that kills pathogenic microorganisms.

glucose oxidase An enzyme used to coat electrodes when measuring glucose.

gmw See *gram molecular weight*.

gram molecular weight (gmw) A chemical measurement for the mass of a chemical equal to the atomic weight of its chemical components (expressed in grams); sometimes called the *combining weight*.

gram-negative Having the pink color of the counterstain used in Gram's method of staining microorganisms. This property is a primary method of characterizing organisms in microbiology.

gram-positive Retaining the violet color of the stain used in Gram's method of staining microorganisms. This property is a primary method of characterizing organisms in microbiology.

Gram stain The method of staining microorganisms by using a violet stain and an iodine solution; decolorizing with an alcohol or acetone solution; and counterstaining with safranin. The retention of either the violet color of the stain or the pink color of the counterstain is a primary means for the identification and classification of bacteria. Also called *Gram's method*.

graphics A visual representation of monitored parameters, such as pressure, volume, and flow per unit time. See also *scalars*.

gravitational potential energy The potential energy an object can gain by falling, as a result of gravity.

Guedel airway An upper airway device (oropharyngeal airway) used to provide air passage distal to an obstructing tongue.

H

Haldane effect The influence of hemoglobin saturation and oxygen on carbon dioxide dissociation.

hardware The mechanical, magnetic, and electronic design, structure, and devices of a computer. Compare this with the term *software*.

heart blocks A group of arrhythmias in which impulses fail to propagate in a normal manner because of an increased refractoriness of one or more conductive paths in the heart (e.g., atrioventricular blocks).

heart sounds A normal series of sounds produced within the heart during the cardiac cycle that can be heard over the precordium.

heat and moisture exchanger (HME) A passive, disposable device that humidifies and warms incoming gases in patients receiving mechanical ventilation by using the principles of condensation and evaporation. Also called an *artificial nose*.

heated blowby humidifier A type of pass-over humidifier that exposes gas flow to a heated water reservoir, where heat and moisture are transferred into the gas stream.

heated wire See *heated-wire circuit*.

heated-wire circuit A type of ventilator circuit in which the inspiratory tubing is heated to reduce water vapor "rain-out" (condensation).

heliox A low-density therapeutic mixture of helium with at least 20% oxygen; used in some institutions as part of large airway obstruction treatment.

Henderson-Hasselbalch equation The chemical formula relating pH, pKa, and the ratio of the conjugate base (bicarbonate) to the weak acid (carbonic acid).

HFFI See *high-frequency flow interrupter*.

HFJV See *high-frequency jet ventilation*.

HFO See *high-frequency oscillation*.

HFV See *high-frequency ventilation*.

high breathing rate alarm A ventilator warning system that indicates rapid respirations exceeding the desired rate.

high-frequency flow interrupter (HFFI or HIFI) A type of high-frequency ventilator that provides rapid gas pulses to the airway (up to 30 Hz) by periodically interrupting a high-flow gas stream.

high-frequency flow interruption See *high-frequency flow interrupter*.

high-frequency jet ventilation (HFJV) A type of high-frequency ventilator that provides a jet gas pulse to the airway via a small-lumen catheter within the endotracheal tube at rates of approximately 100 to 200 pulses/min.

high-frequency oscillation (HFO) A type of high-frequency ventilator that cycles at rates of 60 to 3000 times per minute.

high-frequency oscillatory ventilation (HFOV) See *high-frequency oscillation*.

high-frequency percussive ventilation (HFPV) Ventilation that incorporates the beneficial characteristics of a conventional positive-pressure ventilator and a jet ventilator. Can be compared with time-cycled, pressure-limited ventilation, in which high-frequency pulsations (up to 100 to 225 cycles/min, or 1.7 to 4 Hz) are injected into the airway through a Venturi during the inspiratory phase.

high-frequency positive pressure ventilation (HFPPV) A mode of ventilatory support with rates from 60 to 100/pulses/minute and small tidal volumes (often approaching anatomic dead space) that uses a low-compliance patient circuit.

high-frequency ventilation (HFV) A method of ventilation at rates >80 times per minute. See also *high-frequency jet ventilation* and *high-frequency oscillation*.

high-level disinfection The use of chemical sterilants at reduced exposure times (less than 45 minutes) to kill bacteria, fungi, and viruses. High-level disinfection does not kill a high level of bacterial spores. Compare intermediate-level disinfection and low-level disinfection.

Holter monitoring Making prolonged (usually 24 hours) electrocardiograph recordings on a portable tape recorder while the patient, wearing appropriate monitoring leads, conducts normal daily activities.

hood An environmental control device that covers the head and regulates the humidity, gas concentration, and temperature of inspired gases.

hot film anemometer A flow-sensing device used in some ventilators that works by measuring the temperature of the gas flow. Similar to hot-wire flow transducers.

humidity The amount of water vapor in a system expressed as weight/volume (e.g., grams/liter). Also water in the molecular form.

humidity deficit A condition in which the available humidity is less than the potential humidity; that is, the percentage relative humidity is less than 100 (e.g., the humidity deficit at a body temperature of 37° C is compared with its capacity of 44 mg/L).

hydrogen bonding The attractive force of compounds in which a hydrogen atom covalently linked to an electronegative element (e.g., oxygen, nitrogen, or fluorine) has a large degree of positive character relative to the electronegative atom, thereby causing the compound to have a large dipole.

hydrometer A device that determines the specific gravity or density of a liquid by comparing its weight with that of an equal volume of water. A calibrated, hollow, glass device is placed in the liquid being examined, and the depth to which the device settles in the liquid is noted.

hydrophobic The property of repelling water molecules.

hygroscopic The property of attracting and binding water molecules.

hyperbilirubinemia Above-average amounts of the bile pigment bilirubin in the blood; often characterized by jaundice, anorexia, and malaise.

hypertonic A solution of water and chemicals in which the solute-to-solvent ratio exceeds that of normal body fluids. For salt water, this is greater than 0.9% NaCl.

I

ideal gas A gas acting as if it exactly follows all of the gas laws.

I : E ratio control A ventilator control that regulates the proportions of inspiratory and expiratory time during a respiratory cycle.

I : E ratio limit control A mechanism that prevents high–inspiratory-to-expiratory (I : E) ratios; usually more than 1 : 1.

impedance cardiography A noninvasive technique for measuring cardiac output based on the principle of impedance plethysmography. In this technique, two sets of electrodes are placed on the thorax to measure electrical impedance.

impedance plethysmography A technique for detecting blood vessel occlusion that determines volumetric changes in an area of the body (e.g., limb blood flow) by measuring changes in its girth as indicated in the electrical impedance of mercury-containing polymeric silicone (Silastic) tubes in a pressure cuff.

IMV (pressurized breaths) See *intermittent mandatory ventilation.*

incisura A notch or indentation that appears on the aortic pressure tracing. It is thought to be associated with retrograde flow of blood from the aorta back toward the left ventricle at the end of ventricular systole.

indirect calorimeter A device used for measuring energy expenditure. With a closed-circuit calorimeter, the patient breathes into and out of a container prefilled with oxygen. Oxygen consumption is determined by measuring the volume of oxygen the patient uses. With an open-circuit calorimeter, the volume of oxygen is determined by measuring the volumes of inspired and expired gases, along with the fractional concentrations of oxygen in the inspired and expired gases. The volume of oxygen is then determined by calculating the difference between the amount of oxygen in the inspired gas and the amount in the expired gas.

indirect contact Contacting a susceptible host with a contaminated intermediate object (usually inanimate) in the patient's environment.

indirect-drive piston A ventilator power mechanism in which the power gas is driven by a piston but does not go to the patient. For example, the power gas may compress a bellows that contains the patient gas volume.

inertia The tendency of objects to resist changes in position unless acted upon by an outside force (from Newton's laws).

inertial impaction The deposition of particles by collision with a surface; the primary mechanism for pulmonary deposition of larger particles (usually more than 5 m in diameter). Large particles tend to travel in a straight line and collide with surfaces in their pathway (e.g., airway branches, baffles).

infection surveillance The procedures of a hospital or other health facility to minimize the risk of spreading of nosocomial or community-acquired infections to patients or staff members.

inflating port An orifice through which ventilating gas flows.

injector A device that adds a quantity of liquid or gas to a main flow source. See also *jet.*

inspiratory controls Mechanisms that determine the length and timing of inspiratory gas flow.

inspiratory flow rate control A ventilatory mechanism that sets the gas volume delivered per unit of time during inspiration.

inspiratory hold (plateau) A ventilatory maneuver in which delivered volume is held in the lungs before exhalation. Inspiratory gas flow stops, and the expiratory valve is maintained briefly in the closed position, thus keeping the delivered volume (and pressure) in the lungs. Commonly used to measure plateau pressure for the calculation of static compliance.

inspiratory interrupter switch A control device that terminates inspiration.

inspiratory pause See *inspiratory hold.*

inspiratory positive airway pressure (IPAP) The pressure measured in a patient circuit during inspiration. A parameter that can be set during bilevel positive airway pressure (BiPAP) ventilation and governs pressure delivery during inspiration.

inspiratory pressure calibration control Allows the inspiratory pressure limit to be set.

inspiratory pressure level The maximum amount of pressure allowed during mechanical ventilation.

inspiratory pressure-relief control A device that sets the "pop-off" pressure on a mechanical ventilator.

inspiratory pressure-time product (PTP) The integration of the area within the curve during inspiration on a pressure/time graph.

inspiratory time (T_I) See *inspiratory time control.*

inspiratory time control Sets the length of inspiration either directly or as a fraction of the I : E ratio.

inspiratory time percent The proportion of the respiratory cycle time devoted to inspiration.

inspiratory timer A control that determines the time allowed for inspiration.

insulator A nonconducting substance that is a barrier to heat or electricity passage.

intensive care unit (ICU) A hospital unit in which patients requiring close monitoring and care are housed for as long as necessary.

intermediate-level disinfection Removing vegetative bacteria, tubercle bacteria, viruses, and fungi, but not necessarily killing spores. Compare high-level disinfection and low-level disinfection.

intermittent mandatory ventilation (IMV) (pressurized breaths) A time-triggered ventilatory mode that permits spontaneous ventilation and intersperses required pressurized breaths at predetermined intervals. See also *synchronized intermittent mandatory ventilation.*

intermittent (inspiratory) positive-pressure breathing (IPPB) A treatment modality in which the inspiratory pressure is elevated above atmospheric but is allowed to return to atmospheric during exhalation. Another term applied to mechanical ventilation.

intermittent positive-pressure ventilation (IPPV) Intermittent positive-pressure breathing done continuously as a form of mechanical ventilation.

internal battery A direct current power source sometimes used by ventilators as an alternative power supply when an AC source is not available.

internal demand valve A device that is triggered to provide gas flow when patient effort decreases pressure or flow below a certain baseline.

internal mechanism A device inside a ventilator or piece of equipment that functions in the operation of the equipment.

internal regulator A device inside a ventilator for adjusting pressure delivery.

International 10-20 EEG system The standard pattern for electrode placement on the scalp to record electroenchephalograms (EEGs) during sleep studies.

intrinsic positive end-expiratory pressure (PEEPi) The level of pressure in the airway as a result of pressure trapped in the lung at the end of exhalation. Also called *auto-PEEP*.

invasive Characterized by a tendency to spread or infiltrate. Also refers to the use of diagnostic or therapeutic methods that require access to the inside of the body.

inverse-ratio ventilation (IRV) Ventilation in which inspiratory time exceeds expiratory time. See also *pressure-controlled inverse ratio ventilation* and *volume-controlled-inverse ratio ventilation*.

in vitro Occurring in a laboratory apparatus (said of a biological reaction).

in vivo Occurring in a living organism (said of a biological reaction).

IPPB flow Gas flow during IPPB breaths.

iron lung A negative-pressure ventilator. Also called a *tank ventilator*, *artificial lung*, or *Drinker respirator*.

isolation procedures Infection control measures that combine barrier-type precautions (e.g., hand-washing and the use of gloves, masks, and gowns) with the physical separation of infected patients in specific disease categories to disrupt the transmission of pathogenic microorganisms.

isolation techniques See *isolation procedures*.

isothermic saturation boundary (ISB) The point at which gases reach body temperature and full saturation.

isotonic A solution of water and chemicals in which the solute concentration equals that of plasma.

isovolumetric contraction The period of ventricular systole that occurs during the period between closure of the AV valves and opening of the semilunar valves.

isovolumetric relaxation The period of ventricular diastole that occurs during the period between closure of the semilunar valves and opening of the AV valves.

J

jet A device using a gas-entrainment mechanism to mix gases or add aerosols to a mainstream gas flow.

jet humidifier A humidifier that uses the jet principle to add water vapor to the main gas flow.

jet nebulizer A nebulizer that uses the jet principle to add water droplets to the main gas flow; contains a baffle.

jet Venturi A jet used to produce a pressure drop for entraining gas or fluid.

joule A unit of energy or work in the meter-kilogram-second system. It is equivalent to 10^7 ergs, or 1 W-second.

Joule-Kelvin effect A physical phenomenon in which the rapid expansion of a gas without the application of external work causes a cooling of the gas. Used in the liquefication of air to produce oxygen and nitrogen. Also called the *Joule-Thompson effect*.

Joule-Kelvin-Thompson method See *fractional distillation of liquid air*.

Joule-Thompson effect See *Joule-Kelvin effect*.

junctional escape rhythm Rhythm that is characterized by the AV node becoming the pacemaker of the heart (i.e., intrinsic rate of 40 to 60 beats/min). This type of rhythm typically occurs in cases of sinus block or sinus arrest.

K

K-complexes Large vertical slow waves with amplitudes of at least 75 μV with an initial negative deflection.

Kelvin (K) An absolute temperature scale calculated in centigrade units from the point at which molecular activity apparently ceases ($-273.15°$ C). To convert Celsius degrees to Kelvin, add 273.15 to the Celsius temperature.

kilowatt Unit of measure of electrical power (1000 W).

kinetic activity Molecular motion uses energy and produces heat as a by-product.

kinetic energy The energy a body possesses by virtue of its motion.

kinetic flowmeter A flow-regulation device that incorporates a spindle or plunger in place of a floating ball as a flow indicator.

Korotkoff's sounds Sounds heard during the taking of blood pressure when a sphygmomanometer and stethoscope are used.

kymograph A device for graphically recording lung volume changes during spirometry. See also *spirometer*.

L

laryngeal mask airway (LMA) A custom-formed, soft mask with a hollow tube fitting into the pyriform sinuses directly above the larynx. Used to establish and maintain a patent upper airway.

laryngoscope An endoscope for examining the larynx.

latent heat The amount of heat needed for a substance to change its state of matter.

leaf-type valve See *leaf valve*.

leaf valve A thin membrane that overlays an orifice and that when closed prevents fluid (gas or liquid) transmission through the opening.

Levy-Jennings charts The most common method of recording quality control data. These charts allow the operator to detect trends and shifts in performance and thus can help prevent problems associated with reporting inaccurate data caused by analyzer malfunction.

light-emitting diode (LED) An electronic component that emits light when exposed to current flow. Used in instruments to display digital data.

limiting variable An element of breath delivery including flow, volume, pressure, or time given a set maximum value by the operator that cannot be exceeded during the breath.

linear-drive piston A piston with movement governed by linear (straight line) movement of a shaft that is connected to the piston head. See also *direct-drive piston*.

liquefaction The conversion of a substance into its liquid form.

liquid-crystal A type of data display surface that indicates data by turning parts of the display on (dark) or off (light).

liquid-crystal display See *liquid-crystal*.

lock-out cartridge A control that inhibits (locks out) the functions of other controls or systems.

loop A circlelike graphic display of two variables plotted on the X-axis (horizontal) and Y-axis (vertical). Pressure/volume and flow/volume loops are most commonly used.

low-battery alarm A warning that the power (charge) remaining in a battery is below acceptable limits.

low inlet gas alarm A warning that system pressure is below optimal pressure standards.

low-level disinfection Killing most vegetative bacteria, some fungi, and some bacteria. Compare high-level disinfection and intermediate-level disinfection.

low-pressure reducing valve A pressure-regulating system designed to operate below 50 pound-force per square inch gauge (psig).

low-pressure regulator A low-pressure–reducing valve combined with a flowmeter.

low-residual volume, high-pressure cuff A type of endotracheal or tracheostomy tube seal that uses low volumes at high pressures to achieve an airtight seal.

low-resistance/high-compliance system A system in which the forces resisting flow are low and the volume change per unit of pressure exerted is high.

Luer-Lok A glass or plastic syringe with a simple screw-lock mechanism that securely holds the needle in place. Also called a *Luer syringe.*

M

Macintosh blade A curved laryngoscope blade, as opposed to a straight Miller type of blade.

macroshock A shock from an electric current of 1 mA or greater that is applied externally to the skin.

magnetic valve resistors A type of threshold resistor containing a bar magnet that attracts a ferromagnetic disk seated on the expiratory port of a pressurized circuit.

magnetic PEEP valve A valve that maintains a positive end-expiratory pressure by means of a magnetically activated component.

magnetism The branch of physics dealing with magnets and magnetic phenomena; also called *magnetics.*

main solenoid The master control device governing flow in a gas delivery system.

mainstream capnograph See *capnograph.*

mainstream nebulizer A nebulizer that introduces the jet stream into the main gas flow.

mandatory breath A breath initiated and ended by the mechanical ventilator. Mandatory breath delivery is completely determined by the ventilator.

mandatory minute ventilation (MMV) A closed-loop (servo-controlled) mode of ventilation that guarantees delivery of a set minute volume by monitoring the patient's spontaneous minute volume and supplementing breaths as necessary to achieve the set minute volume.

mandatory minute volume See *mandatory minute ventilation.*

manifold A system of interconnected devices (e.g., a gas manifold). Two or more cylinders connected to regulators and a metering device or a breathing manifold. The externally mounted exhalation valve, tubing, and nebulizer, which make up a portion of the ventilator circuit.

manometer ports Orifices from which pressure readings are obtained by connecting pressure manometers.

manual trigger A device in which the function is activated by hand.

mass median aerodynamic diameter (MMAD) Regarding aerosol particles, the diameter at which the mass is equally divided. That is, 50% of the particles are lighter than the MMAD and 50% are heavier.

mass spectrometry A sophisticated analysis technique used to analyze the composition of substances by examining a stream of charged particles to separate elements on the basis of atomic mass.

maximum expiratory flow A pulmonary function measurement of the patient's ability to exhale quickly and forcefully (in liters/second).

maximum inspiratory time control The mechanism that determines the length of inspiration allowed.

maximum motor current The highest electrical current the motor will tolerate.

maximum pressure control Sets the highest-allowable ventilator pressure. Also called *pressure-limit control.*

maximum pressure limit (P_{max}) The upper pressure value that can be delivered during inspiration. In the Hamilton GALILEO, the P_{max} setting also establishes a reference point for pressure delivered during servo-controlled modes of ventilation.

maximum voluntary ventilation (MVV) The maximum volume of air that a person can breathe over a one-minute period.

mean airway pressure (MAP) The average pressure occurring in the airway during a complete respiratory cycle. Mathematically, the area below the pressure/time curve for one breathing cycle divided by the breath cycle time.

measured variables One or more of the four elements of a breath (pressure, flow, volume, and time) monitored during ventilation.

mechanics The branch of physics dealing with the motion of material bodies and the phenomena of the action of forces on them.

melting point The temperature at which solids begin to turn into liquids.

membrane concentrator An oxygen concentrator that separates oxygen from air by means of a selectively permeable membrane.

mercury barometer A device for measuring atmospheric pressure by the change in the height of a mercury column.

message window A monitoring screen on the front panel of a ventilator; it is used to display messages.

metered-dose inhaler (MDI) A small, pressurized cartridge that contains a propellant and a medication. When the cartridge is activated, a precise amount of aerosolized medication is delivered.

microcuvette A small transparent tube or container with specific optical properties. The chemical composition of the container dictates the vessel's use (e.g., Pyrex glass for examining materials in the visible spectrum or silica for those in the ultraviolet range).

microprocessor A small, compact computer designed to monitor and control specific functions.

microprocessor-controlled Regulated by a small, compact computer.

microshock A shock from a usually imperceptible electrical current (<1 mA) that is allowed to bypass the skin and follow a direct, low-resistance pathway into the body.

microswitch Small control device that institutes or halts processes.

Miller blade A straight laryngoscope blade, as opposed to a curved Macintosh blade.

mini-fluid amp A device that increases the strength of a fluidic signal.

minimal occluding volume (MOV) The least amount of air needed to achieve a seal in a cuffed endotracheal or tracheostomy tube.

minimum minute volume See *mandatory minute ventilation*.

minute ventilation The total ventilation per minute. The product of tidal volume and respiratory rate, as measured by expired gas collection for 1 to 3 minutes. The normal value is 5 to 10 L/min. Also called *minute volume*.

minute volume control The mechanism that sets the minute volume delivered by a ventilator.

mixed sleep apnea Repeated episodes of complete airflow cessation for more than 10 seconds during sleep, with characteristics of both obstructive sleep apnea and central sleep apnea. In mixed sleep apnea, the central event usually precedes the obstructive event.

mixer A device that blends or mixes two gases to provide a precise mixture (concentration) of the gases.

mixture A substance composed of ingredients that are not chemically combined and do not necessarily occur in a fixed proportion.

molecular sieve A term used to describe components of a type of oxygen concentrator that filters air and chemically removes nitrogen and some trace gases from the air.

molecule The smallest unit that exhibits the properties of an element or compound. A molecule is composed of two or more covalently bonded atoms.

monitor To observe and evaluate a body function closely and constantly. Also, a mechanical device that provides a visual or audio signal or a graphic record of a particular function (e.g., a cardiac or fetal monitor).

monoplace hyperbaric chamber A hyperbaric unit rated for single occupancy.

monostable A fluidic device or element that can direct gas flow to only one outlet unless the gas flow is acted upon by a separate gas pulse.

multiplace hyperbaric chamber A walk-in hyperbaric unit that provides enough space to treat two or more patients simultaneously.

multistage reducing valve See *multistage regulator*.

multistage regulator A pressure-reducing valve that has more than one level of pressure reduction between system pressure and working pressure.

murmur A gentle blowing, fluttering, or humming sound, such as a heart murmur.

mustache cannula A type of reservoir nasal cannula that can reduce oxygen supply use from that of a continuous-flow nasal cannula.

myocyte A muscle cell.

N

nasal cannula An oxygen-delivery device characterized by small, hollow prongs that are inserted into the external nares.

nasal catheter An oxygen-delivery device consisting of a narrow, hollow tubing that is inserted through the nose into the nasopharynx.

nasal trumpet A type of artificial airway. Also called a *nasal*, or *nasopharyngeal*, *airway*.

nasopharyngeal airway A type of artificial airway inserted through the nose with the distal tip in the posterior part of the oropharynx. Also called *nasal trumpet* or *nasal airway*.

nasotracheal intubation The use of the nose as the entry point for placement of tubes or catheters in the trachea.

nebulization controls Devices on ventilators that regulate the time and intensity of the flow output from a connector used to power a nebulizer.

nebulizer A type of aerosol production device that consists of an "atomizer," or jet, and a baffle or baffles.

nebulizer controls See *nebulization controls*.

nebulizer solenoid A switch mechanism that turns the nebulizer on or off.

nebulizer system The parts of a device that produce, control, and deliver aerosols to the patient.

negative end-expiratory pressure (NEEP) See *negative expiratory pressure*.

negative expiratory pressure A mode of ventilation in which a small amount of suction pressure is exerted during expiration to assist expiratory flow, reduce mean airway pressure, and decrease expiratory time.

negative extrathoracic pressure A subatmospheric pressure applied to the external chest wall. Used in negative-pressure ventilators.

negative-pressure capability The ability of a device to generate subambient pressures.

negative-pressure control The mechanism that regulates the application of negative pressures in a device.

negative-pressure jet A Venturi or Pitot device that reduces pressure by air entrainment.

negative-pressure Venturi See *negative-pressure jet*.

negative-pressure ventilator A machine that provides ventilation by generating less pressure than ambient (atmospheric) around the thorax while maintaining the upper airway at ambient. The iron lung and chest cuirass are examples.

Nernst equation An expression of the relationship between the electrical potential across a membrane and the concentration ratio between permeable ions on either side of the membrane.

newton A Système International d'Unités (SI) unit of force that would impart an acceleration of 1 m/s to 1 kg of mass.

non–rapid eye movement sleep See *non–REM sleep*.

non–REM sleep Non–rapid eye movement sleep. Four observable, progressive stages of sleep that represent three fourths of a typical sleep period and are collectively called *non–REM sleep*. The remaining sleep time is usually occupied with REM sleep, during which dreaming occurs.

nonconstant flow generator A ventilator that reacts to back pressure and resistance by varying the inspiratory flow pattern.

nonforced vital capacity The maximum amount of air that can be slowly exhaled after a maximum inspiration. See also *slow vital capacity*.

noninvasive Pertains to a diagnostic or therapeutic technique that does not require the skin to be broken or a cavity or organ of the body to be entered (e.g., obtaining a blood pressure reading by auscultation with a stethoscope and sphygmomanometer).

nonlinear-drive piston See *rotary drive piston*.

nonrebreathing valve A valve that opens, allowing gas to flow to the patient, then closes, allowing exhaled air to exit by another route. Examples are spring-loaded and diaphragm valves. Diaphragm valves are further subdivided into duckbill (or fishmouth) valves and leaf-type valves.

normal body humidity At BTPS, 47-mm Hg vapor pressure or 43.8 g H_2O/L of air.

normal flora Microorganisms that live on or within a body, that compete with disease-producing microorganisms, and that provide a natural immunity against certain infections.

normal rate control The system that sets the normal breathing frequency on a ventilator.

normal sinus rhythm A cardiac rhythm characterized by the presence of P waves and an effective ventricular rate of 60 to 100 beats/min.

nosocomial Pertaining to or originating in a hospital (e.g., a nosocomial infection).

O

O₂ relay An electronic or mechanical device that controls oxygen flow into a delivery system.

obstructive sleep apnea (OSA) A condition in which five or more apneic periods (≥10 seconds each) occur per hour of sleep and that is characterized by occlusion of the oropharyngeal airway with continued efforts to breathe. Compare central sleep apnea and mixed sleep apnea.

occlusion pressure (P0.1) or airway occlusion pressure See *P0.1*.

ohm A unit of measurement of electrical resistance. One ohm is the resistance of a conductor in which an electrical potential of 1 V produces a current of 1 A.

one-point calibration Adjusting the electronic output of an instrument to a single known standard to help ensure quality assurance. It should be performed before analyzing an unknown sample, unless the analyzer is programmed to automatically perform a one-point calibration at regular intervals (e.g., every 20 to 30 minutes).

open-loop system A microprocessor-controlled system that provides clinical data or advice but defers to the user, who must then take the appropriate action.

open-top tent An environmental control enclosure used for small children; features an open top to facilitate CO_2 washout.

optical encoder The name of the device on the T-Bird ventilator that sends information about the turbine speed to the microprocessor in order to control the precise flow delivered to the patient.

optical plethysmography A technique for measuring blood volume changes in a specific body part (e.g., a digit or earlobe). These blood volume changes are then used to define systolic and diastolic time periods during the cardiac cycle.

optics A field of study that deals with the electromagnetic radiation of wavelengths that are shorter than radio waves but longer than x-rays.

OR/NOR gate A monostable, fluidic element with one control port and two outlet ports.

oropharyngeal airway An artificial airway that is inserted into the mouth until the distal tip is behind the base of the tongue, providing an open channel to the laryngopharynx.

outflow valve A control device that regulates the gas exiting a system.

outlet manifold Part of the exhalation valve on a ventilator.

outlet valve A safety valve on a piped-gas system that prevents the high-pressure gas from flowing freely.

overpressure alarm A warning that the pressures in a system have exceeded predetermined levels.

overpressure relief A device that allows pressure to be released from a system that has exceeded desired pressure limits.

overpressure-relief valve See *overpressure relief*.

oximeter A device that monitors the amount of oxygen in a (physiologic) system.

oxygen analyzer A device used to determine the concentration of oxygen in a gas mixture.

oxygen blender A device that mixes oxygen with air or other gases to provide precise oxygen concentrations.

oxygen concentrator A device that increases the oxygen content of inspired gas by enriching or concentrating the oxygen in air.

oxygen control A device in a ventilator that regulates the oxygen concentration delivered to the patient.

oxygen controller/blender See *oxygen blender*.

oxygen exhaust port An opening through which oxygen-enriched gas is expelled to the atmosphere.

oxygen inlet regulator A pressure-control device that governs the pressure of the oxygen entering a system.

oxygen percentage control See *oxygen control*.

oxygen percentage valve A metering device that regulates the proportion of oxygen in the delivered gas.

oxygen sensor The monitoring probe of an oxygen analyzer.

oxygen system The equipment and devices that distribute, control, and monitor oxygen from the bulk storage unit to the site of patient use.

P

P0.1 The mouth pressure 100 milliseconds after the start of a patient's inspiratory effort that is measured in a closed (occluded) system; a measure of the output of the respiratory center.

PaCO₂ Partial pressure of arterial carbon dioxide.

PACO₂ Partial pressure of alveolar carbon dioxide.

PaO₂ Partial pressure of arterial oxygen.

PAO₂ Partial pressure of alveolar oxygen.

paramagnetic Of or pertaining to a characteristic that causes a substance to be attracted to magnetic fields.

parameter A value or constant used to describe or measure a set of data representing a physiologic function or system (e.g., the use of blood acid-base relationships as parameters for evaluating the function of a patient's respiratory system).

paroxysmal atrial tachycardia A rapid atrial rate that begins and ends abruptly.

partial pressure The absolute pressure exerted by one gas in a mixture of gases.

partial-rebreathing mask A kind of oxygen mask that allows patients to reinhale the first third of their exhaled breath.

particle filter A device that removes particulate matter from an area or gas stream.

particle inertia The tendency of a particle to maintain a direction and speed of motion unless acted on by another force.

passover humidifier A humidification system in which the patient gas supply flows over a water supply. See also *heated blowby humidifier*.

pasteurization The process of applying moist heat, usually to a liquid such as milk, for a specific time to kill or retard the development of pathogenic bacteria.

pathogenic Capable of producing disease.

patient circuit The portion of the pneumatic circuit consisting of tubing from a ventilator to a patient. Also called *external*, or *ventilator circuit*.

patient-disconnect alarm A system warning that the patient is not connected to the ventilator; a low-pressure alarm.

patient-triggering When pressure, flow, or volume begins the breath; that is, the patient controls the beginning of inspiration.

peak flow A measurement of the maximum amount of gas that can be forcefully exhaled after a maximum inspiration; expressed in liters per minute.

peak flow control A control on the front panel of a ventilator used to set the maximum flow delivered during mandatory inspiration.

peak flow setting See *peak flow control.*

peak flowmeter A device that regulates the maximum flow a ventilator delivers.

peak inspiratory pressure (PIP) A measurement of the maximum pressure in the patient circuit that occurs during the delivery of a mandatory breath from a ventilator. Also called peak pressure (P_{peak}).

peak pressure See *peak inspiratory pressure.*

pedestal ventilator A term used in reference to a Puritan Bennett PR series respirator.

PEEP See *positive end-expiratory pressure.*

PEEP/CPAP pressure-control valve A mechanism that regulates the pressure limits of the PEEP/CPAP device in a ventilator system.

PEEP exhalation valve An exhalation valve fitted with a PEEP device.

pendant cannula A type of reservoir nasal cannula that can reduce oxygen supply use (compared with a continuous-flow nasal cannula). The reservoir is attached as connecting tubing that is a conduit to a pendant, which hangs below the chin.

pendelluft German for "pendulum breath," this term describes the movement of gas, from "fast" to "slow," filling spaces during breathing. Alternatively, the ineffective movement of gas back and forth (accompanied by mediastinal shifting) from a healthy lung to one with a flail segment; caused by a crushing chest injury.

percent pause time A ventilator control that uses a percentage of the inspiratory time to provide a pause at the end of inspiration, usually lengthening inspiratory time and allowing for an inspiratory hold.

pH Abbreviation for potential hydrogen, a scale representing the relative acidity (or alkalinity) of a solution, in which a value of 7.0 is neutral, below 7.0 is acidic, and above 7.0 is alkaline.

pH electrode See *Sanz electrode.*

phase variables During breath delivery, the variables controlled by the ventilator that are responsible for each of the four parts of a breath, including triggering (begins inspiratory flow), cycling (ends inspiratory flow), and limiting (places a maximum on a control variable: pressure, volume, flow, and/or time).

PH₂O Partial pressure of water vapor; 47 mm Hg at BTPS.

phonocardiography The recording of heart sounds and murmurs with an electromechanical apparatus.

photoplethysmography The use of light waves to detect changes in the volume of an organ or tissue. Pulse oximeters use this principle to measure the arterial pulse.

physical analyzer A gas analyzer that uses the principles of physics (heat, electrical flow, and so on) to measure gas concentration.

piezoelectric quality The ability of a substance to change shape in response to and at the frequency of an electrical current, thus changing electrical energy into mechanical energy.

Pin Index Safety System (PISS) A standardized scheme to prevent accidental mismatching of reducing valves and pressurized gases in small-capacity cylinders (E or smaller).

PISS See *Pin Index Safety System.*

piston bag A baglike reservoir that contains a volume of gas to be delivered to the patient when compressed by a piston.

piston compressor A gas source in which a volume of gas is reduced in volume and pressurized by a piston.

plateau pressure (P_plateau) The pressure measured in the patient circuit of a ventilator during an inspiratory hold maneuver. Also the pressure needed to overcome the elastic component of the lungs (static compliance) during breath delivery.

pneumatic Pertaining to air or gas.

pneumatic circuit A series of tubing that directs the gas flow in a ventilator and from a ventilator to a patient.

pneumatic drive mechanism A method of operating a ventilator with pressurized gas as a power source.

pneumatic expiratory timing device A gas-powered device that controls expiratory time (e.g., by using a controlled leak to deflate a diaphragm and open an inspiratory valve).

pneumatic nebulizer A device that produces an aerosol cloud by using a pressurized gas source as the propellant.

pneumatic system An air or gas system.

pneumatic timing mechanisms See *pneumatic expiratory timing device.*

pneumatically powered Energy supplied by high-pressure gas or air.

pneumobelt A corset with an inflatable bladder that fits over the abdominal area. The bladder is connected by a hose to a ventilator that delivers positive pressure at an adjustable rate and pressure. Used to alleviate strain to assist in the respiratory rehabilitation of patients with high cervical injuries.

pneumotachometer A device that measures the flow of respiratory gases. The pressure gradient is directly related to flow, thus allowing a computer to derive a flow curve measured in liters per minute.

pneumotachygraph An instrument that incorporates a pneumotachometer to record variations in respiratory gas flow.

polarographic electrode A device that uses the flow of electric current between the negative (cathode) and positive (anode) electrodes to measure a physical phenomenon such as the partial pressure of oxygen in the blood.

polysomnography The measurement and recording of variations in airflow, EEGs, electro-oculograms (EOGs), and arterial blood gases during sleep. Used in the diagnosis of sleep apnea.

poppet assembly A spool-shaped device used to open or close an orifice in response to pressure differences.

poppet valve See *poppet assembly.*

positive end-expiratory pressure (PEEP) A form of therapy applied during mechanical ventilation that elevates the baseline pressure from which inspiration is delivered. PEEP increases functional residual volume and mean airway pressure (MAP) to improve oxygenation.

positive intrapulmonary pressure A condition in which the pressure in the lungs is maintained at levels above physiologic.

positive-pressure ventilator A device that applies positive pressure to the lungs to improve gas exchange.

POST See *power-on self-test.*

potential energy The energy a body possesses by virtue of its position.

potentiometer An electronic device in which the output signal varies in strength with the strength of the input signal.

potentiometric Refers to measuring voltage.

power A source of physical or mechanical force or energy. Force or energy that can be put to work (e.g., electric power).

power failure alarm A warning device that indicates that the main power source of a piece of equipment has failed. Also known as a *power disconnect alarm.*

power indicators Monitoring lights or diodes that illuminate to give information about a device's power source.

power-on self-test (POST) An essential test started by the microprocessor as soon as the ventilator is turned on and that lasts approximately 5 seconds. The unit must complete this test before it is functional.

power source The origin of physical or mechanical force or energy. Force or energy that can be put to work (e.g., electric power).

power transmission system Gas or electrically powered mechanical devices that generate a pressure gradient to provide all or part of the work of breathing for a patient. Also called a *drive mechanism*.

precision/imprecision In measurement, precision is freedom from random errors; imprecision is inaccuracy caused by random error.

precision metering device See *proportional metering device*.

premature ventricular beats A ventricular depolarization occurring earlier than expected.

premature ventricular depolarizations See *premature ventricular beats*.

preset minute volume The set volume of gas to be delivered through a ventilator in a minute.

preset reducing valve See *preset regulator*.

preset regulator A device that decreases the pressure from a gas supply system to a predetermined lower pressure.

preset working pressure A predetermined pressure at which pneumatically powered devices function efficiently and safely. Usually below 60 psig.

pressure The amount of force exerted per unit of area.

pressure and sensitivity adjustments Mechanisms that let the operator select the pressure and sensitivity values on a mechanical ventilator.

pressure augmentation (P$_{aug}$) A servo-control (closed-loop) mode of pressure-targeted ventilation that guarantees volume delivery on a breath-by-breath basis.

pressure capacitance chamber A device that increases or decreases pressure against a pressure-relief valve in the Bio-Med MVP-10 ventilator.

pressure compartment In the Bird Mark series, the right side of the respirator in which superambient pressures could develop and be transmitted to the patient.

pressure control The mechanism that determines the pressure level generated by the ventilator.

pressure-controlled ventilation (PCV) A mode of ventilation in which the maximum preset pressure is delivered, regardless of the volume achieved.

pressure-controlled inverse-ratio ventilation (PCIRV) Pressure-targeted, time-cycled ventilation in which the inspiratory time exceeds the expiratory time.

pressure differential devices Mechanisms that operate by attempting to balance pressures within the device.

pressure differential transducer A device whose output signal strength depends on the difference between two or more input pressures.

pressure-equalization passage In the Bird Mark series, a hole in the center body that allows for the equalization of pressure between the pressure and ambient sides of the respirator.

pressure-limit control A dial or button that allows the operator to determine the preset maximum pressure a ventilator will deliver.

pressure-limited A descriptive term indicating that a maximum pressure has been set that cannot be exceeded. Also see *pressure-targeted ventilation* and *pressure ventilation*.

pressure-limited resuscitators Emergency ventilation devices that have a preset maximum inspiratory pressure.

pressure-limited ventilation A mode of ventilation in which inspiration is stopped when a selected pressure value is reached.

pressure ramp (Pramp) A ventilator control that determines how rapidly the set pressure is achieved during inspiration. Also called *pressure sloping*.

pressure-regulated volume control (PRVC) The name given to a mode of ventilation on the Servo 300 ventilator that provides pressure-targeted, time-cycled ventilation that is volume-guaranteed.

pressure release Baseline ventilation in which elevated baseline pressures are periodically allowed to fall to baseline or a pressure-relief safety valve is activated.

pressure-relief valve A safety device that vents pressure in excess of a preset value; the pressure is vented to the atmosphere.

pressure sensor A device that detects pressure or pressure changes.

pressure slope A ventilator control that adjusts the rate at which the set pressure is reached during inspiration. Also called *pressure sloping*. See also *pressure ramp*.

pressure support See *pressure-support ventilation*.

pressure-support ventilation (PSV) A mode of ventilatory support designed to augment spontaneous breathing. Patient-triggered, pressure-targeted, flow-cycled ventilation.

pressure swing absorption (PSA) A technique used in some oxygen sieve concentrators to produce an enriched oxygen mixture. In this technique, room air is drawn through one or more filters by a compressor and eventually compressed to a pressure of 15-25 psig and then passed through an air-cooled heat exchanger before entering two or more sieve beds containing a porous material such as zeolite. The PSA method attempts to minimize the problems associated with the accumulation of moisture and other contaminants building up on the sieve bed and allows for the pressurization of one sieve bed while the other bed is purged at a rate of 1 to 5 times per minute.

pressure switch A device that responds to changes in a pressure signal by instituting an action within the ventilator system.

pressure-targeted ventilation A form of ventilation in which the operator selects a specific pressure for the delivery of inspiration.

pressure transducer A mechanism that converts a pressure signal to another form of energy, usually electric.

pressure-triggering Inspiration begins when the ventilator senses a drop in circuit pressure.

pressure ventilation Setting a desired pressure. Also called *pressure-limited ventilation*, *pressure-controlled ventilation*, and *pressure-targeted ventilation*.

pressurized metered-dose inhaler (pMDI) See *metered dose inhaler*.

prokaryotic Of or pertaining to an organism that does not contain a true nucleus surrounded by a nuclear membrane. Characteristic of lower life forms, such as bacteria, viruses, and blue-green algae. Division of the organism occurs through simple fission.

proportional amplifier A fluidic control device that boosts or reduces output signal strength in proportion to the strength of the input signal.

proportional assist ventilation (PAV) A method of assisting spontaneous ventilation in which the practitioner adjusts the amount of work the ventilator will perform.

proportional manifold A mechanism that directs blended gas through a series of solenoids to control flow; it is found in the Infrasonics Infant Star ventilator.

proportional metering device A mechanism used to provide precise mixtures of gases. As the amount of one gas increases at a given total flow, the amount of the second gas decreases proportionately.

proportional solenoid A valve designed to modify gas flow. Typically, an electrical current flows through an electromagnet, creating a magnetic field that controls a plunger. The plunger governs the valve opening and gas delivery.

proportioning valve A system in which two or more valves vary the amounts of the gases they control as these gases enter the gas-delivery system. This dictates the final composition of the gas mixture.

proximal airway pressure gauge A gauge that indicates the proximal airway pressure.

proximal pressure line A line in the patient circuit to monitor airway pressures at the Y connector.

PSV See *pressure-support ventilation.*

PSV$_{max}$ The amount of pressure-support ventilation delivered to achieve a desired volume.

pulmonary vascular resistance The impedance to right ventricular blood flow offered by the pulmonary circulation.

pulse-demand oxygen-delivery system A system that delivers oxygen to the patient only during inspiration (i.e., on demand).

Q

quality assurance Any evaluation of services provided and the results achieved as compared with accepted standards.

quality control A planned, systematic approach to designing, measuring, assessing, and improving performance.

quenching A process of removing or reducing an energy source, such as heat or light. Also, stopping or diminishing a chemical or enzymatic reaction.

quick-connect adapter A device that allows rapid connection and disconnection of compressed gas appliances to high-pressure gas delivery systems.

quick-connect outlet See *quick-connect adapter.*

R

radio frequency interference (RFI) The disruption of the operation of a device due to specific types of radio waves in the vicinity.

rapid eye movement sleep See *REM sleep.*

rapid shallow breathing (RSB) index A weaning parameter mathematically defined as the spontaneous respiratory rate divided by the spontaneous tidal volume.

rate The frequency of occurrence stated in incidents per unit of time (e.g., 16 per minute).

rate control A device that allows the number of breaths per minute to be selected.

ratio light A visual warning indicating that the I:E ratio is not within predetermined limits.

real gas A gas that does not fit all of the kinetic theories, as compared with an ideal gas.

rebreathing mask A gas-delivery system in which expired gases are oxygen-enriched and inhaled again by the patient. Characterized by a reservoir bag and a series of one-way valves.

reducing valve A mechanism that decreases the delivery pressure of a gas to a lower "working" pressure.

reference electric potential A constant electrical voltage against which electrical flow in a sampling chamber is compared during gas analysis.

reference potentiometer A device that compares a predetermined, preset signal with other signals within an electrical or fluidic system.

reference pressure A preset pressure level to which other pressures are compared within a control system.

reference pressure-support bias pressure A condition in the Bear-3 ventilator in which spring tension in the adjustable pressure-support regulator equals the PEEP pilot pressure plus the pressure-support setting. This increases the machine-side pressure in the regulator, maintaining pressure support.

relative humidity The ratio of actual to potential water vapor in a volume of gas (i.e., how much is present as opposed to how much could be present).

relative refractory period The time period during phase 3 of a ventricular action potential in which a depressed response to a strong stimulus is possible.

REM sleep (rapid eye movement sleep) Sleep periods, lasting from a few minutes to half an hour, during which dreaming occurs. REM sleep periods alternate with non–REM sleep periods.

reservoir bag A pliable container that holds a volume of premixed gas for use in succeeding ventilations or as a back-up.

reservoir system A collection of bags or tubes that form a device to contain a supply of gas or liquid for later use.

residual volume (RV) The volume of gas remaining in the lungs after a complete exhalation.

respiration rate control The mechanism that controls the number of respirations per minute in a ventilator.

respiratory mechanics Measurable values used to evaluate the capacity for spontaneous breathing, which includes parameters such as maximum inspiratory pressure (MIP, also called *negative inspiratory force* [NIF]), vital capacity (VC), tidal volume (V_T), respiratory rate (f), compliance (C), and airway resistance (R_{aw}).

respiratory system compliance The distensibility of the lungs and chest wall, which is determined by dividing the V_T by the pressure. Normal compliance averages 0.1 L/cm H_2O.

rheostat An electronic device that allows for variable control of the amount of electrical current flowing from the device.

rhythmicity See *automaticity.*

rocker arm assembly The mechanism that determines piston stroke length to control tidal volume in the Bennett M25A and M25B portable ventilators.

rocking bed A device that rocks a patient from 15 to 30 degrees. Rocking moves the abdominal contents, and the resulting diaphragmatic movement assists lung ventilation.

rotary blower A kind of fan or compressor in which a fanlike device spins at high speeds to produce a pressurized gas flow.

rotary compressor See *rotary blower.*

rotary drive piston A piston that is connected to a wheel-like device, the movement and speed of which govern it. Also called *nonlinear-drive piston.* Compare this term with *direct-drive piston* or *linear-drive piston.*

rotary vane respirometer A volume recording device that measures the movement of a drumlike cylinder with blade-shaped or wing-shaped extensions (air foils).

S

safety valve A device that protects a patient-breathing system from complete closure, leading to suffocation, by allowing access to air. Also, a device that prevents excessive pressure in a patient-breathing system.

sample chamber In gas analyzers, the reservoir in which the observed gas (that to be analyzed) is held and compared with the reference gas.

Sanz electrode The standard electrode that measures pH. Composed of two half-cells that are connected by a potassium chloride bridge.

scalars Graphic displays of pressure, volume, and flow over time.

Schmitt trigger An integrated circuit made up of several proportional devices (three proportional amplifiers and two flip-flop valves) connected in a series. Often used in pressure-cycled fluidic ventilators.

secondary equipment Oxygen-delivery equipment extending from the wall outlet or reducing valve to the patient apparatus.

sedimentation The deposition of insoluble materials at the bottom of a liquid or out of suspension in an aerosol.

semipermeable membrane A biologic or synthetic membrane that permits the passage of certain molecules (e.g., based on size or electrical charge).

sensing port A connection or opening through which gas pressure, flow, or concentrations are sampled or measured.

sensing/servoing Venturi A Venturi device with known pressure gradients, which allows for comparisons with unknown pressures.

sensitivity See *sensitivity setting*.

sensitivity control See *sensitivity setting*.

sensitivity setting A setting on a ventilator that determines the amount of patient inspiratory effort necessary to start inspiration. Also called *trigger sensitivity* and *sensitivity control*.

separation bubble A low-pressure vortex.

sequencing switch Used in the Bird Mark 7A and 8A respirators to regulate flow through control ports. See also *ceramic switch*.

service verification test (SVT) A test procedure used on the T-Bird ventilator to evaluate unit function.

servo-controlled A closed-loop system in which a microprocessor compares a set parameter with a measured parameter and alerts the operator or makes specific changes to the set value based on its findings.

servo-controlled flow valve A servo valve that varies and controls gas flow in response to feedback from a flow transducer.

servo valve A scissorlike device that controls flow through the patient circuit in the Siemens Servo 900 ventilators.

set tidal volume (V_T) The preset or desired volume of a ventilator, usually calculated based on the patient's physical characteristics.

sidestream A gas analyzer that extracts a small sample of gas from the main gas flow for analysis. A nebulizer in which the aerosol cloud is formed outside of the main gas flow.

sidestream capnograph See *capnograph*.

sidestream nebulizer See *sidestream*.

Siggaard-Andersen nomogram A graph for calculating actual and standard bicarbonate, buffer base, and base excess concentrations.

sigh rate The frequency, in sigh breaths per hour, that will be delivered by a ventilator.

sigh system The portion of a ventilator dedicated to the production and timing of sigh breaths.

silica gel A crystalline chemical compound that is reversibly hydrophilic. It absorbs water and water vapor; a drying agent.

simple humidifier A device that uses unsophisticated methods of adding water vapor to inhaled gases (e.g., bubble or pass-over type of humidifiers).

simple mask A device consisting of a gas supply line and a conelike appliance that fits over the mouth and nose of the patient.

SIMV See *synchronized intermittent mandatory ventilation*.

SIMV breaths/min The number of synchronized mandatory respirations delivered per minute.

SIMV cycle time The length of time between mandatory synchronized inspirations.

SIMV system The part of a ventilator mechanism devoted to producing and monitoring SIMV breaths.

SIMV volume ventilator A ventilator that can deliver volume-targeted breaths in the SIMV mode.

sine waveform A graphic representation of the relationship between amplitude and time in which amplitude demonstrates repetitive peaks and valleys.

sine-wavelike curve See *sine waveform*.

single circuit A ventilator whose source gas powers the machine and is also the gas delivered to the patient's airway.

single-circuit ventilator See *single circuit*.

single-stage reducing valve See *single-stage regulator*.

single-stage regulator A pressure-reducing system that lowers primary equipment pressure to working pressure (approximately 50 psig) in one step.

sinus arrhythmia Cardiac rhythm characterized by a waxing and waning of the heart rate. The rhythm appears to be related to the breathing cycle, with heart rate increasing during inspiration and decreasing during expiration.

sinus bradycardia Cardiac rhythm characterized by the presence of P waves preceding each QRS complex with an effective ventricular rate of less than 60 beats/min.

sinus tachycardia Cardiac rhythm characterized by the presence of P waves preceding each QRS complex with an effective ventricular rate greater than 100 beats/min.

sinusoidal Of or pertaining to the shape of a sine wave.

sleep spindles Waveforms with waxing and waning amplitude that occur at a frequency of 9 to 13 Hertz.

slip/stream nebulizer See *sidestream nebulizer*.

slope Any inclined line or surface, position; a slant.

sloping To have an upward or downward inclination. To take an oblique direction, incline, or slant. Also see *pressure slope* and *pressure ramp*.

slow vital capacity See *nonforced vital capacity*.

small-volume nebulizer (SVN) A pneumatic aerosol generator. It may be used with a gas-flow circuit used for IPPB therapy or mechanical ventilation or as a handheld nebulizer powered by low-flow oxygen or compressed air.

smart window The name given to part of the display screen on the Dräger E-4 ventilator that gives information about ventilating parameters.

SmartTrigger The name given to the trigger function on the Bear 1000 ventilator in which the ventilator selects the signal that is most sensitive to the patient's effort with the quickest response.

sniffer's position Extension of the occiput with flexion of the lower cervical spine; the optimal position to establish and maintain a patent upper airway, as well as for oral intubation. Also called *extreme extension*.

software The programs, data, routines, and so on for a digital computer. Compare this term with *hardware*.

solenoid A magnetically operated, electrically powered switching device in which an electrically charged coil moves in a cylinder.

solenoid valve A valve that has its position controlled by a solenoid.

solubility coefficient An expression of the ability of a liquid to hold dissolved solids or gases.

spacer An accessory to enhance aerosol delivery from an MDI.

specific gravity The ratio of the weight of one volume of a substance to the weight of the same volume of water. Usually expressed in grams per liter or grams per cubic meter.

sphygmomanometer An instrument for indirect measurements of arterial blood pressure. It consists of an inflatable cuff that fits around the arm, a bulb for controlling air pressure within the cuff, and a mercury or aneroid manometer.

spinning disk A kind of nebulizer in which a volume of water is broken into particles by the action of a rapidly revolving, toothed disk. Also called a *centrifugal humidifier*.

spirochete Any bacterium of the genus *Spirochaeta* that is motile and spiral-shaped, with flexible filaments. Spirochete organisms include those responsible for leptospirosis, relapsing fever, and syphilis.

spirogram A graphic representation of lung volumes and ventilatory flow rates.

spirometer A device that measures lung volumes and flow rates.

spirometer alarm A low-volume or patient-disconnect warning device.

splitter configuration Part of a fluidic element consisting of an intersection point, toward which the main gas flow is directed. The gas flow hits the splitter, causing the gas stream to split and follow two separate pathways.

spontaneous bag A reservoir device that holds gas to be inhaled during patient-initiated, unassisted respirations.

spontaneous breaths Breaths initiated and ended by the patient with no ventilatory support provided. The ventilatory muscles must assume all responsibility for breathing.

spontaneous indicator (demand indicator) A visual or audio signal denoting patient-initiated breathing.

spring and disk release valve A valve that is opened by a pressure greater than that caused by a spring's pressure on a movable, disk-shaped valve cover.

spring disk A spring of a predetermined tension attached to a flat disk. Used to occlude orifices until the spring tension is exceeded by another pressure source.

spring-loaded bellows A power transmission system for a ventilator that uses a spring to apply force and increase the pressure delivered to the patient.

spring-loaded device A device that functions based on its ability to overcome the tension imposed by a spring.

spring-loaded disk PEEP valve A positive end-expiratory pressure valve that allows for pressure relief when the expiratory pressure exceeds the spring disk's spring tension.

spring-loaded resistors A type of threshold resistor that relies on a spring to hold a disk or diaphragm down over the expiratory port of a pressurized circuit.

spring-loaded valve A valve that functions based on its ability to overcome the tension imposed by a spring.

square-wave flow curve A flow-time diagram that takes the form of a box, indicating a constant flow delivered during inspiration.

square waveform A graphic representation of two variables that form a boxlike shape. Also called a *constant*, or *rectangular*, *waveform*.

standard bicarbonate The plasma concentration of HCO_3^- in milliequivalents/liter that would exist if the PCO_2 were normal (40 mm Hg).

standard precautions Guidelines recommended by the Centers for Disease Control and Prevention (CDC) to reduce the risk of transmission of blood-borne and other pathogens in hospitals. Standard precautions apply to blood and all body fluids, secretions, and excretions (excluding sweat) regardless of whether they contain blood, nonintact skin, or mucous membranes.

Staphylococcus spp. A genus of nonmotile, spherical gram-positive bacteria. Some species are normally found on the skin. Certain species cause severe purulent infections or produce an enterotoxin, which may cause nausea, vomiting, and diarrhea. Life-threatening staphylococcal infections may arise in hospitals.

static compliance A lung characteristic associated with the elastic properties of the lungs such that a delivered volume is associated with a specific delivered pressure under conditions of no gas flow. Mathematically expressed as the change in volume divided by the change in pressure.

Stead-Wells spirometer A type of water-sealed device that uses a plastic instead of a metal bell to measure volume changes in the airway opening.

stepper motor A microprocessor-controlled motor with multiple possible positions. Used to open valves or gas-flow channels for quick response to microprocessor signals.

sterilization The complete destruction of all microorganisms, usually by heat or chemical means.

Stokes' law The physical law governing the rain out of aerosol particles in the lung through sedimentation.

streptobacilli Chains of bacilli.

Streptococcus spp. A genus of nonmotile, gram-positive cocci classified by serologic type (Lancefield groups A through T), hemolytic action (alpha, beta, gamma), reaction to bacterial viruses (phage types 1 to 86), and growth on blood agar. The various species occur in pairs, short chains, and chains. Some are facultative aerobes; some are anaerobic. Some species are also hemolytic, but others are nonhemolytic. Many species cause disease in humans.

subambient overpressure pressure-relief valve (SOPR) See *subambient pressure-relief valve*.

subambient pressure-relief valve In the Bear 5 and Bear 1000 ventilators, a safety bypass system that lets the patient breathe ambient air if ventilator power fails or inspiratory circuit pressure exceeds 120 cm H_2O.

subambient-pressure valve See *subambient pressure-relief valve*.

subambient relief valve An internal antisuffocation valve. If the ventilator cannot provide a breath, the patient can inhale, open the valve, and receive room air.

sublimation The direct transition of a substance from solid to the gas or vapor state.

sulfhemoglobin A form of hemoglobin containing an irreversibly bound sulfur molecule that prevents normal oxygen-binding.

supercooled liquid An amorphous solid (e.g., margarine).

supply pressure The driving or operating pressure of a gas-powered device.

sustained maximum inspiration (SMI) A therapeutic breathing maneuver in which patients are coached to inspire from the resting expiratory level up to their inspiratory capacity (IC), with an end-inspiratory pause.

synchronized intermittent mandatory ventilation (SIMV) A mode of ventilation in which the patient breathes spontaneously with mandatory breaths periodically imposed after an inspiratory effort.

synchronous period The period during which a mandatory breath may be imposed.

system failure alarm A warning device that signals that the mechanism being monitored has ceased functioning.

Système International d'Unités (SI) An internationally accepted scientific system of expressing length, mass, and time in base units (IU) of meters, kilograms, and seconds, replacing the old centimeter-gram-second system (CGS). The SI system includes the ampere, Kelvin, candela, and mole as standard measurements.

systemic vascular resistance The resistance to left ventricular blood flow offered by systemic circulation.

T

tank ventilator Another name for the iron lung.

Taylor dispersion The enhanced mixing of gases associated with the turbulent flow of high-velocity gases moving through small airways and their bifurcations.

temperature A measure of molecular activity or motion. Also a reference to the reactive hotness or coldness of a material.

temperature correction Attaining body temperature within a normal range.

terminal flow control A control on the Bennett PR-2 that lets the operator provide a minimum flow to compensate for leaks during inspiration.

thermal conductivity The physical ability of a substance to conduct heat. This principle is used in oxygen analyzers and flow sensors.

thermal flowmeter A device that measures gas flow by using a temperature-sensitive, temperature-resistive element.

thermodynamics The science of the interconversion of heat and work.

thermometer An instrument for measuring temperature. Usually consists of a sealed glass tube that is marked in degrees Celsius or Fahrenheit and contains liquid such as mercury or alcohol. The liquid rises or falls as it expands or contracts according to changes in temperature.

theta wave One of the four types of brain waves, characterized by a relatively low frequency of 4 to 7 Hertz and a low amplitude of 10 mouse unit (MU). Theta waves are the "drowsy waves" that appear on electroencephalograms when the individual is awake but relaxed and sleepy. Compare this term with *alpha wave*, *beta wave*, and *delta wave*.

Thorpe tube See *Thorpe tube flowmeter*.

Thorpe tube flowmeter A type of flowmeter in which the gas stream suspends a steel ball in a tapered tube. As the ball obstructs a greater proportion of the cross-section of the tapered tube, flow is reduced.

Thorpe tube/reducing-valve regulator A combination of a pressure-reducing valve and a Thorpe tube type of flowmeter that can regulate both pressure and flow.

three-point calibration Adjusting the electronic output of an instrument to two known standards, as in a two-point calibration, and then adding a third standard intermediate to the other

two to ensure linearity of the response. It should be performed every 6 months or whenever an electrode is replaced.

three-way exhalation valve solenoid An electronic device that determines the direction of flow in an expiratory valve.

threshold resistance Usually the amount of pressure needed to overcome resistance to flow.

threshold resistor In positive airway therapy, a device against which a patient exhales. The pressure generated by a threshold resistor can be set to provide specific expiratory pressures independent of flow.

timing flip-flop A fluidic control device that is an on/off switch.

tonicity An expression of the amount of solute in a solution.

total cycle time (TCT) The time required for both inspiration (T_I) and expiration (T_E). Also called *total respiratory cycle* and *ventilatory cycle time*.

total lung capacity (TLC) The total amount of gas in the lungs after a maximum inspiration.

total volume output In ventilators, the sum of nebulizer gas volume and ventilatory gas volume.

tracheal button A device used to provide a temporary seal in a tracheostomy; used to keep the stoma patent.

tracheostomy tube An artificial airway surgically inserted into the trachea through the neck.

transcutaneous electrode A monitoring electrode that measures or indicates changes in physiologic conditions across the skin.

transmission-based precautions In hospitals, safeguards designed for patients documented or suspected to be infected with highly transmissible or epidemiologically important pathogens for which additional precautions (beyond standard precautions) are needed to interrupt transmission. There are three types of transmission-based precautions: airborne precautions, droplet precautions, and contact precautions, which may be combined for diseases with multiple transmission routes. Whether these types are used singularly or in combination, they are to be used in addition to standard precautions.

transport ventilator A mechanical ventilator used to provide ventilatory support while moving a patient from one location to another.

trigger The manner in which a ventilator determines when to begin inspiration (e.g., time-triggering or patient-triggering).

trigger sensitivity The amount of patient effort needed to begin inspiratory gas flow from a ventilator. Usually determined by measured pressure or flow changes.

trigger variable That which begins inspiration. A ventilator may be time-triggered, pressure-triggered, flow-triggered, or volume-triggered.

triple-stage reducing valve A pressure-reducing system that reduces pressure from 2200 to 750 psig, then to 50 psig.

turbine An engine or motor driven by the pressure of steam, water, air, and so forth against the curved vanes of a wheel or set of wheels fastened to a driving shaft.

two-point calibration Adjusting the electronic output of an instrument to two known standards to ensure quality assurance. Usually performed at least three times daily, or approximately every 8 hours.

U

ultrasonic nebulizer (USN) A device that uses high-intensity sound waves to break water into very fine particles.

ultrasonic transducer A mechanism that converts electrical energy into mechanical energy by means of a piezoelectric crystal.

underwater jet humidifier A device that adds water vapor to a carrier gas by injecting a high-velocity gas stream below the surface of a water reservoir, causing a large amount of small bubbles to form and rise to the water surface.

underwater seal resistor A type of threshold resistor in which tubing attached to the expiratory port of a pressurized circuit is submerged beneath a column of water.

universal precautions An approach to infection control designed to prevent transmission of blood-borne diseases, such as human immunodeficiency virus and hepatitis B, in health care settings. Universal precautions were initially developed in 1987 by the CDC in the United States and in 1989 by the Bureau of Communicable Disease Epidemiology in Canada. The guidelines for universal precautions include specific recommendations for use of gloves, masks, and protective eyewear when contact with blood or body secretions containing blood is anticipated.

upper pressure limit The maximum amount of pressure allowed to be delivered by a ventilator. See also *maximum pressure limit*.

user interface The control panel; where the operator sets the controls. Also called the *front panel*.

user verification test (UVT) A ventilator test on the T-Bird AVS that allows the operator to review several ventilator functions, such as a lamp test, a filter test, and a leak test.

V

van der Waals forces Physical intermolecular forces that cause molecules to be attracted to each other.

vapor A transition state between a liquid and a gas during which, through application of pressure/temperature changes, the transition may be reversed.

vapor pressure The force exerted by vapors on a gas or a mixture of gases.

vaporization The process whereby matter in its liquid form is changed into its vapor or gaseous form.

variable-performance oxygen-delivery system Oxygen therapy equipment that delivers oxygen at a flow that provides only part of the patient's inspired gas needs. Also called a *low-flow system*.

variable pressure control A closed-loop mode of ventilation available on the Venturi ventilator, Cardiopulmonary Corp.

variable pressure support A closed-loop mode of ventilation available on the Venturi ventilator, Cardiopulmonary Corp. It is patient-triggered, pressure-targeted, flow-cycled, and volume-guaranteed.

variable restrictor A device that reduces flow by incorporating an adjustable orifice.

vector An animal carrier, especially an insect, of infectious organisms.

vehicle Any substance, such as food or water, that can be a mode of transmission for infectious agents.

ventilator A mechanical device that moves gases into and out of the lungs.

ventilator circuit The portion of the pneumatic circuit consisting of tubing from a ventilator to a patient. Also called *external circuit* or *patient circuit*.

ventilator inoperative alarm See *ventilator inoperative system*.

ventilator inoperative system A system that warns of the nonfunctional status of a ventilator.

ventilatory cycle time The time it takes from the beginning of one inspiration to the beginning of the next inspiration. Also called the *total cycle time (TCT)* and the *total respiratory cycle*.

ventilatory pattern The rate, volume, flow, and pressure characteristics of breathing over a period of time.

ventricular asystole The cessation of ventricular contractions.

ventricular diastole The period of the cardiac cycle that encompasses the filling period for cardiac ventricular muscle.

ventricular systole The contraction period for cardiac ventricular muscle.

ventricular tachycardia Cardiac rhythm that is characterized by at least three consecutive ventricular complexes with a rate of more than 100 beats/min. It usually originates in a focus distal to the branching part of the bundle of His.

Venturi A device that incorporates a jet to create pressure, flow, and admixture changes in a gas stream. Also called an *air-entrainment device*.

vernier A control that can initiate small changes in a system—usually a dial that can be adjusted in small increments.

Vibrio A bacterium that is curved and mobile. Cholera and several other epidemic forms of gastroenteritis are caused by members of this genus.

virucide Any agent that destroys or inactivates viruses.

viscosity The thickness of a fluid; its ability to flow.

vital capacity (VC) The total amount of air that can be exhaled after a maximum inspiration. The sum of the inspiratory reserve volume, the tidal volume (V_T), and the expiratory reserve volume.

volt (V) The unit of electrical potential. In an electric circuit, a volt is the force required to send 1 A of current through 1 ohm of resistance, or the difference in potential between two points on a conductor carrying a charge of 1 A when there is a dissipation of 1 W between them.

voltmeter An instrument, such as a galvanometer, that measures (in volts) the differences in potential between different points of an electric circuit.

volume-assured pressure support (VAPS) A pressure-targeted mode of ventilation that guarantees volume delivery with each breath. It is a servo-controlled (closed-loop) mode that is similar in function to pressure augmentation.

volume conductor The heart is surrounded by tissues that contain ions that can conduct electrical impulses generated in the heart to the body surface where these electrical signals can be detected by electrodes placed on the skin.

volume control A dial or setting that determines the volume to be delivered by a mechanical ventilator.

volume-controlled inverse-ratio ventilation (VCIRV) A volume-targeted, volume- or time-cycled mode of ventilation in which inspiratory time exceeds expiratory time.

volume-displacement device The mechanism by which some ventilators deliver a positive-pressure breath. The device may be a piston, bellow, concertina bag, or similar "bag-in-chamber" mechanism.

volume-displacement incentive spirometer A device that encourages a patient to take slow, deep breaths (as in sighing or yawning) to inspire a preset volume of air. The device measures and visually displays the volume of air that the patient inspires during a sustained maximum inspiration.

volume hold A ventilator control or a maneuver where a volume of gas is held in the patient's lungs for a period of time so static pressure can be read or gas distribution improved.

volume limit A setting that determines the maximum deliverable volume on a ventilator.

volume support A closed-loop mode of ventilation available on the Maquet Servo^i ventilator that is patient-triggered, pressure-targeted, flow-cycled, and volume-guaranteed.

volume-targeted ventilation A form of ventilation in which the operator selects a specific volume for delivery of inspiration.

volume ventilation Setting a desired tidal volume in breath delivery. Also called *volume-limited ventilation, volume-controlled ventilation*, and *volume-targeted ventilation*.

vortex shedding A characteristic of flow systems in which changes in flows that contact air foils are proportionate to the velocity of the gas, thus allowing for pressure, flow, and volume to be determined.

W

water-weighted diaphragm A PEEP device in which a water column placed in contact with the diaphragm of an expiration valve creates a PEEP pressure equal to the height of the water column.

watt A unit of power, equivalent to work done at the rate of 1 J/s.

weighted-ball resistors A type of resistor in which a steel ball is placed over a calibrated orifice that is attached directly above the expiratory port of a pressurized circuit.

Wheatstone bridge A particular arrangement of multiple resistors in an electrical circuit.

wick humidifier A type of humidification system in which the flow is exposed to a water-saturated cloth, paper, or polyethylene membrane.

Wolff-Parkinson-White syndrome Cardiac rhythm that is characterized as a preexcitation syndrome. In this arrhythmia, ventricular depolarizations are initiated when impulses initiated in the atria bypass the AV node and travel through an ancillary Kent bundle, resulting in the presence of characteristic delta waves.

Wood's metal A metal alloy commonly used in fusible plugs.

work of breathing The amount of force needed to move a given volume into the lung with a relaxed chest wall. It can be reduced when applied properly with mechanical ventilation.

Y

Y-connector An adapter shaped like the letter Y that connects the endotracheal tube adapter to the main inspiratory and expiratory lines of a patient circuit used for mechanical ventilation.

Z

zone valve A valve that controls gas flow to specific areas served by a bulk gas system.

Index

Note: Page numbers followed by *b* indicate a box, *f* figures, and *t* tables.

Frequently Used Formulae and Values

GAS LAWS

Definitions of Standard Conditions

	Temperature (°C)	Pressure (mm Hg)	Water vapor
STPD	760		Zero
ATPD		Atmospheric	Zero
ATPS		Atmospheric	Saturated
BTPS		Atmospheric	47 mm Hg

Gas Cylinders

Oxygen cylinder factors for common cylinder sizes

D Cylinder	0.16
E Cylinder	0.28
G Cylinder	2.41
H Cylinder	3.14
K Cylinder	3.14

FLOW RATES, AND MIXING AIR AND OXYGEN

Air-to-Oxygen Ratios and Total Flows of Several Common Venturi Devices

%	Oxygen flow rate (L/min)	Air/oxygen Ratio	Total flow (L/min)
24%	4	25.3:1	105
28%	4	10.3:1	45
31%	6	6.9:1	47
35%	8	4.3:1	42
40%	8	3:1	32
50%	12	1.7:1	32
60%	24	1:1	48
70%	24	0.6:1	38

Formulae Used with Gas Laws

Boyle's law (solving for pressure): $P_2 = \dfrac{P_1 \times V_1}{V_2}$

Boyle's law (solving for volume): $V_2 = \dfrac{P_1 \times V_1}{P_2}$

Charles' law (solving for volume): $V_2 = \dfrac{V_1 \times T_2}{T_1}$

Gay-Lussac's law (solving for pressure): $P_2 = \dfrac{P_1 \times T_2}{T_1}$

Combined-gas law:

$$V_2 = \frac{V_1 \times P_1 \times T_2}{P_2 \times T_1} \text{ (solving for volume)}$$

Combined-gas law:

$$P_2 = \frac{V_1 \times P_1 \times T_1}{V_2 \times T_1} \text{ (solving for pressure)}$$

Combined-gas law:

$$T_2 = \frac{P_2 \times V_2 \times T_1}{P_1 \times V_1} \text{ (solving for temperature)}$$

Combined-gas law:

$$V_2 = \frac{V_1 \times [P_1 - (P_{H_2O} @ T_1)] \times T_2}{[P_2 - (P_{H_2O} @ T_2)] \times T_1}$$

$$\text{Density} = \frac{GMW}{22.4\,L}$$

$$\text{Density} = \frac{[(GMW \text{ of gas} \#1 \times \%) + (GMW \text{ of gas} \#2 \times \%)]}{22.4L}$$

Formulae Used with Cylinders and Liquid Oxygen

$$\text{Cylinder factor} = \frac{\text{cubic feet in full cylinder} \times 28.3}{\text{pressure of full cylinder}}$$

$$\text{Duration (minutes)} = \frac{\text{gauge pressure (psig)} \times \text{cylinder factor}}{\text{oxygen flow rate (liters/minute)}}$$

$$\frac{\text{Duration of liquid}}{\text{oxygen cylinder (min)}} = \frac{\text{liquid } O_2 \text{ capacity (L)} \times 860 \times \text{gauge reading (\%)}}{\text{oxygen flow rate (L/min)}}$$

$$\text{Duration (min)} = \frac{\text{weight of liquid } O_2 \text{ remaining (pounds)} \times 344}{\text{oxygen flow rate (L/min)}}$$

Formula Used When Mixing Air and Oxygen

$$O_2 (\%) = \frac{(\text{air flow} \times 21\%) + (O_2 \text{ flow} \times 100\%)}{\text{total gas flow}} \times 100$$

Formulae Used When Calculating Humidity

$$RH (\%) = \frac{\text{content}}{\text{capacity}} \times 100$$